D1449248

www.wadsworth.com

wadsworth.com is the World Wide Web site for Wadsworth and is your direct source to dozens of online resources.

At *wadsworth.com* you can find out about supplements, demonstration software, and student resources. You can also send email to many of our authors and preview new publications and exciting new technologies.

wadsworth.com
Changing the way the world learns®

Sooyearno

016-606-5995.

2003. 8. 19. 타

학관서점부.

PRINCIPLES
OF
NEUROPSYCHOLOGY

Eric A. Zillmer

Drexel University

Mary V. Spiers

Drexel University

William C. Culbertson, Contributor

Drexel University

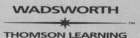

WADSWORTH

™

THOMSON LEARNING

Australia | Canada | Mexico | Singapore | Spain | United Kingdom | United States

WADSWORTH
THOMSON LEARNING™

Psychology Publisher: Vicki Knight
Development Editor: Penelope Sky
Assistant Editor: Jennifer Wilkinson
Editorial Assistant: Julie Dillemuth
Marketing Manager: Marc Linsenman
Marketing Assistant: Megan Hansen
Signing Representative: Ron Shelly
Project Editor: Lisa Weber
Print Buyer: Mary Noel
Permissions Editor: Robert Kauser
Production Service: Greg Hubit Bookworks

Text Designer: Rita Naughton
Art Editor and Photo Researcher: Terri Wright
Copy Editor: Linda Purrington
Illustrators: Lotus Art, Precision Graphics
Cover Designer: Stephen Rapley
Indexer: Joanne Rohrbach
Cover Image: Courtesy of Erin Bigler
Cover Printer: Phoenix Color
Compositor: Thompson Type
Printer: Maple-Vail, New York

COPYRIGHT © 2001 Wadsworth, a division of Thomson Learning, Inc. Thomson Learning™ is a trademark used herein under license.

ALL RIGHTS RESERVED. No part of this work covered by the copyright hereon may be reproduced or used in any form or by any means—graphic, electronic, or mechanical, including photocopying, recording, taping, Web distribution, or information storage and retrieval systems—without the written permission of the publisher.

Printed in the United States of America

3 4 5 6 7 04 03 02

For permission to use material from this text, contact us:

Web: http://www.thomsonrights.com
Fax: 1-800-730-2215
Phone: 1-800-730-2214

Exam View® and Exam View Pro® are trademarks of FSCreations, Inc. Windows is a registered trademark of the Microsoft Corporation used herein under license. Macintosh and Power Macintosh are registered trademarks of Apple Computer, Inc. Used herein under license.

Library of Congress Cataloging-in-Publication Data
Zillmer, Eric.
   Principles of neuropsychology / Eric A. Zillmer, Mary V. Spiers, William C. Culbertson.
      p. cm.
   Includes bibliographical references and index.
   ISBN 0-534-34144-6
   1. Neuropsychology. I. Spiers, Mary. II. Culbertson, William C. III. Title.
QP360 .Z55 2001
612.8–dc21   00-049954

Wadsworth/Thomson Learning
10 Davis Drive
Belmont, CA 94002-3098
USA

For more information about our products, contact us:

Thomson Learning Academic Resource Center
1-800-423-0563
http://www.wadsworth.com

International Headquarters
Thomson Learning
International Division
290 Harbor Drive, 2nd Floor
Stamford, CT 06902-7477
USA

UK/Europe/Middle East/South Africa
Thomson Learning
Berkshire House
168-173 High Holborn
London WC1V 7AA
United Kingdom

Asia
Thomson Learning
60 Albert Street, #15-01
Albert Complex
Singapore 189969

Canada
Nelson Thomson Learning
1120 Birchmount Road
Toronto, Ontario M1K 5G4
Canada

Endpaper Exhibit 6 (top) from Ragland, J. D., Gur, R. C., Raz, J., Schroeder, L., Smith, R. J., Alavi, A., & Gur, R. E. (2000). Hemispheric activation of anterior and inferior prefrontal cortex during verbal encoding and recognition: A PET study of healthy volunteers. *NeuroImage, 11,* 624–633.

This book is dedicated to my teachers of psychology:
Mentors, colleagues, friends

Frank M. Webbe
Robert P. Archer
Jeffrey T. Barth

E.A.Z.

This book is dedicated to my father.
His guidance as a psychologist and personal struggle with Parkinson's disease
have brought some of my greatest lessons.

M.V.S.

BRIEF CONTENTS

CONTENTS

Part Three   # THE DEVELOPING BRAIN   **225**

Chapter 7   # Developmental Disorders of Childhood   227

PREFACE

How can behavior make neuropsychological sense? That is the question we try to answer when we teach neuropsychology to our students. Like many teachers, we have had the experience of observing instructors and examining books on the topic of neuropsychology that presented the material in an esoteric manner removed from real-life situations. Neuropsychology is an exciting and dynamic field that readily stimulates and inspires students and teachers alike. It was with this goal in mind that we have written a progressive and accessible text on the study of neuropsychology.

The goal of *Principles of Neuropsychology* was to write an undergraduate or beginning graduate-level psychology textbook that teaches brain function in a clear, interesting, and progressive manner. The guiding thesis of *Principles of Neuropsychology* was that all interactions in daily life, whether adaptive or maladaptive, can be explained neuropsychologically. Thus the text challenges the reader to consider behavior from a broader biological perspective. This, in turn, leads to the conceptualization of a more neuropsychologically oriented discipline within psychology. In this respect, the text covers the role of the brain in behavior as simple as a reflex and as complex as personality. *Principles of Neuropsychology* stresses the following specific ideas:

1. An emphasis on human neuropsychology, experimental and clinical

Human neuropsychology is most appealing to psychology students, given that approximately half of all professional psychologists identify with a clinical or counseling specialty. A major focus of *Principles of Neuropsychology* is to integrate the relatively new field of human clinical neuropsychology and compare it with what is known about the normal brain.

Rather than focus on a purely cognitive organization, which characterizes brain functioning and behavior according to specific aspects or components such as memory, attention, or executive functioning, we chose to focus on disorders. Because neurologic disorders are multifaceted and usually involve overlapping and interacting cognitive components, we feel it is most useful for aspiring practitioners and researchers to obtain a comprehensive view of each neurologic disorder with its multiple cognitive components.

2. An emphasis on integrating theory and research

The integration of theory with studies of neuroanatomic structure and functioning is central to a dynamic understanding of neuropsychology. In this respect, *Principles of Neuropsychology* reviews general theories of brain function and specific theories of higher cortical functioning. A conceptual understanding of brain function is important because it provides a foundation on which to base the study of complex behavioral syndromes as they correspond to brain regions and neuronal networks. Otherwise, nothing more than the memorization of brain anatomy and corresponding behavioral correlates is achieved, and an integrated understanding of neuropsychology remains out of reach.

3. An emphasis on behavioral function

We give special attention to presenting the function of specific neuroanatomical structures. Students often fail to absorb the tremendous amount of information presented in similar texts because the material is presented in isolation, out of a psychological context. In this text, we present basic neurobiology as it relates specifically to behavior. Using such a functional approach facilitates both the absorption and comprehension of the material.

4. A focus on presenting real-life examples

To facilitate the reader's understanding of complex material and to augment specific points, *Principles of Neuropsychology* includes numerous examples of clinical and normal cases, procedures, and classic research findings at strategic places in the text. Like many other teachers, we find that didactic information is better understood when "real-life" situations are used. Many of the cases and procedures draw on our clinical and research experiences, which we accumulated in a variety of settings and services including state psychiatric hospitals, sleep centers, psychiatry departments, rehabilitation hospitals, and neurology and neurosurgery services. Throughout the text, we feature case examples and Neuropsychology in Action boxes, written by over 20 prominent neuropsychologists, that focus on interesting current issues related to brain functioning.

5. The presentation of didactic aids

Principles of Neuropsychology differs from other texts on the didactic dimension, because it uses unique aids to facilitate learning. Those include an *Instructor's Manual,* which provides outlines, class exercises, additional reference materials, and didactic information; a *Study Guide,* which includes practice exams, exercises, and additional reference materials; over 200 illustrations in the text; 11 color illustrations called *exhibits;* boldfaced Key Terms throughout the text; Key Terms are listed after each chapter and again in the Glossary at the end of the text; a Keep in Mind section at the beginning of each chapter and Critical Thinking Questions at the end of each chapter; and annotations on web sites, called Web Connections, at the end of each chapter.

In summary, the intent of *Principles of Neuropsychology* is to discuss brain functions, neurophysiology, and neuroanatomy in an integrated and accessible format. To facilitate a dynamic understanding of the field, the text emphasizes theory, functional process, case examples, and research, related to what has been learned about normal as well as neuropathological functioning. Approaching the field from this perspective challenges the student to examine the field of neuropsychology as a framework for behavior.

ACKNOWLEDGMENTS

This book could not have been written without the cooperation, assistance, and support of numerous individuals. Many students, scholars, and friends listened to us, offered suggestions, and provided encouragement along the way. The following reviewers helped shape the book from beginning to end, and we are most grateful for their generous contributions: Timothy Barth, Texas Christian University; Richard Bauer, Middle Tennessee State University; Gary Berntson, Ohio State University; Thomas Fikes, Westmont College; Michael R. Foy, Loyola Marymount University; Kenneth F. Green, California State University, Long Beach; Gary Hanson, Francis Marion University; Barbara Knowlton, University of California, Los Angeles; Paul Koch, St. Ambrose University; Mark McCourt, North Dakota State University; James Rose, University of Wyoming; Lawrence Ryan, Oregon State University; Bennett Schwartz, Florida International University; Michael Selby, California Polytechnic Institute; and Frank Webbe, Florida Institute of Technology.

We would also like to acknowledge those scholars who have contributed Neuropsychology in Action boxes to this text. All of them are prominent neuropsychologists who have, going beyond the call of duty, given valuable time to make *Principles of Neuropsychology* "come alive." They are, in order of appearance in the text: Antonio E. Puente, Elkhonon Goldberg, Erin D. Bigler, William C. Culbertson, Jane Holmes Bernstein, Bruce Pennington, Lamia P. Barakat, Carol L. Armstrong, Ronald M. Ruff, Jeffrey T. Barth, Carrie Hill Kennedy, Jeffrey L. Cummings, Barbara L. Malamut, Allen J. Rubin, J. Catesby Ware, Thomas L. Bennett, Jim Hom, George P. Prigatano, Tessa Hart, Douglas L. Chute, and Cecil R. Reynolds.

Drexel University psychology students played an important role in this project. They read initial chapters and provided feedback, were willing to use early versions of the manuscript as their textbook in class, and provided important research assistance. Simply put, this project could not have been accomplished without their diligent efforts. Psychology undergraduate students who provided valuable research support included Barbara Holda, Priti Panchal, Dan Rosenberg, and Holly Giordano.

Special recognition goes to Carrie Kennedy, the principal author of the *Study Guide*. Carrie did an excellent job in communicating complex material to the reader and in providing an excellent student companion text to *Principles of Neuropsychology*. Stephanie Cosentino deserves acknowledgment for proofreading and editing the Study Guide. Recognition is also extended to Melissa Lamar and Cate Price, who wrote and edited the *Instructor's Manual*. Melissa and Cate spent many hours completing the *Instructor's Manual* and assembling modules written by other neuropsychologists. A special thank you goes to my assistant Maureen Finnegan, who provided clerical support on this project.

Appreciation also goes to my colleagues Sepp Zihl and Karin Muenzel, both from the Ludwig-Maximilians University, Institute für Neuropsychologie, in Munich, Germany. Sepp and Karin allowed me to teach neuropsychology in an international forum. Our discussions on neuropsychology have been most stimulating and inspiring, and have provided a springboard for many issues discussed in this text. I also want to acknowledge my colleagues Mark Chelder and Joelle Efthimiou, who have assisted me in the development of the Assessment of Impairment Measure (AIM), which I have used extensively throughout the text to demonstrate the principles of neuropsychological assessment.

My friend Carl Pacifico played a special role in this venture. He reminded me of how important it is to think about brain-behavior functioning within the context of evolution. Carl, ever the pragmatist, also shaped my thinking about the functional and applied aspects of neuropsychology. I especially welcomed the occasions when we discussed neuropsychology and its relationship to culture, religion, and philosophy.

Special recognition goes to key administrators at Drexel University. Our former department head Anthony Glascock played an important role in allowing Mary and me to make neuropsychology a focus in our department. Former Dean of the College of Arts and Sciences Thomas Canavan provided encouragement for our doctoral program in neuropsychology at Drexel and assistance for the successful APA-accreditation process. Senior Vice President Anthony Caneris allowed me to merge administration and academics, and our President, Constantine Papadakis, should be acknowledged for revitalizing our university. Our department faculty served as an important discussion group and sounding board; whether it was around the copying machine, in the hallways, or over lunch, they allowed us to argue over the role of the brain and its relationship to behavior. Thanks to Doug Porpora, David Kutzik, Tom Hewett, Elizabeth Petras, Arthur Shostak, Doug Chute, Lamia Barakat, and Anthony Glascock.

Neuropsychology in the 21st century has gone high-tech. Jonathan "Yoni" Nissanov, Research Professor of Biomedical Engineering and Science at Drexel University, provided MRI pictures. Dorota Kozinska, at the University of Warsaw, Poland, taught me the three-dimensional imaging of brains and provided state-of-the-art brain electrical activity mapping (BEAM) pictures.

Erin D. Bigler, Professor of Psychology, and Tracy Abildskov, both from Brigham Young University, generously provided three-dimensional images of the brain, including the one on the cover of this book. Ruben C. Gur and his research group at the Department of Psychiatry, University of Pennsylvania, allowed us to use cerebral blood flow study pictures. Peter Groesbeck, from Drexel University graphics, created the chapter-opening artwork of "Neuroman."

Any scholar with a family knows what it means to write a book and attempt to maintain a normal family life. We are grateful to my wife Rochelle and my daughter Kanya, to Mary's husband Sean and Bill's wife Nancy, for their patience and understanding.

Special recognition belongs to my coauthor Mary Spiers. First and foremost, she put up with my hypomanic ideas, unreasonable time lines, and other hysterical behavior to move the text along. Mary has a true talent for bringing out the essence of neuropsychology and for that I am very grateful to her. Over my 12 years at Drexel University, she has been my close friend and trusted colleague. Together, we forged an unprecedented approach to doctoral training in neuropsychology, which served as the foundation of teaching neuropsychology at Drexel University and, in fact, of this book in the first place. Without her calm approach to the most demanding tasks, this book would not have been completed. Bill Culbertson wrote two chapters on pediatric neuropsychology. I am most grateful to him for helping us out. Bill is a consummate gentleman, a critical thinker, and a most loyal supporter of neuropsychology at Drexel University. He is the best pediatric neuropsychologist I know.

I can't think of having had better editors to work with than Penelope Sky and Vicki Knight at Wadsworth Publishing. They took our project seriously and forced us to focus on finishing a product of the highest quality. Their expertise in the area of pedagogy and their willingness to create a different neuropsychology textbook was most refreshing and enjoyable. Many of the unique resources in the book should be credited to them. I also want to thank Greg Hubit, Lisa Weber, and Jennifer Wilkinson for assisting with the editing process, and Terri Wright for helping with the art and photo editing.

The assistance of many individuals has enabled us to publish this book. We are grateful to all of them and have benefited from their understanding, criticism, and advice. Thank you.

Eric A. Zillmer
Drexel University
Zillmer@Drexel.edu

ABOUT THE AUTHORS

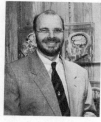

Dr. Eric A. Zillmer is Pacifico Professor of Neuropsychology at Drexel University where he teaches courses in neuropsychology, abnormal psychology, psychological assessment, and sports psychology. He received his doctoral degree from Florida Tech, had internship training at Eastern Virginia Medical School, and completed a two-year postdoctoral fellowship in neuropsychology at the University of Virginia Health Sciences Center. Dr. Zillmer, a licensed clinical psychologist, is a Fellow of the College of Physicians of Philadelphia, the American Psychological Association, the Society for Personality Assessment, and the National Academy of Neuropsychology. He has written extensively in the area of neuropsychology and psychological assessment, having published more than 100 journal articles, book chapters, and books, including *Neuropsychological Assessment and Intervention* (with Mary Spiers) and *The Quest for the Nazi Personality: A Psychological Investigation of Nazi War Criminals.* He is the coauthor (with William Culbertson) of the widely used Tower of London^{DX} test and the d2 Test of Attention. Dr. Zillmer is on the editorial boards of *Assessment,* the *Journal of Personality Assessment,* and the *Journal of Forensic Neuropsychology.* He currently is the Director of Athletics at Drexel University.

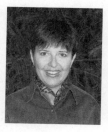

Dr. Mary V. Spiers is an Associate Professor of Psychology at Drexel University. She is a clinical psychologist and neuropsychologist, licensed in the state of Pennsylvania. She received her Ph.D. in clinical psychology from the University of Alabama at Birmingham, where she specialized in medical psychology and neuropsychology. She is currently the director of the Graduate Program in Clinical Psychology, which emphasizes clinical neuropsychological training. She teaches courses in neuropsychology, neuropsychological assessment, tests and measurement, ethics and professional issues in psychology, models of memory in neuropsychology, and health psychology of women. Her areas of research and publishing include normal and disordered aging and memory, practical aspects of memory involved in medication taking, the role of olfaction on mood in memory, and the role of hormonal influences on cognition in women. This is her second book in collaboration with Dr. Zillmer.

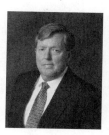

Dr. William C. Culbertson is a clinical neuropsychologist in private practice and specializes in the assessment and treatment of children and adolescents, particularly those with attention-deficit hyperactivity disorder. Dr. Culbertson has published in the field of neuropsychology, presented at professional conferences, and teaches at Drexel University, both at the undergraduate and graduate level. He is the coauthor (together with Eric Zillmer) of the Tower of London^{DX}, a neuropsychological measure of executive function.

GUEST CONTRIBUTORS TO NEUROPSYCHOLOGY IN ACTION BOXES

Carol L. Armstrong, Ph.D., Department of Neurology, University of Pennsylvania, and The Joseph Stokes Research Institute, Children's Hospital of Philadelphia *(Box 10.2: The Neuropsychology of Treatments for Individuals with Brain Tumors)*

Lamia P. Barakat, Ph.D., Assistant Professor of Psychology, Department of Psychology, Drexel University *(Box 10.1: Family and Child Adjustment to Cognitive Aspects of Cancer in Children)*

Jeffrey T. Barth, Ph.D., John Edward Fowler Professor of Psychology, University of Virginia Medical School *(Box 10.5: Mild Head Injury in Sports)*

Thomas L. Bennett, Ph.D., Professor of Psychology, Colorado State University; Clinical Director, Brain Injury Recovery Program, Fort Collins, Colorado *(Box 13.4: Epilepsy and the Case of the Sweeping Lady)*

Jane Holmes Bernstein, Ph.D., Director, Neuropsychology Program, Children's Hospital, Boston/Harvard Medical School *(Box 7.2: Principles of Assessment in Pediatric Neuropsychology)*

Erin D. Bigler, Ph.D., Professor of Psychology, Brigham Young University *(Box 6.2: Diagnostic Neuroimaging and Neuropsychology)*

Douglas L. Chute, Ph.D., Professor of Neuropsychology, Drexel University *(Box 16.6: Bits and Bytes in Rehabilitation)*

Jeffrey L. Cummings, M.D., Professor of Neurology and Psychiatry, School of Medicine, University of California at Los Angeles *(Box 12.1: Understanding Subcortical Dementia)*

Elkhonon Goldberg, Ph.D., New York University School of Medicine *(Box 5.2: The Frontal Lobes)*

Tessa Hart, Ph.D., Clinical Neuropsychologist, Drucker Brain Injury Center, MossRehab; Institute Scientist, Moss Rehabilitation Research Institute *(Box 16.2: The Traumatic Brain Injury Model Systems Project)*

Jim Hom, Ph.D., Editor, *Journal of Forensic Neuropsychology* and cofounder, The Neuropsychology Center, Dallas, Texas *(Box 15.1: Forensic Neuropsychology: Application of Brain-Behavior Relationships in the Legal Arena)*

Carrie Hill Kennedy, Ph.D., Lieutenant, Medical Service Corps, United States Naval Reserve, Naval Medical Center, Portsmouth, Virginia *(Box 10.6: Consensual Sex After Traumatic Brain Injury: Sex as a Problem-Solving Task)*

Barbara L. Malamut, Ph.D., Private Practice *(Box 12.2: Pallidotomy Surgery: A Case Report)*

Bruce Pennington, Ph.D., Department of Psychology, Director of Developmental Cognitive Neuroscience Program, University of Denver *(Box 8.1: Genetics of Learning Disabilities)*

Antonio E. Puente, Ph.D., Professor of Psychology, University of North Carolina at Wilmington *(Box 1.6: The History of Modern Clinical Psychology)*

George P. Prigatano, Ph.D., Chair, Section of Neuropsychology, Barrow Neurological Institute, Phoenix, Arizona *(Box 16.1: Speed of Finger Tapping, Recovery, and Rehabilitation Outcome After Stroke)*

Cecil R. Reynolds, Ph.D., Department of Educational Psychology, Texas A&M University *(Box 16.7: It's More Than a Black Box)*

Allen J. Rubin, M.D., Private Practice *(Box 12.5: The Neurologic Exam for Dementia)*

Ronald M. Ruff, Ph.D., Director of Neurobehavioral Rehabilitation, St. Mary's Medical Center, Associate Adjunct Professor, Department of Neurosurgery and Psychiatry, University of California at San Francisco *(Box 10.4: Can a Concussion Change Your Life?)*

J. Catesby Ware, Ph.D., Professor, Departments of Internal Medicine and Psychiatry, Eastern Virginia Medical School; Director, Sleep Disorders Center for Adults and Children, Sentara Norfolk General Hospital, Norfolk, Virginia *(Box 13.2: Sleep, Memory, and Sleeping Pills)*

TIME LINE OF SIGNIFICANT DEVELOPMENTS IN NEUROPSYCHOLOGY

2,000 B.C.: Early Brain Hypotheses
  Peruvian and central European cultures practice trephination.

6th–4th Centuries B.C.: Ancient Greek Influences
  Heraclitus (6th century B.C.): The mind is an unreachable, enormous space.
  Pythagoras (580–500 B.C.): The brain is the center of human reasoning.
  Hippocrates (460–377 B.C.): The brain controls all sense and movements.
  Plato (420–347 B.C.): The brain is the closest organ to the heavens.
  Aristotle (384–322 B.C.): The heart is the source of all mental processes.

3rd Century B.C. to Middle Ages: The Cell Doctrine
  Alexandrian school (3rd–4th century B.C.): Made advances in physiology and anatomy.
  Galen (Italian, A.D. 130–201): Suggested ventricular hypothesis and role of humors in health.

Medieval and Renaissance Europe: Anatomic Discoveries and the Spiritual Soul
  Albertus Magnus (German, about 1200): Deemphasized the role of the ventricles.
  Andreas Vesalius (Italian, 1514–1564): Corrected many historical mistakes about brain anatomy.
  René Descartes (French, 1596–1650): Proposed a strict split between mental and physical processes.
  Thomas Willis (English, 1621–1675): Made contribution to understanding the brain's vascular structure.
  Giovanni Lancisi (Italian, 1654–1720): Highlighted the role of the corpus callosum.

18th and 19th Century: Phrenology
  Franz Gall (Austrian, 1758–1828): Personality is related to different sizes of specific brain areas.
  Johann Spurzheim (Austrian, 1776–1832): Intellectual capacity is related to brain size.

19th-Century Europe: The Era of Coritcal Localization
  Paul Broca (French, 1824–1880): Motor speech is located in a small region of the left, frontal lobe.
  Carl Wernicke (German, 1848–1904): Understanding of speech is located in the temporal lobe.

19th- and 20th-Century Critics of Cortical Localization
  Sigmund Freud (Austrian, 1856–1938): Coined the term *agnosia*.
  Pierre Flourens (French, 1794–1867): Early advocate of an alternative to localization theories.
  Hermann Munk (German, 1839–1912): Coined the term *mind-blindness*.
  Joseph Babinski (English, 1857–1932): Introduced the term *anosognosia*
  Karl Lashley (American, 1890–1958): Formulated the principle of mass action in equipotentiality.

Late 19th- and 20th-Century Theories of Brain Function
  Hughlings Jackson (English, 1835–1911): Said behavior exists on different levels in the nervous system.
  Alexander Luria (Russian, 1902–1977): Formulated the concept of functional systems of behavior.

Modern Neuropsychology
  Karl Kleist (German, about 1930s): Refined localization approach to neuropsychology.
  Ward Halstead and Ralph Reitan (American, about 1940s): Pioneered neuropsychological testing.
  Donald Hebb (American, about 1950s): Published classic *The Organization of Behavior.*
  Henry Hécean (French, about 1950s): Pioneered the role of the right hemisphere in neuropsychology.
  Arthur Benton (American, about 1960s): Continued to advance the role of the right hemisphere.
  Oliver Zangwill (British, about 1960s): Examined neuropsychology with traumatic brain injury.
  Norman Geschwind (American, about 1970s): Founded behavioral neurology.
  Edith Kaplan (American, 1970s): Pioneered the process approach.
  Muriel Lezak (American, about 1970s): Refined clinical assessment in neuropsychology.

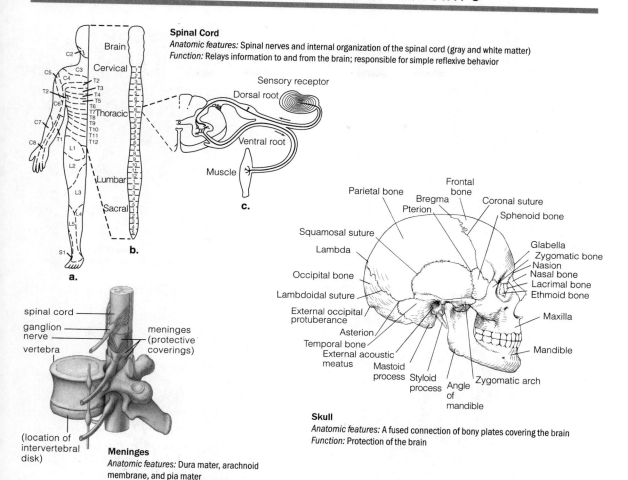

Spinal Cord
Anatomic features: Spinal nerves and internal organization of the spinal cord (gray and white matter)
Function: Relays information to and from the brain; responsible for simple reflexive behavior

Meninges
Anatomic features: Dura mater, arachnoid membrane, and pia mater
Function: Protective covering of the central nervous system, location of venous drainage, and cerebrospinal fluid absorption

Skull
Anatomic features: A fused connection of bony plates covering the brain
Function: Protection of the brain

Ventricular System
Anatomic features: Lateral (1st and 2nd), 3rd, and 4th ventricles, choroid plexus, cerebral aqueduct, and arachnoid granulations
Function: Balancing intracranial pressure, cerebrospinal fluid production, and circulation

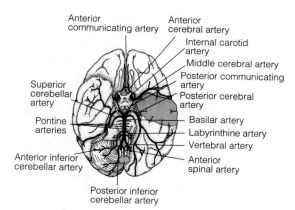

Vascular System
Anatomic features: Arteries, veins, circle of Willis
Function: Arteries: nourishment; supply of oxygen and nutrients
Veins: carrying away waste products

(continued)

STRUCTURE-FUNCTION RELATIONSHIPS

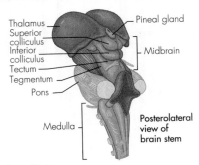

Posterolateral view of brain stem

Lower Brain Stem
Anatomic features:
Hindbrain: medulla oblongata (myelencephalon), pons (metencephalon)
Midbrain: tectum and tegmentum, cranial nerves, reticular activating system
Function: Relays information to and from the brain; responsible for simple reflexive behavior

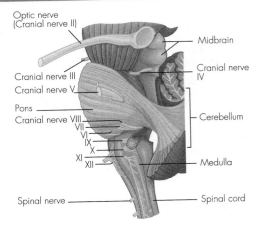

Cranial Nerves
Anatomic features: Located within the brain stem
Function: Conducting specific motor and sensory information

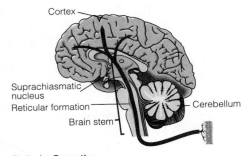

Reticular Formation
Anatomic features: Neural network within the lower brain stem connecting the medulla and the midbrain
Function: Nonspecific arousal and activation, sleep and wakefulness

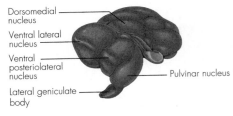

Thalamus
Anatomic features: Thalamic nuclei and thalamocortical connections
Functions: Complex relay station—major sensory and motor inputs to and from the ipsilateral cerebral hemisphere

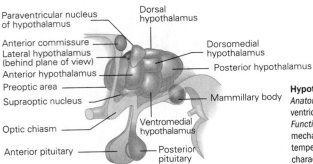

Hypothalamus
Anatomic features: Hypothalamic nuclei, major fiber systems, and third ventricle
Function: Activates, controls, and integrates the peripheral autonomic mechanisms, endocrine activity, and somatic functions, including body temperature, food intake, and the development of secondary sexual characteristics

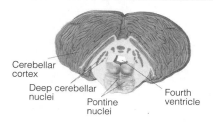

Cerebellum
Anatomic features: Cerebellar cortex, cerebellar white matter, and glia
Function: Coordination of movements, posture, antigravity, balance, and gait

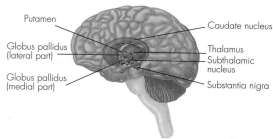

Basal Ganglia
Anatomic features: Structures of the caudate nucleus, putamen, globus pallidus, substantia nigra, and subthalamic nuclei
Function: Important relay stations in motor behavior (such as the striato–pallido–thalamic loop); connections form part of the extrapyramidal motor system (including cerebral cortex, basal nuclei, thalamus, and midbrain) and coordinate stereotyped postural and reflexive motor activity

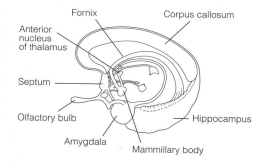

Limbic System
Anatomic features: Structures of the amygdala, hippocampus, parahippocampal gyrus, cingulate gyrus, fornix, septum, and olfactory bulbs
Function: Closely involved in the expression of emotional behavior and the integration of olfactory information with visceral and somatic information

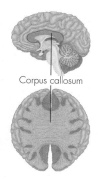

Hypothalamus
Regulates basic biological functions, including hunger, thirst, temperature, and sexual arousal; also involved in emotion.

Thalamus
Switching station for sensory information; also involved in memory

Amygdala
Involved in memory, emotion, and aggression

Hippocampus
Involved in learning, memory, and emotion

Cerebellum
Controls coordinated movement; also involved in language and thinking

Medulla
Controls vital functions such as breathing and heart rate

Spinal cord
Transmits signals between brain and rest of body

Corpus Callosum
Anatomic features: A large set of myelinated axons connecting the right and left cerebral hemispheres
Function: Information exchange between the two hemispheres

Cerebral Hemispheres
Anatomic features: Structures of the frontal, parietal, occipital, and temporal lobes
Function: Higher cognitive functioning, cerebral specialization, and cortical localization

Part One

INTRODUCTION

Chapter 1

THE HISTORY OF NEUROPSYCHOLOGY

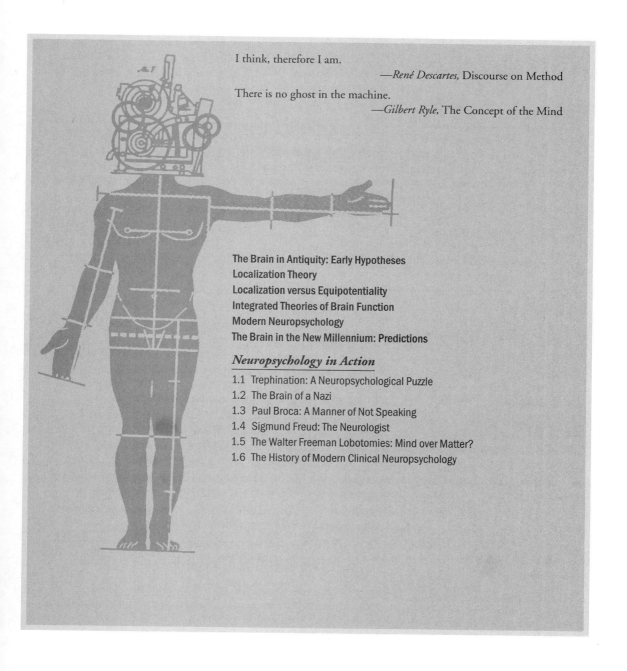

I think, therefore I am.

—*René Descartes,* Discourse on Method

There is no ghost in the machine.

—*Gilbert Ryle,* The Concept of the Mind

The Brain in Antiquity: Early Hypotheses
Localization Theory
Localization versus Equipotentiality
Integrated Theories of Brain Function
Modern Neuropsychology
The Brain in the New Millennium: Predictions

Neuropsychology in Action

1.1 Trephination: A Neuropsychological Puzzle
1.2 The Brain of a Nazi
1.3 Paul Broca: A Manner of Not Speaking
1.4 Sigmund Freud: The Neurologist
1.5 The Walter Freeman Lobotomies: Mind over Matter?
1.6 The History of Modern Clinical Neuropsychology

Keep in Mind

■ Does our brain constitute a major aspect of who we are?

■ Is the brain the source of all behavior?

■ Where do we go when our brain dies?

■ What is a soul?

Overview

All the preceding questions concern the functions of the brain. The brain has evolved to play a particularly significant role, not only in sustaining life, but also in all thought, behavior, and reasoning. It is the only organ completely enclosed by protective bony tissue, the skull, and it is the only organ that we could not transplant and still maintain the person's self. How does brain tissue generate and constrain mental events?

Efforts to understand mind–body relationships and their relative contributions to health and well-being extend back at least to Plato, Descartes, and Kant. Like many other sciences, neuropsychology has evolved from related fields, most notably psychology, neurology, and neuroscience (see Table 1.1). **Psychology** is the study of behavior; specifically, it seeks to describe, explain, modify, and predict human and animal behavior. **Neuropsychology**, a subspecialty of psychology, is the study of how complex properties of the brain allow behavior to occur. Neuropsychologists study relationships between brain functions and behavior; specifically, changes in thought and behavior that relate to the brain's structural or cognitive integrity. So neuropsychology is one way to study the brain by examining the behavior it produces.

Table 1.1   *Professionals Who Study the Brain*

Psychologists study behavior. Education includes an undergraduate degree in psychology and a doctoral degree (Ph.D. or Psy.D.) in an area of psychology.

Neuropsychologists are psychologists who study brain–behavior relationships. Education includes a doctoral degree in psychology and specialty (postdoctoral) training in neuropsychology.

Neurologists identify and treat clinical disorders of the nervous system, emphasizing the anatomic correlates of disease. Training includes a premed major at the college level, a doctoral degree from a medical school (M.D.), and residency training in neurology.

Neuropsychiatrists are medical doctors who have had residency training in psychiatry and are mostly concerned with the organic aspects of mental disorders, such as schizophrenia or bipolar disorder.

Neurosurgeons are medical doctors who have specialized in the surgery of nervous structures, including nerves, brain, and spinal cord.

Neuroscientists are researchers and/or teachers who have completed doctoral training in biology or related fields. They are primarily interested in the molecular composition and functioning of the nervous system.

Humans read and write, compose music, and play sports. You would expect an organ that coordinates and mediates all activity to have a huge number of components. And in fact the brain contains billions of cells, or **neurons,** and an *infinite* number of possible connections among individual neurons, allowing us to exchange very complex information. This amazing pattern of connections determines how and what the brain does. Understanding this network of neurons is the central focus of neuropsychology.

Neuropsychology has grown tremendously over the last 30 years, and in the 1990s was the fastest growing subspecialty within psychology (see Table 1.2). Neuropsychologists lead the study of brain–behavior relationships and are involved in the design and development of technologies to treat diseases of the brain. They are involved in patient care and research on the brain, work in universities, research institutes, hospitals, correctional facilities, the armed forces, and private practice.

The study of neuropsychology is today shaping our understanding of all behavior. But this has not always been true. Many past ideas about how the brain functions do not derive from scientific evidence. In general, two doctrines have emerged. The first, **vitalism,** suggests that many behaviors, such as thinking, are only partly controlled by mechanical or logical forces—they are also partially self-determined, and separate from chemical and physical determinants. Extreme proponents of vitalism argue that spirits or psychic phenomena account for much observable behavior. The second theory, **materialism,** suggests that logical forces, such as matter in motion, determine brain–behavior functions. Materialism, in its simplest form, favors a mechanistic view of the brain (as a machine). The history of neuropsychology is shaped by these two opposing principles.

This introductory chapter provides a grounding in the historical, theoretical, and philosophical aspects of neuropsychology. By charting the work of noted scholars, the chapter traces the development of neuropsychology.

The Brain in Antiquity: Early Hypotheses

Evidence from as long ago as the time of cave drawings shows that people have long been aware of brain–behavior relationships. The earliest neuropsychological investigations recognized how diseases and blows to the brain affect behavior. For example, **trephination** is an ancient surgical operation that involves cutting, scraping, chiseling, or drilling a pluglike piece of bone from the skull. This procedure relieves pressure related to brain swelling. Archaeologists have recovered several thousand such skulls worldwide. Many who underwent trephination clearly survived the operation, because many of the skulls show evidence of healing (new callus tissue). Others show no signs of healing—the patient died during or shortly after the operation. In some cases, the same skull was trephined more than once. One recovered skull was found with seven bore holes, at least some of which were made on separate occasions.

ANCIENT GREEK PERSPECTIVES

Classical Greeks wrote the first accounts of brain–behavior relationships. Heraclitus, a philosopher of

Table 1.2	*Major Neuropsychology Journals*

Assessment

Applied Neuropsychology

Archives of Clinical Neuropsychology

Behavioral Brain Research

Brain and Cognition

Cortex

Journal of Clinical and Experimental Neuropsychology

Journal of Forensic Neuropsychology

Neuropsychology

Neuropsychologia

Neuropsychology in Action 1.1

Trephination: A Neuropsychological Puzzle

by Eric A. Zillmer

Why did our ancestors perform trephination? (See Figure 1.1.) Did they have a reasonable understanding of the brain and its relationship to behavior? Did they use this procedure for medical reasons, such as trauma with swelling, or for other reasons? Did practitioners avoid certain areas of the brain because they knew that permanent behavioral problems or death were more likely to follow?

Much debate focuses on the reason for trephinations. Researchers have suggested that some cases may have involved a medical reason, such as a skull fracture. Such injuries presumably occurred during hand-to-hand fighting with stone-headed war clubs or perhaps as a result of a fall unconnected with warfare. On some skulls, however, people performed trephination on intact crania

with no sign of violence. Thus some investigators suggest that trephination was a "magical" form of healing, perhaps for displays of bizarre behaviors, including what we would recognize as epilepsy or schizophrenia (Lisowski, 1967).

Of course, no one wrote down the exact reasons for the high number of trephinations among ancient cultures. J. Michael Williams, a neuropsychologist

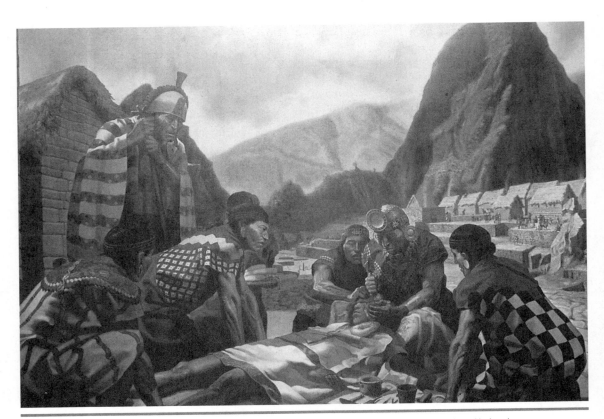

Figure 1.1   Trephination scene in Peru. (Reprinted with permission from Department of Anthropology, National Museum of Natural History, Smithsonian Institution, Washington, D.C. Photo courtesy of the San Diego Museum of Man)

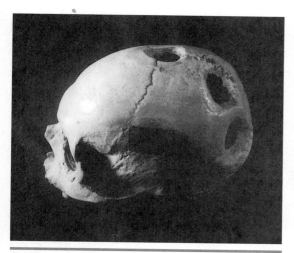

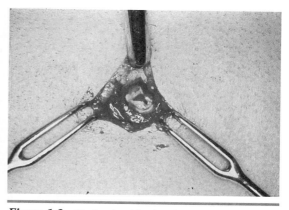

Figure 1.3 Modern trephination. A surgical hole is opened in the skull to relieve the intracranial pressure often associated with consequences of head trauma. (Jeffrey T. Barth, PhD, University of Virginia)

Figures 1.2 Trephination on adult male skull, showing multiple trephinations by the scraping method. Evidence of inflammation indicates temporary survival. (Mütter Museum, College of Physicians of Philadelphia)

at Hahnemann Medical University in Philadelphia, systematically examined trephined skulls to see if they showed specific patterns. Williams and John Verona, a leading anthropologist at the Smithsonian Institute's National Museum of Natural History, collected data on more than 750 skulls from the central highlands of Peru. They assembled data on trephination technique, location, size, healing, association with skull fracture and other pathology, and frequency by age and sex.

Verona and Williams (1992) concluded that the ancient Peruvians did trephine some children and adult females, but that they focused mainly on adult males (see Figure 1.2). They also found no left or right side predominance. Instead, the practitioners did most trephinations equally on both sides and primarily in the frontal and upper parietal regions, which are most exposed to injury. Interestingly, the pattern suggested that the practitioners avoided the muscles around the side of the head

and the sinuses. Although some trephined skulls showed signs of injury from falls or other accidents, most had fractures consistent with damage from blows by clubs and sling-stones—weapons widely used in the Andes in pre-Columbian times. Thus most trephinations clearly correlated with skull injury. Verona and Williams postulated that the practitioner was trying to elevate depressed fractures, remove bone fragments, smooth broken edges, and evacuate bleedings that may have resulted from head trauma. Their research revealed an impressive surgical record among the Inca practitioners of the southern highlands.

Similar operations are important in modern neurosurgery (see Figure 1.3). Surgeons widely use two procedures. The first, similar to the ancient Peruvian technique of drilling a number of small holes, involves drilling a hole next to a depressed skull fracture, to facilitate the elevation and removal of depressed bone fragments. (Incidentally, modern neurosurgeons still use manual drills, which

allow them more control during the operation.) The second surgical procedure drains internal bleeding after a blow to the head (see Chapter 10). With a special drill bit, the surgeon makes a hole over the site of the bleed. Then the surgeon screws a precisely machined bolt into the skull, allowing excessive blood to drain from within the cranium. This procedure reduces the intracranial pressure that is a major cause of death after a head injury.

The fact that surgeons today use an ancient surgical technique that even modern doctors once thought controversial underscores that people have often misinterpreted the historical context in which ancient scientists proposed certain ideas about the brain or performed specific procedures. Most ideas about the brain make more sense when we consider them within the societal and cultural context in which people originally developed them.

the sixth century B.C., called the mind an enormous space whose boundaries we could never reach. A group of scholars, including the geometer **Pythagoras** (about 580–500 B.C.), were the first to suggest that the brain is at the center of human reasoning and plays a crucial role in the soul's life. They described what is now called the **brain hypothesis:** the idea that the brain is the source of all behavior.

Hippocrates (460–377 B.C.), a Greek physician honored as the founder of modern medicine (Figure 1.4), also believed the brain controls all senses and movements. He was the first to recognize that paralysis occurs on the side of the body opposite the side of a head injury (following the areas governed by the right and left hemispheres of the brain). Hippocrates suggested that pleasure, merriment, laughter, and amusement, as well as grief, pain, anxiety, and tears, all arise from the brain (Haeger, 1988). Furthermore, Hippocrates argued that epilepsy, once considered the "sacred disease" (because people thought the patient was possessed by gods or spirits), is in fact no more divine or sacred than any other disease, but has specific characteristics and a definite medical cause. These were bold propositions at a time when people thought behavior was mostly under divine control. Hippocrates and his associates could not, however, discuss exactly how such brain–behavior relationships arose, perhaps because it was then sacrilegious to dissect the human body, especially the brain.

Plato (420–347 B.C.) suggested in *The Republic* that the soul has three parts: appetite, reason, and temper. This may have served as the model for Freud's psychoanalytic subdivision of the psyche into the id, ego, and superego (discussed later in this chapter). Plato thought the rational part of the tripartite soul lay in the brain, because it is the organ closest to the heavens. Plato also discussed the idea that health is related to harmony between body and mind. Thus, historians credit him as being the first to propose the concept of mental health.

Not all ancient philosophers believed in the importance of the brain to behavior. **Aristotle** (384–322 B.C.), a disciple of Plato, was a creative thinker in fields as varied as ethics, logic, psychology, poetry, and politics, and he founded comparative anatomy.

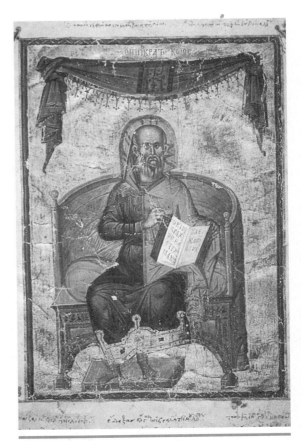

Figure 1.4 Hippocrates suggested that all thoughts and emotions originated in the brain, not the heart, as Aristotle had believed. The ancient Greek physician here opens his book to one of his favorite axioms, "Life is short, and the art is long." (DY/Art Resource, NY)

Aristotle, however, erroneously believed the heart is the source of all mental processes. He reasoned that because the heart is warm and active it is the locus of the soul. Aristotle argued that because the brain is bloodless it functions as a "radiator," cooling hot blood that ascends from the heart. You can still see, in words such as "heartbroken," the influence of Aristotle's so-called **cardiac hypothesis** proposing the heart as the seat of such emotions as love and anger. Nevertheless, Aristotle's view of nature and his anatomical findings dominated medical thinking and methods for the next 500 years.

THE CELL DOCTRINE

In Egypt, during the third and fourth centuries B.C., the so-called Alexandrian school reached its height. Well-known scientists worked in physiology and anatomy. They gained considerable knowledge of the nervous system and neuroanatomy from performing public dissections, which the Ptolemaic rulers encouraged. There are reports of scientists actually vivisecting subjects—condemned criminals were at the scientists' disposal. These dissections allowed scientists to notice different anatomic details, and they hypothesized that specific parts of the brain control different behaviors. Furthermore, they broke new ground by distinguishing between ascending (sensory) and descending (motor) nerves, and demonstrating that all nerves connect with the central nervous system.

An interesting development during this time was the erroneous suggestion that ventricular cavities within the brain control mental abilities and movement (we describe the ventricular system in more detail in Chapter 3). The **ventricular localization hypothesis** postulated that mental as well as spiritual processes reside in the ventricular chambers of the brain. Indeed, gross dissection of the brain shows that the lateral ventricles are the most striking features. Thus brain autopsies may have led investigators to conclude that these cavities contain animal spirits and are in large part responsible for mental faculties. This hypothesis subsequently became known as the **cell doctrine** ("cell" meaning a small compartment or ventricle), a notion that endured for 2000 years. **Leonardo da Vinci** (1452–1519), an Italian painter, sculptor, architect, and scientist, was a keen observer of anatomy. However, many of his early drawings were not guided by his keen scientific acumen, but instead by the inaccurate medieval conventions of his times. Figure 1.5 shows his drawing based on a common, but inaccurate belief about spherical ventricles. According to the cell doctrine, the foremost was the cell of common sense, where people thought the soul resided, and which connected to nerves leading to the eyes and ears.

Today, people know that the cell doctrine is entirely inaccurate. The ventricles are actually the anatomic site through which cerebrospinal fluid passes. This fluid protects the brain and facilitates the disposal of waste material. It plays no role in thinking; in fact, a neurosurgeon friend of ours conceptualizes it poetically as "the urine of the brain." The cell doctrine was scientifically important precisely because it was in error and thus presented an obstacle to further inquiry that people did not overcome until centuries later. However, it did focus the medical community on the brain and stimulated discussion of how behavior, thought processes, and brain anatomy may be related.

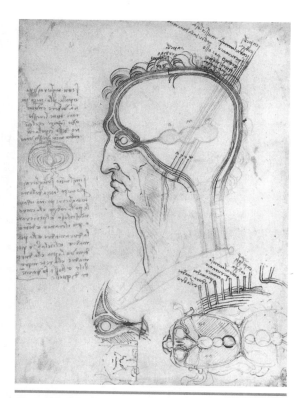

Figure 1.5 Drawing by Leonardo da Vinci demonstrating, inaccurately, the placement of three spherical ventricles in accordance with the cell doctrine. (The Royal Collection © 2000, Her Majesty Queen Elizabeth II)

Along with Hippocrates, **Galen** (A.D. 130–201), a Roman anatomist and physician, stands out as a supreme figure in ancient medicine (see Figure 1.6). Galen was undoubtedly the greatest physician of his time. By significantly advancing the anatomic knowledge of the brain, Galen distinguished himself as the first experimental physiologist and physician. He identified many of the major brain structures and described behavioral changes as a function of brain trauma. It was Galen's misfortune, however, that during his life the Roman authorities forbade autopsies. He therefore based much of his clinical knowledge on his experience as a surgeon appointed to gladiators; he remarked that war and gladiator games were the

greatest school of surgery. Contemporary neuropsychologists have also made significant advances during periods of war, including World Wars I and II, and the Korean and Vietnam conflicts, by studying the behavioral effects of wounds to the brain.

Galen suggested that the brain is a large clot of phlegm from which a pump forced the psychic pneuma out into the nerves. Perhaps he was comparing the brain to a major technological achievement of his time, the Roman system of aqueducts, which relied on hydraulic principles. Although Galen felt the frontal lobes (see Figure 1.7) are the location of the soul, he supported the ventricular localization hypothesis, describing in detail how he imagined human ventricles

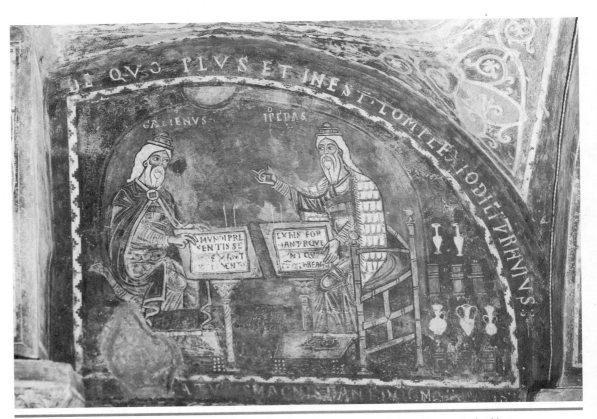

Figure 1.6 Galen learns from Hippocrates. Later, however, he was rather cynical about Hippocrates' writings, stating that they ". . . have faults, and lack essential distinctions his knowledge of certain topics is insufficient, and he is often unclear as the old tend to be. In sum: he prepared the way, but I have made it passable" (Haeger, 1988, p. 59). (Scala/Art Resource, NY)

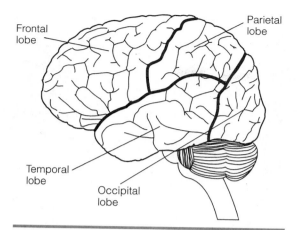

Figure 1.7 The lobes of the brain. (Adapted from Kathryn Wolff Heller, *Understanding Physical, Sensory, and Health Impairments,* Pacific Grove: Brooks/Cole, 1996, p. 51, Figure 4.5)

to look and function, on the basis of his studies of the pig and the ox. Galen believed that all physical function, including the brain as well as the rest of the body, depends on the balances of bodily fluids or **humors,** specifically blood, mucus, and yellow and black bile, which he related to the four basic elements—air, water, fire, and earth—respectively. Given that people thought the agent causing sickness resides in blood, doctors often bled patients as a curative procedure. Galen's view of humors became so ingrained in Western thought that physicians barely elaborated on the role of the brain and other organs, which remained largely unquestioned for nearly the next thousand years. We still say "good humor" or "bad humor" to describe someone's mental disposition. Terms such as *melancholic* (having frequent spells of sadness), and *choleric* (having a low threshold for angry outbursts), also remain in our vocabulary (see Figure 1.8).

ANATOMIC DISCOVERIES AND THE ROLE OF THE SPIRITUAL SOUL

During the 13th century, scientists began to take initial steps away from the ventricular theory. For example, **Albertus Magnus,** a German Dominican monk, the-

orized that behavior results from a combination of brain structures that includes the cortex, midbrain, and cerebellum (see Figure 1.9).

Not until scientific inquiry by **Andreas Vesalius** (1514–1564), however, were Galen's anatomic mistakes corrected, particularly those related to the role of the ventricles and their effect on behavior. (Galen had initially demonstrated the similar relative size of the ventricles in animals and humans, whereas Vesalius placed more emphasis on the relatively larger overall brain mass of humans as responsible for mediating mental processes.) Through continual dissections and careful scientific observations, Vesalius demonstrated that Galen's views were inaccurate. Vesalius also pioneered the anatomic theater—a sort of performance dissection, where medical students and doctors could watch from a circular gallery. Despite a climate of political and religious restrictions, Vesalius performed the first systematic dissections of human beings in Europe. Clearly, many opposed and objected to his experimental predilections. After all, the church retained authority over the soul, which was not subject to direct investigation. But Vesalius proceeded to revolutionize medicine through precise drawings of human anatomy (see Figure 1.10a and 1.10b). For the first time surgeons could see what they were dealing with.

By the 17th century, scientists were looking for a single component of the brain as the site of mental processes. **René Descartes** (1596–1650), for example, proposed a strict split or schism between mental processes and physical abilities. He hypothesized that the mind and body are separate, but interact with each other. Descartes theorized that mental processes reside in a small anatomic feature, the pineal gland. He reasoned that because the pineal gland lies in the center of the brain and is the only structure not composed of two symmetric halves, it was the logical seat for mental abilities. It is also close to the ventricular system and thus the "flow of the spirits" might influence it. Today, the function of the pineal gland is something of a mystery and is perhaps related to light–dark cycles and the production of sleep-enhancing melatonin.

Descartes has had an important philosophic influence on the study of the brain, precisely because

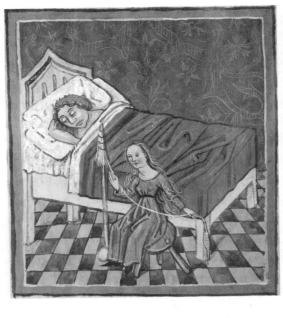
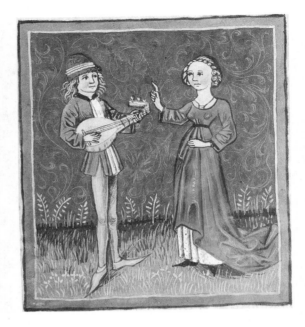
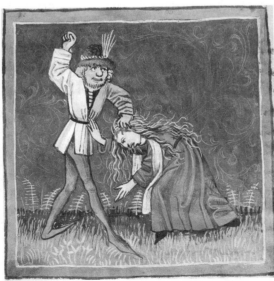
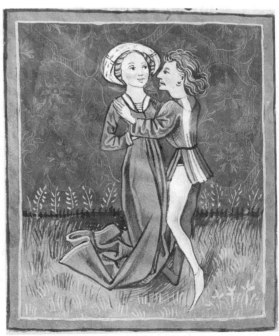

Figure 1.8 Ancient physicians took interest in humors, which served medieval notions of health and disease. Clockwise, excess black bile was responsible for a patient suffering from melancholy (depression); blood impassioned a lutist to play; phlegm is responsible for a slow response to a lover; and yellow bile results in anger. (Zentralbibliothek Zürich)

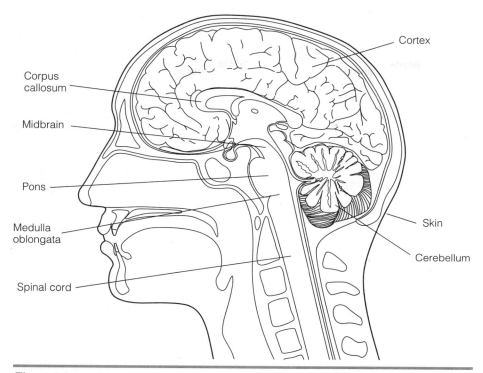

Figure 1.9 Basic anatomy of the brain. (From Kathryn Wolf Heller, *Understanding Physical, Sensory, and Health Impairments,* Pacific Grove: Brooks/Cole, 1996, p. 50, Figure 4.4)

dualist thinking opposes the idea that we can explain psychological states and processes in terms of physical phenomena. In fact, historians often call Descartes the founder of body–mind dualism. If he were correct, it would be hopeless to search for an explanation of mental processes in terms of brain states. However, people have sometimes misunderstood Descartes. He proposed a conception of bodily movement, such as the eye blink, that reflected the mechanistic concepts of his time, such as the functioning of clockworks and water fountains (see Figure 1.11). He generally believed the body to be a machine. Reflexes stem not from the intervention of the soul, but from nerves or message cables to and from the brain. Voluntary actions require a rational, nonmaterial soul and the free exercise of will. The church, however, steadfastly endorsed the idea that animal spirits and vital forces are nonmaterial and that all nervous ac-

tivity requires such vital forces. Descartes, a devoted Catholic, barely remained respectable in the scientific community because of his constant warnings that he was probably incorrect. His work *Treatise on Man* (1664), from which Figure 1.11 is taken, was not published until 14 years after his death, for he feared being charged with heresy.

By the 17th and 18th centuries more precise models of the brain became possible. This advance was in part related to the conviction that people could explain everything in terms of mechanics. English anatomist **Thomas Willis** (1621–1675), best known for his work on blood circulation in the brain, theorized that all mental faculties reside in the corpus striatum, a structure deep within the cerebral hemispheres. Others suggested that most mental faculties reside in the white matter of the cerebral hemispheres. **Giovanni Lancisi** (1654–1720), an Italian

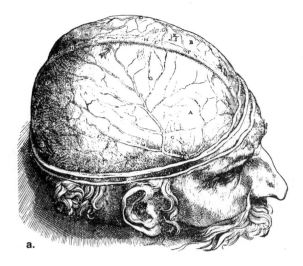

a.

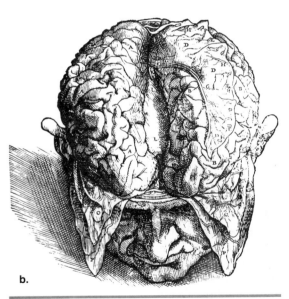

b.

Figure 1.10   Vesalius's drawings of the human brain. In his attempt to learn about anatomy, Vesalius initially depended on the work of others. Later he wanted to see for himself, performing the first systematic dissections of human beings done in Europe. (National Library of Medicine)

clinician who contributed greatly to our knowledge of the aneurysm (an abnormal blood-filled ballooning of an artery in the brain, see Chapter 9), selected the corpus callosum, a band of fibers that joins the left and right cerebral hemispheres, as the seat of mental functions.

Early investigators were preoccupied with identifying the one precise part of the brain that was the seat of the mind, but they based their discussions primarily on speculation and, in fact, conducted relatively little experimentation. Nevertheless, they were part of a movement that would become stronger in the centuries to come.

NON-WESTERN ATTITUDES

Although Western ideologies predominantly shaped the behavioral sciences, non-Western cultures also developed theories to explain behavior. Although some of these theories certainly must have involved the role of the brain, we know little about how advanced people such as the Egyptians and Eastern cultures approached the brain, because we lack detailed written accounts.

Common to eastern Mediterranean and African cultures was the belief that a god or gods sent diseases. For example, Egyptians viewed life as a balance between internal and external forces. As a result, they treated many mental disorders as integrating physical, psychic, and spiritual factors (Freedman, Kaplan, & Sadock, 1978). They conceptualized the brain as different from the mind. As in Aristotelian theory, they considered the heart the center of mind, sensation, and consciousness. In India, one of the earliest and most important medical documents, the **Atharva-Veda** (700 B.C.), proposed that the soul is nonmaterial and immortal.

During the Middle Ages, Arab countries demonstrated a humanist attitude toward the mentally ill, partly because of the Moslem belief that God loves the insane person. Because of this, the same treatments were available for the rich and poor. The treatment of mental patients was humanist and emphasized diets, baths, and even musical concerts especially designed to soothe the patient.

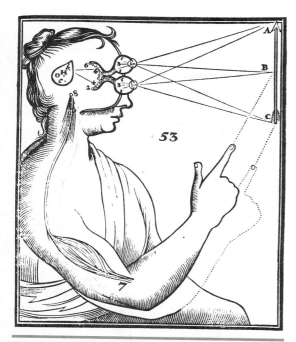

Figure 1.11 Seventeenth-century philosopher René Descartes here illustrates the mechanistic view of how light transmits images to the retina, stimulating nerves in the arm to produce movement. Descartes proposed that the mind interacts with the brain at the pineal gland. (National Library of Medicine)

Ancient Chinese medical texts also discussed psychological concepts and psychiatric symptoms. For example, Chinese medical practitioners endorsed a mechanistic view of mental processes. They conceptualized many mental health disorders as illnesses or vascular disorders, as opposed to the prevailing European belief in demonic possession. The ancient Chinese medical textbook *The Yellow Emperor's Classic of Internal Medicine* (about 1000 B.C.) refers to dementia, convulsions, and violent behavior. Confucian writings reflected early Chinese philosophical thought in proposing that mental functions are not distinct from physical functions and do not reside in any part of the organism, although giving the heart special importance as a guide for the mind. Surgeons practiced trephination in eastern Mediterranean and North

African countries as early as 4000 to 5000 B.C. There is no evidence of trephination in ancient Japan, China, or Egypt.

Because contributions to the development of neuropsychology by non-Western scholars remain unknown, we are left to wonder whether there may have been great discoveries or, alternatively, many of the same fallacies that Western cultures endorsed about the role of the brain on behavior.

Localization Theory

PHRENOLOGY AND FACULTY PSYCHOLOGY

Not until the 19th century did modern neuropsychological theories on brain function begin to evolve. Thinkers in part formulated them from a need not only to recognize the brain as responsible for controlling behavior but more importantly, to demonstrate precisely how the brain organizes behavior. Early in the century, Austrian anatomist **Franz Gall** (1758–1828), borrowing perhaps from the concept of geography (the notion of borders, at a time when people were discovering and mapping new continents), postulated that the brain consists of a number of separate organs, each responsible for a basic psychological trait such as courage, friendliness, or combativeness. Gall, a distinguished Viennese physician and teacher, suggested that mental faculties are innate and depend on the topical structures of the brain. His theory sought to describe differences in personality and cognitive traits on the basis of the size of individual brain areas. He hypothesized that the size of a given brain area is related to the amount of skill a person had in a certain field. Craniology was the study of cranial capacity in relation to brain size, which indicated intelligence.

Gall's work, however, was severely limited by faculty psychology, the predominant psychological theory of that time, which held that such abilities as reading, writing, or intelligence were independent, indivisible faculties. Such specific brain functions, then, were carried out in isolation from functional systems in other parts of the brain. Gall also lacked statistical or methodological theory that would have let him reliably measure the basic skills of interest to him. By assigning specific functions to particular places in the cerebral cortex, Gall formulated the basis of the **localization theory** of brain function (see Table 1.3). Although Gall was wrong on most counts, he did help shape how we perceive brain–behavior relationships today. For example, Gall correctly suggested that because their complexity is greatest in humans, the most intellectual parts of the brain are the frontal lobes. He also argued that the brain is the organ of the mind and that functions are grouped within it.

From Gall's basic theory of localization, the "science" of **phrenology** was born. This theory held that if a given brain area is enlarged, then the corresponding area of the skull will also be enlarged. Conversely, a depression in the skull signals an underdeveloped area of the cortex. It is generally accurate that skull configurations closely follow brain configurations. Phrenology, in its most popular form, involved feeling the cranial bumps to ascertain which cerebral areas were largest (see Figure 1.12). Sophisticated me-

chanical equipment was developed, such as the phrenology cap (see Figure 1.13), to accurately identify bumps and indentations on the skull in order to make "precise" predictions about psychological strengths and weaknesses.

Although Gall made remarkable discoveries in neuroanatomy, the theory of phrenology was entirely inaccurate. In Vienna and Paris, critics accused Gall of materialism and ultimately forced him to leave teaching. His student **Johann Spurzheim** (1776–1832) carried on his phrenology teachings, lecturing extensively on phrenology in the United States. As a result, phrenology societies sprang up in the United States, and the movement became increasingly popu-

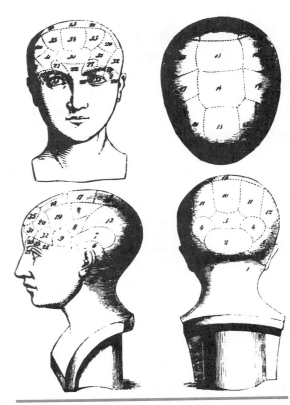

Figure 1.12   Phrenology head. Specific locations on the skull were thought to correspond to specific abilities. (National Library of Medicine)

Table 1.3   *Definition of the Organs*

Selected "interpretations" corresponding to specific locations on the skull.

1. **Amativeness:** love between the sexes, desire to marry

2. **Parental love:** regard for offspring, pets, and so on

3. **Friendship:** adhesiveness, sociability, love of society

4. **Inhabitiveness:** love of home and country

5. **Continuity:** one thing at a time, consecutiveness

6. **Combativeness:** resistance, defense, courage, opposition

7. **Destructiveness:** executiveness, force, energy

8. **Alimentiveness:** appetite, hunger, love of eating

9. **Acquisitiveness:** accumulation, frugality, economy

10. **Secretiveness:** discretion, reserve, policy, management

Source: Wells (1869), p. 35.

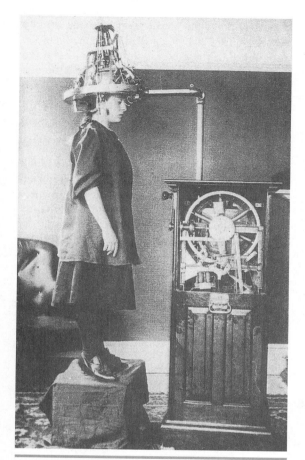

Figure 1.13 Phrenology machine (about 1905) was intended to measure "bumps" on the skull and correlate those with specific human attributes. (Copyright © Museum of Questionable Medical Devices)

lar. To this day people sometimes make attributions about an individual solely on the basis of specific physical characteristics.

Gall also played an important role in developing deterministic thought about the functions of the brain and the mind, but in the final analysis his critics accused him of having made the most absurd theories about the faculties of human understanding. Phrenology, in its simplistic form, had followers who made sweeping statements about the brains and minds

of men and women. Men, they suggested, have larger brain areas in the social region, with a predominance of pride, energy, and self-reliance, compared to those of females, which reflect "inhabitiveness" (love of home) and a lack of firmness and self-esteem. Phrenologists also attempted cross-cultural comparisons, suggesting that the skulls of races and nations differ widely in form. Erroneously, phrenologists (largely Caucasian) suggested that the skulls of Caucasians were superior, indicating great intellectual power and strong moral sentiment. The skulls from "less advanced races" did not fare as well, because those virtues were thought to be almost invariably small in "savage" and "barbarous tribes" (Wells, 1869).

The promise of finding anatomic differences that could explain even complex social and intellectual behaviors is, for some scientists, still very tempting. A controversy has developed whether the brains of murderers and geniuses are indistinguishable or are different. Scientists in the former Soviet Union preserved and studied the brains of famous communists in order to identify their "intellectual superiority." In the United States, Albert Einstein's brain is floating in formaldehyde, and convicted serial killer Jeffrey Dahmer's brain is in storage for later analysis. Einstein's brain, the focus of several studies, may be larger in strategic areas that may partly explain his uncommon ability for conceptual and multidimensional thinking (Witelson, Kigar, & Harvey, 1999). Most neuroscientists, however, agree that the idea of explaining a person's personality and abilities from neuroanatomical evidence is premature. (See Figure 1.14.)

Faculty psychology and discrete localization theory continued to develop for a century. Many factors were erroneous and simplistic, but three major developments represented significant progress. First, scientists were reluctant to accept a single part or component of the brain as responsible for all behavior, as had proponents of earlier theories. Second, they placed more emphasis on the role of the cortex, which until then had not been seen as functioning neural tissue but as relatively unimportant protective "bark" ("cortex" in Latin). Third, and perhaps most important, scientists focused their study of behavior and the mind on the brain.

THE ERA OF CORTICAL LOCALIZATION

Before the 19th century people knew little about the cortex of the brain. Almost completely unexplored as to their functions, cerebral convolutions were not considered the least bit interesting. Scientific evidence supporting a localization position was not available until 1861, when **Paul Broca** (1824–1880) announced to the medical community that motor speech was specifically located in the posterior, inferior region of the left frontal lobe. Before Broca's time, what he called this "grotesquely shaped, fast-decaying, and unmanageable organ" had attracted only very few investigators.

Broca's accomplishments in his short 56 years of life are impressive. Even nonhistorians know about his work in surgery, neuroanatomy, neurophysiology, and neuropathology. Broca, who was sympathetic to Charles Darwin's concept of evolution by natural selection (*On the Origin of Species,* 1859), was also the founder of French anthropology. In fact, because of his stature in that field, he was one of the first to have been presented with a trephined skull recovered from a Peruvian burial site. Broca dismissed the evidence, however, as merely a "hole in the head," because he was biased about "primitive" cultures and their ability for intellectual thought.

Broca's landmark contribution was in understanding the origins of **aphasia**. In Paris, he was a professor of surgery, but contributed most to advancing the field of brain anatomy. Broca presented two clinical cases to support his proposal for the locus of speech. Both individuals had fairly extensive injuries, involving lesions in the left posterior frontal lobe, corresponding paralyses on the right side, and motor speech deficits, but in other respects seemed intelligent and normal. From his investigations he described the condition of aphasia (often called *Broca's aphasia* or *nonfluent aphasia*), an inability to talk be-

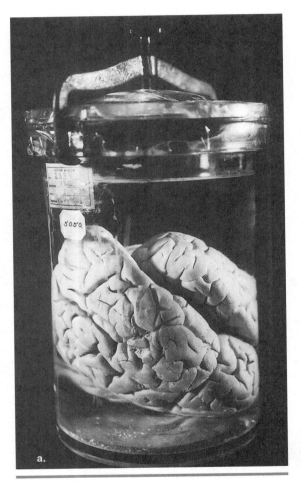

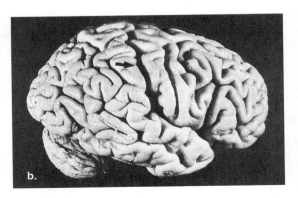

Figure 1.14 (a) Preserved brain of murderer John Wilson. In a widely publicized case in 1884, Wilson admitted to killing Anthony Daly in a fit of rage. Wilson attacked the former butcher with a cleaver to the forehead and then dismembered him. Phrenologists argued that murderers "generally have the forehead villainously low." (Mütter Museum, College of Physicians of Philadelphia) (b) Brain of Albert Einstein. There is much controversy whether the physicist's brain is in any way superior anatomically to that of normals. (Witelson/Kigar/Harvey/*The Lancet*)

Borrowing on ideas of Gall and Spurzheim, the Nazi propaganda leadership suggested that natural biological traits decide the total being of a person and challenged those who sought to explain personality on any basis other than a biological or racial one. Of course, the Nazis erred in refusing to recognize complex contributing environmental and social influences that also shape and determine behavior. But U.S. armed forces leadership were also invested in the same fallacy, trying to demonstrate that there was something biologically wrong with the Nazis. For example, in 1945 the U.S. Army ordered a postmortem autopsy of the brain of Robert Ley, a high-ranking Nazi Labor Front boss, after he had committed suicide while waiting to stand trial at the International Military Tribunal in Nuremberg. Allied doctors argued that deterioration in Ley's frontal lobes as a result of an old head injury explained his criminal behavior, which included violent anti-Semitism and ostentatious vulgarism. Army pathologists concluded that "the [brain] degeneration was of sufficient duration and degree to have impaired Dr. Ley's mental and emotional faculties and could well account for his alleged aberrations in conduct and feelings" ("Dr. Robert Ley's Brain," 1946, p. 188).

The fact that the U.S. Army and the American public had an investment in the pathology of Ley's brain is ironic, because the Nazis themselves expended much effort to demonstrate, through pseudomedical research using principles based on phrenology, that the skulls of *Untermenschen* ("subhumans") were biologically inferior. In a morbid display of unethical medicine, Nazi doctors at concentration camps routinely sent postmortem specimens of the targeted groups to Berlin to exhibit and demonstrate "inferiority" (Lifton, 1986). In the same way the American public and media were very invested in viewing the Nuremberg "gang" as biologically and psychologically abnormal. Following World War II, British and U.S. psychiatrists went so far as to suggest that one could detect a Nazi by phrenology. Rudolf Hess, Hitler's deputy, they argued had specific anatomic features, including an "extreme primitive skull formation and misshapen ears," which could serve as possible warning signals in spotting future Nazis (Rees, 1948).

The neuropathologic evidence that Ley's brain was abnormal turned out to be very weak and undoubtedly distorted by the significant external pressure to find something wrong with the Nazis at Nuremberg. Interestingly, after the execution of the 11 high-ranking Nazi leaders at Nuremberg, scientists asked to perform additional autopsies, particularly histological studies of the Nazis' brains (Zillmer, Archer, & Castin, 1989; Zillmer, Harrower, Ritzler, & Archer, 1995). The authorities denied this request, however, because the bodies were to be cremated at the Dachau concentration camp and the ashes disposed of secretly. Today, the remains of Ley's brain are kept at the U.S. Army Institute of Pathology in Washington, D.C.

Although a variety of functional and organic disturbances may lead to aggression and violent behavior, most violence is committed by people suffering from no diagnosable brain impairment. Phrenology has always been a tempting theory, because it reduces complex racial views to simple physical observations. For example, when my mother studied physics at the University of Vienna during the early 1940s the authorities did not have much interest in the study of individual differences. A required course during the Nazi occupation was Rassenkunde (Racial Theory), which replaced psychology and philosophy.

---

cause the musculature of speech organs do not receive appropriate brain signals. Broca's announcement, hailed by many as a major breakthrough, led to numerous investigations into the localization of other higher cognitive functions. Broca, of course, supported other localizationists by proposing that behavior, in this case expressive speech, is controlled by a specific brain area. It was also one of the first discoveries of a separation of function between the left and right hemisphere of the brain. But most important, it was one of the first indications that specific brain functions exist in particular locales in the brain. There is a connection, or so it seemed, between the anatomy of the brain and what the brain does.

Neuropsychology in Action 1.3

Paul Broca: A Manner of Not Speaking

by Eric A. Zillmer

Paul Broca identified a specific area on the convoluted surface of the human brain, approximately 1 cubic centimeter (cm^3) in size, as the central organ for expressive speech. Broca's famous discovery came at a time when he viewed the convolutions of the brain as distinct organs. The evidence for this was, however, particularly weak, and phrenology was receiving some criticism. Thus, it was not a coincidence that Broca made such a discovery. He had been searching for some time for a patient just like Monsieur Leborgne. In May 1861 Broca presented the brain of Leborgne, alias "Tan," a 51-year-old man who had died on the previous day under Broca's care.

I found one morning on my service a dying patient who 21 years ago had lost the faculty of articulate speech. I gathered his case history with the greatest care because it seemed to serve as a touchstone for the [localization] theory of my colleague. The patient died on April 17 [1861] at 11 A.M. The autopsy was performed as soon as possible, that is to say within 24 hours. The brain was shown a few hours later in the Société d'Anthropologie, then immediately put in alcohol.

The abolition of speech is a symptom of sufficient importance, that it seems useful to designate it by a special name. I have given it the name aphemia [the term was later changed to *aphasia* by a colleague of Broca's, Professor Trousseau]. For what is missing in these patients is only the faculty to articulate words.

Although I believe in the principle of localization, I have been and still am asking myself, within what limits may this principle apply? If it were demonstrated that the lesions which abolish speech constantly occupy the same convolution then one could hardly help admitting that this convolution is the seat of articulated speech. (Schiller, 1982, pp. 177–178, 180, 182)

Probably no other single, preserved human brain has aroused more attention than the one Broca was describing. Some criticized the manner of its preservation (in an unorthodox erect position) and the damage to the brain involving chronic and progressive softening of the second and third left frontal convolutions, as well as the specimen's unavailability for examination (see Figure 1.15). Broca responded to his critics, "I have refrained from studying the deeper parts

Contemporary research methodology proposes that in order to attribute a precise cognitive function to a specific anatomic section of the brain, research must meet two conditions: The first, which Broca did demonstrate, is that destruction of a localized brain site impairs a specific function, in this case articulate speech. The second, which Broca did not demonstrate, relates to the fact that damage to any other area of the brain—for example, the patient's right frontal lobe—should not result in the same deficit. This second condition is called **double dissociation** (Teuber, 1950) and requires that "symptom A appear in lesions in one structure but not with those in another, and that symptom B appear with lesions of the other but not of the one" (Teuber, 1959, p. 187). Nevertheless, although Broca may not have followed the standards of modern science, articulate speech is in fact to an important extent localized in and controlled by Broca's area.

A decade after Broca's discovery, **Carl Wernicke** (1848–1904) announced that the understanding of speech was located in the superior, posterior aspects of the temporal lobe (Wilkins & Brody, 1970). Wernicke noted that no motor deficit accompanied a loss of speech comprehension caused by damage in this area; only the ability to understand speech was disrupted. That is, the patient was still able to talk, but his speech made no sense and sounded like some unknown foreign language. Such speech was called **fluent aphasia** (Geschwind, 1965). Although Wernicke, who like Broca has an area of the brain named after him (see Figure 1.16), supported localizationists by locating a specific area important for word comprehension, he also demonstrated that language is

(of the brain), in order not to destroy the specimen which I thought should be deposited in the (Dupuytren) museum" (Schiller, 1982, p. 180).

Tan's history has often been told, but his basic disease has never been satisfactorily diagnosed. Broca's acquaintance with this patient lasted barely a week. Neither the history nor the appearance and description of the brain allow a confident clinical and pathological interpretation in modern terms. Leborgne had been epileptic since his youth and became aphasic at the age of 30. He showed progressively weakening on his right side since the age of 40, first in the arm. He became hemiplegic and was bedridden for seven years. Leborgne deteriorated gradually, losing his intellect and vision, and finally died at age 51 of cellulitis with gangrene of the paralyzed right leg. His early history of epilepsy arouses the suspicion that successive thrombotic infarcts may have not been the correct diagnosis, and that perhaps a form of degenerative disease may be more plausible. He was also known to have cursed when he was disturbed,

which may also suggest that aphasia may have been the least of his problems (however, as we discuss in later chapters, cursing and grunts may be actually controlled by the right hemisphere, which does not dominate speech). In retrospect, Leborgne's history suggests that many other symptoms accompanied his aphasia. It now seems Leborgne was a poor choice for being selected as the prototype for Broca's aphasia. If Broca had had a statistical consultant, he would have been advised not to make such sweeping conclusions based on only one subject!

Just as Broca preserved Leborgne's brain for safekeeping, he would have been pleased to know that his own brain too has been stored in the Museum de l'Homme (Museum of Man) in Paris. There, deep in the museum in a remote, musty corner among abandoned cabinets and shelves hidden from the public, is a collection of gray, convoluted objects, stored in formaldehyde. Among them is the brain of Paul Broca. If you looks closely, you can detect the small region in the third convolution on the left frontal lobe of the

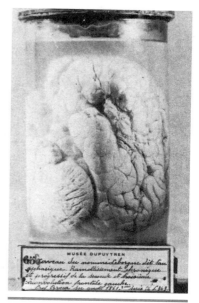

Figure 1.15 Leborgne's brain. Note atrophy in Broca's area. (Museé Dupuytren)

cerebral cortex that made him famous— "Broca's Broca's area"!

not strictly localized. Broca's area, or expressive speech, is in the frontal lobes and Wernicke's area, or receptive speech, is posterior to that, in the temporal lobe. As a result of Wernicke's work, theories of strict localization have become less feasible because speech is not located in one specific location of the cortex, but in two distinct cortical areas.

CRITICS OF CORTICAL LOCALIZATION

Sigmund Freud (1856–1938) is best known as the founder of psychoanalysis. Yet Freud's initial love was for investigating the secrets of the central nervous system. Freud, who made significant discoveries in the area of brain–behavior relationships, never gained the respect that he deserved for his work as a neurologist.

In *Zur Auffassung der Aphasien* (An Understanding of Aphasia) (1891), Freud criticizes Wernicke's and Broca's localization doctrine of aphasia. At the time that Freud wrote this text, many neurologists confronted the task of explaining the many partial and mixed varieties of aphasias. We now know that aphasia comes in a variety of "flavors," including the inability to speak spontaneously, the inability to repeat words, the inability to read words yet being able to read letters, and so on. Wernicke proposed that for each different syndrome there was one corresponding specific lesion in the connections between Wernicke's and Broca's area that would account for the disturbance. The more combinations of aphasic disturbances that he observed, however, the more complicated became Wernicke's diagrams. To simplify Wernicke's diagrams, Freud suggested that various

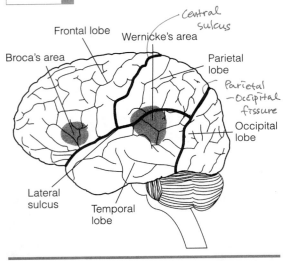

Figure 1.16   Broca's area and Wernicke's area. (Adapted from Kathryn Wolff Heller, *Understanding Physical, Sensory, and Health Impairments,* Pacific Grove: Brooks/Cole, 1996, p. 52, Figure 4.7)

aphasias could be explained by subcortical lesions in less localized association pathways. Freud pointed out, quite correctly, that the Broca and Wernicke centers are little more than nodal points in a general and complicated network of neurons. Freud proposed that the Broca and Wernicke areas were not self-acting agencies and that their significance was simply due to their anatomic location, in the former case to the motor areas of the brain, and in the latter to the entry of the fibers from the acoustic nuclei. Freud also described the distinction between the ability to recognize an object and the inability to name it, **agnosia,** a term that has remained with us ever since.

"Is the whole greater than the sum of its parts?" Clinical observation did not validate the idea that each skill is controlled by a circumscribed part of the brain. Localizationists could not explain findings, reported by numerous physicians, that lesions in widely disparate parts of the brain, not one specific area, impaired the same skill. Moreover, many patients with lesions in a specific brain area could still carry out a skill assigned exclusively to that area.

Pierre Flourens (1794–1867) was the foremost early advocate of an alternative to localization theo-

ries (Krech, 1962). Through an extensive number of experiments and logical arguments, Flourens attempted to disprove Gall's localization theory. To support his beliefs, Flourens developed the **ablation experiment,** in which removing any part of the brain in birds led to generalized disorders of behavior. From his experiments, he reached several general conclusions. Sensory input at an elementary level is localized, but the process of perception involves the whole brain. Loss of function depends on the extent of damage, not on the location. All cerebral material is **equipotential;** that is, if sufficient cortical material is intact, the remaining material will take over the functions of any missing brain tissue. Flourens suggested that the brain operated in an integrated fashion, not in discrete faculties, and that mental functions depend on the brain functioning as a whole. Thus, the size of the injury, rather than its location, determines the effects of brain injury.

Flourens, however, was criticized on a number of different points. First, he used animals with brains so small that any ablation would invade more than one functional area. Second, he observed only motor behavior—that is, behaviors such as eating or wing flapping—whereas the localizationists were mostly interested in more complex faculties such as friendship or intellect. Flourens also erroneously suggested that humans use only 10 percent of the brain, an idea that laypeople still commonly hold today. Despite these scientific problems, many accept Flourens as having refuted localization theory. Nevertheless, the work of Broca and other localization theorists was the predominant view of brain–behavior relationships and was in large part accepted by the scientific community. Consequently, few people supported Flourens's work until the early 1900s, when equipotentialists began to again develop evidence and research to support their position.

 ## Localization versus Equipotentiality

Pierre Marie (1906) challenged Broca's findings by examining the preserved brains of the pa-

Neuropsychology in Action 1.4

Sigmund Freud: The Neurologist

by Eric A. Zillmer

Freud entered the University of Vienna in the autumn of 1873, at the early age of 17 and graduated with a medical degree in 1881. Considering an academic research career in physiology, he went to work in the laboratory of the Brücke Institute. There he took a great liking to laboratory work and, initially, harbored an aversion to the clinical practice of medicine. Beset by financial difficulties, he began working under Meynert, a neurosurgeon and psychiatrist, to gain additional practical experience in May 1883. During this time he came closer to disorders of the brain, but he restricted his laboratory work to dissecting the nervous system. At first Freud investigated the cells of the spinal cord, the part of the nervous system that held his chief interest. For the next two years he concentrated on a specific area of the brain stem, the medulla, that resulted in three published papers. From October 1885 to February 1886, Freud visited Paris to study with the great neurologist Jean-Martin Charcot. Charcot was then at the zenith of his fame. No one, before or since, has so dominated the world of neurology, and for Freud to have been a pupil of his was a passport to distinction.

When Freud went to Paris, his anatomic interests were still more in his mind than any ambition as a clinician. On his return to Vienna, he researched topics of visual field deficits, hemianopsia, in children and its localization. From correspondence we also know that in 1887 and 1888 Freud was working on a book on the anatomy of the brain, which he never finished (Jones, 1981). The next publication in 1891 was Freud's first book *Zur Auffassung der Aphasien* (An Understanding of Aphasia). Freud thought the text the most valuable of his neurologic writings, although it proved not to be the one by which neurological circles remembered his name. Despite Freud's critical and speculative monograph on aphasia, which ultimately achieved acceptance, he did not have much luck with his book. Of the 850 copies printed, after nine years only 257 had sold, and Freud was paid only a total of $62 in royalties (Jones, 1981). The neurological community was not yet ready for his insights, and all historical writings on aphasia omit any reference to the book. Yet his neurologic achievements were remarkable, especially for a young student, and illustrate his biological and genetic outlook.

In retrospect, Freud's psychoanalytic model can be loosely related to brain processes. For example, Freud's id, the unconscious "beast in the basement" that operates on the pleasure principle, may have developed out of the reptilian brain, a product of presocial evolutionary history. Freud's superego, our conscience, is an evolutionarily more recent invention, conceptualized within prefrontal lobe processes that are involved in forming such abstract concepts as morality, guilt, planning, and inhibition. At this highest, most complex level of brain structure, a major function is to inhibit the spontaneous expression of the more biologically programmed patterns of behavior that arise from lower and evolutionary older structures of the brain such as the id. The ego, based on the reality principle, is perhaps related to complex brain processes in the "middle," that is, the cortex, excluding the prefrontal lobes (Wright, 1994). It is often difficult to trace threads between Freud's subsequent focus on unobservable, intrapsychic events and his early investigation of the nervous system. He never did, however, venture too far away from his neurological roots, as demonstrated in his work *On Narcissism* (1959), in which he suggested that all provisional ideas on psychology will one day be explained on the basis of organic substrates.

---

tients Broca had used to support his hypothesis of localization. Marie found that Leborgne had widespread damage, not a specific lesion, as Broca had suggested. Marie attacked Broca's theory, indicating that the patient could not speak because the extensive lesion had caused a general loss of intellect, rather than a specific inability to speak. Other researchers soon expressed support for the equipotentiality position. In general, these researchers proposed that although basic sensorimotor functions may be localized in the brain, higher cortical processes were too complex to confine to any one area.

Two important neuropsychological findings also challenged strict localization theory. In 1881 (cited by Blakemore, 1977), **Hermann Munk** (1839–1912) found that experimental lesions in the association cortex of a dog produced temporary **mind-blindness:** The animal could see objects but failed to recognize their significance (for example, as objects of fear). In the experiment, Munk first had the dogs learn to associate the shape of a triangle with fear by pairing them together with an electric shock. After the learning occurred, he then lesioned parts of the cortex that were not primarily involved in seeing. Afterward, the dogs could see the object, but could not perceive the meaning of the stimuli they were conditioned to before the surgery. In 1914, **Joseph Babinski** (1857–1932), the founder of neurology, introduced the term **anosognosia,** which means "no knowledge of the disease," to describe an inability or refusal to recognize that one has a particular disease or disorder, thereby introducing the phenomenon of unawareness (Babinski & Joltran, 1924). Babinski observed patients who had lesions, most often in the association cortex of the right hemisphere. These patients were capable of seeing and hearing, but denied that anything was wrong with them even when they had severe neurological damage such as hemiplegia.

Karl Lashley (1890–1958), a student of the famous behaviorist John Watson, was a great exemplar of experimental neuropsychology and, according to Hebb (1983), practically its founder. He was one of the first to combine behavioral sophistication in experiments with neurological sophistication. Lashley become America's most eminent early neuropsychologist, highly respected for his ingenuity in devising ways of disclosing the effects of brain operations (Popplestone & McPherson, 1994). Although Lashley accepted the localization of basic sensory and motor skills, he supported equipotential views with experiments on rats similar to those of Flourens on birds (Lashley, 1929; Luria, 1973). Lashley found that impairment in maze running in the rat was directly related to the amount of cortex removed. He stated that the specific area removed made little difference. From his experiments, Lashley formulated his famous principle of **mass action:** The extent of behavioral impairments is directly proportional to the mass of the removed tissue. Lashley also emphasized the multipotentiality of brain tissue: Each part of the brain participated in more than one function (Teuber, Battersby, & Bender, 1960). Lashley felt that his results were highly compatible with a view that brain tissue is equipotential and can be involved in tasks other than those assigned by the localizationists.

In one form or another, localization and equipotentiality have dominated American psychology, although neither approach has enjoyed universal acceptance because neither can encompass all the collected scientific data and clinical observations. Clinical observers of medical patients with very small lesions have often reported marked behavioral deficits, even though the lesion may be microscopic. Thus equipotentiality theory fails to account for the specific deficits often seen in the absence of general impairment in intellect, abstract attitude, perception, or other global ability.

Integrated Theories of Brain Function

JACKSON'S ALTERNATIVE MODEL

Unable to accept either the localization or equipotentiality models of brain function, psychologists and neurologists have searched for other alternative models. The creation of one such model has been credited to the English neurologist **Hughlings Jackson** (1835–1911), whose primary work was written during the second half of the 19th century, but was not published in this country until the 1950s. Jackson, a London neurologist, devoted his research to the investigation of epileptic seizures, and the study of connections between limb movements and specific areas in the brain. Jackson observed that higher mental functions are not unitary abilities, but consist of simpler and more basic skills. He suggested that one does not have a speech center. Rather, one has the ability to combine certain basic skills, such as hearing, discrimination of speech sounds, and fine motor and kinesthetic control of the speech apparatus, in order to create more complex higher skills (Hebb, 1959). Consequently, the loss of speech can be traced to the loss of any one of a number of basic abilities or functional systems. It can be related to the loss of motor control, the loss of adequate feedback from the mouth and tongue, a defect in the understanding and use of the basic parts of speech, or the inability to decide to speak, to name just a few examples.

Thus the loss of a specific area of the brain causes the loss or impairment of all higher skills dependent on that one area. Furthermore, a lesion causing the loss of speech does not necessarily indicate that we have found the brain area responsible for speech. Jackson proposed that localizing damage that destroys speech and localizing speech are two different things. Jackson also believed that behavior can exist on many different levels within the nervous system. Thus, a patient may be unable to repeat the word "no," when asked to repeat it, even though, the patient is capable of saying, in exasperation, "No, Doctor, I can't say no!" (Luria, 1966). In the first instance, the patient cannot say the word voluntarily. When the word is given as an automatic response, however, the patient is able to say it. The ability to say "no" exists as two separate skills; one voluntarily and one automatic. Each ability can be impaired independently of the other. Because of this, Jackson noted, behavior is rarely lost completely unless the damage to the brain is severe (Golden, Zillmer, & Spiers, 1992).

Jackson suggested that given his observations, behavior results from interactions among all the areas of the brain. Even the simplest motor movement requires the full cooperation of all the levels of the nervous system, from the peripheral nerves and the spinal cord to the cerebral hemispheres. In this regard, Jackson pointed toward a more holistic, nearly equipotential view of brain function. But Jackson also argued that each area within the nervous system had a specific function that contributed to the overall system. Thus his views had a localizationist's flavor. In actuality of course, Jackson's views were those of neither school, but reflected an integration of significant empirical data. Jackson's influence can first be seen in British neurology of the early 20th century, although many people overlooked the essential nature of what Jackson proposed. They interpreted his work as more supportive of an equipotentiality view of higher mental functions than it actually was. Since World War II,

many major theorists have presented views compatible with Jackson's. For example, Harlow (1952) concluded from his experimental monkey studies that no cognitive ability is completely destroyed by any limited lesion, although there appears to be some localization, a view entirely consistent with Jackson's. After reviewing much of the literature, Krech also reached two similar conclusions (1962; Chapman & Wolff, 1959). First, no learning process or function entirely depends on any one area of the cortex. Second, each area within the brain plays an unequal role in different kinds of functions. These conclusions, although contrary to either the localization or equipotentiality beliefs, were also in accordance with Jackson's alternative approach.

LURIA'S FUNCTIONAL MODEL

The most detailed adaptation of the principle first suggested by Jackson, has appeared in the work of the Russian neuropsychologist **Alexander Luria** (1902–1977). Luria was responsible for the most profound changes in our approach to understanding the brain and the mind. Luria, who earned doctoral degrees in psychology, medicine, and education, was the most significant and productive neuropsychologist of his time, and he raised the field to a level that could not have been imagined 50 years ago. Luria realized that a viable brain–behavior theory must not only explain data that fit both the localization and equipotentiality hypothesis, but also must account for findings inconsistent with either theories. Luria—building on the work of his mentor and arguably the founder of cognitive psychology, Vygotzky (1965)—and Jackson conceived each area in the central nervous system as being involved in one of three basic functions, which he labeled *units*. The first unit, roughly defined as the brain stem and associated areas, regulates the arousal level of the brain and the maintenance of proper muscle tone. The second unit, including posterior areas of the cortex, plays a key role in the reception, integration, and analysis of sensory information from both the internal and external environment. The third unit, the frontal and prefrontal lobes, is involved in planning, executing, and verifying behavior (Luria, 1964, 1966, 1973).

All behavior requires the interaction of these basic functions. Consequently, all behavior reflects the result of the brain operating as a whole. At the same time, each area within the brain has a specific role in forming behavior. The importance of any one area depends on the behavior to be performed. For example, picking up the receiver when the phone rings—a simple, well-practiced act—requires little arousal, planning, or evaluation. A more complex behavior, such as telling a caller what you will be doing next Tuesday evening, however, requires attention and arousal, as well as planning and evaluation. An injury having little effect on the first behavior might be disastrous for the second, more complex one.

For each behavior, Luria formulated the concept of **functional systems,** which represent the pattern of interaction among the various areas of the brain necessary to complete a behavior. Each area in the brain can operate only in conjunction with other areas of the brain. Furthermore, no area of the brain is singly responsible for any voluntary human behavior; thus each area of the brain may play a specific role in many behaviors. As with the equipotentiality theory, Luria regards behavior as the result of interaction among many areas of the brain. As with the localization theory, Luria assigns a specific role to each area of the brain. The multiple, functional role of the brain is called **pluripotentiality;** any given area of the brain can be involved in relatively few or relatively many behaviors.

Luria suggested that behavior results from several functions or systems of brain areas, rather than from unitary or discrete brain areas. A disruption at any stage is enough to immobilize a given functional system. For example, an individual without injury to what localizationists would call the "reading center" is unable to read if there is damage to any of a number of parts of the functional systems involved in reading. Each functional system, however, has some plasticity and can change spontaneously or through retraining. For example, sensory feedback is necessary for continually knowing the location of one's fingers and arm to direct motor movement. A person who loses sensory feedback from the arm loses an important link in completing fine motor tasks. The functional system, however, can be altered by using visual feedback to locate the fingers of the hand, something not previously needed. The patient can thus reestablish fine motor skills, despite the disruption of the old functional system. Luria's concept of alternative functional systems accounts for the ability of higher-level brain skills to compensate for lower-level skills in brain injury. This concept was clearly demonstrated in an interesting patient we once examined. At age 3 months the patient had undergone a complete left hemispherectomy (removal of a hemisphere). When we saw him at age 7, not only could he walk, but he also spoke fluently. This was undoubtedly related to the plastic nature of the brain, in which the right side of the brain can develop the organization necessary to execute such behaviors.

Luria's hypothesis is particularly attractive to clinical neuropsychologists, because it can account theoretically for most observations of brain-injured patients. The theory also explains the observation that certain lesions generally yield consistent deficits. In addition, through the concept of reorganization, Luria's theory can account for individuals who recover from brain trauma. Finally, the theory suggests ways to establish rehabilitation and treatment programs for the brain-injured patient and provides a strong theoretical basis for understanding clinical neuropsychology.

Modern Neuropsychology

Since Broca made his momentous discovery in the 1860s, a number of major achievements and influential concepts led to the evolution of neuropsychology as a discipline. Nevertheless, until the 1960s and Luria's writings, there was no unifying theory of brain–behavior relationships. In 1933 Kleist published his monumental work on wartime brain injuries. Although his localization approach was accepted in Germany, it was largely unknown outside that country. In the United States and Britain, the findings and conclusions of Lashley, Marie, and Jackson set up a general antilocalization bias. In particular, the field of aphasia remained divided between the "holists" and "diagram makers" such as Wernicke (Benton, 1994). The birth of modern psychosurgery was in 1935, when Moniz and Lima first attempted to alleviate mental suffering by operating on the human frontal lobes. The novelty of his concept and the "quality" of Moniz's results earned him a Nobel prize in medicine in 1949. In the 1940s the apparently favorable effects of the surgery on the majority of severely disturbed patients led to its introduction in the United States by psychiatrist Walter Freeman and his surgical colleague, James Watts. Treating psychiatric patients' with lobotomies is now, however, regarded as a step backward (see Neuropsychology in Action 1.5).

Clinical neuropsychology originally emerged in the medical setting within traditional neurosurgery and neurology services. Early research was mostly concerned with the cortical functioning of patients with penetrating missile wounds or the diagnosis of neurological disorders such as brain tumors or strokes. In the late 1930s neuropsychology engaged the interest of only a few neurologists, psychiatrists, and psychologists. Neuropsychology was loosely organized and no journals at that time reflected a focus interest in this area. But a number of scholars were working on interesting issues that in time made decisively important contributions to the field and shaped neuropsychology as we know it today.

The first neuropsychology laboratory in the United States was founded by Ward Halstead in 1935 at the University of Chicago. Halstead worked closely with neurosurgery patients and developed assessment devices that differentiated between patients with brain damage and those without (see Figure 1.18). Halstead

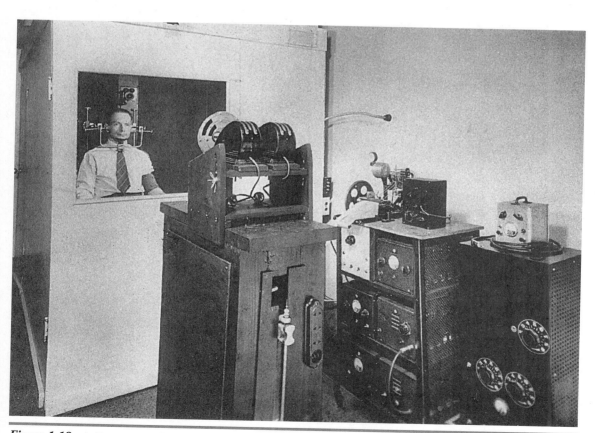

Figure 1.18 In the summer of 1940, Ward C. Halstead is recording eye movements. (Archives of the History of American Psychology, David P. Boder Museum Collection, Encyclopaedia Britannica)

Neuropsychology in Action 1.5

The Walter Freeman Lobotomies: Mind over Matter?

by Eric A. Zillmer

Freeman saw his mission as severing the fibers of a sick mind (Pennebaker, 1982). He felt that most psychiatric patients' mental illness was related to "confused" neurological processes and that an appropriate surgical cut would free the patient of that confusion (Freeman & Watts, 1950). Over the span of 20 years Freeman performed more than 3,500

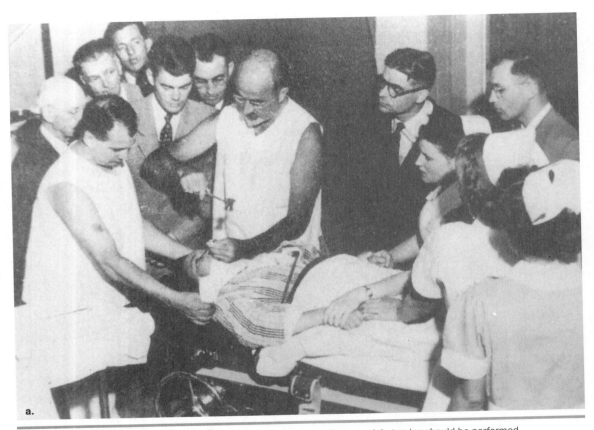

Figure 1.17 (a) Dr. Freeman performing a lobotomy. According to Freeman, lobotomies should be performed in every patient if conservative therapy fails. (Bettmann/CORBIS) (b) Lobotomy leucotome with Freeman's name engraved at the handle. Freeman suggested that, even though the risk for infections was low, different leucotomes be used for the two frontal lobes because of hygienic reasons. (Mütter Museum, College of Physicians of Philadelphia) (c) Electroconvulsive shock apparatus (around the 1950s). Lobotomy patients were anesthetized using electroconvulsive shock to the brain. After an induced seizure the patient was typically in a dazed and confused state, during which the lobotomy was performed. (Mütter Museum, College of Physicians of Philadelphia)

lobotomies across the country and pioneered the transorbital lobotomy. Freeman recommended lobotomies for any patient who had been institutionalized for more than two years, regardless of the patient's diagnosis or response to other therapy. The actual transorbital procedure consisted of initially anesthetizing the patient, typically achieved by electroconvulsive shock, with which the psychiatrist was familiar. Next, the patient's frontal lobes were pierced with a surgical instrument, a leucotome, inserted through the orbital cavity and passed through the orbital plate into the prefrontal region of the cortex. The psychiatrist swung the handle of the surgical instrument laterally and medially, "windshield wiper fashion," to sever the fibers at the base of the frontal lobe (Valenstein, 1973). The complete procedure took approximately 15 minutes and could be carried out in an office by a psychiatrist and one assistant (see Figure 1.17a–c).

(continued)

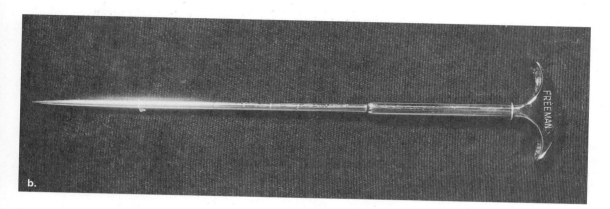

b.

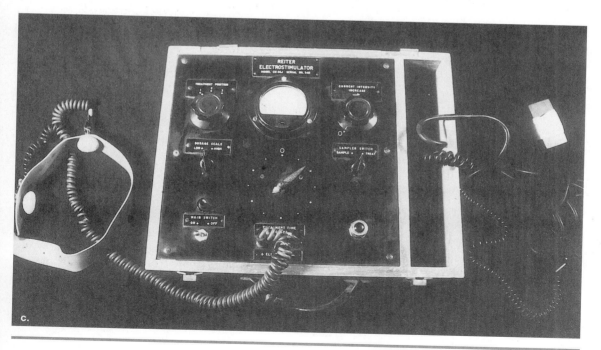

c.

(continued)

Between 1940 and 1954, approximately 40,000–50,000 psychiatric patients, most diagnosed as schizophrenic, underwent prefrontal orbital lobotomies in their doctors' effort to decrease inappropriate behavior while increasing ease of patient management. Although many of these patients subjected to prefrontal lobotomies were claimed as "cured," some died and a large number showed dangerous side effects, including confusion, flat affect, impulsiveness, continued psychotic episodes, and deteriorated intellectual functioning (Glidden, Zillmer, & Barth, 1990). Furthermore, because a major function of the frontal lobes is to inhibit behavior, many lobotomized patients actually developed new symptoms (such as incontinence, inappropriate affect, violent behavior, and so forth). When I was a fellow in neuropsychology, I once evaluated an elderly schizophrenic woman. In reviewing the medical chart, I was surprised to learn that Freeman had operated on the same patient more than 30 years earlier. Freeman's medical note was still in the patient's medical chart, detailing the more gruesome aspects of this so-called treatment:

July 2, 1953 Pre-lobotomy Examination: This patient looks quite a bit younger than her given age of 42. She stands with her head bowed and relatively little change of expression on her face. For the most part, she answers questions with a nod of her head, or a very silent yes, and even though conflicting statements are given, she nods just the same. At times she moves her lips in a way that suggests that she is continuously hallucinating. A story of a long psychotic illness with difficult behavior and brief furloughs since 1929 indicates that the problem is a very tough one. A proposal is made in this case to accompany the transorbital operation with an injection of 10cc. blood on each side into the inferior external aspects of the lobe, in the hope of eliminating to some extent the hallucinatory activities. The outlook for her release from the hospital is not good, but it may be possible that she will be more effectively able to adjust on the ward.

July 2, 1953 Operative Note: This patient presents an exceptionally difficult problem: therefore, after a triple electroshock, the orbitoclasts were driven to a depth of 5 cm. from the lid margin, parallel with the nose and 3 cm. from the midline. The instruments were pulled far laterally then brought back halfway and driven 2 cm. deeper. The handles were touched over the nose, then separated a total of 45 degrees and then elevated as firmly as possible. On the right side, the orbitoclast went through at an angle of about 60 degrees satisfactorily, but on the left side I met with such resistance that I was afraid for the instrument and replaced it with a new instrument, upon which I could apply the utmost in two-handed traction. Finally, the orbital plate gave way, and a cut of something like 75 degrees was achieved on this side. Then I drew 10 cc. blood from the right arm and injected it into the outer lower portion of the frontal lobe on the left side, and a similar quantity on the left side. The patient was coming to by this time, and made known her displeasure by her rather excited praying. When the blood injection had been completed, however, she was apparently in good condition.

—*Walter Freeman, M.D.*

later developed, together with Ralph Reitan, the popular **Halstead-Reitan Neuropsychological Battery,** an empirical approach to assessing brain damage (Halstead, 1947; Reitan & Wolfson, 1993).

The term *neuropsychology* itself is of very recent origin and was most probably first coined by Sir William Osler in 1913, when he first used the word in an inaugural address for a new psychiatric clinic at Johns Hopkins Hospital in Baltimore, Maryland (Bruce, 1985). In 1936, Karl Lashley also used the term *neuropsychology* when he addressed the Boston Society of Psychiatry and Neurology (Bruce, 1985). **Hans-Leukas Teuber** (1916–1977) is credited for first using the term in a national forum during a presentation to the American Psychological Association in 1948, during which he described different aspects of brain–behavior relationships in war veterans with penetrating brain wounds (Teuber, 1950). Then, in 1949, Donald Hebb published his classic, *The Organization of Behavior: A Neuropsychological Theory.* Neuropsychology has enjoyed tremendous growth ever since. The study of neuropsychology has drawn information and knowledge from many disciplines, including anatomy, biology, physiology, biophysics, and even philosophy. Thus, many interdisciplinary professionals, including neurologists, neuropsychiatrists, linguists, neuroscientists, speech pathologists, school psychologists, and others were interested in the field of brain–behavior relationships and contributed to its development.

One of these individuals was **Henry Hécaen** (born 1912), founder and editor of the international journal *Neuropsychologia*. Hécaen, who earned his M.D. degree, made important contributions to brain–behavior relationships in health and disease. One of his discoveries, which has earned him an enduring place in the history of neuropsychology, was his demonstration of the functional properties of the right hemisphere. In the 1940s and 1950s most thought that the left hemisphere dominated the brain, because it plays an important role in the mediation of language. Hécaen and his coworkers generated an irrefutable mass of evidence that the right, supposedly minor, hemisphere played a crucial role in mediating visual-perceptual and visual-constructional processes. Much of his work was not translated into English from French until much later (for example, see Hécaen & Albert, 1978) and as recently as during the early 1960s scientists seldom discussed or researched, issues regarding the role of the right cerebral hemisphere. The U.S. neuropsychologist **Arthur Benton** continued to explore the role of the right cerebral hemisphere in behavior and developed many neuropsychological measures assessing the right hemisphere (Benton, 1972).

Oliver Zangwill (born 1913) founded neuropsychology in Great Britain. Zangwill, who received his M.A. from Cambridge University and saw no necessity to work for the Ph.D. degree, transformed into a clinical neuropsychologist working in the Edinburgh Injury Unit of the British military services during World War II. There he was called on to evaluate hundreds of patients with traumatic brain lesions. Zangwill was also among the first investigators to show that hemispheric specialization for speech in left-handers did not conform to the then accepted rule of right hemisphere dominance (Zangwill, 1960). He also contributed significantly to an understanding of the nature of neuropsychological deficits associated with unilateral brain disease or injury.

Another important neuropsychologist who helped shape his profession's focus and development was **Norman Geschwind** (1926–1984). Geschwind received his M.D. degree at Harvard and later single-handedly founded behavioral neurology. In 1958, he joined the staff of the neurologic service of the Boston Veterans Administration Hospital, where he made many significant contributions to neuropsychology. Among them was his proposal that behavioral disturbances are based on the destruction of specific brain pathways that he called *disconnections*. He presented his idea in his now classic paper "Disconnexion Syndromes in Animals and Man" (1965), which was largely responsible for reemphasizing the important role of neuroanatomy in neuropsychology. Based on his faith that anatomy must play a central role for the description and operation of many complex mental functions, Geschwind set out to prove that the left hemisphere's dominance for speech must have an anatomic basis. He and a young colleague set out to study the morphologic features of 100 brains and determined that indeed there was a strong trend toward a larger auditory association cortex in the left hemisphere (Geschwind & Levitsky, 1968). This finding led to a continuing search for anatomic disparities that might be correlated with functional differences. His premature death at the age of 58 deprived behavioral neurology of its preeminent figure.

Muriel Lezak is one of several neuropsychologists who has pioneered the assessment approach in clinical neuropsychology. Over the last 20 years, neuropsychological assessment has played a major role in the development of clinical neuropsychology. Neuropsychological evaluations have become an important procedure, allowing the generation of useful behavioral, cognitive, and clinical information about diagnosis and the impact of a patient's limitations on educational, social, and vocational adjustment. In addition to the development of new testing methods to meet special needs in diagnostic evaluation, there has been a steadily increasing use of neuropsychological assessment techniques in neurology and psychiatry and an expansion of their scope of application into other fields such as education, behavioral medicine, and gerontology. Lezak proposed that neuropsychological testing is clinically relevant and suggested a flexible approach to assessing the individual patient. She also reminded those neuropsychologists who became interested in a rather narrow subspecialty within psychology, that clinical neuropsychology is firmly rooted in clinical psychology. Her classic text *Neuropsychological Assessment,*

Neuropsychology in Action 1.6

The History of Modern Clinical Neuropsychology

by Antonio E. Puente   Ph.D., Professor of Psychology, University of North Carolina at Wilmington

One of psychology's experimental pioneers, Herman Ebbinghaus (1850–1909) suggested that "psychology has a long past but a short history." This analysis holds true for clinical neuropsychology as well. The history of modern clinical neuropsychology could be subdivided into three phases: before 1975, 1975–1990, and 1990–2000 (the decade of the brain). Each phase added greater impact and breadth with each one yielding increasing complexity and challenges.

Prior to 1975, neuropsychology was often intertwined with various other specialties including clinical psychology, bio- or physiological psychology, and the beginnings of what later became neuroscience. Few practitioners existed, and those involved in the field were primarily researchers, often in what is now considered experimental neuropsychology.

The work of Lashley provides an excellent example of this golden age of brain research.

The second phase is marked by movement from the laboratory to the clinic. During this period, individuals (such as Reitan) began to apply the ideas of their mentors (such as Halstead) to clinical problems encountered in neurology inpatient services. The primary activity was that of assessment with two major test batteries being introduced and later gaining widespread interest and acceptance (the Halstead-Reitan and the Luria-Nebraska). The International Neuropsychological Society (INS) was founded in the mid-1970s, its primary focus being experimental and multidisciplinary. Although initially the membership of INS was small, about 100, and drew from many different fields, it has increased to over 3000

members and now primarily consists of neuropsychologists.

Soon thereafter, two groups were formed with an emphasis on clinical issues. First, the National Academy of Neuropsychology (NAN, 1976) and later the Division of Clinical Neuropsychology (40) of the American Psychological Association (1980), both of which have grown to over 3000 members. During this time most of the important U.S. journals of the discipline were established (for example, *Journal of Clinical and Experimental Neuropsychology, Archives of Clinical Neuropsychology*) and a wealth of important books, again primarily on neuropsychological assessment, were published. Two certification boards came into being during the early 1980s, the American Board of Clinical Neuropsychology (ABCN) and the American Board of Professional Neuropsychol-

originally published in 1976, is now in its third edition (1995). In Chapters 14 and 15 we describe the assessment approach in neuropsychology in detail.

Neuropsychology was first seen as an organized field with the appearance of two international journals, *Neuropsychologia* and *Cortex,* in the 1960s. These two journals uniquely focused on developing a science of human behavior solely based on brain function. This increase in professional organizations did not occur in isolation, but was directly related to developments in other fields, including clinical (for example, behavioral neurology, biological psychiatry, and radiology) and experimental (such as neurosciences and neurochemistry). Although neuropsychology has enjoyed unprecedented growth, it is unclear

whether this remarkable development will continue, given the current economic changes and scientific context (see Neuropsychology in Action 1.6).

 ## The Brain in the New Millennium: Predictions

Neuropsychologists have been at the forefront in studying brain–behavior relationships (Zillmer & Resnick, 1994), as well as in designing and developing technologies to ameliorate disease conditions. Research at the cutting edge of brain study include investigations into the aging process, the causes of schizophrenia, recovery from traumatic brain injury,

ogy (ABPN). The two boards have often reflected broad theoretical, and often personal, differences in the field.

The mid-1990s brought forth the most volatile period so far in modern neuropsychology. This phase is marked with explosive growth in the field as evidenced by increased membership in the professional societies, publication of several new journals and numerous books, and in highly successful conferences and continuing education offerings. This unprecedented growth, which appears to have peaked in the 1990s, has seen several interesting movements. The field has become more cohesive, though probably not enough so, and the political and theoretical divisiveness that previously existed is currently only reflected in isolated instances by those holding to earlier perspectives. Also, there has been unusual acceptance of the field in both the health care and forensic arenas as well as by our psychological colleagues. This acknowledgment has combined with an economic revolution within health care that has spilled over into neuropsychology.

Medicine and the federal government acknowledge the unique role of neuropsychology by allowing the development of specific reimbursement codes for neuropsychological services (CPT, or current procedural terminology codes) outside of psychiatry. This development established, for the first time, a prescriptive authority for considering the field as being more medical than psychiatric. This acknowledgment provided not only a unique role for neuropsychology within health care, but provided greater professional independence and opportunity. Combined with this acceptance was the recent vote by the Council of Representatives of the American Psychological Association for adopting clinical neuropsychology as the first formal "specialty" within psychology.

Current trends, however, suggest that these recent positive experiences may be short-lived. An economic revolution has swept through health care, and the fortunes of our physician colleagues, which we now share more closely than ever, have, in turn, affected clinical neuropsychology. Recent rulings by the federal

government threaten to undermine our training programs, and the downward spiraling reimbursement for all health care services is taking a toll on the profitability and morale of the discipline.

Congress named the 1990s the "Decade of the Brain." Clinical neuropsychology has enjoyed unprecedented growth during this decade and has made important professional and theoretical contributions. However, for the discipline to grow, great cohesion between professional factions must occur. Further, traditional views of doing business (for example, lengthy evaluations, limited ecological validity, limited appreciation for our unique role in health care, lack of cohesive theories, poor understanding of cultural and ethnic minorities, and a preponderance of practice to the exclusion of teaching and research) must be supplemented with newer and more creative paradigms. Not to pursue these alternative strategies will surely place clinical neuropsychology outside the realm of active professional practice and into the history books as a specialty whose time has come and gone.

---

and the role of the brain in personality. What new discoveries will people make about the brain? And will they change how people view themselves?

We offer the following prediction. It seems clear to us that dualism as we know it today will become outdated, and we challenge our students to think outside the paradigm of dualism. The people of the future will accept and embrace brain-based explanations of behavior, even of everyday tasks. They will make no distinction between a medical illness and mental illness. They will conceptualize mental illness as a biological entity related to brain processes. As a result, there will be no differences in health coverage for mental and physical conditions. People will treat and conceptualize schizophrenia as a disease like

pneumonia. It will be acceptable to call in for work sick because of depression.

People will understand that anything, whether a drug, a war experience, or talking therapy, changes the way nerve cells talk to each other. They will accept that in the brain, "hardware" as well as "software" are always changing. They will learn more about the biological foundations of emotion and personality. As a result, the people of the future will rethink the notion of free will in terms of behavior probabilities. They will learn that genes may predispose very specific central nervous system activities, such as temperament and emotion, including neurological disorders such as Alzheimer's, proving that Darwin's axiom "Heredity is law" is more accurate than we perhaps wish it to be. New preventive drugs administered to men and women, for example, before they are exposed to war may block the consolidation of traumatic memories (Zillmer, 1996).

The public will clearly understand that their concept of self depends on an intact functioning brain. Thus, there will be a general awareness of the concept of brain injury and more protection of the brain from possible trauma. Air bags in automobiles will be designed to protect specifically the head and the brain. Finally, neuropsychological theories will have implications for a neurophilosophy of the mind affecting new ways of how people relate to the brain and the mind, and even their sense of self, the soul. This final thought, ironically, brings us full circle to the intellectual ancestors discussed in this chapter. The more things change, the more they stay the same.

Conclusion

Neuropsychology has had a particularly rich history, and the future is promising as well. Philosophical thought, medical practice, and religious dogma have shaped human's relationship with the brain. Understanding "where we came from" and "where we are" shows how neuropsychology evolved as a discipline. Furthermore, recognizing different viewpoints encourages the neuropsychology student to compare and contrast different theories. Knowledge of brain–behavior relationships is a developing science rather than an absolute fact. In addition, we propose that neuropsychology is a paradigm of how to explain and research behavior, not just a body of knowledge. Neuropsychology is also not a separate area of research to be pursued in isolation from other models of psychology. It is distinct from physiology, however, because its direct concern is not with synapses, but with behavior. In 1983 Donald Hebb suggested that "[The] neuropsychologist of the future must be a psychologist as well as a neurologist. The complexities of psychology and the complexities of neurology are the same complexities" (p. 7). Neuropsychology, we propose, is a natural part of psychology.

We still know relatively little about the 3-pound organ that defines us, but many significant advances in recent years have brought the field to a new threshold of knowledge that has allowed researchers to identify many of the anatomic areas and functional systems within the brain that help determine behavior. It is to this complex integration of neuroanatomy and functional knowledge that we turn next.

Critical Thinking Questions

▨ How does localization brain theory differ from equipotentiality brain theory? What is each one's lasting contributions?

▨ Is the quest for the search of the organ of the soul completed?

▨ Why is Luria's functional model of the brain such an important step in understanding brain functions?

▨ In the year 2025, what will the most important future concepts about the brain be, and how will they relate to society?

Key Terms

Neurons	da Vinci, Leonardo	Double dissociation	Jackson, Hughlings
Vitalism	Galen	Wernicke, Carl	Luria, Alexander
Materialism	Humors	Fluent aphasia	Functional systems
Trephination	Magnus, Albertus	Freud, Sigmund	Pluripotentiality
Heraclitus	Vesalius, Andreas	Agnosia	Halstead-Reitan
Pythagoras	Descartes, René	Flourens, Pierre	Neuropsychological
Brain hypothesis	Willis, Thomas	Ablation experiment	Battery
Hippocrates	Lancisi, Giovanni	Equipotentiality	Teuber, Hans-Leukas
Plato	Atharva-Veda	Munk, Hermann	Hécaen, Henry
Aristotle	Gall, Franz	Mind-blindness	Benton, Arthur
Cardiac hypothesis	Localization theory	Babinski, Joseph	Zangwill, Oliver
Ventricular localization	Phrenology	Anosognosia	Geschwind, Norman
hypothesis	Spurzheim, Johann	Lashley, Karl	Lezak, Muriel
Cell doctrine	Broca, Paul	Mass action	

Web Connections

http://NANonline.org
National Academy of Neuropsychology
The official home page of the National Academy of Neuropsychology (NAN). Includes information on doctoral programs in neuropsychology, annual meetings, membership information, and more.

http://www.apa.org
American Psychological Association
The official site of the American Psychological Association (APA) provides links to student information, membership information, PsychNET, and career-planning information.

http://www.biomednet.com/hmsbeagle
HMS Beagle
A newsletter you can subscribe to for free, via email, that provides pertinent articles about graduate training in the social sciences as well as specific topics relevant to the teaching of this course.

http://www.swets.nl/sps/journals/jhn.html
Journal of the History of the Neurosciences
Focuses on an understanding of the principles of how the neurosciences developed since their earliest days. Dedicated to enriching our knowledge of one of the fastest-growing fields of science. Abstracts and contents are online.

Part Two

THE FUNCTIONING BRAIN

Chapter 2

A CLOSER LOOK AT NEURONS

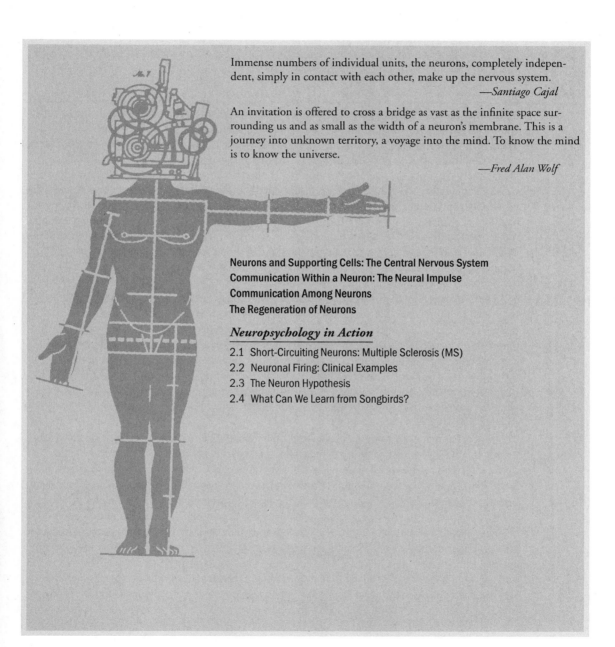

Immense numbers of individual units, the neurons, completely independent, simply in contact with each other, make up the nervous system.

—*Santiago Cajal*

An invitation is offered to cross a bridge as vast as the infinite space surrounding us and as small as the width of a neuron's membrane. This is a journey into unknown territory, a voyage into the mind. To know the mind is to know the universe.

—*Fred Alan Wolf*

Neurons and Supporting Cells: The Central Nervous System
Communication Within a Neuron: The Neural Impulse
Communication Among Neurons
The Regeneration of Neurons

Neuropsychology in Action

2.1 Short-Circuiting Neurons: Multiple Sclerosis (MS)
2.2 Neuronal Firing: Clinical Examples
2.3 The Neuron Hypothesis
2.4 What Can We Learn from Songbirds?

Keep in Mind

■ How does the unicellular neuron differ from a one-celled creature?

■ What are the purposes of different cell types in the central nervous system?

■ How do neurons communicate?

■ Are damaged neurons able to regenerate?

Overview

Evolutionarily old, one-celled creatures such as the amoeba show elementary responses to sensation and have decision-making capabilities. When you look at amoebas under a microscope in their universe of a droplet of water, you can see them move about, locate food, and engulf it. They can differentiate light from dark and warmth from cold. This unicellular organism has complex electrochemical processes, but no nervous system and no brain. As you trace movement up the evolutionary ladder, you can see that complexity of behavior accompanies specialized systems of nerve cells, or neurons, that cannot survive on their own but are essential for specialized communication. The "jellyfish," for example, has a rudimentary nervous system, which allows coordinated movement, but has no brain. The more recently developed human brain has billions of neurons that form exceedingly complex structures. The number of interconnections is mind-boggling. In comparison, the best computer modeling of neuronal systems has approximated only the nervous system of an earthworm.

Understanding the neurologic organization as well as the psychological functioning of the brain is a daunting task. Brain scientists have only just begun to connect the structural hardware—the neurons, neuronal systems, and brain structures—with the software of behavior, thought, and emotions (Damasio, 1991; Goldman-Rakic & Friedman, 1991; Stuss, 1992). In humans, this complexity reaches its apex. Animal research provides important clues to brain functioning, but the focus of this book is on human neuropsychology. In the human brain you can examine the full richness of psychological behaviors such as language and memory. Humans are also more interesting to students who plan to be clinicians. Abnormalities in human neurological functioning offer clues to diagnosis and treatment.

In this chapter we provide an overview of the nervous system and neuronal functioning. We expect you to have some background in physiological psychology, from a basic course. Instead of duplicating detailed explanations of neuronal structures and functions, we refer you to texts that provide detailed coverage of anatomy, physiology, and pharmacology. Neuropsychologists should understand the principles of neurophysiology; in fact, they frequently use physiological methods to study the brain. But neuropsychology is distinct from physiology, neuroanatomy, and neuroscience, because its ultimate concern is not with the functioning of individual features such as the synapse, the neuron, or even the hippocampus, but with the integrity of behavior as a whole. You can study the neuron as a universe unto itself, but human neuropsychology focuses on such problems as what happens to behavior if demylinization interrupts the conduction speed of neurons. The neuron's ability to regenerate is intriguing because of its enormous implications for treatment. In this chapter we emphasize such topics to briefly review the central nervous system and provide basic terminology. We review neuronal structures and their function, describe the supporting cells within the brain, and review the most well-known neurotransmitters.

In the following chapters, we build on an understanding of neuronal and neurotransmitter effects on behavior to establish the role of anatomic structures in functional systems such as memory and language. We give special attention to both brain structure and function, and provide examples of normal and abnormal functioning.

Neurons and Supporting Cells: The Central Nervous System

Neurons are the primary building blocks of the central nervous system (CNS). Like amoebas, they are unicellular, but they do not exist in isolation; that is, they constantly communicate with other neurons. The complexity of neuronal circuitry is astounding. Consider that there are approximately 5 billion people on this planet (1 billion = 10 to the power of 9, or 1,000,000,000). Researchers estimate that the human central nervous system contains billions of cells, of which perhaps as many as one-third are neurons; the rest support the neurons. Approximately 12 to 15 billion neurons are in the cerebral cortex, 70 billion in the cerebellum, and 1 billion in the spinal cord (Williams & Herrup, 1988; see Figure 2.1). The glia cells (Greek for "glue"), which outnumber neurons, provide supportive structure and metabolic function to the neuron. Neurons do not meet in a simple, linear, or one-to-one relationship, but in interconnected networks. For example, even if one neuron connected only to 100 others the emerging network is staggering in its size and complexity. Evidence suggests that the number of connections actually ranges from 1000 to 100,000, averaging about 10,000 (Beatty, 1995; Hubel, 1988).

Neurons fascinate neuropsychologists because of their specific functions and their differences from other cells. Neurons vary in shape and size, but have four common features (see Figure 2.2):

1. A cell body with a nucleus
2. Dendrites
3. An axon with a myelin sheath
4. Terminal synaptic buttons

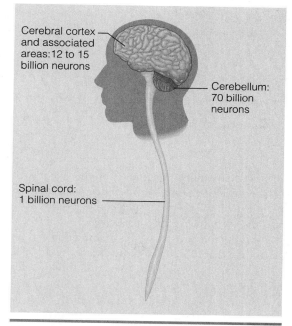

Figure 2.1 Estimated number of neurons in the human nervous system. (From R. W. Williams and K. Herrup, "The Control of Neuron Number," *Annual Review of Neuroscience*, 1988, *11*, pp. 423–453; James W. Kalat, *Biological Psychology*, 6th ed., Pacific Grove, CA: Brooks/Cole, 1998, p. 24, Figure 2.1)

Cerebral cortex and associated areas: 12 to 15 billion neurons

Cerebellum: 70 billion neurons

Spinal cord: 1 billion neurons

The structure of neurons allows them to communicate with each other in a very interesting way. Most body cells communicate with each other or the outside world through energy exchange and intercellular transport, using the cellular membrane. Neurons, however, communicate with each other by a specialized mechanism called *axonal firing*, which allows electrochemical transmission across the synapse, the

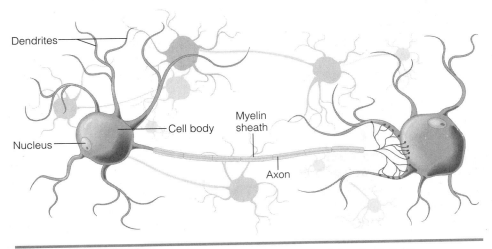

Figure 2.2   Components of a neuron. (From E. Bruce Goldstein, *Psychology,* Pacific Grove, CA: Brooks/Cole, 1994, p. 77, Figure 3.2)

tiny gap between two neurons. The process of such communication releases chemical neurotransmitters, permitting highly sophisticated combinations of reactions that influence neuronal behavior.

Neurons also have properties of formation and regeneration that differ from those of other body cells. Neuroscience has taught us that from shortly after birth, no new neurons form (Cowan, 1990). As important neural connections form in response to learning and maturation, excess neurons that may cause distracting associations die off. An important question is to what extent neurons can regenerate once damaged. Neurons in the periphery can regenerate; for example, if surgeons reattach an amputated finger, the finger may regain some mobility. Neurons in the spinal cord and brain do not show this ability, although some very recent findings in animals suggest that regeneration may be possible. That neurons do not heal spontaneously is most evident in the complete severing of neurons in the spinal cord, which leads to paralysis. Research on reactivating damaged neurons is ongoing, so perhaps one day people will be able to reverse spinal cord damage (Naugle, Cullum, & Bigler, 1998). Later in this section we examine the question of neuronal regeneration and attempts to regain function.

STRUCTURE AND FUNCTION OF THE NEURON

Neurons are specialized to exchange nervous impulses, specifically the reception, conduction, and transmission of electrochemical signals.

Cell Body

The functioning and survival of the neuron depend on the integrity of the cell body that controls and maintains the neuronal structure. Because these cell bodies are gray, the term **gray matter** is used to describe areas of the brain that are dense in cell bodies, such as the cortex. The cell soma contains mitochondria, amino acids, and DNA, and has the same properties of other cells in the body. Protein synthesis cannot take place in the axon, so all axon proteins come from the cell body.

Dendrites

One neuron receives chemical transmissions from another through **dendrites,** feathery extensions that branch from the neuron into the immediate neighborhood of the cell body. There are usually thousands of dendrites per neuron, and they differ in relation to the different functions of the neurons. The profuse branching of dendrites allows them to communicate with a large number of axon terminals. The shapes of dendritic "trees" and spines are often among the most characteristic morphologic features of a neuron (see Figure 2.3). For example, dendrites of **Purkinje cells** (Figure 2.3a), which are found in all areas of the cerebellar cortex, are characteristically spread out in one plane and have thousands of dendritic spines. In contrast, **pyramidal cells** (Figure 2.3c), which are found in all areas of the cerebral cortex, have bodies that are pyramidal or conical. Dendrites are tiny, only visible under an electron microscope, and are usually shorter than the axon, but they

can have up to thousands of synapses or contacts with other neurons. Neuroscientists estimate that the total possible connectivity among neurons in the human brain is approximately 10 to the power of 15, or 10,000,000,000,000,000—more numerous than the known stars in the universe (Beatty, 1995; Williams & Herrup, 1988). Dendrites comprise most of the receptive surface of a neuron.

Axon

The **axon,** the part of the neuron that extends from the cell body, functions similarly in all creatures. Its main function is to transmit electrochemical information

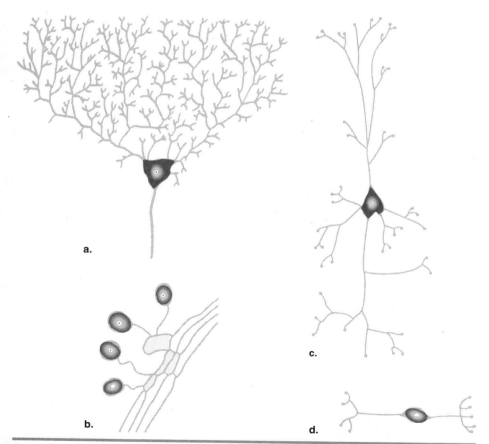

Figure 2.3 Different shapes of neurons: (a) Purkinje cell, (b) sensory neurons, (c) pyramidal cell, (d) bipolar cell. (From James W. Kalat, *Biological Psychology,* 5th Ed., Pacific Grove, CA: Brooks/Cole, 1995, p. 33, Figure 2.8)

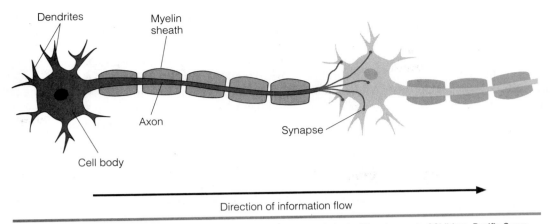

Dendrites

Myelin sheath

Axon

Cell body

Synapse

Direction of information flow

Figure 2.4   The neuron and its axon. (From Faye B. Steuer, *The Psychological Development of Children*, Pacific Grove, CA: Brooks/Cole, 1994, p. 173, Figure 6.10)

from the cell body to the synapse through microtubules along its length (see Figure 2.4). Axons are anywhere from less than 1 millimeter in length to 1 meter or more. Large motor neurons have long axons, some of them reaching from the lower end of the spinal cord to the foot muscles. Other neurons, including those that coordinate activity within a specific region of the central nervous system, have short axons. Unipolar axons proceed from one region in the CNS to another without branching. In bipolar or multipolar axons, the branching is very elaborate.

Many axons are surrounded with a **myelin sheath** that increases the speed of axonal transmission (Beatty, 1995; this is especially important in longer neurons. Myelin is lipoprotein that wraps around the axon like the layers of an onion, giving neurons their characteristic **white matter** appearance. The sheath begins at the first segment of the axon, where the nerve impulse or **action potential** begins. The myelin serves as an electric insulator that increases conduction velocity. The myelin sheath is formed by **oligodendrocytes** in the CNS and by **Schwann cells** in the PNS. Gaps called the **nodes of Ranvier** interrupt it at regular intervals (see Figure 2.5). Oligodendrocytes and Schwann cells are nonneural cells. The projections of the surface membrane of each of those cells fan out and coil around the axon of neurons to form myelin sheaths. Because the nerve impulse jumps from node to node, the length of the myelin segment is of con-

siderable importance. The longest axon fibers, which can have a conduction velocity of up to 100 meters per second, may have myelin segments of more than 1 mm in length.

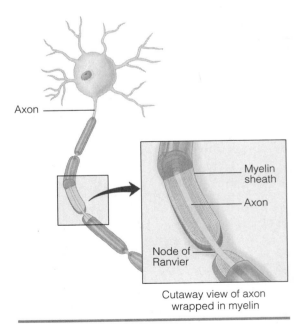

Axon

Myelin sheath

Axon

Node of Ranvier

Cutaway view of axon wrapped in myelin

Figure 2.5   Myelinated axon. (From James W. Kalat, *Biological Psychology*, 6th ed., Pacific Grove, CA: Brooks/Cole, 1998, p. 42, Figure 2.19)

Neuropsychology in Action 2.1

Short-Circuiting Neurons: Multiple Sclerosis (MS)

by Eric A. Zillmer

The destruction of the myelin sheath around the axon can result in significant and often striking behavioral changes, including blindness and paralysis. Such conditions are called *demyelinating disorders,* of which multiple sclerosis (MS) is the best known. MS is the most common neurologic illness in the United States, affecting every 50 out of 100,000 young adults. Symptoms are most often first noticed between the ages of 20 and 40. Because MS is more frequent in certain geographic locations than in others (the extreme south and north), an environmental agent is assumed to be implicated in the etiology of the disease,

perhaps one related to a demyelinating slow virus or an autoimmune process (Ebers & Sadovnick, 1993).

Although the contracting factor of MS remains an enigma, the course of the disease is known, and is related to the localized loss of myelin in the white matter of the brain and subsequent neuronal death. The loss of myelin initially results in "scrambled" electrical impulses, so neuronal information slows or never reaches its target. The symptoms vary according to where the hardened patches known as *sclerotic plaques* lie in the brain and spinal cord, but most manifest visually (sudden unilateral blindness),

in the brain stem and cerebellum (wide-based gait, intention tremors), and in the spinal cord (spastic gait, loss of position sense, and paraplegia). Relapses are usually acute and persist for several weeks. Postmortem studies of MS patients have revealed hundreds of lesions smaller than 1.5 cm (Adams & Victor, 1993). Furthermore, there is little potential for regrowth of myelin.

There is no known effective treatment or cure for MS. The prognosis is a gradual deterioration of the patient's condition over many years. Death can result if the demyelination affects vital centers of the brain.

Myelination begins soon after birth and continues for many years. You can easily observe the importance of the myelin sheath in young children who are unable to control their bladder and bowel functions: This is caused by insufficient myelination of neurons, and therefore children cannot be toilet-trained before about age 2 or 3. In adults, a breakdown of the myelin sheath is a consequence of multiple sclerosis (see Neuropsychology in Action 2.1)

The speed of neuronal conduction is important in the adaptation of all species to potentially dangerous events in the environment. Because in some cases the built-in conduction speed is not fast enough, the nervous system has evolved to process important sensory data at levels closer to their origin. The knee reflex is an example. The sensory information that you are about to fall is sent to your spinal cord, which relays it directly back with "instructions" to extend your knee. This occurs without any higher cognitive processing. If the same sensory information traveled to the brain, the relay would take too long to process, which could result in a fall. Another example is the

reflex arc in response to pain, such as a burn. The sensation is relayed to your spinal cord, which gives the appropriate response, "withdraw finger" (see Figure 2.6). The information also reaches your brain, of course, although somewhat later; it is then processed at that higher level: "Did I burn my finger?"

The alert neuropsychology student may wonder how very large animals, such as the dinosaurs, were affected by neuronal conduction speed. To compensate for the relatively long distances sensory and motor neurons had to travel, large dinosaurs had a small additional brain at the level of the pelvis. Presumably, the brain integrated many sensory and motor functions at this level so the dinosaur could respond adaptively to the environment.

Terminal Buttons

Near the end of the axon are branches with slightly enlarged ends called *axon terminals* or **terminal buttons.** The site of interneuronal contact, where neurochemical information transmits from one neuron to another, is called a **synapse;** we discuss it in detail

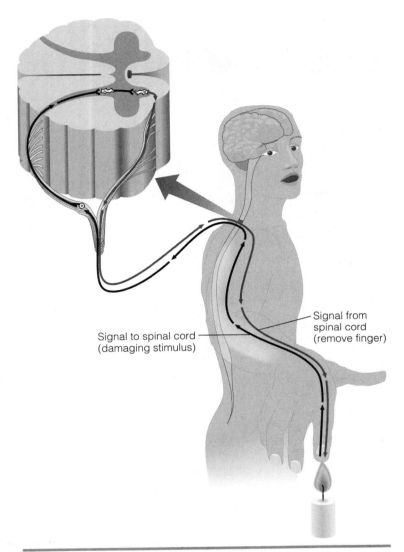

Figure 2.6   Example of a spinal cord reflex. (From E. Bruce Goldstein, *Psychology,* Pacific Grove, CA: Brooks/Cole, 1994, p. 83, Figure 3.7)

later in this section. The terminal button is the presynaptic portion of the synapse, the place where electrical nerve impulses cause the release of a neurotransmitter. This chemical in turn affects another neuron or muscle in either an excitatory or an inhibitory manner. Signals that travel along the axon are electrical, and the transfer of neurotransmitters across synapses, from one neuron to another, is chemical. Researchers can therefore study and analyze the brain through electrical means—for example, using the electroencephalograph (EEG), evoked potential, or electrical stimulation—or through biochemical or metabolic techniques such as positron emission tomography (PET) (see Chapter 6).

Neuron Classification and Terminology

Neurologists commonly classify neurons either by morphology (shape) or by function. The three principal classes of neurons are defined by the number of axons emanating from their cell bodies. Most are **multipolar neurons,** with more than two axons. **Bipolar neurons** have two axons. **Monopolar** or unipolar **neurons** have a single axon. Neurons with short axons or no axons are called **interneurons;** they integrate neural activity within a specific brain region.

In classifying neurons by their function, **motor neurons** make muscles contract (see Figure 2.7) and change the activity of glands; **sensory neurons** respond directly to changes in light, touch, temperature, odor, and so on. The majority of neurons are interneurons or "between" neurons, because they receive input from and send output to other neurons.

That neurons are organized in collective structures means that behavior arises from the firing of many neurons, not a single neuron. As we noted, there are two kinds of neural structures in the nervous system, those composed primarily of gray cell bodies and those composed primarily of white axons. The myelin sheath of the axon appears white because its lipid content is over 60%, so that the areas of the brain that contain mainly bundles of myelinated axons are called *white matter.* These bundles—large collections of axon—are known as **tracts, pathways,** or **fibers** in the CNS and **nerves** in the PNS. The three major types of fibers all primarily consist of white matter:

1. **Intracerebral** (or *association*) **fibers** connect regions within one hemisphere.
2. **Intercerebral** (or *commissural*) **fibers** connect structures in the two hemispheres.
3. **Projection fibers** connect subcortical structures to the cortex and vice versa.

Anatomists often discuss pathways in terms of the direction of the projection and the systems they connect (England & Wakely, 1991). For example, the corticostriatal pathway is where fibers connect cortical areas to the striatum. Likewise, the hypothalamocerebellar tract projects from the hypothalamus to the cerebellum.

Aggregations of cell bodies—predominantly dendrites and terminal buttons—are grayish; their actual color in the living state is pink. As noted, gray matter is typically found on the surface of the cerebral cortex, the center of the spinal cord, and on large subcortical nuclei (for example, in the thalamus). In the central nervous system, clusters of gray cell bodies are called **nuclei** (singular, *nucleus*), a term often used to designate a group of nerve cells in direct relationship to the fibers of a particular nerve. In the peripheral nervous system, clusters of gray cell bodies are

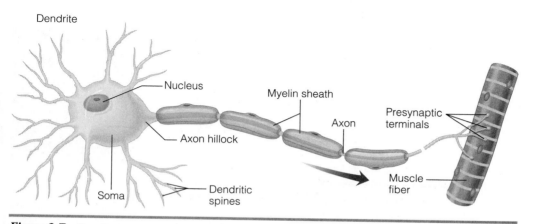

Figure 2.7   A motor neuron. (From James W. Kalat, *Biological Psychology,* 6th ed., Pacific Grove, CA: Brooks/Cole, 1998, p. 27, Figure 2.4)

called **ganglia** (singular, *ganglion*). The presence of nuclei in the brain is important to neuropsychologists, because nuclei often signal strategic clusterings of nerve cell bodies. Vital integration of neuronal information may be taking place at a specific neuroanatomic location. Often neuropsychologists attribute some functional role to the presence of nuclei. The precise role of any one nucleus is, however, difficult to delineate, because the dendrites and axons may extend for a considerable distance outside of the boundary of the nucleus. In addition, some nuclei consist of different neurons with different neurotransmitters from other neurons, which increases the complexity. As a result, neuropsychologists do not always know the functional localization of nuclei, and so their ability to assess functional properties for the neuroanatomic boundaries of nuclei is limited. In some cases, it may be more useful to conceptualize localization of function according to neuronal regions or networks rather than by nuclei. Nevertheless, mapping and identifying specific nuclei in the brain continue to occupy neuroscientists and neuropsychologists.

NEUROGLIA: SUPPORTING CELLS OF THE NERVOUS SYSTEM

The many supporting cells of the nervous system play an important role in supplying nutrients and oxygen to neurons, which have a very high metabolic rate, but can't store nutrients. More numerous than nerve cells, support cells make up more than half the volume of the nervous system and help the neurons in various ways. They are, however, not directly involved in transmitting nerve impulses.

Glia cells, or "nerve glue," help maintain the functioning of neurons by physically and chemically buffering them from each other. They come in different shapes (see Figure 2.8) and surround neurons to hold them in place. Glia cells insulate neurons from each other so that messages do not get mixed up. They control the supply of oxygen and chemicals, and act as housekeepers, metabolizing and removing the carcasses of neurons destroyed by injury or disease.

Astrocytes are highly branched cells that occupy much space between neurons in the gray matter. These star-shaped cells (*astra* is Latin for "star") have small "feet" that cover nerve cell bodies and dendrites. Their

multiple support functions include supporting neurons by interweaving among nerve fibers, contributing to the metabolism of synaptic transmitters, and regulating the ion balance. Astrocytes, like other glia cells, respond to brain injury by swelling, which

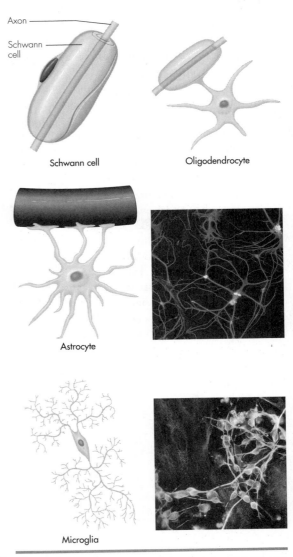

Figure 2.8   Different shapes of glia cells in the CNS. Glia cells are of special interest to neurologists and neurosurgeons because they are the site of the principal tumors of the brain and spinal cord (see Chapter 10). (From James W. Kalat, *Biological Psychology*, 6th ed., Pacific Grove, CA: Brooks/Cole, 1998, p. 30, Figure 2.9. Photos: Nancy Kedersha/UCLA/SPL/Photo Researchers)

may damage other neurons. This potentially life-threatening occurrence is responsible for many symptoms of traumatic brain injuries and can result in coma and death.

Most blood vessels in the CNS have an inside lining of very tightly joined endothelial cells, which the tight astrocyte covering holds in place. This combination permits only very restricted transfer of soluble material between blood and brain. This **blood–brain barrier** allows water, gases, and small lipid-soluble substances to pass across. Certain substances—some drugs, for example—are totally barred from the brain, and other substances require an active transport system across the blood–brain barrier. A most important role of astrocytes is to support the blood–brain barrier by covering the blood vessels in the CNS with

their "feet." Figure 2.9 demonstrates how small, uncharged molecules such as O_2 and CO_2 can cross, but large and electrically charged molecules cannot.

As already mentioned, oligodendrocytes in the CNS and Schwann cells in the PNS are myelin-forming glia cells enveloping axons and neurons. These supporting cells perform a vital function in wrapping the nerve cell with myelin and affecting the speed with which a neuron conducts its impulse along an axon. Within the brain and the spinal cord, the myelin sheath is formed by a type of glia cell called *oligodendrocyte* (*oligo* is Greek for "few"). Outside the brain and the spinal cord, myelin is formed by another type of glia cell, the Schwann cell. Schwann cells myelinate only a single segment of one cell, whereas oligodendrocytes may myelinate several segments of the same axon or several different axons. Microglia are small cells that undergo rapid proliferation in response to tissue destruction, migrating toward the site of injured or dead cells, where they act as scavengers and metabolize tissue debris.

Communication Within a Neuron: The Neural Impulse

The message that travels along the axon from the cell body to the terminal buttons is electrical, but the neuron does not carry it down the axon the way a electrical wire conducts electricity. Rather, chemical alterations in the membrane of the axon result in exchanges of various ions between the axon and the fluid surrounding it, producing an electrical current. This electrical signaling is the foundation of neuronal communication.

THE RESTING MEMBRANE POTENTIAL

As with all living cells, a cell membrane protects the neuron from other matter. Neurons show a **resting potential** or **membrane potential** when they are inactive, a slight electrical imbalance between the inner and outer surfaces of the membrane caused by the separation of electrically charged ions. Neural communication requires the passage of **ions** through tiny channels in the axon wall. Ions are atoms or molecules that have acquired an electrical charge by gaining or

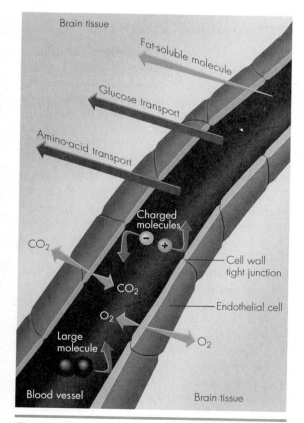

Figure 2.9 The blood–brain barrier. (From James W. Kalat, *Biological Psychology*, 6th ed., Pacific Grove, CA: Brooks/Cole, 1998, p. 32, Figure 2.11)

losing one or more electrons. Four ions are important: sodium (NA⁺), potassium (K⁺), calcium (Ca⁺⁺), and chloride (Cl⁻). Electrophysiological equipment makes it possible to measure the electrical potentials (transmembrane potential) of axons. The inside of the axon is electrically negative with respect to the outside of the neuron, so there is an electrical potential difference between the interior and exterior of the axon that is synonymous with the membrane potential. In the giant axon of the squid, this difference is approximately −70 millivolts. An electrical imbalance can occur because the membrane of the axon is semipermeable to allow the flow of chemicals across the axon membrane (see Figure 2.10). Some molecules, including oxygen and water, flow through the membrane constantly, and other chemicals, such as potassium, chloride, and sodium, cross through gates that control the rate of passage. When the neuron is not firing and the membrane is at rest, the sodium ions (Na⁺) are trapped outside of the neuron. The imbalance in an electrical charge maintains the cell in a state of tension, ready to fire rapidly in response to a stimulus.

The positively charged sodium ions are located in greater concentrations outside the neuron, even though the electrostatic field (negative charges inside the membrane) tends to attract them inside. The biological transport system that exchanges three sodium ions for every two potassium ions across the membrane of the axon is called the **sodium–potassium pump.** Many individual protein molecules in the membrane pump sodium out of the axon. This active transport system exchanges three sodium ions for every two potassium ions that push in, and it consumes considerable energy—up to 40% of the neuron's metabolic resources. The concentration of potassium reflects an equilibrium of competing processes. The pump actively moves potassium into the neuron, expending energy in the process. Concurrently, potassium ions flow passively from an area of greater concentration to an area of lesser concentration by the force of diffusion.

THE ACTION POTENTIAL

To generate a nerve impulse, a cell membrane must first depolarize. Depolarization begins when a sodium channel across the membrane briefly opens and sodium ions pass through it into the cell, reducing voltage. Depolarization occurs only when the membrane achieve a threshold of at least 35 mV of reduction of polarization toward zero. When this occurs, the membrane suddenly opens its sodium gates, permitting a rapid, massive, explosive flow of ions. When sodium enters the cell in this fashion, the neuron fires with an action potential. Subthreshold stimulation does not result in an action potential, but any stimulation beyond the threshold does. Thus neurons fire in an all-or-none fashion. Thus the force of the action potential does not depend on the intensity of the stimulus initiating it, and a neuron cannot send stronger action potentials down its axons. In fact, neurons fire more or less continuously, and the timing and sequences of impulses and pauses determine the message. Figure 2.11 illustrates the varying stages of an electrical potential across a neuron membrane during electrical stimulation. The nerve impulse spreads down the axon, as the voltage-controlled sodium channels open sequentially, like falling dominoes.

Neurons may be in different states of preparedness for firing. Some may be just a few millivolts below

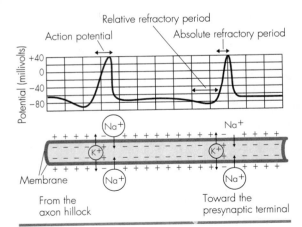

Figure 2.10   During the resting state of the membrane, the unequal distributions of sodium ions (Na⁺) and potassium ions (K⁺) between the inside and the outside of the neuron produced a difference in voltage. (From James W. Kalat, *Biological Psychology*, 6th ed., Pacific Grove, CA: Brooks/Cole, 1998, p. 41, Figure 2.18)

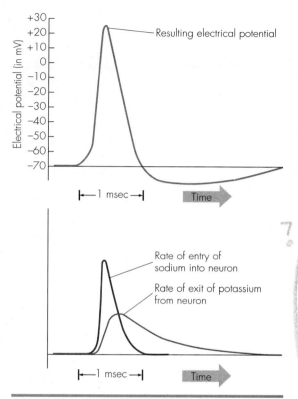

Figure 2.11 The action potential. (From James W. Kalat, *Biological Psychology*, 6th ed., Pacific Grove, CA: Brooks/Cole, 1998, p. 40, Figure 2.16)

excitatory properties of neurons on behavior. The ability to sit quietly and read this book requires many functions, both excitatory and inhibitory. It is very common for patients with generalized brain trauma to have difficulties sitting still, concentrating, and reading for a prolonged period of time (Golden, Zillmer, & Spiers, 1992). Such problems are related to the fact that many of the neuronal collections in the CNS, particularly those of the frontal lobe, serve to inhibit rather than excite behavior. This is of clinical importance because losing inhibitory neurons to trauma or disease may result in impulsivity and inappropriate behavior known as **disinhibition.**

Neurons communicate via one-way conversations. Again, it is the firing rate, not the magnitude of electrical activity of the neuron, that can change; that is, increase. For example, if inhibitory fiber collections increase their rate of firing, inhibition increases and behavior correspondingly decreases. This is why many traumas to the brain often cause both a loss of function, such as the inability to initiate behaviors, and disinhibition, which may include impulsiveness, hypersexuality, and inappropriate expression of emotions such as crying or silliness.

Communication among neurons is the basis of all behavior. Our previous discussion centered on how the individual neuron works. We now turn to how neurons communicate with each other. The anatomic location of this communication is known as the *synapse.* The synapse is the gap between the terminal button and the receptors of the next neuron.

The language of human neural communication is chemical. In fact, almost all mammalian synapses are chemical in nature, although researchers have found electrically transmitting synapses in invertebrates and lower vertebrates. The chemical messengers are called *neurotransmitters.* In simple terms, a chemical message transfers across the synapse from one neuron to another, where it influences the neuron or neurons to fire or not to fire. In reality, this particular exchange is extremely complex, involving many different molecules. The process is so intricate that a neuroscientist can easily dedicate an entire career to the study of one neurotransmitter exchange. But human brains, and minds, are affected not only by internally produced chemical messengers, but also by externally

the critical voltage level, requiring very little additional excitation to reach firing threshold. Others may need to overcome a larger voltage difference between the inside and the outside of the axon in order to generate an action potential. Once a neuron has fired, there is an associated recovery period when the neuron resists re-excitation and is incapable of firing. This **refractory period** lasts one or more milliseconds (msec), during which the membrane cannot produce another action potential in response to stimulation of any intensity.

Neurons communicate through synapses. Chemical messages between neurons are carried by neurotransmitters and have one of two effects on the receiving neuron: excitation or inhibition. Of special interest to neuropsychologists are the inhibitory and

Neuropsychology in Action 2.2

Neuronal Firing: Clinical Examples

by Eric A. Zillmer

The influence of neuronal firing on behavior is easily seen in a variety of related clinical phenomena.

Seizures

Seizures, which are unusual electrical events in the brain, have a wide range of causes, including trauma, tumors, and epilepsy (see Chapter 13). **Seizures** result from massive waves of synchronized nerve cell activation that may involve the entire brain. You can thus conceptualize them as "electrical storms." Seizures may have dramatic behavioral manifestations, including uncontrolled muscle contractions, changes in perception, and alterations in mood and consciousness.

Drugs

Certain drugs and poisons specifically alter the flow of sodium and potassium through the membrane. Most drugs act at the level of the synapse, but several substances influence the axon's firing rate directly, changing the person's perception or mood and in some cases causing death. For example, scorpion and black widow venoms overexcite the nervous system by keeping sodium channels open and closing potassium channels, causing prolonged depolarization that renders the neuron helpless to convey information. As a result, life-sustaining behavior may cease (for example, breathing may stop), or there may be a lack of disinhibition (such as a continuous involuntary flexing of a muscle or tic). Novocain, a topical anes-thetic used by dentists, attaches itself to the sodium gates of the neuronal membrane and prevents sodium ions from entering. Consequently, the action potential is blocked and sensory nerve messages, including pain, cannot reach the brain because the neurons that typically convey this message cannot fire.

Chloroform decreases brain activity by promoting the flow of potassium ions out of the neuron. This reduces the number of sodium ions that spontaneously pass through the cell membrane, and hyperpolarizes the neuronal membrane, which reduces the nervous system's responsiveness. Tetrodotoxin (TTX), a poison found in the Japanese blowfish, directly blocks voltage-gated sodium channels. Lithium, a simple salt extracted from rock, is the most effective treatment for bipolar disorder (manic-depressive illness), which is characterized by severe mood swings (Freedman, Kaplan, & Sadock, 1978). Lithium stabilizes mood most effectively during the manic stage. Its overall effect on brain activity is not clearly understood, but lithium is chemically similar to sodium and may partly take its place crossing the membrane.

Electroconvulsive Therapy (ECT)

Early in the 20th century a physician named Ladislaus von Meduna noted that psychotic patients who had epilepsy improved in mood immediately after each epileptic attack. Reasoning that the electrical storm of neural activity in the brain somehow improved mental activity, Meduna applied a large amount of electricity to the skull of depressed patients, causing the collective firing of neurons; a seizure. **Electroconvulsive therapy** (ECT) sometimes improves severe forms of depression within a few days. Although researchers do not clearly understand the mechanism, today clinicians use ECT when it is important to intervene quickly to prevent a patient from acting on suicidal thoughts.

Death

When is a human considered dead? When the heart stops beating? Or when the lungs stop breathing? Because the brain is the *Zentralorgan* (German for "central organ") that coordinates the beating of the heart and the breathing of the lungs, the clinical moment of death is precisely when the firing of the brain ceases. Thus, in most states once an unconscious patient has been admitted to a hospital the staff monitor brain electrical potential data with an **electroencephalograph** (EEG). As long as there is brain activity, the patient is considered alive. Interestingly, even after a brain has stopped generating action potentials the brain mass itself can hold its own electrical charge for a short time. This can be measured by placing a dead brain slice on an apparatus that is sensitive to small electrical charges.

Neuropsychology in Action 2.3

The Neuron Hypothesis

by Eric A. Zillmer

The neuron hypothesis suggests that (1) all neural function is reflected in behavior, and (2) all behavior has an underlying neural correlate (Pincus & Tucker, 1985). Many have argued in the past that the healthy mature brain produces the mind's range of functions and experiences, which are perfectly correlated to precise biological phenomena. Is there a satisfactory mechanistic explanation for all human activity? Are scientists trying to measure the impossible, or are our instruments just too crude?

Reductionism is a term for investigating complex phenomena by dividing them into more easily understood components. Reductionists think of themselves as cartographers mapping the brain. Everything, they argue, exists at a particular location (Churchland, 1993). Your memories, for example, are nothing else than the chemical and structural relationship among neurons. Proponents of this approach are quick to offer evidence. For example, the voices a schizophrenic "hears" inside the brain relate to an excess of the neurotransmitter dopamine. The planum temporale in the left hemisphere has been associated with auditory processing; it is measurably enlarged in musicians with perfect pitch. Certainly the reductionists have made incredible advances in recent years and their discoveries demand attention. But are all human experiences really ultimately related to biochemical processes?

The brain's potential for receiving and sending messages depends on its structure, which in turn is determined by neurons, its basic components. Consider, for example, that during early pregnancy neurons grow at a rate of 250,000 a minute and that by the end of the sixth month almost a complete set of neurons have developed in the fetus. Neural development is the most sensitive part of fetal growth, and many factors, including maternal smoking and exposure to alcohol or drugs, can prevent such development or damage the neurons. During the next 20 years or so, an increasing number of connections are formed among those neurons. Then the trend reverses, so that by middle age thousands of connections are lost every day. If humans lived 150 years, this normal loss of neural connections would reach a level similar to that seen in Alzheimer's disease. Obviously, neurons have an integral and complex function in the brain and behavior. Thus many propose that no explanation for behavior is useful unless grounded in an understanding of the basic mechanism involved in neuronal processes.

The neuron differs from other cells in that it is specialized for information processing. To some degree all functions that sustain life as well as those that make us human are coordinated and depend on the communication of neurons. Nerve cells are anatomically independent; they come very close to each other but do not touch. The nervous system thus consists of separate units rather than one continuous structure. Scientists increasingly argue about the validity of the neuron hypothesis. Can every human experience be reduced to a physical component? How does the mind arise from matter?

Scientists know that individual neurons send electrical impulses that trigger the release of chemicals or neurotransmitters, which in turn induce an electrical impulse in other neurons. This interaction of electrical and chemical processes is the basis of brain communication. But consider the complexity. For any behavior to occur, millions of neurons must communicate. Although the functioning of the individual neuron is important from a biological as well as clinical point of view, its relevance to behavior is less important.

The electrochemical neuronal process can stimulate growth of new connections through dendritic branching, as we hope is happening in your brain as you read this book! It is difficult, however, to uphold the neuron hypothesis in its classic form, because neurons interact dynamically in very complex networks. This interaction seems highly differentiated. Even though examining the nervous system by analyzing its parts has limitations, scientists traditionally view the big picture neuroanatomically, from the bottom up. However, today scientists are focusing on neural circuits, neural networks, computational models, and even chaos theory in their effort to understand the brain (Turing, 1981). Intelligent behavioral properties can only be understood by studying networks of interacting neurons, rather than individual neurons in isolation.

originating chemicals that find their way to the synapse. Such chemicals are known as *psychoactive drugs* and include caffeine, cocaine, nicotine, and alcohol, among many others.

Chemical transmission is very much at the center of our behavior and emotions. In fact, many of the most fascinating discoveries about the brain concern the chemical nature of neuronal transmission. For example, researchers have established that the very large number of individual nerve cells or units in the nervous system are related to each other through synapses in a more or less continuous fashion, creating what is known as a *network*.

Communication Among Neurons

THE STRUCTURE OF SYNAPSES

Figure 2.12 illustrates the chemical transmission between neurons. The presynaptic neuron delivers an action potential down its axon (Figure 2.12a) until it loses its myelin sheath and divides into many branches called *buttons* or **synaptic knobs.** These swell at the end to increase the area of contact with the postsynaptic neuron. The buttons themselves do not touch the postsynaptic cell, which is covered with myelin and surrounded by glia cells. Between the two neurons lies a very small space known as the *synaptic cleft* or *synaptic gap*. It is so tiny (about 200 to 300 Å) that it is observable only through an electron microscope.

Figure 2.12b shows the typical synapse. Terminal buttons harbor oval structures called the **synaptic vesicles,** which contain neurotransmitters. These vesicles are unique cellular structures that typically cluster close to the presynaptic membrane. Neurotransmitters are synthesized until they are delivered to the **receptor sites** on the postsynaptic neuron (see Figure 2.12c). There are numerous neurotransmitter molecules, each kind shaped differently and with its own key fit to a specific receptor. This mechanism determines how the synaptic endings evoke excitation or inhibition in the postsynaptic neuron. Researchers have identified two major types of receptor

sites (Beatty, 1995): the symmetrical synapse, which seems involved in inhibitory functions, and the asymmetrical synapse, which plays a role in excitatory processes. The anatomic location of the terminal button in relation to the postsynaptic membrane can vary. It may be on the dendrite, the soma, or the axon of the postsynaptic neuron.

SYNAPTIC TRANSMISSION

The synapse includes the presynaptic membrane, the synaptic cleft, and the postsynaptic membrane. When the neural impulse from the presynaptic neuron reaches the button, the vesicles release a specific amount of a neurotransmitter (typically 1000 to 10,000 molecules) into the synaptic cleft (see Figure 2.13). The neurotransmitter passively diffuses across the gap and, after a short synaptic delay of about 0.3 to 0.5 msec, may adhere to receptor molecules on the postsynaptic membrane of the receiving neuron.

Several scenarios are possible after the release of a neurotransmitter. The molecules may not fit a specific receptor site and therefore do not bind to the cell membrane. In this case, the neurotransmitter has no effect on a receiving neuron and no communication takes place. Or neurotransmitters may be released in areas with no immediate postsynaptic receptors. In this case, the transmitter may diffuse over a wider area affecting neurons far from the point of release. If the released neurotransmitter keys into the receptor site, it will bind to the cell membrane, triggering a postsynaptic excitation or inhibition in the receiving neuron. Chemically, the binding of the neurotransmitter changes the ionic permeability of the postsynaptic membrane. For example, as increased levels of Na^+ and Cl^- move into the postsynaptic cell, smaller amounts of K^+ are moving out, depolarizing the postsynaptic cell. This depolarization, known as an **excitatory postsynaptic potential (EPSP),** increases the probability that the postsynaptic cell will reach its threshold. An EPSP makes it more likely that the membrane threshold will reach an action potential and that the postsynaptic neuron will fire.

During an inhibitory exchange, the presence of a neurotransmitter increases the permeability of the postsynaptic membrane, particularly to K^+. This

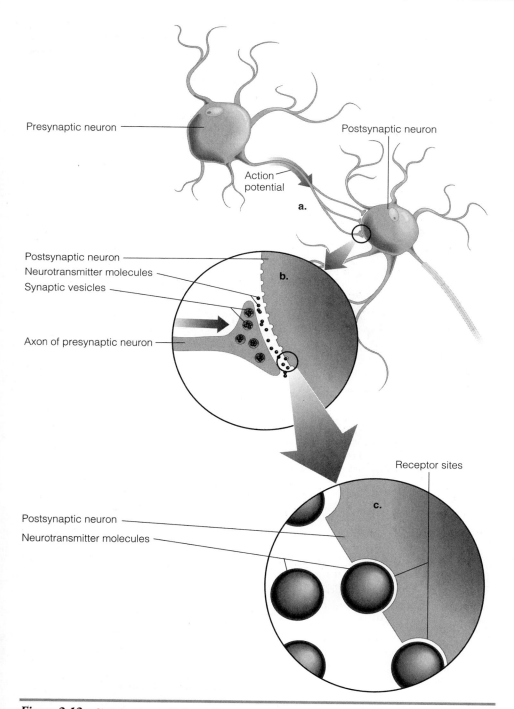

Presynaptic neuron

Postsynaptic neuron

Action potential

a.

Postsynaptic neuron
Neurotransmitter molecules
Synaptic vesicles

b.

Axon of presynaptic neuron

Receptor sites

c.

Postsynaptic neuron
Neurotransmitter molecules

Figure 2.12 Chemical transmission at the synapse. (From E. Bruce Goldstein, *Psychology,* Pacific Grove, CA: Brooks/Cole, 1994, p. 81, Figure 3.5)

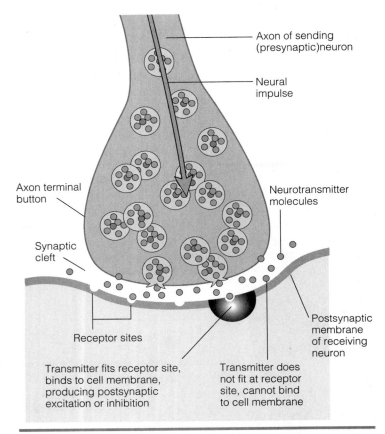

Axon of sending
(presynaptic)neuron

Neural
impulse

Axon terminal
button

Neurotransmitter
molecules

Synaptic
cleft

Receptor sites

Postsynaptic
membrane
of receiving
neuron

Transmitter fits receptor site,
binds to cell membrane,
producing postsynaptic
excitation or inhibition

Transmitter does
not fit at receptor
site, cannot bind
to cell membrane

Figure 2.13 Synaptic transmission involves the release of a neurotransmitter in response to the arrival of an action potential. (From W. Weiten, *Psychology: Themes and Variations*, Pacific Grove, CA: Brooks/Cole, 1998, Figure 3.3,
p. 78)

results in an ionic current that hyperpolarizes the
postsynaptic neuron. Thus greater depolarization
than normal is required to reach an action potential,
which thus becomes less probable. This is an inhibitory postsynaptic potential (IPSP). Next, the
synaptic vesicle either dissipates or is reabsorbed by
the presynaptic membrane, which allows the recycling
of neurotransmitters and completes the cycle. This
summation of EPSPs and IPSPs, analogous to yes/no
messages, is the main principle of neural communication. The nervous system is exceedingly complex,
because one single neuron may have many synaptic
terminals on it that may influence the action potential of thousands of other neurons.

NEUROTRANSMITTERS

Neurotransmitters permit the exchange of information among neurons and between neurons and other
cells. Neurotransmitter types (see Table 2.1) are classified according to molecular size. For example, the
biogenic amines and amino acids are small-molecule

Table 2.1	*Neurotransmitters*
BIOGENIC AMINES	Acetylcholine (ACh)
	Serotonin (5-HT)
CATECHOLAMINES	Dopamine (DA)
	Norepinephrine (NE) (noradrenalin)
	Epinephrine (EPI) (adrenalin)
AMINO ACIDS	GABA
	Glycine
	Glutamate
	Aspartate
PEPTIDES	Vasopressin
	Oxytocin
	Thyrotropin-releasing hormone (TRH)
	Corticotropin-releasing factor
	Substance P
	Tachykinins
	Cholecystokinin

messengers, consisting of fewer than 10 carbon atoms, and the neuropeptides, which are larger molecules. Although smaller-molecule neurotransmitters, such as acetylcholine, serotonin, and the catecholamines, have traditionally received the most study, neuropeptides are more numerous in the brain, with more than 40 different neuropeptides identified so far (Kalat, 1998).

Just as each neurotransmitter has a specific shape, comparable to a key, each receptor site also has a specific structure analogous to a lock. Thus, a specific neurotransmitter will attach itself only to a receptor with an appropriate fit. In some cases, a variety of neurotransmitters can adhere to a single type of receptor molecule: Many different keys may fit the same lock. At times, different neurotransmitters may compete for the same receptor molecule. For example, even though neurotransmitter A may have adhered to receptor Z at one time, in competition with neurotransmitter B, A may fail to activate, because B fits better. This scenario may occur thousands of times even at the individual level of one neuron. Chemical transmission allows tremendous flexibility and refinement.

THE DISTRIBUTION OF NEUROTRANSMITTERS

Many distinct neurotransmitter pathways define the brain chemically and anatomically. The tracing of neuronal pathways along neurotransmitter systems has been at the center of the neurosciences since the development of modern staining methods.

Acetylcholine

Acetylcholine (**ACh**, or choline) was the first neurotransmitter to be identified, in the early 1900s; researchers discovered that it stimulates the parasympathetic nervous system. It plays a prominent role in the PNS, influencing motor control, and in autonomic nervous system functioning. And ACh is a predominant neurotransmitter at the neuromuscular junction, stimulating muscular contraction. In the CNS and brain, ACh affects a wide behavioral repertoire. One of its most important functions may be to influence alertness, attention, and memory.

ACh is a simple chemical structure, but its method of action is complicated and is yet to be fully understood. One component necessary for synthesizing ACh is choline, supplied by foods such as liver, kidneys, egg yolks, seeds, and many vegetables and legumes. It is synthesized in the liver and recycled in the brain. Choline easily crosses the blood–brain barrier. There is evidence showing an influx of choline in the brain after eating and an outflow when plasma choline levels are lower, between meals (see Feldman, Meyer, & Quenzer, 1997). Like other neurotransmitters, ACh binds to a variety of postsynaptic receptor subtypes. The two main subtypes of ACh are **muscarinic choline** and **nicotinic choline,** named after the bitter botanical alkaloids that stimulate the receptors (muscarine from the fly agaric mushroom, *Amanita muscaria,* and nicotine from tobacco, *Nicotiana tabacum*). The implication is that the action of ACh may differ from one receptor subtype to another. Nicotinic receptor binding creates an excitatory response, whereas muscarinic responses may be either excitatory or inhibitory. Therefore, in the PNS, for example, glands and muscles may be either excited or inhibited, depending on the subtype of ACh

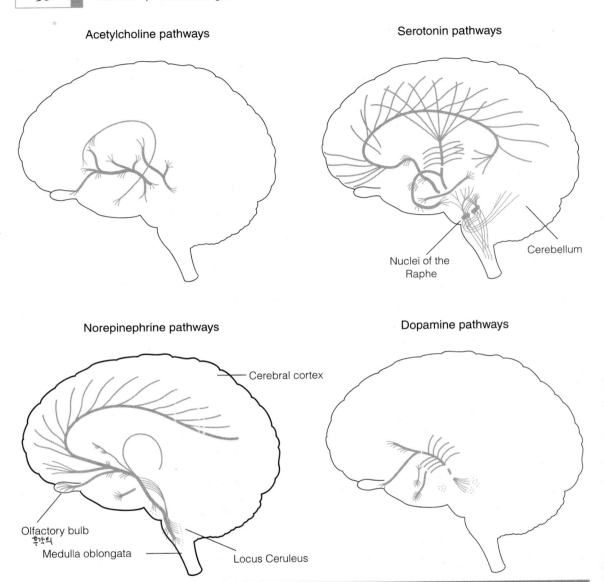

Acetylcholine pathways

Serotonin pathways

Nuclei of the
Raphe

Cerebellum

Norepinephrine pathways

Dopamine pathways

Cerebral cortex

Olfactory bulb
후각의
Medulla oblongata

Locus Ceruleus

Figure 2.14   Major neurotransmitter pathways and their widespread distribution to almost every region in the brain. (From José B. Ashford, Craig W. Lecroy, and Kathie L. Lortie, *Human Behavior in the Social Environment: A Multidimensional Perspective,* Pacific Grove, CA: Brooks/Cole, 1997, p. 41, Figure 2.11)

receptor. Certain drugs act on nicotinic receptors, and others are specific to muscarinic receptors.

As in the peripheral system, distribution of acetylcholine is widespread in the brain, where it has many possible behavioral functions. First, cholinergic (ACh)

neurons in the **striatum,** a collection of brain structures named after their striped or striated appearance, influence motor system functioning. Degeneration of striatal neurons is associated with Huntington's disease (see Chapter 12). Second, ACh functions in arousal and in the sleep–wake cycle. The **reticular activating system (RAS)** (discussed in detail in conjunction with sleep in Chapter 13) is a network of neurons that arises from the brain stem and projects throughout the cortex. One of its primary functions is to regulate brain activation. For example, Sitaram, Moore, and Gillin (1978) revealed that an ACh antagonist such as scopolamine extended the normal interval (about 45 minutes) between REM sleep. Although many neurotransmitter systems are involved in the sleep cycle, ACh seems to play a role in activating the cortex. Increased levels of ACh in the brain stem and **basal forebrain** are associated with increased cortical arousal and wakefulness. Researchers can elicit REM sleep, which is characterized by increased cortical activity, by activating muscarinic ACh receptors.

Third, a major cholinergic system thought to influence attention, memory, and learning emerges from the basal forebrain and projects throughout the cortex and to structures important for consolidating memory, such as the **hippocampus.** An important cholinergic nuclei in the basal forebrain is the **nucleus basalis of Meynert** (named after its discoverer). Its degeneration as a factor in Alzheimer's disease became evident when researchers found that patients suffering from this disorder had measurably lower levels of ACh in their brain than normal (see Chapter 11). Alzheimer's disease is associated with severe memory dysfunction, and this observation led researchers to wonder if ACh plays a role in memory functioning. Scopolamine, a drug that blocks ACh at muscarinic receptor sites, causes deficits in encoding and consolidation into long-term memory (see Polster, 1993). Surgical patients given scopolamine often have amnesia for the events before surgery. These findings led to the development of drugs that serve as acetylcholine agonists binding to the same receptors as ACh and increasing ACh levels for use in clinical trials with Alzheimer's sufferers. However, this intervention was largely disappointing, perhaps in part because Alzheimer's disease involves much more than one neurotransmitter system. It may also be that ACh has a less direct influence on memory, instead functioning to maintain a higher level of cortical alertness and attention that may be a necessary precursor to adequate memory functioning.

Serotonin

Serotonin is widely distributed throughout the brain, but the serotonin system originates in a small area of the brain stem called the **nuclei of the raphe.** The raphe nuclei consist of a collection of neurons throughout the midline of the brain stem. As Figure 2.14 shows, the serotonin pathways of the raphe nuclei branch out toward the cerebellum. Those in the medulla oblongata project toward the spinal cord, and axons of the cells in the rostral group of the nuclei branch out to the forebrain. Ascending projection of serotonergic neurons project to the limbic system, a major collection of subcortical structures involved in the modulations of mood and emotion. Destroying the raphe nuclei leads to insomnia, and serotonin plays a major role in the sleep–wake cycle. Low levels of serotonin are also associated with severe depression. Several studies have demonstrated that depressed individuals are more likely to commit suicide if they have unusually low levels of serotonin produced and released in the brain (Roy, De Jong, & Linnoila, 1989; Träskmann, Asberg, Bertilsson, & Sjöstrand, 1981). Alterations in serotonin also accompany violent and aggressive behavior in animals (Brown & Linnoila, 1990) and humans (Elliott, 1992).

Norepinephrine

Norepinephrine (NE) forms predominantly among neurons and their nuclei in a brain stem site named the **locus ceruleus** (the "blue place"), located below the wall of the fourth ventricle. Norepinephrine pathways innervate many areas in the forebrain, the cerebellum, and the spinal cord. Its functions are complex and widespread. Researchers think that norepinephrine is important in regulating mood, memory, hormones (via the hypothalamus), cerebral blood flow, and motor behavior. NE is implicated in the clinical disorders of depression and anxiety. Researchers have also found that stressful situations can increase the production and release of NE in the hypothalamus in rats (Cenci, Kalen, Mandel, & Bjoerklund, 1992).

Dopamine

The majority of dopaminergic (DA) neurons are in the **substantia nigra,** a collection of neurons and nuclei. Projections ascend to the hypothalamus, the amygdala, the septum, and the frontal cortex (see Figure 2.15). The **dopamine** pathway to the frontal cortex has been implicated in schizophrenia, a mental disorder. The so-called dopamine hypothesis suggests that schizophrenia arises from overactivity of dopaminergic synapses (Davis, Kahn, Ko, & Davidson, 1991; Fibiger, 1991). Researchers think a second pathway to the basal ganglia is responsible for tardive dyskinesia, a movement disorder. The basal ganglia play an important role in organizing motor behavior and thus researchers think dopamine is important to the ability to move.

Amino Acids

Amino acids are the building blocks of protein and are present in every cell in the body. In the brain, amino acids are involved in the basic neuronal transmission that depends on rapid communication among neurons. Of the over 20 amino acids, the most common are **gamma-amino butyric acid (GABA),** which has strong inhibitory properties; and **glutamate,** an excitatory neurotransmitter. In fact, GABA is so common in the CNS that researchers believe one-third of all synapses are receptive to it. Glutamate also occurs in high concentration throughout the nervous system

and is the major excitatory neurotransmitter. The most prominent GABA-ergic projection system consists of the inhibitory Purkinje cells that extend into the deep portions of the cerebellar nuclei. Some of the major projecting systems of the basal ganglia that are also inhibitory are the striatum, the globus pallidus, and the substantia nigra. The inability of patients with Huntington's disease to control their own motor behavior perhaps relates to the loss of inhibitory GABA-ergic neurons in the basal ganglia.

Peptides

Peptides are short chains of amino acid; scientists have identified more than 60. High levels of peptides are present in the hypothalamus and the amygdala, and to a much lesser extent in the cortex, the thalamus, and the cerebellum. Naturally produced peptides with opiate properties are called **endorphins.** Endorphins have received much scientific attention for their analgesic effects and their possible role in a pain-inhibiting neuronal system. Psychologists have always been interested in new procedures to alter the perception of pain, and think that acupuncture and electrical stimulation of the brain stem arouse the pain-inhibiting endorphin system. Of equal interest is the discovery that the nervous system has specific receptor sites that bind the drug morphine and related opiate compounds. The presence of opiate receptors suggests that the brain itself can create opiate neurotransmitters, perhaps to produce a natural high after prolonged physical stress or in the event of a catastrophic injury. Researchers believe that endorphins originate in the brain stem and reach to the spinal cord, where they interfere with pain impulses.

The Regeneration of Neurons

To what extent a patient recovers from an injury to peripheral or central nervous system pathways depends largely on the regenerative capacity of the damaged neurons. The capacity for regeneration in the peripheral nervous system is actually quite good; useful function can often be restored with surgical nerve repair. Surgeons have reattached fingers and even complete limbs, and much sensory and motor function has been restored.

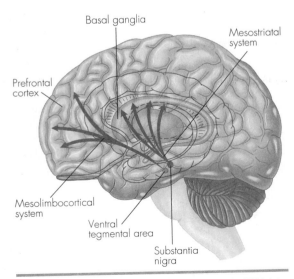

Basal ganglia

Mesostriatal system

Prefrontal cortex

Mesolimbocortical system

Ventral tegmental area

Substantia nigra

Figure 2.15 Dopamine pathways. (From James W. Kalat, *Biological Psychology*, 6th ed., Pacific Grove, CA: Brooks/Cole, 1998, p. 439, Figure 16.17)

Neuropsychology in Action 2.4

What Can We Learn from Songbirds?

by Mary V. Spiers

Can the adult brain form new neurons? The common wisdom has been that at birth the brain has all the neurons it will ever possess. In fact, the brain goes through a necessary process of pruning neurons as learning strengthens certain neural associations and others become unnecessary. There is evidence in some species of songbirds, however, that new brain cells form in conjunction with seasonal changes in mating songs. Researchers Ball and Hulse (1998) have reviewed this literature and reported intriguing findings. Male canaries and sparrows, some of the most studied songbirds, have complex mating songs that show seasonal variation, being most prominent in spring. Neurobiologists have precisely mapped the vocal system of these songbirds and have found a consistent structure function relationship between specific nuclei and singing behavior.

For example, the high vocal center (HVC) is responsible for vocal production and the robust nucleus of the archistriatum (RA) aids in coordinating respiration with singing. Within this circuit of nuclei

are neuroreceptors that are specific for sex hormones, such as androgens and estrogens. Receptors for these steroid sex hormones are not present in the vocal control circuitry of birds that are not songbirds. The complexity of song production differs in males and females, with males singing more songs and more complex songs. Researchers think this greater production in males serves a mating function, to attract females and establish territory. This sex difference in singing behavior corresponds to structural differences in the vocal control systems of males and females. Specifically, in male songbirds the HVC and RA are larger and contain more hormonal receptor nuclei. These differences aroused the curiosity of researchers. Male song production is seasonal, so might there be seasonal changes in the brains of males?

In fact, there were. In male canaries, the HVC had increased in size by nearly 100% in the spring as compared to the fall! The RA had increased by a factor of about 75% (Nottebohm, 1981). The next question was, What was causing this

increase? Was the size or volume of existing neurons changing? For example, might new dendritic connections form during this time? Or were new neurons developing? Evidence showed that the nuclei controlling singing increase in volume when the blood levels of testosterone rise. New staining techniques involving a traceable radioactive tag of newly forming cells indicated that new neurons formed in the ventricles of canaries and migrated to the vocal control system, specifically the HVC and RA (Goldman & Nottebohm, 1983). This was an astonishing finding. Further evidence indicates that adults of other species also generate new neurons and that this co-occurs with learning. Such research has exciting implications for the study of human language. Will the findings of neurogenesis in adult canaries generalize to human language, or other types of learning? And if new neurons can be formed, what is the implication for rehabilitation from brain injury and for lifetime adult learning programs?

The regeneration of neurons in the central nervous system is more complex. Once damaged, neurons do not heal spontaneously after the developmental period. Generally speaking, humans are born with as many neurons as they will ever have. This fact is related, in part, to the structure of the CNS, which is infinitely more complicated than that of the PNS. As a result, the CNS has little of the spontaneous cellular regeneration required to reconnect a damaged axon to its normal target. Most often, the projections of such neurons are lost and so are the targets of other

neurons. We discuss in later chapters why the brain can compensate when neurons are lost and how neuronal plasticity and the reconfiguration of functional systems are important to the developing brain. Most recently a flurry of research activity has focused on establishing procedures that facilitate neuronal growth by injecting chemicals into an injured area.

Injuries and diseases that result in neuronal loss or degeneration are a major health concern and can significantly affect the quality of life in individuals suffering from CNS disorders. For example, over 100,000

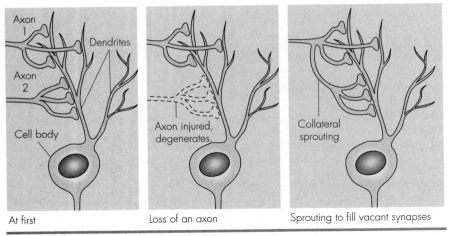

Axon 1
Dendrites
Axon 2
Cell body

Axon injured, degenerates.

Collateral sprouting

At first   Loss of an axon   Sprouting to fill vacant synapses

Figure 2.16   Example of collateral sprouting. (From James W. Kalat, *Biological Psychology*, 6th ed., Pacific Grove, CA: Brooks/Cole, 1998, p. 407, Figure 15.7)

individuals in the United States are afflicted with paraplegia or quadriplegia, a disabling condition resulting from severed neurons in the spinal cord. Head injuries—in which axonal shearing, a form of stretching caused by physical forces is common—affect about three million people. Stroke—neuronal cell death due to insufficient oxygen—affects about two million people, and degenerative diseases such as Alzheimer's, Parkinson's, and Huntington's burden millions more. It is thus very important for neuropsychologists to understand the life cycle of a neuron and what happens when it becomes damaged or diseased. Subsequent chapters cover neuropsychological disorders in more detail.

Some immediate recovery of function can be observed after traumatic or vascular lesions to the CNS. A lesion is any pathological or traumatic discontinuity of tissue resulting in the loss of neurons. Interest-ingly, recovery is related to a reduction of swelling in surrounding brain or spinal cord tissue, not to a spontaneous healing of neurons. A process called *collateral sprouting*, which occurs in nearby intact neurons, may also facilitate functional reorganization (see Figure 2.16). Within the last few years researchers have made great advances in stimulating the growth responses with which the central nervous system typically reacts to trauma, replacing tissue lost to injury or disease with neuronal transplants, and developing assessment, prosthesis, and cognitive rehabilitation techniques for disrupted functional systems. One major finding by neuropsychologists has been that an active training rehabilitation program facilitates recovery of function. It is within this area of assessment and intervention that clinical neuropsychologists have made some of their greatest advances (see Part Five, "Neuropsychology in Practice").

Conclusion

In this chapter we outlined the function of a single neuron and outlined how neurons communicate with each other. Exploring the fundamental structure of the nervous system depends in large part on the development of the microscope and staining techniques. At the microscopic level, the neuron has undergone a spectacular evolution. The total number of neurons in the human brain has increased, and the brain's architecture has become more complex. Neurons exchange information with each other through action potentials analogous to simple yes/no messages. All human behavioral events originate from this basic process mediated by interconnections and fiber systems in different areas of the brain. Thus it is important for neuropsychologists to learn as much as possible about these interconnections of the brain before they interpret brain–behavior relationships. In principle, this complex circuitry defines all brain structures, as we discuss in greater detail in the next section, Chapter 3.

Critical Thinking Questions

■ What are the limitations of the neuron hypothesis?

■ Actor Christopher Reeves has pledged that one day in the future he will walk again, even though he has a severe spinal cord injury that has left him paraplegic. What are the odds that he will fulfill his pledge? Why?

■ What are the anatomic and electrophysiological constraints of a neuron? How can they affect behavior?

■ What is the connection between drugs and neurotransmitters?

Key Terms

Gray matter
Dendrites
Purkinje cells
Pyramidal cells
Axon
Action potential
Terminal buttons
Myelin sheath
White matter
Oligodendrocytes
Schwann cells
Nodes of Ranvier
Synapse
Multipolar neurons
Bipolar neurons
Monopolar neurons
Interneurons
Motor neurons

Sensory neurons
Tracts
Pathways
Fibers
Nerves
Intracerebral fibers
Intercerebral fibers
Projection fibers
Nuclei
Ganglia
Glia
Astrocytes
Blood–brain barrier
Resting potential
Membrane potential
Ions
Sodium–potassium pump
Refractory period

Disinhibition
Seizures
Electroconvulsive therapy
   (ECT)
Electroencephalograph
   (EEG)
Reductionism
Synaptic knobs
Synaptic vesicles
Receptor sites
Excitatory postsynaptic
   potential (EPSP)
Inhibitory postsynaptic
   potential (IPSP)
Neurotransmitter
Acetylcholine (ACh)
Muscarinic choline
Nicotinic choline

Striatum
Reticular activating system
   (RAS)
Basal forebrain
Hippocampus
Nucleus basalis of Meynert
Serotonin
Nuclei of the raphe
Norepinephrine
Locus ceruleus
Substantia nigra
Dopamine
Amino acids
Gamma-amino butyric acid
   (GABA)
Glutamate
Peptides
Endorphins

Web Connections

http://psych.hanover.edu/Krantz/neurotut.html
Basic Neural Processes Tutorials
A good tutorial on the basics of neural processing. Includes a glossary of terms and quizzes on the structure of the neuron and the brain.

http://www.neuroguide.com
Neurosciences on the Internet
A searchable page that provides links to sites in neuroscience.

Chapter 3

FUNCTIONAL NEUROANATOMY

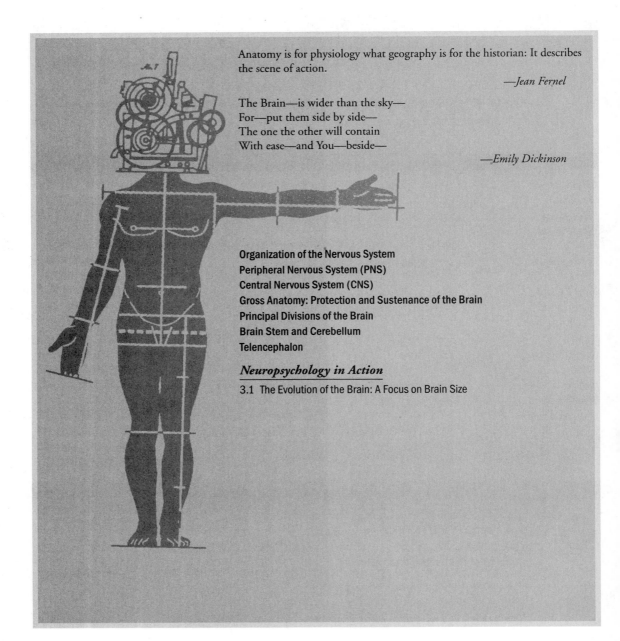

Anatomy is for physiology what geography is for the historian: It describes the scene of action.

—*Jean Fernel*

The Brain—is wider than the sky—
For—put them side by side—
The one the other will contain
With ease—and You—beside—

—*Emily Dickinson*

Organization of the Nervous System
Peripheral Nervous System (PNS)
Central Nervous System (CNS)
Gross Anatomy: Protection and Sustenance of the Brain
Principal Divisions of the Brain
Brain Stem and Cerebellum
Telencephalon

Neuropsychology in Action

3.1 The Evolution of the Brain: A Focus on Brain Size

Keep in Mind

■ How are the subsystems of the brain organized?

■ How does the brain protect and nourish itself?

■ Does brain structure follow brain function?

■ In what ways do the cortical cerebral hemispheres differ from the subcortical structures?

Overview

Neuroanatomy is best understood within a conceptual framework of structure–function relationships. In neuropsychology, a primary goal is to understand the brain's psychological functions and systems. Rather than from memorizing structures for structure's sake, a more meaningful picture emerges from knowing how the subdivisions of the brain are related, and what roles they play in initiating and regulating behavior. Neuroanatomy and neuroscience texts present slightly different variations of organization within the major subdivisions of the brain. Some authors focus on morphology as the organizing scheme, some on physiology, and some on embryonic and fetal development. Despite the daunting array of structures, the basic logic of neuroanatomy is straightforward. The organization we present here shows the relationships among the often confusing terms and groupings. It accomplishes this goal by using the foundation of the developing brain within the context of evolution, which provides a useful picture of functioning from basic to more complex behaviors.

In this chapter we discuss individual structures and terminology, show their location in the brain, and give a brief overview of function. The material covered here is not a detailed review of the content often covered in courses on neuroscience or sensory motor systems, but rather constitutes an illustrated account of the functional anatomy of the major components of the nervous system. With the foundation of the gross anatomy and functioning this chapter presents, you can appreciate the normal and abnormal phenomena associated with brain dysfunction. The structures are the important topographical features on which the various processing systems of the brain depend. This chapter is a stepping-stone for the next chapters related to functional systems, and indeed, for the entire book. We integrate and develop these structures further in examining functional systems and neuropsychological disorders.

The first section of this chapter presents a general overview of the major components of the nervous system. We also introduce the necessary terminology for a common orientation to the geographical locations of structures. Next we present structural features that protect and sustain the brain. Then we discuss principal divisions of the brain, from lower, evolutionarily older structures to higher-order structures.

Organization of the Nervous System

The nervous system is customarily divided into two parts; the **peripheral nervous system (PNS)** and the **central nervous system (CNS)** (see Figure 3.1 and Table 3.1 on p. 66). This division stems from the different properties and functions of neurons and systems within the two systems. The previous chapter discussed neuronal differences, specifically the special properties of neurons within the CNS; this chapter discusses functional differences. The PNS includes

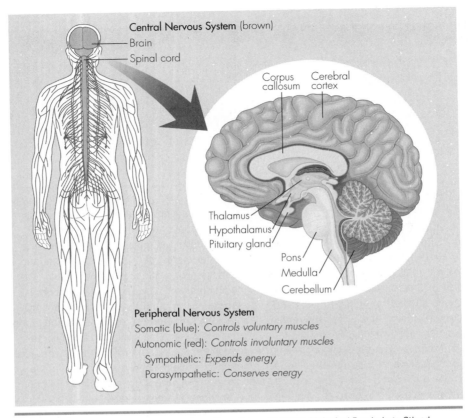

Central Nervous System (brown)
— Brain
— Spinal cord

Corpus callosum   Cerebral cortex

Thalamus
Hypothalamus
Pituitary gland

Pons
Medulla
Cerebellum

Peripheral Nervous System
Somatic (blue): *Controls voluntary muscles*
Autonomic (red): *Controls involuntary muscles*
    Sympathetic: *Expends energy*
    Parasympathetic: *Conserves energy*

Figure 3.1   The human nervous system. (From James W. Kalat, *Biological Psychology,* 6th ed., Pacific Grove, CA: Brooks/Cole, 1998, p. 79, Figure 4.1)

Table 3.1 ***Principal Divisions of the Nervous System***

1. Central nervous system (CNS)
   • Brain
   • Spinal cord

2. Peripheral nervous system (PNS)
   • Somatic nervous system
       Cranial nerves
       Spinal nerves
   • Autonomic nervous system (ANS)
       Sympathetic
       Parasympathetic

all the portions of the nervous system outside the CNS. The PNS consists of the **somatic nervous system,** which interacts with the external environment, and the **autonomic nervous system (ANS),** which participates in regulating the body's internal environment. The ANS has two divisions, the **sympathetic** and **parasympathetic nervous systems.** The PNS and the CNS are in constant communication with each other.

The CNS includes the **brain** and **spinal cord.** It communicates with the PNS by exchanging sensory and motor information via the spinal nerves and cranial nerves. You can imagine the spinal cord as a cable carrying bundles of spinal nerves from the body up to higher processing areas in the brain. It serves as the CNS conduit of the majority of sensory and motor information to and from the body. The **cranial nerves** also carry very specific sensory and motor information directly to the brain, bypassing the spinal cord.

Peripheral Nervous System (PNS)

In principle, all components of the PNS inform the CNS about events in the environment and transmit commands from the CNS to the body. The somatic nervous system consists of **afferent nerves** or sensory nerves that convey messages from the sense organs to the CNS (incoming) and **efferent nerves** carrying motor signals from the CNS to muscles (outgoing). Most nerves of the somatic nervous system project at regular intervals to the spinal cord via the spinal nerves), except for 12 pairs of cranial nerves, which synapse directly with the brain.

The function of the autonomic nervous system is the neural control of internal organs (for example, heart and intestines). The ANS consists of both peripheral and central parts, and includes a sympathetic division that is involved in activities that expend bodily energy. This expenditure most often occurs in response to, or anticipation of, a stressful event. A simplified summary of the role of sympathetic activation is that it prepares the body for action based on the "fight or flight" principle. Sympathetic activity mobilizes the energy necessary for psychological arousal. It includes an increase in blood flow, blood pressure, heart rate, and sweating; and a decrease in digestion and sexual arousal.

The parasympathetic division of the ANS acts to conserve energy and is typically associated with relaxation. It increases the body's supply of stored energy and facilitates digestion, and gastric and intestinal motility. Most autonomic organs receive both sympathetic and parasympathetic input, and are influenced by the relative level of sympathetic and parasympathetic activity. For many bodily functions, the sympathetic and parasympathetic divisions act in opposite directions. You can think of the two branches of the ANS as balancing each other, like two sides of a scale. People generally consider the functions of the ANS automatic, not under voluntary control. Because people think ANS functions are sensitive to stress, these functions form the basis of the lie detector test. However, biofeedback, meditation, hypnosis, and other forms of stress management have shown that these functions are not as "automatic" as once thought, although some controversy has focused on the degree to which humans can control them (Zillmer & Wickramaserkera, 1987).

Although it is useful to divide the nervous system as just outlined, real functional anatomic circuits and systems pay little heed to these boundaries. For example, many nerve cells described as part of the PNS have their cells of origin or their terminal branches actually situated in the CNS. Consider the divisions within the nervous system as somewhat flexible; they follow the organizational need to separate complex phenomena into discrete and less complex units.

Central Nervous System (CNS)

The brain and spinal cord form a continuous communication system of the central nervous system. The CNS has several unique features. First, as previously discussed, the neurons have some properties different from PNS neurons in that, for example, they don't show similar properties of regeneration. Second, you can recognize the importance of the CNS by the fact that the body gives it extra protection. Structurally, it is located within the bony cavities of the skull and the spine. Coverings called the **meninges** protect it, and it is surrounded by and floats in the protective **cerebrospinal fluid (CSF).** The CNS, and especially the brain, is the most well-nourished area of the body, being supplied with an intricate system of arteries designed with "backup" systems. The body gives it priority in receiving nutrients and oxygen, and at the same time gives it more protection, through the blood–brain barrier, from potentially harmful substances circulating in the body.

BRAIN

Anatomically, the brain is continuous with the spinal cord, from which it emerges. From an exterior view the brain appears to be one organ with a left and a right hemisphere. It actually consists of several divisions with many identifiable structures.

How the brain is organized into subsystems that ultimately result in human behavior is a very challenging question, on which the rest of this text focuses. Consider that the brain occupies a relatively small space of about 1000 to 1500 cm^3, roughly the size of a cantaloupe. Within this space function an incredible array of different types of cells. There is also an almost infinite number of possible connections that make up exceedingly complex networks. From this complexity a sense of order and organization emerges that supports basic life, behavior, and consciousness. The human brain represents the most advanced stage of this integration.

Anatomic Terms of Relationship

Because the brain is a three-dimensional structure, neuropsychologists use a number of terms that describe specific parts, planes, and directions. Unfortunately, the terminology is complex and not entirely standardized. This is related, in part, to the fact that we still use nomenclature proposed in Latin or Greek more than a century ago. In some instances anatomists disagree about the boundaries of a specific brain structure, so several terms may describe overlapping brain regions. Early anatomists used names to describe structures, simply because they reminded them of something else. For example, the outer part of the brain was named *cortex*, meaning "bark," because it is a thin mantle or covering for the brain. Thus, whenever we use the original meaning of the names of brain structures to help the reader form associations about the nomenclature of various neuroanatomical structures. We use precise anatomic terms to clear up any resulting confusion and to increase your ability to communicate accurately about the geography and topology of the brain.

Descriptions usually divide the brain into one of the three main planes (using the x, y, and z axes) (see Exhibit 1 inside the front cover). The terms in Table 3.2 offer a way to describe brain anatomy.

Table 3.2 *Planes of the Brain and Directions of Orientation to the CNS*

- Planes bisecting the brain:
  Horizontal Plane
  A plane (x axis) that shows the brain as seen from above or parallel to the ground.
  Coronal Plane
  A plane (y axis) that shows the brain as seen from the front (frontal section). Typically this plane is viewed from behind to provide consistency for right and left directions of the brain and the picture.
  Sagittal Plane
  A plane (z axis) that shows the brain as seen from the side or perpendicular to the ground, bisecting the brain into right and left halves (*sagitta*, Latin for "arrow").

- Directional terms: Most often directions in the human nervous system are related to the orientation of the spinal cord.
  Anterior: toward the front or front end.
  Posterior: toward the back or tail.
  Inferior: toward the bottom, or below.
  Superior: toward the top or above.
  Medial: toward the middle/midline, away from the side.
  Lateral: toward the side, away from the midline.
  Rostral: toward the head.
  Caudal: toward the rear away from the head.
  Proximal: near the trunk or center, close to the origin of attachment.
  Distal: away from the center, toward the periphery, away from the origin of attachment.
  Dorsal: toward the back. The top of the brain is dorsal in humans.
  Ventral: toward the belly. The bottom of the brain is ventral in humans.
  Ipsilateral: on the same side.
  Contralateral: on the opposite side.

SPINAL CORD

Overview

■ *Gross anatomic features:* Spinal nerves, internal organization of the spinal cord (gray and white matter)

■ *Function:* Relay information to and from the brain, responsible for simple reflexive behavior

Structure

The spinal cord is continuous with the brain and extends downward along the back for about 46 cm. Like the brain, it is protected by bone, meninges, and CSF. The spinal cord is physically housed in the spinal column, which consists of alternating bony vertebrae and intervertebral discs made up of cartilage that absorb mechanical shocks sustained to the spinal column. The spinal cord itself is considerably smaller than the vertebral canal and the meninges. Fat, CSF, and veins combine to protect against contact with bony surroundings.

The spinal nerves consist of both sensory and motor neurons. At each of the 30 levels of the spinal cord, a pair of incoming (afferent) dorsal root fibers signals incoming sensory information, and a pair of outgoing (efferent) ventral root fibers controls motor nerves and muscles (see Figure 3.2). These nerves conduct information related to both the somatic and autonomic nervous systems in the periphery. In the spinal cord, white matter (myelinated axons) makes up the outside of the cord, whereas gray matter (cell bodies) is located on the interior. Each area of the spinal cord

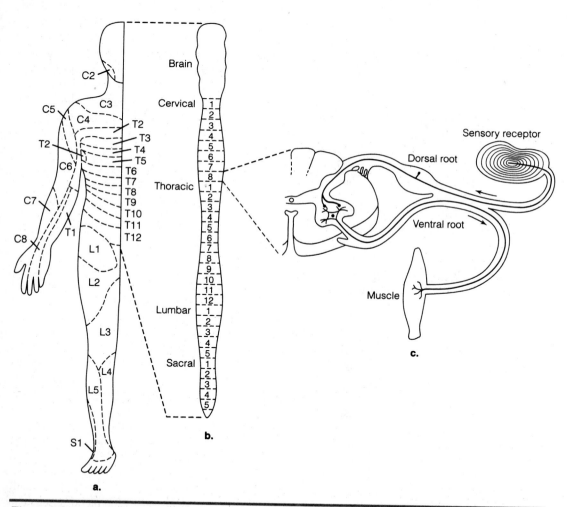

Figure 3.2   Spinal nerves and areas of body innervation. (a) The body segments of spinal innervation are segmented in rings around the body. (b) The divisions of the 30 segments of the spinal cord. (c) Cross-section through a segment of the spinal cord showing sensory input through the dorsal root and motor output through the ventral root. (Adapted from *Fundamentals of Human Neuropsychology*, 4th ed., by Bryan Kolb and Ian Q. Wishaw © 1996 by W. H. Freeman and Company, p. 46, Figure 3.3. Used with the permission of Worth Publishers)

corresponds to a specific body location and controls sensation and movement of the associated body area; skin, muscle and internal organs. There are 1 coccyx, 5 sacral (S), 5 lumbar (L), 12 thoracic (T), and 8 cervical (C) spinal cord levels. The spinal nerves form ringlike innervations around the trunk of the body at each level of the spinal cord. The innervation of the limbs are extensions of the body rings. For example, the nerves to the arms and hands are extensions of C-6, C-7, and C-8 innervations from the trunk.

Function

The spinal cord relays somatosensory information from the trunk and limbs to the brain. The cord also relays simple motor messages from the brain to the trunk and limbs. It does some integration of information that involves basic reflexive behavior. Spinal cord lesions can result in motor as well as sensory impairment. Although in their evaluations, clinical neuropsychologists have often placed less emphasis on spinal cord function compared to lesions of the brain, sensory or motor impairment may reflect brain dysfunction, but may also be related to spinal cord or even peripheral nerve damage. A thorough neurologic evaluation in combination with a comprehensive neuropsychological evaluation often clarifies the location of the dysfunction. Spinal cord injuries frequently co-occur with brain injury caused by whiplash, which may go unnoticed until after the trauma of paralysis has been stabilized.

Gross Anatomy: Protection and Sustenance of the Brain

The body affords extra protection and sustenance to the central nervous system because of its special status. The structural and physiological protections extend to the spinal cord and the brain, although the focus is on the brain. Structurally, bone provides a type of "armor" to surround both the brain and spinal cord. In most cases the skull holds the brain snugly and physically protects it from injury. However, as in closed head injury (see Chapter 10), the gelatinous brain may accelerate and scrape against the skull's bony projections. It is important to understand the skull–brain relationship to understand how the brain may be vulnerable to skull-related damage. Under the hard protection of bone, the protective membranes called *meninges* form a flexible structural but semipermeable protective pad that completely surrounds the brain and spinal cord. The covering of the meninges form another layer of protection. However, certain types of tumors called **meningiomas** may form here and impact on the brain. The CSF circulates around and throughout the CNS via the **ventricular system,** which provides not only an additional structural fluid cushion but also physiological protection through its immunological functions and its ability to act as a "waste disposal" system. The unique **vascular system** of the brain not only supplies nutrients to the energy-demanding brain but adds a layer of protection through the blood–brain barrier.

SKULL

Overview

- *Gross anatomic features:* A fused connection of bony plates covering the brain
- *Function:* Protection of the brain

Structure

The skull consists of the frontal bone (in some individuals, the frontal bone develops in two parts), two parietal bones, two temporal bones, the occipital bone, and the sphenoid bone (see Figure 3.3 on p. 72). The cerebral lobes get their names after the cranial plates of the skull, whose corresponding outline they generally follow. This has led to an imprecise nomenclature of the cortex because the external aspects of the skull are easily differentiated, unlike those of the cortical lobes. The skull provides grooves for blood vessels in the roof (calveria) of the cranium, conspicuous ridges in the base of the skull, known as **fossae,** that hold the brain in place, and more-or-less symmetrical orifices or **foramina** in the base of the skull that provide passage for nerves and blood vessels. The largest of these is the **foramen magnum,** which provides a large median opening in the occipital bone for the spinal cord to pass through to the brain stem.

In the newborn, the skull is a relatively large part of its body, accommodating the disproportionally large brain. At birth, the brain is approximately 25% of its adult size weighing about 500 grams, but will reach about 75% of its mature size by its first year of maturation. Facilitating this rapid development of the brain, the bony plates that comprise the skull are not fused as they are in later years, but are separated by membranous, soft tissue. In the newborn the membranous gaps are largest at the corners of the parietal bone. These soft openings are labeled **fontanelles** ("small fountains") and may fluctuate with changes in intracranial pressure. The largest of these is the anterior fontanelle, located at the top of the head between the frontal and parietal bones. It does not fully close until two years after birth.

Function

The skull completely encases the brain, protecting it from external influences. Although normally the shell of the skull is an asset, in some instances it can actually be a liability. The fact that the skull is rigid can become life threatening when the internal pressure of a swelling, injured brain cannot be released. Because the skull is not smooth on the interior, but rather consists of bony projections designed to hold the brain in place, injury to the areas around the bony projections of the frontal and temporal lobes is common with whiplash and other head injuries, which cause the gelatinous brain to reverberate in the skull. The skull varies in thickness; particularly the areas around the temporal and sphenoid bones are relatively thin and are easily fractured by a blow to the side of the head. Fractures to the base of the skull can lead to serious damage of the brain related to shearing of the cranial nerves, leakage of the cerebrospinal fluid from the nose, and bleeding from the auditory canal.

MENINGES

Overview

■ *Gross anatomic features:* Dura mater, arachnoid membrane, pia mater

■ *Function:* Protective covering of the central nervous system, location of venous drainage and cerebrospinal fluid absorption

Structure

The brain and spinal cord are the only human structures completely enclosed in protective bone. In addition, they are covered by the meninges, a set of thin membranes that hold the brain and spinal cord in place and act as a protective buffer. The meninges of the CNS consist of three meningeal membranes and completely surround the brain and the spinal cord. Inner to outer they can be remembered with the mnemonic PAD: pia mater, arachnoid membrane, and dura mater (or simply dura) (see Figure 3.4 on p. 74). The thin **pia mater** (Latin for "pious mother") directly adheres to the surface of the central nervous system, following its contours closely. The **arachnoid membrane** (spider web–like membrane) overlies the **subarachnoid space,** which contains cerebrospinal fluid. The **dura mater** (Latin for "tough mother") is a dense, inelastic, double-layered membrane that adheres to the inner surface of the skull. The meningeal veins are in the outer portion of the dura. The space between the two dural layers is the **epidural space.** The space between the dura and the arachnoid is the **subdural space.** Cerebral veins crossing the subdural space have little supporting structure and are therefore most vulnerable to injury and bleeding as a result of trauma (for example, **subdural hematoma**).

Function

The meninges provide a protective covering by encasing the brain and spinal cord. They have no function in cognitive activity, but are of importance to neuropsychologists because of clinical complications during injury. For example, a head trauma frequently tears large blood vessels in the subarachnoid space. In addition, the meninges are susceptible to inflammation, usually by bacterial infection, resulting in **meningitis.** Meningitis can be caused by both bacteria and viral infection. The disease is very dangerous because it can progress quickly, within 24 hours, from a respiratory illness, with fever, headache, and a stiff neck, to changes in consciousness including stupor, coma, and death.

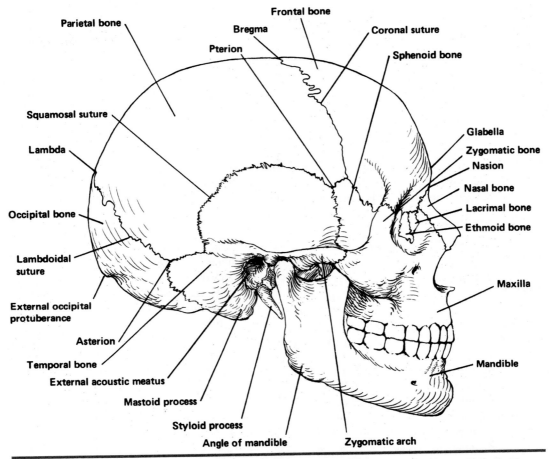

Figure 3.3   Lateral (a) and basal (b) views of the skull. (From J. G. Chusid, *Correlative Neuroanatomy & Functional Neurology*, NY: Appleton & Lange, 1982, p. 256, Figure 19.3 and p. 257, Figure 19.4. Reproduced with permission of the McGraw-Hill Companies.)

VENTRICULAR SYSTEM

Overview

- *Gross anatomic features:* Lateral (1st and 2nd), 3rd, and 4th ventricles, choroid plexus, cerebral aqueduct, arachnoid granulations
- *Function:* Intracranial pressure, cerebrospinal fluid production and circulation

Structure

Within the brain are four interconnected, fluid-filled cavities known as the **ventricles** (see Figure 3.5 on p. 75). There are two lateral ventricles, one in each hemisphere, the third ventricle, and the fourth ventricle. The lateral ventricles are the largest and are easily seen in many types of brain imaging, as they occupy what seems to be a large hollow in each hemisphere. They are connected by a small opening, the **foramen of Monro,** to the third ventricle, which is situated between the two lateral ventricles at the level of the thalamus and the hypothalamus. The third ventricle has a single opening that leads downward through a narrow channel known as the **cerebral (or Sylvanian) aqueduct,** connecting it to the fourth ventricle.

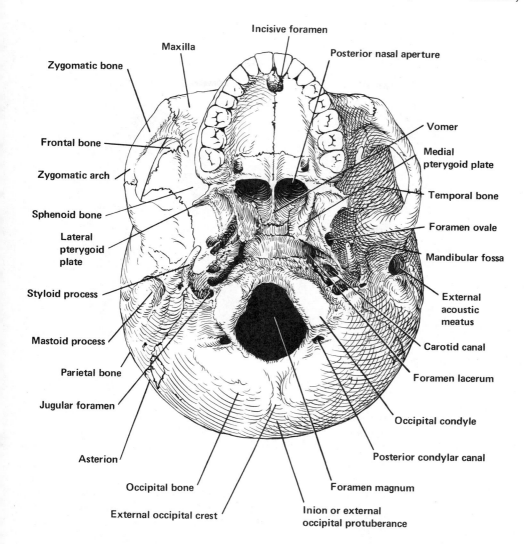

The cerebral aqueduct passes through the midbrain and expands into the fourth ventricle, which lies in the brain stem, just beneath, and anterior to, the cerebellum. Early anatomists such as Leonardo da Vinci were fascinated by the ventricles, which were believed to contain the spirit (see Figure 3.6 on p. 76).

Within these ventricles the **choroid plexus** tissue secretes cerebrospinal fluid (CSF), which flows from the upper to the lower ventricles. The choroid plexus is a highly vascularized network of small blood vessels that protrude into the ventricles from the lining of the pia mater. It continually produces CSF. The CSF circulates through the ventricles and around the spinal cord and brain. In humans, approximately 450 ml (somewhat more than a 12-ounce soft drink can) of CSF is produced every day, mostly by the choroid plexus in the lateral ventricles. Then, after flowing through the interventricular foramen of Monro, CSF volume is increased by fluid produced in the third ventricle.

The fourth ventricle has three openings in its membranous roof, the **foramen of Magendie** and two lateral **foramina of Luschka,** that allow the CSF to flow

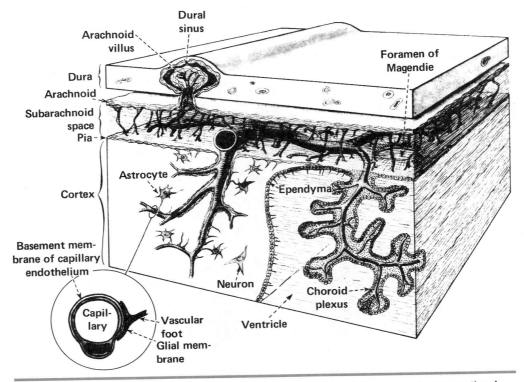

Figure 3.4 Protective covering of the brain. The protective layers of the brain are seen in cross-section. A closeup of a capillary represents the blood–brain barrier. (From Tschirgi, in J. Field and H. W. Magoun, eds., *Handbook of Physiology,* Section 1, The American Physiological Society, 1960, pp. 1865–1890. Reproduced with permission of the McGraw-Hill Companies from J. G. Chusid, *Correlative Neuroanatomy & Functional Neurology,* NY: Appleton & Lange, 1982, p. 57, Figure 1.63)

outside the brain and recirculate. The cycle is completed via the continuous reabsorption of CSF from the subarachnoid space between the arachnoid and the pia mater. From the expansions of the subarachnoid space called **cisterns,** most of the CSF moves upward along pressure gradients to a large sinus called the **superior sagittal sinus** and is reabsorbed into the blood system into larger blood-filled spaces. Within the subarachnoid space are also small pockets of veins, termed **arachnoid granulations.** These cauliflower-like projections serve as pathways for the cerebrospinal fluid to be absorbed and reenter the venous circulation. The fluid recirculates every six to seven hours.

The ventricular system not only boasts some of the most exotic terms of the brain, but it is also important to any study of brain anatomy. The reason for this is that the brain shapes the ventricular system, so that any changes in the anatomy of the brain can distort the ventricular system. The location of the fourth ventricle, for example, near the cerebellum, is important for neuroradiology. When neuroradiologists view two-dimensional pictures of the brain, locating any of the four ventricles helps precisely locate the brain image, because the structure of the surrounding brain defines the ventricles. If brain tissue is distorted, ventricle size and shape are usually distorted.

Function

The ventricles and the cerebrospinal fluid are involved in two principal processes. First, cerebrospinal fluid protects the brain and the spinal cord by acting

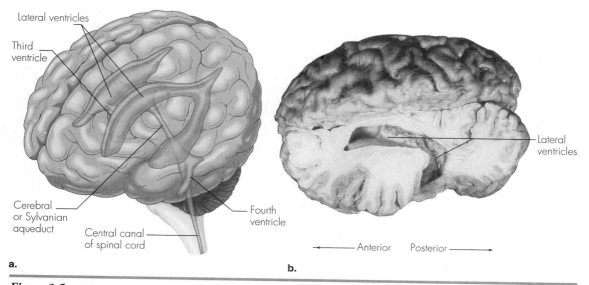

Lateral ventricles

Third ventricle

Cerebral or Sylvanian aqueduct

Central canal of spinal cord

Fourth ventricle

Lateral ventricles

Anterior   Posterior

a.

b.

Figure 3.5   The ventricular system. (From James W. Kalat, *Biological Psychology,* 6th ed., Pacific Grove, CA: Brooks/Cole, 1998, Figure 4.1, p. 89)

as a buffer. The ventricles of the brain, the central canal of the spinal chord, and the subarachnoid spaces all contain cerebrospinal fluid with a normal intracranial pressure of 0 to 15 Torr (a unit of measurement—the pressure necessary to support a column of mercury one millimeter high). The CSF thus floats the central nervous system like a buoy and protects the brain by acting as a liquid buffer or cushion to absorb internal as well as external forces. This is easily appreciated in patients who had some of their CSF drained as part of the now outdated x-ray diagnostic procedure known as *pneumoencephalography* (see Chapter 6). Such patients suffered from severe headaches and stabbing pain with any head movement due to injected air and less support to the brain.

The second function of cerebrospinal fluid is in disposing of waste products from the brain, which are thus absorbed via cisterns into the venous vascular system. Chapter 1 noted that medieval scientists attributed significant mental as well as spiritual processes to the presence of cerebrospinal fluid within the ventricular chambers of the brain. This theory became known as the ventricular localization hypothesis and later formed the basis for the cell doctrine.

On gross dissection of the brain, the lateral ventricles are the most striking features, and thus this theory, although wrong, persisted robustly.

The ventricles have no direct role in cognitive function. However, abnormal intracranial ventricular pressure (greater than 15 Torr) may lead to general cognitive deficits. A sequence of events can occur in which the ventricles become enlarged with fluid, occupying greater space than usual. This results in brain swelling and an increase in intracranial pressure. The squeezing or displacing of brain tissue in turn leads to changes in behavior and cognition. This expansion of the ventricles accompanied by increased intercranial pressure results in a medical condition called **hydrocephalus,** which may be caused by an imbalance in the rate of CSF production or absorption, or by blockage (such as by a tumor) of the circulation. The skull itself may actually swell. If hydrocephalus occurs in childhood before the cranial bones have closed, the skull may enlarge to enormous size (see Figure 3.7 on p. 77). Acute hydrocephalus can be life threatening. Because the fused plates of the skull cannot accommodate the additional space, untreated hydrocephalus among adults and in older

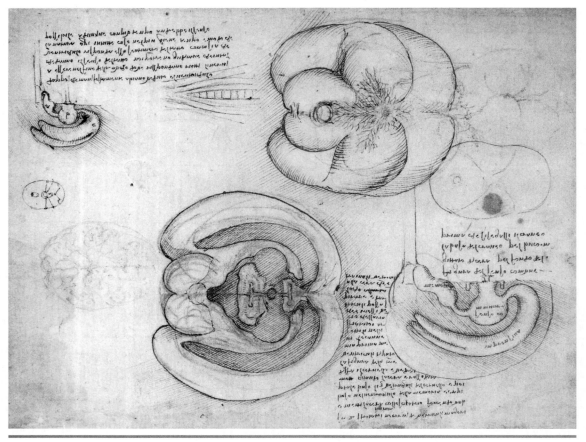

Figure 3.6   Although many of Leonardo da Vinci's (1452–1519) early brain anatomy drawings were inaccurate, he later became a keen observer of neuroanatomy. For this drawing, which presented an anatomic breakthrough, he poured melted wax into the ventricles of an ox, then cut away the brain tissues to determine the true shape of the ventricles. (The Royal Collection © 2000, Her Majesty Queen Elizabeth II)

children results in chronic dilation of the ventricles and a thinning of the cortex.

Because the subarachnoid space extends down toward a small central channel that runs the length of the spinal cord, it is possible to collect a small sample of CSF at the level of the lower back by tapping into the subarachnoid cisterns of the lower lumbar vertebrae. This can be done without damaging the integrity of the spinal cord, using an invasive diagnostic procedure known as a "lumbar puncture" or "spinal tap" (see Chapter 6). The CSF sample can then be exam-ined under the microscope for the abnormal presence of blood, infection, or cancerous cells.

VASCULAR SYSTEM

Overview

■ *Gross anatomic features:* Arteries (see Table 3.2), veins, circle of Willis

■ *Function*
Arteries: nourishment: supply of oxygen, nutrients
Veins: carrying away of waste products

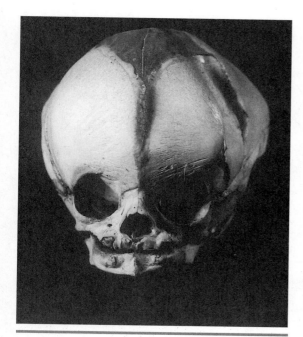

Figure 3.7 Skull of a child with severe hydrocephalus. Note the enlarged fontanelle. (Mutter Museum, College of Physicians of Philadelphia)조구역.정문

To function properly, the brain must receive adequate oxygen and many nutrients (such as glucose) from the blood vessels. If a blood vessel is obstructed or bursts, the brain cells supplied by that vessel cannot function properly and begin to die. When brain cells do not function, neither do the parts of the body controlled by those neurons or other related parts of the brain to which the damaged neurons project (targets). Becoming familiar with the blood supply of the brain can make important vascular disorders such as stroke more understandable.

Arteries Supplying the Brain

All major cerebral arteries and the meninges are supplied by four large arteries to the brain. They are the right and left **internal carotid arteries** as well as the two **vertebral arteries** (see Figure 3.8 and Table 3.3 on pp. 78 and 79). These vessels originate directly or indirectly from branches of the **aortic arch,** which arises

from the left ventricle of the heart. The internal carotid arteries supply the anterior portions of the brain and the vertebral arteries supply the posterior portion.

The two vertebral arteries join together at the level of the brain stem to form the **basilar artery.** The basilar artery divides into the left and right **posterior cerebral arteries.** This vertebro-basilar system provides approximately 20% of the total cerebral blood circulation mostly to the posterior portions of the brain, and, a corresponding 20% of all **cerebrovascular accidents** (CVAs), or strokes, are restricted to this territory.

The Circle of Willis

The cross-brain connections from both the internal carotid and basilar systems form a remarkable vascular structure near the base of the brain, the **circle of Willis,** named after its discoverer, English anatomist and physician Thomas Willis (1621–1675; see Figure 3.9 on p. 80). The circle is formed by the anterior cerebral branches of the internal carotid artery and its connections, the anterior communicating artery, the posterior communicating artery, and the posterior cerebral branches of the basilar artery. The circle of Willis is the most important intracranial collateral blood supply, and allows a certain degree of redundancy among blood vessels and blood supply to the various areas of the brain.

CEREBRAL ARTERIES

The internal carotid artery on each side of the body divides into the **anterior cerebral artery** (which supplies the anterior paramedian cerebral hemisphere) and the larger **middle cerebral artery** (which supplies the lateral hemisphere and most of the basal ganglia). Figure 3.10 on page 81 shows the areas of the brain served by each of the three cerebral arteries. The left and right anterior cerebral arteries are connected by the **anterior communicating artery.** The **posterior communicating arteries** arise from the internal carotid arteries and connect the middle and posterior cerebral arteries. The major cerebral arteries have multiple cortical branches, which we do not discuss in detail here. Disrupting blood supply to any of the

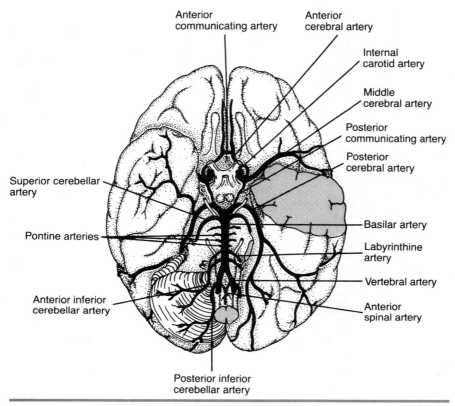

Figure 3.8 Major arteries to the brain. The cerebral arteries are seen from the base of the brain. The left half of the cerebellum and the tip of the left temporal lobe have been removed. (From A. M. Burt, *Textbook of Neuroanatomy,* Philadelphia: W. B. Saunders, 1993, p. 179, Figure 9.8)

cerebral arteries or its branches may cause relative uniform and characteristic symptoms related to each brain area served by the artery. Of the major arteries supplying the brain, blockage of the carotid arteries most often results in a stroke affecting the middle cerebral artery. The anterior cerebral artery is not as commonly involved in stroke because the anterior communicating artery can supply blood.

In the normally functioning brain, there is little arterial crossover from one hemisphere of the brain to the other, or between anterior and posterior arteries. In the event of a stroke to a major artery, other intact blood vessels can take over for injured blood vessels. For example, if the basilar artery is occluded, shutting off blood supply to the posterior communi-

cating artery, the internal carotid arteries may provide blood to posterior circulation via the posterior communicating artery. However, there is much individual variation in the circle of Willis; parts of the system may actually be missing in some people (for example, in 15% of normal brains the posterior cerebral artery is a direct extension of the posterior communicating artery).

VENOUS SYSTEM

The veins are located in the outer portion of the dura and pass blood through vessels back to the heart. Venous drainage starts with the superficial cerebral veins, which originate in the brain substance within the pia

Table 3.3 *Arteries to the Brain*		
Artery Name	**Origin from . . .**	**Distribution to . . .**
Basilar	Junction of right and left vertebral arteries	Brain stem, internal ear, cerebellum, posterior cerebrum
Carotid, common	Brachiocephalic (right), aorta (left)	Internal and external carotid
Carotid, external	Common carotid artery	Neck, face, skull
Carotid, internal	Common carotid artery	Middle ear, brain, choroid plexus of lateral ventricles
Cerebellar, inferior anterior	Basilar artery	Lower anterior cerebellum, inner ear
Cerebellar, inferior posterior	Vertebral artery	Lower part of cerebellum, medulla, choroid plexus of fourth ventricle
Cerebellar, superior	Basilar artery	Upper part of cerebellum, midbrain, pineal body, choroid plexus of third ventricle
Cerebral, anterior	Internal carotid artery	Orbital, frontal, and parietal cortex, corpus callosum, diencephalon, corpus striatum, internal capsule, choroid plexus of lateral ventricles
Cerebral, middle	Internal carotid artery	Orbital, frontal, parietal and temporal cortex, corpus striatum, internal capsule
Cerebral, posterior	Basilar artery	Occipital and temporal lobes, basal ganglia, choroid plexus of lateral ventricles, thalamus, midbrain
Ophthalmic	Internal carotid artery	Eye, orbit, facial structures
Spinal, anterior	Vertebral artery	Spinal cord
Spinal, posterior	Vertebral artery	Spinal cord
Vertebral	Subclavian artery, which arises from brachiocephalic (right), aorta (left)	Neck muscles, vertebrae, spinal cord, cerebellum, cortex

mater and empty into the superior sagittal and transverse sinuses, the deep veins of the brain, and the straight sinus, which connects to the internal jugular vein. As we noted in discussing the ventricular system, the subarachnoid space pockets of veins called *arachnoid granulations* serve as pathways for the subarachnoid cerebrospinal fluid to be absorbed and reenter the venous circulation. Arachnoid granulations first appear in childhood, around age 7, and increase in size and number during adulthood. Unlike the arterial blood supply, the venous system of the brain does not have a right and left system. Thus, there is free circulation within the venous system, which may facilitate the spread of infectious agents from one hemisphere to the other. Chapter 9 gives a detailed description of vascular disorders.

 ## Principal Divisions of the Brain

You can subdivide the brain into three major divisions based on the development of the human embryo. As the embryo's neural tube closes, it begins to differentiate into three bulges. The topmost becomes the **forebrain,** or **prosencephalon,** the middle is the **midbrain** (**mesencephalon**), and the third is the **hindbrain** (**rhombencephalon**). The remainder of

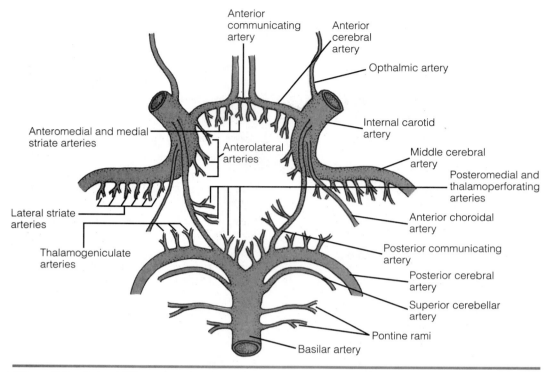

Figure 3.9   Circle of Willis. (From A. M. Burt, *Textbook of Neuroanatomy,* Philadelphia: W. B. Saunders, 1993, p. 179, Figure 9.9)

the neural tube develops into the spinal cord (see Chapter 7 for a detailed discussion of the developing brain). The three major subdivisions of the brain further differentiate into five subdivisions: (1) the **telencephalon,** (2) the **diencephalon,** (3) the **mesencephalon,** (4) the **metencephalon,** and, (5) the **myelencephalon.** This framework organizes the study of the primary structures evident in the adult. Table 3.4 and Figure 3.11 on pages 82 and 83 depict the relationships between the principal anatomic divisions, subdivisions, and major structures of the brain.

Traditionally, neuropsychologists focus on the brain areas of complex processing within the telencephalon, primarily the cerebrum. In fact, the major structures of the telencephalon, including the cerebrum, the basal ganglia and the basal forebrain, comprise about 85% of the brain's weight (Burt, 1993). So although this is only one subdivision of the brain, it covers much area and is of great importance in un-

derstanding higher cognitive abilities. Therefore, a common manner of dividing the brain is to differentiate between the telencephalon and the brain stem. The brain stem includes all the subdivisions below the telencephalon (diencephalon, mesencephalon, metencephalon, and myelencephalon), except for the cerebellum, and mediates many primary regulatory processes of the body. We begin by discussing the major structures of the brain stem and cerebellum and then move to the telencephalon.

Brain Stem and Cerebellum

The brain stem and the cerebellum, in terms of evolution, form the most primitive area of the brain. The **cerebellum,** which looks like a "little brain," connects to the dorsal aspect of the brain

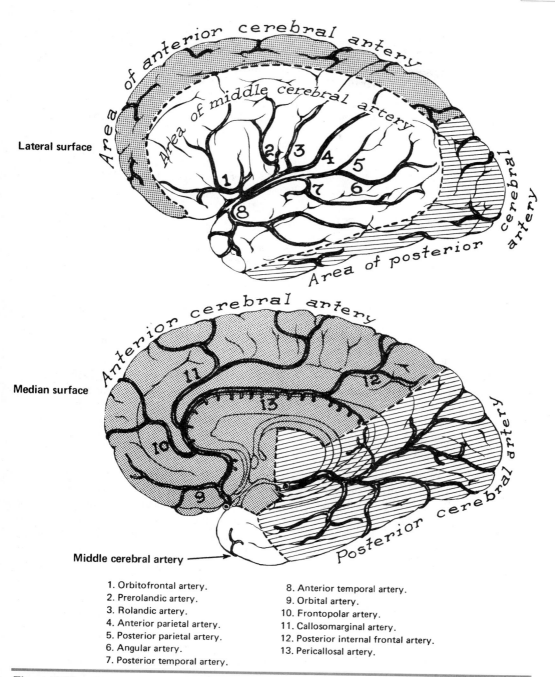

Lateral surface

Median surface

1. Orbitofrontal artery.
2. Prerolandic artery.
3. Rolandic artery.
4. Anterior parietal artery.
5. Posterior parietal artery.
6. Angular artery.
7. Posterior temporal artery.

8. Anterior temporal artery.
9. Orbital artery.
10. Frontopolar artery.
11. Callosomarginal artery.
12. Posterior internal frontal artery.
13. Pericallosal artery.

Figure 3.10   Blood supply to the cortex. Major arteries and areas of cortical profusion. (a) A lateral view shows the middle cerebral artery and its branches. (b) The course of the anterior and posterior cerebral arteries in mid-sagittal view. (From J. G. Chusid, *Correlative Neuroanatomy & Functional Neurology*, NY: Appleton & Lange, 1982, p. 50, Figure 1-54. Redrawn from Bailey: *Intracranial Tumors*, 2nd ed. Thomas, 1948. Reproduced with permission of McGraw-Hill Companies)

Table 3.4   *Principal Anatomic Divisions of the Brain*

Major Division	Subdivisions	Structures	Cavity
Forebrain (prosencephalon)	Telencephalon (endbrain)	Cerebral cortex Basal ganglia Basal forebrain Hippocampal complex Corpus callosum	Lateral ventricles
	Diencephalon (between brain)	Epithalamus Thalamus 시상 Hypothalamus	Third ventricle
Midbrain (mesencephalon)	Mesencephalon (midbrain)	Tectum Tegmentum	Cerebral aqueduct
Hindbrain (rhombencephalon)	Metencephalon	Pons 뇌교 Cerebellum 소뇌	Fourth ventricle
	Mylencephalon	Medulla oblongata 연수	

stem. Figure 3.12 (p. 84) shows the brain stem and cerebellum in relation to the entire brain. The **brain stem** extends from the spinal cord and comprises about 4.4% of the total weight of the adult brain. The cerebellum makes up about 10.5% of the total weight (Burt, 1993). The four parts of the brain stem include the **medulla oblongata** (myelencephalon), the **pons** (metencephalon), the structures of the midbrain (tectum and tegmentum), and the structures of the diencephalon (thalamus and hypothalamus). Although the brain stem and cerebellum account for relatively smaller areas of brain and function more primitively than the telencephalon, this area consists of a number of different structures worth knowing in order to understand the basics of brain functioning. We first discuss the structures of the lower brain stem (medulla, pons, and midbrain), then the upper brain stem (diencephalon), and finish the section by considering the cerebellum.

LOWER BRAIN STEM

Overview

■ *Gross anatomic features*
   Hindbrain: medulla oblongata (myelencephalon), pons (metencephalon)

   Midbrain: tectum and tegmentum
   Cranial nerves
   Reticular activating system

■ *Function:* Relay information to and from the brain; responsible for simple reflexive behavior

Structure

The lower brain stem resembles a road system of neural interconnections. In it, large tracts ferry information between telencephalon and spinal cord, and between cerebellum and brain stem. It also contains smaller groups of nerves such as the cranial nerves, specialized nuclei, and the network of the reticular activating system. The medulla oblongata, pons, and midbrain structures are old structures, from an evolutionary perspective. Interestingly, they are relatively uniform in shape and organization over the range from evolutionarily less complex species such as fish to more complex humans (see Figure 3.13 on p. 85). However, the size of the pons appears to increase in proportion to the degree of neocortical organization across species (Burt, 1993). The medulla is immediately superior to the spinal cord and forms an intermediary zone between the elementary neuronal configuration of the spinal column and the complex

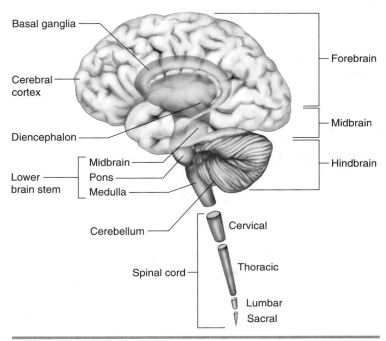

Figure 3.11 The three divisions of the brain. (Adapted with permission from Banich, M. T., *Neuropsychology: The Neural Basis of Mental Function*, p. 13, Figure 1.7. Copyright © 1997 by Houghton Mifflin)

neural organization of the brain. It contains myelinated tracts carrying motor and sensory information between the brain and spinal cord. Here the tracts **decussate,** switching transmission of information from one side of the body to the contralateral side of the brain. From this point upward, the left side of the brain controls the right side of the body and vice versa. The pons ("bridge") resembles two bulbs immediately superior and anterior to the medulla and inferior to the midbrain. The cerebellum connects to its posterior aspect, and information from the cerebellum funnels through the pons by way of large tracts termed the **cerebellar peduncles.**

The midbrain lies between the cerebrum and the pons and is the smallest portion of the brain stem. It merges anteriorly with the hypothalamus and thalamus. Although its beginning and end are not well outlined, it can be divided into the **tectum** ("roof"), and the **tegmentum** ("covering"). Within the roof of the tectum are four small elevations, a pair of **infe-**

rior colliculi, and, above those, a pair of **superior colliculi.** The tegmentum surrounds the tiny cerebral aqueduct, which connects the third and fourth ventricles. The lower brain stem contains many important nuclear groups, including the cranial nerves and important pathways connecting the spinal cord and cerebellum with the telencephalon. The major motor and sensory tracts to and from the cerebral hemispheres all pass through the lower brain stem. The lower brain stem also contains a network of neurons known as the **reticular activating system (RAS)** or reticular formation. We discuss the cranial nerves and the reticular activating system separately, later in this section.

Function

The lower brain stem serves several functions in addition to conducting information from spinal cord to brain. This complex system with many different nuclei and ascending and descending connections

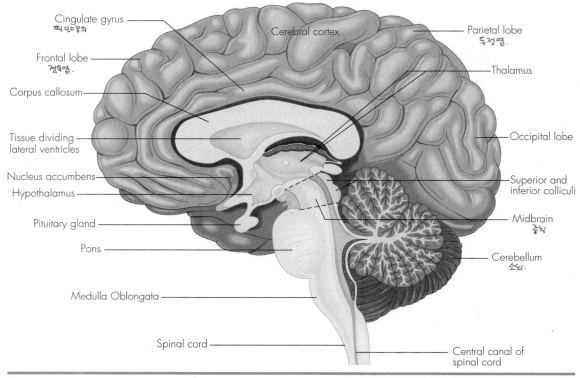

Figure 3.12   The human brain in midline and brain stem. (From James W. Kalat, *Biological Psychology,* 6th ed., Pacific Grove, CA: Brooks/Cole, 1998, p. 87, Figure 4.12)

plays a crucial role in reflexive functions necessary for life as well as in arousal level, auditory processing, visually guided movements, and the control of movement. The medulla mediates vital functions such as respiration, blood pressure and heart rate, and basic muscle tone. Damage to this area can interrupt motor and sensory pathways and threaten life itself. The pons serve as a major juncture for information passing between the structures of the spinal cord, brain, cerebellum, and some of the cranial nerves. It also plays a role in balance, vision, and auditory processing.

Together with the midbrain, the two are composed of structures that play an important role in orienting visual and auditory information. The superior colliculi contain important reflex centers for visual information and contain some retinal fibers via the optic tracts and the visual cortex. The inferior colliculi serve as an important relay center for the audi-

tory pathway. Interestingly, bats have, compared to humans, proportionally enlarged inferior colliculi. This is related to their sonarlike system which allows them to receive echoes and thus determine structures in space. Tracts originating in the colliculi connect to established motor nerve cells and influence the movement of the neck and the head in response to visual and auditory information.

CRANIAL NERVES: STRUCTURE AND FUNCTION

Overview

■ *Gross anatomic features:* Located within the brain stem

■ *Function:* Conduit of specific motor and sensory information

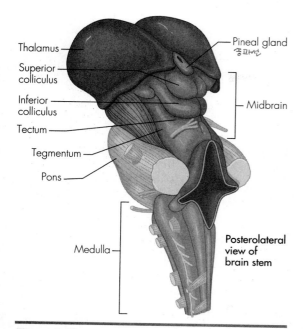

Thalamus

Superior colliculus

Inferior colliculus

Tectum

Tegmentum

Pons

Pineal gland

Midbrain

Medulla

Posterolateral view of brain stem

Figure 3.13 Brain stem structures. (From James W. Kalat, *Biological Psychology*, 6th ed., Pacific Grove, CA: Brooks/Cole, 1998, p. 84, Figure 4.8)

The lower brain stem is also the site of origin of 10 of the 12 cranial nerves. These nerves, which are directly connected to the brain, carry information to muscles or sensory information back to the brain. The cranial nerves were originally numbered by Galen, and each one also has a name associated with it. Cranial nerves I through IV arise from nuclei in the midbrain and forebrain, and nerves V through XII originate from the medulla and pons in the hindbrain (see Figure 3.14 on p. 86).

The cranial nerves integrate sensory information and motor output. Table 3.5 lists the individual cranial nerves and their functions. These nerves are very old from an evolutionary point of view. Some aspects of facial emotional expressions are also organized at this level, suggesting that our basic facial expressions are ancient and consistent across all human cultures. Because cranial nerves have more or less specific sensory or motor responsibilities, neurologists often test them during a clinical exam. For example, difficulties with eye tracking or numbness on one side of the face are a clear symptom of dysfunction with a cranial nerve.

RETICULAR FORMATION: STRUCTURE AND FUNCTION

Overview

■ *Gross anatomic features:* A neural network located within the lower brain stem transversing between the medulla to the midbrain

■ *Function:* Nonspecific arousal and activation, sleep and wakefulness

The reticular formation (see Figure 3.15 on p. 87) is, evolutionarily, one of the oldest systems in the nervous system. The brains of primitive vertebrates are almost exclusively made up of a reticular, or "netlike," formation. Humans retained the reticular formation over the course of evolution, as the more organized parts of the nervous system appeared. The formation has a diffuse arrangement of both ascending and descending neurons that form a system of networks (hence "reticular").

The reticular system is the starting point for the brain's vital activity. Life-sustaining nuclei and widespread connections here lead to the cerebral cortex. The reticular formation plays a role in nonspecific arousal, cortical activation and tone, and regulating sleep and wakefulness. Because of the system's role in arousal, it is often called the reticular activating system (RAS), which may be stimulated by outside, environmental events or by internal events. The reticular system forms the basis of Unit 1 in Luria's conception of the brain (Units 2 and 3 reside in the cerebral hemispheres, see Chapter 1). Defects in the reticular system can lead to a variety of problems. The major deficit, seen in many neurologic disorders, is a change in the level of consciousness, ranging from sleepiness to coma. The role of the RAS in sleep and wakefulness is discussed in Chapter 13.

As we mentioned earlier in discussing the medulla, the medullary levels of the reticular formation contain important respiratory and cardiovascular centers. Injury to these areas can result in death related to impaired respiratory rate, heart rate, and blood pressure. Thus, low-level RAS injuries (or high-level

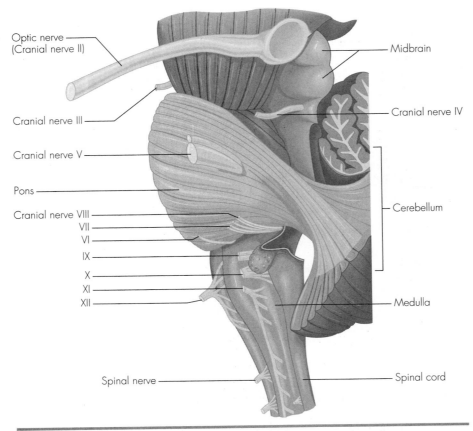

Optic nerve
(Cranial nerve II)

Cranial nerve III

Cranial nerve V

Pons

Cranial nerve VIII
VII
VI
IX
X
XI
XII

Spinal nerve

Midbrain

Cranial nerve IV

Cerebellum

Medulla

Spinal cord

Figure 3.14 The 12 cranial nerves. (From James W. Kalat, *Biological Psychology*, 6th ed., Pacific Grove, CA: Brooks/Cole, 1998, p. 85, Figure 4.9)

spinal cord injuries; for example, C-1, C-2, and C-3) may result in respiratory deficits. One such example is that of actor Christopher Reeves, who fractured his neck at the C-2 level while horse jumping. Not only was he paralyzed after the accident, but he also required an artificial respirator because part of his brain stem, and specifically the reticular formation, was injured.

In addition to the task of arousal, the RAS is also responsible for selective attention. The system must decide what information to let pass on its way to the cortex and what information to filter. This is an important function because there is generally too much competing information at any one point in time for

the brain to analyze it all. Thus, a further deficit or injury to this structure is one of filtering. Such a deficit can be related to RAS injuries that occur at or near birth. In these cases, the ability of the brain to filter information is either increased or decreased to an abnormal level. In the case of decreased filtering, the child is stimulus bound, easily distractible, and more pliable in low-stimulus sensory environments. In the case of increased filtering skills, the child shows symptoms of sensory deprivation. This can result in a complete withdrawal from the external world, similar to the deficit seen in some autistic children.

In general, the brain stem and the RAS in particular play a major and vital role in regulating wakeful-

Table 3.5	*The Cranial Nerves*	
Number	**Name**	**Function**
I	Olfactory	Sensory, smell
II	Optic	Sensory, vision
III	Oculomotor	Sensory, eye muscle; motor, eye movement, pupil constrictions
IV	Trochlear	Sensory, eye muscle; motor, eye movement
V	Trigeminal	Sensory, skin of face, nose and mouth; motor, chewing and swallowing
VI	Abducens	Sensory, sensation from eye muscles; motor, eye movement
VII	Facial	Sensory, taste; motor, facial expression, and crying
VIII	Statoacoustic	Sensory, hearing, equilibrium
IX	Glossopharyngeal	Sensory, taste; motor, swallowing
X	Vagus	Sensory, taste, and sensation from neck; motor, control of larynx, parasympathetic nerves to heart and viscera
XI	Accessory	Motor, movements of shoulder and head
XII	Hypoglossal	Sensory, tongue; motor, movement of tongue

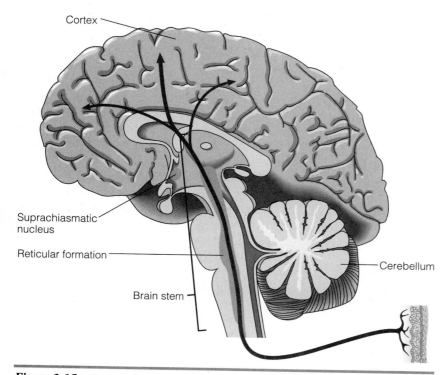

Figure 3.15 The reticular formation. (From E. B. Goldstein, *Psychology,* Pacific Grove, CA: Brooks/Cole, 1994, p. 188, Figure 5.8)

ness and in mediating and filtering ascending and descending sensory and motor information. As such, the brain stem constitutes the starting point of the brain's analysis of information. Disruption of the brain stem and specifically of the RAS affects the level of arousal, orientation, and general awareness of one's surrounding. Neuropsychologists are very interested in the often profound symptoms associated with dysfunction of these areas. Neuropsychologists can systematically assess general arousal when it is important to monitor the progress of people who are recovering from RAS injuries. Individuals with acute brain stem injuries may be placed in inpatient medical care, because such patients may be in a coma and depending on external life support.

UPPER BRAIN STEM: DIENCEPHALON

The diencephalon (also known as the *interbrain* or "between brain") is located at the head of the brain stem connecting the cortex with lower structures of the brain. The diencephalon is part of the larger forebrain and its evolution has paralleled that of the cortex. The diencephalon consists of two prominent brain structures, the **thalamus** and the **hypothalamus,** which contain many nuclei of interest to neuropsychologists because of their functions in regulating behavior. Phylogenetically, the thalamus consists of ancient nuclei that may have originally reacted reflexively to pleasant and unpleasant environmental stimuli before the cerebral cortex evolved. The hypothalamus, part of the limbic system, is considered instrumental in controlling the autonomic system. This system regulates emotional responses and other functions such as thirst, appetite, digestion, sleep, temperature of the body, sexual drive, heart rate, and smooth muscles of the internal organs.

Hypothalamus: Structure and Function

Overview

■ *Gross anatomic features:* Structure of the hypothalamus, hypothalamic nuclei, major fiber systems, third ventricle

■ *Function:* Activates, controls, and integrates the peripheral autonomic mechanisms, endocrine activity, and somatic functions, including body temperature, food intake, and development of secondary sexual characteristics

The hypothalamus is the portion of the diencephalon that forms the floor and part of the lateral wall of the third ventricle. Anatomically, it is defined by the optic chiasm, rostrally, and the mamillary bodies, caudally. The boundaries of the hypothalamus are easily described, but it does not form a well-circumscribed region and extends into surrounding parts. The hypothalamus itself is small in terms of weight (pea size, about 4 g in adults), but contains a grouping of small and complex nuclei located at the junction of the midbrain and the thalamus (close to the roof of the mouth). Within the hypothalamus lie at least a dozen identifiable cell clusters named the *hypothalamic nuclei* (see Figure 3.16). The exact number depends on how the clusters are organized, but is similar in most vertebrates, suggesting that little has changed over time and across species. In general, the hypothalamus has three longitudinal zones, lateral, medial, and periventricular. The adjacent master gland of the brain, the pituitary, is innervated and controlled by neurons from the hypothalamus.

Originally thought of as "a trifling part of the human brain," the hypothalamic nuclei have become known over the last 50 years as an important collection of nuclei, "the brain within the brain." The hypothalamus plays an important role in regulating, activating, and integrating peripheral autonomic processes, endocrine activity, and somatic functions. The pituitary regulates the body through hormones, specialized chemicals carried in the blood to target cells in the body. A properly functioning hypothalamus is essential for the proportional development of body size, differentiation of sex characteristics, and reproductive activities. These include such important functions as body temperature, food intake, and development of secondary sex characteristics. The hypothalamus also plays a role in regulating levels of hormones affecting such functions as digestion, sexual arousal, and circulation (Papez, 1958), and influ-

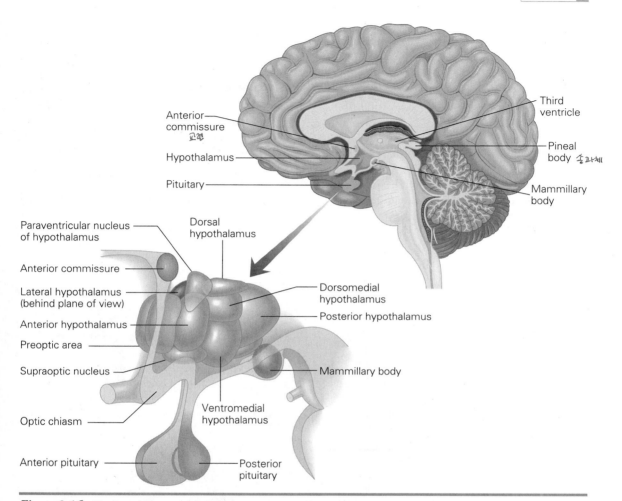

Figure 3.16 The hypothalamus and pituitary. (From James W. Kalat, *Biological Psychology,* 6th ed., Pacific Grove, CA: Brooks/Cole, 1998, p. 272, Figure 10.1)

ences thirst, hunger, and circadian rhythms (Neff & Goldberg, 1960; Symonds, 1966). The medial aspects of the hypothalamus have rich connections with the thalamus. The lateral nuclei have efferent and afferent connections to and from regions outside the hypothalamus, including brain stem fiber systems and preoptic and olfactory areas. The hypothalamus is also an interaction center for several neurotransmitter substances. Thus the hypothalamus is a very complex structure in terms of its interconnectedness, and

no picture can begin to demonstrate the intricate web of dendrites and axons that make up the complexity of this diencephalon structure.

Many pathologic processes can influence the function of the hypothalamus. Of these, tumors are the most frequent, including hypothalamic tumors and the more frequent tumors of the pituitary (see Chapter 9). Disturbances of the medial aspects of the hypothalamus (the ventromedial nucleus) may lead to severe behavioral disorders, because these nuclei have important connections with the frontal cortex and the amygdaloid complex.

Thalamus: Structure and Function

Overview

■ *Gross anatomic features:* Structure of the thalamus, its nuclei, and thalamocortical connections

■ *Function:* Complex relay station, handling major sensory and motor inputs to and from the ipsilateral cerebral hemisphere

The thalamus consists of two symmetric large nuclei embedded in the cerebral white matter toward the base of the cerebral hemispheres superiorly to the hypothalamus (*hypo* is Greek for "beneath"). Each cerebral hemisphere contains half of the thalamus (see Figure 3.17). Each half is a relatively large (about 4 cm in length), ovoid, gray mass that sits partially within the hollow made by the internal capsule and help form the lateral walls of the third ventricle. The word *thalamus* means "bridal chamber," a name that reflects the deep, hidden, and secure location of the thalamus within the two hemispheres. On dissection of the brain, the relatively well-defined thalamus is

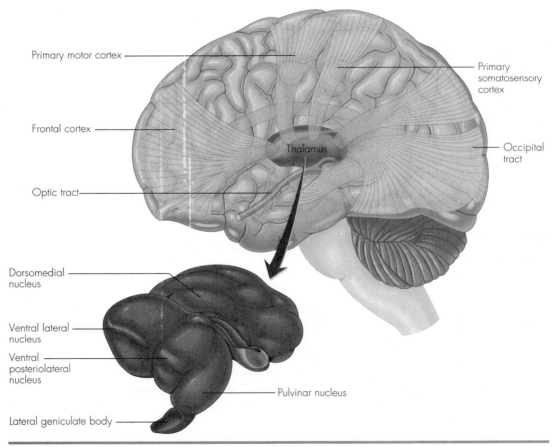

Primary motor cortex

Frontal cortex

Optic tract

Primary somatosensory cortex

Occipital tract

Thalamus

Dorsomedial nucleus

Ventral lateral nucleus

Ventral posteriolateral nucleus

Lateral geniculate body

Pulvinar nucleus

Figure 3.17   The thalamus. (From James W. Kalat, *Biological Psychology,* 6th ed., Pacific Grove, CA: Brooks/Cole, 1998, p. 89, Figure 4.14)

easily visible because of its grayish color, signaling the presence of many nerve endings.

Cortical and thalamic functions are significantly interrelated. The thalamic nuclei consist primarily of gray matter and are connected extensively with most other parts of the CNS. For example, many pathways carrying information from the brain stem to the cortex relay their information through the thalamic nuclei before reaching the cortex. Thus the thalamus plays a central role in processing most information that reaches the cortex. The thalamic nuclei are relatively well-defined geographic areas that can be divided into groups, based on their geographic location within the thalamus as well as their specific function. Some major nuclei of the thalamus are the

pulvinar nucleus (PN), ventral posterolateral (VPL), ventral posteromedial (VPM), medial geniculate (MG), lateral geniculate (LG), ventral lateral (VL), and dorsal medial (DM).

In addition to receiving ascending input, all thalamic nuclei receive descending input from the cerebral hemispheres, principally from the cortical regions to which they project. As such, the thalamus plays a key role in providing a complex "relay station" for all sensory systems except for olfaction that project to the cerebral hemispheres. The thalamus and the hypothalamus together make up an important part of the activities of the limbic system (described in more detail later in this chapter). Figure 3.18 shows the relationship of the thalamus and hypothalamus to other brain structures.

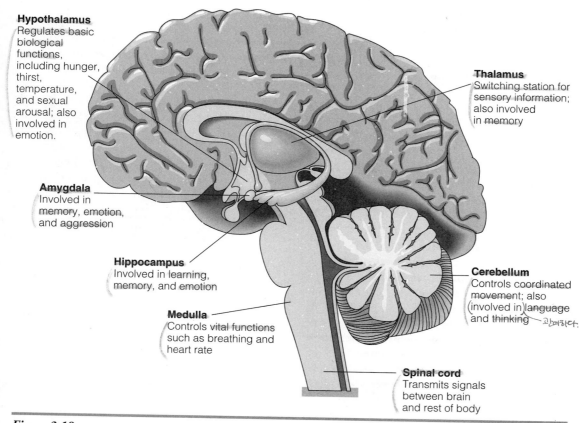

Hypothalamus
Regulates basic biological functions, including hunger, thirst, temperature, and sexual arousal; also involved in emotion.

Thalamus
Switching station for sensory information; also involved in memory

Amygdala
Involved in memory, emotion, and aggression

Hippocampus
Involved in learning, memory, and emotion

Cerebellum
Controls coordinated movement; also involved in language and thinking

Medulla
Controls vital functions such as breathing and heart rate

Spinal cord
Transmits signals between brain and rest of body

Figure 3.18   Subcortical structures of the brain. (From E. B. Goldstein, *Psychology,* Pacific Grove, CA: Brooks/Cole, 1994, p. 89, Figure 3.8d)

As the gateway to the cortex, the thalamus serves as the major pathway for primary sensory and motor impulses to and from the cerebral hemispheres. The one exception is olfactory sensory information (cranial nerve I), which bypasses the thalamus and progresses directly from olfactory receptors to olfactory bulbs, to the cerebral cortex. Other neuronal fibers that do not pass through the thalamus are those that are involved in arousal.

The thalamus is analogous to the concept of a large, busy, commuter train station. It makes preliminary classifications, integrates information, and "sends" it on to the cortex for further processing. Specifically, each half of the thalamus sends information to, and receives information from, the cerebral hemisphere on the same (ipsilateral) side of the brain. In this fashion, the descending projections serve as a two-way system between each cortical region and the corresponding thalamic nuclei.

The nuclei of the thalamus can be divided into two groups on the basis of their structure, connections, and function. The first group include *nonspecific nuclei,* which are primarily located toward the median portion of the thalamus. These nuclei project widely to other brain structures, including other thalamic areas, and to the cortex, particularly its frontal regions. They receive input from the spinal cord and the reticular formation and seem to play a role in monitoring the overall excitability of neurons in the cortex and the thalamus.

The second group of nuclei of the thalamus are referred to as *specific nuclei* and are involved in sensory and motor processing (see Figure 3.19). Specific nuclei project to restricted regions of the cortex. For example, specific sensory nuclei include the *ventral posterolateral (VPL)* and *ventral posteromedial (VPM;* not shown) nuclei, which receive input from somatosensory relay neurons and project directly to the primary and secondary somatosensory cortex. The *lateral geniculate body (LG)* receives input from the optic tract and projects to the primary visual area in the occipital cortex. The *medial geniculate body (MG)* receives input from the auditory relay nuclei and projects to the primary auditory cortex in the temporal lobe. Specific nuclei of the thalamus that are involved in controlling motor activity include the *ventral lat-*

eral (VL) and *ventral intermedial (VI;* not shown) nuclei, which receive input from the cerebellum. The lateral portion of the *ventral anterior (VA)* nucleus receives ascending fiber tracts from the basal ganglia, which are involved in regulating motor behavior. All three thalamic nuclei (VL, VI, and VA) project to the precentral motor areas of the cortex. Finally, the *dorsal medial (DM)* nucleus has many connections to the limbic system, which regulates emotional activity. This list of thalamic nuclei only provides an overview of the neuropsychological function, because the connections of the thalamus are extremely complicated and an understanding of them all lies beyond the scope of this text.

Lesions, particularly vascular accidents, and to some extent tumors, have been most often associated with the thalamic syndrome, marked deficits in gross areas of sensory or motor function. For example, lesions of the left thalamus have been implicated with depressed scores on cognitive-verbal tasks (Vilkki & Laitinen, 1974; Zillmer, Fowler, Waechtler, Harris, & Khan, 1992). Lesions of the right thalamus have been associated with defects in spatial ability (Bundick, Zillmer, Ives, & Beadle-Linsay, 1995; Jurko & Andy, 1973), facial recognition (Vilkki & Laitinen, 1974), and the perception of music (Roeser & Daly, 1974). Consequently, many sequelae of thalamic injury are those you might expect from the interruption of essential relay elements in pathways to and from the cerebral hemispheres. In some thalamic lesions, the symptoms are short lived, indicating that alternate pathways are quickly formed.

CEREBELLUM

Overview

■ *Gross anatomic features:* Cerebellar cortex, cerebellar white matter, and glia

■ *Function:* Coordination of movements, posture, antigravity movements, balance, and gait

Structure

The cerebellum (Latin for "little brain"), surprisingly, contains nearly 50% of the neurons of the brain, even though it makes up only 10% of its weight. On

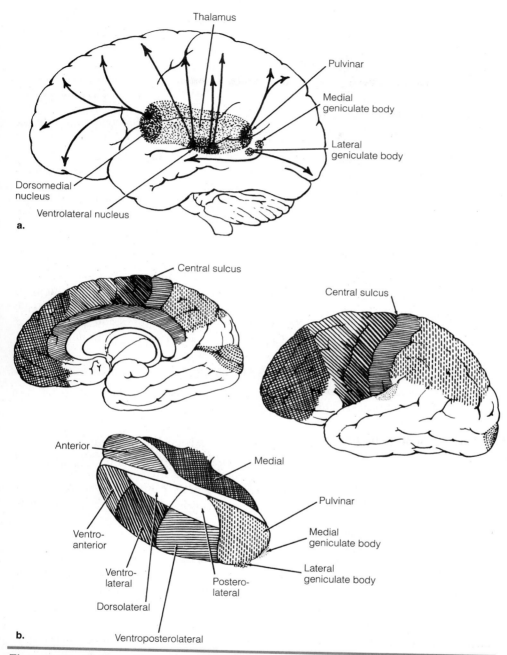

Figure 3.19 Thalamocortical radiations. (a) Principal thalamocortical projections. (b) Relationship of cortical areas to thalamic nuclei. (From J. G. Chusid, *Correlative Neuroanatomy & Functional Neurology,* NY: Appleton & Lange, 1982, p. 19, Figure 1.19 and p. 20, Figure 1.21; [b] reproduced with permission from original drawings by Frank H. Netter, MD; first appeared in Ciba Clinical Symbosia. Copyright © 1950, Ciba Pharmaceutical Co. Reproduced with permission of the McGraw-Hill Companies)

visual inspection, the cerebellum is a spectacular brain structure because of its clearly defined morphology and symmetry (see Figure 3.20). The cerebellar cortex is heavily infolded, and the numerous parallel sulci give it a layered appearance. The cerebellum also has several deep fissures dividing each cerebellar hemisphere into separate lobes. Its histological structure, however, is relatively simple compared with that of the cortex. The neurons appear to be organized in repeating patterns. The cerebellum is located posteriorly and superiorly to the pons and medulla, just inferior to the posterior portion of the cerebral hemispheres. The cerebellum is attached to the brain stem at the level of the pons ("bridge") via the cerebellar peduncle and consists of two large, oval hemispheres connected by a single median portion, termed the **vermis** (Latin for "worm").

Function

The cerebellum is phylogenetically old and may have been the first brain structure to specialize in coordinating motor and sensory information. Observing patients with cerebellar disease makes evident that this is an important center for coordinating movement and postural adjustments. The cerebellum is heavily involved in basic processes necessary for general motor behavior as well as in coordinating movements. The oldest areas of the cerebellum are concerned with keeping the body oriented in space motorically. The cerebellum also helps control muscles keeping the body upright despite the pull of gravity and in monitoring background muscle tone involved in voluntary movement.

Lesions of the cerebellum, depending on location, may cause a variety of disorders, including deterioration of coordinated movement, irregular and jerky movements, intention tremor when attempting to complete a voluntary task, static tremor when resting, impairment of alternating movements, impairment in balance, disturbances of gait, and uncontrolled nystagmic movements of the eyes. There is evidence that people born without a cerebellum can function completely normally, because other brain structures have adapted to take over those functions. Neuropsychologists often erroneously ignore the cerebellum, because no obvious cognitive properties have been

associated with lesions of the cerebellum. However, it now appears that the cerebellum stores memories for simple learned motor responses.

Telencephalon

The telencephalon, or endbrain, consists of the two cerebral hemispheres connected by a massive bundle of fibers, the corpus callosum. The outer layer of the cortex consists primarily of cell bodies (gray matter) and affects thinking, memory, and voluntary behavior as well as regulatory motor behavior. Within each hemisphere is a lateral ventricle and a collection of several large nuclei known as the *basal ganglia,* which contain the cell bodies of motor control neurons. The basal forebrain is also recognized as a prominent division of the **subcortical** (below the cortex) **aspect** of the cerebrum. This area, surrounding the inferior tip of the frontal horn, is strongly interconnected with limbic structures, and some (such as Crosson, 1992), consider it part of the limbic system.

BASAL GANGLIA

The **basal ganglia,** also called the **basal nuclei,** are a collection of deep nuclei of the telencephalon (basal = "lowest level"). (See Figure 3.21.) The basal ganglia communicate with motor regions in the cortex via the thalamus. With their complex interconnections and efferent outputs and afferent inputs, the basal ganglia participate in the control of higher-order movement, particularly in starting or initiating movement.

Overview

- *Gross anatomic features:* Structures of the caudate nucleus, putamen, globus pallidus, substantia nigra, and subthalamic nuclei

- *Function:* Important as relay stations in motor behavior (for example, the striato-pallido-thalamic loop); coordinating stereotyped postural and reflexive motor activity

Structure

Embedded deep within the cortex lie a group of symmetric subcortical gray-matter structures known col-

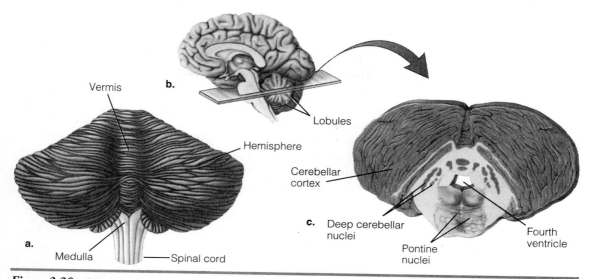

Figure 3.20 Structure of the cerebellum. (a) A dorsal view of the cerebellum, showing the vermis. (b) A midsagittal view of the brain, showing a cerebellar lobe. (c) A cross-section of the cerebellum, showing the deep nuclei. (From M. F. Bear, B. W. Connors, and M. A. Paradiso, *Neuroscience: Exploring the Brain,* Baltimore: Williams & Wilkins, 1996, p. 397, Figure 14.17)

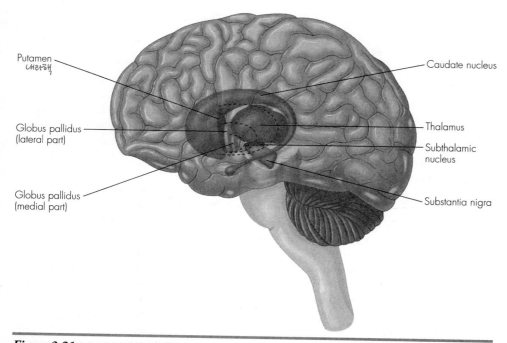

Figure 3.21 The basal ganglia within the cortex. (From James W. Kalat, *Biological Psychology,* 6th ed., Pacific Grove, CA: Brooks/Cole, 1998, p. 226, Figure 8.11)

lectively as the *basal ganglia*. They partially surround the thalamus and are themselves enclosed by the cerebral cortex and cerebral white matter. They have sensory projections to the cerebral hemispheres, interconnections between parts of the cortex, and outflow from the cerebral cortex to other nervous system structures. Neuropsychologists most often conceptualize the basal ganglia within the context of the motor system and thus typically exclude the amygdala (located at the tail of the caudate nucleus) and a large part of the thalamus. However, the substantia nigra and the **subthalamic nucleus** have important motor functions and are usually included as part of the basal ganglia.

The two major structures of the basal ganglia are the **caudate nucleus** and the **putamen,** with the adjacent medial and lateral **globus pallidus.** In general, these structures connect with the cortex, via the thalamus, the reticular formation, and the midbrain, but to a lesser degree with the spinal cord. The caudate nucleus connects to the putamen via the anterior limb of the internal capsule. This conglomeration is so difficult to identify as separate structures that it is usually referred to as the striatum because of its striped or striated appearance.

The precise circuitry of the basal nuclei is not fully understood, but researchers think they act as a relay station between the cerebral cortex via the thalamus. The major output from the basal ganglia targets the thalamus.

One major pathway between different structures comprising the basal ganglia is the *striato-pallido-thalamic loop.* This communication loop greatly interests neuropsychologists because it provides a mechanism for processing and integrating information from different regions of the brain before cortical processing. The input side of the basal ganglia, the striatum, receives information (descending connections) from separate sources, including the motor system, sensory and higher integrative areas of the cortex, the language centers of Broca's and Wernicke's areas, the thalamic nuclei, and the substantia nigra. The **striatum,** in turn, projects to the globus pallidus, which directly projects to the motor areas of the thalamus. The **substantia nigra** plays an important role in basal ganglia function via the dopaminergic *nigro-*

striatal system. Its links to the globus pallidus and the thalamus can influence motor behavior, which is organized by the cortex.

Function

Researchers think the primary activity of the basal ganglia regulates voluntary movements, specifically related to planning and initiating motor behavior. The basal ganglia, together with the red nucleus and substantia nigra of the midbrain and the cerebellum, form what has clinically been termed the **extrapyramidal motor system,** which is responsible for stereotyped postural and reflexive motor activity. The system also acts to keep individual muscles ready to respond. The other major motor system, the **pyramidal system,** originates in the cerebral cortex.

Two general theories of the role of the basal ganglia have been advanced. One suggests that the basal ganglia are mostly integrative in nature and receive input from visual centers, from the balance centers of the brain, and from the muscles and joints of the body. An alternative hypothesis assigns less importance to the basal nuclei, suggesting they are, more or less, a relay station with few integrative properties (Noback & Demarest, 1975). The basal ganglia may also play some language role, specifically motor planning and programming for speech, and perhaps even functions associated with attention and alerting prior to a motor response.

Most understanding regarding the basal ganglia's function is gained from knowledge of movement disorders associated with basal ganglia dysfunction. Such abnormalities, which also include disorders of the cerebellum, have been labeled *extrapyramidal* and are characterized by atypical movements and changes in muscle tone. In contrast, *pyramidal* symptoms involve upper motor neuron disorders of the cortex and are more often associated with a loss of voluntary movement, including paralysis. Two relatively common basal ganglia disorders are Parkinson's and Huntington's disease (see Chapter 12).

Extrapyramidal symptoms have also been observed in schizophrenics who are treated with antipsychotic drugs. Those drugs, including Thorazine, Stelazine, and Haldol, block dopamine transmission. Although this reduces psychotic behavior and hallucinations, it has the side effect of Parkinson-like symptoms, including writhing movements of the mouth, face, and tongue. This neurologic presentation in schizophrenics who develop such symptoms is known as **tardive dyskinesia** and is irreversible. In general, the overall connections and functions of the basal ganglia are not fully understood, although the principal function of this formation is associated with motor behavior, specifically organizing ease and flow of movement.

LIMBIC SYSTEM

The anatomic term *limbic,* from the Latin word *limbus* for "border" was first coined by Paul Broca (Schiller, 1982). Broca noticed that a ring of cortical tissue forms a border around the brain stem and medial aspects of the brain. Broca thought *"le grand lobe limbique"* was primarily involved with olfaction, because of its interconnections with the evolutionarily older **rhinencephalon** or "smell brain." In 1937, James Papez suggested the presence of a more precise circuit or "limbic system," which he suggested was significantly involved in mediating emotional behavior. Indeed, proposing that a set of brain structures might be primarily involved in processing emotions was a bold statement at the time. Since then, however, the limbic system has received much attention for its major role in the expression of emotions as well as in olfaction, learning, and memory.

Overview

- *Gross anatomic features:* Structures of the amygdala, hippocampus, parahippocampal gyrus, cingulate gyrus, fornix, septum, and olfactory bulbs

- *Function:* The limbic system is closely involved in the expression of emotional behavior and the integration of olfactory information with visceral and somatic information

Structure

Broca defined the limbic lobe to include those structures on the medial and basal surfaces of the cerebral hemispheres. Because the limbic lobe is most developed in mammals, it is also known as the mammalian brain. In fact, in some primitive animals, such as the crocodile, the entire forebrain is limbic brain (the limbic cortex is part of the forebrain that developed first in evolution). The primary structures of the lobe include the medial cortex surrounding the corpus callosum, termed the **cingulate gyrus** (see Figure 3.12), and the medial cortex of the temporal lobes, or the **parahippocampal gyrus,** and the **hippocampal formation** (*hippocampus, dentate gyrus,* and *subiculum*). The structures of the **limbic system** are often debated, but usually also include the **fornix,** some brain stem areas, particularly the **mammillary bodies** of the hypothalamus, specific basal forebrain structures, including the **amygdala** ("almond" because of its shape), and the **septum,** (see Figure 3.22 on page 98). Several anatomic circuits have been described that include limbic system structures. The most likely role of the **basolateral circuit,** which centers around the amygdala, is in emotional processing. The **Papez circuit,** which centers around the hippocampus, is perhaps the most well-known loop. We discuss these functional systems further in the next chapter.

Function

The limbic system is a most complex, but important set of brain structures that has fascinated anatomists, neurologists, and neuroscientists for over 50 years. The limbic system is a bit misnamed because there is no one-to-one structure–function relationship as is evident in many sensory systems we discuss in the next chapter. The role of the limbic system in emotions and memory has generated a great deal of interest in neuropsychology. Extensive research has been conducted on several components of the highly interconnected limbic system. However, because of the system's interconnectivity, it is often hard to discern structure–function relationships. For example, the amygdala and hippocampus have specific connections with other brain structures and have also been studied as separate entities. The activities of the limbic system in memory consolidation, emotional behavior, and olfactory processing are topics we elaborate on further in the next chapter.

The limbic system is very closely related to the hypothalamus, which researchers have singled out as the main brain structure for integrating and organizing

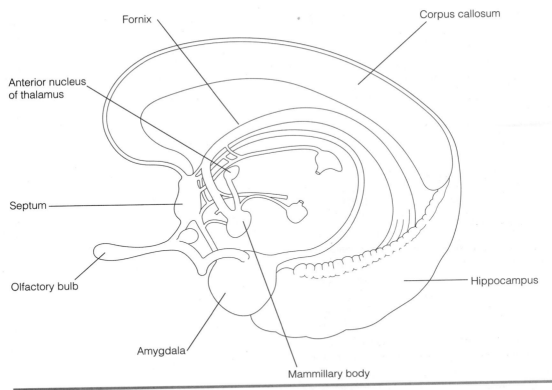

Figure 3.22 The limbic system with cortical area removed. (From K. W. Heller, *Understanding physical, sensory, and health impairments*. Pacific Grove, CA: Brooks/Cole, 1996, p. 54, Figure 4.9)

autonomic processes related to the emotional expression of behavior. In humans, limbic system dysfunction has been associated with a variety of abnormalities, including emotional and behavioral problems (Glaser & Pincus, 1969) and sexual dysfunction (Rosenblum, 1974).

The hippocampal formation has been specifically associated with memory acquisition (Douglas & Pribram, 1966; Penfield & Milner, 1958; Scoville & Milner, 1957). The primary defect, seen after bilateral injury of the hippocampus, involves a difficulty in learning new information. Such patients find themselves unable to retain newly learned information, although immediate and old memories remain relatively intact (Luria, 1971; Milner, 1968). These effects on memory functioning are less profound when only one hippocampal gyrus is affected (McLardy, 1970).

Lesions of the left hippocampal gyrus may cause problems with verbal memory (Russell & Espir, 1961), whereas lesions of the right hippocampal gyrus may cause greater impairment in spatial memory, including maze learning (Corkin, 1965).

The amygdala has ascending as well as descending connections with the cerebral hemispheres, the thalamus, the hippocampus, and even the spinal cord. The amygdala plays a specific role in fear conditioning and in impacting the strength of stored memory (LeDoux, 1994). We discuss this in greater detail in the next chapter.

Numerous psychological disorders are characterized by emotional disturbances, and the limbic system has been implicated in many of them. Extreme violence in patients who exhibit rage attacks and frequent aggressive behavior can follow damage to the amygdala and its connections. In fact, removal of the amygdala (amygdalatomy) has been performed on extremely violent and aggressive patients in an attempt to stem rage reactions. Balasubramanian and Ranamurthi (1970) reported 100 cases of bilateral destruction of the amygdala in patients with behavior disorders.

Another clinical disorder associated with memory function of the limbic system is **Wernicke-Korsakoff's syndrome.** This is typically observed in severe alcoholics who show multiple nutritional deficiencies because they have essentially replaced solid food with alcohol. Such patients may develop a confusional state over time as well as severe motor and new learning difficulties. This syndrome is related to vitamin B_1 (thiamine) deficiency.

Despite the limbic system's popularity among researchers; the complexity of the system's connections, internally as well as to other areas outside of the system; and the disagreement as to what brain structures should be included in the limbic system, it still puzzles modern neuropsychologists. In fact, some scientists suggest that now neuropsychology needs to move away from the concept of the larger "system" of the limbic structures and to define them in more precise terms individually.

CORPUS CALLOSUM

Overview

- *Gross anatomic features:* A large set of myelinated axons connecting the right and left cerebral hemisphere
- *Function:* Information exchange between the two hemispheres

Structure

The most prominent bundle of axons in the brain is a collection of intercerebral fibers, known as the **corpus callosum,** an arched mass comprised almost exclusively of myelinated axon bundles or white matter. The corpus callosum lies in the depths of the space between the two hemispheres called the **longitudinal fissure** and lies immediately inferior to the **cingulum,** a major intracerebral fiber within the **cingulate gyrus** (see Figure 3.23).

Function

In the normal brain, information that enters one hemisphere crosses to the opposite side almost instantaneously (about 7 to 13 milliseconds). This happens via the corpus callosum, but also through smaller intercerebral fibers, the **anterior commissure** and **hippocampal commissure.** Because of the corpus callosum, both hemispheres share information, even though initially only one hemisphere may have received the information. The corpus callosum enables

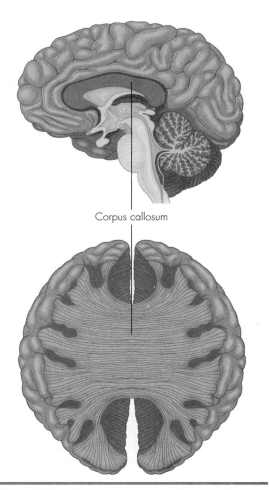

Corpus callosum

Figure 3.23 The corpus callosum. (From James W. Kalat, *Biological Psychology*, 6th ed., Pacific Grove, CA: Brooks/Cole, 1998, p. 374, Figure 14.1)

most communication and exchange of information between left and right hemispheres (Springer & Deutsch, 1993; Sperry, 1958).

An interesting problem for the brain arises if the corpus callosum is severed. This is very intriguing to neuropsychologists, because now information presented to only one side of the body (or brain) is not shared with the other hemisphere. In very young children, cutting the corpus callosum has little apparent effect, because the brain develops alternative pathways to help compensate for the loss. In the adult brain, however, neural pathways have already developed. If the corpus callosum is severed surgically, which is sometimes done as a medical procedure to arrest the spread of seizures between hemispheres, the processing of some sensory information is confined to only one hemisphere. The study of such individuals, also known as *split-brain patients,* has helped provide extensive and interesting data on the independent functioning of the two cerebral hemispheres (Gazzaniga, 1966; Geschwind, 1965; Zaidel & Sperry, 1973). Researchers have learned from such cases that each hemisphere can function and process information in isolation. The idea that the brain might be composed of two independently functioning brain halves, perhaps even having two personalities or separate minds is a question we take up in our later discussion of consciousness (see Chapter 5).

THE CEREBRAL HEMISPHERES

Overview

- *Gross anatomic features:* Structures of the frontal, parietal, occipital, and temporal lobes
- *Function:* Higher cognitive functioning, cerebral specialization, and cortical localization

The cerebral hemispheres represent the most recently evolved brain structure in humans, although they are approximately one to three million years old (see Neuropsychology in Action 3.1). The complexity of the inter- and intrahemispheric connections reflects this degree of evolution, which has allowed humans to use such abstract concepts as symbols, language, and art.

Structure

The largest part of the brain consists of the **cerebrum** or the right and left **cerebral hemispheres** (see Exhibit 2 inside front cover). The two hemispheres form a half globe with a flat basal surface. The hemispheres are separated by a deep midline cleft, the longitudinal fissure, and are connected via the corpus callosum. The surface of each hemisphere folds in on itself in many places, creating grooves along the surface named **sulci** (singular, **sulcus**). Very deep grooves are termed **fissures.** The irregularly shaped ridges between sulci are known as **gyri** (singular, **gyrus**). No two brains are exactly identical in the size or the shape of their gyri, although the general gyral pattern is consistent enough to locate major landmarks. The morphology of the brain's gyri can be thought of as somewhat related to the idea of a face where the features such as the nose, eyes, and mouth are generally localizable but vary in shape according to the person. Perhaps, more like a fingerprint, each person has his or her own "brain print." So much variation is evident between the brains of people that researchers conducting imaging and histological analyses must compensate for interindividual variability by standardizing and transforming formulas rather than by comparing brains directly (Mai, Assheuer, & Paxinos, 1997). Figure 3.24 presents general gyral and sulcal features.

The surface of the cerebral hemispheres are covered by gray matter. As previously described, the gray areas of the central nervous system consist mainly of cell bodies of neurons serving as the brain's functional units. Underlying the cortex is white matter that links structures within the cerebral hemispheres and the central nervous system as a whole. The size, shape, and distribution of the cells and fibers vary from place to place within the cerebral cortex. In principle, there are many connections within the cortex itself, both horizontal and vertical, as well as to subcortical areas.

Four of the major divisions within each hemisphere are the **frontal, parietal, temporal,** and **occipital lobes** (see Figure 3.25 on page 104). The frontal and parietal lobes are separated from the temporal lobe by the **lateral fissure.** The frontal and parietal lobes are separated by the **central sulcus.** The parietal and occipital lobes are separated by the parietal–occipital fissure and its imaginary extension across the lateral surface

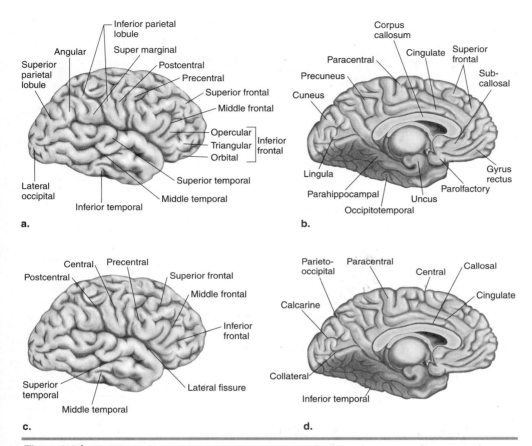

Figure 3.24 Major gyri and sulci of the cerebral hemispheres. (a) Lateral and (b) medial views of gyri; (c) lateral and (d) medial views of sulci. (Adapted from *Fundamentals of Human Neuropsychology*, 4th ed., by Bryan Kolb and Ian Q. Wishaw © 1996 by W. H. Freeman and Company, p. 51, Figure 3.5. Used with the permission of Worth Publishers)

of the hemisphere to the **occipital notch.** The division and naming of the cortex into four lobes is quite arbitrary and related to the names of the cranial plates that provide protective covering just superior to the lobes.

Another way of referring to the topography of the brain is related to the architectural arrangements of neurons in different regions throughout the brain. Brodmann (1909) divided up the cortical surface according to these differences and showed that the anatomic organization of the cortex is similar in all mammals. He divided the brain into 52 sections, which are now referred to as **Brodmann's areas** (see Figure 3.26 on page 105). Correspondence between architectural regions and functional regions is, how-

ever, not precise. In fact, Brodmann's cytoarchitectural scheme is now considered questionable. For example, in humans the cerebral cortex is much more developed than Brodmann's map suggests. The Brodmann system particularly did not do justice to the degree of complexity of the brain's inter- and intrahemispheric connections. Nevertheless, it has been widely used for referring to particular parts of the cortex and is certainly more sophisticated than gross descriptions of the cerebral lobes. The publication of Brodmann's famous map of the human cortex in 1909 was instrumental in clarifying the confusion that until then existed. Using Brodmann's system, for example, Broca's area is called area 44.

Neuropsychology in Action 3.1

The Evolution of the Brain: A Focus on Brain Size

by Eric A. Zillmer

To understand the functioning brain, place it within the context of evolution. Two to three million years ago, humans living in East Africa were making stone tools, perhaps building simple dwellings. Their brains would, in the course of a spectacular evolution, enlarge one day to the size and complexity of today. Humans could not possibly perform the numerous and complex behaviors that they do, without brain mechanisms that have evolved over hundreds of thousands of years. Evolutionary psychology offers a coherent theory that may begin to explain the strategic differences and similarities in the structures and functions of the brain.

Central to the concept of evolution was Charles Darwin's (1809–1882) text *On the Origin of Species* (1859). His historic 1835 trip to the Galápagos Islands laid the foundation of his theory of biological evolution, even though he only stayed for five weeks. Darwin suggested that the mechanism for explaining how species evolve from existing forms is a process based on natural selection. He identified the process of natural selection as the mechanism underlying the evolution of all organisms. He reasoned that some individuals were better able to survive and reproduce than others, and that the characteristics that made these species more successful could then be transmitted to the next generation. Perhaps the most significant legacy of evolution is a powerful brain that has evolved to a degree allowing humans to learn from experiences.

Basic human psychological mechanisms related to brain processes are likely to be species specific. For example, most or all humans share certain psychological processes, including fear of dark-

ness; characteristic emotions such as anger, love, and humor; weapon making; sexual attraction; and probably hundreds more (Wright, 1994). People often call these processes human nature, but they must be related to brain processes. One reason why most humans share many psychological mechanisms relates to the fact that natural selection tends to impose relative uniformity in complex adaptive designs such as the brain. Thus, central to any theory on brain evolution is that certain aspects of the central nervous system remain stable, whereas others must adapt over time. This is most readily apparent at the level of human physiology and anatomy: All people have two arms, a heart, and a brain; that is, they do not vary in possessing basic physiological mechanisms. According to evolutionary psychology, however, the brain must contain a large number of specialized psychological mechanisms, each designed to solve a different or related adaptive problem. Thus, individuals also differ, and fundamental individual differences must be central to any comprehensive brain theory.

One way that the human brain differs, compared to other species, is its size, particularly the size of the neocortex. For example, a general principle of neural organization indicates that the size and complexity of a structure is related to its functional importance of the structure. The brain, through the meninges, is firmly attached to the skull. Anthropologists measure the internal volume of skulls, which is easily preserved over time, to estimate the weight of the brain. Using this technique, researchers estimated the brains of our earliest ancestors,

dated approximately five million years ago, to be relatively small, about 400 cm^3 (Changeux & Chavaillon, 1995). Anthropological evidence suggested that approximately three million years ago the anatomic organization of the central nervous system and its associated functions evolved at a spectacular rate. Although the human's brain was always relatively large, in proportion to the body, and presented a modern organization, the relative size of the brain rapidly increased in size. About one million years ago the occipital lobes began to develop, followed by the frontal, parietal, and temporal lobes. This new biological foundation enabled increased memory capacity, more frequent and specific spoken communication (language), a more elaborate social life, and a more extensive exploration of the environment. Humans no longer depended on gathering rocks, carcasses, and vegetables, but became proficient in animal capture. This evolution in the structural complexity and performance of the brain corresponded directly with the formation and development of diverse cultures.

Neanderthals are thought to have inhabited Europe and the Middle East as early as 100,000 years ago. It is not clear exactly how similar they were to us, but they certainly had an elaborate tool-using culture that included ritual burial (Changeux & Chavaillon, 1995). About 100,000 years ago the growth in brain size started to level off, probably related to the fact that the female pelvis, and the size of the skull that can fit through it, has not kept pace with the evolution of the brain. This has made for a remarkable state of affairs as it relates to brain development in humans. At birth, the brain is approximately 1/4th its eventual size, compared to the rest of the body, which is 1/20th its eventual size. Then, over the next 20 years of a human's life, the brain matures at an amazing rate, developing billions of connections and supporting cells. At age 16, it reaches a level of behavioral control and conscious realm (maturity) that the owner of the brain is allowed to drive him or herself around in an automobile. At age 18 the brain is allowed to render an opinion, a vote, affecting other brains (through culture and society).

The basic brain structures are very similar for all mammals, although brain size may vary considerably among different species. One of the many fascinating aspects of how humans have evolved as a species is related to this extreme and unprecedented growth of the human brain, the cerebral cortex, and specifically the prefrontal cortex, which Luria named the "organ of civilization." To many students, the size of an organism's brain may seem intuitively related to the intellectual properties of a species. Certainly, if you compare animals to humans, there is a relationship between brain size and intelligence. Aristotle commented on the fact that humans had proportionally the largest brains of all animals.

Consider, for example, that gorillas, although physically larger than humans, only have about one-fourth of the brain size. In humans the average adult brain size is about 1300 cubic centimeters (cm^3) weighing about 1500 grams. But a blue whale's brain weighs 6000 grams and an African elephant's brain 5700 grams, much larger than in the human. If, however, brain size is held constant as it relates to body size, humans compare very well. Taking body weight into consideration, the brain of a whale accounts for only 1/10,000ths of its body, the elephant's brain 1/600th, and the human brain 1/40th. Thus, if the range of brain size with body size is held constant, the

human brain is 21,000 times larger and the neocortex is 142,000 times larger than that of the shrew, a very small, mouselike mammal. This means that if a shrew were the size of a human, its brain would only weigh 46 grams. The body/brain weight formula, however, does not work well with all small animals. For example, the ferret's brain makes up 1/12th of its body weight. In fact, the best ratio seems to be between an organism's body surface (not body weight) and brain size. Certainly it is logical to assume that the surface of the body, through which the organism has contact with the environment, is more directly related to brain function than is the total weight in bones and blood. When body surface is taken into consideration, the human comes in first place among all vertebrates, with the chimpanzee and the dolphin following second and third (Changeux & Chavaillon, 1995).

Large brains are not necessarily more efficient or effective; in fact, absolute brain weight has no significance in itself. It may require a larger brain more time to process information than a smaller one. There are even differences in brain size among humans. Big people tend to have larger brains than smaller people. This does not imply that men, who are on average taller and heavier than women, are smarter. After correcting for body size, men and women have brains of approximately equal size.

The size of a brain has been an object of debate and controversy for many centuries. Broca, for one, argued that the size of the brains of human races had to account for something (1861). He proposed that "in general, the brain is larger in mature adults than in the elderly, in men than in women, in eminent men than in men of mediocre talent, in superior races than in inferior races. . . . There is a remarkable relationship between the development of intelligence and the volume of the brain" (1861, pp. 188, 304). As evidence, Broca offered find-

ings that 51 unskilled workers had an average brain weight of 1365 grams, compared to the brain weight of 24 skilled workers, which was an average of 1420 grams. Any student of statistics knows that this finding may not be statistically significant, given the large variation of brain weights in humans and presumably in Broca's sample as well. Furthermore, it is entirely possible that the unskilled workers were malnourished and therefore were smaller in stature than the skilled workers. In any case, Broca's data has not been confirmed by more recent studies, suggesting that his findings were due to chance. But Broca went to great lengths to "prove" his theory. One has to wonder what Gall himself must have thought of this—his brain measured "only" 1100 grams.

The measurement (or mismeasurement) of human intellectual properties according to brain size has been described by the evolutionary biologist Stephen J. Gould in *The Mismeasure of Man* (1981), in which he presented a fascinating historical account of phrenology and other pseudoscientific explanation of the size of the human brain and its relationship to intelligence. What Broca and others did not realize was that body size as well as many other factors relate to the complexity of the brain and the nervous systems of humans and other species. In fact, the complexity of the brain depends on many dimensions beside brain size, including connectivity, cell density, cell morphology, neurotransmitter complements, and perhaps the most important variable, the rate and duration of neuronal sprouting. Among humans, no brain size–intelligence relationship exists.

The brain of Albert Einstein, the Nobel prize–winning physicist, underwent autopsy after his death on April 18, 1955. Gall and Broca would have been surprised to learn that the Princeton professor's brain was normal looking in appearance and of average size.

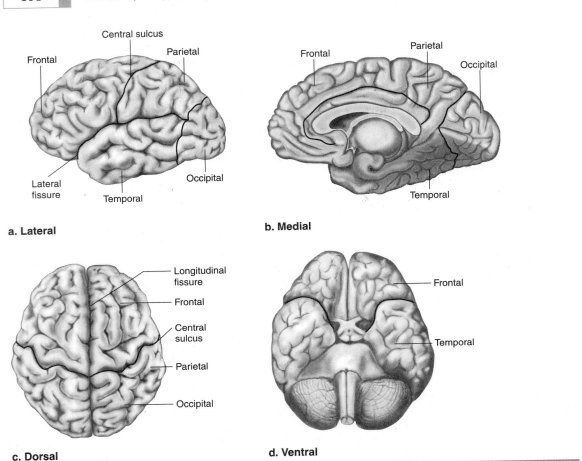

a. Lateral

b. Medial

c. Dorsal

d. Ventral

Figure 3.25   Lobes of the cerebral cortex. Four views of the frontal, temporal, occipital, and parietal lobes of the brain. (Adapted from *Fundamentals of Human Neuropsychology,* 4th ed., by Bryan Kolb and Ian Q. Wishaw © 1996 by W. H. Freeman and Company, p. 52, Figure 3.6. Used with the permission of Worth Publishers)

Function

Because the cerebral hemispheres are responsible for "higher mental functions" in humans, it is not surprising that neuropsychologists have been most interested in these structures. The cerebral cortex is what makes us uniquely human. In general, the cerebral cortex organizes higher cognitive functions, first analyzing input, or processing of elementary sensory information such as touch, sound, or vision; and then sorting through, organizing, integrating, synthesizing, storing, or otherwise using the information. Then it directs output through motor processing, which can range from activities such as walking to speaking.

The greatest one-to-one correspondences between structure and function within the cortex are in the areas of primary sensory input and primary motor output. For example, the **somatosensory cortex,** which occupies the anterior aspect of the parietal lobes, is responsible for receiving primary tactile sensation from the body, and the **primary motor cortex** of the frontal lobe is concerned with initiating, activating, and performing motor activity. These areas are well mapped, and are discussed in detail in the next chap-

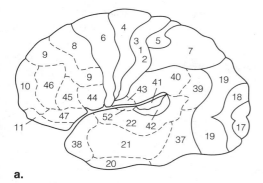

a.

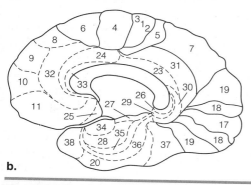

b.

Figure 3.26 Brodmann's map of the human cortex. This map is based on hypothesized cytoarchitectural differences between brain areas. Dashed lines refer to less distinct borders. (a) Lateral view, (b) midsagittal view. (Adapted from *Fundamentals of Human Neuropsychology*, 4th ed., by Bryan Kolb and Ian Q. Wishaw © 1996 by W. H. Freeman and Company, p. 55, Figure 3.3. Used with the permission of Worth Publishers)

ter. As a general rule, within the cortex sensory processing occurs in the posterior aspects (the temporal, parietal and occipital lobes), whereas motor processing is controlled more by the anterior aspects (frontal lobes). The four lobes of the brain are associated with varying and identifiable functions in the primary and secondary processing of sensory information. For example, in addition to the primary somatosensory and motor cortexes, elementary visual processing is associated with the occipital lobe, whereas the temporal lobes are concerned with receiving and interpreting auditory information. In regard to sensory process-

ing, the parietal lobes function somewhat differently to integrate cross-sensory information. The interconnections of the auditory (temporal), sensory (parietal), and visual (occipital) segments of the lobes combine to form complex, highly integrated areas of the cortex called **sensory association areas.** When one cortical area is activated by a stimulus, other areas also respond. This is caused by the rapid activity along a large number of precisely organized, reciprocally acting association pathways, which ensures coordination of sensory input and motor activity, as well as regulation of higher cognitive functions. Some of these neuronal pathways may be very short (for example, intracerebral fibers), linking neighboring areas within the gray area, or they may be long bundles, passing through the white matter connecting different lobes (for example, intercerebral fibers).

The frontal lobe contains the motor cortex and also houses the **prefrontal cortex.** This area is akin to a conductor or executive of the brain, organizing, controlling, and managing behavior, and making high-level decisions about socially appropriate behavior—when to act, and when not to act. The prefrontal cortex makes it possible to perceive, even anticipate, the consequences of your brain's behaviors. It is very much responsible for the many aspects of what makes you unique, your personality and your conscience. Obviously, for such a suprasystem to function it must have many connections to practically every major cortical and subcortical region of the brain. It must constantly be informed about events, both inside and outside the body, and it must overlap with important motor areas to immediately express and change the environment through behavior.

As can be seen, whereas sensory-perceptual and motor processing is more easily associated with certain lobes, higher mental functions such as executive functions, language rule learning, memory, emotion and executive functioning rely on integrative functions and cross-sensory modalities. These functions do not wholly reside within boundaries of a single lobe. For example, although encoding new information into memory is often associated with the temporal lobes, memory can best be conceptualized as a processing system spanning limbic system structures, as well as aspects of the frontal, temporal, and parietal lobes. Aspects of higher mental processing such as memory, executive functioning, emotional processing, language, and consciousness are covered as systems in the next two chapters.

In general, damage to primary receptive areas produces identifiable deficits, whereas lesions in nonspecific or association areas of the cortex may produce a deficit far beyond the functional identity of that particular area, because the complex interconnections beneath that cortical region may also be damaged. For example, lesions of the somatosensory cortex may cause contralateral paralysis and loss of sensory reception. In contrast, lesions of the parietal-temporal-occipital association area often result in a more complex neuropsychological deficit, such as an inability to understand the numeric value of numerals even though the person is able to read them. Damage to the prefrontal area often produces deficits in concentration, ability to solve new problems, and judgment.

Asymmetry, Lateralization, and Dominance

There are well-known differences in hemispheric functioning. This idea has become so popularized, in fact, that many have taken to differentiating people according to a notion of being right-brained or left-brained. We discuss evidence for this later in this section; it suffices to say here that this notion has been greatly oversimplified. We also address the interesting question as to what extent cerebral differences correlate with handedness and gender.

Much of what has been discovered about lateralization of function has come from the study of brains by one of four methods. In the first instance, destroying cortical tissue creates a situation similar to that which Broca encountered, whereby location of a function is inferred if damage to a particular area results in loss of that function. The second line of evidence has come from *split-brain patients* who have undergone the surgical separation of the corpus callosum, leaving the two hemispheres largely unable to communicate with each other. Third, epilepsy patients being considered for surgery typically submit to anesthesia of one cortical hemisphere at a time in a procedure called the **Wada test.** While one hemisphere is "unconscious," neurologists can test the functional abilities of the opposite conscious hemisphere in iso-

lation. Finally, neurosurgeons also electrically stimulate specific cortical areas to delineate boundaries of function before removing brain tissue. These methods have provided valuable converging evidence regarding general brain function and lateralization. However, all these methods seek to measure brain functioning in an "unnatural state." Can it be assumed, from measuring function of an isolated portion of the brain, that functioning will remain the same within the context of whole-brain function? Also, the people being assessed typically have a brain disorder of some type. Dysfunctioning brains, particularly if the disorder has existed over a long period of time, may not behave the same way as intact brains. Now, through newer, noninvasive methods of brain imaging, such as PET (positron emission tomography) and SPECT (single-photon emission computed tomography), which reveal the dynamic workings of the brain (see Chapter 6), researchers can test normal subjects and pinpoint centers of greatest brain activity for any one type of task.

The term **hemispheric asymmetry** relates to the differentiation in morphology and physiology of the brain between the right and left hemispheres. For example, in many people the right hemisphere is larger and heavier than the left, although the left is typically more densely packed with gray matter connections. The terms **lateralization** and **dominance** refer to the differences in functional specialization between the two hemispheres.

Paul Broca first determined that damage to the *frontal operculum* of the left hemisphere resulted in loss of speech. Before his time researchers widely believed that the two hemispheres were redundant in function. Because aphasia was specific to the left hemisphere, neuropsychologists now deduced that speech was primarily a property of the left hemisphere. To say speech is lateralized to the left hemisphere is to say there is a functional dominance of the left hemisphere over the right for speech. Although some structural differences between the hemispheres are known to correspond to functional differences in behavior, the relationship between structure and function has not been entirely worked out. Table 3.6 outlines the differences in morphology between the two hemispheres. Figure 3.27 depicts some of the major hemispheric differences in structure.

On gross inspection, the two hemispheres of the brain do look different. If you first look at the entire brain from the top down, it may appear askew. This is because the right hemisphere often protrudes anteriorly from the frontal lobes and the left hemisphere protrudes posteriorly from the parietal-occipital area.

Turning the brain to the lateral surface of the cerebral hemispheres, it is often the case that the **Sylvian fissure,** which is the large fissure separating the frontal from the temporal and parietal lobes, is steeper in the right hemisphere than in the left. This results in a larger parietal and temporal area in the right hemisphere. It is reasonable to speculate that this allows higher-level integration of visual, auditory, and proprioceptive information in the more spatially oriented right hemisphere. If you look anteriorly, into the frontal lobes to the area of the frontal operculum (Broca's area), the right hemisphere has a larger surface area and the left hemisphere is larger under the surface in the subcortical area. This may reflect differences in language production abilities between the two

Table 3.6 *Anatomic and Physiological Brain Asymmetries*		
	Left Hemisphere	**Right Hemisphere**
SIZE	Greater density	Larger and heavier
LOBES	Parietal-occipital protruberance 우기	Frontal protruberance
FRONTAL	Frontal operculum larger subcortical	Frontal operculum larger surface
TEMPORAL	Larger planum temporale	Larger Heschl's gyrus (often 2)
PARIETAL		Larger area
SYLVIAN FISSURE	Longer and more horizontal slope	Steeper slope

hemispheres. If you remove the top half of the brain, allowing a look from the top down at a horizontal section of the two hemispheres (see Figure 3.27), you

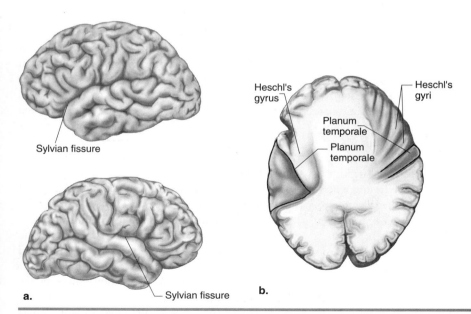

Heschl's gyrus
Heschl's gyri
Planum temporale
Planum temporale
Sylvian fissure
Sylvian fissure
a.
b.

Figure 3.27 Brain hemisphere asymmetries. (a) The sylvian fissure on the right (bottom) has a steeper slope than on the left. (b) View cutting through the top portion of the brain at the level of the temporal lobes. (Adapted from *Fundamentals of Human Neuropsychology,* 4th ed., by Bryan Kolb and Ian Q. Wishaw © 1996 by W. H. Freeman and Company, p. 181, Figure 9.1. Used with the permission of Worth Publishers)

can easily examine the area of the temporal lobes. In the superior temporal lobes is **Heschl's gyrus,** and posterior to that is the **planum temporale.** Heschl's gyrus, which is known as the *primary auditory cortex,* is often larger in area in the right hemisphere, owing to the fact that there are often two gyri present. In the left hemisphere, the planum temporale is larger. The structural differences here may account for functional differences in auditory processing between the two hemispheres: Heschl's gyrus may hold more functional responsibility for nonspeech aspects of language and musical processing, and the planum temporale has a larger role in speech comprehension. In addition to visible structural differences, there are also differences in neuronal architecture and neurochemistry dependent on the side of the brain.

Neuropsychological and Behavioral Cerebral Differences

A number of behavioral differences are evident in the functioning of the two hemispheres. The correspondence between structural asymmetries and functional lateralization depends, in some measure, on the complexity of the behavior. The more simple primary sensory and motor functions show very specific patterns of representation in each hemisphere. In general, except for smell, sensory processing is funneled through the contralateral, or opposite, hemisphere from the site of the stimulus. For example, the somatosensory strip in the parietal lobe of the left hemisphere processes objects placed in the right hand. The primary occipital cortex of the left hemisphere processes information in the right visual field. These two senses are completely crossed, because the neural tracts project only to one hemisphere, opposite from the body site of stimulation. Audition is only partially crossed. Although the majority of information presented to the right ear is processed by the left hemisphere, a portion is processed by the right hemisphere auditory processing area. Olfactory information, which evolutionarily represents a more primitive sense, projects to the same (ipsilateral) hemisphere from each nostril; the right nostril is processed via the right olfactory bulb. On the output side, primary motor processing is also controlled by the primary motor strip in the frontal lobes of the contralateral hemisphere.

Higher-order processing is, by definition, integrative. Depending on the nature of the integration required, more or fewer brain areas are involved. Some may be primarily the domain of a single hemisphere, and some may require both sides of the cortex. For example, language, which is a highly complex function of the brain, requires many subcomponent skills. If a person's left hemisphere is dominant for speech, his or her left hemisphere is the primary processor for spoken words. However, the right hemisphere, then, is usually dominant for the prosody, or melodic intonation, of communication. In most people, both hemispheres contribute to language functioning, albeit in different ways. The usual pattern of language dominance is for left hemisphere mediation of speech, but individuals show a number of variations. Men are more likely to show strongly lateralized speech functions, whereas more women have bilateral representation. This came to attention when researchers noticed that after suffering a left hemisphere stroke, women were less likely to suffer the language impairment seen in men (see Levy & Heller, 1992).

Although neuropsychologists recognize the integrative nature of higher-order skills, some abilities are typically lateralized. As a general way of conceptualizing the differences between the hemispheres, the side that is dominant for verbal abilities (often the left) is usually more proficient in processing both the spoken and written word. It is facile in manipulating the symbols of language, such as letters, words, and numbers. It processes in a more detail-oriented and sequential mode. The right hemisphere, by contrast, typically holds the advantage for emotional, melodic, and visual-spatial processing and tends to "think" in a holistic mode. This visual-spatial processing is concerned with the orientation of one's own body in space (proprioception) as well as the spatial configuration, and orientation of objects.

To understand the difference in styles of right and left hemisphere processing, consider how you would approach the following tasks: When asking for directions, do you prefer verbal instructions directing you to go three blocks to the first stop sign, then turn left and proceed three blocks, then take a right, and so on, or do you prefer a spatial map with directions marked on it? When you complete a puzzle, do you attempt to match individual features or concentrate on overall shapes? When learning or listening to music, are you more attuned to the rhythm or the melody? In math, are you more adept with mathematical calculations and algebra or with geometry? In each of these cases the first style or ability corresponds to verbal-sequential processing typically associated with the left hemisphere, and the second to right hemisphere spatial-holistic processing. The stereotypes of "left-brained" and "right-brained" people have come from the oversimplified notions that one set of hemispheric skills will become dominant in a particular person. Perhaps you feel you use one style more than another. But in a normally functioning brain, all capabilities are used to some degree, although they may be developed to different degrees. Sometimes the contributions of various hemispheric abilities are not even noticed until their loss is made evident through brain damage or disease. When neuropsychologists discuss lateralization and dominance, the reference is to the division of labor for a particular skill in the brain rather than the dominance of "brain traits" in any one person.

Conclusion

This chapter reviewed the major structures and functions of the brain. This anatomy lesson is important for a variety of reasons. It is important to understand the functional aspects of the brain as they relate to brain anatomy. Knowledge of brain structures, in and of itself, is not very useful to neuropsychologists. This is most interestingly demonstrated when students with little neuropsychological knowledge dissect a brain. They proceed in a most rapid manner with the dissection, naming each structure they are able to detect as they go along. Once finished, they are typically perplexed with the mess they have made and how little they have learned. They often ask,"Where has the brain gone?" Novices look at the brain as an anatomic object; neuropsychologists examine it as a functioning organ of interconnected systems.

This chapter serves as an overview of the basic neuroanatomical structures and functions of the CNS (see pp. xxxi–xxxiii). However, it is typically the more integrated behaviors that interest neuropsychologists. Therefore it is necessary to move from discussions of groupings of structures based on ontogeny, to the idea of *plurapoteniality* of structures within functional systems. This concept, first introduced in Chapter 1, often transverses groupings based on migration of structures during brain development. As behavior becomes more complex, it also becomes more dependent on the functional organization of many areas within the cerebral hemispheres. It is to these cognitive systems of higher mental functions of the cerebral hemispheres that we now turn.

Critical Thinking Questions

- To what extent can behavioral functions be localized to specific brain structures?
- What level of brain mapping is most useful to the neuropsychologist?
- If a human was born without cerebral hemispheres, would the resulting behavior be like that of a comparable animal on the phylogenetic scale? Explain.
- Are there adaptive reasons why the cerebral hemispheres would gravitate toward either a bilateral or asymmetrical organization? Explain.

Key Terms

Peripheral nervous system (PNS)	Somatic nervous system (SNS)	Sympathetic nervous system	Brain
Central nervous system (CNS)	Autonomic nervous system (ANS)	Parasympathetic nervous system	Spinal cord
			Cranial nerves

Afferent nerves
Efferent nerves
Meninges
Cerebrospinal fluid (CSF)
Blood–brain barrier
Brain stem
Telencephalon
Cerebellum
Horizontal plane
Coronal plane
Sagittal plane
Anterior
Posterior
Inferior
Superior
Medial
Lateral
Rostral
Caudal
Proximal
Distal
Dorsal
Ventral
Ipsilateral
Contralateral
Meningiomas
Ventricular system
Vascular system
Fossae
Foramina
Foramen magnum
Fontanelle
Pia mater
Arachnoid membrane
Subarachnoid space

Dura mater
Epidural space
Subdural Space
Subdural hematoma
Meningitis
Ventricles
Foramen of Monro
Cerebral (or Sylvanian)
    aqueduct
Choroid plexus
Foramen of Magendie
Foramina of Luschka
Cisterns
Superior sagittal sinus
Arachnoid granulations
Hydrocephalus
Internal carotid arteries
Vertebral arteries
Aortic arch
Basilar artery
Posterior cerebral arteries
Cerebrovascular accident
    (CVA)
Circle of Willis
Anterior cerebral artery
Middle cerebral artery
Anterior communicating artery
Posterior communicating
    arteries
Forebrain (prosencephalon)
Midbrain (mesencephalon)
Hindbrain
    (rhombencephalon)
Diencephalon
Mesencephalon

Metencephalon
Myelencephalon
Medulla oblongata
Pons
Decussate
Cerebellar peduncles
Tectum
Tegmentum
Inferior colliculi
Superior colliculi
Reticular activating system
    (RAS)
Thalamus
Hypothalamus
Vermis
Basal forebrain
Subcortical aspect
Basal ganglia
Basal nuclei
Subthalamic nucleus
Caudate nucleus
Putamen
Globus pallidus
Striatum
Substantia nigra
Extrapyramidal motor system
Pyramidal motor system
Tardive dyskinesia
Rhinencephalon
Parahippocampal gyrus
Hippocampal formation
Limbic system
Fornix
Mammillary bodies
Amygdala

Septum
Basolateral circuit
Papez circuit
Wernicke-Korsakoff's
    syndrome
Corpus callosum
Longitudinal fissure
Cingulum
Cingulate gyrus
Anterior commissure
Hippocampal commissure
Cerebral hemispheres
    (cerebrum)
Sulcus, sulci
Fissure
Gyrus, gyri
Frontal lobe
Parietal lobe
Temporal lobe
Occipital lobe
Lateral fissure
Central sulcus
Occipital notch
Brodmann's areas
Somatosensory cortex
Primary motor cortex
Sensory association area
Prefrontal cortex
Wada test
Hemispheric asymmetry
Lateralization
Dominance
Sylvian fissure
Heschl's gyrus
Planum temporale

Web Connections

http://www.meddean.luc.edu/lumen/MedEd/GrossAnatomy/h_n/cn/cn1/mainframe.htm
The Cranial Nerves
Excellent discussion of the cranial nerves.

http://www.neuropat.dote.hu
Neuroanatomy
This page features links to a number of resources in neuroanatomy.

Chapter 4

SENSORY-PERCEPTUAL AND MOTOR SYSTEMS

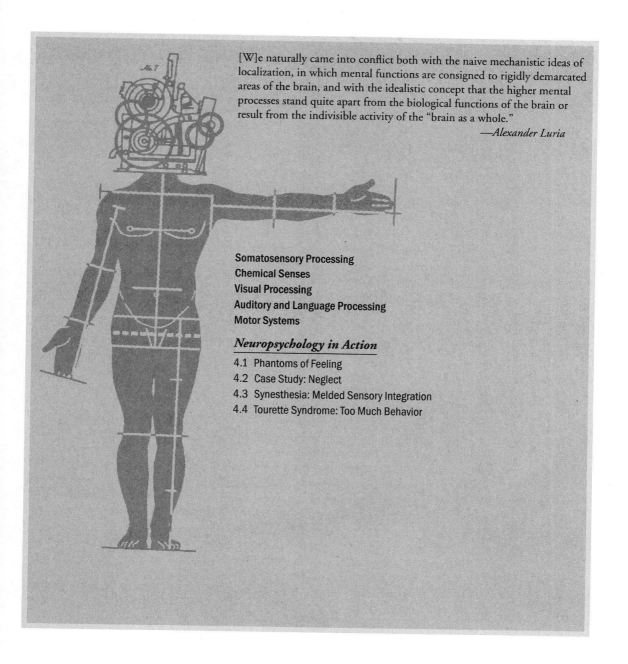

[W]e naturally came into conflict both with the naive mechanistic ideas of localization, in which mental functions are consigned to rigidly demarcated areas of the brain, and with the idealistic concept that the higher mental processes stand quite apart from the biological functions of the brain or result from the indivisible activity of the "brain as a whole."

—*Alexander Luria*

Somatosensory Processing
Chemical Senses
Visual Processing
Auditory and Language Processing
Motor Systems

Neuropsychology in Action

4.1 Phantoms of Feeling
4.2 Case Study: Neglect
4.3 Synesthesia: Melded Sensory Integration
4.4 Tourette Syndrome: Too Much Behavior

Keep in Mind

▪ How does the brain map incoming sensory information?

▪ Is sensory information processed in the same manner by each system?

▪ What happens when brain alteration causes malfunctions of ordinary experiences of perception?

▪ What would it be like to no longer be able to recognize one's friends by their faces?

Overview

A functional system is a circumscribed area of behavior that corresponds to a specific neuro-anatomic pathway or network of pathways. Some systems are well defined and traceable, and others remain incompletely mapped. The sensory systems are generally well defined, especially the visual and auditory systems. For example, the topography of the primary visual cortex includes areas devoted to such specific aspects of visual processing as line, shape, and color. Secondary areas of perception, including object recognition and spatial perception, are also specifically mapped. In contrast, multiple subsystems within the brain serve complex higher-order functional behaviors, such as attention and memory.

At times tracing systems through the brain seems mechanistic, like the "leg bone connected to the thigh bone" routine. Scientists gained their current understanding of the brain by identifying individual functions and attempting to map them to structure hierarchically, from lower- to higher-order functions. However, many structures participate in multiple functions. A complex internet-working of functions is evident in the progression from the sensory and motor systems to higher functional systems where the work involves anatomic networks that are sometimes widely dispersed throughout the brain.

The brain is a dynamic biological network, but a small lesion in a strategic location can have devastating effects on the system. It is therefore impossible to gain.a thorough understanding of systems such as vision or language by studying intact brains only. Russian psychologist Alexander Luria, whose pioneering work made possible our understanding of functional brain systems, argued that although higher mental functions may be disturbed by a lesion in any of the many different links of the system, they are disturbed differently by lesions in different links (Luria, 1966). Luria's research profited greatly from his keen observations of neurological patients. He noticed that anatomically different lesions were possible within the same behavioral syndrome. He also noticed that a lesion in one area could affect a number of different behaviors.

The functional systems we focus on here may be broadly categorized as arising from sensory input and resulting in motor output. Most of this chapter concerns the sensory-perceptual systems, which have multiple input modalities. Although the motor system has fewer output modalities, it is served by both cortical and subcortical systems. We concentrate on how each system operates at the level of central brain mechanisms. Most sensory systems are anatomically mapped to specific cortical areas devoted to primary sensory processing, which provide information that is then routed to secondary processing areas where it is "perceived" and meaning is attached. All sensory systems except smell follow a pathway through the thalamus, where they are directed to primary and secondary cortical processing areas (see Figure 4.1). We ask how each system functions at the level of the brain, and what can happen when behavior goes awry because of injury or disease. In the areas of visual and auditory processing, we progress to higher-order functions such as visual object recognition, visual-spatial processing, and speech and language. These abilities certainly require integration with other higher functional systems, but are best discussed here. In general, we discuss disorders that illustrate a specific breakdown of a system rather than broad-based disorders. (In later chapters we discuss disorders that involve multiple systems.)

Sensation is the body's window to the world. The range of what humans can detect is unique to our species and becomes the raw material of our perceptions and the stuff of our experiences. Information comes in fragments and requires the central processor of the brain to literally "make sense" of the outside environment. Sensation begins with the process of **transduction** (from the Latin *transducere,* meaning to "lead across"). An environmental stimulus activates a specific **receptor cell** creating energy, which is transduced into an electrical stimulus that is then carried to neurons for the brain to process. (Receptor cells are not technically neurons, although they do synapse with neurons.) Sensory receptor cells throughout the body detect numerous stimuli, including sight, sound, pressure, pain, chemical irritation, smell, and taste, to name a few. We hear with our ears and see with our eyes, but if photoreceptor cells were on our hands we would see with our fingers. Some sensory systems are very complex. For example, taste uses multiple transduction processes to detect subtle differences of flavor. The visual system uses two primary types (rods and cones), and the auditory system uses a single basic mechanism.

Agnosia, the inability to recognize the form and/or function of objects and people, occurs in every sensory

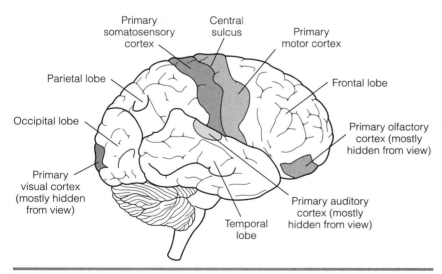

Figure 4.1 The primary sensory and motor cortexes. In general, primary sensory processing lies posterior to the central sulcus and primary motor processing is anterior. The chemical senses of olfaction and taste are the exception. The primary gustatory cortex cannot be seen from this view. (Banich, Marie T., *Neuropsychology: The Neural Bases of Mental Function.* Copyright © 1997 by Houghton Mifflin Company, p. 25, Figure 4.1. Adapted with permission)

The hour is striking so close above me,
so clear and sharp,
that all my senses ring with it.
I feel it now; there's a power in me
to grasp and give shape to my world.

I know that nothing has ever been real
without my beholding it.
All becoming has needed me.
My looking ripens things
and they come toward me, to meet and be met.

—Rainer Maria Rilke

domain. For example, a **visual agnosia** is present if someone is unable to recognize a person or object by sight. **Tactile agnosia,** also called **astereognosis,** is an inability to recognize objects by touch; for instance, failing to recognize a quarter or a pen held in the hand. Agnosia is possible in every sensory domain and can sometimes result in very odd behavior. In his popular book of neurological tales, *The Man Who Mistook His Wife for a Hat* (1987), Oliver Sacks tells the story of a music professor who, coming upon his wife standing next to a coat rack, tried to lift her head instead of his hat. He no longer "knew" people or objects visually, but relied on distinctive voice characteristics and his other senses for identification.

Agnosia is not a single sensory phenomenon. It may strike any sensory domain, but the most commonly studied instances affect the visual, auditory and tactile senses. Olfactory and taste agnosias have not been researched extensively. Agnosias in general are relatively rare, but have received considerable attention in the neuropsychological literature, perhaps because they so strikingly alter consciousness.

Somatosensory Processing

The **somatosensory system** includes two types of sensory stimulation, external and internal. This system can monitor sensations such as cold and heat, whether the sensation comes from handling an ice cube or from a fever. So the system processes external stimulation of touch (pressure, shape, texture, heat) in recognizing objects by feel and is also concerned with the position of the body in extrapersonal space, termed **proprioception.** Of great interest to neuropsychology are sensory dysfunctions that result in proprioceptive disorders of altered sense of bodily sensation or bodily position.

The somatosensory system contains a conglomeration of receptor types and sensory information. Receptors on the skin are attuned to external sensations such as the pressure of a hand, a blast of wind, the pricking of a finger, the vibrational frequency of touch, the burn of a hot stove, and the itching of poison ivy. Somatosensory receptors are also spread internally throughout the body to monitor the stretching of the stomach during eating and digestion, the pain of muscle aches, and the spatial position of arms and legs, to name a few examples. The receptor types and systems we discuss in this section range over widely varying areas of function from mechanical and chemical monitoring to damage and body position monitoring.

The somatosensory system begins at the level of receptors, of which five types are found on the skin and throughout the body. **Mechanical receptors** transduce energy from touch, vibration, and the stretching and bending of skin, muscle, internal organs, and blood vessels. A detailed discussion of subtypes is not necessary, but at least five different types of mechanical receptors exist. For example, hair follicle receptors sense breezes or a brush of fern across the skin. They are essential to animals such as cats and mice in their whisker navigational system. **Chemoreceptors** respond to various chemicals on the surface of the skin and mucous membranes. They range from detecting level of stomach acidity to skin irritations. Smell and taste are special examples of chemoreception that we discuss separately. **Thermoreceptors** detect heat and cold. **Nocioceptors** (from the Latin *nocere,* "to hurt") serve as monitors to alert the brain to damage or threat of damage. They can be mechanical or chemical but are specifically activated by potentially damaging stimulation such as heat or cold, painful pressure or pricking, or chemical damage such as exposure to noxious chemicals. They are present throughout the body, but are noticeably absent in the brain. This is how some types of brain surgery and brain mapping can be done while the patient is conscious and alert. **Proprioceptors** (from the Latin *proprius,* "one's own") on skeletal muscles detect movement via degree of stretch, angle, and relative position of limbs. Proprioceptors on the hands help identify the shapes of objects via touch.

These somatosensory receptors synapse with neurons into two primary pathways that transmit information from the spinal cord to the thalamus (see Figure 4.2 on pages 116–117). In each case sensory information travels to the contralateral hemisphere from the point of origin. The first pathway, the **ascending spinal-thalamic tract** carries sensory information related to pain and temperature and runs in parallel to the spinal cord. It synapses over a wide region of the thalamus and then to the somatosensory cortex. The second pathway is the **dorsal column medial lemniscal pathway** carrying information pertaining to touch and vibration. It is so named because it is routed up the dorsal aspects of the spinal cord to a white matter tract termed the **medial lemniscus,** which courses through the contralateral side of the brain stem through the medulla, pons, and midbrain and then up through the thalamus (ventral posterior nucleus, VP) and on to the primary somatosensory cortex. All stimulation of the face is on a separate system through the large trigeminal nerve (cranial nerve V), which enters the brain through the pons.

The primary somatosensory cortex lies in the parietal lobe immediately posterior to the central sulcus on the post central gyrus (Brodmann's areas 1, 2, and 3; see Figure 4.3 on page 118). It is **somatopically organized;** that is, the distorted figure of the sensory homunculus mapped onto the primary somatosensory cortex represents the relative importance and distribution of touch in various areas of the body rather than the actual size of the body part. Notice that the thumb, fingers, and face represent proportionately the largest areas. These are the areas of most sensitive and discriminating sensation in the body, having the largest proportion of touch receptors. The somatosensory system is organized contralaterally, with the left hemisphere processing tactile sensation from the right side of the body and vice versa. The work documenting the close correspondence of sensation to cortical mapping in the primary somatosensory cortex began in the early days of neurosurgery. In the 1940s Wilder Penfield, a noted neurosurgeon at the Montreal Neurological Institute, started to use electrical stimulation to explore the functions of the cortex in patients undergoing neurosurgery for the relief of epilepsy. Applying electrical stimuli to different cortical areas in over 1,000 fully conscious patients, Penfield mapped motor, sensory, language, and memory functions (see Figure 4.4 on page 119).

From the primary somatosensory cortex, sensory information is then integrated at the next level in the secondary somatosensory cortex which is immediately posterior (Brodmann's areas 5, 7). Here the individual properties of tactile stimuli such as shape, weight, and texture are combined to form the perception of single and whole percepts such as "pencil," "coin," or "key" that can be recognized by feel. Damage to this area may result in astereognosia even though the person may readily recognize objects by sight. In this case, elementary powers of sensation are intact, but the person cannot recognize things placed in the hand contralateral to the lesion. Neuropsychologists usually test for this problem by blindfolding the patient, placing an object in the hand, and asking the person to recognize and name it by touch only (see Chapter 14). Damage interrupting higher-level somatosensory integration in the parietal area, particularly the right parietal lobe, may result in a problem variously referred to as *tactile suppression, tactile extinction,* or *tactile inattention.* In this instance, of right parietal damage, a person does not report the sensation of touch on the left hand (that is, left-sided suppression) when the left and right hands are touched simultaneously, although he or she may accurately report a left-sided touch when that hand is touched in isolation. In this case the problem involves sorting out competing tactile sensations. Left-sided touch is suppressed or extinguished when there is competing sensation from both sides of the body. Table 4.1 gives examples of somatosensory disorders.

Disorders of proprioception represent the second type of tactile disorder in that the sensory problem is one of recognizing the relative position of your own body in space rather than the recognition of objects

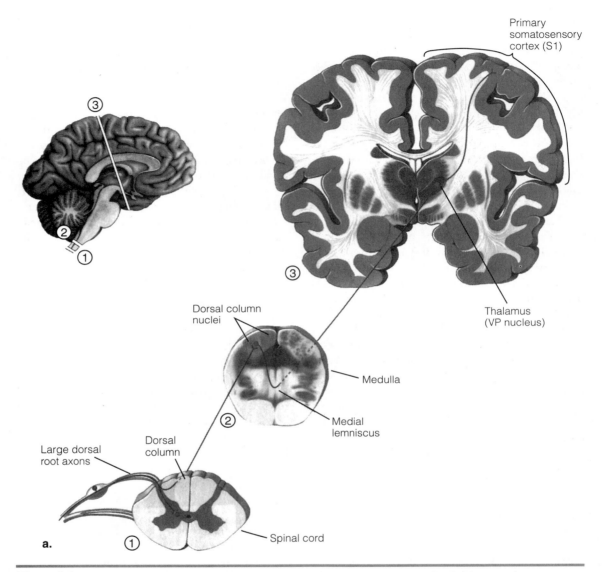

Figure 4.2 The two primary somatosensory pathways. (a) The dorsal column medial lemniscal pathway carries touch and proprioceptive information. (b) The ascending spinal-thalamic tract carries pain and temperature information. (Modified from M. F. Bear, B. W. Connors, and M. A. Paradiso, *Neuroscience: Exploring the Brain,* Baltimore: Williams & Wilkins, 1996, p. 327, Figure 12.15 and p. 328, Figure 12.16.)

external to yourself. This is a problem of tactile integration, which is usually compromised by parietal lobe dysfunction. Because proprioceptors record from the stretching of muscle, what you are receiving as sensory information is feedback from your own motor movements. This sensory information then is available to feed back to fine-tune body movement. Normally a combination of vision, the vestibular organs, and the proprioceptive sense supplies a **kinesthetic sense** of your physical body. Proprioception, like most

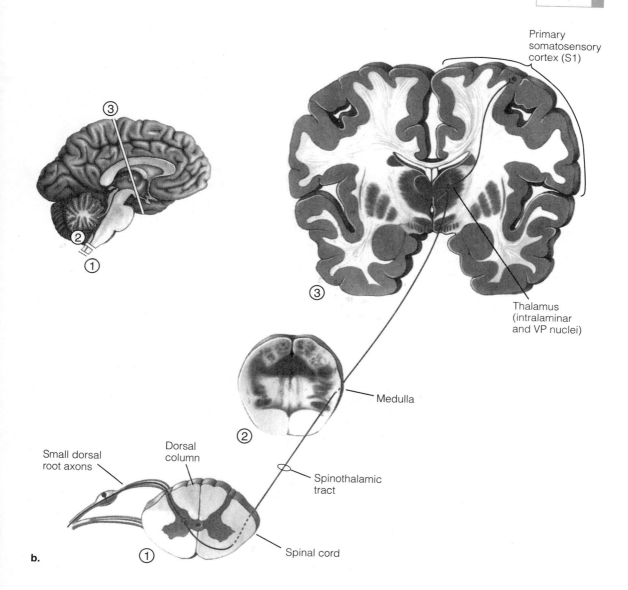

Primary somatosensory cortex (S1)

Thalamus (intralaminar and VP nuclei)

Medulla

Dorsal column

Small dorsal root axons

Spinothalamic tract

Spinal cord

b.

elementary sensations, is so basic and automatic that you take it completely for granted unless it is disrupted or absent. Imagine, however, having no sense of where your hands and legs are, or even of your posture if your eyes are closed. In Oliver Sacks's case of the "Disembodied Lady" (Sacks, 1987), a young woman of 37, suffering a sensory neuritis, had the feeling of "losing" parts of her body if she couldn't see them, the feeling of total disembodiment. Having no natural posture, her movements became a caricature of types, such as a dancer's pose. Quite the opposite problem is expressed in phantom limb pain. People with no external sensation entering the brain still have the curious experience of pain or other sensation. Neuropsychology in Action 4.1 explores this odd phenomenon.

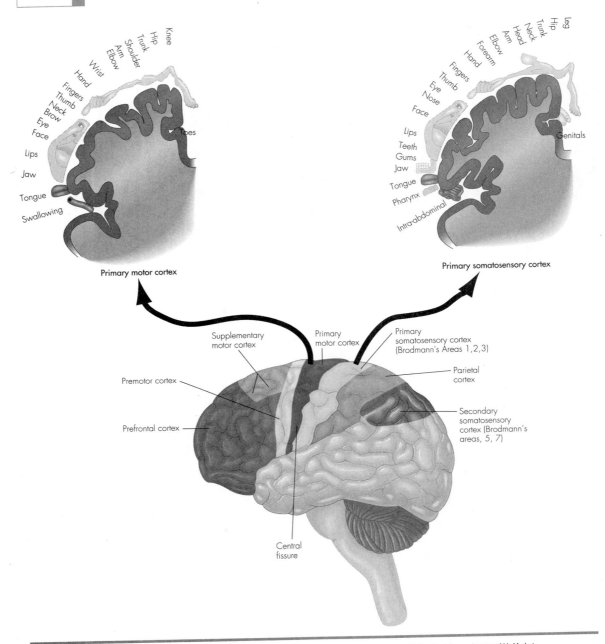

Figure 4.3   The homunculi from the primary motor and somatosensory cortexes. (Adapted from James W. Kalat, *Biological Psychology,* 6th ed., Pacific Grove, CA: Brooks/Cole, 1998, pp. 96, 227)

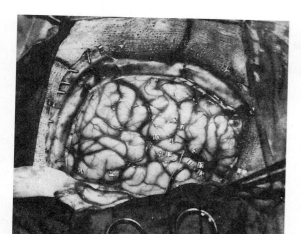

Figure 4.4 Penfield's electrical stimulation experiments. Penfield numbered sections of the open cortex of a conscious patient as he mapped the response to direct electrical stimulation to the brain. (From Case M. M., in Wilder Penfield, *The Mystery of the Mind: A Critical Study of Consciousness and the Human Brain*, with Discussions by William Feindel, *Charles Hendel, and Charles Symonds.* Copyright 1975 by Princeton University Press. Figure 4, p. 24. Reprinted by permission of Princeton University Press)

Table 4.1 *Examples of Somatosensory Dysfunction*
Asteriognosis/tactile agnosia: inability to recognize an object by touch
Finger agnosia: inability to recognize or orient to one's own fingers
Paresthesia: spontaneous crawling, burning or "pins and needles" sensation
Peripheral neuropathy: peripheral nervous system dysfunction causing sensory loss (for example, in diabetes)
Phantom limb pain: a feeling of pain in a nonexistent limb
Proprioceptive disorder: loss of body position sense
Tactile extinction/suppression/inattention: suppression of touch sensation on one side of body

Chemical Senses

Taste and smell are evolutionarily the oldest sensory systems. They work in concert, and to most people appear indistinguishable until a cold or other sinus condition congests and diminishes the sense of smell. People are likely to report that food doesn't "taste" so good or have as much flavor as usual, when it is actually blocked smell that is affecting the pleasurability of food. It is easy to experience this condition by just holding your nose and sampling different foods to see what "tastes" you actually experience. Taste and smell are also the least studied of the senses within neuropsychology and neuroscience. This neglect may be due partly to the fact that other senses such as vision and audition are well developed in humans and so have overshadowed the chemical senses. The idea that the senses of taste and smell may be vestigial and no longer of any real adaptive use to modern humans

has also probably contributed to the lack of interest. However, these chemical senses are enjoying a surge of research attention that is pointing to connections with emotional behavior, hormones, immunology, and identification of neurologic disease states.

TASTE

The tongue contains numerous **papillae** or bumps on which lie from one to several hundred taste buds consisting of between 50–150 taste receptor cells. The bundles of receptor cells resemble onions, with the cilia at the tips of the cells protruding into the surface of the pore. Taste receptors are not neurons, but respond to the chemical qualities in food dissolved in saliva as they wash over the tips of the receptors. In the course of eating, taste receptors endure extremes of temperature, spicy food, and other chemical substances, which may cause damage. Perhaps because of this, taste receptors quickly wear out and are replaced on a cycle of about 10 days.

The traditional theory about how taste functions, presented in most general psychology textbooks, describes the tongue's ability to discriminate four primary taste sensations; sweet, salty, sour, and bitter. This schema is based on specific taste bud receptor ability to detect the chemicals associated with each

Neuropsychology in Action 4.1

Phantoms of Feeling

by Mary Spiers

Phantoms are the experience of external sensory experience in the absence of available sensory input. This sounds strikingly like an hallucination. And perhaps had it not have been for the widespread occurrence of phantoms felt by what are considered otherwise "rational" people, phantoms might have been considered psychosomatic experiences at best and psychotic at worst. People most commonly think of phantoms in respect to phantom limb pain after amputation, but they can and do exist in any sensory modality. The interesting questions here are, How are phantoms experienced, and what are their causes? Finally, understanding phantoms may also provide some clues to understanding certain aspects of brain plasticity and reorganization.

Phantom limbs and phantom limb pain are most commonly associated with amputations. The amputee may feel a lost arm, feel that it swings in coordination with the other arm while walking, or

experience it sticking out so much as to necessitate maneuvering through doors sideways. All the while, objective reality is shouting that it is not there. Cold, heat, pressure, itching, tickling, and sweat can all be experienced in the missing limb. Because as many as 70% of amputees experience pain in the amputated part, psychologists specializing in pain management are striving to understand causes and formulate treatments for this problem.

Phantoms may also be experienced in situations other than amputation and in senses other than tactile. Children born without limbs, people who have suffered paralysis following a spinal cord injury, and even women in labor who have had spinal anesthesia have also "felt" the presence of a limb. Some congenital amputees have reported being able to move nonexistent fingers or to experience the phantom emerge and disappear from consciousness. Phantom seeing and hearing can occur in the

complete or partial absence of vision and audition. Auditory phantoms may be passed off as tinnitus, or ringing in the ears, but some people hear voices or music. Visual phantoms can also range from flashes of light and color to fully formed images of people and objects. In both cases, and perhaps a differentiating factor between these types of "hallucinations" and those experienced by schizophrenics, is that phantoms are quickly judged as separate from normal sensory-perceptual reality.

How can phantoms be described neurologically? Scientists know that phantoms emanate from central brain mechanisms rather than purely peripheral ones, although the exact mechanism for the production of phantoms is still a matter of some speculation. In the case of phantom limbs, amputations leave exposed nerve endings that heal as nodules called *neuromas*. Neuromas continue to generate neural impulses. For this reason, initial treatments fo-

---

taste. For example, certain receptors are attuned to sodium chloride (NaCl) and other salty chemicals, and likewise for the remaining primary taste sensations. Some researchers have suggested a fifth taste, *umami,* from the Japanese word for "delicious." Deliciousness is operationally defined by the activation of l-glutamate receptors that are attuned to glutamate-triggering substances such as monosodium glutamate (MSG). The primary tastes theory implies that in any mixture individual taste sensations, such as saltiness, are identified by specific saltiness receptor types and transmitted to the brain along dedicated pathways, where they are analyzed and labeled

as salty. According to this theory, taste receptors of different types are grouped in various areas of the tongue; the tip is specific for sweetness and saltiness, the sides detect sourness, and the back is most sensitive to bitterness.

The competing pattern theory suggests that taste is best thought of as a pattern of sensation in which individual receptors can process information about more than one taste type. There is strong evidence that individual taste fibers are not exclusive to one taste sensation, although they may roughly focus on one type (Smith & Vogt, 1997). The suggestion from the pattern theory is that the experience of any par-

cused on severing communication between the peripheral sensory input and the spinal cord. However, this does not obliterate phantoms. Consequently, as an attempted treatment surgeons have blocked or cut spinal nerves, and then central pathways feeding the somatosensory cortex from the sensory relay station of the thalamus. But phantoms still exist. Traditional painkilling drugs are also largely ineffective, because phantom pain does not seem to arise from the same pain system.

From where in the brain do phantoms arise? Recent work in this area has lead to rethinking about the supposed lack of plasticity of adult brains. A logical place to start is to understand what happens in the somatosensory strip when the corresponding sensory area on the body ceases to provide input. Researchers have done deep brain electrode recording on monkeys with an amputated finger. Surprisingly, sensory input from adjacent fingers remapped itself onto the somatosensory cortex so that it invaded the area previously serving the amputated finger. This remapping occurred within weeks of the amputation. Neuroscientist Timothy Pons demonstrated this sensory strip encroachment in monkeys who had had their sensory nerves cut

over 12 years previously. In this case, massive territorial invasion was seen; in one case a hand and arm were now mapped onto the face. Recall that we made the point earlier that neurons, once severed, are for all practical purposes dead and unable to regenerate; only partially severed axons can resprout. At least, this has been the common wisdom. Also, no brain reorganization is expected after a certain critical period of development. However, in the case of phantoms there is no damage to neurons in the brain; all the damage is peripheral. Somehow, healthy neurons are reorganizing themselves to take over an area of the brain that the body is no longer using. It is reasonable to expect that healthy brain neurons may more easily reorganize themselves than damaged ones. However, the mechanism by which this is done is still a mystery. One aspect that has puzzled scientists working on this problem is the fact that if neurons were reorganizing themselves on the homunculus of the somatosensory strip itself, their growth would have to cover long distances. This mechanism seems unlikely, given that adult neurons can only sprout over very short distances. One possible explanation is that instead of reorganization at the level of the

somatosensory cortex, reorganization is occurring within the relay station of the thalamus, where all sensory inputs from touch, vision, and audition funnel through in a very tight space. An axon merely has to reach across a very narrow stream in order to remap a finger to the face or to even to the back. Odd as it may seem, this phenomenon is now being demonstrated in human amputees. Ramachandran (Ramachandran, Rogers-Ramachandran, & Steward, 1992) tested a teenager who had recently lost his left arm in an auto accident. As the boy sat blindfolded, Ramachandran touched various parts of his body with a cotton swab. When he stimulated various areas of his lip and lower face, the boy felt his missing thumb and fingers tingle. Sensations from his hand were now remapped onto his face. Because acupuncture has helped some people with phantom limb pain, it seems reasonable to speculate that knowledge of remapping may dampen pain if massage, acupuncture, or other means can be applied to the newly remapped areas of the body. In the case of this boy, odd as it may seem, maybe face massage would alleviate left arm and hand pain.

---

ticular taste, such as saltiness, is carried to the brain, because the fibers are activated to respond mostly to saltiness of the substance in the mixture. The implication is that taste receptors may have multiple potentiality rather than being dedicated to respond to a specific chemical.

Taste receptor cells synapse with sensory neurons that carry information via cranial nerves VII, IX, and X to the medulla of the brain stem (specifically the nucleus of the solitary tract), where they are relayed via the thalamus (ventral posterior medial nucleus) to the primary gustatory cortex (see Figure 4.5). Additional projections run from the thalamus directly

to the somatosensory cortex amygdala, hypothalamus, and orbital prefrontal cortex. The hypothalamus may code for pleasurability of food, because it contains neurons that respond specifically to sweetness of food (Rolls, 1986).

The function of taste appears to be drawing us to certain basic substances that the body needs and repelling us from potentially harmful chemicals. Certain receptors are attuned to sweet and salty foods, which the brain codes as pleasurable. Before the days of candy and fast salty foods, being drawn to sweet foods such as fruit provided needed nutrition. Salt contains the body's necessary sodium. It is also adaptive to be

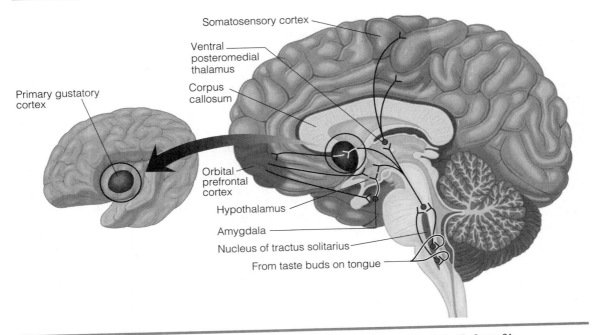

Figure 4.5   Taste pathways in the brain. (From James W. Kalat, *Biological Psychology*, 6th ed., Pacific Grove, CA: Brooks/Cole, 1998, p. 204, Figure 7.21)

repelled by bitter foods, which might be poisonous, and by sour foods, which might be spoiled.

Disorders of taste are rare in comparison to disorders of smell, although as we mentioned earlier, people may report disorders of smell as disorders of taste because the two systems interact in flavor perception. Taste disorders may range from a diminished sense of taste (hypoguesia) to a complete loss of taste (aguesia). Table 4.2 summarizes taste disorders. Phantoguesia is the experience of a taste "phantom" or hallucinatory taste. Taste phantoms often coincide with other disorders of taste. Most disorders of taste seem to be caused by a problem in the central perception of taste, rather than a problem at the level of the taste buds. For example, one of the more common reasons for taste distortion is medication usage. Other etiologies for taste dysfunction include head injury, upper respiratory infection, and in the case of phantoguesia, are sometimes caused by damage to the "taste nerve," the chorda tympani (cranial nerve VII) if it is injured during ear or dental surgery (see Cowart et al., 1997).

Table 4.2	*Disorders of Taste*

Aguesia: inability to recognize tastes

Dysguesia: distorted taste sensation

Phantoguesia: experience of a phantom or hallucinatory taste

Hypoguesia: diminished taste sensitivity

SMELL

Amble through a field on a summer afternoon, and the air is fragrant with smells of wildflowers, grasses, and aromatic herbs. Inhale, and microscopic molecules of scent wafting through the air are gradually taken in by your relatively slow olfactory detection system. The aromas you detect and identify are in part a function of the odorant's ability to dissolve in the moist mucous lining of the nose, but are also affected by age, gender, health, and brain injury. Smell is the least well understood system, perhaps because scientists have considered it of little adaptive value to humans. Certainly it is the oldest sensory system, evolutionarily, and appears much more crucial to animals such as bloodhounds and snakes, which are lower on the phylogenetic scale. What function does scent serve for humans? Is it a vestigial sense? On the one hand, many people seem to function very well in their lives having completely lost their sense of smell. On the other hand, the perfume industry is booming and aromatherapy is becoming a popular naturopathic approach to mood enhancement. In this section we examine the unique neuroanatomy of the primary olfactory system. Unlike other systems, olfactory neurons have regenerative qualities when damaged. Finally, we also reflect on the potential implications of links among mood, memory, and olfaction.

With inhalation (but actually just a sufficient sniff is needed) to send molecules of scent traveling up to the roof of the nasal cavity. These odorants dissolve in the olfactory epithelium, a fine mucous lining consisting of odorant-binding proteins (OBPs), antibodies, and enzymes. Mucus is being continually produced, so that the entire epithelium is replaced about every 10 minutes. Scent molecules bound to OBPs activate the fine, hairlike cilia of olfactory neurons waving within the olfactory epithelium. Researchers have discovered at least 500–1000 odorant-binding protein genes that appear to be coded for different odorants. In humans, the epithelium is small, about half the size of a postage stamp (5–10 cm^2). Dogs, with their keen sense of smell, have an epithelium easily 10 times that of humans (100 cm^2) with 100 times the neurons per square centimeter. Olfactory neurons in the epithelium synapse with the right or left olfactory bulb through the thin cribriform plate of the skull. Here the central olfactory pathway (cranial nerve I) originates. So whereas three cranial nerves subserve taste, smell has only one pathway.

The olfactory system is unique in several ways. Note that we have spoken of receptors when discussing other sensory systems. These receptors then synapse with dendrites of neurons. This is not the case with the olfactory system. The neurons themselves are directly exposed to the environment. The health of the epithelial layer, in which the dangling neurons lie, is crucial because some viruses, such as rabies, take advantage of this direct route to the brain. This system is also interesting in that contrary to the notion that new neural cells do not form in adults, the olfactory neurons compose a uniquely "plastic" system, continuing to reproduce and replace themselves every one to two months throughout adulthood. The olfactory neurons, however, are very susceptible to traumatic injury because they dangle through a opening in the skull, the cribriform plate. A blow to the head can easily sever these neurons. Although the neurons do regrow, they do not always reconnect with the olfactory bulbs (see Figure 4.6).

The olfactory bulbs contain complex circuitry; the two bulbs even communicate with each other. Although the mechanism is not completely understood, micro electrode recordings show that various aromas produce identifiable spatial maps on the bulbs and these mosaics may change even during the sniffing of an odorant. The plasticity of the system has suggested to scientists that experience with smell can easily modify the representational pattern of stimulation on the olfactory bulb. The map on the bulb projects to the areas of the brain that process and encode the scent. It appears that specific odors code specific patterns. It is not clear if these coded representations are invariant, in other words, always stimulating the same brain areas, or if learning can also feed back to modify scent maps when the same scent is later reintroduced.

Another unique aspect of olfaction is its pattern of projection into the brain. All other sensory systems first pass through the thalamus and then into the neocortex. However, the primary projections of the olfactory system innervate the limbic system directly through the amygdala and hippocampal formation. Olfactory information projects into these primitive areas of the brain before passing through the relay station of the thalamus and then into the frontal cortex and onto other areas of the neocortex. Because of this connection, the effect of scent on emotion and mood is instantaneous, and most intensely processed preconsciously. Secondarily, scientists believe that parallel thalamic projections to the frontal lobes are responsible for conscious recognition of scent. The cortex can then elaborate and refine the perception of aroma. The hippocampus,

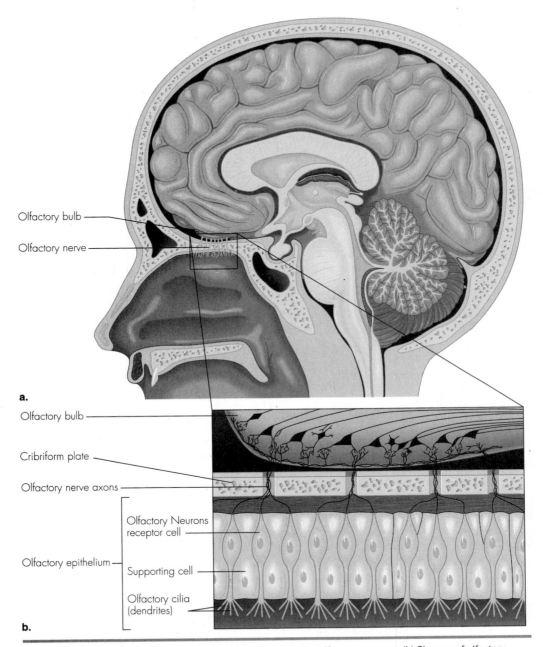

Olfactory bulb

Olfactory nerve

a.

Olfactory bulb

Cribriform plate

Olfactory nerve axons

Olfactory Neurons
receptor cell

Olfactory epithelium

Supporting cell

Olfactory cilia
(dendrites)

b.

Figure 4.6   Olfactory system (a) Odorants are taken up via the olfactory neurons. (b) Closeup of olfactory neurons, which protrude through the cribriform plate. (From James W. Kalat, *Biological Psychology*, 6th ed., Pacific Grove, CA: Brooks/Cole, 1998, p. 205, Figure 7.22)

although not a memory storage center, is responsible for processing and coding memories before they are stored in the neocortex. Together with the amygdala, these limbic system structures appear to be responsible for coding much of the emotional tone of memories. This neural pattern of projection into the brain reflects olfaction's ancient evolution. Considering this brain anatomy, it is no wonder that smell is so strongly tied to emotional memory.

In the early part of this century, Freud suggested that disorders of smell and specific psychological dysfunctions may be connected (for types of olfactory dysfunction, see Table 4.3). This idea remained largely unexamined until a relatively recent resurgence of interest in olfaction occurred as it relates to certain brain diseases such as Alzheimer's disease, Parkinson's disease, and schizophrenia. For some time people have observed that decreased ability to smell (hyposmia) is associated with aging, and that both loss and distortion of smell (dysosmia) are associated with depression. With aging, the ability to perceive sour or bitter odors appears to diminish first, whereas the ability to detect pleasant smells such as sweetness may persist well into old age. Interestingly, recent work has shown that diminution of olfactory ability is an early sign of diseases of accelerated aging, such as Alzheimer's disease and Parkinson's disease (for example, see Doty, 1990). Also, schizophrenics often have a distorted sense of smell. Clinical neuropsychologists are now using scratch-and-sniff tests of odor identification and odor recognition threshold such as the University of Pennsylvania Smell Identification Test (UPSIT) (Doty, Shaman, & Dann, 1984) to test for the presence of olfactory dysfunction in cases where clinicians suspect these diseases.

Table 4.3	*Disorders of Smell*

Anosmia: total loss of smell

Dysosmia: distorted smell sensation

Phantosmia: experience of a phantom or hallucinatory smell

Hyposmia: diminished taste sensation

Partial or complete loss of smell is also a common occurrence after traumatic injury to the brain. As noted earlier, because the olfactory neurons dangle through the cribriform plate, they are easily damaged or sheared off by sudden movements of the brain in relation to the skull. Even though olfactory neurons can regenerate, they often do not reconnect to the olfactory bulbs because they are blocked by scar tissue.

Visual Processing

Visual processing covers more cortical territory than any of the other senses. Approximately one-fourth of the cortex, centered on the occipital, temporal, and parietal lobes, is devoted to visual-perceptual processing. This is not surprising, because the primary mode of sensory information gathering in humans is through sight. Visual information processing is also the most studied and one of the best understood sensory systems of the brain. Furthermore, it represents one of the most complex systems.

No one "master processor" integrates all visual information into perceptible form. Recognition of surroundings, people, faces, and objects is, although seemingly instantaneous, the culmination of separate but locally connected visual-perceptual processes. As a prerequisite to recognizing a friend walking through a crowd, you must first have the necessary visual acuity as well as adequate color and form perception. Visual acuity speaks to the ability to perceive light, contrast between light and dark, resolve a target, and have adequate visual fields. Receptors for form interpret shapes such as roundness or squareness, as well as orientation of lines to each other. Qualities of texture and color such as feathery and blue are processed by yet other primary visual areas. Then, at a higher perceptual level the ventral visual pathway to the temporal lobes serves as the "what" system largely responsible for object and face recognition. The dorsal pathway to the parietal lobes, or the "where" system, is specialized for spatial location. In building a visual percept, some of these processes operate in sequence, and others may operate in parallel.

As complicated as this general characterization may be, the human visual system is actually much more sophisticated. In daily life you see under extremely "messy" visual conditions, through haze, from different perspectives, and from varying distances. Amazingly, visual perception of a tree stays constant, even though sometimes you may see it through a fog, sometimes in the shade, sometimes partially obscured, sometimes seen from the north, sometimes from a distance, and sometimes from underneath. Each time the image of the tree makes a different impression on your retina, yet your brain's perception of "tree" remains constant. Obviously you don't simply match templates for a particular tree—there would be so many as to soon overload the system. The visual-perceptual system must be highly flexible and sophisticated to accommodate a constantly changing visual landscape.

PRIMARY VISUAL PROCESSING

In a general way the eye functions as a type of camera, mapping visual images on the retina, and transmitting the inverted "picture" to a corresponding "retinotopic" map to the primary visual processing area of the cortex. But the eye is much more dynamic and complex in operation; it can constantly adjust focus and adapt to changing visual conditions as well as extract information about images. The visual system operates via two types of photoreceptor cells. The rods and cones transduce the electromagnetic wavelengths of light energy and extract properties of objects. Cones, which detect wavelengths of color, are fewer, and center in the middle of the retina. The more numerous rods surround the cones and are attuned to the shades of gray we experience in low-light and nighttime conditions. Visual stimuli from the right side of space activate receptors on the left side of each retina, and information from the left visual field activates right-sided receptors.

Visual information leaves the eye through the optic nerve's bundle of axons. The retina sends projections to at least 10 brain areas. Some of these areas, such as the pineal gland and the superchiasmic nucleus, are important in regulating long biological rhythms such as migration in birds and the circadian rhythms of sleep and wakefulness (see Chapter 13). Others are involved in controlling eye movement. A small proportion of neurons from the optic tract synapse with the hypothalamus, and a proportion (10%) synapse with the superior colliculus in the midbrain tectum. However, the primary route, consisting of the largest number of axons, funnels information along the visual pathway to the occipital cortex (see Figure 4.7). The route leaving the eye follows the optic nerve to the optic chiasm on the ventral surface of the brain, just anterior to the pituitary gland. Here information from both eyes joins and partially **decussates** (crosses over to the contralateral side). From here on out, the left hemisphere processes information from the right visual field and vice versa. In addition, information from the visual fields also reverses top to bottom. The lower portion of the visual field is now on top, close to the parietal lobes, and the upper portion is on the bottom, next to the temporal lobes. The optic tracts synapse with the thalamus in the dorsal portion at the lateral geniculate nucleus (LGN), then project to the occipital lobes.

Disorders of the visual system, along the pathway from the retina to the occipital lobes depend on where along the pathway a lesion occurs. Because the pathway is topographically oriented, observing visual abilities gives a good clue to lesion location. Figure 4.8 (p. 128) shows a number of variants of visual difficulties, or **anopsias,** possible with lesions to the optic pathways. If a lesion occurs anterior to the optic chiasm, effectively cutting off the visual input from one eye, the effect is blindness in one eye. Both visual fields with full peripheral vision remain in the other eye. If, however, the optic nerve is cut posterior to the optic chiasm, the relay for one visual field in both eyes is destroyed. This condition is technically termed **homonymous** (same-sided) **hemianopsia** (half-blindness), and refers to partial blindness on the same side, or visual field, of each eye. The partial blindness is not related to a malfunction of the eye, but to the brain connection to the occipital lobes. This problem is also attributed to unilateral damage to the right or left occipital lobes. Often right- or left-homonymous hemianopsia occurs as a result of hemorrhage, tumor, or trauma. The result of this condition can be quite hazardous. For instance, a person attempting to ma-

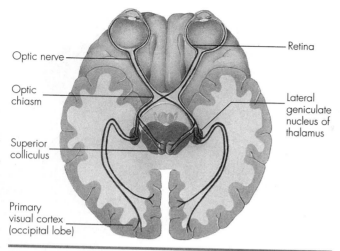

Optic nerve

Optic chiasm

Superior colliculus

Primary visual cortex (occipital lobe)

Retina

Lateral geniculate nucleus of thalamus

Figure 4.7 Visual pathways. The primary visual pathway partially crosses over at the optic chiasm. From there it routes through the thalamus to the primary visual cortex. (From James W. Kalat, *Biological Psychology,* 6th ed., Pacific Grove, CA: Brooks/Cole, 1998, p. 174, Figure 6.6)

neuver across a busy highway may not see traffic on the left side of his or her visual space. This condition is often compounded by other problems, for example, muscle weaknesses of the eyes that prevent a synchronized movement of the eyes across space.

If all visual information reaches the occipital lobes without disruption, the first area of processing corresponds to Brodmann's area 17, which is also known as area V1 (visual area 1) or the **striate cortex,** because of its striated or banded appearance. It lies in the most posterior aspect of the occipital lobes, but a major portion of it extends onto the medial portion of each hemisphere. Functionally, this area is the primary visual cortex (see Figure 4.9, p. 129). The **secondary association,** or **prestriate cortex,** is contiguous and corresponds to Brodmann's areas 18 and 19. Functional visual areas V2 through V5 are present in the prestriate cortex. Reseachers have used various terminology to label these areas; however, the labels of V1 to V5 represent the best correspondence between structure and function relationships. The responsibility for elementary visual interpretation lies in areas V1 to V5, which process primary features of visual information such as light wavelength, line ori-

entation, and features of shape. These represent the building blocks of the eventual composite image.

Area V1 covers a large cortical area and contains the *retinotopic map,* which maintains the same topographic relationships among visual elements as they are mapped on the retina. The primary purpose of this area is to assemble and relay information to prestriate areas of V3–V5. In a reciprocal fashion, V1 also receives back projections from information processed by secondary visual areas within the occipital lobes and seems to continue to play a role in maintaining spatial orientation between local bits of information. Area V2, which is closely related to V1, is also a visual preprocessing area, assembling and mapping information. Damage to area V1 causes cortical blindness, or hemianopia, in the opposite visual field. There are no reports on the effect of damage to V2 alone. If V2 is damaged, V1 is also likely involved, because V2 encircles V1 like a donut.

The remaining functional visual areas in the occipital lobes (areas V3–V5) are organized into four parallel systems having reciprocal integration (Zeki, 1992). The four systems include motion, color, dynamic form (without color), and color plus dynamic

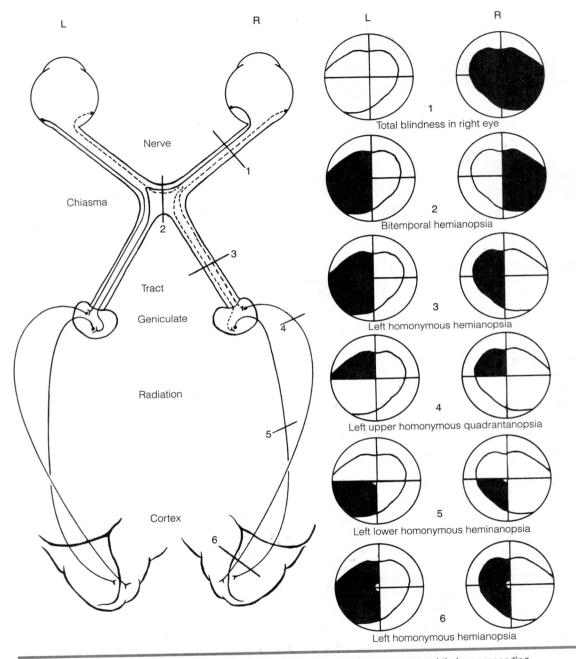

Figure 4.8   Visual field defects. The numbers indicate interruptions of visual pathways and their corresponding behavioral effects. In lesion 4 only the ventral temporal lobe fibers have been severed. In lesion 5 only the dorsal parietal lobe fibers have been severed. (From T. L. Peele, *The Neuroanatomical Basis for Clinical Neurology*, 3rd ed., McGraw-Hill, New York, 1977. Reproduced with permission of the McGraw-Hill Companies)

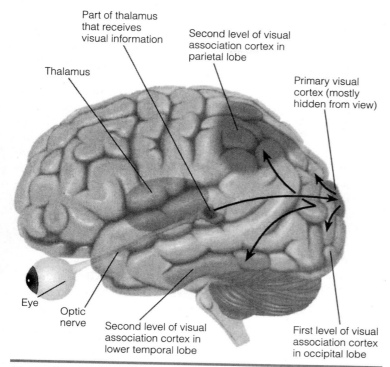

Part of thalamus
that receives
visual information

Second level of visual
association cortex in
parietal lobe

Thalamus

Primary visual
cortex (mostly
hidden from view)

Eye

Optic
nerve

Second level of visual
association cortex in
lower temporal lobe

First level of visual
association cortex
in occipital lobe

Figure 4.9   Cortical visual processing. Information relays from the thalamus to the primary visual cortex (Brodmann's area 17). Visual information passes to the secondary association cortex (Brodmann's areas 18 and 19). From there it is analyzed in parallel streams through the ventral temporal areas ("What") and the dorsal parietal areas ("Where"). (From N. Carlson and W. Buskist, *The Science of Behavior,* 5th ed., Boston: Allyn and Bacon, 1994, p. 201. Reprinted by permission)

form or shape. Area V3 appears specialized for dynamic form, or recognition of moving shapes, but does not code aspects of color. V4 is selective for the electromagnetic wavelengths of color, some aspects of line orientation, and form (color-and-form area). Area V5 (also called area MT) lies on the occipital-parietal juncture and receives input from a number of visual cortical areas. It contains visual motion detector cells, specialized to respond to direction of motion. Columns of cells within the layers of the cortex are responsive to different directions. Damage that targets individual components of these secondary processors leads to very specific deficits in visual behavior. For example, dam-

age to V4 results in **achromatopsia,** the complete loss of ability to detect color. People with this malady live in a black-and-white world. One man, a successful painter of abstract art, experienced this as very different from watching black-and-white TV. (This case is discussed at more length in Chapter 16.) Lesions to area V5 result in a very different problem, **akinetopsia,** or the specific inability to identify objects in motion (Zihl, 1995). Damage to areas V3–V5 can result in a general inability to perceive form. In this situation, patients may be able to make a perfect copy of a drawing, but are totally unable to understand that the connection of lines corresponds to a specific shape or object.

HIGHER VISUAL PROCESSING: OBJECT RECOGNITION AND SPATIAL LOCALIZATION

Neuroscientists have identified at least 20 areas of secondary or higher visual processing. However, for the purposes of this discussion we focus on (1) how visual elements are integrated so that the viewer appreciates the pieces of vision as a coherent whole, or object, and (2) how objects are localized within a spatial framework. These two streams of visual processing are well differentiated neuroanatomically, and are sometimes called the "what" system, or ventral processing stream, of object recognition, in contrast to the "where" system, or dorsal processing stream, of object localization (Mishkin, Ungerleider, & Macko, 1983) (see Figure 4.9). The two anatomically distinct areas of the ventral and dorsal streams are probably coordinated through the thalamus (Peterson, Robinson, & Morris, 1987). In the first part of this section, we discuss the behavioral functions associated with object recognition and object localization and give an overview of the ventral and dorsal processing streams.

One of the best ways to understand the differences between the two systems is to examine the types of disorders that occur if each system is damaged. The disorders evident at this higher level of visual processing and perceptual integration involve the interaction of vision with other sensory-perceptual systems and higher-order systems such as attention, memory, and consciousness. Each of these disorders could thus be included in the next chapter, on higher functional systems. However, because each presents a logical progression of the hierarchy of the visual system, we discuss them here. The problem of visual object recognition is best illustrated by the visual agnosias, and the problem of spatial location can be considered by examining neglect.

The "What" and "Where" Systems of Visual Processing

The ventral processing stream is perceptually specialized for higher aspects of visual object recognition. It helps the person connect the visual perception of shape and form with the representation of that object's meaning. The ventral processing stream contains interconnected regions from the occipital lobes to the temporal lobes. The left hemisphere's visual processing stream is more specific to recognizing symbolic objects such as letters and numbers. The left ventral occipital lobe shows increased blood flow when normal people process strings of letters (Snyder, Petersen, Fox, & Raichle, 1989). The right ventral system is more specific to the global recognition of objects and faces. Damage to this system can result in visual agnosia. We discuss the subtypes of visual agnosia (apperceptive and associate agnosia) in depth in the next section.

The dorsal processing stream is essential for visually localizing objects in space, and for appreciating the relative relationship of those objects to each other. Through reciprocal feedback to the motor system, this "where" system also helps in planning and coordinating motor movements. This stream of integrated structures connects the occipital to the parietal lobes. Disorders of this system contribute to right–left discrimination problems, constructional apraxia, and neglect.

Directional impairment, a form of spatial relations confusion, is usually referred to as a right–left discrimination problem. Patients with this kind of difficulty routinely get lost if left on their own, particularly in a new environment. We discuss apraxia (absence of action) in the section on motor systems. An inability to perform voluntary actions, constructional apraxia is the inability to perform actions that require three-dimensional movement, such as building a tower from blocks.

Disorders of the "What" System: Apperceptive and Associative Visual Agnosia

Agnosia (a term first coined by Sigmund Freud) is a literal absence (1) of knowing (*gnosis*) that can occur in any sensory domain. In the modality of vision, people with **visual object agnosia** may fail to recognize objects at all, or in milder cases, confuse objects that they observe from different angles or in different lighting conditions. The term **prosopagnosia** refers to the special case of inability to recognize people by their faces, even though the person can often recognize people by other means such as gait or tone of voice. Amazingly, people with visual agnosias can see. The disorder is less a pure sensory disorder than a higher perceptual disorder of "knowing." It is literally a "mind-blindness" or *Seelenblindheit*, so named by Munk in 1881 when he observed this phenomenon in dogs with bilateral occipital lesions (reviewed in Chapter 1). In *The Man Who Mistook His Wife for a Hat*, Oliver Sacks describes the affliction of Dr. P, a music teacher who can no longer recognize objects or people by sight. Presented with a red rose, Dr. P "took it like a botanist or morphologist given a specimen, not like a person given a flower. 'About six inches in length,' he commented. 'A convoluted red form with a linear green attachment.'" Dr. P was completely unable to name what he had in his hand until it was suggested to him to smell it. "'Beautiful!' he exclaimed. 'An early rose. What a heavenly smell!' He started to hum [the German tune] "*Die Rose, die Lilie . . .*" (Sacks, 1987, pp. 13–14). Dr. P's affliction was that he was visually unaware of the totality or *gestalt* of objects. He could see and identify form and color but could not combine these aspects into a higher sense of meaning that is a rose. His only visual reality was a mechanistic identification of features. This is typical of how visual agnosia primarily involves the processes necessary for object recognition or object meaning while leaving intact elementary visual processes. Also, Dr. P's agnosia, as is usually the case, was modality specific. Although his visual knowing was impaired, a higher sense of knowing was available through sense of smell. Dr. P also had no problem in recognizing people by their voices.

Cognitive neuropsychologists often differentiate between **apperceptive visual agnosia** and **associative visual agnosia.** The essential difficulty in apperceptive visual agnosia is *object perception,* or the inability to combine the individual aspects of visual information such as line, shape, color, and form together to form a "whole" percept. They seem to see in bits and pieces, like the proverbial blind men feeling the elephant. Their brains are not synthesizing the entire picture. Associative visual agnosics have difficulty to varying degrees in assigning *meaning* to an object. Even though they can, for instance, recognize differences in form between pictures of a pair of scissors and a paper punch by matching the scissors to a like pair in a display of office objects (with which an apperceptive agnosic would have difficulty), they have lost the link between the visual percept and the semantic meaning. In both cases, if shown a pair of scissors neither the apperceptive or the associative agnosic can correctly name "scissors." But although the associative agnosic can pick out a pair of scissors, she or he shows difficulties not only in naming but in explaining or demonstrating the use for scissors.

This distinction provides a useful conceptual framework and is employed here, but in practice the line between apperceptive and associative agnosias becomes cloudy partly because the brain damage likely to cause these problems is often widespread and overlapping.

Apperceptive Agnosia At first glance, those like Dr. P. with the apperceptive form of object agnosia may be thought blind, because they tend to take no apparent notice of objects and people in their vicinity. But on closer examination their sensory functions are clearly intact. Many people with this condition are aware that they can indeed see but have a problem correctly perceiving things. Curiously, others with apperceptive agnosia are strangely unaware of their condition. Only watching for a period of time might you catch them stepping over or avoiding objects. Awareness in this case is not an either/or phenomenon. Apperceptive agnosics may appear to disregard or show no concern for their problem until neuropsychological testing reveals it to them. For example, visual recognition tasks of the type shown in Figure 4.10 (p. 132), in which an object must be identified from fragments, is embedded, or is at an odd angle, are notoriously difficult. Apperceptive agnosics also have difficulty copying objects. Because they only "see" pieces, their drawings are likely to appear as a set of unconnected fragments focusing on the details rather than on the entire gestalt of the object.

The most common site of damage in apperceptive agnosia is the parietal-occipital area of the right hemisphere. Sudden insults to the brain are the most common cause, often from carbon monoxide poisoning, mercury intoxication, cardiac arrest, or stroke.

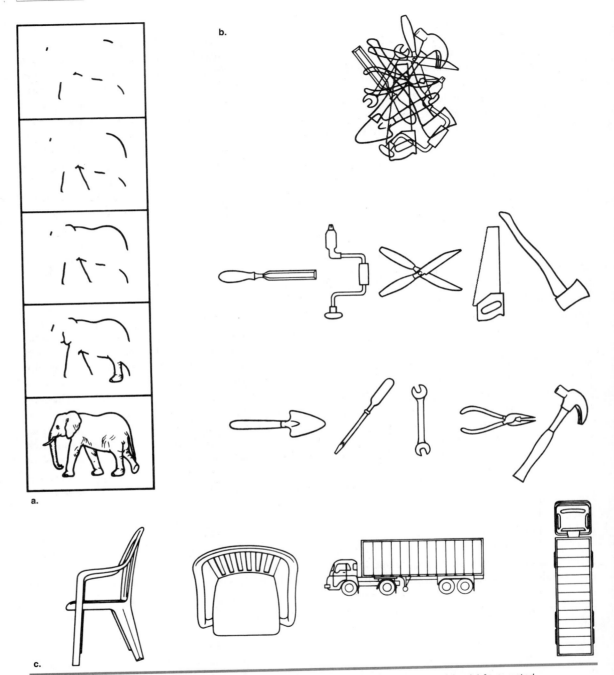

Figure 4.10 Tests for apperceptive agnosia. Apperceptive agnosics have difficulty recognizing (a) fragmented objects, (b) entangled object, and (c) objects seen from unusual views. (Modified from J. L. Bradshaw and J. B. Mattingly, *Clinical Neuropsychology: Behavioral and Brain Science,* San Diego: Academic Press, 1995, [a] p. 90, [b] p. 91, [c] p. 88. Reproduced by permission of the publisher. All rights of reproduction in any form reserved)

In these cases apperceptive agnosia does not usually occur in isolation without other visual-spatial impairment, because these brain insults are likely to affect large areas of the cortex. Some cases of apperceptive agnosia are caused by bilateral cortical atrophy. If both hemispheres are involved, then the patient may show **Ballint's syndrome,** which includes visual agnosia along with other visual-spatial difficulties such as misreaching and left-sided neglect.

Associative Agnosia   Associative agnosia is differentiated behaviorally from apperceptive agnosia in that the primary difficulty is a loss of knowledge of the semantic meaning of objects. Conceptually, the person can "recognize" objects at a perceptual level by picking them out, or correctly copying them, but perception breaks down at a higher level of meaning. For example, some people have very little apperceptive difficulty and can draw or copy pictures of objects in great detail but cannot name them (for example, see Rubens & Benson, 1971). As Figure 4.11 shows, after making an accurate rendition of a bird, the patient tentatively guessed it could be a "beach stump." This represents a pure form of associative agnosia, but many other patients also show aspects of apperceptive agnosia. For example, they may copy objects inconsistently, sometimes drawing them accurately and at other times making perceptual mistakes. However, whereas the perceptual mistakes of the apperceptive agnosic are likely to show inability to recognize the whole, the perceptual mistakes of the associative agnosic may show problems of either recognition of the whole or of an object's details.

The research on the neurocorrelates of associative agnosia is confusing. A lateralized left hemisphere parietal-occipital lesion may be enough to lose meaning, aspects of vision, although associative agnosia may arise in the presence of a unilateral right occipital lesion. Indeed, a number of structural areas may produce associative agnosia. Farah (1990) suggests the variety of sites that produce associative agnosia may lead to heterogeneous perceptual impairments. Because assigning meaning is such a high-level cortical process, different lesion sites producing a similar effect also speaks to the complexity of the perceptual-meaning system. We would venture, as have others,

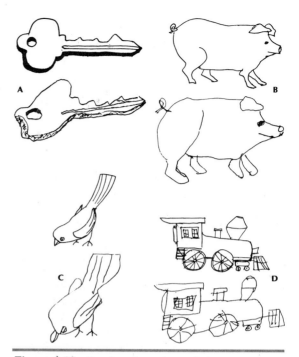

Figure 4.11   Drawings from an associative visual agnosic. These pictures were accurately drawn but mislabeled: (a) "I still don't know"; (b) "Could be a dog or any other animal"; (c) "Could be a beach stump"; (d) "A wagon or a car of some kind. The larger vehicle is being pulled by the smaller one." (From Bauer, R. M., "Agnosia." In Heilman & Valenstein, *Clinical Neuropsychology* (1993), Oxford University Press)

that in general the left hemisphere assigns meaning, whereas the right hemisphere governs the global aspects of perceptual integration.

As stated earlier, many patients show both apperceptive and associative aspects to their visual agnosia. For example, one artist who suffered a stroke resulting in bilateral medial occipital damage could name some objects but not others. Those he could name, he could also draw well. But those he didn't recognize, he could only mechanistically copy, feature by feature, first a square, then a circle, then connecting lines, without any inkling of what they represented (Wapner, Judd, & Gardner, 1978). In sum, the differentiation between apperceptive and associative agnosia is useful for descriptive and conceptual understanding, but does not correspond to strict anatomic correlates that can be readily differentiated or dissociated.

Disorder of the "Where" System: Neglect

Certain types of brain damage can alter body experience. Damage to the right parietal-occipital or inferior parietal area is the most common site of damage for an odd type of inattention termed unilateral neglect, or simply neglect. (*Unilateral spatial neglect* has other aliases, such as *contralesional neglect, hemineglect, visuospatial* or *hemispatial agnosia,* and *visuospatial* or *hemispatial inattention.*) People with neglect lose conscious awareness of an aspect of personal space despite adequately functioning sensory and motor systems. Behaviorally, this problem may first look like the result of a right hemisphere stroke or lesion affecting the motor and somatosensory strips on the contralesional side. The left limbs appear useless and hang limply. On closer examination, the arm or leg can clearly move and feel touch or pain—they are simply being ignored by the conscious mind. This failure of awareness extends beyond the body to the entire left hemispace from the perspective of the afflicted person. It is not unusual for people with neglect to collide with objects and people on their left sides. Also, when reading they may leave out the left side of words or pages. Their copied drawings focus on the right side of pictures. In one respect, neglect can be thought of as a forgetting or lack of conscious attention to the left side, but even more so—it is as if awareness is being *pulled* to the right. When trying to navigate, neglect patients frequently veer rightward and end up traveling in circles. The case study in Neuropsychology in Action 4.2 gives an in-depth illustration of the behavioral manifestations of unilateral neglect. Although not in this case, many people with neglect think that the left-sided part of their body does not belong to them. Protesting that it belongs to someone else, they may fail to dress half of the body, put makeup on only one side of the face, or simply treat the neglected parts as objects with no personal meaning. What are the mechanisms that disable body and spatial awareness? We will return to this question after considering the neuropathological and clinical presentation of neglect.

Neuropathology of Neglect   The classic picture of unilateral neglect that we have been discussing is most likely to occur with lesions in the right inferior parietal lobe or generally in the posterior regions of the cortex. As mentioned, neglect cannot be solely attributed to sensory processing deficits, implying that lesions in the somatosensory strip are not enough to produce neglect. Neglect can also appear with other right hemisphere lesions, and much less frequently, with left hemisphere lesions. Other right hemisphere locations reported to produce neglect include a variety of subcortical structures, the majority implicating the thalamus. Left-hemisphere lesions may also include other than parietal cortical areas.

Classic neglect produces an abrupt alteration of consciousness most commonly occurring as a result of a right parietal stroke, but sometimes coinciding with a traumatic brain injury. In any case the manifestation is typically sudden and rarely seen in slow-growing tumors or disease processes. Temporary and reversible neglect may also occur in conjunction with seizures, electroconvulsive therapy, and intracarotid sodium amytal testing (Wada testing) (see Bradshaw & Mattingly, 1995). Neglect may also stand out against the background of widespread right hemisphere damage. In this instance there are accompanying motor, sensory, or attentional problems. For example, a variety of neglect-type problems are associated with motor weakness. In these cases awareness of left-sided stimuli may be less impaired, but neglect-type symptoms become evident with the inability to perform or sustain motor acts on the side contralateral to the lesion (see Heilman, Watson, & Valenstein, 1993). If we include all the subtypes and derivations, we can best conceptualize neglect as a syndrome or general classification for a number of related problems. However, for this discussion we restrict ourselves to classical unilateral spatial neglect, caused by right hemisphere damage, which is the best example of the neglect phenomenon.

Clinical Presentation   In clinically evaluating cases of unilateral neglect, neuropsychologists must disentangle the contributions of spatial, motor, and attentional factors. This can only be done in a relative fashion, because each of these systems contribute a

Neuropsychology in Action 4.2

Case Study: Neglect

by Mary Spiers

One of the first cases of pure spatial neglect was published by Paterson and Zangwill in 1944. Their patient was a healthy 39-year-old right-handed man who, because of an explosion, was hit by a projectile steel nut that penetrated his skull in the right parietal occipital area. "Stereoscopic X-rays of the skull (28.9.43) showed a metallic foreign body consisting of a hexagonal nut about 1 in. in diameter with a short length of screw-headed bolt projecting from its upper lateral surface" (pp. 335–336). "The upper borders of the supramarginal and angular gyri on the right side were damaged on the surface and their deeper connection interrupted by the in-driven bone fragments to a depth of just over 1 in. The lesion was circumscribed and there was minimal contusional damage" (p. 337). The resultant difficulties, as you would expect, were largely confined to spatial and visual-perceptual functions. This man could perceptually recognize objects, identify colors, and discriminate right and left. He also had no problems in spatial depth perception and size con-

stancy. But the patient himself alerted his doctors that he was having trouble finding his way through the hallways on the way to the bathroom and he was having trouble reading the time. He said he had to read each hand of the clock separately and then figure out the time. Staff observed him to collide "with objects on his left which he had clearly perceived a few moments before. He was liable at table to knock over dishes on his left-hand side and occasionally missed food on the left of his plate. He commonly failed to attend to the left-hand page in turning the pages of a book and reading lines of disconnected words commonly omitted the first word or two" (p. 339). On neuropsychological testing, when asked to draw, his figures showed a "piecemeal perception" typical of right hemisphere spatial problems. Interestingly, he could slowly recognize objects placed in his left visual field but if two designs were presented simultaneously to the right and left visual fields, he did not acknowledge the left-sided design. In setting the time on a clock, he often

transposed the minute hand from the left- to the right-hand side. In a pointing task, the authors arranged objects around the patient in a semicircle. "He was instructed to point to each object in turn. With eyes open no errors were made. With his eyes closed, on the other hand, there was at once a general shift toward the right-hand side. Thus when asked to point to the object on his extreme left the patient often pointed straight ahead" (p. 339). Unlike other cases of neglect, this man did not neglect the left side of his own body, only his extrapersonal space.

This case presents an interesting problem of consciousness. How can this loss of awareness be explained? On one level, the patient was aware of the fact that he now disregarded the left side of space. This shows some insight into his problem. But on another level, no force of will could coax a full knowing of his left-sided spatial world (also see Paterson & Zangwill, 1944).

portion to a sense of body and spatial consciousness. For example, although investigators agree that a functioning attentional system is crucial to spatial awareness, unilateral neglect and severe inattention can be differentiated. With both problems there can be a failure to detect an object, such as an apple, that is placed in the left visual field. However, the inattentive person becomes aware of the apple if forced to orient to it, whereas the person with neglect may continue to insist that nothing is there. Neglect is also dissociable from visual field defects such as hemianop-

sia, in which the person visually explores the left side of space (Hornak, 1992). Neglect may look similar to visual problems, but is actually a problem at a much higher level of integration.

Because neglect is so obviously out of the range of ordinary experience, measures to test for it do not rely on norms, but rather on pathognomic signs. For example, we do not expect neglect to be evenly distributed in the population in the form of a bell-shaped curve, with only a few of us having no neglect, many of us having moderate neglect, and a few of us having profound neglect. Instead, we expect all people with normally functioning brains to be free of neglect. Therefore the detection of neglect and neglectlike symptoms is fairly straightforward by observing per-formance on tasks such as drawings and line bisec-tion tasks. Figure 4.12 shows several clinical exam-ples of neuropsychological tasks performed by peo-ple with neglect. Notice that in the drawings the left

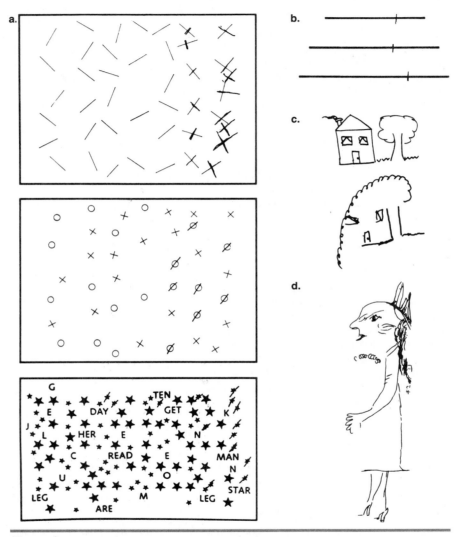

Figure 4.12   Performance of a patient with left neglect. (a) Three cancellation tasks in which the left side of the page has been neglected. (b) A line bisection task that veers to the right of midpoint. (c) A copy of a house that is distorted on the right side. (d) Spontaneous drawing of a woman. (From J. L. Bradshaw and J. B. Mattingly, *Clinical Neuropsychology: Behavioral and Brain Science,* San Diego: Academic Press, 1995, p. 128. Reproduced by permission of the publisher. All rights of reproduction in any form reserved)

side of the picture may be left out, sparse, or grossly distorted. In the line bisection and line cancellation tasks, the midpoint shifts to the right, leaving the left side of the line or the page empty.

It is clear that unilateral neglect patients do not consciously acknowledge stimuli in the left side of space. But does perception or a tacit recognition at an unconscious level exist? Clinical investigations suggest that it does. In an interesting series of studies, Vallar and his colleagues (Vallar, Sandroni, Rusconi, & Barbieri, 1991) tested autonomic responses such as galvanic skin conductance and brain response via evoked potentials. In each case the patients with unilateral left-sided neglect failed to consciously recognize the presence of a stimulus presented to the right side, although autonomic testing revealed the patients were processing the stimulus implicitly at a preconscious level, without reaching awareness. Some clinical studies also suggest that people with neglect may implicitly process at a higher level, indicating acknowledgment of meaning or semantic awareness. In one of the first case studies to suggest implicit awareness in neglect, Marshall and Halligan (1988) gave their patient two pictures of a house, identical except for the fact that in one, the left side of the house was obviously burning. She did not acknowledge any discrepancies between the two houses when asked to describe the pictures, nor did she say they were different when forced to make a same–different choice. Curiously, however, when asked which house she would prefer to live in, she consistently chose the picture of the house that wasn't burning, although she could not explain or give reasons for her choice. It is as though, from her perspective, the only explanation she could give relied on an intuitive sense. Although not all neglect patients show this preservation of semantic knowledge (some actually chose the burning house; see Bisiach & Rusconi, 1990), studies using a variety of methodologies confirm that higher-order processing of various types is possible in some patients with neglect (see Bradshaw & Mattingly, 1995).

Interestingly, the behavior of left unilateral neglect usually resolves somewhat over time if the damaged area remains stable. Afflicted people gradually begin to acknowledge stimuli on the left side of their bodily space. Tests of tactile recognition, in which the researcher touches one hand or the other while the patient is blindfolded, show that he or she is recognizing both hands. However, when both hands are touched at the same time in a specific test of double simultaneous stimulation, residual neglect is often evident in that the patient again suppresses or extinguishes perception of the left hand.

Neglect, as can be imagined, is notoriously difficult to treat in the beginning stages. Patients who don't acknowledge their problem and who may believe their left side does not even belong to them are not motivated to pay attention to their left side. Rehabilitation methods often try to direct attention to the neglected side. Therapists may use various methods such as forcing attention to the left side via gradual movement of objects to the left, or even through the use of prism glasses. These methods do meet with some success but often do not generalize to daily life.

Theories of Neglect There are two primary issues in conceptualizing neglect. The first is understanding the asymmetrical presentation of neglect between the two hemispheres. Why is neglect more prevalent with right hemisphere lesions? Any theory of neglect must explain why the overwhelming majority of cases show left-sided neglect, and why right-sided neglect is so rare. The second issue relates to the higher-order or "conscious" processing problem that is neglect. If neglect is thought of as a network problem rather than as a dysfunction of an individual system, it is easier to make sense of the variety of lesion sites that may produce neglect.

Research has established that the right hemisphere is more specialized for global spatial processing, whereas the left hemisphere has a propensity for decoding specific spatial features. Because the right hemisphere, and particularly the right parietal lobe, plays a role in understanding the gestalt or totality of space, disruptions here are more likely to upset global spatial awareness. Also, the right hemisphere plays a larger role in arousal and attentional levels, which are prime factors in many explanatory models of neglect. However, each of these problems can occur in isolation without the patient losing consciousness of the left side of space. As with the man described in Neuropsychology in Action 4.2, no force of will could coax a "knowing" of his spatial world on the left. Interestingly, it appears that patients may shift their "spatial axis" to the right so that midline is pulled or repositioned within the right side of space relative to the body (Mattingly, 1996). Marcel Kinsbourne (1993) has postulated that this strong rightward orientation is less a function of right hemisphere dysfunction per se than a release of inhibition that lets the left hemisphere assert dominance in the presence of a now weakened right hemisphere. Perhaps some of the prime areas damaged, rendering the right hemisphere spatially ineffective, are locations within the right parietal lobe having to do with personal spatial frames of reference. Body position with respect to space is always egocentric, although people may have multiple frames with respect to bodies, heads, or position in relation to environment. Animal studies support the contention that there are distinct neuronal centers for these spatial frames within the right parietal cortex (for example, see Anderson, Snyder, Li, & Stricanne, 1993).

Do these findings explain why the midline shift in neglect is nearly always to the right? Bradshaw and Mattingly (1995) suggest that each hemisphere plays a specific role in spatial body position processing. The left hemisphere focuses on features and is strongly rightward oriented. The right hemisphere takes a "global view." Normally the two hemispheres hold each other in balance, but when certain spatial positioning aspects of the right hemisphere are damaged, the left hemisphere becomes overbearing, forcing a reorientation to the right side of space. According to this view, if damage to the left parietal lobe produces no corresponding leftward shift because the spatial concerns of the left hemisphere are more feature oriented and language focused, resulting in a "no specialized spatial position" sense within the left parietal lobes. If right neglect does occur, they suggest, along with others (such as Ogden, 1985), that the focus of the left hemisphere lesion would be anterior to the parietal lobes. Unfortunately, partly owing to the rarity of occurrence, no research has explained the mechanisms of right-sided neglect.

Understanding neglect is not only a problem of dominance and asymmetry, it is also an issue of conceptualizing the problem as a higher-order network processing phenomenon. The fact that unilateral neglect can occur with other nonparietal foci of damage is partial testament to this claim. We mentioned earler that the region of the right inferior parietal lobe is the area most commonly damaged in cases of left unilateral neglect. As in other disorders discussed throughout this book, however, absence of function associated with a lesion does not necessarily imply that the lesioned area "contains" the function. Just as the hippocampus does not "contain" or store memory, but is one of the most crucial links in memory processing and consolidation, the right inferior parietal lobe does not in itself contain "body mindfulness" but may be a crucial link. Neuroanatomically, left unilateral neglect also occurs with damage to a variety of subcortical structures, most notably the thalamus (see Bradshaw & Mattingly, 1995). It is reasonable to speculate that neglect results from a disconnection in higher-order processing that involves the coordination of many second-order systems such as visual processing, attention, memory, and possibly others.

A number of theories attempt to provide models for unilateral neglect. They are beyond the scope of this overview, and excellent reviews exist elsewhere (for example, see Bradshaw & Mattingly, 1995). Suffice it to say that most models describe the process of body and hemispace cognition as including visual-perceptual processes, attention, and motor action. Mesulam's neural network model (for example, see 1985b, 1990) is closely tied to neuroanatomic functioning. He identifies three major functional areas that must interact for the body–space system to work normally. Each of these areas corresponds to a cortical site. The parietal lobes control perceptual processing, the premotor and prefrontal cortices mediate exploratory-motor behavior, and the cingulate gyrus directs motivation. In turn, subcortical structures probably coordinate the orchestration of all three areas. The reticular formation directs arousal, and the thalamus (particularly the pulvinar of the thalamus) is postulated to focus and guide attention between spatial locations.

Summary—The visual processing system is indeed the most complex of the sensory systems. Each feature discussed here builds to the next level. The primary visual system, which serves as a "feature analyzer," builds to the higher-order systems of object recognition and spatial localization. Disorders such as visual agnosia and neglect provide good examples of how each of these systems may malfunction. However, with vision there is much reciprocal networking between parallel systems, so what appears hierarchical may not be entirely so. At this point brain science has uncovered much of the structure and many of the functions of the vision road map through the brain. There is also much work to be done in understanding how the brain accommodates to varying visual experiences that represent the same precept. However, brain science is still struggling with how high-level integration of the fragmentary components of visual processing occurs, especially in visual disorders, in which integration may be a product of systems beyond the visual system.

Auditory and Language Processing

The human auditory system is one of the most important sensory systems, because it is the pathway to language, a uniquely human development. In this section we examine the brain's control of auditory processing, speech, and language by exploring the brain structures believed to be principal in language functioning. Because no animal models of language exist, much knowledge of the neuropsychology of language links closely to knowledge about the behavioral effects of aphasia subtypes. Reliance on brain-damaged patients to delineate systems can be tricky because lesions may not indicate site of damage, and many aphasics are stroke patients with a fairly wide area of damage.

PRIMARY AUDITORY PROCESSING

Humans can detect a wide range of sound from the 30 Hz range to the 20,000 Hz range. Difficulties in detecting the features of sound, such as how long a vowel versus a consonant sound might resonate, can result in higher-level language disturbance. One theory of autism considers the idea that autistic people may not be tuned in to the frequency of human speech, but instead have a propensity for lower-frequency environmental sounds such as those made by machines. If human speech is an aversive and even fear-producing noise, then there would be a withdrawal from the sound of human speech. Many difficulties can emerge if the primary building blocks of sound detection and recognition, discussed in this section, are not intact.

The auditory system contains mechanical receptors designed to detect sound frequency. These hair-like receptors are located in the fluid of the long, coiled, snail-like *cochlea* of the inner ear. As the mechanical mechanisms of the middle ear respond to external sound waves they cause vibrations in the fluid of the inner ear, thus vibrating the hairs of the auditory receptors. These receptors synapse with the auditory nerve. The auditory nerve from each ear projects ipsilaterally to the cochlear nuclei of the medulla. From there each pathway branches to project auditory information to both the ipsilateral and contralateral superior olivary nuclei of the medulla. In this way, the auditory system differs from the visual system in that each hemisphere receives input from both ears, resulting in bilateral representation of sound. This may help the person localize sound in space. The auditory pathways then course through the lower brain stem and ascend through the thalamus, where they are projected to the primary auditory cortex (see Figure 4.13).

The primary auditory cortex of each hemisphere lies deep within the temporal lobe, largely on the medial aspect of the superior temporal gyrus, within the valley of the lateral fissure. This area is commonly termed Heschl's gyrus and corresponds to Brodmann's area 41. As mentioned in Chapter 3, Heschl's area is often larger in the right hemisphere, sometimes consisting of two gyri to the left's one. This cortical area processes the "fragments" of sound, much as the visual system processes individual visual stimuli. The primary auditory cortex is organized into frequency-specific bands that parallel the layout of auditory

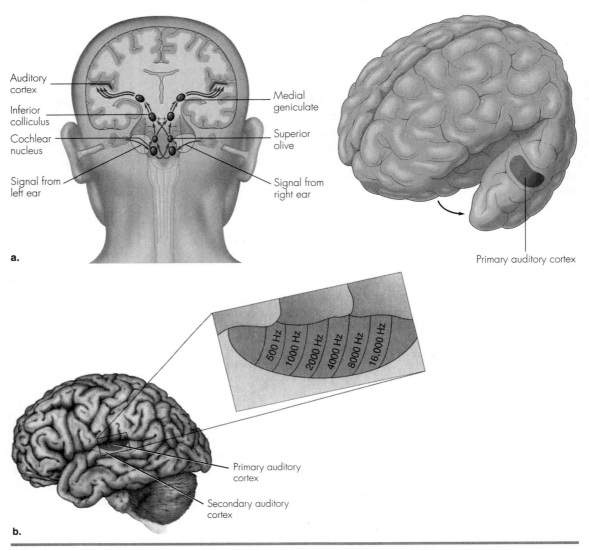

Figure 4.13   Pathway from the ear to the primary auditory cortex. (a) Each ear projects to the ipsilateral cochlea and then projects to the primary auditory cortex in both hemispheres. (b) The primary auditory cortex is organized according to a tonotopic frequency map. ([a] From James W. Kalat, *Biological Psychology,* 6th ed., Pacific Grove, CA: Brooks/Cole, 1998, p. 184, Figure 7.6; [b] modified from M. F. Bear, B. W. Connors, & M. A. Paradiso, *Neuroscience: Exploring the Brain,* Baltimore: Williams & Wilkins, 1996, p. 303, Figure 11.28)

frequency ranges mapped on the cochlea (see Figure 4.13). In this way a **tonotopic map** projects onto the auditory cortex, similar to the retinopic mapping of the visual system. Because the cortical bands can respond to multiple frequencies, there is no strict one-to-one correspondence, but bands are more attuned to certain frequencies than others. The primary auditory cortex processes several elements of sound. In addition to frequency, the features of sound include loudness, timbre, duration, and change.

HIGHER AUDITORY PROCESSING: SPEECH AND LANGUAGE

Speaking requires the ability to differentiate between speech sounds, or phonemes, such as vowels and consonants. For example, in French the brain must hear the fine distinctions between the pronunciation of *tu* and *tous,* the sounds of which are not differentiated in English and only heard as *too.* Vowels have a slightly different frequency from consonants, and different consonants are differentiated from each other. Speech also requires the ability to produce intelligible speech output. Learning a language, as anyone who has tried to master a second language knows, involves much more than being able to understand and articulate words in a spoken fashion. Language also requires putting meaning to word fragments (morphemes), words and groups of words (semantics). Another major requirement of language is knowledge of its syntax or grammatical rules. This requires learning information regarding subject–verb agreement (for example, "girls run"), how to use articles and propositions (for example, *the, to, but, if, and*), and how to put strings of words together to make meaningful sentences.

After the primary auditory cortex processes sound features, they are integrated into understandable speech sounds in the secondary auditory processing area commonly known as **Wernicke's area.** Wernicke's area lies on the posterior aspect of the superior temporal gyrus (see Figures 4.13 and 4.14). It includes the secondary auditory cortex and does not technically involve the adjacent primary auditory cortex (Heschl's gyrus). The secondary auditory processing area serves to connect sound from the primary auditory areas to word meaning stored in the cortex. This is an intermediate step to the full understanding of language. Additional cortical processing areas are required to integrate the comprehension of individual words into grammatically correct phrases and sentences, and to link spoken words with the written symbols of language necessary for reading comprehension. The supramarginal and angular gyri of the inferior parietal lobes are contiguous to Wernicke's area, and the two are closely integrated. These higher association areas serve to bring together visual and spatial information from the occipital and parietal lobes with auditory information. The angular gyrus plays a role in reading comprehension by matching words and word sounds (phonemes such as the sound of /ba/) to written symbols of language (graphemes such as *b*).

Damage to the left hemisphere auditory processing areas results in the partial or total inability to decipher spoken words. This condition is known as **receptive** or **Wernicke's aphasia.** However, those with receptive aphasia can often still recognize the emotional tone of language, because the speaker's intent such as anger, sarcasm, or humor is processed as voice intonation. Conversely, right hemisphere damage has the opposite effect: The patient accepts words at face value, but loses the nuances of jokes and emotional intention. Another hallmark of right hemisphere damage is impaired harmonic and melodic ability. The ability to appreciate musical tunes may be completely wiped out. As an example of a problem with recognition of environmental sounds, one patient with a right hemisphere auditory processing deficit repeatedly had to have starters replaced in her car. She could no longer discriminate the difference in sound between the sound of the starter engaging and the sound of the engine turning over. Speech understanding, therefore, conveys word analysis as well as emotional intentions, through tone of voice, pitch, intensity and rhythm.

Expressive speech links to the **frontal operculum** (Broca's area), located in the left frontal lobe on the posterior portion of the third frontal gyrus (the inferior frontal gyrus). This area is adjacent to the facial area of the motor cortex. The inferior frontal gyrus is a premotor area of the frontal lobes and so is concerned with aspects of speech planning prior to output coordinated by the nearby motor strip. In addition to mediating the fluency of speech, Broca's area plays a role in the grammatical and syntactical arrangement of words. Wernicke's and Broca's areas are linked by a band of white matter fibers called the *arcuate fasciculus.* This allows for close communication between the two areas in expressive output. Words, whether from external sources or from the self, are picked out for meaning in Wernicke's area, and in parallel, the syntax of the phrase is constructed in Broca's area. This is possible because the arcuate

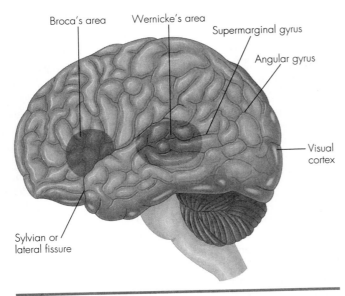

Broca's area   Wernicke's area
Supermarginal gyrus
Angular gyrus
Visual cortex
Sylvian or lateral fissure

Figure 4.14   Major cortical language areas. In most people the left frontal operculum, or Broca's area is specialized for speech production, whereas Wernicke's area is specialized for speech comprehension. (From James W. Kalat, *Biological Psychology*, 6th ed., Pacific Grove, CA: Brooks/Cole, 1998, p. 390, Figure 14.13)

fasciculus permits reciprocal interaction between the two areas (Yeterian & Van Hoesen, 1978). This interaction also makes logical sense, because syntax depends on the words used and the words selected also depend on the emerging syntax of the sentence (Bradshaw & Mattingly, 1995).

The basal ganglia and the thalamus have also been implicated in language functioning via their participation in a cortico-striato-pallido-thalamo-cortical loop (see Crosson, 1992). This loop, or perhaps set of loops, connects the language centers of the cortex to the putamen and caudate nucleus of the striatum, to the globus pallidus, to specific nuclei in the thalamus, and back to the cortical language centers. The current thinking regarding the function of these loops is that they play a role in regulating language, more so in initiating language production than in constructing speech content (Crosson, 1992).

As we discussed in Chapter 3, one hemisphere, usually the left, is dominant for speech. This means that the left cerebral cortex preferentially processes speech sounds, whereas the right processes nonspeech sounds. Not surprisingly, the functional dominance of the left hemisphere for speech corresponds to preferential treatment for speech sound processing in the larger planum temporale of the left hemisphere. Following analysis of sound features, secondary auditory information, such as phonemes, is integrated in the planum temporale, in the temporal area adjacent to the primary auditory cortex (Brodmann's area 42). Although sound from each ear projects bilaterally, there is an opposite hemisphere advantage, in this case meaning the left hemisphere preferentially processes sound from the right ear. Because the left hemisphere shows a preference for analyzing speech in most people, speech sounds processed through the right ear will be understood faster and more accurately than speech sounds processed through the left ear.

The left hemisphere also has a propensity for rhythm of both speech and music as it codes for the sequence of sounds. To check your left hemisphere dominance for rhythm, try keeping a metronome-like beat with your left hand and beat out the rhythm of a familiar tune, such as *Jingle Bells,* with your right hand. Most people find this easy if their left hemisphere, which controls their right hand, is dominant for rhythm. After doing this, try reversing what each hand is doing (right keeps the beat, and left taps out the rhythm) and see if you have more or less difficulty. The secondary auditory cortex of the right hemisphere, by contrast, is specific for aspects of tonality, including the melody of music and the intonation of speech, which is commonly referred to as *speech prosody.* The right hemisphere is adept at recognizing the relationship between simultaneous sounds such as the harmony of chords, or the musical interval between notes. It also shows an advantage for recognizing nonspeech or environmental sounds such as those made by machines and cars as well as animals, birds, the pounding ocean surf, or a babbling creek.

The brain's asymmetry for language processing and production is an extension of speech processing. The left hemisphere specializes in processing word sounds, or morphemes; semantics; and the grammatical rules of language. The right hemisphere, long thought to be "mute," plays a role in the emotional intention of both vocalization and understanding. The right hemisphere may have no speech or understanding of grammatical rules; however, a number of people, and more women than men, have some bilateral representation of speech. The right hemisphere, is nonetheless, capable of considerable comprehension and expression. Although frank aphasia is rare after right hemisphere strokes, there can be linguistic impairments. These include a deficit in comprehending tone and voice, producing similar emotional tone, and understanding metaphors and jokes. We once examined a male adult patient who had undergone a complete left hemispherectomy. Although he was severely aphasic, he could communicate somewhat using "grunts." He was also able to curse, possibly because such communication is more emotional in nature and therefore, in part, controlled by the right hemisphere.

In sum, the complexity of speech and language necessitates specific brain systems, which in most people are lateralized. Beyond the discrete cortical components controlling auditory reception (auditory cortexes and Wernicke's area) and auditory speech production (Broca's area and motor cortex), language requires thought, and therefore extensive interconnections to higher-order planning and memory centers. The supermarginal gyrus and the angular gyrus of the parietal lobes are also important to integrating verbal aspects of language with the visual symbolic components involved in reading. Subcortical neural connections, including portions of the basal ganglia and the thalamus also play a role in language. Finally, cerebral lateralization exists for various language functions.

APHASIA: A BREAKDOWN OF LANGUAGE

Aphasia is a disturbance of language usage or comprehension. It may impair the power to speak, write, read, gesture, or to comprehend spoken, written, or gestured language. Aphasia is a disturbance connecting speaking to thinking and so is differentiated from purely mechanical disorders of speech such as **dysarthria** or **speech apraxia** caused by paralysis or incoordination of the musculature of the mouth or vocal apparatus. Aphasic disorders also do not include pure mutism, disturbances of language caused by severe intellectual impairment or loss of sensory input (such as deafness or inability to see words). Aphasias are most frequently caused by vascular disorders such as stroke, or by tumor or brain trauma. Although cortical damage to the frontal and temporal areas of the left hemisphere causes most aphasias, damage to subcortical structures of the basal ganglia (specifically the corpus striatum) and the thalamus has also produced aphasia.

The two major types of aphasia are commonly referred to as Broca's aphasia and Wernicke's aphasia. Other classifications, subtypes, and combinations exist that may contain slightly different features or a mixture of some features of these two types (see Table 4.4 on p. 144). In seeing aphasia patients, it is quickly evident that very few patients fit neatly into one classification or the other. This is not surprising, because brain lesions, and pre-existing brain anatomy for language varies among individuals, most notably between men and women. Many clinicians find it most useful to describe the features of the aphasia in behavioral terms, describing aphasia according to degree of fluency and the nature of the expressive and receptive problems involved. **Fluent aphasia** is characterized by fluent spontaneous speech with normal articulation and rhythm, or fluency in the repetition of words, phrases, or sentences. **Nonfluent aphasia** is difficulty in the flow of articulation, so that speech becomes broken or halting. **Expressive aphasia** is a disorder of speech output. **Receptive aphasia** implies a difficulty in auditory comprehension.

Often patients experience not only a loss of spoken language, but also a loss of written language and reading comprehension. Writing is one of the most complex of language abilities. If it is disturbed as a result of impairment of the limb to produce letters and words, the disturbance is not thought to be a disorder of language. Rather, words, letters, or numbers may appear foreign or incomprehensible because of an inability to recall the form of letters. Attempts at writing may be filled with real or imagined letters that make no sense to others. With time and training, the person may be able to understand simple written language—for example, single words such as *bath* or *food*—but not more complex written language, such as sentences or paragraphs. The extent of

the recovery in this and other areas largely depends on the degree of damage. Because reading comprehension is based on prior mastery of auditory language, deficits in reading (alexia) often accompany deficits in auditory comprehension. As with auditory defects, impairment in visual comprehension may involve a deficit in recognizing individual letters or words as being letters or words, or an impairment in attaching the correct meaning to the symbols written on a page. Deficits in writing are most often associated with lesions to the angular gyrus, a cortical association area that provides cross-modal integration of visual, tactile, and verbal information. Reading deficits (alexia) are frequently related to lesions of the left fusiform and lingual areas.

Broca's Aphasia

Broca's aphasia is an expressive, nonfluent aphasia characterized by difficulties in speech production but relatively adequate auditory verbal comprehension, as evidenced by the ability to follow spoken commands (such as "point to the cup"). There are many forms of disorders of production, which can range from an inability to form words, to an inability to place words together to form a spoken or written sentence. In simple expressive aphasia, the person knows

Table 4.4	*Aphasia Types*			
	Fluency, Content	**Repetition of Speech**	**Comprehension of Speech**	**Reading and Writing**
BROCA'S	Confluent, agrammatical	Impaired	Normal	Agrammatical, misspelling
WERNICKE'S	Normal, word salad	Abnormal	Poor	Inaccuracies
CONDUCTION	Normal fluency, phonemic errors	Abnormal	Relatively intact	Abnormal
TRANSCORTICAL MOTOR	Halting	Fluent	Normal	Reading normal Writing impaired
TRANSCORTICAL SENSORY	Normal	Normal	Poor	Inaccuracies
ANOMIC	Normal fluency, word-finding errors	Normal	Normal	Normal
GLOBAL APHASIA	Abnormal	Abnormal	Abnormal	Abnormal

what he or she wants to say, but cannot find the words to say it. It's like continually experiencing a situation in which the word or words are on the tip of the tongue, but not quite connected to thought. In mild cases of **anomia,** or word-finding difficulties, only a word or two here and there is lost, and the communication can proceed quite normally. In more severe cases, most or all words can be lost. This problem in word finding is one that virtually all expressive aphasics suffer. Even when the person produces words, he or she takes longer than normal to do so. Difficulty in finding a word often results in the person's deliberately "talking around" a word that approximates the intended idea when he or she cannot find the intended word. For example, an aphasic might say, "I looked through that long pipe thing at the stars" (that is, a telescope). Aphasics may also make phonetic, or like-sounding errors such as "I looked through that telephone at the stars" or semantic meaning–related errors such as "I looked through that barometer at the stars."

Another problem experienced by many Broca's aphasics is one of **articulation,** or the ability to form phonetic sounds of vowels and consonants, which then are placed in different combinations to form words and sentences. People with severe deficits in articulating words often cannot produce simple sounds, even by imitation. If the deficit in articulation is related to a motor impairment of the mouth, tongue, larynx, or pharynx, then it is not aphasia. The aphasic impairment is marked by the person's confusion or deficit in choosing the desired sound from all those available in his or her repertoire. This sometimes results in unintended strange-sounding syllables, words, or phrases (phonemic paraphasias) during the effort to speak, or in noises being produced rather than language. Those with Broca's aphasia may also show poor pronunciation and inappropriate speech rhythm, manifested by dysarthria, stuttering, and effortful speech.

Broca's aphasia most commonly occurs with lesions to the frontal operculum, but typically also includes lesions to the motor cortex (precentral gyrus or motor strip) and underlying white matter and subcortical structures of the basal ganglia. Aphasia seems to resolve quickly if the frontal operculum is the only structure involved, but tends to be more persistent the more surrounding structures are damaged (Bradshaw & Mattingly, 1995).

Wernicke's Aphasia

Wernicke's aphasia is a receptive, fluent aphasia. This implies reduced comprehension of spoken language with the continued ability to produce speech. If you stop to imagine this odd situation, you can see that Wernicke's aphasics, in addition to not understanding what others say, may not be able to understand what they themselves are saying. This problem contributes to speaking in the form of a **word salad** of unconnected words and word sounds. This feature of Wernicke's aphasia is a deficit in putting words together in proper grammatical and syntactical form. This condition, more formally known as **paragrammatism** or **extended paraphasia,** refers to running speech that is logically incoherent, often sounding like an exotic foreign language. That is, a Wernicke's aphasic's speech flows forth without hesitation, and has appropriate intonation. Appropriate social interaction, such as speaking in turn, and gesturing appropriately remains intact. However, the words and phrases spoken are meaningless. Wernicke's aphasics usually don't realize their spoken language is meaningless to others (anosagnosia for speech). It is as if they know exactly what is to be communicated, but their delivery is incoherent.

In mild cases of Wernicke's aphasia, only a word or two here and there sounds garbled or incomprehensible. In this case, communication can generally proceed because the person is able to grasp the essence of the intention based on the context within which the communication takes place. With moderate disability, the patient can understand part, but not all, of the communication. In severe cases, the patient may experience most or all speech as if it were nonsense syllables or a foreign language. It is not uncommon for others to be misattribute behavior problems to people with receptive aphasia. Sometimes noncompliance is actually caused by the fact that the patient has misunderstood the communication in the first place. Thus a patient may act as though a word was not heard at all (so-called word deafness) or as though only fragments of the word were heard. The most common defect, however, lies not in failing to recognize that a word was spoken,

Neuropsychology in Action 4.3

Synesthesia: Melded Sensory Integration

by Mary Spiers

One of the more exotic and seemingly rare (reported by 1 in 500,000) alterations in sensory processing is the "cross-wiring" of senses called *synesthesia*. One woman reported that tasting lemon is like "points pressing against the face" and spearmint feels like "cool glass columns." The most reported form of synesthesia is "audition colorée" or colored hearing, described vividly by the synesthete poet Arthur Rimbaud in his poem "Les Voyelles" ("The Vowels," see insert).

Probably the most completely described case of synesthesia was "S," described by Luria in his book *The Mind of a Mnemonist* (1968). Every sound, including tones, words, music, voices, and other noises, summoned up a vivid visual image. One tone could be a "velvet cord with fibers jutting out on all sides," while another tone conjured up a strip, the color of "old tarnished silver." The sound of a voice could be "crumbly and yellow" or like a "flame with fibers." Seeing sounds could often be so attention grabbing that "S" could not follow the content of what people were saying to him unless they spoke very slowly.

The melding of sensory perceptions appears unique to each person, but the underlying neural processes may be quite similar. Neurologist Richard Cytowic (1993) has suggested that the source of synesthesia emanates from the most primitive reaches of the brain, specifically the limbic system. In his early studies Cytowic used xenon inhalation to study the dynamic blood flow activity within the brain of synesthetes in mid *audition colorée*. Contrary to his initial expectations, neural activity in the cortex did not increase, but actually decreased an average of 18 percent. Surprisingly, it was the limbic system that "lit up." Cytowic hypothesizes that the neocortex "turns off" during synesthetic processing while a more ancient, fundamental processing system takes over. Finding limbic system involvement seems congruent in light of the way Luria's patient S describes his own experiences:

> S: . . . I recognize a word not only by the images it evokes, but by a whole complex of feelings that image arouses. It's hard to express. . . . Usually I experience a word's

---

but rather in failing to attach meaning to the word. In some aphasics, comprehension of individual words is intact, but grammatical constructions are not.

Damage in Wernicke's aphasia includes the secondary auditory cortex (Wernicke's area) and some involvement of surrounding structures. These often include the supramarginal and angular gyri and portions of the middle temporal gyrus.

Other Aphasia Subtypes

The classification of aphasias into receptive and expressive is a useful didactic tool, but many people with left-hemisphere lesions have a combination of both symptoms, because of damage to the left middle cerebral artery, which serves both expressive and receptive areas. In this section we briefly review the symptoms of the various subtypes of aphasia beyond the more common Broca's and Wernicke's aphasias.

Table 4.4 summarizes the behavioral features of the aphasias.

Conduction Aphasia   The behavioral hallmark of conduction aphasia is a problem in repeating what others say. This problem, obviously, may not become apparent except on formal testing. In ordinary conversation, expressive speech is fluent but marked with **phonemic paraphasias,** or errors of word usage of similar-sounding words (such as using the word *bark* for *tarp*). Comprehension is relatively well preserved but may suffer from minor errors. Reading aloud and writing are frequently impaired. Neuroanatomically, conduction aphasia is a result of separation of Broca's area from Wernicke's area by damage of the arcuate fasciculus, the connecting white matter fibers between the two areas. The damage may also include lesions to the posterior portions of the lateral fissure respon-

taste and weight, and I don't have to make an effort to remember it—the word seems to recall itself. But it's difficult to describe. What I sense is something oily slipping through my hand . . . or I'm aware of a slight tickling in my left hand caused by a mass of tiny, lightweight points. When that happens I simply remember, without having to make the attempt. (Luria, 1968, p. 28)

Mood and memory are intimately linked through the limbic system. In the case of S, auditory and visual sensation also appear linked to this system. The final effect was effortless and seemingly unlimited memory capacity. A sound, once experienced, would always recall an image. S went on to use this strange gift as a professional performer of feats of memory, astounding audiences throughout Russia.

Many viewed synesthesia as an abnormal medical oddity. It is different from other "disorders" in that it is not an effect of acquired brain damage. This cross-wiring appears to be "hard-wired" since birth. If, as Cytowic suggests, synesthesia is an evolutionarily more primitive form of processing sensory experience, there may be remnants of synesthesia in many of us. Do you ever feel blue?

Vowels

A black, E white, I red, U green, O blue: vowels,
One day I will tell you latent birth.
A, black hairy corset of shining flies
Which buzz around cruel stench,

Gulfs of darkness; E whiteness of vapors and tents,
Lances of proud glaciers, white kings, quivering of flowers;
I, purples, spit blood, laughter of beautiful lips
In anger or penitent drunkenness;

U cycles, divine vibrations of green seas,
Peace of pastures scattered with animals, peace of the wrinkles
which alchemy prints on heavy studious brows;

O supreme Clarion full of strange stridor,
Silences crossed by worlds and angels:
O, the Omega, violet beam from HIS eyes!

—Arthur Rimbaud

---

sible for aspects of reading and writing, specifically the supramarginal gyrus and the angular gyrus.

Transcortical Motor Aphasia Clinicians can recognize transcortical motor aphasia by the patient's halting, nonfluent spontaneous speech; oddly, however, speech becomes fluent if the person merely must repeat what another says. In many respects, except for the differences in repetition ability, this deficit resembles Broca's aphasia. Speech comprehension is unimpaired, and writing may also suffer. Reading comprehension, however, is generally intact. Lesions to the area anterior or superior to Broca's area are associated with this aphasia type.

Transcortical Sensory Aphasia Severe speech comprehension deficit marks transcortical sensory aphasia. Interestingly, despite being unable to comprehend speech, such aphasics can adequately repeat phrases and sentences presented to them. Lesions in the angular gyrus are the most likely culprits for this aphasia, and thus reading and writing are also affected.

Anomic Aphasia A problem in word finding, or anomia, is the primary, and often only, difficulty in anomic aphasia. This aphasia is a frequent result of widespread brain impairment caused by conditions such as traumatic brain injury and dementias such as Alzheimer's disease. As people age, a very annoying concomitant often reported is a difficulty in remembering people's names or being unable to retrieve a word that is just on the "tip of the tongue." The act of "word finding" seems to be one of the most easily affected aspects of expressive language. Witness even the problem of being "speechless" with anxiety. It is very difficult, therefore to distinguish what might be a temporary word-finding difficulty and a true aphasia.

Global Aphasia   Global aphasia is the most devastating of the aphasia subtypes because of its profound effect across all areas of speech functioning. There is marked disability in speech production as well as speech comprehension. Reading, writing, and repetition are also impaired. This aphasia is caused by a massive lesion encompassing major portions of the left hemisphere.

Summary   Within the primary sensory systems, we have traced the basic connections in a way, but the actual functioning systems are seamlessly interwoven with other functioning systems. It is useful to understand the workings of primary systems and build on these to understand higher systems. You can see sensory-perceptual processing as a bottom-up process of sensory logic, because in each domain the brain seeks to make "sense" of incoming information. A fundamental question of consciousness is how the brain constructs perceptions of integrated wholes, such as an orange, for which you integrate the visual features with the smell and taste. Brain scientists are beginning to ask how the disparate local elements bind to form a unified experience. This is referred to as "the binding problem of consciousness."

A question related to the binding problem concerns how the brain accesses meaning. Some argue that meaning is specific within each sensory system. In other words, there exists a specific visual meaning, auditory meaning, or even olfactory meaning. If this meaning is lost, as in various sensory agnosias, the ability to access it through another sensory modality would be impossible. In discussing the senses, it is quickly evident that basic sensory perception is anatomically and functionally distinct. However, meaning lost in one sensory modality can often be accessed through another. Exactly how an integrated sense of meaning emerges is still unclear. There may be local interconnections between sensory cortexes or some sort of central integrative multimodal processor that allows multiple access from the sensory systems. In Chapter 13 we take up the problems of binding and how the mind constructs meaning. Neuropsychology and neuroscience are still wrestling with the larger questions of how this system operates. Functionally,

however, knowing that sensory-perceptual agnosias are modality specific lets rehabilitation professionals seek alternate "routes" for accessing meaning when one system is damaged (see Chapter 16).

Motor Systems

The sensory systems provide a window to the world, and the motor systems, in turn, provide the means of acting on the world. Whereas control of sensory systems takes place in posterior brain regions, the control of movement is largely anterior. Movement takes several forms, including reflex actions, automatic repetitive actions such as walking, semivoluntary actions such as yawning, and voluntary actions such as deciding to pick up an object (Bradshaw & Mattingly, 1995).

Traditionally, scientists thought the motor system was organized hierarchically. Whereas sensory processing is thought to proceed in a bottom-up fashion, motor processing would follow a reverse path in a top-down manner. Sensory-perceptual processes build up from fragments analyzed in primary processing areas and are synthesized in secondary and higher-order cortexes. Then information that directs motor processing comes into the system in the form of highly integrated sensory information from the sensory association areas, such as the parietal lobes, and the subcortical structures of the basal ganglia and the cerebellum. In addition, internally generated motivation for action also directs movement. The system then directs this information to areas of secondary motor planning and programming before sending it to the primary motor cortex. According to this hierarchy theory, the primary motor cortex sits at the top and funnels all information about movement to the body. However, a competing theory suggests that the system works in a parallel processing mode, with several motor processing circuits working in coordination with the primary motor cortex (Haines, 1997).

CORTICAL MOTOR PROCESSING

Several cortical areas of the motor system are involved in motor processing (see Figure 4.15). The first of

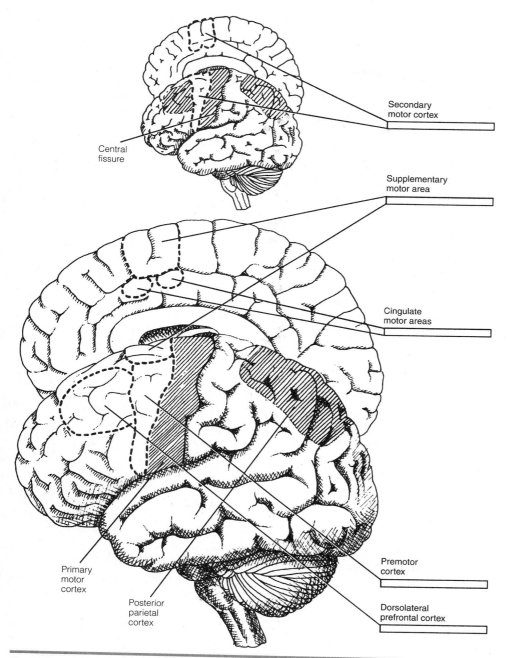

Figure 4.15 Cortical motor processing areas. The primary motor cortex is shaded. The secondary motor cortex areas include the supplementary motor area, the premotor cortex, and the cingulate motor areas. Associative sensory information travels from the posterior parietal cortex to the secondary motor areas. The dorsolateral prefrontal cortex also plays a role in initiation and planning. (Modified from P. J. Pinel and M. Edwards, *A Colorful Introduction to the Anatomy of the Human Brain,* Boston: Allyn and Bacon, 1998, p. 151. Reproduced by permission of the publisher. All rights of reproduction in any form reserved)

these is the primary motor cortex. The next three motor areas are often referred to as the secondary motor cortex and include the supplementary motor area, the premotor area, and the cingulate motor area. Finally, areas of the parietal lobes and the dorsolateral prefrontal cortex are areas of premotor planning.

The role of the **primary motor cortex** is to manage the fine details required to carry out movement. The primary motor cortex lies in the precentral gyrus, or motor strip of the frontal lobes, just anterior to the central sulcus and the somatosensory strip. Neuronal input emanates from the secondary motor areas and from the somatosensory cortex. Neuronal output travels through the internal capsule and on to descending tracts of the spinal cord and ultimately to the muscles of the body. The primary motor cortex, like the somatosensory cortex, is somatopically (or topographically) mapped as a homunculus and allots area according to its degree of motor innervation (see Figure 4.3). If the primary motor cortex is stimulated directly, typically through microstimulation in the course of neurosurgery, corresponding muscles in the body move. For example, stimulating the thumb causes the thumb to twitch or jerk. If the motor homunculus is compared to the sensory homunculus, it is evident that there are many similarities in the cortical mapping for motor control and sensory processing of movement. For example, the acute sense of touch on the fingers is also related to fine finger dexterity. However, some areas have proportionately more motor control abilities, or vice versa, so the maps appear somewhat different. The motor cortex, like the somatosensory cortex, controls the contralateral side of the body.

The primary motor cortex and the somatosensory cortex are in reciprocal communication with each other through a reflex circuit. The primary motor cortex receives feedback from the somatosensory cortex about the effect of movement just initiated. So when your thumb moves across the page to turn it, the sensation of the contact of the thumb on paper is immediately sent to the somatosensory cortex and informs the primary motor cortex of the effect of its movement.

Each area of the **secondary motor cortex** has a slightly different role. The **supplementary motor area** (**SMA,** or **supplementary motor cortex,** or **me-**dial premotor cortex**) functions in organization and sequential timing of movement. The internal intention to move is also a function of this area. The SMA lies on the dorsal and medial portion of each frontal lobe (in Brodmann's area 6). It is posterior to the prefrontal cortex and anterior to the primary motor cortex. The SMA receives input from the parietal lobes (posterior parietal association area), the somatosensory strip, the secondary somatosensory areas and subcortically from the basal ganglia and the cerebellum. It also interconnects with the premotor area. The SMA outputs to the primary motor cortex in both the ipsilateral and contralateral hemisphere. It also outputs back to the basal ganglia and the cerebellum (Bradshaw & Mattingly, 1995). It functions specifically as a planner of motor sequences. Like the primary motor cortex, it is also somatopically mapped to the musculature in the body; however, the mapping is not as tightly organized. Electrical microstimulation of the SMA elicits the *urge* to make a movement, or the feeling of anticipation of a movement (Bradshaw & Mattingly, 1995). Stimulation may also elicit muscle movement. But instead of the single-muscle flexion of the primary motor cortex, this stimulation activates groups of muscles and a sequence of movement, and can activate bilateral movement (Haines, 1997).

Experiments with humans show a **dissociation,** or separation, between the functional contributions of the primary motor cortex and the SMA. In an early method of studying areas of brain activity, before PET scans were available, researchers injected radioactive xenon into the bloodstream. In this way, they could measure increased areas of brain blood flow, and thus brain neuronal activity, as they were occurring. When the researchers asked volunteers to make random finger movements, the primary motor cortex "lit up," but the SMA remained relatively silent. When the experimenters asked volunteers to make a sequence of movements with their fingers, such as drumming their fingers in a certain order, both the primary motor cortex and the SMA were active. Finally, when they asked the participants to only imagine and rehearse the movements in their minds, without doing anything, only the SMA was active (Roland, Larson, Lassen, & Skinholf, 1980). This offered strong evidence for the planning role of the SMA in sequential motor activities.

The **premotor area** (**PMA, or premotor cortex**) also plays a role in motor planning and sequencing and movement readiness. The PMA lies next to the SMA in Brodmann's area 6 of the frontal lobes. Whereas the SMA is more medial, the PMA is more lateral. The PMA receives neuronal input from some of the same general areas as does the SMA; however, from slightly different places. For example, the PMA receives parietal input from posterior parietal areas, rather than parietal association cortex. The PMA receives input from the secondary somatosensory areas rather than from both the primary and secondary somatosensory areas, and receives more cerebellar input. As stated earlier, it is also reciprocally interconnected with the SMA, and projects to the primary motor cortex and the reticular formation (Haines, 1997). The PMA is also somatopically organized. In a general way the PMA carries out similar premotor planning functions as the SMA, such as the sequencing, timing, and proper initiation of voluntary movement, but it may function more in *externally* cued readiness for action, whereas the SMA provides more of an *internal* readiness cue (Bradshaw & Mattingly, 1995). For example, when runners line up for a race and hear the official say "On your mark . . . Get set . . . Go," their PMA is most active between "Get set" and "Go." Studies with monkeys also indicate that the PMA is most active during this interval between *cue* and *go* (see Haines, 1997).

Less is known about the functioning of the third structure of the secondary motor cortex, the **cingulate motor area** (**CMA or cingulate motor cortex**), although it likely plays a role in the emotional and motivational impetus for movement. The CMA is a medial infolding of the frontal area of the cingulate gyrus. Recall that the cingulate gyrus plays a role in the limbic system. The CMA lies next to the cingulate gyrus. The CMA is organized somatopically in relation to the spinal cord. It projects both to the spinal cord and to the primary motor area. Damage to the CMA results in a lack of spontaneous motor activity (Bradshaw & Mattingly, 1995). This apparent apathy is neurologic in origin and not necessarily caused by a depressive state. People may be able to say what they can do or should do, but often do not translate this into action. Together with the supplementary motor area, the anterior cingulate also appears to play a role in the semantic premotor processing, or initiation, of speech.

Two additional cortical areas contribute to motor processing: the posterior parietal lobes and the dorsolateral prefrontal cortex. The posterior areas of the parietal lobes (Brodmann's areas 5 and 7) are important in coordinating spatial mapping with motor programming. These association areas receive input from the somatosensory cortex, the vestibular system, and the visual system. Brodmann's area 7 is involved in the *where* system of spatial location we discussed earlier. Integrated sensory information travels to the supplementary and premotor cortexes regarding the relative spatial position of the body and objects in space.

Much initiation for motor behavior and executive programming for movement originates in the higher-association area of the **dorsolateral prefrontal cortex.** This area lies, functionally, in the prefrontal cortex, which is responsible for orchestrating and organizing many brain functions. The dorsolateral prefrontal cortex is not a "movement center" in and of itself, but it is instrumental in deploying movement. Much input to this area comes from the subcortical motor centers of the basal ganglia.

Apraxia

Impaired cortical motor processing can occur with disease or injury. If the primary motor area in one hemisphere is damaged by stroke or injury, paralysis or partial loss of movement on the contralateral side often results. If the damage affects secondary motor processing areas, then the disorders involve motor planning, organization, and initiation. If the damage impairs spatial organization of motor behavior, the parietal lobes are often implicated (see Table 4.5 on p. 151 for examples of motor dysfunction).

Strictly defined, **apraxia** implies an absence of action, but neuropsychologists most often use it to describe a variety of missing or inappropriate actions that cannot be clearly attributed to primary motor deficits, lack of comprehension, or motivation. Thus, the term *apraxia* refers to an inability to perform voluntary actions despite an adequate amount of motor

Table 4.5	*Examples of Motor Dysfunction*

Apraxia/dyspraxia: an inability or disability in performing voluntary actions

Dysarthria: difficulty formulating words because of a problem with motor control

Dyskinesia: uncontrolled involuntary movement

Tremor: involuntary shaking, usually of a limb, tremors may be resting or occur with intentional movement

strength and control. The adjective "voluntary" is key to understanding this disorder. A patient may be able to spontaneously don a jacket, for instance, but be unable to do so on command. An individual may also have motor apraxia and have the ability to correctly stand up when not thinking about it, but to be unable to do so when asked. Because of this, family members who ask a patient to do something may perceive him or her as being oppositional or stubborn when in fact he or she does not control the skills required to perform the action.

Researchers have proposed many subtypes of apraxia, depending on a number of behavioral variables affecting movement and movement initiation. For example, does the person have more difficulty in generating the idea of movement, sequencing movements to learn a specific task, and using objects appropriately, or does the problem center more on drawing, writing, or speaking?

A specific motor apraxia involving the vocal musculature is dysarthria. Dysarthriacs differ from pure aphasics in that they know what they want to say, but cannot formulate words because of a problem with motor control. The difficulty lies in not knowing what to do with the muscles of the tongue and lips to generate a word. This problem can also make it difficult or impossible for patients to use gestures to communicate needs.

SUBCORTICAL MOTOR PROCESSING

Cortical motor processing is largely concerned with voluntary, conscious movement, whereas subcorti-cal structures, namely the basal ganglia and the cerebellum, function in a more automatic manner to regulate movement. The function of the basal ganglia in movement largely controls the fluidity of overlearned and "semiautomatic" motor programs (Bradshaw & Mattingly, 1995). The basal ganglia reciprocally connect to the PMA and the SMA via the thalamus. Also, an important brain circuit responsible for perceptual-motor learning and adaptation centers on the basal ganglia. Specifically this circuit includes the caudate nucleus, putamen, and globus pallidus. The nuclei of the **striatal complex** (caudate and putamen) receive projected information from cortical sensory areas. From the striatum, information then funnels through the globus pallidus, and then on to the thalamus, where it projects to the premotor and prefrontal areas (Mishkin, Malamut, & Bachevalier, 1984). We futher discuss the behavioral effects of damage to this area in the next chapter, in the context of memory and learning.

Some well-known motor disorders are associated with neurochemical abnormalities affecting the basal ganglia—most notably, Parkinson's disease, which specifically targets the substantia nigra, and Huntington's disease, which attacks the caudate nucleus. Although these two disorders attack structures within centimeters of each other, you can easily distinguish these motor disorders. You can recognize Parkinson's disease by its resting tremor and difficulty in initiating movement, whereas Huntington's patients show characteristic puppetlike jerking and grimacing choreic movements. The motor difficulties in these patients are prominent, but exist within a larger constellation of symptoms. We discuss these two disorders and their specific motor impairments at length in Chapter 12.

The cerebellum permits seamless coordination and unconscious flow of movement. It coordinates reflex action as well as voluntary movement, is concerned with the timing of movement, and can differentiate movement frequency at a rate of 1/1000 of a second. The cerebellum aids in maintaining posture, balance, and muscle tone. It is also implicated in sequential aspects of motor learning such as the steps required to learn the piano. The cerebellum recipro-

Neuropsychology in Action 4.4

Tourette Syndrome: Too Much Behavior

by Eric Zillmer

George was a patient I saw for neuro-psychological evaluation. I knew that George, a 29-year-old, left-handed male, was diagnosed with Gilles de la Tourette syndrome (TS), but I was not prepared for his odd behavior during my administration of the Category test. The Category test measures planning and reasoning. I asked George to match a stimulus to one of four targets. In essence, George had to figure out which abstract category the stimulus fit best. My responsibility was to present each stimulus figure, tell George whether he was correct or not, tell him when the category changed, and keep score. In total, over 200 stimuli cards are presented, which fall into seven categories. The first stimulus card is very easy, and I told George his response, "2," was correct. As soon as I did so, he made a peculiar gesture, a kissing motion, in which he looked directly at me, raised his eyebrows, and shaped his mouth as if "blowing" me a kiss. If this were not odd enough, I was dumbstruck with George's behavior when I told him he had made an error. He made an obscene gesture commonly known as "flipping the bird"!

And so it went for the entire exam. When George was correct, he blew me a kiss, and when he made an error, he "gave me the finger." Like many neuropsychological tests, this one is stag-gered so it becomes more and more difficult. This resulted in George making more errors toward the end, a total of 53. Midway through the exam, I decided to continue with the test, but I did ask George after the evaluation whether he knew he was engaging in these behaviors and if he was somehow angry with me. He informed me that he was aware of what he did, but that it seemed uncon-trollable; "I just had to do it." He also told me that he was not angry with me and, in fact, enjoyed the testing and my company.

TS is a rare and fascinating disorder that has puzzled scientists for over 100 years. TS occurs in less than 1% of the population. Symptoms include facial and bodily tics, usually progressing from the head to the torso and extremities, as well as repetitive verbal utterances, including coprolalia (uncontrollable cursing) in approximately 50% of the cases (New-man, Barth, & Zillmer, 1987). Onset of the disorder is typically before age 10, and symptoms vary in intensity over time and may be exacerbated by stress. Most individuals with TS are male and left-handed.

The specific cause of TS is unknown but the prevailing view is that there is a neurologic basis for the disorder, possi-bly involving subcortical structures that are responsible for motor coordination (Devinsky, 1983; Bornstein, King, & Carroll, 1983). This view is supported by findings of a high incidence of motor asymmetries on clinical neurologic exams, and abnormal EEGs and CT scans (Newman, Barth, & Zillmer, 1987). No consistent or focalized neurologic deficits, however, have yet emerged.

George, adopted in infancy, first displayed bizarre motor symptoms—jerking of his shoulders—at age 2. Later, he developed short barking sounds, repetitive movements of his facial mus-cles and arms, and finally, loud shouting of profanities. The bouts of impulsive and sometimes assaultive behavior became so difficult to manage in the classroom that George was taken out of school in the third grade. Subsequently, he was in and out of psychiatric institutions most of his life. He was in a state psychiatric facility when I evaluated him. He had been hospitalized because he threw a brick at a passing car and chased it with an axe. Somehow he thought that pas-sengers in the car were teasing him. Like George, many patients with TS display peculiar motor symptoms and psychiatric symptoms, including depression and impulsivity. Medications often help patients with TS so that, in most cases, they can lead a productive and symptom-free life.

cally connects to the cortical sensory and motor sys-tems, resulting in a constant feedback loop coordi-nating the two areas. Cerebellar motor disorders are most often caused by structural damage caused by trauma or stroke. They are characterized by irregular, jerky, and poorly coordinated movement. Muscle tone and strength may also decrease as well as motor resistance. Finally, in contrast to the resting tremor seen in Parkinson's patients, cerebellar patients show an intention tremor.

Conclusion

The primary sensory areas receive afferent input through the relay station of the thalamus, except for olfaction, which receives input directly from the olfactory bulbs. In some sensory systems, such as touch and taste, primary sensory reception is completely crossed, coming entirely from the contralateral side of the body. In vision, the contralateral hemispace sends input to each hemisphere. In audition information travels bilaterally. Olfaction has ipsilateral projection to the primary olfactory cortex.

Each sensory system has a primary receiving area in the cortex. In general, sensory information is represented in detailed 1:1 or pattern mapping onto the corresponding primary cortex. In vision, audition, and touch, these are respectively the retinotopic map, the tonotopic map, and the somatotopic maps. The primary mapping for the chemical senses is less well understood but likely occurs in a similar manner.

From the primary sensory cortexes, where information is first labeled, it is then sorted and relayed to the secondary sensory processing areas. These areas are generally contiguous to the primary sensory areas. They receive preprocessed sensory information through reciprocal connections with primary areas. They do not receive sensory information directly. Secondary areas may process only specific qualities of sensory information in a parallel manner, as we have seen with the "what" and "where" visual streams. In other systems, a distributed "maplike" representation may remain. As processing moves into tertiary or association areas, dense reciprocal interconnections both within and between sensory modalities are evident. Language and visual-perceptual processing are examples representing the highest level of processing emerging from individual sensory systems. These systems employ higher-association information within a specific sensory modality while integrating it with other higher-order systems such as memory or executive functioning (discussed further in the next chapter).

The motor system involves both cortical and subcortical areas of processing. The general stream of processing moves from subcortical and secondary motor areas to the primary motor area to output; however, there are many reciprocal interconnections. Some of the coordination and planning of movement takes place in the subcortical areas of the cerebellum and the basal ganglia. The three secondary cortical motor areas add fine planning, sequencing, and motivational aspects. The primary motor cortex, or motor homunculus is responsible for managing the fine details of movement.

It would be difficult to imagine the behavioral oddities that disorders of specific sensory and motor systems present had not nature and odd twists of fate actually presented them. These include descriptions of sensory phantoms, distortions of chemical senses, visual agnosias, neglect, aphasias, and the odd disorder of "miswired" sensation termed *synesthesia*. Although these disorders can be connected to specific sensory modalities, it is at once evident that most afflictions do not stay within the bounds of a single cognitive system.

We briefly reviewed apraxia but reserve discussion of the more wide-ranging motor disorders of Parkinson's disease and Huntington's disease until Chapter 12.

Critical Thinking Questions

■ What does the neuropsychology of sensory-perceptual processing have to contribute to the idea that there is an objective reality related to object perception?

■ In what ways does the study of sensory-perceptual and motor disorders inform us about intact brain functioning? In what instances might the study of damaged brains lead us astray?

■ Do conditions such as phantoms, neglect, and synesthesia represent altered states of consciousness? Explain.

■ Does intact motor processing require intact sensory-perceptual processing? Explain.

Key Terms

Transduction
Receptor cells
Agnosia
Visual agnosia
Tactile agnosia
Astereognosis
Somatosensory system
Proprioception
Mechanical receptors
Chemoreceptors
Thermoreceptors
Nocioceptors
Proprioceptors
Ascending spinal-thalamic tract
Dorsal column medial lemniscal pathway
Medial lemniscus
Somatopic organization
Kinesthetic sense
Astereognosia

Finger agnosia
Paresthesia
Peripheral neuropathy
Phantom limb pain
Proprioceptive disorder
Tactile extinction/ suppression/inattention
Papillae
Aguesia
Dysguesia
Phantoguesia
Hypoguesia
Anosmia
Dysosmia
Phantosmia
Hyposmia
Decussating
Anopsias
Homonymous
Hemianopsia
Striate cortex

Secondary association
Prestriate cortex
Achromatopsia
Akinetopsia
Visual object agnosia
Prosopagnosia
Apperceptive visual agnosia
Associative visual agnosia
Ballint's syndrome
Tonotopic map
Wernicke's area
Wernicke's aphasia
Receptive aphasia
Frontal operculum
Aphasia
Dysarthria
Speech apraxia
Fluent aphasia
Nonfluent aphasia
Expressive aphasia
Receptive aphasia

Anomia
Articulation
Word salad
Paragrammatism
Extended paraphasia
Phonemic paraphasias
Primary motor cortex
Secondary motor cortex
Supplementary motor area (SMA) or supplementary motor cortex, medial premotor cortex
Dissociation
Premotor cortex or premotor area (PMA)
Cingulate motor area (CMA) or cingulate motor cortex
Parietal lobes
Dorsolateral prefrontal cortex
Apraxia
Striatal complex

Web Connections

http://illusionworks.com
Illusion Works
Award-winning site for optical illusions that may help illustrate specific points in this chapter.

http://www.braintricks.com/home.html
Braintricks
Interactive links feature quizzes and humorously points out "brain programs" about various aspects of everyday life.

Chapter 5

HIGHER FUNCTIONAL SYSTEMS

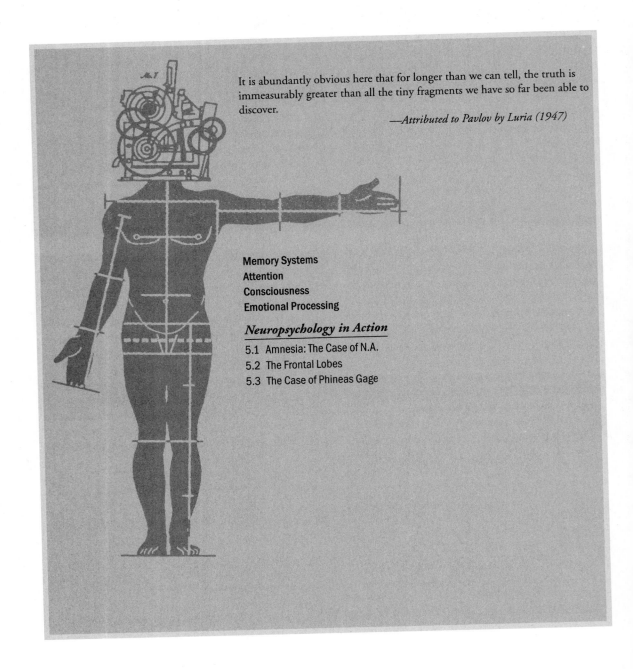

It is abundantly obvious here that for longer than we can tell, the truth is immeasurably greater than all the tiny fragments we have so far been able to discover.

—Attributed to Pavlov by Luria (1947)

Memory Systems
Attention
Consciousness
Emotional Processing

Neuropsychology in Action

5.1 Amnesia: The Case of N.A.
5.2 The Frontal Lobes
5.3 The Case of Phineas Gage

Keep in Mind

◼ What integrative and management functions do higher systems serve?

◼ Does the brain function differently during automatic or "unconscious" processes from the way it functions during conscious or explicit processes?

◼ What effects on behavior do disorders of "management" and "executive" functions have?

◼ Is there a cognitive function that could be considered the highest? Explain.

Overview

This chapter is devoted to higher functional systems that are not specific for sensory modalities. Language and visual perception, which we discussed in the last chapter, are also considered higher functional systems because their full expression depends on additional functional systems such as memory, attention, and executive functioning. However, language and visual perception emerge from sensory-perceptual systems, so it is easier to follow their progression when they are discussed with those systems. The sensory and motor systems represent the building blocks on which other systems are constructed and the raw material from which other systems draw; they are the most straightforward and best mapped systems. The systems we discuss in this section are integrated with the sensory-perceptual and motor systems but do not depend on any one modality. We refer to the systems here as "higher order" systems because, evolutionarily, the expression in humans is complex and highly integrated. You can also think of most of these systems as background management systems. Their functions are important for learning, organizing, setting priorities, planning, self-reflection, and self-regulation.

The systems in this chapter include the classic systems or modules of cognitive neuropsychology, such as memory, attention, and executive functioning. In addition, we consider the brain and mind expressions of consciousness and emotional processing. For each system we discuss the conceptual organization of the system, as well as known structure–function relationships.

◼ Memory Systems

Memory forms the basis of experience and perceptions of self. It is dynamic and malleable. It allows people to travel back in time. How you see yourself, to a large degree, is a product of the experiences of your life, the lessons you've learned, and what you remember as being important. Even what you tell yourself to remember to do in the future must incorporate memory. Memory pervades most aspects of human experience. Stories of your personal and cultural past are stored in memory, so it is a necessary foundation of social communication. In ancient days and the Middle Ages, people relied more on memory than today in daily activities and for transmitting the oral traditions of culture. Today, appointment books, reminder systems, calculators, history books, and other records allow people to "offload" many memories to the environment. They are no longer required to expend mental effort on these bits of information. Does this mean memory has fallen into disuse? In this section we examine how people use the various components of memory and what can happen when aspects of the memory system malfunction.

When memory is working fluidly, there is little need to notice it. But consider the question from a neuropsychological perspective: What do you lose if you lose your memory? One patient we saw, a man in his seventies with Alzheimer's disease, could not remember that his wife had died two years earlier. All his memories were still of her being there. Every time someone mentioned that his wife was dead, he relived the grieving experience. It is scary to imagine waking up not knowing who you are, who your friends are, and what has happened in your life. Consider also what it might be like if you could not encode new information, if you couldn't remember what someone said 10 minutes ago, or if you couldn't register the information you needed to take a test or learn a new skill.

Memory is an umbrella concept, and it is impossible to say categorically that someone has an overall good or bad memory. It is simply not a single system. Memory is parceled into subsystems based on ideas of storage and processing. Neuropsychologists ask how the brain stores information over the long term and how it encodes, organizes, and then retrieves information from memory. In many disorders neuropsychologists see on a daily basis, memory processing is at issue because memory is a "fragile" system, affected by many disorders, including most of the dementias, such as Alzheimer's disease, toxic conditions, loss of oxygen, and head injury.

Scientific understanding of normal memory processing in the brain has profited greatly from the study of people afflicted with various memory disorders, especially the amnesias. However, the term *amnesia* can refer to more than one type of condition. The "soap opera" version of amnesia occurs when one of the characters gets hit on the head and promptly forgets who she is and all the specific episodes of her life. She invariably then wanders off to make a new life for herself, having to develop her identity anew. Perhaps after a time, a startling event occurs or she gets knocked on the head again, and her prior memory and identity floods back. This type of memory deficit is reminiscent of a psychiatric dissociative state caused by severe emotional trauma, but is not what occurs with neurologic injury or disease.

Because neurologic patients acquire their memory problems in conjunction with a brain injury or disease, it is important to have terminology that marks the nature of the patient's memory before the event

and the effect on memory following the event. **Anterograde amnesia** is the loss of the ability to encode and learn new information after a defined event (such as head injury, lesion, or disease onset). **Retrograde amnesia** is the loss of old memories from before an event or illness. For example, one of our patients, L.S., suffered a head injury as a result of a car accident and had moderate anterograde amnesia and mild retrograde amnesia. She had no memory of the car accident and only vaguely remembered the paramedics. She did remember being in the emergency room. After the accident she had difficulty learning new information (anterograde amnesia). She often forgot her doctor's name, and when she returned to college she found it hard to study and do well on history tests for which she had to recall facts and dates. Her mild retrograde amnesia is evidenced by the fact that she remembered driving out of the grocery store parking lot, which was about 5 blocks from the accident. However, she remembered nothing else of the short time preceding the accident. Amnesias of this type are common in closed head injury, a condition described further in Chapter 10. Amnesia can be caused by a number of different problems and take several forms. An example of a circumscribed lesion causing amnesia is the classic case of N.A. (see Neuropsychology in Action 5.1).

A FRAMEWORK FOR CONCEPTUALIZING MEMORY SYSTEMS

Psychology textbooks typically describe memory as having three main divisions; sensory memory, short-term memory, and long-term memory. Sensory memory is fleeting, lasting only milliseconds, but its capacity is essentially unlimited in what may be taken in. **Short-term memory (STM)** is of limited capacity (7 ± 2 bits of information) and degrades quickly over a matter of seconds if information is not held via a means such as rehearsal, or transferred to long-term memory. **Long-term memory (LTM),** theoretically, is of unlimited capacity and relatively permanent except for models that suggest that loss of information through forgetting is possible. Neuropsychologists are most concerned with long-term memory and its disorders because these are the problems most evi-

Neuropsychology in Action 5.1

Amnesia: The Case of N.A.

by Mary Spiers

In 1960, N.A. was 22 years old and in the Air Force, when one day while working on a model airplane he suffered an accident that would affect him for the rest of his life. His roommate, apparently ready for a little rough-housing, took a miniature fencing foil from the wall, tapped N.A. from behind, and as he turned around, thrust forward. Unfortunately for N.A. the tiny foil found the most vulnerable route to the brain through the cribriform plate at the top of his nasal cavity. The foil pierced his third cranial nerve, but more importantly, it made a small lesion in the left dorsomedial nucleus of the thalamus. It was quickly discovered that N.A. had retrograde amnesia for the past two years. This minute injury, however, also left him with a devastating impairment in his ability to register new verbal memories (anterograde amnesia).

To meet him, the casual observer might not at first suspect there is anything wrong. N.A.'s IQ is in the high average range, he has good social skills, is friendly, polite, and has a good sense of humor. But after talking with him for a few minutes, it becomes apparent that he doesn't remember details of just a few minutes ago. If he is distracted by a passing thought or a passing car, the thread of conversation is lost. He has very little recollection of the day's events. If you meet again the next day, he probably won't remember you or what you did together. N.A. likes to keep his room exactly the same at all times and spends much time obsessively arranging things. He becomes very upset at his mother if she moves the telephone or one of his model airplanes. He likes things exactly the same so he has a better chance of finding them. Only after a long period of time, after much repetition, does he remember something. If N.A. saw you every day, after a period of time he might recognize you, but still might not know your name. He has only a sketchy memory of events that have transpired since 1960. For example, he has a vague idea that Watergate was a political scandal in "Washington or Florida" but recalls no other details. Because N.A.'s injury is in the left dorsomedial nucleus, he shows more verbal than visual memory deficits, as expected. Interestingly, when he had to learn a new route from his house to the Veterans Administration hospital for therapy, even after four years he was unable to form a spatial map. He found his way much like an adult returning to a childhood neighborhood after years of absence. As pieces of the visual scenery popped up before him, he decided if the landmark looked familiar and turned accordingly. This haphazard approach of seeing things sometimes required him to back up or retrace his steps until something looked familiar.

N.A. recognizes that he has memory problems and is not confused. He knows who he is and where he is, but may not know the day or year. As would be suspected, he has little social life. He forgot to show up for the one date he made. Also, most of his memories are from the 1950s. In a large sense he remains stuck in time. When he fantasizes, he thinks of Betty Grable. He does not know of the people or events since then. However, N.A. remains optimistic about his situation and rarely uses notes, because he wants to work on his memory.

This case demonstrates that even a very small lesion, strategically placed, can cause a devastating problem of memory. The complete case of N.A. can be found in Kaushall, Zetin, and Squire (1981).

---

denced by patients. Often STM, as measured by neuropsychological tasks, is intact even when there are deficits in LTM, although isolated disorders of short-term memory exist. Neuropsychological conceptualizations of memory generally do not consider sensory memory; rather, it is thought of as a component of sensory processing.

Neuropsychology concerns itself with understanding how memory systems work in correspondence with known brain functioning, An important question concerns the possible existence of anatomically separate systems in the brain for such concepts as short-term memory (STM), long-term memory (LTM), explicit-implicit and episodic-semantic memory. One way in which researchers can support the idea of separate structures is by showing a double dissociation between behaviors. Research can demonstrate strong evidence for different systems if a lesion in an area of the brain affects one system (LTM) but not the other (STM). Evidence is even stronger if researchers can show that a different lesion results in the opposite dissociation (affects STM but not LTM). In this section we focus on conceptualizations of long-term memory and short-term working memory. We explore evidence for different memory subsystems, a division between STM and LTM, and between possible divisions of LTM such as separate declarative/explicit versus procedural/implicit systems. As we explore each subsystem, we also discuss disorders affecting that system.

LONG-TERM MEMORY (LTM)

A problem that is inherently confusing in studying memory is the cornucopia of terms scientists use to describe the possible subcomponents of LTM. Cog-

nitive psychologists, neuropsychologists, neurologists, and the lay public use various—and sometimes conflicting—terms. For example, when referring to long-term memory, the lay public often thinks of the ability to remember information from the distant past. However, neuropsychologists are referring to the specific ability to register information (encode), organize the information in a meaningful way (storage), and recall or recognize the information when needed (retrieval). According to this definition, long-term memory (LTM) is the ability to learn and retain *new* information. **Remote memory,** by contrast, concerns memory for long-past events.

Various theoretical conceptualizations parcel long-term memory into subsystems (see Figure 5.1). Squire (Squire & Cohen, 1984; Squire, 1987) and others have advocated for a structural–functional difference between declarative memory and proce-

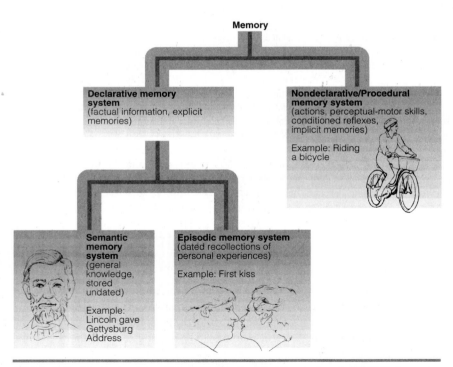

Figure 5.1   Long-term memory taxonomy. Theories of anatomically separate LTM stores have included the noted distinctions. (From W. Weiten, *Psychology: Themes and Variations,* Pacific Grove, CA: Brooks/Cole, 1998, p. 291, Figure 7.28)

dural memory. **Declarative memory** is explicit and accessible to conscious awareness. **Procedural memory** is usually implicit, and a person demonstrates it via performance. Squire maintains that procedural memory's domain is that of rules and procedures rather than verbalizable information, although procedural memory has not been clearly operationally defined and often includes a hodgepodge of tasks such as motor skill learning, mirror reading, and verbal priming. Schacter (1987) differentiates between **explicit** and **implicit memories.** Recall or recognition, through verbal or nonverbal means, directly indicate explicit memories. Conscious awareness is usually implied, as is intention to remember. People demonstrate implicit memory by means in which conscious awareness is not always necessary, such as implicit priming, skill learning, and conditioning. Yet another possible distinction within LTM is between semantic and episodic memory. Researchers consider both of these to be forms of explicit or declarative memory. Tulving (1972) introduced the distinction between an **episodic memory,** which refers to individual episodes, usually autobiographical, that have specific spatial and temporal tags in memory, and **semantic memory,** which refers to memory for information and facts that have no specific time tag reference.

The most neuroanatomically defensible division between long-term memory systems is that of declarative/explicit and nondeclarative memory systems. Some also use the terms *declarative* versus *procedural* or *explicit* versus *implicit* in a nearly synonymous manner. There is much debate over the existence of separate episodic and semantic systems, and in fact although researchers first described these two systems as clearly distinguishable conceptually, they now consider the systems to overlap with other memory concepts.

Declarative Memory

One of the first questions that comes to mind when people begin thinking about memory is "Where is memory stored in the brain?" This often implies the search for a "center" for memory storage in the brain. It also implies that if this center is removed then all memory is removed. This would be like erasing the

entire hard disk of a computer. If all remote memory were removed from the brain, a person would be unable to remember his or her language, facts, episodes, names of people, or any other information previously encoded. From studies of brain-injured individuals, we know that this doesn't happen. People may lose pieces of remote memory, but their brains are not "erased." There is no one memory storage center. Rather, most neuropsychologists think of memory as being ultimately stored in the area where it was first processed (for example, see Squire, 1987). This would imply, for example, that auditory memories are stored in primary, secondary, or auditory association areas and likewise for other functional systems.

The function of the declarative memory system is to process information in such as way as to tag it or consolidate it for storage in the brain. According to this model, when new declarative learning is taking place, information from various cortical areas funnels into the structures responsible for declarative memory. After it is processed, return neural pathways transmit information back to specific cortical areas. Research has implicated three major constellations of brain structures in declarative memory. The first centers around the *medial temporal lobes,* the second around the *diencephalon,* and the third in the *basal forebrain.* These three areas interconnect and play a role in consolidating information into LTM as it passes through circuits or subsystems of memory.

The medial temporal structures important for long-term declarative memory center around the hippocampus and medial temporal lobes. The well-documented case of H.M. (Milner et al., 1968; Scoville, 1968) best exemplifies what occurs in the absence of these structures. H.M. became amnesic in 1953 following bilateral removal of his hippocampus and portions of the surrounding area which included the hippocampal formation (see Figure 5.2 on p. 162). The surgery was an effort to control his intractable seizures. The hippocampal formation, or hippocampal complex, includes the hippocampus, the dentate gyrus, and the subiculum. In cross-section the hippocampus has a distinctive "seahorse" shape. Information funnels into the hippocampus via the entorhinal

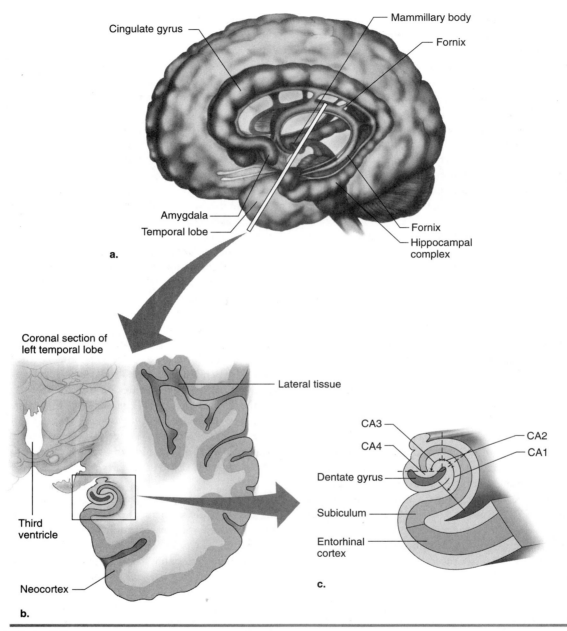

Cingulate gyrus

Mammillary body

Fornix

Amygdala
Temporal lobe

Fornix
Hippocampal complex

a.

Coronal section of left temporal lobe

Lateral tissue

CA3
CA4

CA2
CA1

Dentate gyrus

Subiculum

Entorhinal cortex

Third ventricle

Neocortex

b.

c.

Figure 5.2 The hippocampal complex. (a) The hippocampal complex is located on the medial surface of the temporal lobe. (b) A coronal section shows the hippocampus as a deep infolding of the temporal lobe. (c) A closeup reveals the structures in relationship. The hippocampus consists of four parts (CA1–CA4). The pathway to the hippocampus from the cortex leads through the entorhinal cortex. ([b] Adapted from Pinel, P. J. & Edwards, M., *A Colorful Introduction to the Anatomy of the Human Brain,* p. 169, Figure 10.1. Copyright © 1998 by Allyn & Bacon. Reprinted by permission; [c] adapted from A. M. Burt, *Textbook of Neuroanatomy,* Philadelphia: W. B. Saunders Co., 1988, p. 488, Figure 20-7)

cortex. Neuropsychologists also believe the perirhinal and parahippocampal cortexes adjacent to the hippocampal formation have a role in memory. H.M. probably lost most of these areas. Like N.A., he suffered a profound amnesia for most ongoing events, an amne-sia that persisted in spite of above-average intelligence. H.M's amnesia was even more profound in that he also had difficulty in learning new visual-spatial information.

The structures of the diencephalon involved in memory center around specific nuclei of the thalamus and the mammillary bodies of the hypothalamus (see Figure 5.3 on p. 164). The thalamus consists of several nuclei, with the dorsal medial nucleus of the thalamus most often implicated in memory disorders. Damage to the dorsal medial nucleus of the thalamus is often implicated in Korsakoff's syndrome and in some cases of specific amnesia, such as N.A.'s (see Neuropsychology in Action 5.1).

The basal forebrain is the third area implicated in long-term declarative memory processing. As Chapter 3 describes, this area is a subcortical part of the telencephalon surrounding the inferior tip of the frontal horn and is strongly interconnected with limbic structures, and some consider it part of the limbic system (for example, see Crosson, 1992). The basal forebrain represents a major source of cholinergic output to the cortex. Some have suggested that extensive damage of basal forebrain structures may be needed to affect memory (Zola-Morgan & Squire, 1993), so looking at an individual nucleus's contributions to memory is probably not as profitable as regarding the system as a network. Because of its location surrounding the inferior tip of the frontal horn and the fact the inferior communicating artery perfuses this area, stroke easily affects the basal forebrain. This area is important to memory not only for the nuclei within but for the fibers that traverse the area. The basal forebrain also contains numerous connections to the medial-temporal area.

The basal forebrain structures implicated in memory include the nucleus basalis of Meynert, the medial septal nucleus, the nucleus of the diagonal band of Broca, and the substantia innominata (see Figure 5.4 on p. 165). The nucleus basalis of Meynert includes a group of large neurons interspersed within the sub-

stantia innominata. The substantia innominata is a gray and white matter area separating the globus pallidus from the inferior surface of the forebrain. It interconnects with the frontal, parietal, and temporal cortexes. An important tract coursing through the substantial innominata is the ventral amygdalofugal pathway, connecting the amygdala to the dorsal medial nucleus of the thalamus. The medial septal nucleus lies at the precommisural end of the fornix and projects to the hippocampus through the fornix. It most likely affects memory when damage disrupts information flow to the hippocampus. The nucleus of the diagonal band of Broca is a white matter and cell body area located near the nucleus basalis. It also projects to the hippocampus through the fornix. Researchers think these structures are important cholinergic memory structures.

The major declarative memory system is the Papez circuit. Papez originally thought this looping pathway was specific for emotional processing. He noticed that the clinical presentation of intense emotional symptoms in animals with rabies (Latin for "rage") was associated with lesions in several limbic system structures, specifically the hippocampus. Today, researchers know this loop has more to do with consolidating information in memory than as a primary emotional processor. Information from the cortex and higher cortical association areas enters the circuit through the cingulate gyrus, moves to the parahippocampal gyrus, and then into the hippocampus through the hippocampal formation. The major output system of the hippocampal formation is the fornix. It contains nearly 1 million fibers and is comparable in size to the optic tract (Nauta & Feirtag, 1986). The fornix rises out of the hippocampal complex and arches anteriorly under the corpus callosum. The fornix relays information to the mammillary bodies (specifically the medial mammillary nucleus) of the hypothalamus. From there information is projected to the anterior nucleus of the thalamus along the mamillo-thalamic tract, from where it then goes to the cingulate gyrus to complete the circuit. Figure 5.2 shows the anatomic location of the structures. Figure 5.5 (p. 166) shows a schematic of the loop.

It is readily apparent by examining amnesia cases such as H.M. and N.A. that a break in the memory

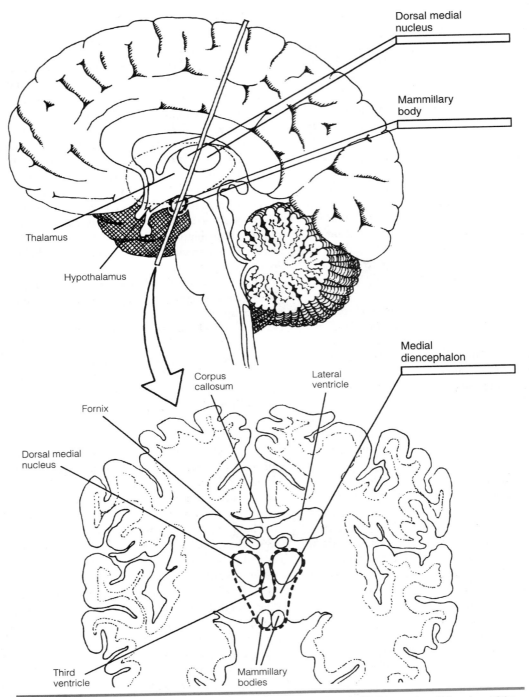

Figure 5.3   The medial diencephalon, comprising the mammillary bodies and the dorsal medial nucleus of the thalamus, is located on both sides of the third ventricle. (Adapted from Pinel, P. J. & Edwards, M., *A Colorful Introduction to the Anatomy of the Human Brain*, p. 175, Figure 10.4. Copyright © 1998 by Allyn & Bacon. Reprinted by permission)

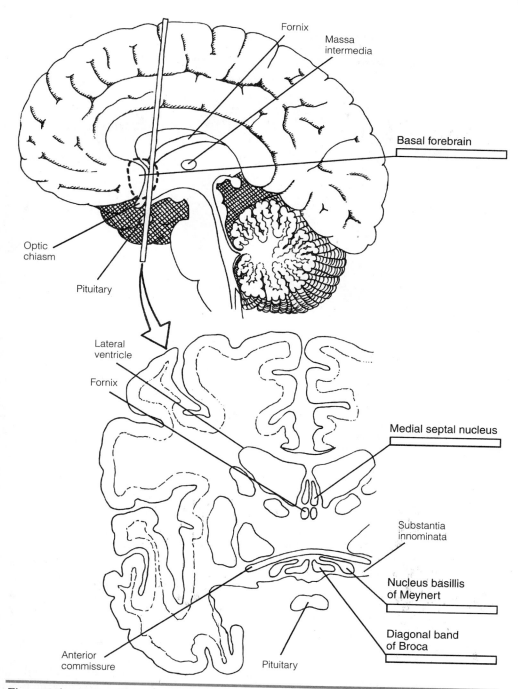

Figure 5.4 The basal forebrain consists of a set of structures at the base of the forebrain. The four implicated in memory include the medial septal nucleus, the nucleus basilis of Meynert, the nucleus of the diagonal band of Broca, and the substantia innominata. (Adapted from Pinel, P. J. & Edwards, M., *A Colorful Introduction to the Anatomy of the Human Brain,* p. 177, Figure 10.5. Copyright © 1998 by Allyn & Bacon. Reprinted by permission)

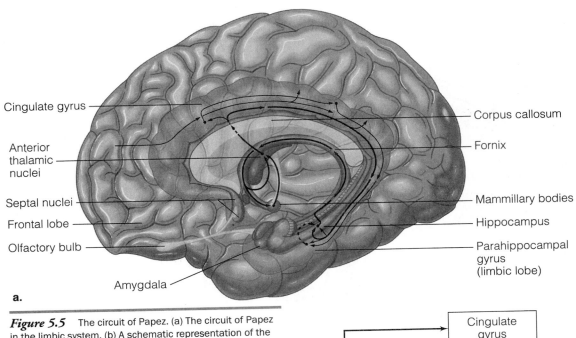

Cingulate gyrus

Anterior
thalamic
nuclei

Septal nuclei

Frontal lobe

Olfactory bulb

Amygdala

Corpus callosum

Fornix

Mammillary bodies

Hippocampus

Parahippocampal
gyrus
(limbic lobe)

a.

Figure 5.5   The circuit of Papez. (a) The circuit of Papez in the limbic system. (b) A schematic representation of the circuit of Papez. The pathway proceeds from the hippocampus to the mammillary bodies (MB) via the fornix. It then projects to the anterior nucleus (AN) of the thalamus, around the cingulate gyrus and back to the hippocampal complex. (From [a] James W. Kalat, *Biological Psychology,* 6th ed., Pacific Grove, CA: Brooks/Cole, p. 324, Figure 12.1. [b] B. Crosson, *Subcortical Functions in Language and Memory,* New York: Guilford Press, 1992, p. 166, Figure 5.5)

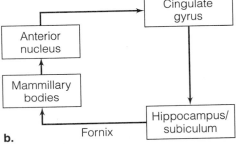

b.

consolidation circuit can disrupt memory in a manner similar to direct removal of the hippocampus, which neurologists typically consider the most crucial structure in the system.

Nondeclarative Memory

The term *nondeclarative memory* does not refer to a discrete memory system as much as it acknowledges that some memory functions operate outside the limbic circuitry of explicit or declarative memory. Researchers have variously referred to the opposite of limbic circuitry–based memory as "habit memory" (Mishkin, Malamut, & Bachevalier, 1984), "proce-

dural memory" (Cohen, 1984), and "implicit memory" (Graf & Schacter, 1985). The variety of memory functions this term encompasses most likely reflects a collection of different abilities, not necessarily mutually exclusive, and perhaps dependent on different processing systems. For example, implicit memory implies influence by prior experience without conscious awareness of the event. Procedural learning concerns the learning of procedures, rules, or skills manifested through performance rather than verbalization, although conscious awareness may aid procedural learning. Because these terms do not by themselves encompass the whole range of nondeclarative memory, researchers prefer the less specific term (see also Squire, 1994). Neurologists also know that a single lesion cannot erase all nondeclarative memory, as it may for declarative new learning. Although it is premature to present a neuroanatomic classification scheme, scientists can describe some aspects of nondeclarative memory with respect to brain structures, particularly subcortical basal ganglia areas.

Researchers observing H.M. noticed that despite severe amnesia for declarative information, H.M. improved with practice on perceptual motor tasks such as the pursuit rotor and cognitive problem-solving exercises (such as the Tower of Hanoi) (Milner et al., 1968; Scoville, 1968). He was learning with practice despite no conscious ability to recognize this. If his amnesia had been total, examiners would have expected that each presentation of the task would be performed as if it were brand new. One area of nondeclarative memory concerns perceptual motor adaptation and skill acquisition. Many amnesiacs such as H.M. show a normal learning curve as they practice the pursuit rotor, and reverse mirror-reading tasks. The pursuit rotor requires the examinee to keep a stylus on a spinning disk, much like having to hold a place on a record on a turntable. Reverse mirror reading requires him or her to trace a maze while looking at it through a mirror. Perceptually, amnesiacs also show normal adaptive behavior when wearing visual prisms. Because prisms distort visual input, simple acts such as reaching for an object are misdirected at first. The visual motor system must quickly learn to "retune" the system so that it again correctly targets reaching according to the new visual information. Interestingly, amnesiacs can do this performance learning and adaptation despite severe declarative amnesia.

Researchers also noticed that severely amnesic Korsakoff's patients showed a phenomenon known as **implicit priming.** For example, in the word stem completion priming paradigm, a list of words is first presented (for example, *church, parachute, clarinet,* and so on) Because of the severe amnesia, the person's memory is very poor when examiners demand recall in a declarative task. Examiners then give patients three-letter word stems (for example, *chu____, par____, cla____*) and ask them to make a word by completing the stems. "Primed" Korsakoff's patients were more likely to complete the stem with a word they had already seen than were unprimed examinees, despite the same level of declarative amnesia for the words. Perceptual priming also appears in the quicker recognition of fragmented objects (such as those we presented in Chapter 4 for testing apperceptive agnosics) or of words (see Figure 5.6 for examples of priming stimuli).

In a parallel vein, Mishkin introduced the idea of "habit" memory (Mishkin et al., 1984), which he saw as not depending on the limbic system circuitry needed for explicit or declarative memory. This type of memory is evolutionarily much older and generally operates on the idea of learned associations. Researchers can demonstrate that even animals with no hippocampus can learn simple stimulus–response associations. For example, planaria can learn a light–shock pairing and recoil from the light when they subsequently encounter it alone. This suggests that

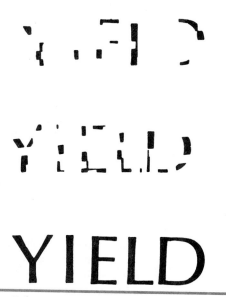

Figure 5.6 Amnesiacs who have deficient declarative memory may still have intact implicit memory as they demonstrate by quickly recognizing fragments of previously presented words. (From R. A. McCarthy and E. K. Warrington, *Cognitive Neuropsychology,* San Diego: Academic Press, 1990, p. 302, Figure 14.3)

some very basic and primitive aspects of associative conditioning are operating. Human amnesiacs produced corroborating evidence for this associative learning. An amnesic who meets a doctor on one occasion does not remember the doctor's name on the next meeting. But (demonstrating the power of associative conditioning) if that doctor pricks the patient with a pin while shaking hands on the first meeting, on the second meeting amnesiacs have been known to withdraw their hand when that hand is again extended to them, even though they may not consciously recall the association between shaking hands with the doctor and being pricked by a pin.

Whether the same brain circuitry governs all aspects of nondeclarative memory is not clear. However evidence suggests that structures supporting nondeclarative memory are probably evolutionarily and ontologically older and more primitive. We stated earlier that even simple animals with no hippocampal systems can learn associative information. Also, preverbal babies show perceptual-motor learning. Infants between 2 and 5 months of age quickly learn that they can kick to move a mobile attached to one leg (Rovee-Collier, 1993). Many brain structures involved in movement, including the cerebellum, the basal ganglia, and the motor strip, are implicated in motor learning. The cerebellum aids in sequential motor learning such as the steps required in learning the piano. An important brain circuit centered on the basal ganglia is responsible for perceptual-motor learning and adaptation. We discussed this circuit (see Figure 5.7) in Chapter 4 (see the section on subcortical motor processing). Behaviorally, Huntington's disease best portrays the effect of caudate nucleus dysfunction of the basal ganglia. Huntington's disease develops as a progressive subcortical dementia (for a thorough description, see Chapter 12), but caudate nucleus degeneration is the hallmark of Huntington's disease and is one of the first structural changes that CT scans identify. The atrophic imaging change appears at the onset of the choreic movement disorder. The effect of this change seems to target perceptual-motor learning tasks. In a series of studies spearheaded by Nelson Butters (for review, see Squire & Butters, 1984), Huntington's patients

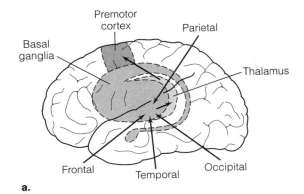

a.

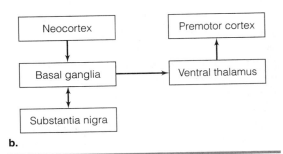

b.

Figure 5.7   (a) The circuitry of nondeclarative perceptual-motor learning. (b) Schematic of information flow from the neocortex through the basal ganglia to the premotor cortex. (Adapted from Petri and Mishkin. Behaviorism, cognitivism and the neuropsychology of memory. *American Scientist* 82:30–37, 1994)

showed a dissociation in performance from Korsakoff's amnesiacs and Alzheimer's patients. On declarative verbal memory tasks Huntington's patients performed relatively better than Korsakoff's and Alzheimer's patients. However, on motor learning tasks the two cortically impaired groups outperformed the Huntington's patients. This double dissociation in functioning prompted the initial suggestion for separate cortical and subcortical memory structures. Since that time, animal studies and imaging studies with normals performing motor learning tasks have added evidence for the role of the basal ganglia in memory.

SHORT-TERM MEMORY (STM) AND WORKING MEMORY

There seems to be a presence-chamber in my mind where full consciousness holds court, and where two or three ideas are at the same time in audience, and an ante-chamber full of more of less allied ideas, which is situated just beyond the full ken of consciousness. Out of this ante-chamber the ideas most nearly allied to those in the presence chamber appear to be summoned in a mechanically logical way, and to have their turn of audience.

—*Francis Galton* (1883)

A moment in time. In the case of amnesiacs such as H.M. and N.A., this is everything they had. But normal people also travel from moment to moment in a "presence-chamber" of the mind, using this workspace to assemble information for storage and to connect and reconnect information retrieved from LTM (long-term memory), to solve problems or make new associations. The difference is that N.A. could no longer connect moments and store aspects of the present as new memory in LTM. The limited capacity and short time frame of short-term memory (STM) does not accommodate more than a few thoughts, ideas, or bits of information at a time. As new bits arrive, they may take the place of others or simply degrade. If there is no linkage between STM and LTM, STM floats as an island with only a small area of possible habitation.

Researchers interested in memory have debated the question of the relationship of short-term memory to long-term memory. Cognitive tasks illustrate that the two appear to measure different areas of memory. STM is a limited-capacity rapid-access input-and-retrieval system analogous to computer RAM (random-access memory). LTM has unlimited capacity but with a restricted rate of input and retrieval much like ROM (read-only memory). The two systems are also coded differently. STM uses phonological coding, relying on an acoustic code, whereas LTM heavily uses semantic coding, or the associative meaning value of information to be remembered (for review, see Baddeley, 1986). Even though the two seemingly measure different aspects of memory functioning, a unitary view of memory functioning would argue that LTM depends on STM. In other words, these two systems are actually two components of one system linked in a serial fashion, so information entering LTM must inevitably flow through STM. In contrast, a separate system view would argue that LTM and STM are dissociated, so someone could have an LTM deficit with intact STM, whereas another person could have an STM deficit but maintain adequate LTM. Patients with amnesia, with severe LTM deficits, often show intact STM. On formal testing they can repeat increasingly longer series of digits and do well on other tasks presumed to test STM. However, other patients have a specific STM deficit with preserved LTM. This is some of the most convincing evidence that STM and LTM are anatomically separate.

Patients with a pure STM deficit are rare. However, researchers have reported cases with exactly this problem (for example, see Shallice & Warrington, 1970; Basso, Spinnler, Vallar, & Zanobio, 1982). Shallice and Warrington reported the case of a K.F., a patient who suffered a left posterior temporal lesion that left him with a greatly reduced short-term memory capacity for verbal information. He had a profound STM deficit, having a digit span length of about two, rather than the usual seven bits of information. As you would imagine, he also had a conduction aphasia whereby he could not repeat sentences. Surprisingly, K.F. showed a normal verbal learning curve with practice, indicating intact storage of information in LTM. It is difficult to explain K.F.'s performance with theories in which verbal STM and LTM use the same anatomic structures in different ways. Such theories also make less plausible the serial model of the relation between STM and LTM, and support a model in which verbal STM and LTM have parallel inputs.

The notion of STM as a component of LTM has gradually given way to ideas that now refer to **working memory** (Baddeley, 1986) as a distinct system encompassing some of the capacity limitations of STM, but that is a dynamic system also influencing aspect of attention and executive functioning. In this concept, which Alan Baddeley popularized, working memory directs the temporary storage of incoming information in any range of tasks from reading to math to problem solving. Researchers conceptualize

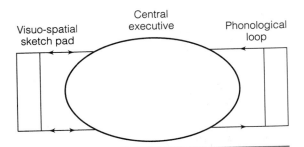

Visuo-spatial sketch pad — Central executive — Phonological loop

Figure 5.8 A simplified representation of Baddeley's working memory model. (Adapted from Alan Baddeley, *Human Memory: Theory and Practice,* Revised Edition © 1998, Boston, Allyn & Bacon, 1998, p. 71, Figure 4.2)

working memory as having three components (see Figure 5.8). The **central executive** is an attention-controlling system; it supervises and coordinates slave systems and is the proposed deficit in Alzheimer's disease. There are also two modality-specific "slave" systems. The **articulatory phonological loop** stores speech-based information and is important in the acquisition of vocabulary. The **visual-spatial sketch pad** manipulates visual and spatial images.

Neuropsychologically, the phonological loop and the visual-spatial sketch pad link to lateralized modalities in the brain and to frontal lobe executive processes. The phonological loop involves auditory-verbal processing and depends on language-based left hemisphere processes. Likewise, the visual-spatial sketch pad is associated with the right hemisphere. Goldman-Rakic's (1988) groundbreaking work in primate models of working memory points to the dorsolateral prefrontal cortex as the area that holds information "on line" while it is processed. In these studies, Goldman-Rakic tested monkeys' abilities to recall the position of food in one of two food wells after a short delay of several seconds. Figure 5.9 shows the general paradigm of the study. Simultaneous recordings from neurons in the dorsolateral prefrontal area continued to fire during the delay until the action of food selection was completed. Since her work, PET and fMRI studies have supplied confirmation in humans that the prefrontal cortex activates during working memory tasks (Jonides et al., 1993).

The move from conceptualizing STM as a storage capacity system to working memory as a dynamic integrated system reveals a greater understanding of the interrelated nature of brain systems. Attentional and executive processes are both crucial to the adequate functioning of working memory. Other memory processes such as prospective memory, or the memory for future intention, also rely on frontal lobe and executive functioning processes.

Attention

Moving about the world, people confront a flood of information that the nervous system cannot treat equally. Your brain must target or "spotlight" specific material to process and tune out the irrelevant. For example, when you stop to talk to a friend in a hallway, you may hear competing sounds of others talking and people walking down the corridor. You may also be preoccupied by your own inner thoughts. Nonetheless, if you "pay attention" you can orient to a small sample of the incoming information and to ignore most of the other input. In this way attention operates as a gateway for information processing. Attention allows orienting to, selecting, and maintaining focus on information to make it available for cortical processing.

The neuropsychology of attention has historically been an amorphous subject because there are so many subsets of attentional processing and many possible definitions of attention. The term *attention* can refer to general level of alertness or vigilance; a general state of arousal; orientation versus habituation to stimuli; the ability to focus, divide, or sustain mental effort; the ability to target processing within a specific sensory arena (such as visual attention or auditory attention); or a measure of capacity. Researchers have also asked whether attention implies a general state of cortical tone or energy, or functions as a network or set of specific structures or networks within the brain. Attentional processing does not imply a unified system, but most researchers now see it as a multifaceted concept that implies multiple behavioral states and cortical processes that various subsets of cerebral structures control.

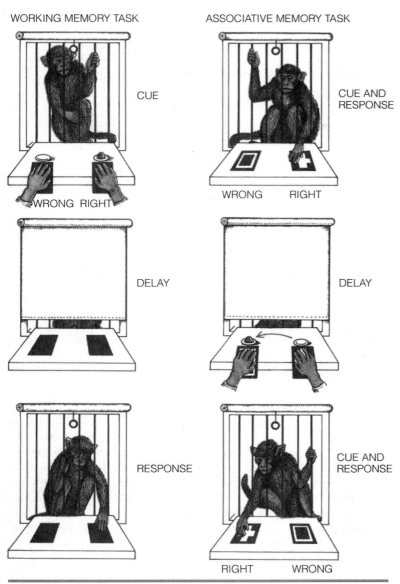

WORKING MEMORY TASK

ASSOCIATIVE MEMORY TASK

CUE

WRONG RIGHT

CUE AND RESPONSE

WRONG RIGHT

DELAY

DELAY

RESPONSE

CUE AND RESPONSE

RIGHT WRONG

Figure 5.9 In Goldman-Rakic's working memory task (left), the target food stimulus is placed and the monkey must remember the position during a brief delay. This contrasts with an associative LTM task (right) in which the monkey has to learn the association of the plus sign with food. (Courtesy of Patricia J. Wynne/Tody Press, New York. From P. Goldman-Rakic, "Working Memory and the Mind," in *Mind and Brain: Readings from* Scientific American. New York: W. H. Freeman, 1993, p. 69)

In many types of brain dysfunction, efficiency of the brain to process information diminishes. Sometimes people cannot sustain attention to one particular stimulus for longer periods of time or cannot select information (selective attention) from competing sources. This impairment may be minimally present and can only be detected with formal neuropsychological testing, or may be profound and easily noticeable by any observer.

Neuropsychological theories of attentional processing (for example, see Mesulam, 1981; Posner & Petersen, 1990) usually consider the role of the reticular activating system in cortical arousal, subcortical and limbic system structures (particularly the cingulate gyrus) in regulation of information to be attended to, the posterior parietal lobe system in focusing conscious attention, and the frontal lobes in directing attentional resources. They also give the right hemisphere prominence as an attentional processor. Theorists have not yet worked out any one-to-one correspondence between levels of attentional behavior and brain structures or networks. Rather, they can describe general subsets of brain systems related to attentional functioning. Figure 5.10 presents a useful framework for conceptualizing attention, which Mesulam (1985a) developed.

SUBCORTICAL STRUCTURES INFLUENCING ATTENTION

The reticular activating system (RAS) regulates the level of cortical activation or arousal—a necessary first step in attentional processing. With its genesis in the midbrain and its ability to project to large cortical areas, the RAS sets a general cortical tone. Researchers can observe and categorize this arousal into brain wave types (beta, alpha, theta, and delta) by their frequency as measured by an EEG. In a general way, sensory input "charges" the RAS. If the brain stem is processing sensory input, the RAS maintains high cortical activation. However, lack of sensory input does not necessarily make one drowsy. In fact, even with constant sensory input there can be habituation. Those who live on a noisy street grow accustomed to the sound, but a sudden silence will cause the brain to orient to the change in sound pattern-

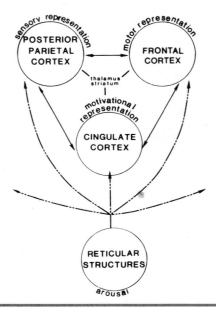

Figure 5.10   A theoretical schematic of the attentional system. (From M. M. Mesulam, *Principles of Behavioral Neurology*, Philadelphia, E. A. Davis, 1985. Reprinted from R. A. Cohen *The Neuropsychol of Attention*. NY: Plenum, 1993, p. 334, Figure 14.2, with permission)

ing. Daily biorhythms of 90 minutes of relatively higher and lower alertness also cycle throughout the day and circadian rhythms control the sleep-wake cycle through the RAS. We discuss these changing levels of cortical tone further in our discussion of sleep (see Chapter 13). If a person is awake and alert, general level of arousal is more of a background issue than a central one in the neuropsychology of attentional processing. However, the RAS also plays a role in anticipatory responding. Researchers have hypothesized that the RAS may send a preparatory signal to the cortex to alert it to receive stimuli and so put it in a heightened state of readiness to receive. Lesions to the RAS can result in lowered alertness or coma.

Researchers know the basal ganglia best for their role in motor functioning but have also recognized their role in the sensory selection of material for further attentional processing. Van Zomeren and Brouwer (1994) have likened the role of the basal ganglia to that of a clearinghouse of competing stimuli, selecting some information for further processing and ignoring others.

THE CEREBRAL CORTEX AND ATTENTION

The attentional issues of most interest to human neuropsychology generally concern the higher levels of attentional processing coordinated by the cerebrum, including focused attention, the ability to alternate and divide attentional processes, and the ability to sustain attention. **Focused attention** is the ability to respond and pick out the important elements or "figure" of attention from the "ground" or background of external and internal stimulation. Focused attention also implies a measure of concentration or effortful processing. A basketball player who can concentrate on making a free throw while tuning out the crowd is a good example of high focus. However, even the most ordinary event of noticing requires cognitive focus. People are frequently called on to alternate and divide attention in the course of daily activities. For example, a receptionist who must switch back and forth between answering the phone and talking with customers must employ **alternating attention** while mentally holding a place to return to the other activity. **Divided attention** requires partialing out attentional resources at the same time rather than switching back and forth, however quickly. A good example is driving a car, listening to a radio, and talking with a passenger. Researchers have debated whether divided attention is in fact possible or if people just manage to shift their attention quickly between different stimuli. However, some evidence indicates that people can divide attention to some degree. **Sustained attention** is the ability to maintain an effortful response over time. It is related to the ability to persist and sustain a level of vigilance. People who work as air traffic controllers or on assembly-line jobs must have excellent abilities for sustaining attention.

Posner and his colleagues (for example, see Posner & Petersen, 1990) have studied the posterior parietal lobe system extensively in the realm of visual attentional processing. The posterior attentional network centers on the parietal lobe, the lateral pulvinar of the posteriolateral thalamus, and the superior colliculus. This system plays a role in conscious attention to portions of your visual-spatial field and then directs the attention of your eyes to the point in space. The posterior parietal lobe mediates conscious attention to spatial targets, the superior colliculus plays a role in directing the eyes from one position to another, and the pulvinar of the thalamus is an area that, like the basal ganglia, helps select and filter important sensory information for processing. People with lesions to the right posterior parietal lobe frequently fail to attend to the opposite visual field, although they can detect visual input. We introduced this problem, termed *neglect,* in the section on visual disorders in Chapter 4, because it certainly affects the visual system. However, it is also a problem of inattention (see Figure 5.11 on p. 173). Posner (Posner & Petersen, 1990) describes this as a problem of engaging, moving, and disengaging focus to objects in the contralateral field of vision. In this view, the patient loses attention to a visual field partly because the problem affects covert orientation and partly because of difficulties in returning attention to previously examined locations. The term *covert orientation* refers to a spatial engagement of attention to a target area before the nervous system directs the eyes to move. In this case the system does not direct the eyes and the brain to attend to, or engage, the left side of space, or to disengage attention from the right side of space.

The posterior parietal lobes have rich interconnections to specific regions within the lateral and medial frontal cortex (Goldman-Rakic, 1988). This neural highway courses through the cingulate. The cingulate gyrus contains alternating neuronal bands, some of which project to the posterior parietal lobe and others that project to the dorsolateral prefrontal cortex (Goldman-Rakic, 1988). One role for the anterior cingulate is in target detection (Posner & Petersen, 1990). Recall, also, that the cingulate is also important in language processing, so it may play a larger attentional role beyond visual processing. The role of the frontal cortex in attention relates to aspects of attentional planning, shifting of attentional set (alternating and dividing attention) and sustaining attention versus becoming distracted. Patients with frontal lobe damage often complain of being upset or easily

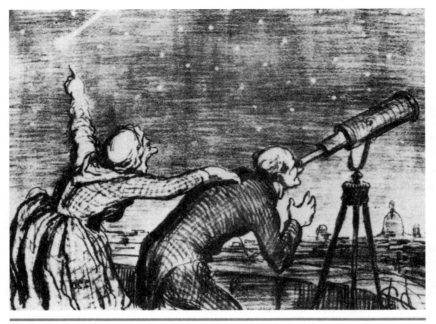

Figure 5.11   A case of "hemispatial inattention." (From Honoré Daumier, "M. Babinet prevenu par sa portiere de la visite de la comete," *Le Charivari,* 1858. Reprinted from R. A. Cohen, *The Neuropsychology of Attention,* New York: Plenum Press, 1993, frontispiece, with permission)

led off track by distractions. They may find it difficult to listen and take notes at the same time, to sequence the steps of a meal if interrupted by talking with someone, or to watch a movie without drifting off.

The attentional systems and structures we have presented here are skewed toward visual attentional processing because this is the best understood and most widely studied sensory processing system in relation to attention. Less is known about auditory attention, but some have suggested that where the superior colliculus plays a role in directing visual attention, the inferior colliculus plays a similar role in auditory attention. Also, researchers have identified the right hemisphere as having a special role in attentional processing. It may have its most important role in maintaining alertness and vigilance. In split-brain patients, tests that present information to one hemisphere indicate that vigilance is lower in the left hemisphere. Norepinephrine (NE) is one of most important neurotransmitter systems in maintaining alertness and attention (Posner & Petersen, 1990) because of its widespread innervation in the posterior attention system (posterior parietal lobe, pulvinar, and superior colliculus). Also, animal studies with rats show that right hemisphere lesions deplete NE in both hemispheres. Finally, drugs that affect NE also impact attentional level.

The problems presented thus far indicate how specific or localized damage to attentional networks can affect attentional processes. Attentional dysfunction, however, is often a concomitant of more generalized cerebral impairment. Table 5.1 provides a partial listing of disorders that include attentional dysfunction as a prominent component of the symptom pattern. The range of disorders illustrates that attentional processes are somewhat "fragile" and thus are easily compromised by a number of neurologic, metabolic, and psychiatric disorders. Fatigue, or inability to sustain attention to an activity, frequently appears across a number of more generalized neuropsychological dis-

Table 5.1	*Disorders Showing Prominent Attentional Dysfunction*

Attention Deficit Disorder

Neurological Disease
    Multiple sclerosis
    Alzheimer's disease
    Parkinson's disease

Head Trauma

Seizure Disorders

Metabolic Disorder
    Hypoglycemic encephalopathy
    Hyperthyroidism

Psychiatric Disorders
    Depression
    Mania
    Schizophrenia

Right Hemisphere Stroke: Unilateral Neglect

orders. Patients with neurologic disease, as well as patients who have suffered a closed head injury, often complain of mentally wearing out when engaged in tasks that require persistent effortful attention. People with affective disorders frequently complain of attention and concentration problems. Depressed people often complain of drifting off or "spacing out," so that even when driving they may miss an exit. Mania is associated with concentration problems of another sort. Manic people may become so energetic with a relentless "flight of ideas" passing through the mind that they cannot accomplish anything, because they cannot concentrate on one thing at a time.

Attentional deficits are also a common concomitant of schizophrenia. These include perseveration of thought and action, inability to disengage attention, problems in sustained attention or vigilance, distractibility, and an almost random tendency to orient to both external and internal stimuli. This set of deficits may give rise to the loose associations in thought processes that schizophrenics commonly show. Close to half of schizophrenics show no galvanic skin conductance response, which is ordinarily considered an orienting response to novel sensory stimuli (Dawson &

Nuechterlein, 1984). Neuropsychologists call this subgroup of schizophrenics *electrodermal nonresponders*. Nonresponders are more likely to show the negative symptoms of schizophrenia including apathy, emotional and social withdrawal, and blunted affect. Nonresponders are also more likely to have cortical atrophy than schizophrenic galvanic skin responders. Interestingly, the failure of a psychophysiological skin conductance orienting response to sensory stimulation comes against a background of chronic elevation of autonomic responses, which implies a generalized hyperarousal in this subgroup. Some have suggested (see Cohen, 1993, for review) that the attention deficit in schizophrenia may be a primary cognitive dysfunction.

EXECUTIVE FUNCTIONING

The prefrontal lobes are unique in organization and function among all other areas of the cortex. For a long time neuropsychologists only knew what the frontal lobes did *not* do. The functions of the temporal, parietal, and occipital lobes follow straightforward principles of organization built around sensory system processing. But the frontal lobes seemed "silent," largely because injury did not result in obvious disability. Frontal lobe pathology does not result in primary disorders of sensation or perception, motor disability, memory, or language. But the frontal lobes are richly interconnected with all posterior and subcortical areas. If the brain is a symphony, the frontal lobes act as the conductor. The term "executive functioning" is apt in describing that aspect of cortical functioning that has to do with managing, structuring, and directing behavior. It deals with planning, flexible problem solving, and at the highest levels, the self-monitoring and self-assessment of behavior. Executive functioning is not a single behavior but a category of behavior that is orchestrated primarily by different aspects of the frontal systems on the rest of the brain. Executive functioning impairments become most evident in the most complex aspects of human conscious activity, or those activities of higher problem solving, reasoning, abstraction, critical self-awareness, and social interaction that make us human (see Neuropsychology in Action 5.2).

Stuss and Benson (1986) have proposed a useful model of executive functioning in relation to general brain functioning (see Figure 5.12). At a basic level of brain functioning, they suggest, operations such as memory, language, sensory, and motor functions operate according to well-defined and automatic programs (they can function without much conscious intention). However, to be executed at the right time and in the right place, higher levels of behavior require planning and integration of these functions. Luria (1990) gives an example of the problem-solving difficulties of Patient U, who suffered from a progressive frontal lobe tumor:

The patient gets the problem: *One ABC book and one pen cost 37 cents. One ABC book and two pens cost 49 cents. How much do one ABC book and one pen cost separately?*

The patient repeats the problem correctly but does not begin to solve it.

What should you do to solve the problem?
"37 and 49 . . . then it's 86 all in all . . ."
What did you add them for?
"To learn how much they paid all in all."
What should you do next?
"Next . . . I don't know what next. . . . There is nothing else. . . ."

In order to draw the patient's attention to the final question and help him distinguish the main solution elements, the statement is presented in writing in the form of the following equations:

One ABC book + one pen = 37 cents
One ABC book + two pens = '49 cents
The question *How much do one ABC book and one pen cost separately?* is repeated.

The patient reads the equation, draws a line underneath and writes down the result of simple summation:
"Two ABC books + three pens = 86 cents" saying "I've learned how many pens and ABC books, how much everything costs."

It is evident that our attempt to show the difference between the two equations and to prompt the proper logical sequence ended in failure. . . . [T]he investigator gives him the initial element of the respective logical chain.

First 37 cents were spent, then 49 cents. What is the difference accounted for?
"It is accounted for by one pen! Then, 49 − 37 = 1 pen."
What should you learn?
"How much do an ABC book and a pen cost separately."
So?
So, a pen costs 12 cents. Now an ABC book . . .
49 − 24 = 25 cents. One ABC book costs 25 cents. (Luria, 1990, pp. 106–107)

In this example, U knows the arithmetic operations necessary to solve problems but cannot discern the important aspects of the problem without external structure. In fact, at first he cannot initiate any response. His first, rather impulsive response is simply to sum the numbers. He rigidly adheres to this strategy and is too cognitively inflexible to think of other possibilities. However, when he is guided, when the

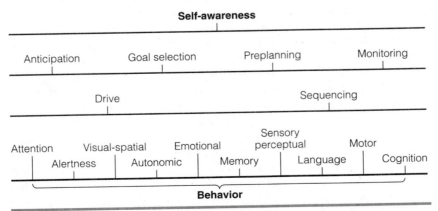

Figure 5.12 A hierarchical model of brain functioning. (From D. T. Stuss and D. F. Benson, *The Frontal Lobes*, Philadelphia: Lippincott-Ravens Publishers, 1986)

Neuropsychology in Action 5.2

The Frontal Lobes

by Elkhonon Goldberg Ph.D., New York University School of Medicine.

Over the last few decades it has become clear that the prefrontal cortex is particularly vulnerable to a broad range of neurologic and psychiatric conditions, and that it plays a pivotal role in the neural control over cognition. Neuropsychologists presume that the prefrontal cortex is central in formulating goals, intentionality, and plans subordinate to the goals; selecting goal-appropriate cognitive routines; providing sequential access to these routines; and evaluating the outcome of the actions. Some authors refer to the functions of the prefrontal cortex as "executive," by analogy with a corporate CEO (chief executive officer). An analogy with the orchestra conductor may be even more appropriate. The literature links two types of cognitive operations to the prefrontal cortex particularly often. The first operation concerns the organism's ability to guide its behavior by internal representations. In a poetic vein, David Ingvar referred to such representations as "memories of the future." This capacity is at the core of goal-oriented behavior.

The ability to guide behavior by internal representations links to working memory. Working memory involves accessing goal-appropriate internal representations in a changing cognitive context. The prefrontal cortex plays a crucial role in these processes. For example, an organism must be capable of shifting cognitive sets when demands change (Goldman-Rakic, 1987a). And a dynamic balance must exist between guiding behavior by internal represen-

tations and shifting cognitive sets, controlled by the frontal lobes (Milner, 1982). Various forms of frontal lobe pathology may upset this balance, leading to extreme cognitive symptoms: perseveration and environmentally dependent behavior.

Most real-life situations are intrinsically ambiguous. There is nothing inherently correct in wearing a blue suit as opposed to a gray suit, ordering steak as opposed to lamb chops, or attending medical school as opposed to law school. Such choices reflect an interaction between the properties of the external situation and the goals, motives, and personal history of the actor. Recent research has demonstrated the central role of the prefrontal cortex in resolving ambiguity (Goldberg, Podell, Harner, Lovell, & Riggio, 1994). Another important role of the frontal lobes is in its relationship to novelty. The frontal lobes seem to be crucially engaged when the organism faces a novel situation. Conversely, when the organism encounters a routine situation, the role of the frontal lobes is less prominent. Neuroimaging studies show that prefrontal activation accompanies the introduction of a novel task (Raichle et al., 1994).

Recent research suggests that the functional organization of the frontal lobes is sexually dimorphic. In males the frontal lobes are strongly lateralized: the left prefrontal system adopts a more context-dependent response selection bias, and the right hemisphere a more context-independent response selection

bias. In females the frontal lobes are less lateralized, both exhibiting a more context-independent response selection bias (Goldberg et al., 1994). The prefrontal cortex is implicated in an exceptionally broad range of neurologic, neuropsychiatric, neurodevelopmental, and neurogeriatric disorders. It appears that in many conditions frontal lobe dysfunction, documented through physiological or cognitive means, is evident although there is no morphologic damage. This has led some authors to conclude that the frontal lobes have a particularly low functional breakdown threshold (Goldberg, 1991).

Reticulo-frontal disconnection is an important mechanism producing a frontal lobe syndrome without a frontal lobe lesion (Goldberg, Bilder, Hughes, Antin, & Mattis, 1989). It entails neurodevelopmental or acquired abnormality of the nuclei found in the ventral brain stem and/or pathways projecting from these nuclei into the frontal lobes. These structures involve the ventral tegmental area and the mesocortical dopamine projections emanating from it. Thus a neurodevelopmental aberration of these pathways has been implicated in schizophrenia, and an acquired aberration in closed head injury. As you can see, people's lives are full of ambiguity and frontal lobes help them make choices— one hopes, the right ones. If their frontal lobes are injured or are not functioning correctly, people's choices usually become inaccurate, and unusual; maladaptive, or dangerous behavior may result.

interviewer provides the important aspects of the problem for him, he can arrive at the correct answer. According to the Stuss and Benson model, U's primary programs for math algorithms are intact, and they act in a fairly automatic or stereotyped manner. Unless organized by higher-order executive functions, problem-solving behavior becomes chaotic, sometimes failing to initiate, sometimes having to logical sequence, or sometimes perseverating on the first problem-solving strategy that comes to mind.

At the top of the hierarchy, perhaps the most high-level function of all is the ability to self-monitor and self-regulate behavior; in other words, to notice one's own behavior and modify it as the circumstances dictate. This includes monitoring internal states as well as monitoring response to external feedback. Others often describe people who have suffered frontal lobe injury as having suffered a personality change (see Neuropsychology in Action 5.3). The individual may also feel the loss of a sense of self. The specific psychosocial difficulties co-occurring with frontal lobe injury, which others often perceive as a personality change, are impulsivity, disinhibition, lack of initiation, rigidity, loss of abstract attitude, poor social judgment, and loss of personal and social awareness. In addition, neuropsychologists usually attribute to various manifestations of frontal lobe difficulties the common perception that individuals with closed head injuries have an "egocentric" or "unempathic" attitude (for example, see Grattan & Eslinger, 1989). Specifically, researchers suggest that the inability to take the role of another is either a result of cognitive rigidity or is related to cognitive rigidity in some other manner.

One of our patients, a man in his fifties provides a classic example of impulsivity following a frontal lobe injury. Before his injury T.J. was a successful businessman who traveled around the region making sales calls. After the injury, one day he was to arrive at our office within a major medical center at 9 A.M. He drove around the parking garage trying to find a parking space. Being unsuccessful in finding an empty spot he became frustrated. Finally he was stuck behind a car whose driver was waiting for someone else to back out. Impulsively, T.J. rammed the car ahead of him. Relating this story, T.J. expressed dismay at himself for acting in a way he felt was wrong. Yet he felt that

at the moment, he just couldn't help himself. Most of us have been frustrated, and many have felt like lashing out at such times. But for the most part we inhibit these impulses. Impulsivity, a lowered frustration tolerance, and disinhibition also manifest in sexually or socially inappropriate comments. The psychosocial impact of self-monitoring difficulties often represents the heaviest burden for patients and families and are probably most influential for reintegration into family and society (for example, see Bond, 1976). Failures of self-monitoring often contribute to the loss of jobs and relationships.

Consciousness

What is consciousness? What makes human consciousness different from that of other animals? What sorts of brains or brain activity are necessary for conscious experience? Is self-awareness a mind process, as William James thought, or a mind state? These questions have tantalized philosophers, theologians, and scientists throughout time. Brain science has relatively recently taken up the challenge of deciphering consciousness. This was once the domain of psychology, spearheaded by Wilhelm Wundt and the early structuralists at the turn of the century; the strong behavioral movement in American psychology later cast aside the study of consciousness as too subjective for serious study. Observable behavior was now paramount, and the brain was merely a "black box." Psychologists now know that consciousness is fundamentally important to understanding the human condition. Conscious experience, however, is difficult to measure and observe because of its highly private nature. Nobel prize laureate Francis Crick (Crick and James Watson discovered the structure of DNA) admonishes scientists to not worry too much over aspects of the problem that they cannot solve scientifically or, more precisely, cannot solve solely by using existing scientific ideas. Perhaps the only sensible approach is to press the experimental attack until scientists confront dilemmas that call for new ways of thinking (Crick & Koch, 1990).

Here we are concerned with defining the concept of consciousness, the mind–brain relationship, and

Neuropsychology in Action 5.3

The Case of Phineas Gage

by Mary Spiers

In 1848 Phineas Gage was 25 years old, a foreman employed by the Rutland and Burlington Railroad. On an autumn day in Vermont, he and his crew were blasting through a rocky section when an accidental explosion sent a long metal bar, a tamping iron, shooting through his head. The pointed end of the rod entered under his left cheek and exited near the top middle of his skull, near the coronal and sagittal sutures. The rod was launched with such force that it landed 30 meters away from him. Amazingly, although Gage was knocked flat, he was able to get up, and walk to the ox cart on which he sat while being driven into town. During the ride he chatted and made an entry into his logbook. Because he survived such a freakish accident, the case of Phineas Gage is arguably one of the most famous in the early history of neuropsychology.

Before the accident Gage was seen as well balanced emotionally and mentally, healthy and active. Immediately after the accident, he fought postinjury infection to recover physically. He could walk and converse, he recognized his friends and family, and appeared rational. To some he seemed fully recovered. But changes in his behavior soon emerged. His doctors noted, "Remembers passing and past events correctly, as well as before the injury. Intellectual manifestations feeble, being exceedingly

capricious and childish, but with a will as indomitable as ever; is particularly obstinate; will not yield to restraint when it conflicts with his desires" (Harlow, 1868, in Macmillan, 1996, p. 246). As time went on this behavior did not abate but endured. Six months later his doctor, John Martin Harlow, summarized his condition:

> The equilibrium or balance, so to speak, between his intellectual faculties and his animal propensities, seems to have been destroyed. He is fitful, irreverent, indulging at times in the grossest profanity (which was not previously his custom), manifesting but little deference for his fellows, impatient of restraint or advice when it conflicts with his desires, at times pertinaciously obstinate, yet capricious and vacillating, devising many plans of future operation, which are no sooner arranged than they are abandoned in turn for others appearing more feasible. A child in his intellectual capacity and manifestations, he has the animal passions of a strong man. Previous to his injury, although untrained in the schools, he possessed a well-balanced mind, and was looked upon by those who knew him as a shrewd, smart businessman, very energetic and persistent in executing all his plans of operation. In this regard his mind was radically changed so decidedly that his friends and acquaintances said he was

"no longer Gage." (Harlow, 1868, in Macmillan, 1996, p. 247)

Gage certainly suffered extensive damage to his left frontal lobe and probably also suffered damage to his right frontal lobe. Damasio and her colleagues (Damasio, Grabowski, Frank, Galaburda, & Damasio, 1994) have attempted to reconstruct the trajectory and site of damage based on three-dimensional computer modeling of the brain and skull. Their best estimate is that the tamping rod impacted "the anterior half of the orbital frontal cortex . . . the polar and anterior mesial frontal cortices . . . and the anterior-most sector of the anterior cingulate gyrus." Some right hemisphere damage was also implicated. It is interesting that Harlow implied Gage could no longer "execute" his plans. Many behaviors Gage exhibited are characteristic of people who have problems of executive functioning. Although his basic abilities to process information were intact, he showed low frustration tolerance and impulse control and a loss of ability to structure and follow through on plans—so much so, in fact, that he was seen as a changed person.

Source: The historical references for this case were summarized from M. Macmillan, "Phineas Gage: A Case for All Reasons," in C. Code, C, Wallesch, Y. Joanette, and A. R. Lecours (eds.), *Classic Cases in Neuropsychology* (Sussex, England: Psychology Press, 1996, pp. 243–262).

current theories related to how the brain represents consciousness. After considering the "how" of consciousness, we turn to theorist David Chalmer's question related to the "why" of consciousness. Even if we can explain how the brain represents conscious experience, we need to know *why* this is important to human functioning. Why are we not unthinking and unfeeling automatons?

To begin, most people agree that consciousness implies awareness. This is the primary dictionary definition. The term *consciousness* also refers to a certain level of mental alertness and attention. It also connotes what one's inner self knows or feels. Consciousness is above all a subjective and highly personal reckoning of both external and internal events. Measuring it has also relied largely on the person's ability to manifest internal experiences through verbal expression. The issue of awareness raises interesting questions for the neuropsychologist. If the mind is the subjective experience of brain states and processes, then the mind reflects awareness of brain and body functioning. Because of either external or internal stimulation, sometimes the mind may be able to show more awareness whereas at other times it seems totally oblivious to the workings of the physical brain and body. One of the main questions that brain science must answer (to put it in what is now the common vernacular) is, What distinguishes the conscious mind from the subconscious or unconscious mind?

MIND AND BRAIN

Popular culture often represents the brain in mechanistic terms, like a type of giant computer, reminiscent of Newtonian physics. However, machines can self-regulate their behavior, but do not have self-awareness or a subjective experience of consciousness. An interesting theoretical question relates to whether computers will someday imitate the human brain, and presumably become conscious. This concept, known as *artificial intelligence (AI),* underlies the imagined character HAL, the supercomputer in the science fiction movie *2001: A Space Odyssey.* During a space shuttle to Mars, HAL starts to display "his" own awareness and decision-making capability, finally killing off the shuttle crew.

Conceptualizing the brain as a computer has only limited usefulness. After all, brains have built computers, not the other way around. It seems more useful to conceptualize the brain as attached to the person, as a biological entity. The level of consciousness of biological entities partly responds to biological and cosmic rhythms, as evidenced in the sleep–wake cycle and the rhythm of the sun. Consciousness also changes in response to internal physiology and chemistry, with inputs from food and drugs. People use the term "mind" to reflect subjective experience, and therefore consciousness, of the emanations of the brain and the body together. They assume that every state of mind links to a brain state, and every state of brain reflects a mind state, be it conscious or unconscious.

Scientists have often wondered if split-brain patients, who have had the two hemispheres of their brain surgically disconnected, are "of two minds." In an older method of treating seizures, surgeons cut the half-billion axons that allow interhemispheric cross-talk in many patients with intractable seizures. Are these two hemispheres still conscious of each other? Do split-brain patients retain one consciousness, or do two separate realities or even two separate personalities exist? Immediately after surgery some split-brain patients report having two competing hemispheres. When getting dressed, the right hand may reach for a blue shirt while the left hand is grabbing a red shirt. These apparently competing programs, however, usually resolve within a matter of weeks. After that, split-brain patients typically report a unified conscious experience. In daily life their actions are not recognizably different from their presurgery state. Only specialized testing that can present information to only one hemisphere at a time continues to reveal differences. In effect, this testing appears to reveal more differences between right and left hemisphere processing than it shows a fundamental division of consciousness in those who have had a split-brain operation.

The stumbling block is that we usually document awareness via our ability to verbalize, a province largely of the left hemisphere. In individuals with an intact corpus callosum, the right hemisphere—and therefore the consciousness of the right hemisphere—is accessible to left hemisphere verbalizations. Split-brain patients must reformulate a sense of completeness by making their experiences accessible to both halves of their brains through external cross-talk. They can largely do this by moving their eyes to capture both visual fields and verbalizing out loud so that each hemisphere hears what is available to the other hemisphere. Within all people many brain and body processes are either automatic or unavailable and so typically remain unconscious to the mind. For split-brain patients the hemispheres are physically unavailable to each other. The brain is not communicating internally, but the subjective experience is of one mind. The challenge for the split-brain patient is to consciously integrate each half of the cerebral hemispheres that have been made surgically unconscious of each other.

Most people with intact brains agree that large areas of potential experience remain below the level of conscious experience. The common saying "We only use 10% of our brain" (see discussion of Flourens in Chapter 1) might be better thought of as "Our conscious mind may be only aware of a percentage of what our brains do and are capable of." Our brains control and monitor the entire nervous system of our bodies and respond to physiological mechanisms in the body, such as those of the endocrine system, to maintain a state of brain–body homeostasis. Many of these processes are automatic and reflexive. They are unconscious. But they can be brought into awareness via techniques such as biofeedback and can then be modified by the conscious mind. Many have wondered what might be possible if aspects of the unconscious mind became conscious. What hidden potential could people then develop, such as becoming conscious during the "unconscious" state of sleep or developing senses and perception beyond what is now commonly thought possible? This may sound like the stuff of science fiction, but researchers have documented lucid dreaming, which we discuss later in Chapter 13. It is also reasonable to assume that scientists will find ways to study the limits of sensory-perceptual experiences. Boundaries between the concepts of the conscious mind and the unconscious mind are blurring. The challenge now before brain science is to understand the workings of these aspects of mind and to relate them to brain states and processes.

ANATOMIC CORRELATES OF CONSCIOUSNESS

How are states of consciousness represented in brain anatomy and physiology? Descartes thought the pineal gland was the center of conscious experience, but researchers have found no single location for consciousness. After several hundred more years, this question may still be somewhat premature, because brain science has not yet clearly defined the operations and boundaries of consciousness. Different areas of the brain may play roles in specific aspects of conscious perception and alertness. Brain science is also now providing interesting clues as to how the brain "binds" disparate fragments of information from different cortical and subcortical regions into a subjective sense of coherent unity.

The candidates for brain regions and or functional areas having a role in conscious behavior have, depending on the behavior in question, included numerous areas of the brain, both cortical and subcortical. The various definitions of consciousness suggests that different brain correlates are implicated depending on whether the focus is on notions of awareness or perception, notions of alertness or attention, or notions of what is felt or known by one's inner self. Perceptual awareness, "knowing," and therefore perceptual consciousness, build up through modality-specific sensory systems of vision, audition, proprioception, olfaction, and taste. The brain correlates of sensory-perceptual consciousness depend on the integrity of each of these systems. Therefore, it is possible for one sensory modality to block access to "knowing," while still showing awareness through other sensory modalities. Such is the case with the agnosias, which can follow damage to any of the sensory systems (see Chapter 4). When speaking of level of consciousness, or alertness, researchers often identify the reticular activating system in the midbrain as responsible for arousal. Finally, if the self-referential, self-evaluative, and metacognitive aspects of consciousness are the focus, then researchers can consider aspects of executive system and frontal lobe functioning. Only the cerebellum seems to have no identified role in current discussions of the neuropsychology of consciousness.

Brain researchers and theorists have been most intrigued by how the brain creates a unitary experience of consciousness at one particular moment in time. They call this the *binding problem*. What is the mechanism that binds disparate neural elements together? A unitary experience of consciousness is an operation of the highest order and therefore requires a cortex. Thus the more sophisticated the cortex, the greater the ability for subjective experience and self-awareness.

Let's examine the role of the cortex in consciousness more closely. Neuroscientists commonly describe experiences represented in the cortex as stable spatial patterns. For example, vision is a complex constructional process resulting in object recognition by building and binding elements related to color, form, movement, and spatial position. This binding may occur as a simple structural pattern. Experience in seeing your grandmother increasingly "hard-wires" the synaptic conjunctions between the neurons from various cortical areas, forming the pattern that defines "grandmother." This way of thinking is an advance over conceptualizations that first postulated the existence of single "grandmother" cells in which the recognition of grandmother, although the culmination of many processes, was ultimately embodied in one neuron or neuron group. Brain scientists soon realized that the model of single cumulative grandmother cells was grossly inefficient, because separate cells would have to be available for every possible combination and permutation of people and objects. Even though the brain consists of billions of neurons, it would soon run out of neurons for every possible permutation of a memory. Having grandmother represented in a large cortical neuronal assembly is a more efficient conceptualization in terms of processing. Individual neurons can participate in different assemblies, one representing grandmother, another father, another a teacher, and so on. The firing pattern within the web of neurons takes precedence over any individual neuron. If the pattern is disrupted at crucial points, the brain loses recognition of the person.

The neocortex unquestionably plays a major role in evaluating external and internal experience, but subcortical structures, and particularly the thalamus, may play a crucial role in orchestrating the higher cortical symphony. Francis Crick and Christof Koch (1990), in their study of visual consciousness, have postulated that the upper layers of the cortex are largely unconscious, while the pyramidal neurons in layer 5 may be "conscious." Their reasoning is that this is the only layer that "projects right out of the cortical system." Layer 5 also shows an unusual propensity to fire in bursts. Others have also noted this important observation that groups of neurons fire together in bursts, which appears to be an important clue to the binding problem. Researchers know that many cell assemblies throughout the brain fire in synchronous oscillations. For example, in the motor system the inferior olive of the brain stem sends information in packets of bursts at an oscillation of 10 cps (cycles per second) to the cerebellum. Much as with frames of a movie, the movement only appears fluid because we cannot discriminate the fine breaks in continuity.

The thalamus, the sensory relay station of the brain, may play one of the most crucial roles in synchronizing cortical processes. In an alert state, an EEG records in the gamma frequency range (35 to 80 cps) averaging 40 cps from the cortex. This normal frequency decreases with relaxed wakefulness to 8 to 10 cps and with deep sleep and coma to 1/2 to 4 cps. Faster frequencies are asynchronous, whereas slower frequencies become increasingly synchronized and rhythmic. Rodolfo Llinas of New York University (Llinas, in Becker & Seldon, 1985) postulates that the EEG frequency represents a binding wave that continuously sweeps the cortex like a huge radar arm. As the wave scans the brain, the brain synchronizes and interprets all information in that sweep as a unified experience. This action, then, could bind packets of information from widely distributed and noncontiguous regions of the cortex by synchronizing them in time. The implication is that more hard-wired spatial patterns of neurons do not act as the prime binding mechanism. Researchers have postulated this theory as a general explanation for how consciousness operates, as well as a specific explanation for how aspects of visual consciousness such as visual object recognition work (Bressler, Coppola, & Nakamura, 1993; Crick & Koch, 1990).

If there is a "binding wave," from where does this frequency emanate? It appears as if the intralaminar nucleus of the thalamus generates the cortical binding signal every 12.5 thousandths of a second (Llinas, in Becker & Seldon, 1985). As previously mentioned, nearly all sensory and motor systems route through the thalamus. The thalamus is in constant two-way communication with the cortex through a feedback system of millions of thalamocortical loops. Many investigators believe this system, which reaches throughout the cortex, is intimately involved with conscious experience. Because nearly all information channels through the thalamus, it can act as the integrator, selecting, packaging, and tagging information that occurs together in time from all areas of the brain, and sending it back for the cortex to record as an object or an event. The thalamus and the thalamocortical projection system play an important role in arousal, sleep, and seizure disorders. It may also play a role in remapping phantom sensations as discussed in Chapter 4. A temporal binding system, whether through the thalamus or other structures, would be highly efficient, because it could register any number of novel neural code combinations together and be experienced instantly without relying on the hardware of contiguous, linear cortical connections. These findings suggest that indeed there is no single organ of consciousness; instead, the frequencies of temporal binding may coordinate experience. This would indicate that the whole brain can contribute to awareness depending on which systems activate at any one time to signal the effect of an experience. This view implies a dynamic quality to the brain and conscious experience that is infinitely more flexible than former conceptualizations.

According to theorist David Chalmers (1996), the "how" question of consciousness is not the hard question. The hard question is not how conscious processes bind together, but how a subjective experience of mind arises from the functioning brain and its synchronized and bundled oscillations. By looking deeper into peoples' direct subjective experiences, some of which are explicit and some of which are implicit, researchers will learn more about the relationship of brain to mind.

People customarily link consciousness of external events with the tangible. Even our vocabulary reflects this: "I know something to be true because I saw it with my own eyes, I can feel it, I can sense it." Most of what people experience they know by way of senses of smell, taste, sight, sound, and touch: the springtime smells of lilacs and freshly mown grass, the sight of children running across the yard, the sound of laughter, and the squeeze of a hand. But external realities exist that most of us cannot perceive directly through our senses. At the turn of the last century, people were just becoming aware that sound could travel through long distances, even through bodies, yet people cannot perceive such sound directly without a little box called a radio. In the animal world, whales, dogs, and bats communicate within their species on different frequencies than humans can "consciously" perceive. People now know that low- and high-frequency sound exists, because they now

have instruments that can measure and transmit these "unconscious" ranges of sound. In the same vein, people know that electrical fields and microwave energy exist. In 1933 Enrico Fermi, a physicist, predicted the presence of neutrinos, or energy particles, which permeate the universe and freely flow through bodies without leaving a trace. In 1956 physicists definitively identified neutrinos. What else may exist that people cannot consciously perceive? Modern science may be just beginning to unravel the mysteries that lie beyond limited human sensory abilities.

The Western empirical, materialistic tradition of science takes the stance that if something cannot be observed and measured it does not exist. To study the full range of consciousness, this archaic and human-centered view must give way to the possibility that the range of reality extends beyond ordinary human sensory-perceptual experience. Brain dysfunction can truncate, extend, or otherwise bend sensory-perceptual experience. Many cases we present in this book certainly stretch the bounds of ordinary conscious experience. Supersensory abilities may also be possible. Some Chinese health practitioners diagnose and heal by working only with the energy fields of the body. Fortunately, new technologies may bring into awareness many aspects of sensory experience that are out of range to the "naked senses." Scientists may now experimentally verify awareness of both pathologically altered and exceptional sensory perception, although few studies have considered these issues.

Previously, the limited means of measuring subjective experience have hampered scientists in studying consciousness. Primarily, they have had to rely on direct experience of the senses and on language to reveal consciousness. In other words, people could demonstrate awareness if they could hear, see, taste, smell, or touch something and be able to describe it. Because the left hemisphere is more specialized for spoken words, some have characterized it as the seat of consciousness. But that simplistic notion equates awareness with an ability to describe the phenomenon. Many people can probably recall experiences in which they had a sense of knowing without the ability to verbalize or touch what they felt.

Also, some processes that are now implicit may be made explicit. People can demonstrate implicit knowledge through their actions based on that knowledge.

Scientists also know that subliminal sound and scent, under the level of detectable awareness, can affect brains in a predictable manner. Similarly, scientists will also be able to determine if some individuals can detect electrical energy fields of which most are not conscious. On the internal side of the coin, many of what are considered *automatic processes,* such as breathing and heart rate, churn along without conscious awareness or control. But the means already exist to bring many of these processes into conscious awareness through various biofeedback technologies such as heart-rate monitoring, galvanic skin response measurement, and EEG (electroencephalography). Although these technologies present a recent tool for more conscious body and mind control, masters of meditation have long exerted amazing control over many brain and body states. Given the increased ability to gain a window into automatic and subconscious processes through vivid functional brain-imaging techniques, whole new areas of research are opening up that may now allow neuropsychologists to learn not only about the workings of the brain, but also how to consciously control various brain states. The possibilities available for extending the range of normal conscious experience represent an exciting frontier in brain science.

In Chapter 13 we visit disorders of consciousness. What happens when the fundamental experiences of consciousness run amok because of brain dysfunction? The daily rhythms of alertness and arousal people all move through from waking to sleeping and dreaming provide directions for studying the limits of normal brain alterations of consciousness. Disrupted flow of these brain rhythms can cause a variety of sleep disorders, of which one of the more interesting is narcolepsy. Finally, seizures represent an alteration of consciousness that also affects level of alertness—an internally generated brainstorm of synchronized activity.

Emotional Processing

Brain processing of emotion is an area that neuropsychology has largely ignored until recently. This neglect is partly a holdover from philosophical traditions of rational empiricism, and from conceptualizations of the body and brain as machinelike. People saw emotions as peripheral to understanding cognition, as being of a lower order of evolutionary development, perhaps even vestigial. In other words, humans had evolved to become rational logical beings somehow above emotion. Moreover, it is difficult to study subjective feeling states. Such research is not straightforward, as is presenting a visual or auditory stimulus and recording activation of corresponding brain regions. Also, animal models can provide only limited information, because they can't verbalize their feelings, and researchers must rely on motor behaviors to infer the such expression of emotions as rage and fear. The emotional repertoire of humans is enormous, subtle, and much more complicated than a response to external threats to physical safety, such as embodied in the fight-or-flight response.

Today, science views emotions as necessary for higher evolutionary adaptation. In television's *Star Trek* (and its spinoffs), the ultralogical characters Mr. Spock, Data, and Seven of Nine show being human entails having "emotional equipment." People who are out of touch with emotions and who have autistic-like qualities—like Temple Grandin, who describes herself as an "anthropologist on Mars" in Oliver Sacks's book of the same name (1995)—have expressed a sense of alienation from other humans on these grounds. Humans live in a social context in which self-understanding and social skills are some of the most crucial factors in determining success in society. Witness the surging interest in "emotional intelligence," which stresses the ability to understand mood and emotion in self and others, to understand self and one's own character, and then to act effectively on that knowledge. Researchers suggest that emotional intelligence accounts for just as much, or more, variance in determining success in life as traditionally measured general cognitive intelligence.

One of the more interesting questions related to understanding emotions is to ask whether emotional processing is a type of cognitive processing the cortex initiates, or whether emotion emerges without conscious thinking, and only secondarily becomes labeled. This dichotomy is a variation on an old debate emanating from the early 20th century. The **James-**

Lange theory of emotion, promoted by American psychologist William James and Danish psychologist Carl Lange (Lange 1922), postulated that people consciously experience emotion as a reaction to physical sensory experience. In other words, we feel fear because our hearts are racing; we are sad because we are crying. Although others saw this as an overstatement, the James-Lange theory did insist that sensory and cognitive experiences were intimately entwined and inseparable from each other. In other words, if all the physical sensations of fear disappeared, so would the cognitive experience of fear. The opposing theory of the time was the **Cannon-Bard theory** (Cannon, 1927). Walter Cannon, and later Philip Bard, argued that the conscious emotional experience is separate from bodily sensation or expression. Although today most scientists agree that cognitive experience of emotion corresponds to sensory experience, much variation exists among types of emotion, emotional intensity, and individual variation.

Joseph LeDoux (1992, 1994) describes emotion as a subjective state of awareness and suggests that only because people have a cortex can they label emotion and think about it rather than just react to it as other animals might. Someone walking along in a forest might be startled by something that looks like a snake. It is adaptive if the mind signals the body in an immediate response of danger. Some scientists have suggested that certain emotional responses, such as reactions to certain movements and noise, may be genetically "hard wired" as a protective mechanism. According to LeDoux (1994), after that initial lower-order automatic processing the cortex receives and further processes the information, perceiving the object as a snake or a stick, weighing options, and directing the body to take further action. The competing view argues that the person must first recognize something cognitively as a threat for the emotion to develop. LeDoux and others have amassed convincing research suggesting that basic fear conditioning can occur without a cortex. Some animals with their cortex removed still show basic fear responses. In this scenario, thought does not necessarily precede emotion. However, in addition to subcortically initiated emotion, is it also possible to initiate an emotional response just by thinking? Certainly the experience of most people would confirm this. Considering an upcoming speech, thinking about running into a snake, feeling socially embarrassed, or anticipating a joyful reunion can all produce emotional responses in the body separate from immediate external threats or joys. In this section we examine both types of emotional response, subcortical limbic and cortical responses.

BRAIN ORGANIZATION OF EMOTION

There is no one discrete emotional system in the brain. Emotional processing varies according to type of emotion and according to the manner in which the emotion arises. It also appears subject to individual, cultural, and gender differences. Subsystems of emotion are responsible for processing specific emotions. These emotional subsystems ultimately tie into the limbic system. It is useful to conceptualize emotional processing in humans along two lines, one devoted to primary emotions that people share with other vertebrates, and one devoted to social emotions that (reasonably) depend on higher cognition and cultural influences.

Primary Emotions

Primary emotions are automatic, preorganized, arise from sensory experience, and are processed through the limbic system before or parallel to being recognized consciously. Emotions such as fear, disgust, surprise, anger, and joy appear universal, as people express and recognize them across all cultures of the world. Damasio (1994) suggests that these emotions are innate and primarily controlled by the amygdala and anterior cingulate of the limbic system. As we have discussed, sensory information first funnels through the thalamus, and then is relayed to the cortex. After this it travels to the subcortical limbic system. Because of this anatomy, the general consensus was that conscious perception of an emotion preceded emotional limbic response. But LeDoux, who has studied fear conditioning, has suggested that projections from the thalamus to the amygdala provide a "shortcut" allowing the amygdala to process information directly, bypassing the cortical loop. This allows for an immediate, automatic, preconscious, and nonconscious emotional response.

Fear is a well-researched primary emotion. In the hope that the knowledge of fearful emotions can aid in treating secondary emotions such as human anxiety and posttraumatic stress disorders, Joseph LeDoux, who has done extensive work in the area of fear conditioning with animals, has studied how primary fear interacts with memory. The neuroanatomy of the primary conditioned-fear response centers on the amygdala. Fearful behaviors are easily conditioned to a tone via shock, trauma, or loud noise. Researchers have long known that severing connections between the subcortical areas of the brain and the cortex does not eliminate the conditioned-fear response. Learning and maintaining fear conditioning must therefore take place in the subcortical structures. Researchers then demonstrated that lesioning the amygdala in certain places did interfere with fear conditioning. Most notably, if they destroyed the central nucleus of the amygdala, animals no longer showed an autonomic fear response when presented with a tone (which had previously been associated with shock). The expected increase in heart rate, respiration, and vasodilation did not occur. LeDoux could then conclude that the cortex is not necessary to condition fear, but the amygdala is crucial. He then showed that the sensory systems that pass through the thalamus have a direct route into the amygdala, while the cortex is also processing them in a parallel fashion. LeDoux proposed that the pathway for learned fear operates so that information from the sensory systems (such as sound) relays through the thalamus to the basolateral nuclei of the amygdala. From there some circuits project to the central nucleus, which in turn sends information to various brain regions that can alter cognition of emotion, behavioral, and autonomic nervous system response (see Figure 5.13).

Secondary Emotions

Secondary emotions require higher cortical processing, and according to Damasio (1994), are primarily orchestrated by prefrontal cortical networks. There is also a hemispheric asymmetry to higher emotional processing. People acquire secondary emotions through learning and experience. The perception of these states is highly personal and individual. Social emotions such as embarrassment, pride, shame, and anxiety are highly dependent on learning and interact with one's cognitive perception of the social environment as it pertains to oneself. Secondary emotions do not necessarily imply a separate "feeling" experience in the body. The feeling of emotional experience remains linked through the limbic system. The difference is that secondary emotions are first generated through higher cortical processes and arrive at the limbic system over a different route from that taken by primary emotions generated through sensory experience. Once in the limbic system, the brain processes the experience of primary and secondary emotions in a similar manner.

Secondary, or social, emotions mediated by the cerebral hemispheres show lateralization of functioning. If a face is considered closely, you soon see that it is not symmetrical. In 1902, before the days of computer morphing, the German scientist Hallervorden (cited in Borod, Haywood, & Koff, 1997) cut pictures of faces in half at the midline. Taking the left half, he recreated the whole face by using the original and its mirror image. He did the same with the right half. Among other descriptors, he saw right-sided faces as more "lucid," "sensible," and "active," and left-sided faces as more "perceptive" and "affective." Because the right hemisphere controls the left side of the lower face, and vice versa, lateralized facial differences in emotion basically reflect the activity of the contralateral hemisphere. The general consensus across subsequent studies confirms some of the early observations in that the left side of the face (left hemiface) is more emotionally expressive than the right hemiface. In general, the right hemisphere seems to be dominant for emotional expression (for a review of the literature, see Borod et al., 1997). The picture, however, is not completely cut and dried. Faces have an amazingly complex ability for emotional expression. The amount of space devoted to facial control on the motor homunculus attests to this. Just in variations of smiles, there may be more than 18 different types. Psychologist Paul Ekman has described the cocktail party smile, the smile of relief, and the miserable smile, to name just a few. Some theorize that each hemisphere may be specifically attuned to emotional type. Perhaps positive emotions emanate from the left hemisphere and negative emotions from the right (for review, see Borod et al., 1997). The structure–function picture for emotion is complex, but many neuroanatomic theorists continue to assert that the right hemisphere plays the major integrative role in emotional processing. People with right hemisphere damage caused by stroke are usually less accurate at producing emotions when compared to those with left-sided damage or normal controls (Borod, 1993).

Observations of neurologically impaired patients have provided clues to an interesting issue in emotional processing, the anatomic differences between spontaneous and posed smiles. Posed facial expression appears largely controlled by contralateral cortical structures in the motor cortex. Spontaneous smiles and laughter, however, appear to be largely a function of subcortical limbic system structures, including the cingulate gyrus, thalamus, and some structures of the basal ganglia (such as the globus pallidus). Left hemisphere stroke patients, with damage to the left motor cortex, have difficulty smiling for the camera because

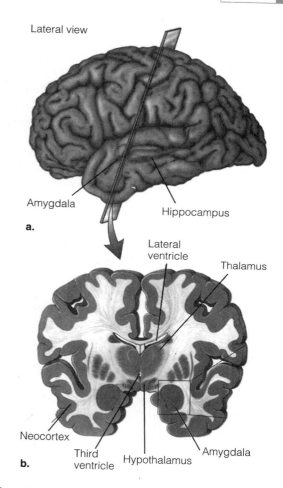

a.

b.

Figure 5. 13 The amygdala and fear conditioning. (a) A lateral view showing the amygdala through the temporal lobes. (b) A coronal section showing the amygdala. (c) A closeup of the nuclei of the amygdala showing the pathways of the conditioned fear response to emotional auditory stimuli. (From M. F. Bear, B. W. Connors, and M. A. Paradiso, *Neuroscience: Exploring the Brain*, Philadelphia: Lippencott, Williams & Wilkins, 1996, [a, b] pp. 444, Figure 16.5, [c] p. 445, Figure 16.6)

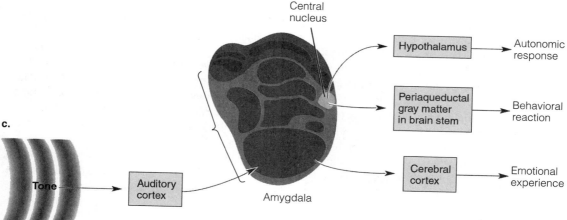

c.

their facial muscles malfunction in response to the brain command to produce a willful or social smile. The smile pulls to the left. A quite different picture emerges if the person laughs spontaneously. The smile appears natural. The limbic system and other subcortical structures, including the basal ganglia, control the spontaneous smile (see Figure 5.14). In any person, an observer can easily see a difference between these two types of smiles. The true smile of enjoyment activates the orbicularis oculi muscles around the eyes; a fake smile does not. Another way of putting this is that smiling eyes show an activated limbic system. People with subcortical disorders, such as Parkinson's disease, show the opposite problem of stroke patients. Although they can show willful emotion, much of their spontaneous emotion is dampened by a "masklike" face.

Emotional dysfunction often appears in conjunction with neurologic disorder, sometimes as a normal reaction to loss of function and sometimes as a direct result of brain dysfunction. For example, depression is a common reaction to life-altering injury or disease, but depression also is more common in people with right hemisphere dysfunction and in some subcortical disorders such as Parkinson's disease. A frontal executive system called amotivational syndrome often appears behaviorally as indifference, apathy, or depression. On the other side of the emotional spectrum, euphoria or inappropriate labile emotional responses can also occur with frontal and subcortical syndromes.

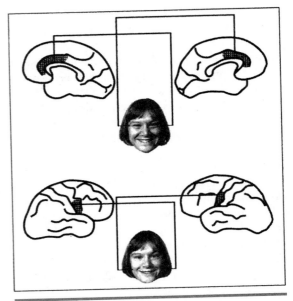

Figure 5.14 The limbic cortexes control a spontaneous smile (top) whereas the motor cortex controls a posed smile (bottom). (From A. R. Damasio, *Descartes' Error,* New York: Putnum's, 1994, p. 141)

Conclusion

The systems presented in this chapter represent the highest level of brain integration. They depend on the input of processed sensory information and to a large extent manage, organize, manipulate, and store this information for further use. Many of the processes of these systems operate automatically or unconsciously without apparent verbal awareness. Subcortical brain regions control many "unconscious" processes. The more explicit, and therefore more seemingly conscious aspects of higher-order processing are represented in the cortical areas, most notably the frontal lobes. Perhaps the most abstract and least well understood system is that of consciousness. This frontier, into which neuropsychology has recently ventured, presents some of the most intriguing puzzles of the human mind.

This chapter, as well as the previous chapters in this part of the book, provide the foundation for the clinical examples presented later in the book. Whereas here we have considered functions and disorders by subsystem we next examine cases of disorders that cut across functional areas.

Critical Thinking Questions

■ Do the higher cognitive functions discussed in this chapter represent more intelligent thought processes than those functions discussed in previous chapters? Explain.

■ Are animal minds other than humans also conscious? Explain.

■ Do disorders of higher cognitive functioning represent a greater disability for humans than sensory-perceptual and motor disorders? Why or why not?

■ Do emotions represent a higher cognitive function, or a lower basic function? Explain.

Key Terms

Anterograde amnesia	Procedural memory	Working memory	Alternating attention
Retrograde amnesia	Explicit memory	Central executive	Divided attention
Short-term memory (STM)	Implicit memory	Articulatory phonological	Sustained attention
Long-term memory (LTM)	Episodic memory	loop	James-Lange theory
Remote memory	Semantic memory	Visual-spatial sketch pad	Cannon-Bard theory
Declarative memory	Implicit priming	Focused attention	

Web Connections

http://www.lycaeum.org/drugs/other/brain
Mind-Body
Great source for links to topics related to theories of the mind.

http://www.nimh.nih.gov/events/prfmri2.htm
Working Memory
Site provides graphics for three-dimensional MRI reconstruction of subject's brain, including parietal and frontal areas, while holding a series of letters in working memory.

http://www.exploratorium.edu/memory/index.html
Memory Web Site
Features online exhibits and articles and lectures on memory. Page also shows demonstration of memory for common objects such as a penny. The page asks the user to click on the penny that actually looks like one.

Chapter 6

METHODS OF INVESTIGATING
THE BRAIN

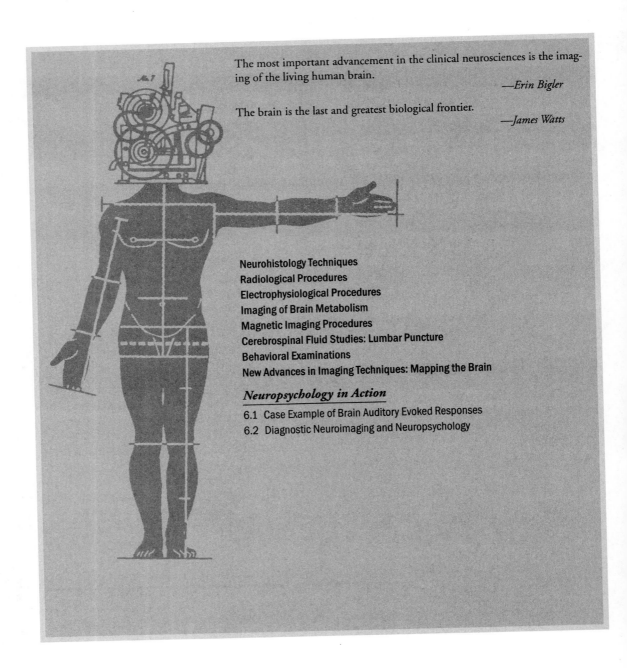

The most important advancement in the clinical neurosciences is the imaging of the living human brain.

—*Erin Bigler*

The brain is the last and greatest biological frontier.

—*James Watts*

Neurohistology Techniques
Radiological Procedures
Electrophysiological Procedures
Imaging of Brain Metabolism
Magnetic Imaging Procedures
Cerebrospinal Fluid Studies: Lumbar Puncture
Behavioral Examinations
New Advances in Imaging Techniques: Mapping the Brain

Neuropsychology in Action

6.1 Case Example of Brain Auditory Evoked Responses
6.2 Diagnostic Neuroimaging and Neuropsychology

Keep in Mind

- What is the difference between a CT scan and a MRI?
- What does an EEG measure?
- What is functional imaging?
- What is the difference between an invasive and a noninvasive procedure?
- Are modern imaging techniques dangerous to the brain? Explain.

Overview

The primary constraint in unlocking the secrets of the brain has been the limits on available techniques and examination procedures for investigating the brain. This was certainly true for early scientists, who struggled with how inaccessible the living brain is to direct visualization. Short of performing in vivo neurosurgical procedures or postmortem examinations immediately after death, they simply could not examine the living brain. As a result, study of the brain was largely speculative and inferential, and researchers have made many errors (see Chapter 1). Because of such difficulties, many famous psychologists, including William James and B. F. Skinner, insisted that the brain is not the province of psychologists. They suggested that the brain is like a "black box"—researchers cannot study the brain itself, but can associate certain inputs with specific outputs of behavior.

Over the last 100 years an explosion in technology has allowed more precise examination of the brain. During the end of the 19th century, researchers developed staining techniques by which they could visualize neurons. In the early part of this century x-ray technology and pneumo-encephalography allowed scientists to visualize the skull and the ventricles. The brain, however, remained elusive. This all changed in the 1970s, during which researchers introduced computed transaxial tomography (CT) and then, in the mid-1980s, magnetic resonance imaging (MRI). These two procedures, although crude in their initial stages of development, were soon refined so that visualizing specific and detailed brain structures became possible, including visualizing asymmetries in the living brain. At the same time other technologies, including electroencephalography (EEG), single-photon emission computed tomography (SPECT), and positron emission tomography (PET) advanced, allowing clinicians to view the brain from structural, metabolic, and electrophysiological perspectives. For example, using PET it is now possible to measure, with three-dimensional resolution, biochemical and physiological processes in the human brain. These recent advances in neuroimaging dramatically changed how scientists are investigating neural correlates of human behavior. These spectacular new developments are akin to changing filters in a camera, resulting in new and different images of the same picture. A "window to the brain" has opened, and so has our understanding of the brain.

Modern advances in medical examination procedures of the brain directly relate to an unprecedented development in computer technology capabilities that resulted in high spatial resolution of brain structures, allowing for a more precise diagnosis of brain functioning and pathology. The term *spatial resolution* refers to the smallest distance between adjacent regions for which a structure or activity can be distinguished. Technology has advanced so remarkably that scientists have not universally established a standard or systematic method for analyzing images. Clinical diagnosis once depended on clinical rating schemes or the clinician's interpretation. This led to the next paradigm shift in imaging technology, related to the actual volumetric measurement of specific brain structures in the normal and pathological brain (Bigler, Yeo, & Turkenheimer, 1989). This computational technology gave birth to quantitative imaging. Using computer-automated algorithms, in the 1990s researchers became capable of segmenting the brain into different components (such as white matter, gray matter, and cerebrospinal fluid) to calculate the size of each of those elements. Next, three-dimensional (3-D) segmentation of the brain became possible, allowing clinicians to view a tumor or the results of a stroke in 3-D. This was particular useful for evaluating brain pathology, which clinicians often found difficult to appreciate in a two-dimensional perspective.

The most recent development in imaging technology has been the integration of different evaluation modalities such as PET, MRI, and EEG to obtain a more complete picture of the brain. This integration includes new technology that allows the interfacing of multiple and quantitative analysis of brain images using different examination methods. For example, MRI technology together with PET data on the same brain renders images of the brain that capture both structure and function quantitatively and simultaneously. Scientists can use such approaches to examine a brain while the person is performing a neuropsychological task, such as completing a memory test. Using this procedure for specific neuropsychological functioning, researchers can establish baselines of healthy brains, which are then compared to pathological brains, for example, of schizophrenics. Looking at gender differences has shown often striking differences in how men and women process information. Current technology has de facto taken the neuropsychological test into the MRI scanner to test brain function. Research into the functional and structural properties of the living human brain is now the most important advancement in the neurosciences (see Bigler, 1996).

In this chapter we summarize the major technological methods of examining the brain. We discuss advantages and disadvantages for each procedure, particularly as they relate to understanding brain–behavior relationships and disease processes. This chapter provides the neuropsychology student with background on the various investigation procedures he or she will likely encounter in the literature, research laboratory, or in clinical practice. Neuropsychologists should familiarize themselves with the basic information these techniques can provide. In fact, neuropsychologists play an important role in advancing this technology and are working side by side with radiologists and neurologists to unlock the secrets of the brain.

"Eric, your brain looks OK!" announces Dr. Jonathan "Yoni" Nissanov, Research Professor of Biomedical Engineering and Science at Drexel University. It is 11:30 P.M., and I am lying in a magnetic resonance imaging (MRI) scanner at Thomas Jefferson University Hospital in Philadelphia. Yoni has reserved the million-dollar diagnostic tool for research he is conducting on functional imaging. I have agreed to be one of his test subjects. Because using the machine is expensive, research time is only allotted at night. I have been looking forward to this procedure, not only because I am interested in how such technology works, but also because I am ready to relax a little bit and lie down. It's been a long day at the office.

MRI is a relatively new diagnostic procedure and has only been available for routine brain imaging since the mid-1980s. So I am not surprised by the up-to-date, modern look of the facility. I work my way past the security guard to the heart of the center, a space age–looking control station. Yoni and his research assistant, who are operating the complex computerized machinery, greet me. I know my brain will be exposed to a very strong magnetic field, so I must remove all metals that are on me, including my credit cards. The procedure is completely safe, I am being reassured. Yoni goes through his protocol: "You don't have a pacemaker, you don't have an aneurysm clip, is there any shrapnel in your head, metal plates in your skull?"

Just as I am ready to enter the imaging suite, Yoni smiles at me and asks, "You know the risks?" Yes, as a neuropsychologist I know them all too well. The risks Yoni is referring to are related to the possibility that I may find out something about my brain that I do not necessarily want to know. The MRI will produce textbook-quality anatomy pictures of my brain. Although the probability is small, there is the outside chance that the diagnostic procedure may reveal a tumor or some other abnormality of my brain. Just a month ago a research colleague of mine learned that she had a malformation of her venous system in her brain. She was also one of Yoni's research participants. I repress these thoughts as I enter the imaging suite. The layout of the MRI scanner consists of two rooms, which are connected via intercom. The first one is the control room, which features a rectangular window overseeing the second larger room, where an oversize, doughnut-shaped machine is placed. The control room has an assortment of electronic gadgetry, the centerpiece being a large TV-type console that controls the imager and provides immediate visual feedback of the results. This is where Yoni and his assistant will remain during the procedure.

"We're out of earplugs, Eric." Great, so much for getting my much deserved rest. I lie on a stretcher-like surface, and at the push of a button I am whisked via electrical motors headfirst into the center of the large electromagnet. I remember Yoni asking me earlier if I was claustrophobic, and now I understand why. There is only about an inch of space around my head, which is placed approximately four feet within the center of the imager. "This is very tight," I whisper to myself as I try to relax by slowing my breathing.

The small confines of the MRI machine are a significant problem for patients who suffer from claustrophobia. I have once been told that such people are referred to the animal MRI at the Philadelphia Zoo, which can accommodate large animals. As I lie in the imager waiting, I wonder if this story is true and think what it must be like to go to the zoo as a patient: "Yes, you're next, right after we image the hippo." I'm grateful there is a small mirror positioned in an oblique angle right over my head, which gives me the illusion of space, because I can look out through the narrow opening toward my feet. I can see Yoni behind the window in the control room. "OK, we're ready to start." His voice reverberates through the intercom as a loud clicking noise begin.

For clinical diagnostic studies, the procedure takes about 15 minutes, during which the patient must remain as stationary as possible. But Yoni wants to go through a series of experiments during which I, on command, will clench my fists, right and left alternately, to see how the MRI machine detects functional activity in my brain. Yoni will then superimpose the functional MRI data, which reflect changes in blood oxygenation in my motor cortex, over the structural images of my brain. So I must keep my head still all the time. Yoni constantly reminds me of this over the intercom. I've agreed to be in the imager for over 90 minutes. Given the confines of the space and the incredibly loud, jackhammer-like, staccato noise, all of a sudden this does not seem like such a good idea after all. The first task for Yoni is to establish a traditional MRI study of my brain, a baseline. The loud clicks I hear are bombardments of radio frequency on my brain, which has been placed under a high magnetic field. The radio frequencies realign the magnetic fields of billions of hydrogen protons in my brain. The MRI machine is tuned into the frequencies that my water molecules in my brain emit after the external radio frequency stops. The deflection or realignment of this hydrogen map to the magnetic field can be detected, amplified, and recorded, and is the basis of the MRI process. Amazingly, I do not feel anything.

To be honest, I've thought about my MRI results for some time. As a neuropsychologist, I know that my personality, my intellect—essentially who I am, depends on the integrity of my brain. What if they find something wrong? Wouldn't a small change in the organization of my brain almost guarantee an altered sense of my reality? Haven't I been acting rather eccentric lately? How would they break the news to me? Would a team of summoned doctors rush in to announce, "There is a problem with your brain"? I find myself wondering how much training in psychology physicians receive for sharing diagnostic test results with patients and their families.

After 15 minutes Yoni steps into the imaging room to deliver his personal analysis of my brain. Although Yoni is a biomedical engineer, I am greatly relieved when he announces that my brain, on visual inspection, looks "OK." I have to remain in the increasingly uncomfortable same position for the next 75 minutes as Yoni goes through a series of studies. But now I am excited about the thought of actually seeing anatomic pictures of my brain for the first time. I can hardly wait until the procedure is over and Yoni shows me the coronal images on the control screen. Yes, everything is there, lateral ventricles, brain stem, cerebellum, and most importantly, my frontal lobes! I am a happy neuropsychologist as I leave the hospital at 1:30 A.M., with computer disk in hand, on which Yoni loaded an electronic copy of my brain images.

Neurohistology Techniques

On visually inspecting brain tissue under a microscope, one can find order to the anatomic arrangement of neurons. For example, pyramidal cell bodies in the cerebral cortex and hippocampal tissue "line up" to process neural information. For neuroscientists, the key to understanding the structures that make up the brain lies in technology that facilitates visualization of different aspects of neural tissue. One of the first ways to study neural processes involves stains; chemicals that attach themselves to specific cell structures and thereby make it possible for researchers to examine them visually and even count them. For over a century, neuroscientists have developed several staining techniques to help visualize mapping fiber connections. Initially, the light microscope, invented in the 1890s, gave birth to the pioneering works of Cajal (1937) and Brodmann (1909) in cellular neuroanatomy. The introduction of the powerful electron microscope in the 1950s made it possible to analyze in detail the synaptic con-

tacts between individual neurons. Next we outline this remarkable progress for several classic histologic techniques.

GOLGI STAIN

One of the most remarkable developments in the neurosciences came with a discovery made by **Camillo Golgi** (1843–1926). Golgi, an Italian physician, discovered in the early 1870s that silver chromate stained dead neurons black. This remarkable breakthrough allowed, for the first time, visualization

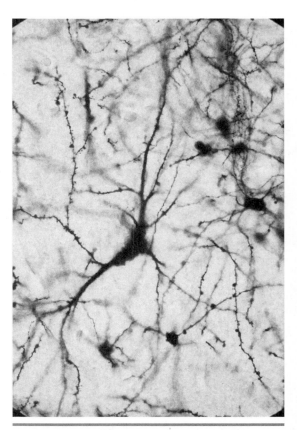

Figure 6.1   Golgi-stained neurons at 400 magnification. (From James W. Kalat, *Biological Psychology,* 6th ed., Pacific Grove, CA: Brooks/Cole, 1998, p. 104. Photo by Martin Rotker/ Photo Researchers)

of individual neurons (see Figure 6.1). The Golgi method enabled detailed study of cell process, often allowing a three-dimensional view of the cell and its processes. Practically overnight, the basic building blocks of the nervous system became visible. More recently researchers have even been able to stain single neurons in a Golgi-like fashion and visualize many of the different cells that make up the brain. Using this method, they found that Purkinje cells reside in the cerebellum and have a remarkably differentiated dendritic tree (see Chapter 2). The Golgi method also led to the classification of neurons based on the length of their axon. Golgi Type I neurons, for example, have long axons that transfer information from one region of the brain to another. In contrast, Golgi Type II neurons are those with short axons. The Golgi method has remained in use for over 100 years to characterize specific cell types in different regions of the nervous system.

NISSL STAIN

One drawback of the Golgi stain is that it provides little information about the number of neurons in a specific brain region, because it only affects a few neurons. It also permits only a view of neural tissue in silhouette and does not allow visualization of the neuron's inner structure. In the 1880s **Franz Nissl** (1860–1919), a German histologist, discovered that a simple dye will selectively stain cell bodies in neurons. As a result, researchers adapted several different stains, originally developed for dyeing cloth, for histological purposes. Methylene blue, for example, is a neural stain that has an affinity for the inner structures of neural cell bodies. One of the most popular dyes is cresyl violet, a cell body stain that is not selective for neural cell bodies, but stains all CNS cells. Cresyl violet facilitates the differentiation of fiber bundles, which appear lighter, and nuclei, which appear darker. Using the Nissl stain technique, scientists could then count the number of Nissl-stained dots representing neurons in any area of the brain.

The Nissl method has become the classic microscopic method for studying the cell body and one of the most valuable techniques for studying neurons in both normal and pathological states. The Nissl stain outlines all cell bodies and selectively stains the nucleus but not the axon. Furthermore, Nissl patterns vary among different types of neurons. For example, motor neurons have larger Nissl bodies, and sensory neurons have smaller ones. The appearance of the Nissl substance also varies with cell activity; that is, Nissl bodies disintegrate when the axon of the neuron is injured.

OTHER STAINING TECHNIQUES

The Nissl and Golgi methods are selective in their affinity for specific characteristics of neurons. The Nissl method reveals the cell body, specifically, the cell nucleus. Thus it maps cell density. The Golgi method is particularly useful for investigating the distribution of dendrites and axons in individual neurons, which appear pitch black. Scientists have developed other staining procedures specifically for studying axons. For example, **myelin staining** selectively dyes the sheaths of myelinated axons. As a result, white matter, which consists of myelinated axons, is stained black, whereas other areas of the brain consisting mostly of cell bodies and nuclei are not (see Figure 6.2 on p. 196).

Over the last two decades researchers have introduced new tracing methods based on the principle of axonal transport to chart previously unexplored regions and circuits of the brain. For example, in the 1970s they introduced the **horseradish peroxidase method** (**HRP** is an enzyme found in horseradish roots). They inject HRP into a region of the nervous system, and surrounding cell bodies and axon terminals take it up. In neurons that have incorporated HRP, axonal transport carries the enzyme to other interconnected cell bodies, where researchers can detect it with a simple staining procedure. Using the axonal transport technique, neuroscientists can study the tracing of pathways in the brain. Staining remains a viable method for studying the cellular function of the nervous system and helps neuroscientists in studying the specialized contacts among neurons and their complex and often puzzling arrangements. Table 6.1 on page 196 summarizes the different staining techniques used in neuroscience.

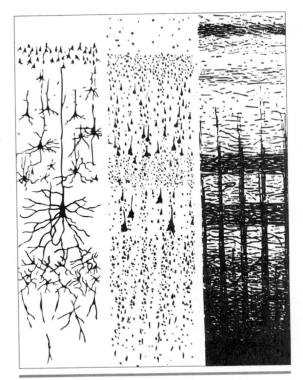

Figure 6.2   Different staining techniques of the human cortex highlight different aspects of nerve structures. Left, a Golgi stain visualizes individual cortical cells. In the middle, a Nissl-stained section reveals only the cell bodies. Right, a myelin-stained section of the human brain shows the myelin coating of the axon of neurons. (Adapted from A. Brodal, *Neurological Anatomy in Relation to Clinical Medicine*, 3rd ed., New York: Oxford University Press, 1981, p. 25, Figure 2.7)

Table 6.1	*Different Staining Techniques*
NISSL STAIN	A dye that stains the cell body of the neuron. This method is particularly useful for detecting the distribution of cell bodies in specific regions of the brain.
GOLGI STAIN	A method of staining brain tissue that marks a few selected individual cells, differentiating the cell body as well as its extensions.
MYELIN STAIN	Reveals the myelin coating of axons, rendering it useful for mapping pathways in brain tissue.
HORSERADISH PEROXIDASE	Allows mapping of neuronal pathways using axonal transport mechanisms. This technique works in both directions, that is, from the axon back to the cell body, and vice versa.

Radiological Procedures

From the initial x ray of the head and the practically extinct air encephalogram to sophisticated computerized tomography, the rapid progress of radiology has made a significant impact on the field of clinical neurology and neuropsychology. This section discusses the technique involved in neuroradiology, with special emphasis on computed tomography and angiography.

SKULL X RAY

Wilhelm Conrad Röntgen (1845–1923), a physicist, made a remarkable discovery that changed the science of medicine forever and that earned him the 1901 Nobel prize in physics. Röntgen (or Roentgen, to transliterate the German *ö* into English) quite serendipitously produced an invisible ray that, unlike heat or light waves, could pass through wood, metal, and other solid materials. This ray, also called the **x ray**, gave rise to radiology. The principle of x-ray technology is the generation of Roentgen rays, electromagnetic vibrations of very short wavelength that can penetrate biological tissue and can be detected on a photographic plate. At the basis of its medical application was the principle that the diagnostic rays travel through the body at different rates according to the density of organs. The resulting picture would show clear contrast between bones and, to a lesser degree, soft parts. Researchers discovered that x rays pass easily though low-density tissue (water) but are absorbed by high-density tissue (bone). In addition, they found that the harmful possibilities of x rays could destroy diseased tissue, a discovery that gave rise to radiotherapy.

Diagnostic x-ray films are very useful for clinical work on various parts of the body, because they reveal the presence and position of bones, fractures, and foreign bodies. A clinical disadvantage of x-ray films, specifically of the head, is that they are two-dimensional. Thus positive diagnosis of a three-dimensional clinical pathology is difficult. Secondly, an x-ray film of the head shows little differentiation between brain structures and cerebrospinal fluid, making clinical use of this procedure ineffective, with the exception of very large and vascularized brain tumors or massive bleeds. Furthermore, x rays are dangerous, because they are cumulatively absorbed by high-density tissue. Thus x-ray exposure entails a minor danger. The advantage of head x-raying is that it uses universally available technology, is inexpensive, and provides good visualization of the skull. Thus, if there is the possibility of a skull fracture, x-ray technology remains a useful diagnostic tool (see Figure 6.3).

AIR ENCEPHALOGRAPHY (PNEUMOENCEPHALOGRAPHY)

An **air encephalogram,** or **pneumoencephalogram,** is the radiographic visualization of the fluid-containing

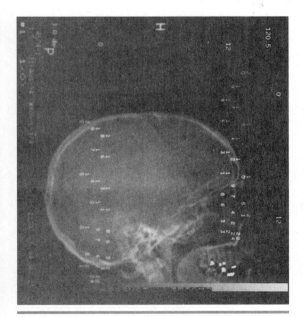

Figure 6.3 X-ray film of the head. (Eric Zillmer)

structures of the brain, the ventricles, and spinal column. It is similar to x-ray visualization, but it involves withdrawing cerebrospinal fluid (CSF) by lumbar puncture (described later in this chapter); the CSF is then replaced with a gas such as air, oxygen, or helium. The gas rises and enters the ventricular system, specifically the four interconnecting cavities of the brain. Once the gas has filled the ventricles, a technician takes a standard x-ray film of the head. Because the gas is of much lower density than the surrounding brain, the ventricles appear as a dark shadow on the x-ray film and clearly outline the surrounding brain tissue. Using this approach, a clinician can make a clinical diagnosis. The air encephalogram was an advance on the standard x-ray film, because it allowed visualization of the ventricular system.

However, patients did not tolerate the procedure well. Attendants had to turn patients in various positions, often awkwardly, and invert them in three-dimensional space to advance the gas to a specific ventricle before the technician could take an x-ray film. Because gas had replaced the CSF, the cushioning aspects of the CSF had been compromised, which often resulted in excruciating headaches that could last for several days before the gas was reabsorbed. Today, the more modern CT scan has replaced both the traditional x-ray image and the pneumoencephalogram.

COMPUTED TRANSAXIAL TOMOGRAPHY (CT SCAN)

Computed transaxial tomography (CT) is based on the same principle as the x-ray examination. The medical community has widely embraced it, making it the standard technology for examining the brain.

History

CT scanning was invented in Great Britain in 1971 and introduced to the United States in 1972 (Haeger, 1988). Physicists developed the first model of transaxial tomography partly building on dramatic advances in computer technology. Since then, CT technology has progressed from detecting only gross brain features to visualizing highly refined structural features.

Prior to this new technology, precise neuropathological diagnosis was difficult and psychologists played a large role in diagnosing brain lesions, including stroke and tumor. For example, a friend and mentor of ours, Molly Harrower, professor emeritus at the University of Florida and inventor of the Group Rorschach, was routinely asked in the 1930s to evaluate "organic patients." In her autobiographical essay "Inkblots and Poems" (1991), she describes how as a research fellow of noted neurologist Wilder Penfield at the Montreal Neurological Institute, she was asked to perform regular diagnostic workups using the Rorschach test. "I was assigned to examine all incoming patients suspected of tumor, with re-testing 14 days postoperatively" (p. 141). Today neuropsychologists play a smaller role in diagnosing neurologic disorders (see Chapter 15) but an important part in evaluating functional impairment, prognosis, and recovery.

Technique

After placing the patient's head in the center of the CT scanner, the technician revolves an x-ray source around the head as detectors monitor the intensity of the x-ray beam passed through the brain. The technician does not take the images at a perfect horizontal perspective of the head. Rather, he or she slightly tilts the images at a 20-degree angle to avoid scanning the air-containing sinuses, which produce distortion because of the combination of low (air) and high (bone) density (see Figure 6.4). The first (lowest) image selected is usually at the level of the foramen magnum, the base of the brain. Multiple sequential images reveal the ventricles, basal ganglia, thalamus, and cerebral cortex. Multiple transaxial images of the brain are obtained from many different angles. This requires a large apparatus or x-ray tube, which can rotate 360 degrees around the patient's head (see Figure 6.5). The detectors, which either rotate with the x-ray scanner or are placed in a circle around the patient, are more sensitive than the traditional x-ray film. For comparison, x-ray film can detect difference of 10 to 15% in the density of soft tissue, whereas CT can measure variations as little as 1%, often pinpointing density changes as little as 2 mm in diameter.

In contrast to the traditional x-ray visualization, in CT the head is scanned using a very narrow beam.

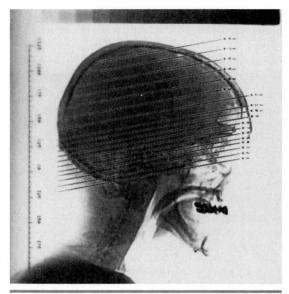

Figure 6.4   X-ray image of the head demonstrating the various "slices" of which the images are calculated. Note the absence of any differentiation of this patient's brain using x-ray technology. The 20-degree angle of the cuts is implemented to avoid having rays pass through the brain sinuses at the front of the brain, which often causes distortion. (Eric Zillmer)

This allows for the segmentation of the brain into many different slices. Depending on the nature of the study, the slices of the brain range from thin (2 mm) to thick (up to 13 mm). The information obtained by the CT scanner is entered into a computer, which then calculates, in three-dimensional space, cross-sections of the brain within the plane of the horizontal x-ray beam and the available density information of the brain. From these data, the computer generates a picture of the brain that can be in any orientation (sagittal, horizontal, or coronal). The complicated calculations the computer performs use the mathematics for computing solid three-dimensional structures based on data from a two-dimensional source. In principle, the procedure is similar to examining any three-dimensional structure—for example, a soft drink can—from many different angles, and then drawing it from a different perspective.

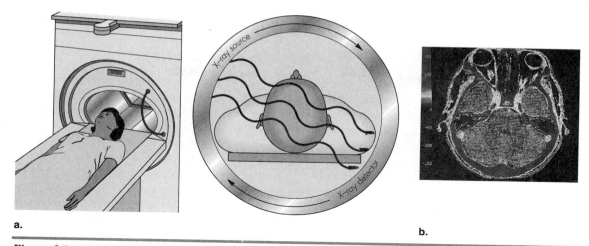

a.

b.

Figure 6.5 CT scanner. (a) The head of the subject is placed in the scanner, which is then subjected to a rotating source of x rays that pass through the brain at various angles. (b) A computer constructs the final image of the brain. (From James W. Kalat, *Biological Psychology*, 6th ed., Pacific Grove, CA: Brooks/Cole, 1998, p. 106, Figure 4.28. Photo by Dan McCoy/Rainbow)

Interpreting the CT Scan

The final product of CT technology is to produce a visualization of brain structures. This can take any form, including numbers or colors, but radiologists, not surprisingly, have favored an end result looking like the familiar x-ray film, with black-and-white shadings that reflect structure density. Accordingly, bone is white and cerebrospinal fluid is dark. Dense collections of cell bodies, gray matter, and nuclei look darker. In contrast, myelinated pathways or white matter look lighter. Neuroradiologists complete the interpretation of CT images, which they relate to their examination of the general symmetry of the brain. Marked asymmetries of brain structures typically signal a pathological process. The neuroradiologists also closely examine the scans for sites of abnormal densities, both **hypodensity** (associated with low density and perhaps an old lesion) and **hyperdensity** (typically signaling an abnormal density such as in tumor or a bleed). In this way they examine the general distribution of white versus gray matter (see Figure 6.6).

Enhanced CT

Soon after the introduction of CT, reseachers realized that the brain could be x-rayed more clearly by using

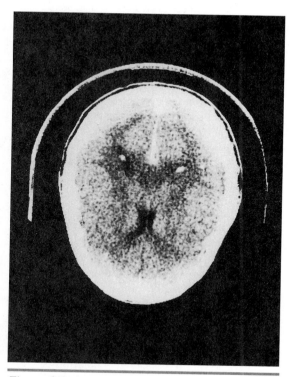

Figure 6.6 Early-generation CT scan (horizontal). (Eric Zillmer)

a contrast material, which would absorb the rays better. Thus, the **enhanced CT** scan, which involves intravenously injecting an iodinated contrast agent, reveals more contrast of brain structures. In the intact cardiovascular system, the contrast agent does not enter the brain, because it remains contained in the vascular system. But if there is a lesion, increased vascularization (as in an arteriovenous malformation or in a tumor), or a defect in the blood–brain barrier, that area shows increased contrast.

The refinement of the CT scan has made available a new generation of brain images that before then were only possible on autopsy. The CT scan has become a very useful diagnostic tool because alterations caused by pathologic processes or deformation of brain structures are easily visible, even to the untrained eye. The routine availability of CT has also increased the diagnosis of specific disorders, almost overnight. For example, small strokes, previously undetectable with x-ray technology, were all of a sudden easily diagnosed, which increased in the prevalence of diagnosed multi-infarct dementia.

ANGIOGRAPHY

Angiography is the roentgenographic visualization (x-raying) of blood vessels in the brain after introducing contrast material into the arterial or venous bloodstream. Consistent and sufficient blood supply is essential for a healthy brain, and angiography has become a standard procedure for examining the integrity of the brain's vascular system. Because the blood vessels of the brain reflect the surrounding brain tissue, angiography is a technique based on the x-ray procedure of examining the brain through its vascular system. Angiography is particular important in diagnosing structural abnormalities in the blood vessels themselves or in their arrangement. As a result, angiography has become a very useful tool in the early identification of aneurysms (a ballooning of an artery; see Chapter 9) and the subsequent prevention of stroke. To a lesser extent, clinicians can also identify other pathologies such as tumor, because they depend on increased vascularization or blood supply. The procedure can also detect shifts in cerebral arteries, which may indicate a mass-occupying lesion.

Technique

Femorocerebral angiography, developed in the mid-1950s, introduces a catheter into the arterial system. In the past physicians injected the contrast material directly into an artery, such as the internal carotid artery, but it is safer to insert a catheter via the femoral artery. The specialist passes the preshaped, semirigid catheter through a needle inserted in the femoral artery and then guides it up the aorta to the aortic arch with the assistance of x-ray and television monitoring. He or she can then place the catheter into any of the three major arteries arising from the aortic arch; the brachiocephalic artery, which leads to the common right carotid artery or the right vertebral artery; the left common artery, which leads to the left internal and external carotid artery; or the left subclavian artery, which connects to the left vertebral artery (for a more detailed discussion of the vascular system of the brain, see Chapter 9). Using this technique, the specialist can position or "park" the catheter tip at various strategic places of blood supply to the brain, in order to examine anterior or posterior cerebral arteries. Next an automatic injector sends an iodinated contrast agent through the catheter. At the same time, a technician takes rapid, serial x-ray films of the head over an 8- to 10-second interval in the frontal and lateral plane, providing visualization of the injected vessels and their complex intracranial branches.

Digital subtraction angiography, compared to conventional film angiography, is particularly effective in enhancing visualization of blood vessels, including the morphological and physiological states of the arterial, capillary, and venous phases of the cerebral circulation (see Figure 6.7). In this procedure, after the images of the contrast material have been acquired, the computer stores and subtracts the x-ray image of the brain. The resulting visualization of the vascular system is easily distinguished from that of brain tissue.

Intravenous angiography is somewhat more complicated than femorocerebral angiography, and there-

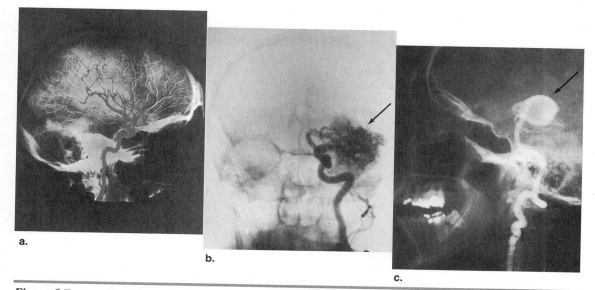

Figure 6.7 Examples of angiography. (a) Normal lateral view angiogram; (b) arterial-venous malformation from coronal perspective; (c) aneurysm from lateral perspective. ([a] SPL/Custom Medical Stock Photo, [b] English/Custom Medical Stock Photo, [c] English/Custom Medical Stock Photo)

fore clinicians do not use it as routinely. In intravenous angiography, the specialist inserts the catheter in the patient's arm, but must pass it through the heart, then the lungs, and then to the left side of the heart before it reaches the aortic arch. Thus larger amounts of contrast medium must be used, increasing the risk of renal toxicity to the patient.

Clinical Use

Angiography allows, from the puncture of a single artery, the maximum radiographic detail for diagnosing intracerebral lesions. Angiography is an invasive procedure, yet is relatively safe and well tolerated by the patient, who is awake but slightly sedated. The risk from the procedure is related to the possibility of the catheter loosening plaques in the arteries that may then separate and travel to a smaller location in the arterial system, where they can block the flow of blood, leading to an embolism. This is of concern in a patient suffering from arteriosclerotic vascular disease. Very few patients are allergic to the contrast medium, and thus the procedure is contraindicated for them.

In general, for initial diagnosis clinicians prefer noninvasive techniques, including CT scan and ultrasound (see Chapter 9 for a description of ultrasound used to examine the carotid arteries). Angiography is, however, the most accurate diagnostic procedure for evaluating vascular anatomy and its abnormalities. Thus, it is particularly useful in diagnosing cerebrovascular disorders.

SODIUM AMYTAL INJECTIONS (WADA TECHNIQUE)

The **Wada technique,** named after its developer, is similar to the angiogram in that the examiner places a catheter, typically in the left or right internal carotid artery. Then, a barbiturate sodium amytal is injected, which temporarily anesthetizes one hemisphere. Only one hemisphere is affected, even though vascular structures connect the two hemispheres (Wada & Rasmussen, 1960). This difference is related to the fact that the pressure gradients along cerebral arteries in both hemispheres are the same and thus there is no

Table 6.2	*Overview of Radiological Procedures*

Skull X-Ray

Two-dimensional representation of the head. Disadvantages include low resolution of brain anatomy. Advantages include low cost, availability, and its use in the diagnosis of skull fractures, which are easily seen using this technique.

Air Encephalogarphy (Pneumoencephalography)

The radiographic visualization of the fluid-containing structures of the brain, which have been filled with gas. An improvement over the skull x ray, but because of its invasive nature and side effects it is not used in contemporary medicine.

Computed Transaxial Tomography (CT scan)

Computed transaxial tomography renders an anatomic image of brain density based on multiple x-ray images of the brain. CT, which is readily available and can be used with almost anyone, provides a 3-D perspective of the brain with acceptable differentiation of brain structures. Its disadvantages include the use of penetrating radiation and the fact that CT does not provide as much spatial resolution as does MRI.

Enhanced CT

A CT scan that involves injecting a contrast agent to provide better visualization of brain structures, particularly bleeds. The disadvantages are that it is invasive and some patients may not tolerate the contrast agent well.

Angiography

The roentgenographic visualization of blood vessels in the brain after introducing contrast material into the arterial or venous bloodstream. Angiography is the most useful technique for examining the blood supply to and from the brain. One disadvantage is that a catheter must be inserted into the patient's bloodstream, which requires an invasive medical procedure.

Sodium Amytal Injections (Wada technique)

The injection of sodium amytal temporarily anesthetizes one hemisphere. Primarily a research technique. Used clinically to determine the lateralization of language before temporal lobectomy is performed. A complicated medical procedure that requires placing an arterial catheter.

---

cross-filling (or crossover) of blood from one hemisphere to the other, except if there is a stroke or other damage to the vascular system. In this way neuropsychologists can study the precise functions of one hemisphere while the other "sleeps." We discuss the Wada technique in more detail in Chapter 13. Table 6.2 provides an overview of the radiological procedures discussed in this section.

Electrophysiological Procedures

ELECTROENCEPHALOGRAPHY (EEG)

One of the most widely used techniques in neurology is **electroencephalography,** or **EEG.** The electroencephalogram is a recording of the electrical activity of nerve cells of the brain through electrodes attached to various locations on the scalp. The Austrian psychiatrist Hans Berger first discovered in 1924 that patterns of electrical activity can be recorded using

metal electrodes placed on the human head (Brazier, 1959). Initially, Berger was interested in finding physiological evidence for telepathy, the scientifically unverified phenomenon of a mind communicating with another by extrasensory means. Berger was, however, frustrated in his search to find support of mental telepathy, but he discovered that the electrical activity of the sleeping brain differed fundamentally from that of the awake brain. Researchers have used the resulting electroencephalogram ("electrical brain writing") to investigate distinct patterns of electrical activity in both the normal and pathological brain. Its potential use for identifying EEG correlates of behavior and personality made it a popular research tool among behavioral scientists. Thus, EEG became the first dynamic way to measure of brain function.

Technique

To record an EEG, the technician places small metal electrodes or leads on the scalp and connects them via wires to the electroencephalograph machine, which amplifies the electrical potential of neurons recording their activity on moving paper, a polygraph. In the past, the electrodes were small needles that were inserted just below the skin of the scalp. Modern electrodes used with conductive gel have proven just as effective. In principle, each pair of electrodes can act as its own recording site, measuring the electrical activity of millions of neurons close to the scalp. The neuronal activity of deeper subcortical structures are not as easily evaluated using EEG. Also, surface electrodes are placed at electrically inactive sites on the head, such as the mastoid bone behind the ear (electrode placement A1 and A2), which act as ground leads. The EEG itself is generated primarily by neuronal activity immediately below the cortex. Pyramidal nerve cells, which have somewhat conical cell bodies, make up about 80% of neurons in that region and exist in all areas of the cerebral cortex. Thus, EEG is mostly a measure of cortical nerve cells of the pyramidal type.

To measure the electrical signal of the neuron, its electrical signal must penetrate through different tissues to reach the electrodes, including the meninges, cerebrospinal fluid, blood, the skull, and the scalp. Each neuron's electrical contribution is tiny, and it takes many thousands of neurons firing in concert to generate any electrical signal large enough for EEG to detect. Thus the most easily visible EEG wave patterns depend on the synchronicity or the working together of millions of neurons.

In general, brain wave patterns are either rhythmic or arrhythmic. Neurons typically fire in a rhythmic or synchronous pattern leading to alpha, beta, theta, and delta waveforms. In epilepsy, however, many neurons fire at once, or in a burst or "spike," which corresponds with the amplitude that the EEG record shows. In principle, each electrode measures the summed signal of electrical activity of groups of neuronal dendrites. You can think of the EEG as analogous to holding a microphone over New York City to estimate the traffic by measuring the amount of noise from automobiles. Thus, EEG is a diagnostic tool more sensitive to the "forest" than to the individual "tree."

Electrode Placement

The pattern of electrode placement on the scalp—the International 10–20 System—is relatively stan-

dard in clinical practice. The exact points of measurement are the differences between any of two electrodes produced by brain activity. One pair of electrodes produces a single channel of recording. A standard EEG typically has eight channels, which are recorded on a pen recorder (see Figure 6.8). One of the more fascinating and complex parameters in EEG involves switching the pairs of electrodes or channels to a different direction. For example, during one portion of the EEG recording, a horizontal pattern may be used to measure activity in the right brain crossing over to the left brain. Then the clinician switches the pairs of electrodes to an anterior–posterior pattern (or montage), and compares it to the first pattern.

Overview of Brain Wave Activity

Brain wave activity may differ in polarity, shape, and frequency. The amplitude typically ranges from 5 to 100 microvolts and is a measure of the signal strength of neural activity. The EEG records frequency of the waveforms from 1 to 100 Hz (signal frequency per second), meaning that neural activity oscillates in a particular frequency. The specific shape of the waveform also interests the electroencephalographer. For example, during light sleep the EEG shows a characteristic spindle activity and vertex (V) waves. Researchers have established a system of dividing brain wave activity that is based on its frequency and amplitude. To the neuropsychology student, frequency

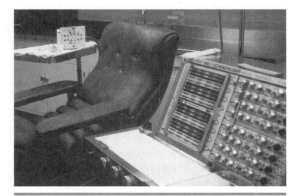

Figure 6.8 Electromechanical EEG recorder of the type used in the mid-1980s. (Jeffrey T. Barth, University of Virginia)

subdivisions of the EEG may appear somewhat arbitrary, but they correlate in general with distinct divisions of subjective experience of attention and arousal. Several different basic types have been established that vary according to whether a person is alert, wakeful, drowsy, or sleeping (see Table 6.3).

The pursuit of a specific brain state is a goal in itself. Because alpha and theta waves are characteristic of a person being relaxed, isolation flotation tanks and relaxation audio cassette tapes, among other tools, have proven effective in helping achieve such brain states. In athletics, researchers have clearly demonstrated that peak performance is associated with specific cortical arousal levels (Van Raalte, & Brewer, 1996). Alpha, in contrast, is incompatible with being alert and focused. Thus, it is advantageous for the competitive athlete to be in mid-beta when a difficult task is required, such as in ice hockey when the goalie faces a breakaway, or in baseball when the batter steps to the home plate to face a pitch. During beta the cortex is most actively engaged via complex sensory input and external processing. The activity rate of cortical neurons should be high, but also unsynchronized, because neurons may be involved in different aspects of complex neuropsychological tasks. During beta, neurons fire rapidly, but not in concert with each other. However, it is difficult to sustain beta for long periods of time, so successful athletes are very skilled in switching from alpha to beta and back "on command."

Seizures and EEG

Neurons can organize their rate of electrical activity in two fundamental ways. First, groups of neurons can fire in synchronized oscillations by taking cues from other cells, also known as *pacemaker cells* or *k neurons* (k for constant). Cortical neurons also take cues from other brain structures such as the thalamus, which can act as a powerful pacemaker, even when there is no external sensory input. For example, during non-REM sleep (nonrapid eye movement or nondream sleep) the thalamus generates rhythmic, self-sustaining discharge patterns that prevent organized information from reaching the cortex. Thus one's brain is asleep, demonstrating large, rhythmic delta waves. Second, neurons may fire in a consistent rhythmic pattern in response to collective behavior, like a large group of people clapping in a synchronized way without a cheerleader being present.

Seizures are the most extreme form of synchronous brain activity, during which the whole brain (as in a grand mal seizure) or large portions of the brain (as in a partial seizure) fire with a defined and pronounced synchrony that never occurs during normal behavior (see Figure 6.9). During seizures most, if not all, cortical neurons participate in excitation. Behavior is disrupted, and often consciousness is lost. Seizures themselves are best conceptualized as a symptom, not unlike a fever, and may be triggered by dozens of different causes. It is unlikely that seizures have one underlying etiology. The lifetime prevalence for a single seizure is very high, approximately 10%. Drugs that block gamma-amino butyric acid (GABA) receptors increase the possibility of a seizure. GABA has strong inhibitory properties and plays a major role in the basic type of neuronal transmission that depends

---

Table 6.3   *Brain States and Associated Subjective Experience*

Gamma activity (35+ Hz) is a low-amplitude fast-activity wave. Gamma rhythms are the fastest and are often associated with peak performance states and hyperarousal.

Beta is a low-amplitude, fast-activity wave with a frequency of more than 12 Hz. Beta is often divided into high beta (18 to 35 Hz), typically associated with a narrow focus, overarousal, and anxiety; mid-beta (15 to 18 Hz), often correlated with being active, alert, excited, or focused; and low beta (12 to 15 Hz), which has been associated with relaxed, external attention.

Alpha activity (8 to 12 Hz) is the predominant background activity in wakeful persons. Alpha is most often associated with quiet, passive, resting, but wakeful states.

Theta activity ranges from 4 to 7 Hz, and is most indicative of drowsiness, deeply relaxed, and inwardly focused states.

Delta activity is the slowest frequency, of less than 0.5 to 4 Hz. High-voltage, slow-frequency delta waves are never present in a wakeful, healthy person, but mostly occur during NREM (nondream) deep, stage 4 sleep.

on rapid communication among neurons. Conversely, drugs that prolong the inhibitory action of GABA (barbiturates or benzodiazepines; for example, Valium) suppress the possibility of seizures. The brain is potentially always close to having a seizure, because runaway excitation is possible given the brain's redundant feedback circuitry and its delicate balance between inhibitory and excitatory potentials. Multiple seizures, however, are typical of a disorder known as *epilepsy*, which we discuss in more detail in Chapter 13.

In patients with intractable (incurable) epilepsy, one intervention is neurosurgery to remove, if possible, the precise site or origin of the pathologic electric discharge. In such cases a more precise EEG measure-

ment is needed, which can be obtained by placing electrodes directly on the surface of the brain. This form of EEG, known as **electrocorticography** or **ECoG**, is often performed during temporal lobectomy surgery to isolate a precise location of brain pathology. In addition, a surgeon can place depth electrodes in the brain close to the projected area of interest while the patient is awake and being monitored via 24-hour closed-circuit television. This is usually done to correlate seizure activity with EEG data. Depth electrodes and ECoG are invasive techniques and entail risks, including infection. These methods are only used when the medical benefits greatly outweigh the risks to the patient. Thus, surface scalp electrode placement is the first and least

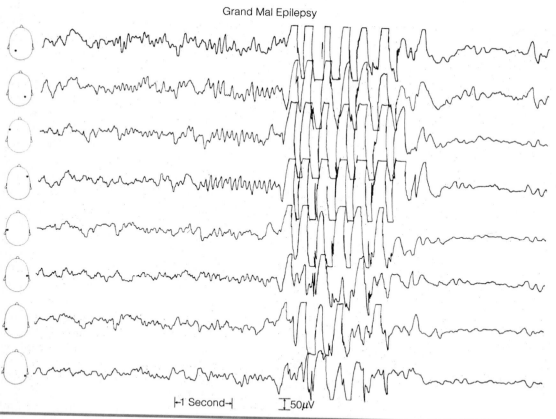

Grand Mal Epilepsy

|-1 Second-| |50µV

Figure 6.9   Electroencephalogram example of spiking activity that accompanies epilepsy. (Eric Zillmer)

invasive electrophysiologic study of the brain. EEG is also relatively inexpensive compared to CT and MRI procedures, and is readily available.

Clinical Use of EEG

The primary referral for a clinical EEG is to help with diagnosis of a seizure disorder, sleep disorder, level of coma, or presence of brain death. In fact, EEG is the primary tool in diagnosing epilepsy and can often pinpoint the type and location of seizure disorder. EEG is also very useful in diagnosing sleep disorders, because specific sleep states are associated with particular forms of electrical activity. The primary abnormality seen on EEG recordings is a slowing of activity as well as the presence of epileptiform activity. For example, it is abnormal to find delta activity in a wakeful person. Typically the slower the frequency in an awake subject, the more severe its abnormality. People with partial seizures often have EEG activity slowing to 3 Hz. Epileptiform EEG activity consists of sharp waves (spike-and-wave discharge), which indicate a seizure disorder. EEG diagnosis of epilepsy, however, produces frequent Type II errors (misses). Thus, a normal EEG may not indicate a normal brain.

Unfortunately, the EEG also demonstrates Type I errors (false positive or false hits). That is, a mildly abnormal EEG may not necessarily reflect an abnormal brain unless the EEG indicates the specific profile of epilepsy, which, if present, has very few false positives. Interpreting the EEG recording is something of an art because so many different variables are introduced. These include amplitude configuration of the polygraph, speed of recording paper, different electrode montages, a high incident of artifact caused by muscle movement that contributes to electrical activity, and inadequate electrical shielding of the examination room. Thus different electroencephalographers often disagree on interpreting borderline abnormal EEGs, although they easily diagnose the more definite epileptic EEG patterns.

When a diagnostician suspects seizure disorder, several techniques can provoke epileptic discharges during the EEG recording, which is the absolute positive sign of epilepsy. These methods include administering an EEG during the patient's sleep or when sleep deprived; that is, after the patient stays awake for one night the diagnostician administers the EEG in the morning. Other activation techniques that provoke epileptic discharges during the EEG recording include hyperventilation and photic stimulation. The latter is the presentation of a strobe light, right in front of the closed eyes, that is set at different frequencies to influence the base rate activation pattern of occipital neurons. Diagnosticians also use serial EEGs and 24-hour EEG recordings to monitor brain wave patterns over time. Once epilepsy is identified, doctors most commonly treat it with anticonvulsant medication to reduce spiking activity.

EEG and Neuropsychology

EEG is a safe, painless, and relatively simple procedure. Its use in neuropsychology has been disappointing and limited historically by a lack of relationship between EEG parameters and behavior, specifically indices of higher cortical functioning. In fact, complex EEG waveforms do not change very much during different kinds of sensory input, but seem to be most sensitive to the general arousal level of the brain (Penfield & Jasper, 1954). This lack of convergence between EEG activity and behavior is probably caused by the fact that the EEG is a relatively nonspecific measure of the underlying brain activity. Thus, using the traditional eight-channel EEG, researchers have established only general relationships related to right versus left hemisphere differences, or to posterior and anterior regions of the cortex.

EEG does not give an account of "what" a person is thinking; rather, it tells us *if* the person is thinking. Over recent years more sophisticated recording equipment and computer analysis have refined the EEG. Investigators have been using increased numbers of electrodes (64, 128, and even up to 256) placed over the subject's entire head to correlate specific neural networks involved in a particular neuropsychological task. Such enhanced EEGs have greatly improved signal quality and localization.

One invention that examines the more dynamic aspects of electrophysiological activity in the brain is brain electrical activity mapping, or BEAM (Duffy, 1989). CT shows the structure of brain tissue and, as we will see, PET scans let researchers and clinicians examine the pattern of brain biochemistry and metabolism. BEAM, in contrast, uses computer technology to provide color-coded mapping of the brain's electrical activity in real time, that is, as quickly as it is occurring in the subject's brain. In general, BEAM is nothing more than a way of enhancing the amount of information available on a standard EEG. Using an automated, integrated approach to EEG, the computer can calculate color-coded maps of electrical brain activity (see Exhibit 4 in the front of the book). Then it codes computed EEG parameters as topographic displays showing neuroelectric activity across the cortex while the subject is performing a neuropsychological task. BEAM is much more sensitive to electrical correlates of cognitive tasks than the traditional EEG. Quantitative EEG analysis has also shown some promise in the diagnosis of clinical disorders such as dyslexia, a reading disorder.

Other improvements in EEG technology entail merging EEG's temporal resolution with MRI's anatomic detail or PET's ability to localize function. Such coregistration of different approaches to representing the functioning brain has resulted in multimodal approaches to neuroimaging, often providing new insights as well as corroborating established findings. For example, schizophrenics show abnormal, less active, BEAMs as well as PET scans (less metabolism) in the frontal regions of the brain. Exhibit 4 shows a comparison of conventional BEAM presentation (left) with the presentation of the BEAM and three-dimensional MRI image using the individual's brain surface (right).

EVOKED POTENTIAL (EP)

A further electrophysiological diagnostic test is **evoked potential** or **EP** (also called *event-related potential* or *ERP*). EP involves artificial stimulation of sensory fibers that, in turn, generate electrical activity along the central and peripheral pathways as well as the specific primary receptive areas in the brain. In contrast to EEG, EP is dependent on a stimulus, and is most useful for assessing the integrity of the visual, auditory, and somatosensory pathways at specific regions of the brain. EEG technology can record the electrical activity in response to a stimulus or event. During the traditional EEG, the overall background activity of the cerebral cortex hides specific sensory stimuli. In evoked potential, a computer makes it possible to visualize the changes in EEG responses to a specific stimulus (visual, auditory, or somatosensory), canceling out random electrical activity but displaying electrical activity related to the potential evoked by the stimulus. The resulting evoked potential consists of a series of positive and negative changes lasting about 500 milliseconds after the stimulus ceases. The diagnostician analyzes the EP according to amplitude, latency, and the location of the specific brain region where the stimulus is processed.

Brain Stem Auditory Evoked Response (BAER)

In brain stem auditory evoked response (BAER), the examiner presents clicks to each ear individually via headphones. In response to the auditory stimulus, the auditory pathways generate an electrical signal along the central auditory pathways. EEG recording consists of five distinct waves representing different latencies related to five nuclei groups where the auditory signal is being integrated. Although this delay is short, the examiner can measure and amplify it. Abnormal delays in responses, measured in milliseconds, can often pinpoint specific lesions, but only along the pathways measured. The BAER can diagnose a malfunction of the auditory nerve at the cochlear nucleus, the superior olive, the lateral lemniscus, and the inferior colliculus (see Figure 6.10 on p. 208).

In BAER, five characteristic waves are recorded. Wave I reflects activity of the vestibular nerve; wave II, the cochlear nucleus; wave III, the superior olivary complex; and wave IV and V, the pons or lower midbrain. Decreased amplitudes, the absence of a wave, or prolonged interwave latencies may point to abnormal brain stem responses.

Approximately 50% of patients with multiple sclerosis demonstrate a pathologic BAER typically at the level of the brain stem. Brain stem auditory evoked response has also aided in diagnosing patients with acoustic neuromas (tumors). Research using EP indicated that schizophrenics, compared to normals, demonstrate an abnormality that may indicate a deficit in the "sensory gating" at the brain stem level, which

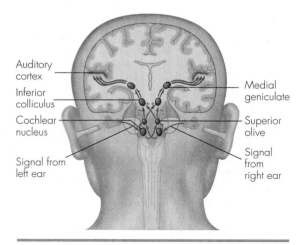

Auditory cortex

Inferior colliculus

Cochlear nucleus

Signal from left ear

Medial geniculate

Superior olive

Signal from right ear

Figure 6.10   Auditory pathways from receptors in the ear to the auditory cortex. Note the different nuclei along the pathways that form the basis for measuring integration delays, which can be measured and amplified using evoked potential and EEG technology. (From James W. Kalat, *Biological Psychology,* 6th ed., Pacific Grove, CA: Brooks/Cole, 1998, p. 184, Figure 7.6)

may result in impaired attention (Cullum et al., 1993). Researchers can then confirm the finding using neuropsychological measures of attention, sustained concentration, and digit vigilance (for example, digit cancelation). As with many of the other imaging techniques featured in this chapter, there are interesting implications and a promising future in the interrelationships between neurophysiological and neuropsychological indices of brain function. Neuropsychology in Action 6.1 reviews a case example using brain stem auditory evoked response technology.

Visual Evoked Response (VER)

Similarly to the auditory evoked response procedure, in visual evoked response (VER) the examiner presents a visual stimulus to each eye separately. An alternating light-and-dark reversing checkboard pattern provides the visual stimulus. EEG responses are recorded from electrodes over the parietal and occipital regions. One wave originates in the receptive visual cortex and is measured using EEG technology. A normal delay from the presentation of the visual stimulus to the registration of the electrodes over the occipital cortex is about 100 msec. Lesions along the visual nerve pathways result in abnormal delays and/or decreased amplitude of the recorded response.

Somatosensory Evoked Response (SER)

In somatosensory evoked response (SER), the examiner stimulates peripheral nerves via an electrode placed over the median nerve at the patient's wrist. In addition, the examiner places three electrodes for purposes of measurement, with the first two measuring peripheral electrical activity of sensory pathways at the level of the patient's arm and spinal cord. The third electrode is placed over the patient's contralateral somatosensory cortex. Abnormalities in amplitude or latencies at the first two points of measurement suggest peripheral nerve involvement. Delays at the third wave suggest central sensory pathway involvement.

Exhibit 5 shows the graphic results of a sensory evoked response examination to evaluate somatosensory pathways in three dimensions. The technician delivers pulses transcutaneously via a cup electrode to the median nerve at the subject's wrist. He or she adjusts the intensity of the stimulus to determine a painless muscle twitch of the thumb. Collected data are then transmitted to a computer for analysis.

ELECTRICAL STIMULATION

Historically the electrical stimulation of nerve tissue is one of the oldest ways of investigating the living brain. Initially, scientists hoped that use of this technique could chart a precise map of the cortex that would outline, akin to phrenology, the behavioral and cognitive properties of the brain and specifically the topography of the cortex. Surprisingly, however, this technique, which has been largely confined to the primary and sensory areas of the cortex, has elicited very few positive responses (the generation of a measurable behavior). However, scientists found a great number of negative responses (disruption of function) as a result of electrical stimulation of the cortex.

Neuropsychology in Action 6.1

Case Example of Brain Stem Auditory Evoked Response

by Eric A. Zillmer

The patient is a 38-year-old man who was employed as a mechanic. Previously he had worked as a tile layer for 6 months, during which he reported he was exposed to epoxy, alcohol, and other possibly toxic solvents. Since then he has complained of symptoms of dizziness and short-term memory loss. Physicians subsequently diagnosed him with chronic solvent intoxication. An audiogram showed normal hearing bilaterally. An audiologist performed brain stem auditory evoked response testing. Specifically, the tester presented monoaural click stimulation in each ear at 70 dB using click rates of 11.4 per second and 57.7 per second, with 2000 and 4000 repetitions respectively. Absolute and interpeak latencies in milliseconds at slow rate of 11.4 per second were as follows for waves I, III, and V.

	I	III	V	I–III	III–V	I–V
RIGHT	1.50	3.90	5.87	2.40	1.97	4.37
LEFT	1.60	4.14	6.10	2.54	1.87	4.42

Absolute interpeak latencies in milliseconds at a fast rate of 57.7 per second were as follows:

	I	III	V	I–III	III–V	I–V
RIGHT	1.79	4.40	6.25	2.26	2.21	4.46
LEFT	1.74	4.28	6.40	2.54	2.11	4.66

Note that the delays in milliseconds increase the further the signal is measured from its initial detection in the ear (e.g., at nuclei I, the vestibular nerve, the latency is 1.5 ms for the right ear; but at nuclei III, the superior olive, the signal was measured 3.9 ms after it was introduced to the right ear). Also, note the symmetry between right and left auditory processing routes. BAER testing revealed normal absolute and interpeak latencies at slow and fast rates in the right ear for waves I through III. Findings for the left ear revealed delayed absolute latencies for waves III and V at the fast and slow rates. The audiologist measured interpeak delays at I–III for the slow and fast rates, and III–V and I–V for the fast rate. Interear absolute and interpeak latency differences lay within normal limits. Even though there were minor variations among the brain wave recordings, the audiologist concluded that the test results suggested a normal brain stem auditory evoked response not consistent with brainstem dysfunction. Subsequent neuropsychological testing did show neuropsychological impairment on various tasks of new learning and memory. BAER, however, ruled out the possibility that those were related to brain stem impairment, and they were thus most likely related to cortical dysfunction.

For example, researchers easily demonstrated aphasia, a disruption of language functions, by numerous stimulations in different locations of the left hemisphere (Ojemann, 1980).

More recently, neurologists have introduced electrical stimulation in treating Parkinson's disease, based on the advances of stereotaxic operations and knowledge of specific associations between electrical stimulation and subcortical regions of the brain. Obviously, direct electrical stimulation of the brain is not a routine diagnostic procedure, because of its invasive nature. Primarily, researchers use it experimentally in clinical cases in which other interventions have not been successful. It can, however, provide great theoretical and clinical value in understanding the functions of the brain (see Chapter 12).

ELECTROMYOGRAPHY (EMG)

Electromyography (EMG) is the electrical analysis of muscles. In EMG, diagnosticians perform a nerve conduction study of a specific muscle to diagnose neuromuscular disorders. Patients undergoing EMG receive deep needle stimulation of a muscle, which the technician measures electrophysiologically ventral (closer to the spinal cord) to the stimulation. The technician delivers an electrical potential to a muscle, using a wire inserted within a hollow needle. The electrical activity is amplified and displayed graphically via an oscilloscope. At the basis of EMG is the fact that a relaxed muscle is electrically silent. During voluntary contraction, muscle action potentials are present.

EMG is an important medical diagnostic technique that aids in diagnosing peripheral nerve damage, because it can isolate the dysfunction to a specific sensory-motor unit, including a motor or sensory neuron, neuromuscular transmission, or the muscle cell itself. The procedure also helps substantiate the presence of intact sensory-motor pathways—for example, when hysteria or malingering is suspected. If Sigmund Freud had had this diagnostic test available, he could have proven that Anna O., the subject of his first famous published case study, was truly hysterical and did not suffer from a neuromuscular disorder as she complained. (Anna O. actually saw Freud's mentor Breuer, but Freud wrote up her case.) Anna O.'s motor functioning was normal, even though she complained of partial paralysis. Freud suspected this normality anyway and concluded that Anna produced the paralysis of the arm hysterically, because of her unconscious wish to remain in the role of a patient and to receive daily visits by famous doctors. Nevertheless, using EMG technology he could have diagnosed this much more efficiently, without needing to develop elaborate psychoanalytic theories.

A variation on the preceding techniques is recording an electric shock stimulus of a peripheral nerve and measuring the subsequent muscle contraction. This technique can test both motor and sensory

nerves. Results assist in the differential diagnosis of muscle disease and peripheral nerve damage. For example, in carpal tunnel syndrome, a relatively common peripheral nerve disorder with accompanying sensory deficits in the first three digits and weakness of the thumb, there is a characteristic latency of muscle and nerve action potentials. Although most patients tolerate this procedure well, EMG is mildly uncomfortable, because pain accompanies the insertion of the needle into the muscle. Table 6.4 reviews the most popular electrophysiological procedures in use today.

Imaging of Brain Metabolism

Over the last several decades, researchers have developed techniques for analyzing the brain that focus on measuring parameters of regional brain physiology. Such techniques are related to the biological fact that neurons have an active metabolism, which the cerebral blood supply provides. Specifically, the delivery of oxygen and glucose to neurons depends on cerebral blood flow. If the metabolic needs of the active neurons are high, the rate of cerebral blood flow is correspondingly higher. In this manner, neurologists can study regional blood flow while the patient is performing neuropsychological tasks. In contrast to CT, which provides a static representation of brain structures, measuring regional blood flow provides dynamic data on cerebral blood flow and metabolic activity. The imaging of brain metabolism, then, permits a completely different approach to examining the brain.

REGIONAL CEREBRAL BLOOD FLOW

Blood flow in the cerebral hemispheres varies with metabolism and activity. It can be a very sensitive index of the changes in cellular activity in response to cognitive tasks (Andreasen, 1988). The amount of blood flowing through different regions of the brain can indicate that region's relative neural activity. In the 1940s researchers introduced a technique in which the patient inhaled nitrous oxide (N_2O), which circulates through the brain. Using this technique, sci-

| Table 6.4 | *Electrophysiological Procedures* |

Electroencephalography (EEG)

Electroencephalography, or EEG, is one of the oldest brain-monitoring techniques. It measures the general electrical activity of the cortex. It is most useful in assessing, in real time, the overall arousal state in a person. Increased electrode placements and computer integration capabilities have resulted in high-resolution EEG and BEAM (brain electrical activity mapping), a promising assessment and research tool of the electrical activity of neurons.

Evoked Potential (EP)

Evoked potential or event-related potential (ERPs) is similar to EEG, in that it assesses an electrical signal, but it is related to a specific auditory (brain stem auditory evoked response, or BAER), visual (visual evoked response, or VER), or sensory event (somatosensory evoked response, or SER). Evoked potential assessment provides, not an evaluation of general brain activity, but a millisecond-by-millisecond record of a specific sensory process.

Electrical Stimulation

Researchers have used electrical stimulation of nerve tissue to empirically map pathways of the cortex. More recently, clinicians have introduced electrical stimulation in treating Parkinson's disease. Direct electrical stimulation of the brain, a very invasive medical procedure, is only used in those cases in which other interventions or diagnostic procedures have not succeeded.

Electromyography (EMG)

EMG is the electrical analysis of muscles, a diagnostic procedure useful in diagnosing peripheral nerve damage. The procedure is, however, uncomfortable, because it accompanies insertion of a needle into the muscle.

entists were able to measure total cerebral blood flow per unit weight of brain per minute. The procedure, however, had disadvantages. It was invasive and could only provide a measure of overall cerebral blood flow (Kety, 1979).

Lassen and Ingvar pioneered regional cerebral blood flow (rCBF) in living and awake subjects (Haeger, 1988). These researchers developed a special radioactive isotope known as xenon 133 (^{133}Xe), which emits a low gamma radiation and stays in the bloodstream for approximately 15 minutes. Isotopes are a species of atoms of a chemical element with the same atomic

number and position in the periodic table and nearly identical chemical behavior, but with differing atomic mass numbers and different physical properties. Thus, isotopes are highly unstable. Initially researchers injected this tracer intra-arterially into the bloodstream (via the internal carotid artery). The blood supply then carried the ^{133}Xe to either hemisphere, over which researchers placed special scintillation detectors that recorded the number of gamma rays the tracer emitted. In this manner scientists could determine the rate of clearance of ^{133}Xe from various regions of the brain. From this information they could quantify the rCBF with considerable accuracy. Cerebral blood flow studies corroborate many brain–behavior relationships established in the literature (see Exhibit 6). Occipital areas are more involved when a subject examines moving stimuli, and auditory areas are involved when speech is initiated. The most interesting aspects are anterior–posterior comparisons of blood flow in the brain, rather than right–left differences. For example, the ^{133}Xe technique reliably showed that the anterior brain regions have an increased rCBF in the resting subject (Gur et al., 1982).

One of the findings regarding rCBF relates to an absence of measurable information in the deepest regions of the brain. Furthermore, the ^{133}Xe technique can only measure one hemisphere at a time. In the 1970s researchers developed a special noninvasive technique in which subjects inhaled an air-xenon mixture through a face mask. Using this technique, researchers can study both hemispheres at the same time. The amount of detail for measuring specific brain region blood flow depends on the number of detectors. Initially this number was 8, then 16, and more recently 254 detectors. A computer then analyzes the data and provides a color-coded visualization of the findings (see Figure 6.11 on p. 212).

SINGLE-PHOTON EMISSION COMPUTED TOMOGRAPHY (SPECT)

A technique for the three-dimensional imaging of rCBF is **single-photon emission computed tomography,** or **SPECT.** SPECT is similar to PET, which uses radionuclides, but unlike positron emission, SPECT does not require an expensive cyclotron (a

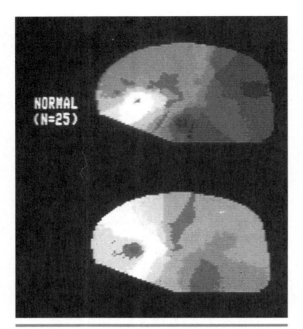

Figure 6.11   Topographic display of resting regional cerebral blood flow (rCBF) using an early system. Darker areas signaled high rCBF, and lighter areas suggested low areas of rCBF. (From James W. Kalat, *Biological Psychology*, 6th ed., Pacific Grove, CA: Brooks/Cole, 1998, p. 109, Figure 4.33. Courtesy of Karen Berman and Daniel Weinberger, NIH of Mental Health)

device that can generate radioactive chemicals with a short half-life, also known as *radioactive isotopes*) for their production. Radiologists can label biochemicals of interest with a radioactive compound whose gamma rays can be picked up by detectors surrounding the brain. Using SPECT, it is possible to three-dimensionally image the distribution of a radioactively labeled contrast agent. As in CT, a computer analyzes the data and reconstructs a three-dimensional cross-section of the emissions pattern. The tracer is injected intravenously and crosses into the brain tissue based on cerebral blood flow. Using this technique, analysts can estimate cerebral blood flow and blood volume. Researchers can study subjects undergoing SPECT while they are engaged in a neuropsychological task, although the tracer has a long half-life and it is difficult to keep a subject in the same mental state

for long. A further limitation is that the tracer takes approximately two days to clear from the brain, so it is only possible to obtain a single exposure of the brain using SPECT. An advantage of SPECT is that it is relatively inexpensive (it is referred to as "the poor person's PET"). A further advantage is that individuals can be imaged while they are sleeping or sedated, a useful option with young children or unmanageable patients. Thus, imaging studies that require multiple conditions are typically investigated by using the more costly **positron emission tomography** or **PET** technique.

POSITRON EMISSION TOMOGRAPHY (PET)

Emission tomography is a new visualization technique that detects a diverse range of physiologic parameters, including glucose and oxygen metabolism, in addition to blood flow, by distributing a radioactively labeled substance in any desired cross-section of the head. The method of PET technology is intravenous injection of a radioactive tracer (specifically positron-emitting substances) and subsequently scanning the brain for radioactivity. In contrast to SPECT, the radioactive isotopes injected with the PET procedure have a very short half-life and can attach to specific agents, such as glucose. Glucose, the body's fuel, mixes with blood to reach the brain. As already mentioned, the metabolism of the human brain varies in relation to its activity. The more active a specific area of the brain is, the more glucose it uses. Thus, the resting brain differs metabolically from the active brain. PET is the only procedure by which researchers can examine three-dimensionally the regional cerebral glucose use and oxygen metabolism in the living brain. PET analysts do not view the brain as a static structure, but investigate the dynamic properties of the brain (Raichle, 1983).

Technique

In the PET procedure, technicians administer radionuclides intravenously that the subject's brain tissue takes up. The radionuclei are unstable, because they have an excess positive charge. When the radioactive tracer decays, it emits a positron that then travels a

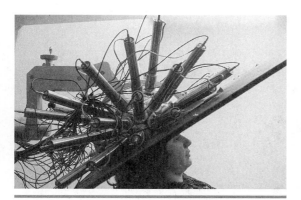

Figure 6.12 An early version of a PET scanner in which detectors around the scalp measure energy caused by the emission of photons. (Burt Glinn/Magnum)

very short distance (a few millimeters) before colliding with an electron. This collision results in the emission of two photons traveling in opposite directions, generating energy that detectors around the scalp can measure (see Figure 6.12). When two detectors calculate photon absorption at the same approximate time, the computer assumes they originate from the same collision and can then calculate the exact position showing neural "hotspots." PET functions on the basis of calculating millions of counts from detectors and estimating their origin. Using a subtraction technique, investigators can isolate blood flow patterns related to specific mental tasks. Computed tomography allows researchers to calculate a count and the locations of these collisions (depending on the type of radionuclide used, such as carbon 11, nitrogen 13, oxygen 15, or fluorin 18) to generate a visual representation of radionuclide uptake. In this manner, researchers can obtain varied physiologic parameters, including glucose and oxygen metabolism, blood flow, and receptor density of neurotransmitters for specific anatomic regions of interest (ROIs). For example, PET has shown different glucose uptake during various cognitive tasks (see Figure 6.13 on p. 214). The major disadvantage of using PET clinically is the cost involved, principally related to the need for an expensive cyclotron, which can produce the short-lived radioactive isotopes. As a result, PET technology is often only available in large medical centers associated with research institutes.

PET and Neuropsychology

Can PET technology detect changes occurring during cognitive activity? Or are the changes in metabolic activity too small to be detected? Measuring glucose metabolism rate is a more direct measure of neuron function than is cerebral blood flow. New tracers with a shorter half-life (such as positron-labeled oxygen, O^{15}) have led to investigating neuropsychological functions using PET, often with remarkable findings. Researchers use O^{15}, which readily crosses the blood–brain barrier, as a reference point for approximate blood intake of various regions in the brain. PET research demonstrates that the effects of cognitive effort on regional brain activity can be detected and measured (for example, a verbal task corresponds to the left hemisphere and a spatial task to the right hemisphere). PET is also sensitive to individual differences, such as gender, that affect the direction and degree of hemispheric specialization for specific neuropsychological abilities. Thus, studies using imaging technology indicate that there is a relationship between brain activity and behavior, and that PET can detect those associations (Gur, Levy, & Gur, 1977).

A major finding using PET technology is that metabolic activity is suppressed in patients with a history of head trauma, brain tumors, and stroke, even though structural representation of the brain, using MRI or CT, suggests intact brain anatomy. Thus metabolic imaging of the brain can lead to a clearer understanding of the functioning brain, specifically where the pathology is unclear, as in schizophrenics or epileptics. Although PET remains mostly a research tool because of its cost, it has proven an important technique in measuring physiologic activity in the normal and damaged brain at rest or while engaging in behavior.

One of the most interesting research aspects of PET concerns subjects performing various mental activities. Experimenters have taken PET scans of female and male adult brains when subjects were either resting or solving a rotating figure problem, a rather difficult spatial puzzle (Gur et al., 1982). Females not only scored lower than males, but there was a gender

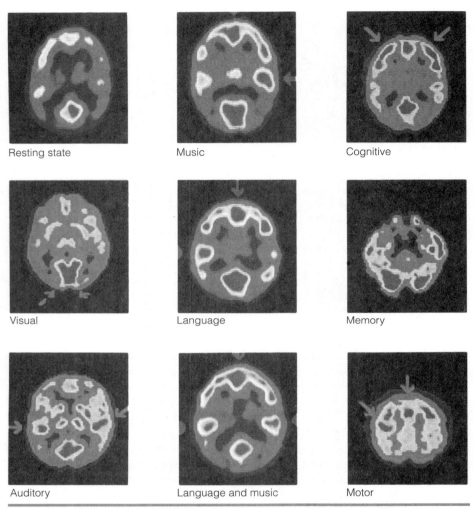

Resting state　　　Music　　　Cognitive

Visual　　　Language　　　Memory

Auditory　　　Language and music　　　Motor

Figure 6.13 PET images obtained during different cognitive tasks. Regions of highest metabolism are gray. (From James W. Kalat, *Biological Psychology,* 6th ed., Pacific Grove, CA: Brooks/Cole, 1998, p. 108, Figure 4.31. Courtesy of E. Phelps and John C. Mazziota, UCLA School of Medicine)

difference on the PET results. Even though the PET scans were not different while resting, when solving the rotating figure problem male brains showed maximum neural activity in the right frontal area, whereas female brains demonstrated maximum activity in the right parietal-temporal lobe. This suggests that men outperform women on the rotation problem and that there may be a neural reason for this. There are, of course, tasks at which women outperform men. For

example, women are generally faster on tests that require perceptual speed and score higher than men on a test of verbal fluency in which one must list as many words as one can that begin with the same letter (Lezak, 1995).

PET studies have generated a lot of controversy regarding sex differences in the brain. Are there really functional differences in the brain that arise from being male or female? The most recent studies suggest there are. Some theorists suggest an evolutionary perspective by which sex differences in the brain may have come from different skills needed by early humans. Males with good spatial skills, they argue, had an advantage in hunting, and females with good communication skills had an advantage in child rearing (Springer & Deutsch, 1993).

But researchers have not established whether sex differences are related to differences in socialization and learning experiences that are different for males and females, or whether the brains of females and males are organized differently and therefore function differently. This controversy is not easily decided, but PET may shed light on this puzzle. Table 6.5 reviews the most frequently used imaging techniques based on brain metabolism.

 ## Magnetic Imaging Procedures

MAGNETIC RESONANCE IMAGING (MRI)

MRI, or **magnetic resonance imaging,** is based on the work of Felix Bloch and Edward Purcell, who won the Nobel prize in physics in 1952 for their development of a new method of nuclear magnetic precision measurement. This led to the medical application of this technology called magnetic resonance imaging (MRI), during the early 1970s. Whereas CT uses penetrating x-ray radiation and PET uses radioactive isotopes, MRI is based on a fundamentally different process, namely, the fact that the hydrogen nucleus, which is present in high concentration in biologic systems, generates alterations in a small magnetic field, which can be measured. MRI provides pictures of anatomy superior to CT (see Figure 6.14), particularly for diagnosing underlying pathologic disorders (Pykett, 1982).

Technique

The principal technique involved in MRI is based on patterns similar to the pattern a magnet makes on surrounding metal flakes. The metal flakes align themselves according to the magnetic field. Similarly, when the head is subjected to a strong magnetic field, hydrogen protons magnetize and align in the direction of the magnetic field. A proton, which is an elementary

Table 6.5	*Imaging of Brain Metabolism*

Single-Photon Emission Computed Tomography (SPECT)

Single-photon emission computed tomography measures blood flow, a correlate of brain activity. Because the radioactive tracer takes almost two days to be eliminated from the body, researchers cannot use SPECT to monitor the brain's mental activity "moment to moment."

Positron Emission Tomography (PET)

Positron emission tomography tracks blood flow, which is associated with brain activity. It is mostly used to assess brain physiology, including glucose and oxygen metabolism, and the presence of specific neurotransmitters. The disadvantages of PET are that it is expensive, involves radiation, renders low spatial resolution, and data must be averaged over time (PET is not based on real time). The most promising use of PET has been its combined application with structural imaging techniques, which can provide a remarkable tool for mapping brain location and function.

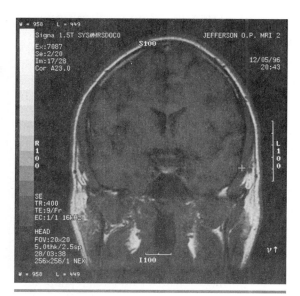

Figure 6.14 Normal MRI (coronal view). Note the symmetry of the lateral ventricles and density differences between white and gray matter in the cortex. (Eric Zillmer)

particle present in all atomic nuclei, has a positive charge equal to the negative charge of an electron. A strong radio frequency (RF) signal applied at a right angle to the magnetic field can alter the alignment of the hydrogen protons. This radio wave sets the aligned hydrogen atom oscillating. The RF specifically selects only aligned hydrogen atoms; other atoms will not react. Once the RF ceases, the hydrogen "spins back" to its original orientation as determined by the magnetic field, which remains active.

The emission of a small radio frequency signal accompanies this deflection or spin back to equilibrium. That is, the hydrogen atoms' return to their previous orientation generates a magnetic field, which researchers can amplify, measure, and record. Computer analysis can then present a visualization of hydrogen density in various regions throughout the brain. Because water is present in most biological tissue, this procedure can generate a strikingly accurate picture of the brain, or any other anatomy.

The principle of MRI is that the hydrogen atom resonates as a result of the combined effect of the radio waves and the magnetic field. This frequency is specific for a given nuclear species in a magnetic field and allows scientists to determine the origin of a given RF signal in space. For example, one measure of RF signal amplitude is hydrogen density. Thus variation of number of protons returning the RF signal is unique for different biological molecules, including fat, brain tissue, bone, and blood. This variation contributes to the MRI contrast, allowing spatial detection of signal data in three-dimensional space. As a result, researchers can very accurately calculate brain tissue densities and can generate a computer-constructed image, which is so spatially precise that it can visualize structures as small as 1 mm.

There is one more major determinant of signal amplitude, namely the magnetic relaxation times, also known as T1 and T2. These are the time intervals necessary for a nucleus to magnetize when placed in a magnetic field and the delay before returning to its original equilibrium. Protons with short T1 values (solids) emit higher signal intensities and appear white on the MRI, whereas those with longer T1 values (fluids) appear dark. T2 measures the loss of the magnetic orientation (or spin) after RF perturbation. On T2-weighted images, nuclei with relatively long T2 val-ues retain their signal strength, emit a higher-intensity signal, and appear brighter. Sometimes the difference in T1 and T2 values may provide additional visual information as in differentiating tumors and surrounding edema (swelling). More recently, three-dimensional images of the brain have been produced, based on MRI technology. MRI images are used as a starting point; specifically, MRI pixels in the X–Y plane resolution of the subject's original images. Using mathematical algorithms, a computer can generate a surface model of the scalp as well as the brain. The algorithms assume that a rigid body transformation of objects can be matched. In this way it is suitable to align MRI data sets into one whole object (Exhibit 7). The result is an exact model of the brain in three dimensions.

Clinical Use

MRI of the central nervous system has provided behavioral scientists and neuroradiologists with revolutionary quality of brain images in all planes (coronal, sagittal, and horizontal). As a result, MRI has become a very important diagnostic tool for detecting disease processes. This usefulness is related to the fact that MRI is very sensitive to tissue alteration, including those seen in diseases associated with demylination (such as multiple sclerosis), hemorrhage (bleeding), and tumor. Because of its increased clinical use, MRI has become readily available, and mobile units have even been built that travel to remote hospitals.

MRI is a complex procedure based in part on molecular physics and the mathematics of imaging three-dimensional objects in space. The principles underlying MRI sound complicated, and they are. Its scientific basis lies in physics and computer science, and thus an exact understanding of the procedure is not necessary for the neuropsychology student. But neuropsychologists are participating in the research using this technology because of their expertise in the functional aspects of neuroanatomical structures, their knowledge of neuropsychological tests, and their background in scientific methodology and design (see Neuropsychology in Action 6.2 on pp. 218 and 219).

Functional MRI (fMRI)

Traditional MRI measures the frequencies of magnetically perturbed water molecules and provides a structural representation of the brain. More recent advances have focused on detecting frequencies emitted from other molecular species associated with cerebral metabolism. Efforts have concentrated on reconstructing images from glucose metabolism and changes in blood oxygenation. A recent finding has been that oxygenated blood has slightly different magnetic properties that special-sequence MRI scans can detect. In this manner, researchers can measure motor activity and neuropsychological tests. The data from fMRI can then be superimposed (cross-sectioned or coregistered) over the structural MRI for a precise mapping of structure and function. This combined use of MRI and fMRI may revolutionize the study of the activated brain, because it can provide almost continuous real-time data on cerebral activity (Cohen, Noll, & Schneider, 1993).

The advantage of fMRI over SPECT, PET, and CT is that there is no radiation exposure. Therefore, fMRI is less invasive. However, scientists do not completely know the effects of exposure of the brain to high magnetic fields, which is higher in fMRI because molecules other than hydrogen are assessed. Furthermore, resolution of fMRI is better than in PET images, which are reconstructed from thousands of calculations averaged over 90 seconds, the half-life of the tracer. In contrast, fMRI can provide independent images every few seconds or as frequently as the RF is turned on and off. This capability gives investigators a better picture-by-picture account of the neural correlates involved in specific tasks.

MAGNETOENCEPHALOGRAPHY (MEG)

Magentoencephalography, or **MEG,** involves measurement of changes in magnetic fields that are generated by underlying electrical activity of active neurons. Neuronal activity generates not only electrical fields, but also magnetic fields. When neurons fire, the magnetic changes resulting from the electrical fields, which reflect neural activity, can be measured. Recording the magnetic fields that accompany the electrical activity of neurons is known as magnetoencephalography, or MEG. MEG is the magnetic equivalent of EEG. The magnetic field of neurons is very small, and requires special superconducting coils, housed in elaborate magnetically shielded rooms, to detect and measure the weak magnetic fields. This specialized detector is called the *superconducting quantum interference device (SQUID),* which is capable of measuring tiny magnetic fields of the brain. MEG has traditionally used systems with one to seven SQUID sensors, although recent technology has made larger sensor arrays possible. The response of the brain to different stimuli, similar to the evoked potential technique, results in measurable alterations in the magnetic field. A computer can then calculate a three-dimensional location based on the source of the magnetic field in the brain. The physical location of the magnetic source can be improved by projecting the MEG onto MRI images. MEG is more elaborate than EEG, but it can better localize the source of activity using isocontour maps of magnetic fields.

MEG is expensive; the SQUID is immersed in liquid helium to keep the system at a low temperature, which is necessary for superconductivity, and relies on complex technology. At this time MEG is experimental and is not used for routine clinical diagnostic studies, although MEG is an added diagnostic tool in epilepsy, because it provides more accurate seizure diagnosis than EEG technology can (Hari, 1994). Table 6.6 reviews current magnetic imaging procedures.

Table 6.6 *Magnetic Imaging Procedures*

Magnetic Resonance Imaging (MRI)

Magnetic resonance imaging can provide the most detailed images of brain structures. The obtained images are of excellent clarity, but individuals who have metal in their bodies are contraindicated for the procedure. Recent research has focused on the functional mapping of blood flow or oxygenation using MRI. The advantage of functional MRI over other functional procedures such as PET is that it provides good spatial resolution and images in very short time periods or "real time."

Magnetoencephalography (MEG)

The magnetic equivalent of the EEG, in which a computer can calculate a three-dimensional magnetic field of the brain. Superconducting quantum interference devices (SQUIDs) detect the small magnetic fields in the brain that are a marker of neural activity. A disadvantage of MEG is related to the fact that it is expensive and not readily available for clinical applications.

Neuropsychology in Action 6.2

Diagnostic Neuroimaging and Neuropsychology

by Erin D. Bigler Ph.D., *Professor of Psychology, Brigham Young University.*

Contemporary neuroimaging represents a very remarkable scientific breakthrough. Prior to the advent of computed transaxial tomography (CT) scanning around 1975, there was no way to visualize actual brain structure except during neurosurgery or in cases where skull trauma exposed the brain. In one technique, pneumo-encephalography, technicians would remove cerebral spinal fluid from the brain, replace it with air, and take a standard x-ray image. But that method only outlined the ventricular system (internal cavity) of the brain and did not provide any actual direct image of brain tissue. Also, radioisotope scans would measure uptake of a radiopharmaceutical, but could not visualize actual tissue. Thus in the early history of neurology and neuropsychology, the clinician had to rely on the powers of inference to make conclusions about underlying brain pathol-

ogy and neurologic disorders, because the brain could not be directly viewed. Before the current state of neuroimaging, knowing the patient's history, an in-depth knowledge of brain anatomy and pathology, and examining the patients on standard neurologic and neuropsychological tests, allowed clinicians to make an inference about particular brain regions that might be involved (damaged) or what type of disease process might be present. All this changed radically with the advent of modern brain-imaging techniques. The CT scan was the forerunner for the development of magnetic resonance imaging (MRI), which uses an entirely different technology. In scanning with computerized tomography (CT) technology, an x-ray beam passes through the head and various computer computations create an index of tissue density. These tissue

density values are then used to form an image of the brain on a gray scale. MRI employs radio frequency waves that permit a reconstruction of the brain essentially mimicking gross anatomy. The beauty of magnetic resonance imaging is that scientists can use it to acquire images of the brain in any plane and in any angle or orientation.

For example, the first set of images shown in Figure 6.15 (upper right) are of my brain (that's me, holding a brain, in the upper left). Viewing my brain in the horizontal (axial) position, you can see that the brain is a symmetric organ and, therefore, a view of one side should mirror the other side. In comparison, just below my MRI scan is one from a patient who sustained a very severe traumatic brain injury in a motor vehicle accident, with penetrating damage to the frontal lobe. The lower left-hand quadrant shows

---

Cerebrospinal Fluid Studies: Lumbar Puncture

The **lumbar puncture** or spinal tap is a medical technique to collect a sample of cerebrospinal fluid (CSF) surrounding the spinal cord for diagnostic study. The patient lies on his or her side in a fetal position, and the physician administers a local anesthetic. A long (3- to 3.5-inch) puncture needle is inserted perpendicular between the third and fourth (or fourth and fifth) lumbar vertebrae. The needle penetrates the dura and enters the spinal canal. Then the physician collects CSF, and checks CSF pressure (normal range = 100 mm). In some cases the physician administers radiopaque material or medication

through the needle, in which case the CSF withdrawn is equal to the volume of fluid introduced. At the end of the procedure, the physician withdraws the needle quickly. The lumbar puncture is a relatively easy and routine way by which to obtain a CSF sample. Yet lumbar puncture is invasive and painful, requiring a local anesthetic, and infection is always a concern.

On visual inspection, normal CSF is colorless and does not coagulate. After a subarachnoid hemorrhage (for example), the CSF may be blood stained. Technicians typically examine the CSF sample in a laboratory for cell count, glucose levels, and protein content, to detect CSF abnormalities. The lumbar puncture is a useful diagnostic aid for a variety of neurologic conditions in which the CSF has been "contaminated,"

the three-dimensional MRI reconstruction of the person's head. You can see the residual scars about the face and nose and the indentation that is in the frontal region where the rear view mirror stand penetrated the skull and brain. Looking at the horizontal (axial) view of this individual's brain in the lower right hand corner and applying the principle of symmetry, you can see the frontal (top) region of the brain, on the right-hand side of the picture (the left side of the patient), a large area of degeneration in the frontal pole (areas in black). This indicates necrosis or wasting of the brain. From the neuropsychological standpoint, because the patient has predominantly a frontal injury, you would expect difficulties with complex reasoning, decision making, change in temperament and personality, as well as alterations in memory functioning. In fact, the patient's neuropsychological studies demonstrate such deficits. This is an excellent example of how brain imaging technology can interface with neuropsychological test findings to establish the most accurate and specific assessment of behavioral and cognitive changes in a patient with TBI.

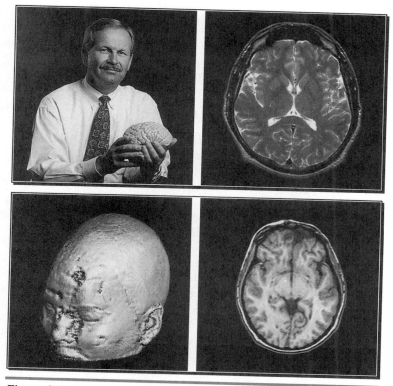

Figure 6.15 Dr. Erin D. Bigler and imaging examples. (Erin Bigler, Brigham Young University)

including acute and subacute bacterial meningitis, viral infections, brain abscess or tumor, multiple sclerosis, and hemorrhage.

 Behavioral Examinations

NEUROLOGIC EXAM

The **neurologic exam** is a routine introductory evaluation that a neurologist performs. A neurologist is a physician who has specialized in evaluating and treating neurologic disorders. Although there are many variations, in principle the neurologic exam involves a detailed history of the patient's medical history and a careful assessment of the patient's reflexes, cranial nerve functioning, gross movements, muscle tone, and ability to perceive sensory stimuli. The neurological exam typically includes a number of brief cognitive procedures. Those include language function, memory (for example, remembering digits or memory for words), visual-spatial function (drawing), attention (reverse counting), and mental status (that is, an assessment of the patient's understanding of where he (or she) is, what time it is, who he is, and why he is there). The neurologic exam is not as detailed as a neuropsychological evaluation, because it is difficult to obtain an accurate comprehensive assessment of higher cortical function during a brief examination. More recently, a special focus in neurology, on behavior and higher cortical function (behavioral neurology), has overlapped more with neuropsychology. In general, the domains previously held by neurologists and by neuropsychologists are getting much closer, and both disciplines have much to learn from each other.

NEUROPSYCHOLOGICAL EVALUATION

Whereas neurologists are interested in changes in the nervous system that occur within the clinical context (such as lesions, disease, and trauma), neuropsychologists are primarily interested in higher cognitive functioning. Luria suggested (1973) that neuropsychology is the most complex and newest chapter in neurology, without which modern clinical neurology would be unable to exist and develop. The **neuropsychological evaluation** provides additional information about the patient's health, and is used, in conjunction with other pertinent information, for diagnosis, patient management, intervention, rehabilitation, and discharge planning. In the last part of this text, (Chapters 14 through 16), we give a detailed account of the role of the neuropsychological evaluation, its purpose, and its applications.

After reading this chapter, the student may wonder if modern imaging technology will soon replace neuropsychology. We strongly suggest that imaging technologies and neuropsychology are compatible. In fact, we are now in an era in which data from CT, for example, should be used routinely with that of neuropsychology information. Note that even though modern imaging technology has had spectacular success in depicting the brain's anatomy, neuropsychological findings appear more sensitive to the progression of degenerative diseases than either CT or MRI. Modern imaging technology is most useful in concert with neuropsychological studies. For example, consider a CT scan that reveals a large, marble-size tumor in the patient's right parietal hemisphere. From a neurobehavioral view, we may make certain assumptions about what cognitive functions may be compromised, based on the CT data. Such assumptions, however, would be only hypothetical, and one would need to assess the precise neurobehavioral sequelae using neuropsychological techniques. In addition, no imaging tool yet developed can indicate how

patients' will adapt with a specific neurologic disorder, whether they will be able to work, or what quality of life they will have.

New Advances in Imaging Techniques: Mapping the Brain

SUBTRACTION PROCEDURES

Researchers often use the subtraction technique in imaging studies to isolate brain characteristics that are relevant during a specific neuropsychological task. In principle, the procedure uses two sets of data. The first set is obtained using the control condition. For example, to use PET in studying the neuronal aspects of a calculus task in the control condition, researchers would ask subjects to recite numbers that have no meaningful relationship to each other. In the task condition, researchers obtain brain images while subjects are performing calculus problems. The logic behind reciting numbers in the control task is that both tasks involve the neural mechanism of using numbers, but only one condition uses numbers in a meaningful way. After researchers subtract the image of the noncalculus condition from the second image they obtained during the calculus condition, the new picture should show brain regions involved in the mathematical effort of using numbers in meaningful relationship to each other.

IMAGE ANALYSIS AND QUANTIFICATION (3-D)

Recent advances in computer software have allowed three-dimensional computer reconstruction of specific brain structures. Because of recent advances in calculating volumetric analysis of specific brain structures, scientists applied segmentation methods to construct 3-D images, in order to visualize a specific structure of the brain (such as ventricles) or a known pathology (such as hemorrhage). Such 3-D images advance the understanding of pathologic conditions as well as brain structures, because scientists can now visualize the site of the lesion from any angle or perspective. The ventricular system is difficult to appreciate in a two-dimensional perspective, but in a 3-D model it can be easily visualized. More recent quantitative imaging techniques have automated the evaluation of definable regions of interest throughout the brain. Because normative data are not yet available, serial quantitative image examinations of individual cases have proven very useful. The correlation between quantitative neuroimaging findings and neuropsychological indices of brain function has only been moderate.

One procedure focuses on using volumetric MRI analyses to estimate brain volume and ventricle-to-brain ratio (VBR). A normal VBR is approximately 1.5%; that is, about 1.5% of a normal, healthy, adult brain is dedicated to cerebrospinal fluid. Increased VBR has been particularly consistent in subjects following traumatic brain injury, who have much higher VBR ratios, up to 4% (Johnson, Bigler, Burr, & Blatter, 1994). This increase is related to brain atrophy following the injured brain, with a corresponding increase of its ventricular space.

Furthermore, researchers can now digitize and superimpose serial MRI sections to create a 3-D picture of the entire head or brain or specific brain structures. This current technology can use 3-D representation of any isolated brain structure (Bigler, 1996). Other methods, including SPECT, PET, quantitative EEG, and MEG, can also be used to generate 3-D images.

After establishing image analysis and quantification, the next step was to address the interfacing of different imaging technologies to further explore structure and function in brain–behavior relationships. For example, the high detail of MRI-based images of the brain can be superimposed over images derived from those obtained by PET. In this way researchers can examine both structure and function simultaneously. As technology develops further, it will be possible to increase the combination and integration of imaging techniques. Thus, one key focus in current imaging research is integrating multifaceted data to understand regional brain function. In this manner, topographic information from CT and MRI about the integrity of brain regions can complement information on regional brain physiologic activity derived from EEG, SPECT, and PET (see Exhibit 8). However, as with any research, neuropsychological theory is needed to guide explorations of how brain activity relates to behavior.

FUTURE DIRECTIONS

One of the greatest uncharted territories before the human species is the functional mapping of its own brain. The cartographers are scientists who use powerful technology to examine the living brain right through the skull. The task is formidable: 100 billion neurons with a seemingly infinite number of interconnections. The human brain is the most complex structure known in the entire universe. To make sense of this three-pound "jungle" of cells, will it be enough to take pictures of the brain? Any new approach to brain mapping must move beyond simply visualizing structure. The challenge before the cartographers of the new millennium is to map function; what brain structures do what, and when. True, neuropsychologists have identified many regions that specialize in particular cognitive jobs. But they have gained much of this knowledge from people with brain pathology or injury. The new imaging technologies are capable of examining the normal, healthy functioning brain. We stand on the brink of learning how the living, normal brain performs sophisticated mental functions.

The most exciting use of neuroimaging, we propose, is in combination with neuropsychological procedures. The fact that neuroimaging measures and neuropsychological studies depend on shared neuroanatomy needs to be further studied. Thus, it is likely that scientists will combine measures of neurophysiology and neuropsychology to unlock the secrets of how the human brain functions. Furthermore, imaging technologies will continue to be refined, with specific regard to the functional and structural aspects of the brain. It will be soon be possible to perform biochemical dissections on the human brain, to pinpoint the concentration of a neurotransmitter receptor within the brain of a living subject. It will be possible to examine the effects of treatment of diseases known to be associated with disturbances in neurotransmitters or its receptors (for example, schizophrenia, Parkinson's disease, and Huntington's chorea).

New advances will also demonstrate brain activity from moment to moment in real time with precise localization. The integration of different imaging technologies is only in its infancy. Scientists have yet to fully explore interrelationships among different neurodiagnostic procedures. The greatest potential of these tools may lie in assessing the neuropsycho-logical functions *during* neurophysiological procedures. The tools that seem most valuable at this time appear to be fMRI, MEG, quantitative EEG, PET, and SPECT. This direction will lead to a multidimensional and increasingly comprehensive approach to the functioning of the brain, bridging the gap between psychology and biology.

Conclusion

The neuropsychology student may feel that the level of technology is so sophisticated that behavioral techniques add very little to the overall information about a human being. This is true to some extent, particularly in the area of diagnosis. The presence of tumors, stroke, and hydrocephalus is most easily, efficiently, and accurately discerned by modern imaging techniques. However, some diagnoses are so subtle and diffuse that only comprehensive neuropsychological tests can identify them. Although the neuropsychologist's role in diagnosis has shrunk, behavioral techniques still play a major role in diagnosing early stages of dementia or attention deficit disorder. Furthermore, sophisticated medical examination procedures cannot provide a functional assessment of an individual, and certainly not an understanding of the patient's quality of life or perception thereof. A functional assessment is most effectively conducted by neuropsychologists using behavioral tools.

Moreover, remember that most of the outlined procedures provide a static picture of the brain, and that neuropsychological dysfunction may extend considerably beyond the pathology that modern imaging techniques uncover. No doubt the alphabet soup of new imaging technologies has become a powerful tool in the study of brain–behavior relationship. But will this new technology fulfill what the phrenologists were unable to do, that is, create a precise functional map of the brain? Probably not. Many constraints hinder the use of functional imaging in studying the human brain. For example, ultimately the image rendered is not a direct representation of the mechanism involved in the mental activity, but some correlate. Furthermore, functional imaging captures brief moments, most suitable for analyzing a neuroimage or process involved in sensory-motor operations or a specific neuropsychological task. But it is doubtful that imaging technology will ever be able to assess a thought or investigate personality.

One of the most exciting advances in the imaging of the living brain is the collaboration among different disciplines, including biomedical engineers, psychiatrists, neurologists, neurosurgeons, and neuropsychologists, to define and differentiate between the normal and the malfunctioning brain. We turn next to the developing brain and its often complex behavioral sequelae.

Critical Thinking Questions

■ What are the differences among electrical, magnetic, and metabolic technologies in imaging?

■ Why is coregistration, that is, the use of multiple assessment using different technologies, an important advance in neuropsychology?

■ Which medical technology examine to your brain would you volunteer for? Why?

■ Will neuropsychology be outdated by the increased use of sophisticated brain imaging technology? Why or why not?

Key Terms

Golgi, Camillo
Nissl, Franz
Myelin staining
Horseradish peroxidase
  (HRP)
Röntgen, Wilhelm Conrad
X rays
Air encephalography, or
  pneumoencephalography

Computed transaxial
  tomography (CT)
Hypodensity
Hyperdensity
Enhanced CT
Angiography
Femorocerebral angiography
Digital subtraction
  angiography

Wada technique
Electroencephalography (EEG)
Electrocorticogram (ECoG)
Evoked potential (EP)
Single-photon emission
  computed tomography
  (SPECT)
Positron emission
  tomography (PET)

Magnetic resonance imaging
  (MRI)
Magnetoencephalography
  (MEG)
Lumbar puncture
Neurologic exam
Neuropsychological
  evaluation

Web Connections

http://www.med.harvard.edu/AANLIB/home.html
The Whole Brain Atlas
Harvard University site that provides neuroimaging primer, and overview of brain anatomy and physiology including images of CT, MRI, PET, MPEG movies, and SPECT. This site can be used as a general reference for exploring the latest in brain imaging.

http://www.bic.mni.mcgill.ca/brainweb
Brain Web: Simulated Brain Database
Contains simulated brain MRI data based on two anatomic models. Full three-dimensional volumes have been simulated using a variety of slice thickness. Data are available for viewing in three orthogonal views.

Part Three

THE DEVELOPING BRAIN

Chapter 7

DEVELOPMENTAL DISORDERS OF CHILDHOOD

CONTRIBUTED BY WILLIAM C. CULBERTSON

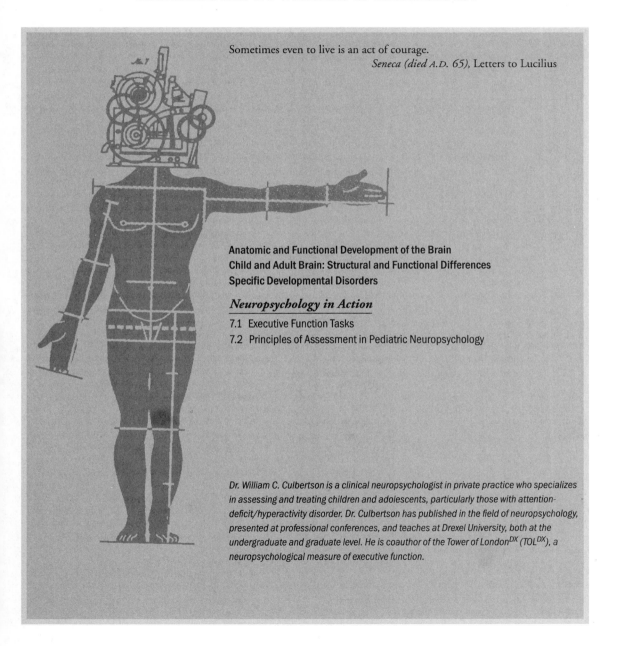

Sometimes even to live is an act of courage.

Seneca (died A.D. 65), Letters to Lucilius

Anatomic and Functional Development of the Brain
Child and Adult Brain: Structural and Functional Differences
Specific Developmental Disorders

Neuropsychology in Action

7.1 Executive Function Tasks
7.2 Principles of Assessment in Pediatric Neuropsychology

Dr. William C. Culbertson is a clinical neuropsychologist in private practice who specializes in assessing and treating children and adolescents, particularly those with attention-deficit/hyperactivity disorder. Dr. Culbertson has published in the field of neuropsychology, presented at professional conferences, and teaches at Drexel University, both at the undergraduate and graduate level. He is coauthor of the Tower of London^{DX} (TOL^{DX}), a neuropsychological measure of executive function.

Keep in Mind

■ How is the development of brain structure related to the emergence of function?

■ What differences in the impact of brain injury are there for children as compared to adults?

■ Is the brain of a child merely a small replica of the adult brain, differing only in terms of size, or do the two brains differ in significant ways?

■ Can children with fetal alcohol syndrome outgrow their cognitive deficits?

Overview

The first part of this chapter provides an overview of the prenatal and postnatal development of the human brain. This is a significant developmental period when you consider that the rate of neuronal development is estimated at 250,000 neurons per minute, for a total, at birth, in excess of 100 billion (Cowan, 1979). Despite this astonishing rate of early brain development, the process is both orderly and systematic. That is, the brain develops in accordance with genetically predetermined templates or "blueprints" that guide the unfolding of structure and function. The developmental process does not stop and wait for better conditions such as optimal maternal health and nutrition, nor does it reverse direction to repeat developmental stages that are compromised by insults such as trauma, drugs, or environmental toxins. So it is not surprising that negative events during this process account for significant numbers of childhood neurological disorders.

In addition, we discuss the vulnerability and plasticity of the young brain, and compare the child and the adult brain. These two issues are particularly significant in evaluating and predicting the immediate and long-term effects of brain insult or injury. Finally, we examine a number of developmental disorders to highlight the unfortunate consequences of anomalies in brain development. Specifically, we look at the developmental disorders with regard to prevalence and manifestations, neuropsychological pathogenesis and assessment, and current interventions to halt or ameliorate negative effects.

Anatomic and Functional Development of the Brain

ANATOMIC DEVELOPMENT

Beginning as a hollow tube, the brain develops steadily through temporally distinct stages to its final anatomic and functional state of well-delineated cellular layers and regions. The development of the central nervous system, brain, and spinal cord is orderly and systematic, generally unfolding from head (cephalic) to tail (caudal), from near (proximal) to far (distal), and from inferior (subcortical) to dorsal (cortical). The earliest stage of brain development, **neurogenesis,** involves the proliferation of neurons of the neural tube and the migration of these cells to predetermined locations. Subsequent stages include the growth of axons and dendrites, formation of synaptic junctures, myelination of axons, and synaptic reorganization involving strengthening or loss of synaptic connections. In examining these stages, we give special attention to the development of the cortex, because of its central role in supporting higher-order cognitive processes such as attention, memory, language, and problem solving.

Neurogenesis and Cellular Migration

The central nervous system (CNS) and peripheral nervous system (PNS) develop from the midline ectoderm layer of the fertilized egg at approximately 18 days after conception. Ectodermal tissue (neural plate) rises, and subsequently folds and fuses to form the **neural tube** surrounding a fluid-filled cavity (see Figure 7.1). The cavity of the neural tube gives rise to the ventricular system of the central nervous system, and the cells lining the wall of the neural tube, termed **precursor** or **progenitor cells,** create the neurons and glia (astrocytes and oligodendrocytes) of the brain (Martin & Jessell, 1991). Developing cells do not proliferate at the same rate along the expanding neural tube. The timing and location of these cells are genetically predetermined, and relate to their final placement and function in the mature brain. Once the proliferation of a specified group of neurons is complete, they begin to migrate outward toward their genetically determined destination. As the cells reach their destination, they begin to develop the characteristics of the cell types that are intrinsic to that particular brain region (Kolb & Fantie, 1997).

The open ends of the neural tube close at approximately the 25th day of gestation, with the anterior end subsequently giving rise to the brain, and the posterior end forming the spinal cord (Spreen, Risser, & Edgell, 1995). The process of forming and closing the neural tube is called **neurulation.** Failure of the neural tube to close during development can cause a number of developmental disorders. For example, neuroscientists believe that **spina bifida,** a congenital developmental disorder characterized by an opening in the spinal cord, results from a disruption of the proliferation rate of neural cells, or from the failure of these cells to differentiate properly in the neural tube. In contrast, when the anterior end of the tube fails to close, the brain fails to develop anatomically, producing a condition termed **anencephaly.** In this condition the brain is a vascular mass and the infant fails to survive.

The development of the cortex, **corticogenesis,** begins in the 6th embryonic week. The rapidly proliferating cells along the wall of the neural tube migrate outward at different predetermined times. The neurons migrate in sheets (laminae) along nonneuronal (glial) fibers that span the cortical wall. Ultimately these neuronal sheets constitute the six laminated layers of the cortex. The inner layer forms first, followed by the development of the outer layers of the cortex. Each successive generation of migrating cells passes through the previously developed

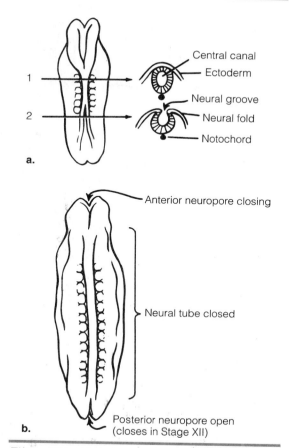

Figure 7.1 Formation and closure of the neural tube. (a) Start of neurulation, two cross-sectional views. (b) Late stage of neurulation, showing the anterior and posterior closing. (From R. J. Lemire, J. D. Loeser, R. W. Leech, and E. C. Alvord, *Normal and Abrnormal Development of the Human Nervous System,* Philadelphia: Lippincott, Williams & Wilkins, 1975. Reprinted with permission)

neuronal cells. Thus the cortex develops from inside out, with migration beginning earlier for the more anterior and lateral areas of the cortex (Rakic & Lombroso, 1998). By the 18th week of gestation, virtually all cortical neurons have reached their designated locations.

Disruption in the migratory process can cause significant and extensive damage to the developing brain. For example, abnormalities of cell migration can produce developmental anomalies of the corpus callosum and other subcortical structures. Relatedly, disruption of cell migration during the first trimester of development is associated with malformations of the cerebral cortex. An example is the condition of **agyria,** or **lissencephaly,** a disorder that occurs during the 11th to 13th weeks of gestation, and is characterized by the underdevelopment of the cortical gyri (Hynd, Morgan, & Vaughn, 1997). Severe neurologic problems accompany this condition, such as severe mental retardation, motor retardation, seizures, and reduced muscle tone. Most infants with agyria fail to survive beyond age 2.

Axon and Dendrite Development

As the neurons migrate along the glial fibers, axons begin to rapidly form and travel to other neurons of the brain, allowing for cortical–cortical, cortical–subcortical, and interhemispheric communication. The intercommunications afforded by axonal connections are crucial to the integrative functioning of the brain. As the migrating neuronal cells reach their designated positions, dendrites begin to sprout in a process called *arborization.* Subsequently, little extensions called **spines** begin to extend out from the dendrites. The dendrites and dendritic spines create synapses for gathering information to be sent to the neuron. Dendritic growth begins prenatally and proceeds slowly, with the majority of arborization and spine growth actually occurring postnatally. The most intensive period of dendritic growth occurs from birth to approximately 18 months. The development of the dendrites and spines is highly sensitive to the effects of environmental stimulation. This sensitivity, on the one hand, fosters the growth and differentiation of the brain, yet, on the other hand, increases its vul-

nerability to damage. An example of the latter is the discovery, for certain groups of mentally retarded children, of abnormalities of the dendritic spines that cannot be attributed to genetic factors. In these cases, neuroscientists suspect some form of environmental insult of having produced the anomaly.

Synaptogenesis

Paralleling the growth of the axons and dendrites of the brain is the formation of synapses, that is, **synaptogenesis.** At the 28th gestational week, synaptic density is low in all cortical regions, particularly the prefrontal cortex. Whereas the occipital lobe begins developing prior to birth, and rapidly achieves near adult-level synaptic density between ages 2 and 4, the more slowly developing prefrontal cortex does not reach adult levels until late adolescence or adulthood. Likewise, the synaptic development of the motor speech cortex (Broca's area) follows a slow trajectory paralleling that of the prefrontal cortex (Huttenlocher & Dabholkar, 1997). Regional increases in synaptic density accompany the emergence of function. For example, a rapid increase in synaptic density of the frontal lobes during the latter part of the first year of life correlates with the emergence of rudimentary executive functions such as delayed response performance (see section on development of executive functions in this chapter).

Myelination

As cellular migration nears completion, glial cells begin to encircle the axons, providing a protective white, insular sheath called **myelin.** The process of myelination begins in the spinal cord, proceeds through the subcortical regions, and finally completes the cortical circuitry. The cortical regions myelinate at different times, beginning in the posterior regions of the brain and moving anteriorly, with the parietal and frontal lobes completing the process last. The myelination of the latter two regions begins following birth, and in the case of the frontal regions, continues into adolescence and adulthood. The significant increase in brain weight in the postnatal years is primarily a function of the brain's increased myelination. Further, the myelination of regional circuitry generally correlates with the emergence of function. Thus, like synaptic density, myelination is a "marker" of the functional maturity of brain circuitry. For example, myelination of the optic nerve begins at birth and is completed by the third month, consistent with the emergence of vision.

Pruning

During the early months of neurodevelopment, the neurons and synaptic processes of the cortex are initially overproduced. Researchers believe that the synaptic connectivity of the neurons is not completely genetically preprogrammed, and many of the initial connections may be random. Subsequent development eliminates, or **prunes,** large numbers of neurons, with the process often beginning at the sites of the dendritic spines. Pruning does not appear to be random, but seems to be a purposeful sculpting of the brain. That is, synaptic connections that are strengthened through sensory input and motor activity are spared. In contrast, pruning eliminates weakly reinforced or redundant connections, thus promoting neural efficiency. Economy in structure and function appears to be an overarching principle of evolutionary development. This process is exemplified by the development of speech and language specific to one's culture. At birth, the infant is sensitive to the range of sounds that are evident in all languages. However, the reinforcement of speech sounds unique to one's culture results in the loss of sensitivity to sounds *not* evident in the language. Neuroscientists speculate that neurons and synaptic processes representing the understimulated sounds are pruned. Functionally, this pruning potentially accounts for the greater difficulty encountered in learning a second language at an older age, in contrast to learning the language at an earlier age.

Pruning is primarily a postnatal process, eliminating 40% of the brain's cortical neurons during childhood. The remaining neurons are eliminated during adolescence, and possibly into early adulthood. Pruning of cortical regions proceeds at different times and rates. Thus, reduction of the synapses in the visual cortex begins at 1 year of age and is completed by age 12, whereas pruning of the prefrontal region proceeds from 5 to 16 years of age (Pfefferbaum et al., 1994).

Regional Development

As previously noted, the anterior, cranial end of the neural tube expands to form the brain, and the posterior end evolves to form the spinal cord. Before neurulation is complete, three vesicles (dilations or expansions) develop at the anterior end. These vesicles subsequently form the forebrain (prosencephalon), midbrain (mesencephalon), and hindbrain (rhombencephalon). In the 5th week of development, the forebrain and hindbrain each subdivide, while the third vesicle, the midbrain, maintains its regional structure. These subdivisions, in combination with the spinal cord, ultimately give rise to six global regions and the inherent neural structures of the mature CNS. Figure 7.2 (p. 232) presents the regional development of the brain.

Lobular and Convolutional Development

As the cerebral cortex moves forward in development, it first expands anteriorly to form the frontal lobes, then dorsally to form the parietal lobes, and finally posteriorly and inferiorly to form the temporal and occipital lobes. The posterior and inferior expansion pushes the cortex into a C shape. As a result, this C form also shapes many of the underlying structures, including the lateral ventricles, the head of the caudate of the basal ganglia, the hippocampus and fornix, and the cingulate and parahippocampal gyri (Martin & Jessell, 1991).

In the initial stages of prenatal development the brain surface is smooth, lacking both gyri and sulci. Then the major sulci dividing the cerebral lobes appear, with the gyri within the lobes emerging later. At approximately 14 weeks of gestation, the longitudinal fissure dividing the two cerebral hemispheres and the Sylvian (lateral) fissure demarcating the border of the parietal and frontal lobes, are visible. Gyrification continues in an orderly and symmetrical fashion through gestation, and by birth the gyral patterns of the adult are present (Hynd & Hiemenz, 1977). Table 7.1 details this progression.

The gyri and sulci patterns of the cortex form after neuronal migration, and reflect the processes of neuronal specialization, dendritic arborization, synaptic

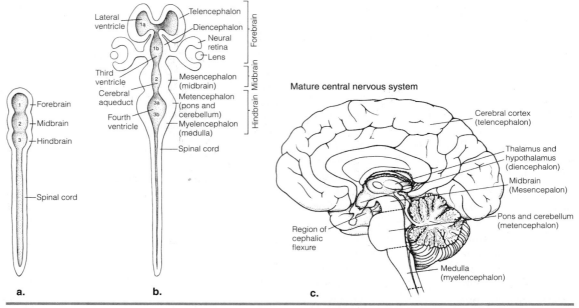

Figure 7.2   Regional development of the brain. (a) Three-vesicle stage of the neural tube in early development of the brain and spinal cord. (b) Five-vesicle stage of the brain and spinal cord at a later stage of development. (c) The regions of the mature central nervous system (spinal cord not shown). (From J. H. Martin and T. M. Jessell, "Development as a Guide to the Regional Anatomy of the Brain," in E. R. Kandel, J. H. Schwartz, and T. M. Jessell, eds., *Principles of Neural Science,* 5th ed., New York: Elsevier Science, 1991, pp. 298–299. Reproduced by permission of the McGraw-Hill Companies)

Table 7.1   *Embryonic Development of the Cortical Gyri in Humans*

Gestational Age (weeks)	Gyrus
16–19	Gyrus rectus, insula, cingulate
20–23	Parahippocampal, superior temporal
24–27	Pre- and postrolandic, middle temporal, superior and middle frontal, occipital
28–31	Inferior and transverse temporal, medial and lateral orbital, angular, supramarginal
32–35	Paracentral
36–39	Anterior and posterior orbital

Source: Adapted from Benes (1997), p. 217. Used by permission.

formation, and pruning. The formation of the gyri signals that intracortical connections are established. Although the gyri and sulci patterns of each person differ slightly, unusual or extreme alterations suggest deviations in cortical connections and potential cognitive and behavioral deficits (Hynd & Hiemenz, 1997). For example, an insult to the brain (such as intrauterine infection) during the 5th and 6th month of gestation can produce **polymicrogyria,** a condition characterized by the development of small, densely packed gyri. This anomaly is associated with learning disabilities, mental retardation, and epilepsy (Hynd et al., 1997).

Ventricular Development

As the CNS matures, the cavities within the cerebral vesicles of the neural tube subsequently form the ventricular system and the central canal of the spinal cord. The cavities of cerebral vesicles differentiate into (1) the two lateral ventricles, formerly called the first and second ventricles of the forebrain; (2) the narrow cerebral aqueduct, or aqueduct of Sylvius, of the midbrain; and (3) the fourth ventricle of the hindbrain (Martin & Jessell, 1991). The remaining caudal cavity forms the spinal canal.

Cerebrospinal fluid (CSF) is produced in the ventricles, cushions the brain and spinal cord within the skull and vertebral column, and removes waste products from the brain. Excessive accumulation of CSF in the ventricular system during pre- or postnatal development can lead to extensive damage to the brain and expansion of the cranium, a condition termed *hydrocephalus* (see section on hydrocephalus in this chapter).

Postnatal Development

During the last three months of prenatal life and the first two years of postnatal development, the brain changes very rapidly. At birth a baby's brain is one-quarter the weight of its final adult weight of approximately 1,300 to 1,500 grams (Majovski, 1997). By age 2 the brain has achieved three-quarters of its eventual adult weight. In addition, the cortical surface area of the hemispheres doubles, reaching adult dimensions by age 2. During this rapid growth period, significant synaptic and dendritic interconnections form and myelination occurs. Other maturational processes are also evident during this period, including increases in neurotransmitters and related biochemical agents, and changes in electroencephalographic (EEG) wave patterns. Primitive neural reflexes emerge, and subsequently become inhibited, as subcortical and cortical centers integrate.

EMERGENCE OF NEUROPSYCHOLOGICAL FUNCTION

The relationship of brain development and maturation to the emergence of function is very complex and remains poorly understood. However, advances in neuroscience and related disciplines are beginning to unlock the secrets of brain–behavior relationships.

We next discuss three examples of the relationship of brain development and higher-order behavior, specifically, the emergence of language and speech, cognition, and executive functions.

Language and Speech Development

The postnatal functional development of the posterior regions, such as the visual and auditory cortexes, is rapid compared to the emergence of function in the anterior regions. The motor cortex develops slowly between the 3rd and 12th month, and parallels the emergence of basic voluntary motor functions such as reaching, sitting, and walking. The emergence of language is evident in the first to second years of life and coincides with development of the anterior region of the brain.

In a series of postmortem studies of infants and children ranging in age from 3 months to 6 years, Scheibel (1990) investigated the correlation of emerging speech with cortical development of the anterior region. Specifically, Scheibel traced the pattern and nature of dendritic growth of the Broca's regions of the left and right hemispheres, and the orofacial regions of the motor cortexes. The Broca's areas constitute the higher-order speech zones, whereas the orofacial regions (mouth and face) represent the motor, or output zones of language function. The cortical development of the Broca's area and the orofacial regions occurs in a leapfrog trajectory, with each area experiencing periods of both faster and slower development as compared to the other.

At 3 months of age, both the left Broca's area and the corresponding region of the right hemisphere are developing at approximately the same rate, suggesting that there is minimal differential activity in the higher-order speech areas during the first few months of life. During the next 9 months, growth in the speech and orofacial areas of the right hemisphere exceeds that of the left hemisphere. This growth pattern is consistent with the early emergence of nonverbal expressive language (for example, gestures), in contrast with later developing verbal language. It also supports speculation that the right hemisphere is intimately involved in the affective and **prosodic** aspects of communication, that is, the conveyance of meaning through intonation, tempo, pitch, word stress, fluency, and rhythm of speech.

Between the ages of 12 and 15 months, dendritic growth of the left Broca's area exceeds that of the right, although the dendritic systems of the motor areas of both hemispheres continue to exceed those of the higher-order speech zones. The expanded development of the left Broca's area correlates with the onset of spoken language. The rapid dendritic development of the left and right Broca's speech regions continues, with both regions exceeding their respective motor areas by 2 to 3 years of age. The emergence of more complex language parallels this growth spurt. By 6 years of age the dendritic complexity of the left and right Broca's areas has significantly exceeded that of the motor areas, with the left Broca's area surpassing all regions. The left Broca's area now resembles that of the adult, suggesting that speech has lateralized. The preeminence of the left Broca's area correlates with the significant increase in language complexity evident during this period of development.

N e u r o c o g n i t i v e   D e v e l o p m e n t

The development of cognition, or knowing, involves the unfolding of biologically determined brain structures and functions in interaction with environmental forces. The matching of developing cognitive abilities to the emergence of structures and neural networks continues to be a focus of study in neuropsychology. The recent advent of sophisticated neuroimaging and electrophysiological measures has enabled neuroscientists to gain a better understanding of neurocognitive development. For example, Hudspeth and Pribram (1990, 1992) and others (Thatcher, 1991, 1997) have sought to map, via electroencephalographic (EEG) procedures, the maturation of the brain. Further, researchers have made efforts to relate these maturational findings to stages of cognitive development. Hudspeth and Pribram analyzed the QEEG (quantified electroencephalogram) data drawn from 561 normal Swedish subjects (1 to 21 years of age) by Matousek and Petersen (1973). QEEG is the quantitative computer analysis of electroencephalographic data in the assessment of brain functioning. The analysis revealed five distinct, but irregular stages

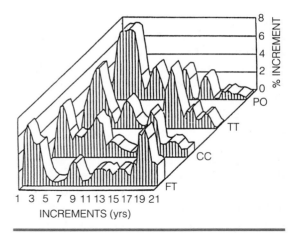

Figure 7.3 Incremental curve for the five stages in QEEG brain maturation. The maturational patterns can be compared to the cognitive stages as suggested by Piagetian theory. PO = parieto-occipital, TT = temporo-temporal, CC = centro-central, FT = fronto-temporal. (From W. J. Hudspeth and K. H. Pribram, "Stages of Brain and Cognitive Maturation," *Journal of Educational Psychology, 4,* 1990, p. 882. Copyright © 1990 by the American Psychological Association. Reprinted with permission)

of brain maturation (see Figure 7.3). Interestingly, the age of peak brain activity at each of the five stages approximates the developmental stages of cognitive maturation as proposed by Jean Piaget (1971). Briefly, Piaget identified four stages of cognitive maturation that he termed the *sensorimotor, preoperational, concrete,* and *formal operation* stages. Neo-Piagetians (such as Kramer, 1983) have proposed a fifth stage labeled *postformal,* or *dialectic,* that begins at approximately 17 years of age and extends into adulthood.

Table 7.2 presents the relationship of emerging cognitive functions to maturational cycles of the brain. The maturation of the cortical regions is characterized by abrupt changes of electrical activity in specific brain regions. Rapid brain maturation is evident across all cortical regions during the Piagetian sensorimotor stage (birth to 2 years of age). The preoperational stage (2 to 7 years of age) is associated with accelerated brain activity in the centro-central, parietal-occipital, and temporo-temporal regions. The concrete operations period (7 to 12 years of age)

Table 7.2   *The Parallel of Piagetian Stages of Cognitive Development and QEEG Maturation Cycles*

Stage 1

Sensorimotor (birth–2 years). The infant changes from being a reflexive responder to being an operator on the environment. Intentional behavior emerges. The understanding of object permanence develops such that "out of sight" is no longer "out of mind."

Maturation Cycle (1–6 years, peak at 2.5 years). Synchronous maturation of centro-central, parieto-occipital, temporo-temporal, and fronto-temporal brain regions.

Stage 2

Preoperational (2–7 years). The child develops the ability to use symbols to represent people, places, objects, and activities that are not present. The child does not understand the concept of conservation (a change in appearance does not necessarily mean that all aspects of an object alter).

Maturation Cycle (6–10.5 years, peak at 7.5 years). Accelerated growth in the centro-central, parieto-occipital, and temporo-temporal regions.

Stage 3

Concrete Operations (7–12 years). The child begins to use symbols to carry out mental activities such as thinking logically. However, the child's ability to think with symbols is limited to the "here and now." Two major achievements of this stage are the development of the abilities to decenter (to focus on two or more dimensions of a task at the same time) and conserve.

Maturation Cycle (10.5–13 years, peak at 12.5 years). Rapid maturation across all cortical regions.

Stage 4

Formal Operations (12+ years). The individual develops the ability to think logically without being bound to the "here and now." Abstract thought, hypothetical-deductive reasoning, and related cognitive operations emerge. The individual can project into the future, consider possibilities, and think differentially.

Maturational Cycle (13–17 years, peak at 15 years). A new period of parieto-occipital and temporo-temporal growth.

Stage 5

Dialectic Operations (18–21 years). The individual can identify contradictions embedded in opposing ideas and integrate these findings to produce new understandings.

Maturation Cycle (17–21 years, peak at 18.5 years). Marked maturational activity in the fronto-temporal regions.

From Papalia, D. E. and Olds, S. W., *Human Development, 6th Ed.*, 1995. Reprinted by permission of the McGraw-Hill Companies.

---

correlates with significant cortical maturation in regions underpinning sensorimotor, visual-spatial, auditory, visual-auditory and executive functions. Subsequently, rapid cortical maturation takes place in the parietal-occipital and temporo-temporal regions during the stage of formal operations (12+ years of age). Finally, the dialectic period (17 to 21 years of age) correlates with increased brain activity in the frontal regions that support executive functions.

Although the temporal periods that Piaget outlined do not precisely match the maturation cycles, the cognitive operations specific to each of the stages are relatively consistent with the maturational patterns of the cortical regions. Further, theorists such as Thatcher (1994) hypothesize that cognitive development proceeds in spurts, rather than in a smooth and continuous unfolding of abilities. The finding of distinct advances in underlying maturation cycles of the brain supports this position.

Development of Executive Functions

For over a century, controversy, confusion, and speculation have existed over the function(s) of the frontal lobes. Speculations have included conceptualizations of the frontal lobes as structures that are silent (having limited function), support a singular or global function (abstract thinking), or maintain a multitude of heterogenous behaviors (impulse control, judgment, creativity, personality, and moral judgment). Fortunately, a consensus is emerging on the role of the frontal lobes as serving supervisory or control functions. These are labeled **executive functions,** because higher-order regulatory and integrative processes

Neuropsychology in Action 7.1

Executive Function Tasks

by William C. Culbertson

Diamond (1991) adapted a number of tasks that Jean Piaget initially employed in studying cognitive development to investigate executive functions. In her study of infants, Diamond endeavored to relate the development of executive functions to the maturation of the underlying frontal circuitry.

Contiguous Object Task

The contiguous object task involves the use of a transparent box, open at the top (see Figure 7.4). The experimenter places a toy block behind the wall of the box and prompts the infant to pick up the toy block. Infants of 7 months can reach the block behind the wall if a single straight movement is required (frame A). However, if the placement of the block necessitates a two-directional reach (two sequential movements), the infant cannot accomplish these movements until approximately 10 months (frame B). Also, prior to 10 months, the infant cannot inhibit the reflexive grasping of the edge of the box when his or her hand comes in contact with it.

Hidden Object

Piaget noted that the infant 5 to 7 months of age would not reach or search for an object hidden from view, that is, "out of sight, out of mind." The hidden object task involves showing the infant a toy, and then covering it with a blanket or placing a screen in front of it to block the child's view (see Figure 7.5). Diamond's research suggests that the infant of 5 to 7 months does, in fact, realize that the object is hidden, but cannot demonstrate this knowledge by executing a motor response. That is, the infant is unable to organize and execute a means–end action sequence such as removing the blanket from the hidden object. However, by 7½ to 8 months, the infant is capable of executing the necessary action sequence.

A not B (Delayed Response Task)

The A not B task involves placing two "wells" in front of the infant (see Figure 7.6) in which a toy can be hidden. The infant observes the researcher hide a toy in one of the wells, and then after a short period (2 to 5 seconds) is allowed to reach for the toy. Then the researchers hides the toy in the opposite well, and after a delay again allows the infant to reach for the toy. An infant younger than 8 months will reach for the well that contained the previously retrieved toy, even though he or she has seen the researcher place the toy in the opposite well.

In Figure 7.6, the infant has already successfully retrieved the toy from the well to the viewer's right. The researcher then placed the toy in the opposite well. In the first two frames (top left and right), the infant is looking at the well containing the toy. However, when allowed to reach for the toy, the infant uncovers the well that contained the toy on the previous trial (bottom left and right). Success on this task requires the emergence of working memory capability and the ability to inhibit a previously reinforced response.

Detour Reaching Task

In the detour reaching task, the experimenter requires the infant to detour around a barrier in order to reach and retrieve an object. The task involves a small transparent box that the experimenter places in front of the infant with one of its sides open (see Figure 7.7). If they can see the toy through an open side, infants 6½ to 7 months of age will reach in to retrieve a toy. However, if the

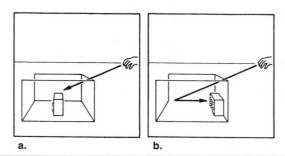

a.   b.

Figure 7.4   Contiguous object task. (a) Single, straight-line reach for the block. (b) Two-directional reach movement for the block. (From A. Diamond and J. Gilbert, "Development as Progressive Inhibitory Control of Action: Retrieval of a Contiguous Object," *Cognitive Development, 12,* 1989, pp. 223–249. Presented by A. Diamond, "Neuropsychological Insights into the Meaning of Object Concept Development," in S. Carey and R. Gelman, eds., *The Epigenesis of Mind: Essays on Biology and Cognition,* Hillsdale, NJ: Erlbaum, 1991, p. 72, Figure 3.2)

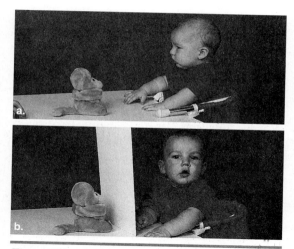

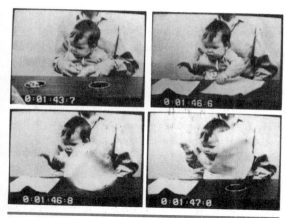

Figure 7.5   Hidden object task. (a) The infant is gazing at a toy. (b) The toy is shielded by a screen, and the infant does not search or reach for the object. (Courtesy of Rutgers University)

Figure 7.6   A not B task. In the top frame, the infant is gazing at the toy in the well. In the following frames, the infant continues to gaze at the well holding the toy, yet lifts the cover from the well that contained the toy on the previous trial. (From A. Diamond, "Neuropsychological Insights into the Meaning of Object Concept Development," in S. Carey and R. Gelman, eds., *The Epigenesis of Mind: Essays on Biology and Cognition,* Mahwah, NJ: Lawrence Erlbaum Associates, Inc., 1991, p. 86, Figure 3.4)

experimenter places the toy directly in the child's view, but behind a closed side, the infant repeatedly and unsuccessfully tries to reach through the closed side. The infant is unable to inhibit reaching straight for the toy. Also, the infant is unable to raise the box with one hand and reach, at the same time, with the other hand. In Figure 7.7, the child has lifted the box and is establishing a direct line of sight to the toy. As one hand moves down to reach into the box (second frame), the other hand holding the box also moves down. At this point (third frame) the toy is in the child's direct line of sight through the top of the box. The child withdraws her hand from the opening and tries, unsuccessfully, to reach for the toy through the closed top of the box. Between 8 and 12 months, the child develops the ability to look through one side of the box while reaching though another side. Similarly, the child can raise the box with one hand, while simultaneously reaching in with the other.

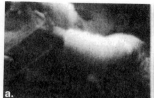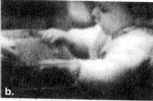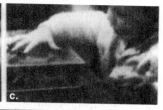

Figure 7.7   Detour reaching task. (a) The child has lifted the box and is looking in at a toy. (b) As the child begins to reach for the toy, the box lowers. The toy is now in the child's line of sight through the top of the box. (c) The child removes the hand from the box, and tries to reach for the toy through the top of the box. (From A. Diamond, "Retrieval of an Object from an Open Box: The Development of Visual-Tactile Control of Reaching in the First Year of Life," *Society for Research in Child Development Abstracts, 3,* 1981, p. 78. As presented in "Neuropsychological Insights into the Meaning of Object Concept Development," in S. Carey and R. Gelman, eds., *The Epigenesis of Mind: Essays on Biology and Cognition,* Mahwah, NJ: Lawrence Erlbaum Associates, Inc., 1991, p. 90, Figure 3.5)

are involved (Samango-Sprouse, 1999). Although disparities exist with regard to the specific cognitive and related operations that fall under the umbrella of executive functions, a common core is discernible. Included in this grouping are planning, mental flexibility, attentional allocation, **working memory,** and **inhibitory control.** Disruption of executive functions results in significant cognitive, emotional, and social impairment. An example of the pervasive effects of executive function disruption is detailed later in this chapter (see Neuropsychology in Action 7.2).

The maturation of executive functions is crucial to psychological adaptation and adjustment across the life span (Eslinger, Biddle, & Grattan, 1997). Unfortunately, understanding of the development of executive functions lags behind that of the maturation of other cortical functions such as intelligence. The lag relates, in part, to the belief in early neuropsychology that prefrontal functions did not emerge until late childhood or early adolescence. This belief delayed the initiation of active study and research of childhood executive functions until relatively recently. Emerging empirical studies (Levin et al., 1991; Welsh, Pennington, & Groisser, 1991) suggest that basic executive functions develop early in life and follow a protracted, multistep trajectory to maturity in adulthood. The early appearance of rudimentary executive functions and the later development of more complex functions, such as abstract reasoning and judgment, parallel the lengthy development of the prefrontal cortex. Interestingly, the emergence of rudimentary executive functions correlates with the periods of maximum synaptic density of the frontal lobes. However, more complex functions continue to evolve long after maximum synaptic density is reached, and reflect a host of other developmental advances such as synaptic pruning and sculpting, axonal myelination, and neurochemical and neurophysiological changes.

Important advances in understanding the development of executive functions are due to the remarkable investigations of Goldman-Rakic (1987) and Diamond (1991). Goldman-Rakic studied the relationship of prefrontal development to the emergence of the cognitive operation of **object permanence,** that is, the capacity to store in memory a representation of an object, for the purpose of guiding future behavior, that is removed from view. Using a delayed response task (see Neuropsychology in Action 7.1), the experimenter required rhesus monkeys to maintain in memory the spatial location or features of an object over delays ranging from zero to 10 seconds. By the age of 2 to 4 months, the rhesus monkeys could perform the memory tasks at delay intervals of 2 to 5 seconds. During this 2- to 4-month period, researchers observed maximum synaptic density in the prefrontal lobes of the rhesus monkeys. The corresponding period of synaptic density in the human infant occurs between 8 and 24 months (Huttenlocher, 1990). The latter time interval also correlates with the infant's ability to perform a delayed response task (see Neuropsychology in Action 7.1), suggesting that the executive function of working memory has emerged.

Diamond (1991) carried out a series of infant studies that have helped clarify the development of executive inhibitory control and other functions as they relate to the maturation of the frontal cortex. She presented infants from 5 to 12 months of age with tasks involving detour reaching, contiguous objects, hidden objects, and delayed response ("A not B") to determine the emergence of frontal functions (see Neuropsychology in Action 7.1). Her findings revealed that the ability to inhibit reflexive reactions to contact (elicitation of the grasp reflex when touching an object) and to combine two or more actions into a behavioral sequence, develops between the 5th and 8th months. These two functions are contingent on the maturation of the supplementary motor cortex (SMC) of the frontal lobes.

Between 8 and 12 months, the baby develops the ability to inhibit a response that is primed for release, and to relate information over time delays and spatial separation. The baby's successful performance of the delayed response task ("A not B") and the detour reaching task, respectively, reflects the development of the ability to relate information across time and space. The performance of these tasks requires inhibitory control and working memory capabilities, functions that the dorsolateral prefrontal cortex supports (Goldman-Rakic, 1987). Finally, the ability of the infant to simultaneously coordinate two different movements appears between 8 and 12 months of age. That is, the infant can execute an action with one hand while simultaneously carrying out a different action with the other. These hand movements require both coordination and inhibition of movements. That is, the action of each hand must coordinate with the other, but each is inhibited from performing the same movement as the other. This complex set of actions requires the maturation of the corpus callosum that joins the SMC areas of each hemisphere. The interhemispheric communication of the SMC regions is necessary for coordinating bilateral actions.

Other researchers have also made notable contributions to the identification of emerging childhood executive functions (Denckla, 1996; Levin et al., 1991; Pennington, 1997b). For example, Welsh and coworkers (1991) traced the development of executive functions in normal children, ages 3 to 12, and young adults. The investigators determined that subjects achieved adultlike performance at three different age levels, 6 and 10 years of age, and during adolescence. Simple functions such as visual search (searching an array of stimuli for targets) emerge early, followed by more complex inhibitory skills and, finally, the most advanced abilities as demonstrated in complex planning.

Similarly, Culbertson and Zillmer (2000, 1998a, 1998b) used the Tower of London-Drexel (TOL^{DX}) test to assess age-related changes in the executive planning of normal children and children with an attention-deficit/hyperactivity disorder (ADHD). Executive planning, as assessed by the TOL^{DX}, involves the development of a "mental template" to guide the sequential movement of colored beads across three pegs to match a pattern presented on the examiner's model (see Figure 7.8). The examiner asks the child to replicate a series of bead patterns of increasing difficulty while adhering to specific problem-solving rules. The goal is to solve each pattern in a minimum number of moves without violating the rules. Children who fail to plan, or plan superficially, require additional moves to reproduce the target patterns.

Culbertson and Zillmer selected ADHD children for study in an effort to determine whether deficits in executive planning were associated with the disorder (see Chapter 8 for a discussion of ADHD). The researchers hypothesized that the ADHD children would perform less efficiently on the TOL^{DX}. Figure

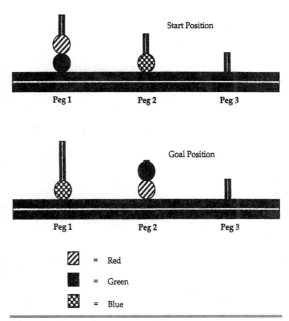

Figure 7.8 Tower of London^{DX}: Start and goal positions. (From W. C. Culbertson and E. A. Zillmer, "The Tower of London. A Standardized Approach to Assessing Executive Functioning in Children," *Archives of Clinical Neuropsychology, 13,* 1998, p. 289. Copyright © 2000 Elsevier Science, Ltd. Reprinted with permission of the authors and the publisher)

7.9 shows the TOL^{DX} total move scores of the two groups of children. Noteworthy is the steady improvement in executive planning from 7 to 12 years of age, with the normal and ADHD children showing a parallel trajectory. However, the children with ADHD, as predicted, performed in a significantly less efficient manner than the normal children. The poorer TOL^{DX} performance of ADHD children is consistent with emerging research (Pennington, 1997b) suggesting that the disorder is developmental in origin and potentially a consequence of impaired executive functions. Further analysis of the children's TOL^{DX} performance revealed that the younger children, both normal and those with ADHD, (1) spent less time planning before attempting to solve the bead patterns, (2) solved fewer bead patterns in a minimum number of moves, and (3) violated a greater number of problem-solving rules than the older normal and

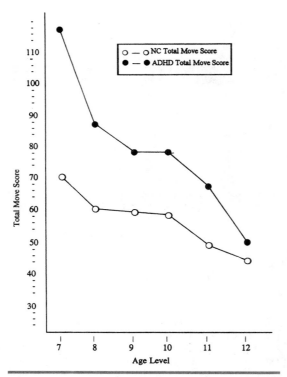

Figure 7.9   Mean TOL^{DX} total move score by age level for attention-deficit/hyperactivity disorder (ADHD) and normal control (NC) children. (From W. C. Culbertson and E. A. Zillmer, "The Tower of London. A Standardized Approach to Assessing Executive Functioning in Children," *Archives of Clinical Neuropsychology, 13,* 1998, p. 291. Copyright © 2000 Elsevier Science, Ltd. Reprinted with permission of the authors and the publisher)

ADHD children. Clearly, the maturation of executive planning involves the advance of a number of component cognitive skills.

Research has also focused on the relationship between the development of emotional regulation and maturation of the frontal region. Bell and Fox (1994) found that changes in EEG activation associated with emotional expression appear early in infant development. When a stranger approached, 10-month-old infants exhibited right frontal EEG activation, but the opposite pattern was evident when the mother approached—that is, greater left frontal activation. Similarly, infants who appeared sad or distressed, as assessed by facial expressions, showed greater right

frontal activation, whereas those expressing joy demonstrated greater left frontal activation. Of importance was the finding that comparable frontal EEG activation patterns continue to be evident in childhood and adulthood (Davidson, 1994).

Case studies of children who sustained damage to the frontal cortex provide further insight into frontal lobe development and the regulation of emotional and social behavior. In a review of cases with varying ages of lesion onset (ranging from prenatal to age 16), Eslinger et al. (1997) found that the children demonstrated impairments in emotional regulation and interpersonal relations, regardless of the age at which the damage occurred. Both immediate and delayed deficits were observed, suggesting that the development of socioemotional regulatory control was ongoing. The progressive emergence of delayed deficits indicated that the damaged frontal system could not negotiate the increasing cognitive, social, and emotional demands of adolescence and adulthood. For example, a boy who suffered damage to his right frontal lobe at age 3 appeared to recover fully, although the mother did note alterations in his personality following the insult. During his early school years he demonstrated problems in visual-spatial performance, attentional focus, impulse control, and establishing friendships. By adolescence he exhibited limited facial expressions and modulation of voice, interrupted the conversation of others, had not developed friendships or dated, and often failed to understand the gist of intended communications. His social deficits reflected an inability to empathize or reciprocate emotionally with others, to understand social cues and the pragmatics of language, and to accurately evaluate his own social strengths and weaknesses.

VULNERABILITY AND PLASTICITY OF THE DEVELOPING BRAIN

The brain may fail to develop structurally and functionally as a consequence of genetic anomalies and environmental insults. With regard to the former, brain disorders, such as **phenylketonuria (PKU),** a genetic metabolic disorder, can be inherited or result from alterations of cellular material, as evident in Turner's syndrome. Environmental causes relate to damaging agents (such as alcohol) that preclude, alter, or halt natural brain development. The degree to which a brain can recover from damage is complex, and not fully understood. Neuroscientists do know, however, that the plasticity of the brain allows recovery of function under certain conditions.

Teratogens are agents that, if introduced or present during certain periods of prenatal development, can produce central nervous system defects. The defects can include **agenesis,** the failure of an organ to develop, or **dysgenesis,** the abnormal development of an organ. Further, the damaging effects of the teratogens can be focal or diffuse and can result in minimal to complete loss of function. Examples of potential teratogens are general diseases (such as rubella, influenza, and mumps), sexually transmitted diseases (such as syphilis, AIDS, and genital herpes), drugs (such as alcohol, barbiturates, and vaccines), environmental toxins (such as mercury, carbon monoxide, lead, and PCBs), and radiation (such as from x rays and exposure to radioactive materials).

The precise impact of the teratogen on the unborn fetus varies with the nature of the insult and its proximity to a particular period of rapid brain growth, the genetic makeup of the child/mother, the quality of the intrauterine environment, and the "dosage" and extent of exposure (Spreen et al., 1995). The prenatal brain appears most vulnerable to structural damage during the 3rd through 8th weeks of development, a period that correlates with the rapid proliferation and migration of cells. However, the brain continues to be vulnerable to damage throughout the prenatal period (see Figure 7.10 on p. 242).

Dangers to the developing brain are not limited to prenatal teratogens. Potential dangers also threaten the perinatal process of birth, including anoxia, medications introduced during labor and delivery, and mechanical injury to the skull and brain caused by trauma during delivery. Mechanical injury can lead to intracranial hemorrhage and tissue damage (Spreen et al., 1995). Babies of low birth weight are at particular risk for central nervous system damage. Further, a wide range of potential dangers threaten postnatal development. Traumatic head injury, toxins, radiation, malnutrition, tumors, infections, and stroke can all cause significant injury to the developing brain.

Yet there is a resilience to the damaged brain, related in part to protective factors such as a responsive, nurturing, and stimulating postnatal environment.

The term *plasticity* refers to enduring changes in neural activity that accompany learning or the recovery of behavioral functioning after brain injury or disease (Frackowiak, 1996). Neuroscientists hypothesize that the brain's plasticity is greatest during developmental periods when synaptic density is highest, that is, when excessive numbers of synapses exist, many of which have not committed to function. These periods of maximum synaptic density differ across cortical regions due to differential rates of neuromaturation. Thus, the window of plasticity for the visual cortex is smaller than for the prefrontal cortex. In the former case, synaptic density extends until 5 years of age, whereas in the latter case maximum density extends into late childhood (Huttenlocher & Dabholkar, 1997).

Initially, neuroscientists believed that the likelihood of recovery from a brain insult was greater if the injury was incurred early, rather than late in development. They later named this principle the **Kennard principle,** in honor of its originator, Margaret Kennard (Kolb, 1995). The Kennard Principle suggested that the immature brain was more plastic than the mature brain. Although some forms of insults do seem to follow this principle, the opposite effect is generally evident. That is, the earlier the damage, the more pervasive and disruptive the impact on developing functions. Early damage may initially appear to have minimal effect if the cognitive or behavioral functions that the damaged region subserves do not emerge until a later point in development. As this point is reached, significant functional impairment surfaces. For example, early damage to the auditory cortex may adversely affect later language development.

The effect that a lesion has on the developing brain varies with regard to the age of insult. Lesions occurring before age 1, including prenatal development, typically correlate with more global and lasting impairment than later injuries. Some degree of neural reorganization and sparing of function is possible with lesions occurring between 1 and 5 years of age, depending on the nature, severity, and region of damage. During this period most cortical regions

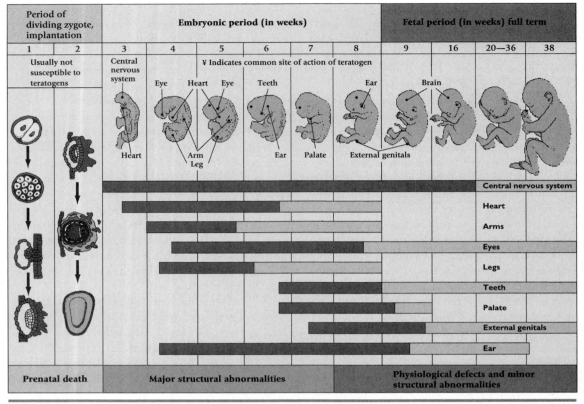

Period of dividing zygote, implantation		Embryonic period (in weeks)						Fetal period (in weeks) full term			
1	2	3	4	5	6	7	8	9	16	20—36	38

¥ Indicates common site of action of teratogen

Figure 7.10   Teratogens and prenatal vulnerability of developing human systems. (From K. L. Moore and T. V. N. Persaud, *Before We Are Born: Essentials of Embryology and Birth Defects,* 4th ed., Philadelphia: W. B. Saunders Co., 1993, p. 130, with permission)

reach maximum synaptic-dendritic density. Finally, injuries after age 5 generally predict minimal recovery of function (Kolb & Whishaw, 1996). Thus, there appears to be a "window" for optimum recovery extending from the toddler through the preschool years.

Child and Adult Brain: Structural and Functional Differences

Neuroscientists are learning more and more about the maturation of the central nervous system. An important realization is that the child's brain differs in many significant ways from the adult brain. We discuss several of these differences here to clarify this basic, though often forgotten, principle of the relationship between brain and behavior.

The adult brain is anatomically, physiologically, and functionally mature, whereas that of the child is still developing. Accordingly, the effects of lesions to the immature and mature brain differ significantly. In the former case, injuries disrupt the acquisition of developmental abilities; in the latter case, previously acquired abilities break down (Eslinger et al., 1997). With the achievement of brain maturity comes greater stability and predictability of behavior. In comparison, the cognitive and behavioral functions of the developing brain can vary dramatically. This variability depends on the current developmental stage and on the nature and quality of the child's social-psychological-physical environment.

With lesions of the mature brain, assessing the degree of functional loss and potential for recovery often involves examining the adult's premorbid history. Young children have an obviously abbreviated history from which to draw variables necessary for prediction. Likewise, the young child has not developed a host of higher-order functions such as reading and writing, thus severely hindering efforts to determine which functions are spared or compromised, both in the present and in the future (Spreen et al., 1995).

Many pathological signs of adulthood brain injury are developmentally appropriate if the developing child exhibits them (Bernstein & Waber, 1997). For example, the primitive neural reflexes of the infant are obviously normal, but in adulthood they are signs of frontal lobe or related neural damage. Likewise, early childhood damage to one cortical region may impact the development of other brain regions— a phenomenon not observed with adult injury. For example, Eslinger and coworkers (1997) reported that childhood lesions to the left prefrontal cortex can disrupt development of the right prefrontal regions, an effect these researchers did not observe with comparable damage to the mature brain.

The immature cortex is diffuse in organization, with increasing specification of structure and function emerging with development. Progressive differentiation of cognitive and other functions correlates with the brain's organizational development. Accordingly, injury to the diffusely organized brain tends to have a global impact across brain regions with greater disturbance of function than later occurring lesions. Focal lesions to the differentially developed adult brain more often correlate with relatively specific and circumscribed deficits.

One of the most striking examples of how the child's brain contrasts with that of the adult's is the differing response to lesions in the language areas of the left hemisphere. Young children who experience such injury rarely show aphasia in later life (Kolb, 1995). But adults subjected to similar lesions show a high prevalence of aphasic disorders. Investigators attribute the difference to the brain's plasticity, as language often reorganizes or transfers to the opposite

hemisphere. Unfortunately, the transfer of language has a cost, because many of the children showed visual-spatial deficits and significant drops in intellectual performance. Researchers believe that the functional losses relate to a crowding effect. That is, language "crowds" into the neural space of the right hemisphere at the expense of other functions.

The impact of adult injury is generally apparent soon after the lesion occurs, whereas the effects of injury to the immature brain are less straightforward. Studies of primates suggest that early lesions to the prefrontal and temporal cortexes can produce both immediate and delayed presentation of impairments. Goldman-Rakic (1987) conducted a series of studies to investigate the effects of damage to the prefrontal cortex. Lesions in the prefrontal dorsolateral region of the brain of mature monkeys impaired performance on a delayed response task (see Neuropsychology in Action 7.1), whereas infant monkeys with comparable lesions did not show immediate impairment. However, as the infant monkeys matured, a significant deficit emerged in delayed response performance. In contrast, lesions of the prefrontal orbital cortex produced delayed response deficits regardless of age at injury. Thus age and region of prefrontal cortex damage interacted to determine immediate or delayed impairment.

Similarly, case studies of children (Eslinger et al., 1997) with early prefrontal damage suggest that immediate and delayed impairments of cognitive and socioemotional executive functions can result. The emerging deficits in adolescence appear most prominent in the development and regulation of socioemotional behaviors such as social awareness, interpersonal sensitivity, perspective taking, friendship skills, and close emotional relationships. These emerging deficits appear more disruptive to adjustment than similar deficits occurring in adulthood. The relationships of immediate and late appearing deficits to age, affected hemisphere, specific cortical region of damage, and other mediating variables remain unclear and warrants further study.

Information on the anatomic and functional development of the brain, its vulnerability and plasticity, and its difference from the adult brain serves as a basic framework for understanding the neuropsychological assessment of childhood disorders. Jane Bernstein

Neuropsychology in Action 7.2

Principles of Assessment in Pediatric Neuropsychology

by *Jane Holmes Bernstein* Ph.D., Director, Neuropsychology Program, Children's Hospital, Boston/Harvard Medical School.

Case Presentation

I was asked to assess T.A., a 17-year-old right-handed girl who was having academic difficulties at the 11th-grade level. In reporting her difficulties, T.A. focused on specific skills: Math was a major problem, and she read very slowly and had to reread constantly for comprehension.

T.A.'s history revealed unremarkable development until she was about 3½ and diagnosed with acute lymphocytic leukemia (ALL). The illness was treated with chemotherapy and cranial irradiation over a 2-year period. Currently T.A. has a half-time job, talents in dancing and teaching dance to young children, and friends at school (with whom, however, she did not socialize elsewhere).

A review of neurobehavioral systems found that T.A. had generally intact attention, behavioral modulation and self-regulation, interpersonal skills, memory abilities, communicative skills, vocabulary use, linguistic units, speech and voice parameters, spatial processing, and motor capacities. Her overall cognitive abilities lay at the low end of

the average range. Her comprehension was insecure because of slowed information processing. To ensure comprehension, she frequently needed people to modify (slow, repeat, or rephrase) speech directed to her. Her goal-oriented problem-solving (executive) skills were variable: T.A. had difficulty with mental flexibility and often failed to "clear the display," carrying over information from one task to the next. She failed to initiate behavior independently; however, with cueing, her planning, organizing, and monitoring skills were adequate.

Overall, T.A. had interpersonal skills and was socially perceptive. She did well on tasks that were structured, tapped her knowledge of social information, allowed hands-on problem solving, and did not require speedy responses. She had difficulty with tasks that taxed her limited verbal knowledge base, involved abstract verbal concepts, had to be completed under time constraints, or depended on processing multiple elements or using multiple processes, more or less concurrently. Although the assessment focused

on T.A.'s academic adjustment, emotional issues proved to be of serious concern. Her mother reported that T.A. tended to argue, cry, eat poorly, and feel she had to be perfect. Personality measures elicited themes of distress, including loneliness, sadness, anger, and the inability to initiate actions on her own behalf. However, T.A. also had a strong sense of herself as an individual, well-developed values, hopefulness about the future, and emotional strength. She derived great satisfaction and feelings of self-worth from her talents in dance and her dance work with children.

The diagnostic formulation highlighted a neurobehavioral disorder that manifested in slow processing of information and executive control processes, and in emotional distress and erosion of self-esteem. The management plan included educating T.A. about the nature of her difficulties and developing interventions that would address her processing and executive issues as they applied to high school curriculum demands and real-life situations.

---

presents a case study of a pediatric neuropsychological evaluation (see Neuropsychology in Action 7.2) that elucidates many neuropsychological principles discussed in this chapter.

 ## Specific Developmental Disorders

In this section we review several groups of developmental disorders that frequently come to the

attention of neuropsychologists. These include abnormalities of anatomic development, genetic and chromosomal disorders, and acquired cerebral insults and diseases. We discuss a sample disorder from each of these groups to acquaint the student with the clinical presentation, neuropsychological pathogenesis, and treatment of the disorder. The first disorder, hydrocephalus, frequently co-occurs with many other disorders of anatomic malformation. Next, Turner's syndrome is one of the most commonly seen chromosomal disorders. Finally, fetal alcohol syndrome is

Commentary

A neuropsychological analysis involves examining the possible role of brain variables in behavioral functioning. In adults, brain–behavior relationships are well established and relatively stable. In children, the relationship between brain and behavior changes dynamically. Thus clinical analysis of a child's behavioral repertoire must include a review of the child's developmental course to date. A brain does not operate in isolation, however; it and the behavior it supports are built and maintained by experience. Thus, at any point the impact of environmental or contextual variables must be evaluated.

T.A.'s early childhood disorder is crucial to her diagnosis and management. Radiation treatment has a toxic effect on brain structures, especially the white matter connections that route information around the brain. Thus it is likely to undermine the speed and efficiency of information processing (rather than to disrupt reasoning skills), and to result in behavioral "late effects" that center on problems in processing information (Waber & Tarbell, 1997).

Life-threatening disease is likely to change one's value system. This is not necessarily negative in itself, but at particular stages in life, notably adolescence, it may lead to detachment from peers, who may be involved in social explorations that do not seem important. This was the case for T.A., and her isolation and loneliness compounded the impact of her academic struggles.

Context interacts with development throughout childhood: One cannot be evaluated without reference to the other. In a developing child, perturbations in brain or experience at any point becomes part of the developmental course thereafter (Segalowitz & Hiscock, 1992). Atypical processing of information was thus an intrinsic part of T.A.'s thinking: All her skills had developed around this anomaly. More than 10 years after her disease was successfully treated, it affected both school performance and life adjustment.

At the high school level, environmental demands on T.A. were discrepant with her capacities. People with information-processing problems depend more on structure in the environment than do others of the same age, and also are more at risk for information overload. This can negatively affect other cognitive skills. High school demands increasing independence on the part of students, and does not provide the support and structure of earlier grades. Students may cope well enough until they suddenly fail under the pressure of high school demands. The interaction of developmental and contextual factors (Rudel, 1981) easily leads observers to assume that the problem is psychological or motivational, rather than a biologically based late effect of early neurologic disruption.

Summary

This case highlights the range of expertise required of a pediatric neuropsychologist: knowledge of (1) normal and atypical psychological, neurological, and neuropsychological development, (2) the effects of medical, behavioral, and psychiatric childhood disorders on behavioral functioning, and (3) measurement methodology, including investigative design and the construction and administration of psychological tests. The clinician's particular expertise is in drawing on this knowledge base to understand the experience of the individual child and family and to create an integrated "portrait" (Matarazzo, 1990). An accurate portrait will result in interventions that promote the child's adjustment and progress. The task is frequently challenging, sometimes humbling, but almost always rewarding and can make a real difference to the well-being of children and their families.

---

a relatively common and destructive disorder. Of the three developmental disorders, fetal alcohol syndrome is completely preventable.

ABNORMALITIES OF ANATOMIC DEVELOPMENT

A vast number of conditions exist that reflect anomalies of neurodevelopment. Hynd and Willis (1988) divide these disorders into five groups, presented in Table 7.3. Each category reflects a malformation of brain tissue with concurrent disruption of function. Several of these are incompatible with life (for example, anencephaly and hydranencephaly), whereas others do not necessarily compromise the child's survival, but do significantly impair or alter neuropsychological functioning. In many cases a given disorder may have multiple etiologies; in others, the pathogenesis is quite specific. However, the origin of most of the disorders is undetermined.

The extensiveness and severity of damage to the developing brain tends to reduce life expectancy of

Table 7.3   *Anatomic Disorders*

Malformation	Description	Clinical Manifestations
Abnormalities of bulk growth		
Micrencephaly	Subnormal brain size associated with abnormally small head (<2 SD below mean for age and gender)	Size of face near normal; folded scalp, possible epilepsy, and most typically intellectual retardation
Megalencephaly	Abnormally large brain from overproduction of cerebral parenchyma. Males > females	Associated with mental subnormality, normality, or (hypothetically) giftedness. Epilepsy may occur
Dysplasias of cerebral hemispheres		
Holoprosencephaly	Two hemispheres fail to develop. A large fluid-filled cavity results. No interhemispheric fissure present. 1:13,000 live births	Faciocerebral dysplasias, cebocephaly, apnea spells, severe mental retardation, hypotelorism, and other systemic deformities. Usually incompatible with life.
Agenesis of the corpus callosum	Complete or partial failure of the corpus callosum to develop. Males > females	Occasionally asymptomatic or found in association with spina bifida, facial and ocular deformities, micrencephaly, and hydrocephalus. Epilepsy and mental retardation may occur
Malformations of the cerebral cortex		
Agyria/pachygyria	Smooth lissencephalic surface of brain. Few coarse gyri may be present	Commonly found in association with agenesis of corpus callosum, micrencephaly, epilepsy, severe mental retardation, and early death
Polymicrogyria	Development of many small gyri. Microscopically, they may form an overlapping folded cortex	Found in association with learning disabilities (dyslexia), severe mental retardation, and epilepsy. Also appear asymptomatically
Focal dysplasia	Focal abnormalities in the cortical architecture usually consisting of disordered cells and layering of cortex	Reported in cases of epilepsy and learning disabilities (dyslexia)
Malformations associated with congenital hydrocephalus		
Dandy-Walker malformation	Malformation of the cerebellum associated with a dilation of the fourth ventricle. Males > females	Hydrocephalus, agenesis of the corpus callosum, Klippel-Feil and DeLange syndromes, and severe psychomotor retardation

children with anatomic brain malformations. Surviving children show a high rate of mental retardation, speech and language delays, learning disabilities, motor impairments, physical anomalies, and epilepsy. Children with severe and global neuropsychological deficits often require lifelong supervision and assistance. We turn first to a relatively frequent anomaly of the brain that can result in minimal to severe neuropsychological deficits.

Hydrocephalus

Clinical Presentation and Prevalence   Hydrocephalus (HC) can occur during any developmental period and seriously damages the developing brain, disrupting both subcortical and cortical functions. This condition results from an excessive accumulation of cerebrospinal fluid (CSF) in the brain's ventricles (see Figure 7.11 on p. 248). The increased volume of CSF produces a concomitant increase in intracranial pressure and expan-

Malformation	Description	Clinical Manifestations
Malformations associated with congenital hydrocephalus *(continued)*		
Arnold-Chiari malformation	Congenital deformation of the brain stem and cerebellum	Congenital hydrocephalus, spina bifida, and severe psychomotor retardation
Stenosis of the aqueduct of Sylvius	Obstruction of the aqueduct and CSF circulation	Often insidious onset of symptoms associated with hydrocephalus. Shunted children may suffer learning/behavioral problems. Nonverbal IQ < verbal IQ
Abnormalities of the neural tube and fusion defects		
Spina bifida occulta	Usually asymptomatic lesion discovered incidentally	Can be associated with lipoma, dermal sinuses, and dimples
Spina bifida cystica	Spinal defect that includes a cyst-like sac which may or may not contain the spinal cord	Hydrocephalus a frequent complication. Cognitive deficits related to extent of hydrocephalus. Arnold-Chiari malformation not uncommon
Cranium bifidum and encephalocele	Fusion defects of skull referred to as *cranium bifidum;* myelomeningoceles or meningoceles on the skull are referred to as *encephaloceles.* Males < females	Many associated difficulties with hydrocephalus including ataxia, cerebral palsy, epilepsy, and mental retardation
Anencephaly	Vault of skull absent and brain represented by vascular mass. Face is grossly normal. 1 male: 4 female	Condition incompatible with life
Hydranencephaly	Cerebral hemispheres replaced by cystic sacs containing CSF	Difficult initially to distinguish from hydrocephalus. Hypnoatremia, eye movement disturbances, and death
Porencephaly	Large cystic lesion develops on the brain. May occur bilaterally or unilaterally	Occasionally asymptomatic but typically associated with mental retardation, epilepsy, and other neurodevelopmental malformations

Source: Modified and updated from Hynd and Willis (1998), p. 45. Adapted with permission of Plenum Publishing Corporation from *Handbook of Clinical Child Neuropsychology, 2nd Ed.*

sion of the ventricles. As the ventricles expand, cerebral tissue is compromised and the cranium distorts. If untreated, the child may die or suffer severe mental retardation. The actual incidence of HC is unknown because it is frequently associated with other congenital disorders. However, it is estimated that 27 per 100,000 newborns suffer from the condition (Kolb & Whishaw, 1996). The prevalence of HC of mixed etiologies appears greater for boys (62%) than girls.

Neuropathogenesis HC is a disorder that occurs secondary to other pathological events or processes. This pathogenesis can be either prenatal, perinatal or postnatal in origin. Congenital (prenatal) disorders such as spina bifida, Dandy-Walker malformation, Arnold-Chiari malformation, and stenosis of the aqueduct of Sylvius often result in HC (see Table 7.3). In contrast, the most common cause of perinatal and postnatal HC is **intraventricular hemorrhage (IVH)**

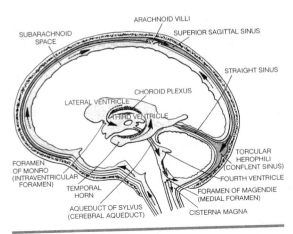

Figure 7.11   Ventricles of the human brain. (From S. Gilman and S. W. Newman, "The Cerebrospinal Fluid," in Manter and Katz, *Essentials of Clinical Neuroanatomy and Neuropsychology*, 9th ed., Philadelphia: F. A. Davis, 1996, p. 260. Reprinted by permission of F. A. Davis Co.)

that occurs in premature infants (see discussion later). Other etiologies of HC, both prenatal and postnatal, include infections (meningitis and encephalitis), vascular abnormalities, tumors, cysts, and other disease processes (Fletcher et al., 1996).

Physiological Dynamics of Hydrocephalus   Any one of three underlying causes can produce an abnormal increase in the volume of ventricular CNS. These causative factors include oversecretion of CSF, obstruction of CSF passages, and impaired absorption of CSF (Rowland, Fink, & Rubin, 1991). Oversecretion of CSF is rare, and generally a consequence of a secreting tumor of the choroid plexus, the primary producer of CSF in the lateral ventricles.

The second cause of HC occurs within the ventricular system and involves obstruction of the CSF pathways as a result of congenital malformation, tumors, or scarring. HC of this etiology is termed **obstructive** or **noncommunicating** (Brookshire et al., 1995). The aqueduct of Sylvius, also called the cerebral aqueduct of the third ventricle, is the most commonly obstructed ventricular pathway, because of its long, narrow structure. Conditions obstructing the aqueduct of Sylvius include (1) congenital nar-

rowing (stenosis) of the aqueduct, (2) a thin membrane lying on the aqueduct, (3) constriction of the aqueduct by pressure from an adjoining tumor, and (4) herniation of the cerebellum and displacement of the fourth ventricle, as in Arnold-Chiari malformation (Hynd et al., 1997). However, the pathogenesis of obstructive or noncommunicating HC may be idiopathic (unknown), and research findings suggest that different familial forms may exist (Hynd & Willis, 1988).

The third form of HC results from disrupted reabsorption of CSF into the bloodstream caused by obstruction in the basal subarachnoid cisterns or in the arachnoid villi (Fletcher et al., 1996; see Figure 7.11). When spina bifida is excluded, the most common cause of HC in early development is intraventricular hemorrhage (IVH), a condition that occurs in 40% to 50% of premature infants with birth weights less than 1,800 grams (Fletcher et al., 1992; Willis, 1993). As a result of breathing problems or pressure on the brain during the delivery process, vessels in the germinal matrix (area around the ventricles) rupture and bleed into the ventricles. Blood and cellular debris clog the arachnoid villa (which is responsible for reabsorbing CSF into the blood stream) and CSF volume and pressure increase, although its outward flow into the spinal canal is not blocked. HC of this form is known as **nonobstructive** or **communicating.**

Obstructive or noncommunicating hydrocephalus is a congenital disorder that develops early in gestation and is associated with an ever expanding impact on subsequent brain development. In contrast, nonobstructive or communicating HC is primarily a consequence of perinatal and postnatal insults to a brain that heretofore had developed normally (Hynd & Willis, 1988).

The Impact of Hydrocephalus on the Developing Brain   If unchecked, HC can have a devastating impact on the developing brain and skull (see Figure 7.12). As CSF volume increases, and the ventricles progressively enlarge, brain anatomy and function are disturbed. The ventricle lining suffers focal damage, cerebral blood vessels distort and become dysfunctional, neurons are injured, and the concentration of neurotransmitters

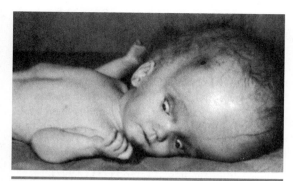

Figure 7.12 Hydrocephalus in a 14-month-old infant. (From J. G. Chusid, *Correlative Neuroanatomy & Functional Neurology*, NY: Appleton & Lange, 1982, p. 303, Figure 24-9. Reproduced with permission of the McGraw-Hill Companies)

and cerebral fluids alters (Dennis & Barnes, 1994). Further, the cortical mantle thins, often damaging the cortex. Cortical damage often compromises cognitive functions. However, cortical thinning without damage to the cortex generally spares higher-order cognitive functions.

Increasing pressure extensively damages underlying white matter of the brain. Specifically, the corpus callosum stretches and thins, midline projection fibers that connect the hemispheres to the diencephalon and caudal regions stretch and distort, the internal capsule (fanlike white fibers separating regions of the basal ganglia and dorsal thalamus) displaces, and the periventricular white matter (white matter adjacent to the lateral ventricles) is damaged (Del Bigio, 1993; Dennis & Barnes, 1994; Fletcher et al., 1996). Destruction of white matter can cause a number of functional deficits, particularly those involving nonverbal cognitive abilities and motor skills.

As the ventricles continue to distend, the cerebral hemispheres mold into a balloon shape. Because sutures in the cranium of the fetus and infant have not yet fused, increasing pressure enlarges the skull to accommodate the increased CSF volume. Once the sutures close, however, cranial volume is invariant, and the HC develops further at the expense of brain tissue (Rowland et al., 1991).

Most children with symptoms of HC receive a **shunt**. This medical procedure drains excessive CSF away from the ventricular system into the stomach. A shunt that fails, or needs adjustment, may necessitate additional surgeries during the child's life. Each surgery increases the risk of ventriculitis, or infection of the ventricles. Further, introducing the shunt involves causing a lesion to the brain, typically through the parietal lobe of the right hemisphere. The shunt track can irritate the surrounding brain tissue and increase the potential for seizures (Willis, 1993).

Although cognitive, motor, and sensory (visual) impairments frequently associate with HC, the precise symptom presentation is highly individualistic. The period of developmental onset, the presence of other congenital disorders and anomalies, surgery to introduce or adjust a shunt, and the nature of the child's environmental context are several variables affecting the array, severity, and form of symptoms the child will experienced.

Neuropsychological Assessment Neuropsychological assessment of the child with HC focuses on clarifying both spared and compromised functions. The extent and degree of impaired or spared cognitive functions differ for each child. In general, greater overall impairment of higher-order cognitive abilities accompanies more advanced cases of HC. However, interaction of HC with other moderating variables, such as age, intelligence, and socioeconomic status can, potentially, lead to differential effects on cognitive functioning.

Before widespread use of the shunt, only a quarter of untreated HC children survived to adulthood, and many survivors were profoundly retarded (Hynd et al., 1997). In contrast, the cognitive performance of early shunted children is significantly higher, spanning the range of abilities from below to above average. Some suggest that children with HC uncomplicated by other structural disruptions (such as multiple shunt operations) are likely to demonstrate age-appropriate cognitive functioning (Willis, 1993). Yet despite relatively preserved overall intelligence, shunted HC children tend to demonstrate verbal and nonverbal memory deficits relative to healthy control children (Scott et al., 1998). These memory failings reflect possible compression of the hippocampal region and white matter tracts of the brain. HC may also affect the development of other specific skills that are relatively independent of intelligence. For example, HC children tend to demonstrate age-appropriate word recognition, but markedly lower reading comprehension abilities. Even HC children of average to above-average intelligence demonstrate this disparity (Dennis & Barnes, 1994). Similarly, HC children often exhibit age-level social behavior, but are hyperverbal (behavior also termed **"cocktail party syndrome"**). This communication style is characterized by excessive verbiage that lacks clarity, organization, and relevance—a form of speech that resembles the "fluent, but empty" speech patterns associated with receptive aphasia, a communication disorder involving impaired language comprehension (Dennis & Barnes, 1994; Willis, 1993).

A particularly interesting finding concerns the relationship of cognitive functioning to early and late occurring HC. Children with prenatal obstructive HC are prone to exhibit average verbal and language abilities and below-average visual-spatial and visual-motor abilities. This profile is similar to that of the nonverbal learning disability syndrome (see discussion in Chapter 8). In contrast, children with HC resulting from perinatal and postnatal insults (such as IVH) are likely to show comparable verbal and performance abilities, although both generally fall within the low-average range (Willis, 1993).

Generally, the performance and neuropsychological deficits of HC children can be summarized as follows:

[HC children] are likely to have difficulties with visual-spatial and tactile perception tasks; tasks involving rapid, precise, or sequenced movement; arithmetic calculation, spelling, reading comprehension, and tasks that involve "executive control" functions governing the ability to establish and sustain one's focus of concentration, to inhibit inappropriate or irrelevant behaviors, and to shift flexibly among responses or modulate one's behavior according to situational demands. (Wills, 1993, p. 260)

Treatment The prognosis for HC children was dire before the development of shunting. However, the advent of shunting markedly increased the number of children who both survive and escape the significant destruction of their cognitive functioning. Children with HC uncomplicated by the presence of other anomalies who have received early shunting often exhibit few, if any, cognitive impairments. **Ultrasonography,** a procedure that uses sound waves to image internal structures, has enabled medical personnel to identify HC in utero by measuring the ventricular expansion that precedes the later developing enlargement of the cranium. From birth until age 2, HC is fairly easy to diagnose because the cranium enlarges quickly, developmental delays are evident, and eye movement abnormalities are present (Hynd et al., 1997).

CHROMOSOMAL AND GENETIC DISORDERS

This section explores chromosomal and genetic disorders. Chromosomal disorders are a consequence of malformation, deletion, addition, and/or dislocation of chromosomal material during the development of the oocyte or spermatocyte, or during conception and germination of the egg (Spreen et al., 1995). For example, Turner's syndrome is produced by a missing or abnormal X chromosome (female) that occurs at the time of conception. Although there are a significant number of chromosomal disorders, the three most frequently studied are Turner's syndrome, Klinefelter's syndrome and Trisomy X syndrome (Rovet, 1993). Genetic disorders, in contrast, are caused by the transmission to the offspring of genes coded to produce the disorders; that is, the disorders are inherited. For example, Lesch-Nyhan disease is a male, sex-linked, genetically transmitted disorder (Harris, 1995). Genetically transmitted disorders typically result in some form of metabolic abnormality. To date, researchers have identified more than 100 genetically transmitted disorders that, if untreated, can produce a number of significant neuropsychological and physical deficits. Fortunately, diet or other medical interventions can treat many of the metabolic disorders. Table 7.4 lists a sample of genetic and chromosomal disorders that can adversely impact neuropsychological functioning.

Turner's Syndrome

Background and Clinical Presentation In 1938, Turner presented a syndrome characterized by a failure to

Table 7.4	*Genetic and Chromosomal Disorders*
Genetic	**Chromosomal**
Adrenoleukodystrophy	Angelman syndrome
Friedreich's ataxia	Cornelia de Lange syndrome
Galactosemia	Down's syndrome
Hyperphenylalaninemia	Fragile X syndrome
Krabbe's disease	Klinefelter's syndrome
Lafora's disease	Prader-Willi syndrome
Lesch-Nyhan disease	Sotos syndrome
Mucopolysaccharidosis	Trisomy X syndrome
Phenylketonuria	Tuberous sclerosis complex
Williams syndrome	Turner's syndrome

From *Developmental Neuropsychiatry, Vol. II: Assessment, Diagnosis, and Treatment of Developmental Disorders* by James C. Harris. © 1995 by Oxford University Press, Inc. Reprinted by permission of the publisher.

develop secondary sexual characteristics, short stature, webbed neck, and **cubitus valgus** (an increased carrying angle at the elbow). The disorder was subsequently named **Turner's syndrome (TS).** A previous case of the disorder had also been reported by Otto Ullrich (1930) and therefore the syndrome is occasionally known as Ullrich-Turner syndrome. TS was recognized as a chromosomal disorder affecting females in 1959 when Charles Ford and colleagues identified a missing X on the 45th chromosome. The **karyotype**—a visual representation of the configuration of a chromosome—is designated as 45,XO, although there are other variations.

Consistent with Turner's earlier description of the disorder, an essential characteristic of TS is gonadal dysgenesis, as evident in either the absence of the ovaries or the presence of **vestigial ovarian streaks** (White, 1994). Short stature is another distinguishing characteristic, with the child's height often falling below the third percentile. Moreover, the mean height of the adult with TS is approximately 57 inches (Harris, 1995). Physicians often identify infants with TS at birth due to characteristic edema of the hands and feet and loose skin folds at the nape of the neck. In

childhood, physicians observe webbing of the neck, low-set ears, shield chest, deformed nails, cardiac and kidney malformations, and other features. Table 7.5 (p. 252) presents a sample of the physical characteristics and medical problems associated with TS. A distinctive cognitive profile for TS has been proposed and is discussed later in the section on neuropychological assessment.

Prevalence and Comorbidity TS is one of the most common chromosomal disorders, with an estimated female birth prevalence of 1 in 2,500 to 5,000 (White, 1994). Researchers believe it occurs at conception, and 99% of the affected fetuses spontaneously abort. The life expectancy of the individual with TS is not affected, although a number of physical conditions accompany the disorder (see Table 7.5).

There are suggestions that girls and female adolescents with TS are prone to depression, feelings of inadequacy, difficulties in concentrating, poor peer relationships, anxiety over sexuality, and relationships with males. The factors accounting for these difficulties are unclear, but the small stature and sexual limitations of the individual with TS likely contributes to social difficulties and negative emotionality (Harris, 1995).

Chromosomal Defect TS is the result of an anomaly of the female sex chromosome. The XX chromosome defines the developing embryo as female. In TS, the second X is either missing (monosomy X or 45,XO) or otherwise abnormal in formation or location. A wide variety of karyotypes appear in liveborn TS children with 45,XO evident in approximately 50% of the cases (Temple, Carney, & Mullarkey, 1996). **Isochromosome,** the duplication of one arm of the X chromosome with the loss of the other arm, constitutes 10% to 20% of the cases (Temple & Carney, 1993). **Mosaic karyotypes** appear in 30% to 35% of children with TS (Temple et al., 1996). The mosaic karyotypes are characterized by the presence of normal chromosomes in some cells (46,XX) and abnormal chromosomes in others (Rovet, 1993). The mosaic karyotype, 45,X/46,XX, is associated with milder and less pervasive anomalies than the other karyotypes. At birth these children exhibit few distinguishing

Table 7.5   *Physical and Medical Problems of Turner's Syndrome*

Anatomic Abnormalities	Cardiovascular
Short stature	Aortic narrowing
Webbed neck	Mitral valve prolapse
Cubitus valgus	Septal defect (defect of the wall separating chambers of the heart)
Broad chest	
Prepubertal ovarian failure	Partial anomalous venous blood return
Growth	
Decreased mean birth weight	**Renal**
Lack of pubertal growth spurt	Horseshoe kidney (abnormal tissue connecting the kidneys) or ptotic kidney (abnormal location in the pelvis)
Skeletal	
Curvature of the spine	
Genu valgum (knock-knee)	Unilateral failure to develop or underdeveloped kidney
Wrist deformity	
Short hand and feet bones	Unilateral double ureter
Craniofacial	**Lymphatic**
Premature closure of the skull sutures	Dilation of the lymph vessels
	Congenital swelling of the hands/feet
Small jaw	
Strabismus (cross-eyes)	**Hair and Skin**
Inner ear defects	Low posterior hairline
	Multiple moles
Malrotation of ears	Finger/toenail deformities
High arched palate	

From White, B. J. (1994). "The Turner Syndrome: Origin, cytogenetic variants, and factors influencing the phenotype," in S. H. Broman, & J. Grafman (eds.), *Atypical Cognitive Deficits in Developmental Disorders* (pp. 183–196). Mahwah, NJ: Lawrence Erlbaum.

features, and short stature may be the first presenting symptom. Note, however, that the TS physical phenotype appears in children with apparently normal karyotypes.

Neuropsychological Assessment   The intellectual functioning of children with TS is generally within the low-average to average range. A smaller proportion of children falls within either the below-average or above-average range of intelligence (Swillen et al., 1993). A number of researchers have suggested that children with TS demonstrate a relatively distinct neurocognitive profile. The profile is characterized by intact verbal abilities in contrast to deficits in visual-spatial and visual-motor performance (Romans, Roeltgen, Kushner, & Ross, 1997). Table 7.6 summarizes the types of visual-spatial and visual-motor deficits identified. Note that these deficits generally accompany right parietal or diffuse right hemisphere dysfunction (Reiss, Mazzocco, Greenlaw, Freund, & Ross, 1995). Relatedly, investigators have drawn a parallel between the neurocognitive profile of TS and that of the nonverbal learning disability syndrome (see discussion of the syndrome in Chapter 8). Alternatively, Pennington et al. (1985) contend that the performance of individuals with TS suggests diffuse brain injury, rather than injury specific to either the right or left hemisphere. Increasingly, investigators are realizing that children with TS are at greater risk for developing specific deficit patterns (such as visual-spatial), but these deficits are not universal for all children with TS.

Neuroimaging provides support for right hemisphere (particularly posterior region) involvement in the pathogenesis of TS. A recent positron emission tomography (PET) study (Elliott, Watkins, Messa, Lippe, & Chugani, 1996) of children with TS and normal children revealed significant bilateral parietal region hypometabolism (reduced metabolism) for the TS group. The researchers also observed a trend toward hypometabolic activity of the occipital region. They found that visual-spatial and mathematic deficits associated with TS stemmed from parieto-occipital hypoactivation. In a related study of identical twins, one affected by TS and the other without the disorder, magnetic resonance imaging (MRI) results revealed significant regional and global brain differences between the twins (Reiss et al., 1993). Specifically, the right frontal, parietal, and occipital regions; the midline structures of the posterior fossa (cranial vault supporting the cerebellum); and the left parietal perisylvian cortical regions (adjacent to the Sylvian fissure) were markedly dissimilar. In addition, the CSF volume in the twin with TS was 25%

Table 7.6 *Visual-Spatial and Visual-Motor Deficits Associated with Turner's Syndrome*

Dysfunctions of:

Arithmetic	Mental rotation	Visual discrimination
Design copying	Motor learning	Spatial working memory
Directional sense	Part-whole perception	
Extrapersonal space		Visual sequencing
Left-right discrimination	Route finding	Visual-motor integration
	Spatial reasoning	
Maze performance		Visual memory

From Buchanan, L., Pavolic, J. & Rovet, J. (1998). *Developmental Neuropsychology, 14,* 341–367. Mahwah, NJ: Lawrence Erlbaum.

greater, and gray matter was reduced, suggesting generalized hypoplasia. In a more recent MRI study of TS and control children, Reiss and coworkers (1995) determined that the ratios of gray to white matter for the right parietal areas were significantly lower for the TS participants. The finding of reduced tissue volume for parietal and parietal-occipital areas is a relatively consistent finding across studies of females with TS.

Although posterior regional circuitry has received much empirical attention, some research indicates that the frontal system may also play a pathogenic role in TS. Preliminary research suggests that children with TS may suffer from deficits in verbal fluency, planning and organization, impulsivity, strategic memory organization, cognitive flexibility, and attentional control (Reiss & Denckla, 1996; Romans et al., 1997; Rovet, 1993; Temple et al., 1996). Further research will determine whether a specific pattern of executive deficits characterizes TS.

Developmental Course   The incidence of prematurity for children with TS (45,XO) is high, with more than 25% of the infants born 2 to 4 weeks early, and approximately 30% born more than 4 weeks before their due dates (Harris, 1995). The body length of the infant at birth is below average. Measures (blood assays) of **gonadotropins** assist in diagnosing the disorder. In the female, gonadotropins are hormones that stimulate the functions of the ovaries. The majority of children with TS are diagnosed before school age.

During the preschool years, children with TS are described as immature, overactive, distractible, and having difficulties sustaining attention. With increasing age, activity appears to slow and many children with TS later become normally active or hypoactive. The young child with TS does not exhibit behavioral problems and is generally accepted by, and involved with peers. However, by school age, the peer interactions of many children with TS have lessened, and involvement in solitary activities has increased. Children affected with TS tend to be compliant, unassertive, and conforming in their interactions with caretakers and peers. Peer interactions, however, continue to decline, and many youngsters with TS report feelings of being alone and alienated (Swillen et al., 1993). With the onset of adolescence, teenagers with TS date less frequently and are involved in fewer romantic and sexual relationships than their age mates. Some suggest that they may not be proficient at reading social cues, which can negatively impact on their efforts to relate to peers. Growth retardation, physical anomalies (such as webbing of the neck), medical problems, social difficulties, and an awareness of their sexual difference likely contribute to diminished self-esteem (Bender, Linden, & Robinson, 1994). In light of these factors, it is not surprising that teenagers with TS are at risk for developing anxiety, insecurity, and depression. Despite deficits in the visual-spatial and visual-motor areas, most children affected by the disorder (90%) attend regular school programs, although they may need remedial interventions. Further, because of the physical problems frequently associated with the condition (see Table 7.5), they often need medical services.

Treatment   It is essential that adolescents with TS receive estrogen therapy due to their gonadal dysgenesis. Without proper medical interventions, youngsters with the disorder do not mature sexually, which can cause significant distress. Further, the short stature associated with TS often requires growth hormone therapy. Psychological or counseling services may be needed, because the risk for teasing and lack of peer acceptance appears high for children with TS (Rovet,

1993). TS children and adolescents with inattention, impulsivity, and hyperactivity encounter significant difficulties within the classroom. Specialized educational interventions and, in many cases, the introduction of psychostimulant medications may assist the student. In addition, spatial, executive, and academic weaknesses (mathematics) must be addressed to ensure appropriate progress. We discuss additional educational recommendations relevant to the needs of the child with TS in the section on nonverbal learning disability syndrome in Chapter 8.

ACQUIRED DISORDERS

The number of agents, events, and processes that can potentially injure the prenatal and postnatal brain is staggering. Environmental toxins, radiation, infections, anoxia, malnutrition, tumors, and traumatic head injuries can result in anomalies of the developing brain. Of these agents, traumatic head injuries, such as concussions, lacerations, and contusions, account for the vast majority of brain damage in children and adolescents. Regardless of the nature of the insult, a one-to-one relationship between brain disturbance and behavior is not evident. The prediction of functional outcomes is contingent on a host of fac-

tors including the (1) age at which the lesion is incurred; (2) type, severity, and status (static or progressive) of the lesion; (3) premorbid personality and intelligence of the child; (4) quality and timeliness of medical attention; and (5) accessibility of acute and long-term services.

Fetal alcohol syndrome is a specific condition reflecting the devastating effects of prenatal exposure to alcohol. Initially it was suspected that impairments associated with fetal alcohol syndrome were restricted to mothers who chronically abused alcohol or were "binge" drinkers. Increasingly, it is being realized that the prenatal fetus is at risk even with social drinking.

Fetal Alcohol Syndrome

Clinical Features and Prevalence   **Fetal alcohol syndrome (FAS)** is a long-lasting and debilitating disorder recognized in the medical and neuropsychological fields for approximately two decades. Lemoine, Harrowsseau, Borteryu, and Menuet (1968) are credited with being the first to describe the effects of alcohol on a group of children of alcoholic parents. Jones, Smith, Ulleland, and Streissguth (1973) later identified the anomalies and characteristics that have come to define FAS.

Children with FAS frequently exhibit intrauterine growth retardation; characteristic facial features of

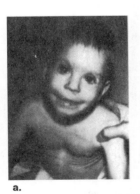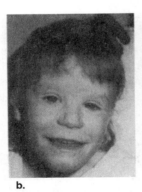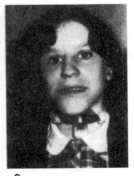

a.   b.   c.

Figure 7.13   The facial features of the developing FAS child (a–c): Unique features are the widely spaced eyes, shortened length of eyelids, low nasal bridge, short and flattened nose, elongated midface, and thin upper lip. ([a, b] From Hanson, J. W., Jones, K. L. & Smith, D. W. (1976). *Fetal Alcohol Syndrome: Experience with 41 patients.* Journal of the American Medical Association, 235 (14), 1459; reprinted with permission of the American Medical Association, copyright 1976; [c] from A. Streissguth, *Fetal Alcohol Syndrome,* Baltimore: Paul Brookes, 1997, p. 53)

widely spaced eyes, shortened length of eyelids, elongated midface, flattened nose, and underdeveloped upper lip (see Figure 7.13); and deficits associated with central nervous system involvement (Streissguth, 1997). Central nervous system deficits include microcephaly (abnormally small head, see Table 7.3), infantile irritability, seizures, tremors, poor coordination, poor habituation (difficulty in tuning out repeating stimuli), and reduced muscle tone. In addition, below-average intelligence, inattention, hyperactivity, learning disabilities, and poor behavioral regulation commonly characterize children with FAS (Steinhausen, Willms, & Spohr, 1993; Kerns, Don, Mateer, & Streissguth, 1997). Although FAS is one of the most well known causes of mental retardation, not all children affected with it are retarded. Table 7.7 presents physical and medical characteristics associated with FAS.

Children who are exposed to alcohol in utero, but who fail to exhibit growth deficits or other physical abnormalities of FAS, may still show functional impairments similar to those of FAS. That is, the exposed children may manifest sensory and sensory-motor impairments, speech and language delays, cognitive and learning weaknesses, and regulatory deficits such as inattention, impulsivity, and hyperactivity (Jacobson, Jacobson, Sokol, Martier, & Ager, 1993). These features are called **fetal alcohol effects (FAE)** or **alcohol-related neurodevelopmental disabilities (ARND).**

Prevalence　Estimates of the frequency of FAS in the general population range from .26 to 2.29 per 1,000 live births (Abel, 1995). Researchers consider the prevalence significantly higher if children suffering from fetal alcohol effects are included, possibly as high as 10 per 1,000 live births (Streissguth, Barr, Bookstein, Sampson, & Carmichael Olson, 1999). The incidence of FAS and FAE among alcoholic mothers is markedly higher, with estimates of 25 per 1000 and 90 per 1000, respectively (Jenkins & Culbertson, 1996).

Neuropsychological Pathogenesis　FAS is a consequence of alcohol use by the pregnant mother during the baby's prenatal development. The relationship of the

Table 7.7　*Physical and Medical Conditions Associated with Fetal Alcohol Syndrome*

Growth	Skeletal *(continued)*
Decreased fat tissue	Pectus excavatum (abnormally depressed sternum)
Prenatal and postnatal growth deficiency	Tapering terminal fingers, deformities of finger/toenails
Cardiac	Union of the radius and ulnar bones
Atrial septal defect (defect in the wall between the atria)	**Other**
Ventricular septal defect (defect of wall between the ventricles)	Abnormal thoracic cage
Craniofacial	Abnormally small eyes
	Anomaly of the sex organs
Abnormally small jaw in adolescence	Cleft lip and/or cleft palate
Microcephaly (abnormally small head)	Dental malocclusion
	Epicanthal folds
Ptosis (droopy eyelid)	Excessive hair in infancy
Short upturned nose	Hearing loss, protuberant ears
Shortened eyelid length	Hernias of diaphragm, umbilicus, or groin
Underdeveloped lip features	
Underdeveloped upper jaw	Myopia, strabismus (cross-eyes)
Skeletal	Renal deformity
	Small teeth with faulty enamel
Altered palm crease patterns	Strawberry hemangiomata (blood-filled birthmarks or benign tumors of small blood vessels)
Cervical spine abnormalities	
Foot position defects	
Joint alterations	

Source: From *Developmental Neuropsychiatry, Vol. II: Assessment, Diagnosis, and Treatment of Developmental Disorders* by James C. Harris. © 1995 by Oxford University Press, Inc. Reprinted by permission of the publisher.

teratogenic effects of prenatal alcohol exposure to intake variables (amount, frequency, and drinking patterns) and the timing of introduction during pregnancy remains poorly understood. The teratogenic effects of alcohol, as revealed in animal and human studies, suggest a continuum of negative effects determined, in part, by a dose–response relationship, that is, increasing amounts and frequency of alcohol ingestion correlate with greater injurious effects (Carmichael Olson et al., 1997). The children of mothers who consumed relatively low levels of alcohol (social drinking) did not exhibit either physical or structural stigmata, but experienced behavioral disturbances, social maladjustment, and cognitive deficits that extended into adolescence. An increased risk for physical and structural damage, in conjunction with disturbances in functionality, accompanied higher levels of consumption. At the most severe end of the continuum, characterized by very high levels of alcohol abuse, full-blown FAS disorder was likely to appear. Originally, researchers thought more severe cognitive and behavioral deficits were specific to FAS. However, increasing evidence indicates that FAE children can display comparable functional deficits. In a recent study of children with FAS and FAE (Mattson, Riley, Gramling, Delis, & Jones, 1998) who underwent a comprehensive neuropsychological evaluation, researchers found both groups to be impaired in language skills, verbal learning and memory, academic skills, fine-motor speed, and visual-motor integration. Of significance was that FAE children showed a pattern of deficits comparable to those of FAS children, except in visual-motor integration and nonverbal concept formation. Thus, significant neuropsychological deficits can appear in children who are exposed prenatally to excessive alcohol use, even though they may appear physically normal.

The risk to the developing fetus seems much greater in alcoholic mothers who chronically abuse alcohol or "binge" (multiple drinks consumed in a relatively short period of time) during pregnancy. Also, alcohol consumption seems to do greater damage during the early months of pregnancy, but there may be no period in pregnancy when the developing child is completely risk free (Carmichael Olson et al., 1997). Further, fraternal twin studies suggest that genetic factors may play a role in determining the vulnerability of the embryo or fetus to FAS. That is, maternal alcohol use can significantly affect one twin more than the other twin, despite their sharing the same prenatal environment. Other factors, such as how efficiently the mother metabolizes alcohol, the physical condition of the fetus, and the mother's health and use of other substances (such as cigarette smoking) may contribute to the development of FAS, severity of symptoms, and potential for postnatal recovery (Sigelman & Shaffer, 1995).

Investigators have identified a number of neuroanatomical changes in the brains of FAS children that potentially reflect the destructive impact of alcohol on the developing brain. Specifically, children with the disorder frequently present either dysgenesis or agenesis of the corpus callosum, hippocampal damage, reduced basal ganglia volume, cerebellar anomalies, and expanded ventricles (Mattson, Riley, Sowell, Delis, Jernigan, Sobel, & Jones, 1996; Randall, 1996). The high proportion of FAS children with microcephaly indicates that brain size is reduced. Moreover, executive dysfunctions appear, thus implicating disturbance of the frontal circuitry.

Neuropsychological Assessment   The myriad of behavioral, adaptive, and neuropsychological characteristics of the child with FAS signal the need for a multidisciplinary approach. Because of the increased risk for cardiac, skeletal, and other physical conditions (see Table 7.7), medical consultation is certainly warranted. Further, a comprehensive neuropsychological evaluation is needed to identify and interpret the cognitive, behavioral, and adaptive dysfunctions that characterize the child. Finally, contingent on the child's presenting issues, the evaluative services of a speech and language pathologist, educational specialist, social worker, and occupational/physical therapist may be warranted.

Children with FAS exhibit a broad spectrum of neuropsychological deficits. In addition to mental retardation, common FAS deficits are evident in attention, response inhibition, complex problem solving, spatial and object memory, language skills, verbal learning and memory, speed of information processing, consistency of task performance, cognitive flexibility, planning, and academic performance (Korkman, Kirk, & Kemp, 1998; Mattson, Riley, Delis, Stern, & Jones, 1996; Streissguth et al., 1999). Further, the array of deficits that accompanying FAS often exceeds what might be predicted based on intelligence, suggesting that limited cognitive ability alone cannot explain these impairments (Kerns et al., 1997).

Clearly, the breadth of deficits associated with FAS imply that many different neural regions and systems are involved in the pathogenesis of the disorder. The interaction of alcohol intake variables, the point in the brain's development when alcohol is introduced, and other pertinent factors, such as the mother's nutrition, likely account for the heterogeneity of implicated brain systems and cognitive dysfunctions. For example, introducing alcohol during neurogenesis may account, in part, for disturbed cortical cell migration, resulting in global cognitive deficits, whereas later prenatal exposure may produce cognitive deficits that are more specific in nature. Interestingly, the ratings of parents and teachers suggest that the primary behavioral difficulties of children affected with FAS, both in the home and school, relate to attention deficits and social relationship problems (Steinhausen et al., 1993).

Developmental Course   Longitudinal studies (Streissguth, 1997) have revealed that the cognitive, behavioral, and adaptive deficits of FAS children do not fully resolve with age. Thus, the negative effects of intrauterine exposure to alcohol often endure. Infants with FAS often present low birth weight, feeding and sleep disturbances, poor habituation and high levels of irritability (Jenkins & Culbertson, 1996). By 4 years of age, deficits appear in attention, memory, achievement, reaction time, and gross and fine motor skills. In addition, **enuresis** (age-inappropriate bedwetting) and communication disorders are very frequent. By elementary school age, ADHD symptoms of inattention, impulsivity, and hyperactivity, coupled with poor organization, communication deficits, behavioral problems, and disturbances of basic functions (sleeping, eating, and elimination) disrupt the adaptive efforts of FAS children (Steinhausen et al., 1993). Cognitive deficits, microcephaly, small physical stature, and poor socialization skills often interfere with peer acceptance. Children affected by FAS with significant intellectual and learning deficits are often identified in their preschool to elementary years and provided with specialized education services.

With the advent of adolescence, communication disorders and disturbances of basic functions decline, although other cognitive and behavioral deficits persist. Of considerable concern are reports that teenagers with FAS tend to manifest high rates of antisocial behaviors and substance abuse. Unfortunately, the multiple cognitive, behavioral, and adaptive deficits of FAS appear to continue into adulthood.

Treatment   It goes without saying that the best form of treatment for an acquired disorder is prevention. Eliminating or significantly reducing alcohol consumption during pregnancy markedly decreases or reduces the risk of FAS for the unborn child. Although public awareness prevents many mothers from drinking during pregnancy, the alcoholic mother is of special concern. The physician, or other personnel who encounter a pregnant woman who abuses alcohol, should immediately apprise her of the risks to the fetus and refer her to the appropriate persons or agencies for assistance. Parents of FAS children often need assistance in understanding the nature and developmental course of the disorder and potential intervention strategies available for the condition. As previously noted, a comprehensive, multidisciplinary evaluation is warranted, including a neuropsychological evaluation to pinpoint the child's strengths and weaknesses across cognitive, learning, and adaptive domains.

FAS children who are mentally retarded generally require specialized educational services either within the public schools or in a residential setting, depending on the severity of retardation and particular learning needs of the child. Higher functioning children affected by FAS, despite average or above-average intelligence, may also need supplemental or specialized educational services because of specific cognitive and achievement weaknesses (Kerns et al., 1997). Further, FAS children with communication deficits should have appropriate speech and language therapy. Behavioral management systems are often needed within the home and school, particularly if the child also displays an ADHD. Medications can be introduced to help regulate the child's ADHD, particularly if the symptoms of inattention, impulsivity, and hyperactivity disrupt the child's learning, family, and peer relations. Social skills training may help improve peer acceptance. The aforementioned interventions will need to be continued into adolescence, and modified in accordance with the changing learning and behavioral needs of the teenager.

Conclusion

The human brain, a marvel of evolution and adaptation, develops in a dynamic and orderly manner, beginning as a primitive tube and moving through temporally defined stages to its final state of anatomical and functional maturity. The developing and mature brain are distinctly different, paralleling the behavioral and functional differences of the child and the adult. The anatomic unfolding of the central nervous system can be viewed from a molecular and a molar perspective. Regarding the former, stages of development include neurogenesis and cellular migration, axon and dendrite development, synaptogenesis, myelination, and pruning of neurons and synaptic connections. At a molar level, the progression of cortical, subcortical, and ventricular formation can be traced.

Functionality emerges concurrent with postnatal development. Exemplifying this emergence are three behavioral domains. Two of these domains, language-speech and cognitive skills, represent relatively early maturing systems; whereas the third, executive function, involves a protracted period of development extending into adolescence and early adulthood. The developing brain is vulnerable to a myriad of insults that can lead to damage and dysfunction. Yet a degree of plasticity allows limited compensation, or return of function, following cerebral insults. However, the dynamics of this recovery process remain poorly understood. The clinical presentation, neuropathogenesis, neuropsychological assessment, and treatment of HC, Turner's syndrome, and fetal alcohol syndrome illustrate the brain–behavior relationships that characterize each of these developmental disorders.

Critical Thinking Questions

- In light of the devastating effects of many of the genetic and chromosomal disorders, do you think that potential parents should seek genetic counseling prior to having children? Explain.
- Why are executive functions important in adaption?
- In recent years, an increasing number of teratogens have been identified in the environment. Are our children at greater risk for brain anomalies than children of earlier generations? Why or why not?
- What steps could be taken to prevent FAS?

Key Terms

Neurogenesis	Spines	Inhibitory control	Intraventricular hemorrhage (IVH)
Neural tube	Synaptogenesis	Object permanence	Obstructive or noncommunicating hydrocephalus
Precursor or progenitor cells	Myelin	Phenylketonuria (PKU)	
Neurulation	Pruning	Teratogens	
Spina bifida	Polymicrogyria	Agenesis	Nonobstructive or communicating hydrocephalus
Anencephaly	Prosody	Dysgenesis	
Corticogenesis	Executive functions	Kennard principle	
Agyria or lissencephaly	Working memory	Hydrocephalus (HC)	

Shunt	Karyotype	Fetal alcohol syndrome (FAS)	Enuresis
"Cocktail party syndrome"	Vestigial ovarian streaks	Fetal alcohol effects (FAE) or	
Ultrasonography	Isochromosome	alcohol-related	
Cubitus valgus	Mosaic karyotypes	neurodevelopmental	
Turner's syndrome	Gonadotropins	disabilities (ARND)	

Web Connections

http://www.med.upenn.edu/meded/public/berp
University of Pennsylvania Educational Page
This site provides in-depth information about central nervous system development from the earliest stages from fertilization to birth. Includes text, pictures, and movies.

http://www.turner-syndrome-us.org
Turner's Syndrome Society of the United States
Facts and information on Turner's Syndrome.

http://www.patientcenters.com/hydrocephalus
Hydrocephalus Center
Provides information about hydrocephalus and its treatment.

http://www.nofas.org
National Organization of Fetal Alcohol Syndrome (FAS)
Page dedicated to raising the public awareness of FAS; includes definition and strategies for working with children with FAS.

Chapter 8

LEARNING AND NEUROPSYCHIATRIC DISORDERS OF CHILDHOOD

CONTRIBUTED BY WILLIAM C. CULBERTSON

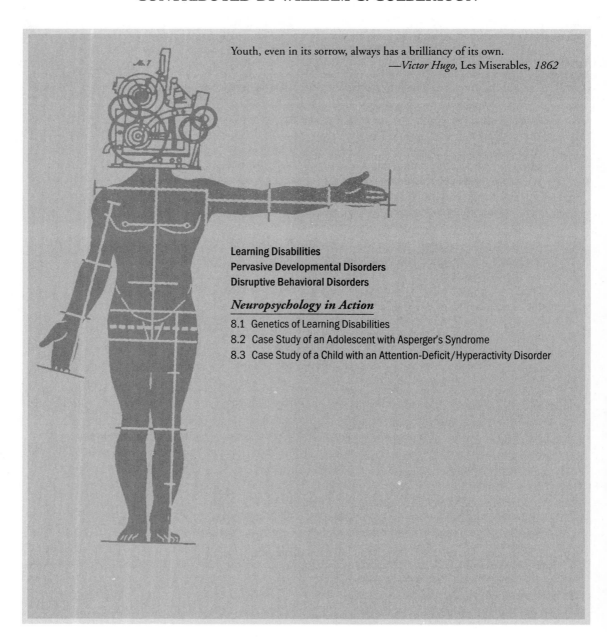

Youth, even in its sorrow, always has a brilliancy of its own.
—*Victor Hugo*, Les Miserables, *1862*

Learning Disabilities
Pervasive Developmental Disorders
Disruptive Behavioral Disorders

Neuropsychology in Action

8.1 Genetics of Learning Disabilities
8.2 Case Study of an Adolescent with Asperger's Syndrome
8.3 Case Study of a Child with an Attention-Deficit/Hyperactivity Disorder

Keep in Mind

■ What are the specific neurocognitive assets and deficits of children with verbal and nonverbal learning disabilities?

■ Can a nonverbal learning disability directly disrupt a child's socioemotional adjustment?

■ Is Asperger's syndrome a separate disorder, or merely high-functioning autism?

■ What treatment interventions are effective for children with ADHD?

Overview

This chapter discusses learning, pervasive developmental, and disruptive behavioral disorders of childhood. These three classes of disorders can significantly hinder a child's developmental progression and adaption and often coexist with other conditions that further compromise the child's functioning. Although the pervasive developmental disorders occur less frequently, the impact of these conditions is profound, generally precluding self-sufficiency and independence, and necessitating lifelong supervision.

The developmental disorders reviewed in the previous chapter are often considered as biological rather than psychological in origin because prominent brain anatomic defects and physical stigmata often accompany the disorders. Moreover, the etiology of these disorders is generally traceable to prenatal disruption or genetic/chromosomal defects. In contrast, the etiologies of childhood learning and neuropsychiatric disorders are not as easily linked to congenital anomalies. Accordingly, theorists have often proposed psychological factors as determinants of these disorders. However, ongoing research and advances in neuroimaging are providing evidence that brain disturbances may, in fact, play a prominent role in the etiology of both learning and neuropsychiatric disorders.

This discussion examines, in detail, three specific disorders that represent learning, pervasive developmental, and disruptive behavioral disorders. The first disorder, nonverbal learning disability syndrome, reflects a major contribution of neuropsychology to the study of learning disabilities. Byron Rourke, through his extensive research, has identified a unique disorder, nonverbal learning disability syndrome, characterized by a specific pattern of neurocognitive assets and deficits. The second disorder, autism, is a pervasive developmental disorder that has attracted a voluminous body of research (Bailey, Phillips, & Rutter, 1996). Despite this research, the etiology and neurobehavioral relationships of autism remain poorly understood. Finally, I review attention-deficit/hyperactivity disorder, one of the most prevalent of childhood disruptive behavioral disorders, comprising about 50% of the population of child psychiatric clinics (Cantwell, 1996). Similar to autism, attention-deficit/hyperactivity disorder is the focus of considerable research that transverses diverse fields of study. Neuropsychology has identified a number of brain–behavior relationships of attention-deficit/hyperactivity disorder that are enhancing the understanding of the disorder.

Learning Disabilities

Learning disabilities adversely affect the ability of the child to communicate and meet the challenges of education. Children with learning disabilities constitute between 7% and 15% of the school population (Gaddes & Edgell, 1993) and comprise one of the largest childhood groups referred for neuropsychological services (Culbertson & Edmonds, 1996). Controversy persists regarding the definition, diagnosis,

Neuropsychology in Action 8.1

Genetics of Learning Disabilities

by **Bruce Pennington** Ph.D., *Department of Psychology, Director of Developmental Cognitive Neuroscience Program, University of Denver.*

When I finished graduate school in clinical psychology in 1977, there was considerable controversy about the validity of the construct of learning disabilities. Some said the construct was a middle-class myth to excuse the poor performance of some children. Another possibility, offered by the psychoanalytic paradigm that dominated clinical work at that time, reduced learning problems to largely unconscious motivational problems. One supervisor I had only half-jokingly interpreted problems with addition as representing conflicts over oral issues, problems with subtraction as representing castration anxiety, and so on. Partly because I had minored in cognitive development in graduate school, I was quite curious about whether learning disabilities existed, and if they did, how to understand and treat them.

Serendipity played a major role in focusing my curiosity. My first job after graduate school was to help with a longitudinal study of children with abnormal sex chromosome numbers (the 45X, 47XXX, 47XXY, and 47XYY karyotypes) initiated by Dr. Arthur Robinson, a pediatric geneticist. These children had been followed since birth, and they were now of school age. It very soon became clear that these children had higher rates of learning disabilities than either their siblings or children with abnormal numbers of sex chromosomes in only some of their cell lines (mosaics). Most interestingly, the type of learning disability a child exhibited was largely karyotype specific. These children provided strong evidence that some learning disabilities were influenced by genetic factors and that different genetic factors affected different aspects of cognitive development and academic skill.

Suddenly a whole new vista opened on the question of how valid the construct of learning disabilities was. The fact of differential genetic etiology for at least some learning disabilities convinced me of their validity, and also gripped me with an intense curiosity to understand in detail how the genetic alteration lead to the alteration in cognitive development. It was very clear to me that one of the missing links in this causal chain was the brain, and so I set out to learn all that I could about neuropsychology, as well as genetics. My new question was, How do the genetic alterations change brain development to cause specific changes in cognitive development? I also wondered if genetic influences on learning disabilities are rare

etiology, and remediation of learning disabilities. Generally, professionals define learning disabilities as impairments of one or more academic skills, that cannot be accounted for by sensory or motor deficits, mental retardation, emotional disturbance, or environmental, cultural, or economic disadvantage (Hooper, Willis, & Grant, 1996). Common learning disabilities involve impairment of reading (**dyslexia**), arithmetic (**dyscalculia**), and written expression (**dysgraphia**). Moreover, a newly identified subtype of learning disorder, **social emotional learning disability,** has been proposed (Culbertson & Edmonds, 1996). This disorder is believed to relate to cognitive deficits that directly produce socioemotional disturbance.

Verbal learning disabilities, such as dyslexia, have received significantly more research and theoretical attention than the nonverbal learning disability syndrome that focuses on deficits in mathematics. We briefly discuss dyslexia to help clarify, by contrast, the nonverbal learning disability syndrome. The expanded coverage, in this chapter, of the nonverbal learning disability syndrome acknowledges its greater disruptiveness to the child, relative to verbal learning disabilities, and the availability of a specific neuropsychological model to guide identification and treatment of the disorder (James & Selz, 1997).

VERBAL LEARNING DISABILITY: DYSLEXIA

Dyslexia can be acquired by insult to a previously normal functioning brain or be developmental in origin. Generally, examiners use a discrepancy between current reading achievement and grade level or intelli-

and limited to infrequent syndromes, such as abnormalities in sex chromosome number, or if they played a substantial role in the etiology of learning disabilities that had no currently known cause.

An opportunity to answer this second question soon presented itself. Herbert Labs and Shelley Smith, both medical geneticists, invited me to help with their study of familial dyslexia by helping to define its cognitive phenotype. They had taken quite seriously Hallgren's (1950) classic study, which had demonstrated a possible dominant gene influence on dyslexia, and were studying genetic linkage in extended families with dyslexia to find such genes. In 1983, we published a paper in *Science* that presented evidence for a gene influencing dyslexia located near the centromere of chromosome 15. That same year, Shelley Smith and I published in *Child Development* a review of what was then known about genetic influences on learning disabilities and speech and language disorders. Subsequently, I published a number of papers on the cognitive phenotype in familial dyslexia, finding that it was characterized by dysphonetic spelling

errors and an underlying deficit in phoneme awareness.

It eventually became clear that a large proportion of the children who present clinically with dyslexia have affected relatives and that the recurrence rate among first-degree relatives is quite high, about 35–45%. This means that if a parent is dyslexic, the risk of having a dyslexic child is about eight times higher than the general population risk. So genetic influences on learning disabilities are not rare, but instead account for a substantial portion of the etiology of the most common learning disability, dyslexia.

The search for genes influencing dyslexia has continued. Shelley and I soon joined forces with John DeFries and colleagues at the Institute for Behavioral Genetics in Boulder, Colorado, who had independently conducted important family and twin studies of dyslexia. Together we eventually identified the approximate location of a second gene influencing dyslexia, this time on the short arm of chromosome 6. Cardon et al. reported this discovery in *Science* in 1994. Three years later, a separate team at Yale and Bowman Gray medical

schools essentially replicated both our linkage results, those on 15 and 6, in an independent sample of families with dyslexia (Grigorenko et al., 1997). Taken together, these findings are essentially the first replicated genetic linkage results for a complex behavioral disorder.

So some but not all of the questions I began with are answered. Learning disabilities exist in much the same way that other complex medical phenotypes (such as obesity or heart disease) exist. There are genetic influences on them and a substantial portion (about 50% according to twin studies) of the variance in the most common learning disability, dyslexia, is attributable to genes. The approximate locations of two of these genes influencing dyslexia are now known. Other disorders have shown us that understanding genetic mechanisms can illuminate the brain mechanisms underlying learning disabilities. The challenge for the future (and for future developmental neuropsychologists) is to better understand both genetic and brain mechanisms in dyslexia and other learning disorders.

---

gence to classify a child as dyslexic. Approximately 4% to 9% of school-age children are affected by the disorder, with boys outnumbering girls 3:2 (Culbertson & Edmonds, 1996; Rumsey, 1996a). Dyslexia tends to run in families, suggesting a genetic etiology. As Bruce Pennington reports in his discussion of the genetics of learning disabilities (see Neuropsychology in Action 8.1), a child with parents affected with dyslexia is eight times more likely to exhibit the disorder than children of parents who are not reading disabled.

Visual Processing Model of Dyslexia

Despite a long history of research and investigation, the study of dyslexia continues to be fraught with divergent diagnostic criteria and a myriad of theoretical explanations. However, a review of the research and

theoretical models reveals increasing convergence on two basic subtypes. The first subtype encompasses children with significant reading deficits caused by possible visual and visual-perceptual anomalies, whereas the second relates to children whose reading impairment stems from auditory-language dysfunction (Spreen et al., 1995). Regarding the first subtype, researchers have studied eye movements and speed of visual processing (Eden, Stein, Wood, & Wood, 1995). Specifically, reading-disabled children and adults show slower **flicker fusion rates** when presented images of low spatial density and contrast (brightness). Flicker fusion rate is the speed at which two separate visual images fuse into a single image when rapidly presented. The magnocellular visual system controls the processing of this form of visual input, prompting the magnocellular-deficit theory of dsylexia.

The magnocellular-deficit theory centers on the two visual pathways of the human visual system, namely the magnocellular and parvocellular pathways. Each of these pathways processes information from the retina and, in turn, transfers the information to the visual cortex for further processing (see Figure 8.1). The **magnocellular visual system** consists of large cells that are located in the inferior region of the lateral geniculate bodies and are highly sensitive to movement, rapid stimulus change, low contrast, and spatial location; the **parvocellular visual system** involves smaller cells that are dorsally located in the lateral geniculate bodies and are responsive to stationary objects, color, high contrast, and fine spatial details (Skotun & Parke, 1999). The former system is believed to be activated during rapid **saccadic eye movements,** whereas the latter system is stimulated during eye fixation and is extensively involved in discriminating and identifying printed/written symbols. In reading, the individual makes a series of brief fixations, separated by saccadic eye movements. Scientists hypothesize that the magnocellular visual system inhibits the parvocellular system at the time of each saccade, ensuring that the previous eye fixation image is terminated. In dyslexia, the magnocellular visual system may fail to appropriately inhibit the parvocellular system, resulting in a prolonged afterimage that interferes with reading; that is, letters seen in one fixation blur into the next fixation.

Preliminary support for anomalies of the magnocellular system in dyslexic persons stems from investigations (Galaburda & Livingstone, 1993) of the lateral geniculate bodies of normal-reading and reading-disabled adults. Brain autopsies revealed that the parvocellular cells of the two groups were similar, but the magnocellular cell bodies were generally smaller and more variable in size and shape in the dyslexic group. The investigators proposed that the structural differences in magnocellular cells is consistent with slower visual processing.

Phonological Model of Dyslexia

Although dyslexia as a consequence of underlying deficits in visual processing has received attention, impairment in phonological processing as the central feature of the disorder has received much more support (Swanson, Mink, & Bocian, 1999). The term **phonological processing** refers to the application of rules for translating letters and letter sequences into their corresponding speech–sound equivalents. This processing is supported by phonological awareness, the awareness of, and ability to differentiate between, individual phonemes, or speech sounds (Rum-

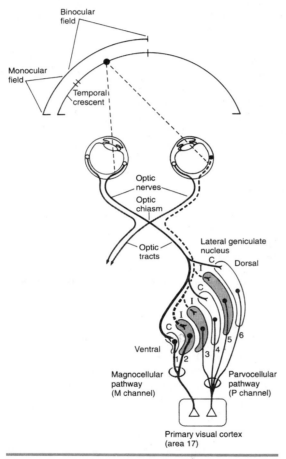

Figure 8.1 Magnocellular and parvocellular visual systems. The ventral magnocellular pathways are designated 1–2, and the dorsal parvocellular pathways are indicated by 3–6. (Adapted from C. Mason and E. R. Kandel, "Central Visual Pathways," in E. R. Kandel, J. H. Schwartz, and T. M. Jessell, eds., *Principles of Neural Science,* 3rd ed., New York: Elsevier Science, 1991, p. 425, Figure 29-6. Reproduced by permission of the McGraw-Hill Companies)

sey, 1996a). Dyslexic children exhibit deficits in translating letter strings into word sounds, also called *word decoding*. Deficits in this process cause reading to be slow and nonautomatic, disrupting efforts to identify and comprehend presented words (Pennington, 1991). The word recognition deficits of the dyslexic are most evident when the child must read novel or unfamiliar words, that is, when the determination of letter–sound associations is most critical. Relatedly, dyslexic children often have problems spelling because they can't efficiently translate the phonological representation of a word to its visual configuration, a process that is the converse of what reading requires. Despite these deficits, dyslexic children frequently demonstrate preserved "listening comprehension" when someone reads material to them.

Individuals with severe dyslexia continue to show reading deficits into adolescence and adulthood, suggesting that reading deficits are often a lifelong problem. Interestingly, adults who were dyslexic as children, but show good reading outcomes in adulthood, continue to exhibit phonological deficits. For example, they continue to experience significant decoding deficits when required to read or spell nonwords, such as *yite*. Researchers believe their improvement in reading reflects a compensatory expansion of their sight vocabulary.

The primary emphasis of neuropsychological research concerning dyslexia has focused on the language cortex of the left hemisphere of right-handed individuals. The **planum temporale** of the left posterior temporal lobe (see Figure 8.2) is one of the neural regions implicated in phonological processing (Hynd & Hiemenz, 1997). For most people, the planum temporales of the left and right hemispheres are asymmetric, the left planum temporale being larger than the right (L > R). Neuroimaging reveals that dyslexic subjects often exhibit left–right planum temporale symmetry (L = R) or reversed normal asymmetry (R > L). However, the nature of the reversed asymmetry differs across studies (Hynd & Hiemenz, 1997). Regional anomalies of the brains of dyslexic individuals have also been found associated with differences in brain activation as revealed by cerebral blood flow. For example, a positron emission tomog-

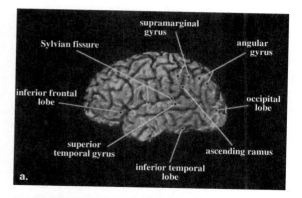

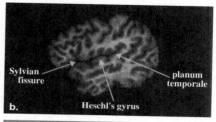

Figure 8.2 Brain regions implicated in dyslexia: (a) lateral view of the left hemisphere of the brain, (b) parasagittal slice through the left hemisphere. (From J. M. Rumsey, "Neuroimaging in Developmental Dyslexia," in G. R. Lyon and J. M. Rumsey, eds., *Neuroimaging: A Window to the Neurological Foundations of Learning and Behavior in Children,* Baltimore: Paul H. Brookes, 1996, p. 61. Reprinted by permission of Brookes Publishing Company)

raphy (PET) study by Rumsey et al. (1992) revealed less activation of the left posterior temporal and temporoparietal cortexes of dyslexic subjects relative to normal reading controls in performing a task sensitive to phonological awareness, namely rhyme detection. A related PET study (Flowers, Wood, & Naylor, 1991) of dyslexic and normally reading children found that cerebral blood flow to both the Wernicke's area (region surrounding the planum temporale) and the angular gyrus related to reading performance. Finally, postmortem investigations of the brains of dyslexic individuals revealed neuronal **ectopias** (small loci of abnormally placed neurons sometimes referred to as "brain warts") and **cytoarchitectonic dysplasia** (focal pathologic changes of cortical architecture) of the left plenum temporale, suggesting abnormal neural development, most likely between the 5th and 7th months of fetal gestation (Hynd & Hiemenz, 1997). During this period the gyri are rapidly forming, suggesting that the origin of developmental dyslexia, whether genetically determined or a consequence of an insult, can be traced to a period of fetal development. However, not all studies have replicated the finding of atypical planum temporale development (Filipek, 1996), suggesting that other neural regions/systems may be involved in the etiology of dyslexia.

Two other neural regions have received attention in the study of dyslexia, the corpus callosum and frontal cortex. Investigations produce contradictory findings regarding the structural anomalies of the corpus callosum of dyslexic individuals. These studies found that the anterior (genu) and posterior (splenium) portion of the corpus callosum of dyslexic individuals either differed from, or were comparable to, the same regions of subjects who were not reading disabled (Hynd et al., 1995; Larsen, Hoien, & Odegaard, 1992). Causal explanations for the relationship of corpus callosum to dyslexia, when structural differences were identified, centered on increased or decreased interhemispheric communication, or inappropriate inhibition of one hemisphere by the other. These conditions are believed to disrupt the flow and integration of information between the two hemispheres necessary for reading.

The frontal cortex has also received attention, with researchers observing tentative differences between proficient and disabled readers. Children with either dyslexia or ADHD presented bilaterally smaller frontal cortexes than normal control children (Hynd, Semrud-Clikeman, Lorys, Novey, & Eliopulos, 1990). Moreover, the children with dyslexia differed from the other two comparison groups by exhibiting greater symmetry of the anterior region due to the smaller width of the right frontal lobe (R = L). Similarly, in a recent pilot study (Semrud-Clikeman et al., 1996), the smaller width of the right anterior frontal cortex was one of several anatomic variables that discriminated among dyslexic, ADHD, and normal control children. The relationship of the anatomic difference of the frontal lobe to dyslexia is unclear. However, the frontal lobes mediate a number of functions, such as mental shifting and allocation of attention that are crucial to reading (James & Selz, 1997).

Although the left posterior temporal and temporoparietal regions are primarily implicated in the support of language and reading, it is simplistic to attribute dyslexia solely to anomalies in these areas. Reading is an exceptionally complex process entailing letter identification, phonological, and grapheme skills, sequencing skills, and **working memory** (a form of short-term memory). Further, the **lexicon stores,** our "internal dictionaries," must be accessed to determine the meaning of words, both singularly and in combination with other words (Kolb & Whishaw, 1996). These multiple functions warrant support by a variety of neural regions, including the temporal, parietal, occipital, and frontal regions of both hemispheres (Rumsey, 1996a; Shaywitz et al., 1996).

The next section explores the nonverbal learning disability syndrome. Children exhibiting the nonverbal learning disability syndrome potentially manifest distinctly different neuropsychological profiles from those with verbal learning disabilities. Whereas verbal learning disabilities are generally attributed to left hemisphere dysfunction and are implicated in reading disturbances, the nonverbal learning disability syndrome is attributed to right hemisphere dysfunction, and is associated with deficits in mathematics. It is to a unique learning disability featuring dyscalculia that we now turn our attention.

NONVERBAL LEARNING DISABILITY SYNDROME (NVLD)

Clinical Presentation and Prevalence

The concept of nonverbal learning disability syndrome (NVLD) as a neuropsychological disorder has been developed by the ongoing investigations of Byron Rourke, who has attempted to identify the neurocognitive, psychosocial, and adaptive characteristics of children with learning disabilities. His investigative efforts revealed two basic subtypes of learning disability; one labeled R-S, for reading and spelling disability, and the other NVLD, for nonverbal learning disability syndrome. R-S children demonstrated weak psycholinguistic skills with relatively preserved skills in visual-perceptual, tactile-perceptual, psychomotor, and nonverbal/novel problem solving (see Table 8.1). Reading and spelling skills were poor, with greater competency evident in mechanical arithmetic, although this was still below age expectancy. Rourke, (1993) hypothesized that the neuropsychological deficits of the R-S group were associated with left hemisphere dysfunctions.

In contrast, children in the NVLD group presented essentially the opposite pattern of strengths and deficits as the R-S group (see Table 8.2). That is, the NVLD group showed relatively poor skills in visual-perceptual, tactile-perceptual, psychomotor, and nonverbal/novel problem-solving skills coupled with strengths in the psycholinguistic domain. They showed major academic weaknesses in basic arithmetic, but they demonstrated preserved linguistic skills such as sight word reading (Harnadek & Rourke, 1994). Note that both groups exhibited comparable deficits in actual arithmetic achievement; however, Rourke (1993) attributed the poor performance of the R-S group to verbal deficits, and the low performance of the children with NVLD to weaknesses in visual-perceptual and nonverbal reasoning.

Researchers estimate the prevalence of the NVLD syndrome within clinic populations at 5% to 10% (Rourke, 1989). Further, the NVLD syndrome represents between 0.1% and 1.0% of the entire learning disability population, with an overall ratio of male to female of approximately 1.2 to 1.0 (Pennington, 1991).

Neuropsychological Pathogenesis

Rourke (1993) considers that the NVLD syndrome reflects right hemisphere (particularly posterior) damage, or dysfunction, whereas R-S deficits more closely reflect problems in the left, language-dominant, hemisphere system. Rourke adopted Goldberg and Costa's (1981) theorization of brain functioning in conceptualizing the neuropathogenesis of the NVLD syndrome. Goldberg and Costa proposed that the right hemisphere, relative to the left, is more diffusely organized, has more association regions, and shows greater

Table 8.1 *Core and Clinical Features of the Reading and Spelling Group*

Neuropsychological Assets	Neuropsychological Deficits
Primary assets	*Primary deficits*
Motor and psychomotor	Auditory perception
Novel material	
Tactile perception	
Visual perception	
Secondary assets	*Secondary deficits*
Tactile attention	Auditory attention
Visual attention	Verbal attention
Tertiary assets	*Tertiary deficits*
Concept formation	Auditory memory
Problem solving	Verbal memory
Tactile memory	
Visual memory	
Verbal assets	*Verbal deficits*
Pragmatics	Phonology
Prosody	Verbal association
Semantic > phonology content	Verbal output (volume)
Verbal associations function	Verbal reception
	Verbal repetition
	Verbal storage
Academic assets	*Academic deficits*
Reading comprehension (late)	Comprehension (early)
Mathematics	Graphomotor
Reading	Mechanical arithmetic
Science	Reading
	Spelling
	Verbatim memory
	Word decoding
Socioemotional/adaptive assets	*Socioemotional/adaptive deficits*
Activity level	Undetermined
Adaptive to novelty	
Emotional stability	
Social competence	

Source: Rourke and Fuerst (1996), p. 282. From *Assessment 3*. Reprinted by permission of the publisher.

specialization for *interregional* integration of information. Because of its capacity to integrate input from multiple brain regions, the right hemisphere is more adept at processing complex, novel, or ambiguous information. In contrast, the left hemisphere is more

Table 8.2 *Core and Clinical Features of the Nonverbal Learning Disability Syndrome*

Neuropsychological Assets	Neuropsychological Deficits
Primary assets	*Primary deficits*
Auditory perception	Complex psychomotor
Rote material	Novel material
Simple motor	Tactile perception
	Visual perception
Secondary assets	*Secondary deficits*
Auditory attention	Exploratory behavior
Verbal attention	Tactile attention
	Visual attention
Tertiary assets	*Tertiary deficits*
Auditory memory	Concept formation
Verbal memory	Problem solving
	Tactile memory
	Visual memory
Verbal assets	*Verbal deficits*
Phonology	Oral-motor praxis
Verbal association	Phonology > semantics content
Verbal output	Pragmatics function
Verbal reception	Prosody
Verbal repetition	
Verbal storage	
Academic assets	*Academic deficits*
Graphomotor (late)	Graphomotor (early)
Spelling	Mechanical arithmetic
Verbatim memory	Reading comprehension
Word decoding	Science
Socioemotional/adaptive assets	*Socioemotional/adaptive deficits*
Undetermined	Activity level
	Adaptive to novelty
	Emotional stability
	Social competence

Source: Rourke and Fuerst (1996), p. 281. From *Assessment 3.* Reprinted by permission of the publisher.

focally organized, presents greater modality-specific cortical regions, and shows greater specialization for *intraregional* integration of input. The specialization of the left hemisphere is hypothesized to relate to the routine application of previously acquired cognitive strategies. The two hemispheres complement one an-other with the right hemisphere showing prominence in establishing new rules, routines, or strategies, and the left storing and applying these newly established computations in similar situations, or with comparable tasks in the future (Fisher, Deluca, & Rourke, 1997).

Rourke (1995) maintains that the primary deficits of tactile-perceptual, visual-perceptual, and psychomotor abilities of the NVLD syndrome are consistent with damage or dysfunction of right hemisphere interregional integration; whereas, assets of auditory-perceptual and verbal skills suggest a relatively intact left hemisphere. He also sees deficits such as poor problem solving in novel situations, or in the face of complexity, weaknesses in conceptual thinking, and impaired socioemotional skills as emanating from right hemisphere involvement.

Rourke suggests that although right hemisphere damage is *sufficient* to produce the NVLD syndrome, it is the destruction of the white matter required for interregional integration that is *necessary* for producing the disorder. That is, the development of the NVLD syndrome can be caused by damage to white fibers (1) accessing the right hemisphere, (2) connecting cortical regions within the right hemisphere, or (3) linking cortical to subcortical regions within the right hemisphere (Rourke, 1995). Interestingly, Rourke hypothesizes that damage to these different communicating fibers accompanies diverse disorders in association with the NVLD syndrome. For example, early damage to the association fibers of the right and left hemispheres could potentially cause both the primary features of the NVLD syndrome and the global linguistic deficiencies that characterize autism.

Although Rourke emphasizes the posterior right hemisphere as playing an important role in the pathogenesis of the NVLD syndrome, he proposes that the anterior brain regions may also be involved. For example, children with NVLD performed in a less efficient manner than children with verbal learning disabilities in carrying out higher-order mental operations such as conceptual thinking and mental flexibility (Fisher et al., 1997). Moreover, Rourke (1995) indicates that the frontal system is necessary for (1) integrating lower-level systems (such as sensorimotor) to formulate higher-order levels of abstraction, (2) responding to novelty and complexity, and (3) **metacognition,** that is, the ability to understand the operation of one's own cognitive processes. Rourke believes that damage to the interconnecting white matter tracks between the frontal lobes and the posterior regions of the right hemisphere contributes to the deficits of higher-order cognition evident in the NVLD syndrome.

Many disorders and brain insults accompany the NVLD syndrome, spanning genetic, chromosomal, structural, and environmental anomalies. Table 8.3 presents a partial list. Although these disorders and insults represent a varied and seemingly dissimilar set of etiologies, clinical presentations, and developmental courses, Rourke and Del Dotto (1994) suggest that each shares a common pathway to the NVLD syndrome, namely dysfunction of the white matter (myelinated circuitry) of the brain. These disorders represent a spectrum of neurodevelopmental conditions that vary in the severity of expression of the NVLD syndrome, ranging from disorders that present virtually all the assets and deficits of the NVLD syndrome (such as hydrocephalus and Asperger's syndrome), to those that display a majority of the assets and deficits (such as FAS and TS), and finally, to those that exhibit only a subset of the assets and deficits of the NVLD syndrome (such as autism). Thus, varying numbers of assets/deficits of the NVLD syndrome are comorbid manifestations of these disorders caused by damage to the white matter (Rourke, 1995).

Neuropsychological Assessment

Harnadek and Rourke (1994) attempted to identify the primary neuropsychological deficits of the NVLD group. They presented selected groups of NVLD, R-S, and normal control (NC) children with a battery of neuropsychological measures recommended for diagnosing the NVLD syndrome (see Table 8.4 on p. 270). Of the full battery of 13 measures, two sets of tests statistically differentiated the NVLD, R-S, and NC groups. The first set of four measures (Target Test, Trail Making Test-B, Tactual Performance Test, and Grooved Pegboard Test) assesses visual-spatial or-

Table 8.3 **Brain Disorders and Insults Associated with Nonverbal Learning Disability Syndrome**
Asperger's syndrome
Autism
Callosal agenesis (absence of the corpus callosum)
Congenital hypothyroidism
Cranial irradiation
Fetal alcohol syndrome
Hydrocephalus
Insulin-dependent diabetes mellitus
Intracranial tumors
Metachromatic leukodystrophy (genetic metabolic disorder)
Myelomeningocele (neural tube defect)
Sotos syndrome (growth disorder)
Traumatic brain injury
Triple X syndrome (genetic neurodevelopmental disorder)
Turner's syndrome
William's syndrome (genetic neurodevelopmental disorder)

Source: Adapted from Tsatsanis and Rourke (1995), *Syndrome of Nonverbal Learning Disabilities: Neurodevelopmental Manifestations.* Reprinted by permission of The Guilford Press.

ganization, tactile-perceptual, and psychomotor skills, and the second set of tests (Wide Range Achievement Test and Speech Sounds Perception Test) is sensitive to academic (reading) and auditory-perceptual skills. These two sets of measures accurately classified the children in their respective groups at an overall classification rate of 98%. Whether the six measures are sufficiently sensitive to be employed for individual diagnosis, thus reducing the need for the full battery, awaits additional study.

As previously noted, children with NVLD frequently exhibit arithmetic deficits. Rourke and Conway (1997) hypothesized that during the initial learning of arithmetic skills in childhood, the novel, visual-spatial, and conceptual nature of the content

Table 8.4 *Neuropsychological Measures for Nonverbal Learning Disability Syndrome*

Neurocognitive

Auditory Closure Test (Kass, 1964)

Category Test (Reitan & Davison, 1974)

Grooved Pegboard Test (Klove, 1963)

Reitan-Klove Sensory-Perceptual Exam (Reitan, 1984)

Sentence Memory Test (Benton, 1965)

Speech Sounds Perception Test (Reitan & Davison, 1974)

Tactual Performance Test (Reitan & Davison, 1974)

Target Test (Reitan, 1966)

Trail Making Test (Reitan & Davison, 1974)

Verbal Fluency Test (Rourke, Bakker, Fisk, & Strang, 1983)

Wechsler Intelligence Scale for Children–Revised (Wechsler, 1974).

Academic

Peabody Picture Vocabulary Test (Dunn, 1965)

Reading, Spelling and Arithmetic (Jastak & Jastak, 1965)

Wide Range Achievement Test

Source: Harnadek and Rourke (1994). From the *Journal of Learning Disabilities, 27,* 144–154. Reprinted by permission of the publisher.

recruits mainly right hemispheric systems. Once these skills are learned, however, function shifts to the left hemisphere because of its greater facility in processing and retrieving automatic information (Dool, Stelmack, & Rourke, 1993).

Examining the mathematical performance of children with NVLD, researchers identified seven overlapping errors (Rourke, 1993). These included (1) errors in spatial organization, (2) misreading or omitting required mathematical symbols, (3) failure to apply or misapplication of mathematical procedures, (4) poorly formed or spaced numbers, (5) failure to remember number facts or arithmetic rules, (6) difficulties shifting from one set of arithmetic operations to another, and (7) poor arithmetic judgment and reasoning. The latter error involves production of

unreasonable solutions, or failure to generalize solutions, strategies, or plans for new or different arithmetic problems. Although children with other forms of learning and neuropsychological deficits can show errors involving spatial and retrieval deficits, several of the errors, particularly those due to poor judgment and reasoning, discriminated children with NVLD from other learning-disabled children. Errors in cognitive shifting, judgment, and reasoning potentially implicate deficits in executive function.

Socioemotional Characteristics

A broad set of adaptive and socioemotional disturbances accompany the NVLD syndrome. Rourke believes these deficits are a direct consequence of the core deficits of the disorder (see Table 8.2). Of these deficits, the most prominent lie in the communication and interactional domains. The communication deficits appear in both verbal and nonverbal behaviors. At the verbal level, children and adolescents with NVLD tend to talk excessively, present tangential contents, and show a poor understanding of the **pragmatics of language,** that is, the emotional and social content of a message. Moreover, they find it difficult to understand the nonverbal behavior of others and to convey information through their own nonverbal behaviors (Rourke, Fisk, & Strang, 1986).

Regarding social behavior, deficits in social sensitivity, interactional skills, social problem solving, and judgment seriously hinder the efforts of individuals with NVLD to relate to others. They are prone to misread, or fail to appreciate the social intents, perspectives, or feelings of others. In addition, they do not accurately assess social cause-and-effect relationships (Rourke & Fuerst, 1996). Social problem solving is particularly compromised in new, changing, or complex social situations, often resulting in rigid or stereotypic responses that are inappropriate to the demands of the situation. Because of poor social judgment, caretakers and peers view the individual with NVLD as lacking in common sense. Frequently the child or adolescent encounters difficulties generalizing social skills learned in one situation to another, even though the new situation is similar to the original learning context. Social conventions, such as maintaining eye contact and appropriate social distance, are often violated. Finally, the poor psychomotor skills and clumsiness that children with NVLD exhibit can elicit teasing and taunting from peers.

Although prone to acting-out behaviors and symptoms of ADHD while young (Voeller, 1996), children with NVLD tend to become shy and withdrawn with increasing age. Assessment by their mothers reveals that children with NVLD often present internalizing symptoms such as anxiety, depression, withdrawal, and poor social skills. Whether this is a direct response to their failures within the social sphere is unclear, although it is likely that social failings contribute to the emotional distress of children and adolescents with NVLD.

Neuropsychological Model

Rourke's model of learning disability, with regard to subtypes such as NVLD and R-S, is summarized as follows:

Subtypes of LD [learning disabilities] are manifestations of distinct profiles of neuropsychological assets and deficits; the subtypes of LD may lead to specific problems in academic functioning, psychosocial functioning, or both; and, the relationship between profiles of neuropsychological assets and deficits, LD, and academic and social learning deficits can be understood fully only within a neurodevelopmental framework that takes into consideration the changing nature of the academic, psychosocial, and vocational demands that humans in a particular society confront. (Rourke & Fuerst, 1996; p. 278)

A hierarchical organization is evident, with primary neurocognitive assets and deficits leading to predictable and differential patterns of neuropsychological functioning (secondary, tertiary, and linguistic) that, in turn, directly affect academic, socioemotional, and adaptive functioning (see Tables 8.1 and 8.2). Thus, the adequacy of the child's sensorimotor development sets the stage for subsequent levels of cognitive development. The young child experiences the world through touch, movement, and vision. Contacting and exploring the environment through the basic sensory modalities fosters the development of increasingly complex and higher-level mental structures. The NVLD child with early deficits in tactile-perceptual, visual-perceptual, and psychomotor domains is limited in the sensorimotor learning necessary for forming the basic building blocks of more advanced mental structures. Rourke and others believe these early limitations bias the later development of conceptual thinking, creative problem solving, communication skills, and socioemotional interactions. As the child moves into adolescence and developmental tasks become increasingly complex, the functional deficits become more apparent. Unfortunately, the impairments of the adult are even more pronounced, as evident in the common finding of marginal adaptive success across behavioral domains.

Little (1993) indicates that the primary deficits and assets of the NVLD syndrome are a robust finding in the studies of learning disabilities. However, support for the socioemotional aspects of the disorder is less compelling.

Developmental Course

The developmental course of the NVLD syndrome is somewhat similar to the natural history reported for Turner's syndrome and higher-functioning autistic/Asperger's syndrome children (see section later on pervasive developmental disorders). For the NVLD infant-toddler, exploratory behavior and motor skills lag behind language development. With increasing age, delays hinder the development of self-help skills, and the child tends to depend too much on caretakers. Increasingly, the child encounters difficulties in the social domain, with playmates being either younger or older than the child with NVLD.

In the elementary years, children with NVLD are prone to act out, respond impulsively, exhibit hyperactivity, and encounter problems in sustaining attention (Rourke et al., 1986). Despite relatively advanced verbal skills, communication patterns (both verbal and nonverbal) are often inappropriate. Misperceptions of social situations, impaired social problem solving and judgment, and poor social skills compromise efforts to relate successfully with peers. The child develops few, if any, close friendships and, during adolescence, peers often avoid teenagers with NVLD. Increasingly, NVLD adolescents become socially withdrawn and isolated, and show internalizing symptoms of anxiety and depression. Developmental patterns for adults with NVLD await clarification. Unfortunately,

NVLD adults show elevated rates of psychopathology, and their risk for depression and suicidal behavior appears high.

Treatment

Because of the communication and social deficits often associated with the NVLD syndrome, the child needs help developing verbal and nonverbal communication skills, basic social skills (such as greeting), and more advanced social skills (social awareness, friendship skills, and social problem solving). Early and ongoing interventions focused on the development of communication and social skills may improve the child's acceptance by peers. The young child with NVLD who exhibits ADHD symptoms may benefit from increased structuring of home and school activities, and from psychostimulant or related medications. Further, the parents can profit from learning management techniques to foster greater self-help skills and independence by the child.

Children with NVLD are at risk for developing psychological difficulties. Parents and professionals should be aware of this risk and prepare to provide early interventions if psychological problems arise. They should pay particular attention to the NVLD youngster with depressive symptoms that might signal an increased risk of suicide.

Rourke and Del Dotto (1994) developed a comprehensive intervention program for children and adolescents with NVLD. The program actively involves the caretakers from its inception. A set of general principles organizes and guides treatment, with each program requiring individualization to accommodate the strengths and deficits of each child. Initially, the program provides the caretakers with information that helps them understand the nature and extent of the child's disorder and develop realistic expectations. Then the program provides interventions that will help the child: (1) understand, learn, and generalize cognitive and social problem-solving strategies; (2) develop necessary communication skills; (3) engage and interact appropriately with others; (4) explore and experience his or her environment; (5) use available aids (such as a digital watch for learning time concepts); and (6) gain a realistic view of his or her strengths and weaknesses.

School-age children who suffer from NVLD are at risk for academic difficulties, particularly if spatial reasoning or executive deficits are severe. Subjects that commonly produce difficulties include handwriting and mathematics. As it is highly unlikely that children with NVLD will outgrow these deficits, programs should direct interventions toward helping them develop compensatory skills and strategies. For example, children with NVLD often dislike writing because of spatial and motor deficits. Accordingly, parents and professionals should encourage them, at an early age, to develop word processing skills. Similarly, adolescents with NVLD need help in developing realistic academic and career goals in light of their individual strengths and visual-spatial and mathematical weaknesses.

Pervasive Developmental Disorders

Pervasive developmental disorders encompass a set of very severe neuropsychological deficits that are evident early in childhood and have a poor prognosis for achieving normal adaptive functioning. To varying degrees, each of the pervasive developmental disorders involves impairment in one or more of the following domains of development: social interactions, verbal and nonverbal language, range of interests and activities, and flexibility of behavior. The behaviors manifested in these domains are age inappropriate and are disproportionate to the child's intelligence and age, even though mental retardation is frequently a correlate of the disorders. Researchers hypothesize that a myriad of central nervous system abnormalities play roles in the etiology of the pervasive developmental disorders. However, in many cases the origin of the disorder remains unknown. Table 8.5 summarizes the primary pervasive developmental disorders and associated behavioral and related features.

AUTISM

Background and Clinical Presentation

Leo Kanner and Hans Asperger are credited with the identification, first theoretical conceptualization, and labeling of the developmental disorder **autism** (Frith,

Table 8.5   *Distinguishing Features of Pervasive Developmental Disorders*

Autistic Disorder

Impairment or delays in the domains of social interactions and communications (including symbolic and imitative play), and repetitive and stereotyped patterns of behavior, interests, and activities, with age of onset evident before age 3.

Asperger's Disorder

Symptom presentation similar to autism with regard to delays in developing age-appropriate social interactions and repetitive and stereotyped patterns of behavior, interests, and activities. Unlike autism, few significant developmental delays in language, cognitive, adaptive (other than social), self-help, and exploratory behaviors are evident.

Rett's Disorder

Initially, normal psychomotor development with normal head circumference. Between 5 and 48 months head growth decelerates, accompanied by the loss of acquired hand motor movements, diminished social interest, emergence of poorly coordinated gait or trunk movements, and severely impaired language development with psychomotor retardation. Present only in female children.

Childhood Disintegrative Disorder

Normal development across behavioral domains is evident until 2 years of age or later. Previously acquired skills deteriorate in two or more of the following domains: language, social or adaptive behaviors, elimination control, play, or motor skills. The emergence of autistic-like symptoms in social relatedness, communication, and repetitive and stereotypic behavior is evident. The loss of skills can plateau or continue to decline if accompanied by a degenerative neurologic disorder. Present in male and female children, with greater prevalence in males.

Source: Adapted with permission from American Psychiatric Association (1994), from the *Diagnostic and Statistical Manual of Mental Disorders, 4th Ed.,* © 1994 APA.

1989). Autism entails severe impairments in social relatedness and language development, and the presentation of unusual, repetitive, and/or stereotypic patterns of behavior. Kanner, working in Baltimore, and Asperger in Vienna each studied a group of very disturbed children for whom there was little recognition, much less understanding. Independently, each published their classic papers (Asperger, 1944/1991; Kanner, 1943) without consultation or reported awareness of the other. Remarkably, both employed the term *autistic* in characterizing the disorder. Asperger's work, largely ignored until recent years, is often associated with a higher-functioning level or subtype of autism, **Asperger's syndrome,** in which near normal to normal functioning is evident in several behavioral domains (Frith, 1991).

The first area of disturbance in autism, impairment in the ability to relate to others, particularly with regard to understanding and entering into reciprocal social relationships, is the cardinal symptom of the disorder. Kanner (1943) referred to this very dramatic aspect of behavior as **"autistic aloneness,"** a psychological state of profound separation and disconnection from other people. At a behavioral level, the autistic child exhibits this social disconnection by displaying (1) a limited awareness of, or interest in, the desires, needs, distress, or presence of others; (2) an emotional remoteness or aloofness; (3) a failure to share activities, pleasures and achievements with others; (4) a lack of understanding of social convention; (5) an impairment in social perspective and empathetic role taking; (6) a restricted repertoire of social skills, such as greeting behavior; and (7) awkward or stereotypic responses to others (Bailey et al., 1996). Moreover, autistic children often show deficits in **joint attention** (reciprocal attention between the child and another), poor conversational skills, lack of eye contact, unusual body postures or gestures, and inappropriate facial expressions (Charman, 1997; Pennington & Ozonoff, 1996).

The second core characteristic of autistic behavior, deficits in communication, appears in impairments of language expression and comprehension (Minshew, Goldstein & Siegel, 1995). Spoken language may be delayed in onset or fail to develop altogether, and the child makes little effort to compensate through nonverbal behaviors such as gestures or facial expressions. When language is present, the child may restrict it to the repetitive use of stereotypic or idiosyncratic content. Caretakers see deficits in the understanding and use of pragmatics of language (Rumsey, 1996b), and deviant forms of language such as **echolalia** (repeating the words or phrases of others), pronoun reversal, and **neologisms** (invention of words). The ability to understand language is often impaired and limited to the comprehension of simple, literal contents.

The ability to initiate and enter into symbolic, pretend, or imitative play is minimally developed (McDonough, Stahmer, Schreibman, & Thompson, 1997). Initially, the child shows little interest in toys, suggesting delayed or poor comprehension of the symbolic meaning of toys (Minshew, 1997). As interest develops, the child manipulates toys repetitively as objects without symbolic or imaginative connotations. Insofar as pretend play is considered necessary for the development of social and communication skills, the autistic child can rarely partake in complex, imaginative, or cooperative play.

The third core feature of autism relates to one or more of the following unusual behavioral patterns: (1) preoccupation with specific areas of interest, objects, or qualities of objects; (2) demands for environmental or behavioral sameness; and (3) stereotypic body movements or abnormalities of posture (American Psychiatric Association, 1994).

A fascination with and abnormal focus on areas of interest (such as geography), objects (fans, vacuum cleaners, and so on), parts of objects (such as buttons), movement of objects (such as spinning toys), or activities (such as drawing) can dominate the child's daily pursuits. Moreover, the child may demand the maintenance of constancy (for example, the child's room cannot be altered), order (toys must be lined up in a certain manner), or routine (the child must always walk the same route to the playground). Interference or disturbance of the child's involvement in areas of interest or the child's efforts to maintain constancy can prompt a range of responses from irritation, to overwhelming anxiety, to thunderous rage. Finally, disturbances of motility can encompass a wide range of movements such as rocking, spinning, twisting, or hand flapping (see Figure 8.3). A variety of unusual postural movements may also be evident. Examples of these are a tendency to walk on tiptoe, holding the hands in an awkward manner, and walking without moving the arms.

Demographic and Comorbid Conditions

Researchers estimate the prevalence of autism at 4 to 20 affected children per 10,000, with males outnumbering females by a ratio of 2 to 6 males for every 1

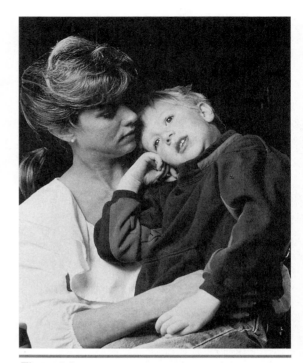

Figure 8.3   An autistic boy with stereotyped behaviors involving pulling on his ears and biting his hand. (Robert Fish/Monterey County Herald)

female (Fein, Joy, Green, & Waterhouse, 1996). Many autistic children (50% to 80%) function within the retarded range of intelligence, as evident in IQ scores below 70 (Bailey et al., 1996; Ornitz, 1992). However, some autistic individuals demonstrate average to above-average intelligence. An inverse relationship exists between IQ and severity of autistic symptoms. That is, the higher the level of intelligence, the less severe the autistic symptoms. Circumscribed abilities and skills of exceptional levels (such as **hyperlexia,** or early acquisition of reading skills without comprehension) may appear within the context of severe mental retardation. The rate of **savant skills**—extraordinarily developed skills within the context of limited cognitive capability—in autism is estimated to be 10 times that of the normal population (Waterhouse, Fein, & Modahl, 1996). The risk for seizure disorders is high in autistic groups, with rates ranging from 20% to 30% and even higher for autistic children with IQs less than 50 (Fein et al., 1996).

High-Functioning Autism or Asperger's Syndrome?

Currently, there is controversy over whether the two primary representatives of pervasive developmental disorders, autism and Asperger's syndrome, are separate disorders, overlapping subtypes, or one disorder with Asperger's syndrome representing autistic individuals who are higher functioning, both cognitively and adaptively. Before considering this controversy, we will review the symptom presentation of Asperger's syndrome.

The term *Asperger's syndrome* refers to a group of children or adults who exhibit autistic-like symptoms, but fail to strictly fulfill the autism criteria. The criteria for autism and Asperger's syndrome of the American Psychiatric Association (APA, 1994) reveal a significant overlap in symptoms related to impairments in social interactions and preoccupations with narrow, repetitive, and stereotypic patterns of behavior, interests, and activities. Despite this overlap, the APA proposes several differences. Specifically, children with autistic-like behavior are *not* to receive the diagnosis of Asperger's syndrome if they exhibit (1) significant impairment in verbal and nonverbal communication skills, (2) a lack of developmentally appropriate symbolic or imaginative play, (3) delayed language development or absence of language, (4) cognitive deficits, (5) impairment in self-help and adaptive skills (excluding those involving social interactions), and (6) limited or absent exploratory curiosity (Bailey et al., 1996). These exclusionary criteria are consistent with Asperger's original behavioral description of children exhibiting the disorder. That is, these children display poor social skills, odd and eccentric behaviors, and restrictive patterns of interests and activities, without significant delays in cognitive or language abilities.

A recent study (Eisenmajer et al., 1996) sought to further clarify the differences between Asperger's syndrome and autism. Children diagnosed as exhibiting Asperger's syndrome, as contrasted with autism, showed a greater (1) desire for social contact and friendship; (2) willingness to participate in play with other children centered on their special interest, such as dinosaurs; (3) likelihood of normal onset of language development and an absence of echolalia; (4) use of odd words of speech, pedantic speech, and one-sided, repetitive conversations; (5) tendency to pursue narrow and limited areas of interest, such as preoccupation with clocks; and (6) likelihood of being inattentive, impulsive, and overactive.

Despite the findings of behavioral differences, the separation of the two disorders poses several challenges. First, varied definitions and differential selection criteria artificially blur the boundaries between the two disorders, hindering efforts to identify commonalities and differences in cognition and behavior, etiology, and responsiveness to differential treatment. Second, the reported difference between autistism and Asperger's syndrome may reflect the level of intellectual or language development of the two disorders. By definition, one criterion for differentiating Asperger's syndrome from autism is the relative absence of language and cognitive impairment in Asperger's syndrome. Thus, children with Asperger's syndrome may simply be brighter autistic children who show fewer language deficits. Third, younger, higher-functioning autistic children frequently exhibit behaviors consistent with Kanner's characterization of autism. With maturity, however, they often show fewer autistic symptoms (Szatmari, Archer, Fisman, Streiner, & Wilson, 1995). Accordingly, Asperger's syndrome may merely reflect the changing presentation, over time, of higher-functioning autistic individuals.

The case study of Tom Z. familiarizes the student with Asperger's syndrome (see Neuropsychology in Action 8.2). The study details the symptoms, evaluative data, and family history of Tom Z., and some rather surprising neuroimaging findings.

Neuropsychological Pathogenesis

Various researchers attribute the development of autism to a host of etiological factors. There are indications that the disorder is familial and genetic in origin; however, the finding of high rates of perinatal complications in the history of autistic children also implicates environmental factors. There is some evidence for an autistic diathesis, that is, a genetically

Neuropsychology in Action 8.2

Case Study of an Adolescent with Asperger's Syndrome

Tom Z. is a tall, stocky 15-year-old. He was born following an uncomplicated pregnancy, and subsequent developmental milestones were achieved within normal limits. Tom talked before he walked. He taught himself to read by age 3 and was reading adult-level books by age 4. By the age of 2½ years he had atypical interests that were pursued to the exclusion of other activities. Over the years these interests have included stop signs, arrows, storm drains, windmills, clocks, mathematics, and computers.

In nursery school he had poor peer relations, talked incessantly about topics of interest only to himself, failed to listen to the comments of others, and was often oppositional and impulsive. A clumsy and poorly coordinated child, he often seemed markedly odd. A preschool psychological assessment recommended special education placement, and the parents tried various programs with limited success. They finally moved him to homebound education. Despite precocious academic achievements, Tom continued to have significant problems with social interaction and in controlling his behavior.

At his first formal evaluation, when he was 9½ years old, Tom had no friends, poor interpersonal skills, and signs of depression. His fascination with clocks pervaded all conversation. His poor social judgment was clearly evident, particularly in his description of interactions with peers. He showed limited nonverbal social behaviors, such as gestures, facial grimaces, emphasis of voice, and nonliteral communications. Interestingly, Tom's father had a history

of similar problems. For example, Mr. Z. carried a small notebook to write down the names of important people he met because, "I can never remember people's faces; I can only remember names when I write them down."

Tom was evaluated again when he was 12 years old. He continued to show a markedly eccentric social style and engaged in one-sided conversations about computers and mathematical concepts in a loud, poorly modulated voice. His very limited awareness of social conventions was evident in his one-sided conversational style, his tendency to belch and pass gas in public, and his use of graphic expletives without apparent intention to shock others. He was preoccupied with the subject of girlfriends and his sexual needs.

Tom's clinical presentation and assessment results were extreme in many respects. There was a significant discrepancy between his Wechsler Intelligence Scale for Children–Third Edition (WISC-III; Wechsler, 1991) verbal and performance abilities (Verbal IQ = 139 and Performance IQ = 127). He had superior scores in verbal reasoning, except for tasks involving social comprehension. Although able to describe social demands, he could not translate this knowledge into appropriate conduct. He also exhibited significant deficits in visual-motor skills, speed of processing, and motor functioning. Moreover, a large difference existed between his very superior intelligence score and his ratings on a measure of adaptive skills. His adaptive rating score was significantly below average, indicating very severe

deficits in meeting the demands of everyday life.

Neuroimaging

Father and son underwent magnetic resonance imaging (MRI) of the brain. The father's sagittal brain images showed a large V-shaped wedge of missing tissue in the dorsolateral frontal region of the brain (see Figure 8.4a). This region of tissue loss appeared in the same location of both hemispheres, but was somewhat larger in the left. Given the absence of a history of trauma, the tissue loss likely represented an area of focal dysmorphology of unknown origin.

Tom showed a similar, but noticeably smaller region of structural anomalies in exactly the same area of both hemispheres. His abnormality, however, was somewhat larger on the right, the reverse of the father's (Figure 8.4b). In addition, he showed decreased tissue in the anterior-mesial region of the left temporal lobe (Figure 8.4c). The similarity of abnormalities in Mr. Z. and Tom indicated potential familial transmission.

Discussion of MRI and Psychological Testing

A three-dimensional rendering of the father's brain showed his neurodevelopmental abnormality to be in the region of the middle frontal gyrus (Figure 8.4d). The deficit was a recessed area of absent tissue. Further, the three-dimensional image revealed an abnormality that did not show on the two-dimensional images: both right and left frontal lobes showed an abnormal pattern of gyri and sulci. Normally, the frontal lobe consists

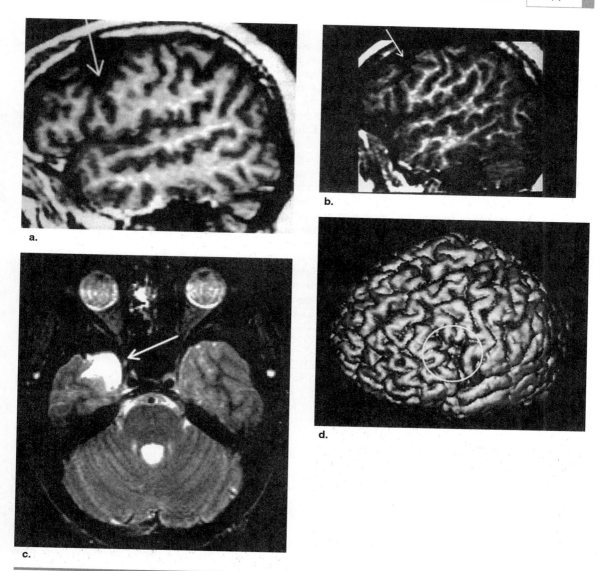

Figure 8.4 (a) Sagittal image of the father's brain, showing a triangular region of missing tissue in the dorso-lateral aspects of the left frontal lobe. (b) Sagittal image of the son's brain, showing a similar by smaller abnormality in exactly the same location as the father's. (c) Axial view of the son's brain. The arrow points to the anterior mesial aspects of the left temporal lobe, where a pocket of CSF fills a region of decreased brain tissue. (d) Three-dimensional reconstruction of the father's brain images. The circle encompasses the region of missing tissue first seen in two dimensions in (a). (From F. R. Volkmar, A. Klin, R. Schultz, R. Bronen, W. D. Marans, S. Sparrow, and D. J. Cohen, "Asperger's Syndrome," *Journal of the American Academy of Clinical and Adolescent Psychiatry, 35,* 1996, p. 121, Figures 1 and 2; p. 122, Figures 3 and 4. Reprinted by permission of Lippincott, Williams & Wilkins.)

(continued)

(continued)

of three prominent horizontal gyri (the superior, middle, and inferior gyri) that run in parallel from anterior to posterior. Although the father's superior frontal gyrus appeared normal, the middle frontal gyri were vertical in both hemispheres. This aberrant pattern of surface structure may have originated from an abnormal prenatal developmental process.

Because of movement artifacts, a clear three-dimensional representation of Tom's brain was not possible. However, researchers reconstructed coronal images by computer methods to evaluate his left temporal lobe abnormality. The images revealed a large region of missing tissue and also an asymmetry of the lateral ventricles.

Any single case report must be interpreted with caution, yet it is of interest that Tom's neuropsychological deficits are understandable in light of his brain abnormalities and other studies of individuals with autism, Asperger's syndrome, and similar disorders (for example, see Piven et al., 1990). As described earlier, Tom's psychological testing revealed significantly higher WISC-III Verbal IQ relative to Performance IQ. Consistent with his greater nonverbal difficulties, Tom's frontal lobe abnormalities were more prominent on the right than left side. The right hemisphere is more prominently involved than the left hemisphere in regulating language prosody and pragmatics (Kolb & Whishaw, 1990), two areas in which Tom performed poorly. Moreover, the volume of his left hemisphere was somewhat larger

than that of the right. In a study published several years ago, Willerman, Schultz, Rutledge, & Bigler (1992) found that a larger left than right hemisphere predicted a higher Verbal IQ than Performance IQ in males.

The frontal lobe findings may clarify Tom's motor difficulties and conceptual inflexibility. The structural abnormality was at the juncture of the primary motor strip, premotor area, and dorsolateral convexity, thus potentially affecting the functions mediated by each of these regions. The dorsolateral prefrontal cortex is known to be involved in the executive functions of working memory and shielding of cognitive operations from disruption by unwanted distractions (Goldman-Rakic, 1987a).

Source: Adapted from Volkmar et al. (1996).

---

mediated vulnerability for autism that interacts with an early environmental insult to produce the disorder (Pennington, 1991).

Further support for a familial/genetic component of autism is the finding of relatively high rates of the disorder in the siblings of autistic children. The rate is approximately 3% to 6%, which is significantly higher than the incidence in normal populations (Frombonne, Bolton, Prior, Jordon, & Rutter, 1997). Heritability studies of identical twins reveal co-occurrence rates of 36% to 96%, whereas rates for fraternal twins range from 0% to 24% (Bailey et al., 1996; Fein et al., 1996). The substantial co-occurrence rates for identical twins suggest that genetic factors play a significant role in the etiology of autism.

The neural substrates considered to produce autism are numerous, but none have received unanimous support. Anatomic abnormalities, hypothesized or identified in autistic samples, have included most cortical and subcortical regions of the brain. In addition, empirical studies reveal differences in brain volume, metabolism, and cellular migratory patterns of the cortex (Lainhart et al., 1997; Piven, Arndt, Bailey, &

Andreasen, 1996; Rumsey, 1996b). The neural regions and systems receiving the most consistent attention are the cerebellum, hippocampus, amygdala, and other limbic nuclei (Fein et al., 1996). I discuss the relationship of anomalies of these neural regions/systems to the behaviors of autism in a later section on the comprehensive neurofunctional model in this chapter.

Studies have also implicated abnormalities involving neurotransmitters as pathogenic of autism, with serotonin receiving the most attention. Serotonin (5-HT) is involved in regulating a number of brain functions, including learning, memory, sleep, pain responsiveness, affect, and inhibitory processes. In addition, there are indications that excessive 5-HT can disrupt social affiliation and attachment (Chamberlain & Herman, 1990). Approximately 30% of autistic children exhibit hyperserotonemia (excessive 5-HT), although the precise role of 5-HT in the production of autistic symptoms is unclear. Even more troublesome are studies showing that elevated levels of serotonin are not specific to autism, with other disorders such as mental retardation also exhibiting hyperserotonemia (Fein et al., 1996).

Neuropsychological Assessment

The diagnosis of autism requires a careful review of the child's developmental history and observations of the child with family members, teachers, and peers. In addition, a complete medical evaluation and review of pertinent medical records should be standard practice because of the potential presence of genetic and chromosomal abnormalities, the high likelihood of co-occurring medical conditions (such as seizures) and the association of autism with other neurodevelopmental disorders. Moreover, assessments by other disciplines (such as speech and language) may also be needed to augment the evaluation.

The neuropsychological evaluation of the autistic child should involve a comprehensive assessment of cognitive and related behaviors. The selection of measures depends heavily on the unique presentation of the child. For example, the evaluation and selection of measures may be quite different for the child who has failed to develop language than for the child who has rudimentary language.

Cognitive Profiles Although Asperger's syndrome children often exhibit near normal intelligence and show facility in verbal problem solving, they often encounter difficulties when confronted with learning tasks requiring visual-spatial or visual-motor problem solving (Ehlers et al., 1997; Minshew, 1997). The problem-solving profile associated with Asperger's syndrome is consistent with that of the nonverbal learning disability syndrome (Rourke & Conway, 1997; see the earlier section on nonverbal learning disability syndrome in this chapter). This pattern is opposite of that identified for autistic children, who demonstrate strength in visual-perceptual and visual-spatial problem solving, although performing significantly below average on tasks requiring verbal processing. Further, the intelligence of the autistic child is often found to be within the retarded range.

Autistic children may exhibit deficits in abstract reasoning, simultaneous performance of multiple operations, and complex language and memory abilities (Minshew, 1997). A similar deficit pattern is revealed in the academic arena. That is, weaknesses affect the performance of complicated language tasks, with preserved performance on contents involving basic procedural or rote operations such as spelling, word decoding, and vocabulary. The high rate of hyperlexia in autism exemplifies this disparity. The autistic child with hyperlexia learns to read (decode) early, but fails to comprehend what is read. Interestingly, the cognitive and learning profile of autism is the converse of learning disabilities such as dyslexia. The dyslexic child cannot decode words, but shows preserved listening comprehension when another person reads the material aloud.

Executive Function Similarities in the behaviors of autistic individuals and patients with prefrontal damage have prompted speculation that executive dysfunctions may have etiological significance in autism. Empirical efforts to determine the validity of this speculation, and to identify differential patterns of executive performance, are growing. Ozonoff, Pennington, and Rogers (1991) sought to determine whether (1) executive deficits are a common dysfunction of high-functioning autistic and Asperger's syndrome individuals, and whether (2) differential patterns of strengths and weaknesses in executive function and social-cognitive performance characterize the two disorders. They targeted two areas of social-cognitive behavior, **emotional perception** and **theory of mind,** for investigation. Emotional perception involves the identification and comprehension of feeling states, such as accurately perceiving emotions as represented in facial expressions, whereas theory of mind relates to understanding that others have mental states that determine their behavior.

Ozonoff et al. (1991) found that the autistic and Asperger's syndrome groups were comparably impaired in the executive functions of planning and mental flexibility relative to normal individuals. However, the autistic subjects presented a distinct profile of inferior executive functions and theory-of-mind performance. In contrast, the Asperger's syndrome subjects showed deficits in executive functions and emotional perception but unimpaired theory-of-mind performance. These findings suggest that autism and Asperger's syndrome present unique cognitive profiles, while at the same time sharing a common deficit, namely executive dysfunction. Consistent with this line of investigation, Hughes, Russell, and Robbins (1994) determined that autistic children perform in an inferior and differential manner on executive measures, compared to control children. Specifically, the autistic group exhibited poorer complex planning and mental shifting performance, and manifested a specific type of executive deficit termed, **"stuck in set" perseveration.** The researchers interpreted the concept of "stuck in set" perseveration as a failure to disengage the current attentional focus from ongoing cognitive operations (Ciesielski & Harris, 1997). Such disengagement is necessary if the person is to shift attentional focus to a new set of demands, activities, or goals.

There is additional evidence that autistic children may present a distinct executive function profile relative to other clinical groups. Pennington (1997b) compared the performance of children with autism, ADHD, and **fragile X** (a genetic disorder associated with cognitive deficits) on measures of four executive factors. These factors included mental shifting, working memory, **executive planning,** and **response inhibition.** Executive planning involves complex, means–end problem solving to achieve a behavioral goal, and response inhibition is the ability to delay a response. The children with autism and fragile X demonstrated deficits in executive planning, verbal working memory, and mental flexibility, but not in response inhibition. In contrast, children with ADHD displayed impairments in executive planning and response inhibition, but not in mental shifting or verbal working memory.

In summary, autistic children demonstrate executive deficits, particularly as related to planning and mental flexibility. In addition, children with autism and Asperger's syndrome seem to present distinct cognitive profiles. However, these latter findings are preliminary and require additional investigation. Relatedly, not all researchers support the finding of executive dysfunction, and some implicate other neural circuitry or physiological dysfunctions.

Comprehensive Neurofunctional Model

Multiple theories and models are available to account for the behavioral manifestations, core deficits, and etiology of autism. These conceptualizations focus on impairments of attention (shifting and selective), theory of mind, social attachment, socioemotional perception, memory, language, and executive function (Fein et al., 1996). The majority of these theoretical efforts are rather narrow with regard to the specific autistic behavior that is interpreted or predicted. Accordingly, most fail to account for the multiple behavioral manifestations and proposed neural impairments of autism.

Recently, Waterhouse and coworkers (1996) proposed a comprehensive model to account for the heterogeneity of symptoms and etiologies of autism. The comprehensive model rests on a series of assumptions relating human social behavior to brain functioning. It proposes four neurofunctional impairments that, in interaction, account for the social and related behavioral disruptions of autism:

1. **Canalesthesia** involves the fragmented processing of incoming information from the different sensory modalities. As a consequence of this fragmentation, sensory information in consciousness, working memory, and declarative memory fails to integrate properly, resulting in distorted representations of the information.

2. **Impaired affective assignment** is the disrupted linking of appropriate emotional meaning or significance to novel and social stimuli. This disruption impairs appropriate responses to new situations and the social actions of others.

3. **Asociality** is a profound disturbance of normal social attachment and interdependence with others. Social interest and bonding motivation are minimal, or lacking altogether.

4. **Extended selective attention** is an overextended attentional focus and inordinate delay in shifting attention, resulting in a variety of inappropriate responses such as hypersensitivity to sensory input and perseverative behaviors.

Waterhouse and associates link each of the aforementioned neurofunctional impairments to relatively distinct neural regions and circuitry. That is, dysfunction of the hippocampus and amygdala of the temporal lobes produces canalesthesia and the impaired assignment of affective significance, respectively. Asociality relates to the aberrant functioning of three interrelated neurochemical systems: oxytocin and vasopressin neuropeptide, endogenous opiate, and serotonin. Finally, the researchers view extended selective attention as a consequence of disruption to the temporal and parietal association areas. Although each of these supporting neural regions and circuitry links to specific broad functions, they interact and overlap in producing the deficits that the autistic child displays. Interestingly, Waterhouse and associates view brain stem, cerebellum, and frontal lobe damage—all of which other researchers and theorists have considered of etiological significance in autism—as only secondary causes or by-products of aberrant input from other neural systems.

An impressive body of supporting research based on neuroimaging, electrophysiology, neuropathology, and animal studies supports the four neurofunctional impairments as pathogenic of autism. An autistic individual can present all four of these impairments. However, some individuals present three or less impaired neurofunctional systems. In such cases, the number and form of the symptoms exhibited relate to the individual system, or group of systems, that is damaged. For example, if only the oxytocin-opiate system is damaged, the model predicts that most of the autistic symptoms will be absent, except for those behaviors associated with disrupted social attachment and affiliation with others. Although the validity and utility of the comprehensive model requires further empirical verification, it represents a bold effort to integrate the theories and empirical findings of autism.

Developmental Course

Autism is a chronic, lifelong disorder that parents and professionals generally detect before the child reaches age 3. A number of distinguishing characteristics appear as the autistic child develops, although individual differences are evident. In infancy, the autistic baby may be passive and unresponsive to being held and cuddled. Social or interactive behaviors directed to the infant by caretakers often fail to elicit recognition or interest.

As the autistic child moves into the toddler and preschool years, the onset of speech and language is often delayed, or may fail to develop altogether. More-over, as language develops, echolalia, reversed pronouns, and neologisms may emerge. Self-help skills lag in development. The autistic child is less likely than normal children to imitate the gestures or vocalizations of adults (Sigman, 1994), and has only a limited desire or ability to communicate with others.

The play of the autistic child lacks sophistication in both structured and unstructured situations. The developmental stages of parallel and cooperative play are delayed, or not attained at all. Stereotypic motor behaviors, unusual interests or preoccupations, demands for order and sameness and other peculiar behaviors may dominate the child's daily activities. Unusual reactions, such as hypersensitivity to specific environmental stimuli (such as noise) or advanced abilities or skills (such as hyperlexia), may also be apparent.

During the toddler and early preschool years, the parents begin to realize their child is not developing appropriately. Professional services are typically sought, and the child is involved in a series of medical, psychological, speech, language, and related evaluations. At this point autism is often diagnosed for the first time, and comorbid conditions, such as mental retardation, are identified. Subsequently, the parents often enter the child into a preschool special education or treatment program with supportive services.

Autistic behavioral excesses and deficits continue to be evident during the child's elementary school years. However, as previously discussed, improvement across behavioral domains begins to be evident with increasing age, particularly for the higher functioning autistic child. Despite this improvement, the child remains developmentally delayed and continues to exhibit unusual behavioral patterns. The vast majority of the children cannot enter a normal educational program. Academic achievement is variable and poor, particularly if cognitive or intellectual deficits are pronounced. Peer interactions are minimal, and most autistic children never develop a close friendship.

Continued improvement may be evident with the advent of adolescence, particularly for the higher-functioning autistic child. However, most continue to exhibit deficits in one or more of the core impairment areas and, unfortunately, some autistic teenagers regress (Piven et al., 1996). Low-functioning autistic adolescents often need continued training in the more basic life skills and placement in a program, such as a sheltered workshop, that emphasizes the development of rudimentary vocational skills. Higher-functioning autistic teenagers, despite relative success in academics, are not readily accepted by peers because of their ongoing difficulties in social relations, understanding social decorum, communicating effectively, and reducing unusual interests and patterns of behavior.

Approximately 80% of autistic individuals are unable to move fully into the workforce and up to one-half require lifelong residential care (Pennington, 1991). Others can function effectively in a sheltered workshop or higher level of employment if the work environment is supportive. Higher-functioning individuals may be capable of life in a group home or other assisted living program in the community. Only about one-third achieve independent living.

Treatment

Currently, the most significant treatments for autism and other pervasive developmental disorders include behavioral interventions, special education, and, occasionally, pharmacotherapy. Despite early intervention and application of currently available treatment options, autistic and related disorders generally do not fully resolve.

Caretakers generally employ behavior modification as an intervention in an autistic child's comprehensive treatment program (Harris, 1995). Several investigators consider behavior modification one of the more effective treatment options for autistic children. Generally the use of behavioral interventions involves a functional analysis of targeted behaviors to determine the relationship of environmental antecedents and consequences to the child's behavior. Using this analysis, psychologists develop a behavioral plan to generate behaviors (such as social skills), strengthen appropriate actions (such as increased eye contact), and reduce or eliminate maladaptive behaviors (such as aggression or self-injury). Caretakers use both rewarding and aversive behavior interventions to bring about desired change. Positive reinforcement and token systems are two examples of rewarding interventions used to produce or strengthen target behaviors. Aversive behavioral techniques incorporate the use of corrective feedback, time-out, **response cost,** and **overcorrection** to reduce inappropriate behaviors. Response cost involves the loss of a reinforcer contingent on the child demonstrating an inappropriate behavior, whereas overcorrection involves having the child practice a positive response that is incompatible with an inappropriate behavior. Overcorrection is particularly effective in reducing self-stimulating behaviors, such as repetitive mouthing of objects.

Insofar as deficits in language and communication skills are often very dramatic, initial treatment efforts focused on increasing language acquisition and production. That is, the interventions centered on prompting speech and reinforcing the child's verbalizations. Although verbalizations increased, the child's actual ability to communicate did not necessarily improve. The realization that verbal production does not equate with communication has prompted a shift in treatment focus to increasing the child's spontaneous, communicative language. Relatedly, social skills training is receiving increased attention as a treatment modality. These interventions target one of the central deficits of autism, the impaired ability to relate to others. Finally, some autistic children benefit from pharmacological interventions for reducing specific autistic symptoms such as self-injurious behaviors, hyperactivity, ritualistic behaviors, and aggression. However, a number of the medications (such as Haloperidol) require careful monitoring for potentially serious side effects.

In summary, autistic children frequently require special educational services tailored to their individual learning, social, and adaptive needs. In addition to academic and daily living skills, many require ancillary services such as speech, language and physical therapy. Vocational training and supervised job placement, often in a sheltered workshop environment, provide meaningful employment and the opportunity for social and recreational activities for the autistic individual.

Disruptive Behavioral Disorders

The American Psychiatric Association (1994) currently classifies disruptive, or externalizing behavioral disorders as psychiatric disorders. These disorders feature a variety of poorly controlled or acting-out behaviors that are developmentally inappropriate or violate societal dictates for acceptable behavior. The three primary representatives of this category are attention-deficit/hyperactivity disorder (ADHD), oppositional defiant disorder (ODD), and conduct disorder (CD). As a developmental disorder, ADHD has generated an enormous number of theoretical and empirical studies over the last 20 years. It is to this disorder, the most prevalent of childhood disruptive disorders, that we turn our attention next.

ATTENTION-DEFICIT/ HYPERACTIVITY DISORDER

Clinical Background and Presentation

The clinical manifestations of children exhibiting **attention-deficit/hyperactivity disorder (ADHD)** are variable, although clinicians generally agree that the core symptom patterns include age-inappropriate inattention, impulsivity, and hyperactivity. These symptom patterns are chronic, cross-situational in presentation, and developmental in origin (American Psychiatric Association, 1994). Thus, the behavioral symptoms of ADHD are not transient in presentation and generally continue into adolescence and adulthood. Further, these symptoms are typically observed before school age and across multiple contexts such as home, school, and the community.

Since its inception in 1980, the diagnosis of attention-deficit/hyperactivity disorder has undergone several revisions (see Table 8.6). These revisions involve introducing different diagnostic models, changing exclusionary criteria, and delineating specific subtypes. Despite these modifications, the diagnosis retains the core symptoms of inattention, impulsivity, and hyperactivity, although the combinations, relationships, and definitions of these symptom patterns have altered.

Demographic and Comorbid Conditions

Currently, ADHD accounts for one-third to one-half of all referrals for psychological services (Richters et al., 1995). Prevalence rates of 3% to 7% for childhood populations are commonly cited (Barkley,

Table 8.6 *Changing ADHD Criteria*

DSM III (1980)	Symptom Presentation
Attention-deficit with hyperactivity	Inattention, impulsivity, and hyperactivity
Attention-deficit without hyperactivity	Inattention and impulsivity
DSM III-R (1987)	
Attention-deficit/hyperactivity disorder	Inattention, impulsivity, and hyperactivity
Undifferentiated attention-deficit disorder	Inattention
DSM IV (1994)	
Attention-deficit/hyperactivity disorder—combined type	Inattention, impulsivity, and hyperactivity
Attention-deficit/hyperactivity disorder—inattentive type	Inattention
Attention-deficit/hyperactivity disorder—impulsive-hyperactive type	Impulsivity and hyperactivity

Source: Adapted with permission from American Psychiatric Association (1980, 1987, 1994), from the *Diagnostic and Statistical Manual of Mental Disorders, 3rd Ed.,* 1980; *3rd Rev. Ed.,* 1987; *4th Ed.,* 1994 APA.

1997b; Hinshaw, 1992). The breakdown of ADHD figures by gender reveals that boys, as compared to girls, are more frequently diagnosed as exhibiting ADHD, with cited ratios ranging from 3:1 to 9:1 (Pennington, 1997a). However, some suggest that females are underrepresented, in part because of the greater likelihood that males will present with higher levels of overactivity and aggressive behaviors that quickly draw the attention of caretakers.

There is a growing recognition that ADHD frequently coexists with other psychiatric and psychological disorders. Oppositional defiant disorder (ODD) and conduct disorder (CD) are the most prevalent comorbid conditions of ADHD, with reported rates of occurrence ranging from 40% to 65% (Barkley, 1990). ODD is characterized by chronic, age-inappropriate angry mood and resistant, stubborn behaviors, and CD involves the repeated violations of the rights of others or of societal norms. Assaultive behaviors and illicit drug use are examples of the types of violations CD children exhibit. The basis for the high rates of comorbidity of ODD/CD with ADHD is unclear. However, the evidence suggests that social factors such as family sociopathy, rather than genetic determinants, are contributors to the pathogenesis of these disorders.

ADHD also covaries with anxiety and depressive disorders at rates ranging from 13% to 51%, depending on the childhood population sampled for study (Biederman et al., 1996; Eiraldi, Power, & Nezu, 1997; Jensen, Martin, & Cantwell, 1997). Finally, from 15% to 20% of children with ADHD also exhibit learning disabilities (Richters et al., 1995). The high rates of comorbidity have led to speculation that ADHD is one disorder within a spectrum of related disorders.

Neuropsychological Pathogenesis

Neuropsychologists consider ADHD a neurobiologically based developmental disorder that responds to specific types of environmental and pharmacological interventions. However, the etiology of ADHD is currently unknown. We review areas of investigation that are expanding our knowledge of the pathogenesis and symptoms of ADHD.

Familial and Genetic Influence   Accumulating evidence suggests that ADHD is a familial disorder, possibly inheritable. The familial nature of the disorder is clear from the elevated rates of ADHD in first- and second-degree relatives. The presence of familial ADHD does not necessarily signal that the disorder is genetically determined, because little is known of the psychosocial environmental transmission of ADHD across generations. The finding of significant parental discord and psychopathology in families of children with ADHD suggests that environmental factors may be of etiological significance. However, the high rate of concordance of ADHD for identical twins (Stevens, 1992), and the discovery of a potential linkage between ADHD and genetic markers tips the balance in the direction of a genetic component as the primary determinant of the disorder. Regarding the latter, researchers have linked a thyroid gene to a narrow subgroup of children with ADHD (Hauser et al., 1993) and have recently identified a relationship between ADHD and chromosomes 5, 6, and 11 (Cook et al., 1995; Warren, Odell, & Warren, 1995).

Neural Substrates   Numerous neural substrates have been implicated in the etiology and neuropsychological manifestations of ADHD, including most major cortical and subcortical systems, regions, and axes of the brain. Currently, three cortical-subcortical brain regions are the focus of study. The first relates to possible abnormalities in the structure of the corpus callosum. Such anomalies are believed to disrupt the transmission of impulses between the cerebral hemispheres, thereby interfering with the communication necessary for integrated behavioral control. However, neuroimaging studies of the genu (anterior portion) and splenium (posterior portion) of the corpus callosum of children with ADHD have produced inconsistent results, with subjects displaying anatomic differences in both regions, in only one region, or in neither region, relative to normal control children (Hynd et al., 1991; Giedd et al., 1994; Semrud-Clikeman et al., 1994).

The second neural substrate considered of pathological significance for ADHD is the frontal lobes. The parallel between the symptom patterns of patients with acquired frontal lobe damage and those of children identified as ADHD has fostered speculation that disruption of the frontal lobes may contribute to the etiology of the latter disorder (Bensen, 1991). Recent neuroimaging investigations have provided some support for this speculation. The majority of these investigations (Castellanos et al., 1994; Filipek et al., 1997; Hynd et al., 1990) have found a lack of normal asymmetry (R > L) in the frontal lobes of children exhibiting ADHD, with the right prefrontal region being anatomically smaller, and therefore symmetrical with the left prefrontal lobe (R = L). The right frontal lobe contributes to the control of attentional functioning, and the finding of atypical symmetry suggests a relationship to ADHD. However, studies have not always replicated these findings of structural differences, nor have they determined differences in the prefrontal lobe to be specific to ADHD. For example, Hynd et al. (1990) also identified atypical symmetry (R = L) of the prefrontal lobes in children exhibiting dyslexia.

Studies of cerebral blood flow within the frontal lobes have revealed differences between individuals with ADHD and normal individuals. Zametkin and coworkers (1990), in a positron emission tomography (PET) study of adults with ADHD, discovered that the participants exhibited hypofrontality in glucose use/cerebral blood flow. Hypofrontality can reflect a disruption in executive inhibitory control of behavior. However, subsequent studies of children and adolescents with ADHD have not consistently replicated these findings, particularly when contrasting male and female adolescents (Ernest et al., 1994; Ernest, Cohen, Libenauer, Jons, & Zametkin, 1997; Zametkin et al., 1993).

The third focus of study asks, How significant is disruption of the frontal-basal ganglia circuitry to the etiology of ADHD? The basal ganglia are subcortical nuclei embedded below the frontal lobes. The prefrontal lobes send projections to the basal ganglia that, in turn, direct projections back to the prefrontal lobes via thalamic nuclei, forming neural circuits. Figure 8.5 (p. 286) portrays the basal ganglia circuitry.

Early investigations suggested that the basal ganglia are primarily involved in motor control (Denckla & Reiss, 1997). Increasingly, investigators are realizing that the basal ganglia may play a role in cognitive functioning, although the precise nature of this role remains unclear. Neuroscientists have posed many and varied speculations as to the cognitive role of the basal ganglia, with most suggesting an inhibitory function that parallels, or serves to augment executive control of the frontal lobes.

Neuroimaging of the frontal-basal ganglia circuitry of children with ADHD has identified decreased cerebral blood flow in several of the basal ganglia nuclei (Castellanos, 1997). Different nuclei have been associated with decreased blood flow with most being specific to the right hemisphere. Similarly, there is evidence of a reduction in the size of basal ganglia nuclei in individuals with ADHD (Aylward et al., 1996). Unfortunately, inconsistent findings exist regarding whether volumetric differences are specific to the right or left hemisphere (Casey et al., 1997; Castellanos et al., 1994, 1996; Hynd et al., 1993). Finally, stimulant medication, a psychotropic known to significantly reduce the core symptoms of ADHD, can

increase, or normalize the blood perfusion of the basal ganglia (Teicher et al., 1996), providing additional evidence for the involvement of this structure in the etiology of ADHD.

In summary, support for dysfunction of the corpus callosum or frontal lobes in the etiology of ADHD remains equivocal. A greater consensus exists for disruption of the frontal-basal ganglia circuitry as pathogenic to ADHD, with anomalies more frequently evident in the right prefrontal-basal ganglia circuitry.

Neuropsychological Assessment

The heterogeneity of children diagnosed as ADHD; the failure to delineate sensitive, specific, and verifiable neuropsychological markers of the disorder; and the inability to identify the underlying pathogenesis of the disorder have hampered assessment. This state of affairs has resulted in a diagnosis by exclusion. That is, clinicians must first rule out all other disorders that could account for the child's inattentive, impulsive, and overactive behaviors before they can diagnose ADHD. This process becomes even more muddled when the child identified as ADHD exhibits comorbid psychological disorders such as ODD.

An assessment to determine whether a child is displaying ADHD warrants the integration of information drawn from developmental data and school records; systematic interviews with the parent, child, and other significant adults; behavioral observations and rating scales completed by the parent, teacher, and child; and a comprehensive battery of neuropsychological measures. Often a team approach enables professionals from a variety of disciplines (for example, neuropsychologist, physician, social worker, and educators) to answer specific questions concerning the child's functioning.

Executive Functions The current focus on frontal-basal ganglia dysfunction as a cause of ADHD has prompted efforts to assess the executive functions attributable to these neural circuits. Investigators have found that children with ADHD perform in a differential manner on measures of executive function (see Chapter 14 for neuropsychological measures). Pennington and

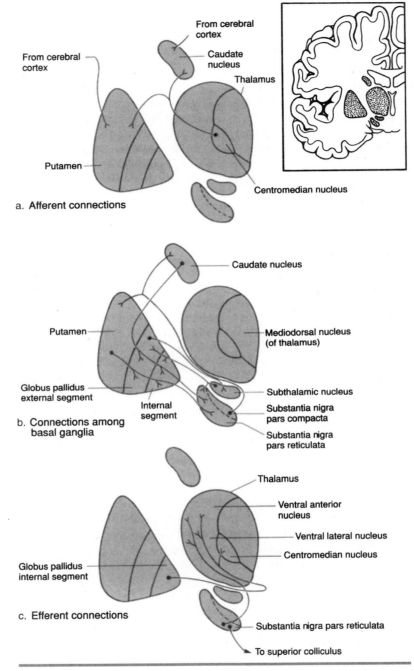

From cerebral cortex

From cerebral cortex

Caudate nucleus

Thalamus

Putamen

Centromedian nucleus

a. Afferent connections

Caudate nucleus

Putamen

Mediodorsal nucleus (of thalamus)

Globus pallidus external segment

Subthalamic nucleus

Internal segment

Substantia nigra pars compacta

b. Connections among basal ganglia

Substantia nigra pars reticulata

Thalamus

Ventral anterior nucleus

Ventral lateral nucleus

Centromedian nucleus

Globus pallidus internal segment

c. Efferent connections

Substantia nigra pars reticulata

To superior colliculus

Figure 8.5 Circuitry of the frontal-basal ganglia. (a) The caudate and putamen receive almost all afferent input to the basal ganglia. (b) The internuclear connections between the nuclei of the basal ganglia. (c) Efferent connections from the basal ganglia to the thalamus.The output from the thalamus returns to the cortex, including the frontal lobes. (From L. Cote and M. D. Crutcher, "The Basal Ganglia," in E. R. Kandel, J. H. Schwartz, and T. M. Jessell, eds., *Principles of Neural Science,* 3rd ed., New York: Elsevier Science, 1991, p. 649, Figure 42-2. Reproduced by permission of the McGraw-Hill Companies)

Ozonoff (1996) reviewed 18 studies that sought to assess the executive functions of children with ADHD. Table 8.7 lists the executive measures that most markedly and consistently differentiated children exhibiting ADHD from normal control children. Of these measures, the Tower of Hanoi (TOH) was the most sensitive to ADHD. The TOH is a complex measure that purportedly assesses executive planning, working memory, and inhibitory control (Welsh, Pennington, & Groisser, 1991).

Researchers report executive deficits for a variety of disorders, including Turner's syndrome, fragile X, autism, **phenylketonuria (PKU,** a genetic metabolic disorder), and **Gilles la Tourette syndrome** (a tic disorder characterized by vocal and motor tics). Thus, impairment of executive performance may be a common impairment of developmental disorders. This does not, however, rule out the possibility that a specific executive function (such as cognitive flexibility) or set of executive functions (such as planning and working memory) may be unique to ADHD. Several investigators (Barkley, 1998; Pennington, 1997b) have proposed that a deficit of inhibitory control may be central to ADHD.

To familiarize the student with the neuropsychological assessment of ADHD, Neuropsychology in Action 8.3 provides a case study. As will soon become evident, the case study reveals significant impairments in several executive functions that have been implicated in ADHD.

Neuropsychological Models

Several neuropsychological models of attentional functioning have evolved that are relevant to the understanding and treatment of ADHD. The next sections briefly review the representative models of Allan Mirsky (1995, 1996), Michael Posner (1988, 1992), and Russell Barkley (1997a, b, c).

Mirsky's Model Allen Mirsky, of the National Institute of Mental Health, developed a neuropsychological model that identifies the possible elements of attention, and relates these elements to neuropsychological measures and underlying neural systems. Mirsky (1996) proposed that there are three elements of attention: focus-execute, sustain, and shift. He compiled a battery of neuropsychological measures considered

Table 8.7 *Consistency of Differences and Average Effect Size of Executive Measures in ADHD*

Measures	Consistency[a]	Average *d*
WCST perseverations	4/10	0.45
TMT B time	4/6	0.75
MFFT		
Time	4/6	0.44
Errors	5/5	0.87
Stroop Test time	4/5	0.69
Mazes	3/4	0.43
TOH	3/3	1.08
Motor inhibition tasks	6/6	0.85

[a]Number of studies finding a significant group difference divided by the number of studies employing the measure. WCST = Wisconsin Card Sorting Test (Heaton, 1981); Stroop Test (Golden, 1978); TMT B = Trail Making Test B (Reitan & Davison, 1974); MFFT = Matching Familiar Figure Test (Kagan, 1964); TOH = Tower of Hanoi (Welsh, 1991).

Source: Pennington and Ozonoff (1996), p. 63. From the *Journal of Child Psychology & Psychiatry,* 37. Reprinted by permission of Cambridge University Press.

sensitive to attentional functioning (see Table 8.8) and administered it to adult neuropsychiatric patients and normal controls. The test data revealed four factors, three of which corresponded with the elements of attention Mirsky proposed, and an additional element labeled *encode.* Subsequently, the battery was extended to normal children with measures appropriate to the younger age group. Once again, four factors were identified, each similar to the elements of attention identified in the adult studies.

Table 8.8 presents the four elements of attention, and their hypothesized supportive neural substrates:

1. **Focus-execute attention** involves selective attention and rapid perceptual-motor output.
2. **Shifting attention** is the ability to move or change attentional focus in a flexible and adaptive manner.
3. **Sustain attention** is the attentional function of vigilance.
4. **Encode attention** is the capacity to briefly maintain information in memory ("on line"), while performing other related computations or actions.

Neuropsychology in Action 8.3

Case Study of a Child with an Attention-Deficit/Hyperactivity Disorder

by William C. Culbertson Psy.D.

B.C. is a 10-year-old boy with a history of school and home difficulties. The parents and regular class teacher were concerned about his inconsistent academic performance and poor behavioral control. The teacher reported that B.C. frequently failed to complete his assignments, appeared distracted, failed to follow directions, and rarely checked his work. Further, he was prone to call out in class, leave his seat, walk about the room, and squirm when required to remain seated. Despite his classroom difficulties, his group achievement test scores revealed average to above-average skill development.

At home, he was "always on the go," could not sit quietly unless playing Legos, and rushed when completing chores or homework. It was very difficult for B.C. to initiate or focus on his homework unless a parent sat with him to guide his efforts. His ability to plan and organize activities (for example, picking up his toys, organizing game activities with friends, and so forth) was described as very poor. Despite his behavioral difficulties, he was characterized as a gentle child who was rarely aggressive or noncompliant.

Neuropsychological Findings

Behavioral rating scales were completed by the teacher and parents regarding B.C.'s behavior. These ratings revealed very high rates of inattention, impulsivity, and hyperactivity. Formal neuropsychological results revealed that B.C. was functioning within the average range of intelligence. Verbal and performance intelligence were both comparably developed in the average range. Relative weaknesses were evident on subtests sensitive to attentional weaknesses. His memory performance was age appropriate. However, he demonstrated very poor sustained attention and high rates of impulsivity on auditory and visual measures of continuous performance. Relatedly, he performed poorly on measures sensitive to selective attention and response inhibition, goal persistence and impulse control, and cognitive flexibility.

B.C. manifested very poor executive planning on the Tower of London[DX] (TOL[DX]; Culbertson & Zillmer, 2000, 1998a, b)

relative to the performance of his age mates. His planning attempts were quick, without adequate forethought or reflection. From a qualitative perspective, his problem-solving approach was impulsive, rigid, and comparable to that of a much younger child.

The integration of the developmental, rating, and neuropsychological findings supported the diagnosis of an attention-deficit/hyperactivity disorder, combined type. The neuropsychologist developed behavioral interventions with B.C.'s teacher and family. These interventions focused on B.C.'s inattention, impulsivity, hyperactivity, and planning deficits. Although he was responsive to behavioral interventions, his behavioral disinhibition remained high, and the neuropsychologist sought medical consultation to determine the feasibility of stimulant therapy. Stimulant medication was introduced and gradually titrated to therapeutic levels. A significant additive effect (behavioral interventions and medication) was evident, with attention, impulse, and activity control showing marked improvement.

Recently, a fifth component of attention, **stable**, was identified (see Table 8.8), which represents the consistency of attentional effort. Mirsky believes the five elements of attention are supported by relatively distinct neuroanatomical regions (see Table 8.8) that interconnect to form an attentional system. This attentional system is distributed widely throughout the brain. Accordingly, it is quite vulnerable to disruption following brain injury, yet it is also resilient. A specific attentional function may be compromised by injury, but undamaged neural regions can provide some degree of compensation.

Although the usefulness of Mirsky's model for identifying and understanding ADHD awaits empirical verification, support for the value of the model is emerging. Of special interest is a recent study (Lowther & Wasserman, 1994) that contrasted the performance of children with ADHD and normal children on a battery of attentional measures selected to represent each element of attention. Each element of at-

Table 8.8	*Mirsky's Elements of Attention*				
	Factor 1 **Focus-Execute**	**Factor 2** **Shift**	**Factor 3/5** **Sustain/Stable**	**Factor 4** **Encode**	
ADULT	WAIS-R Digit Symbol, Stroop Test, Letter Cancellation and TMT A & B	WCST	CPT	WAIS-R Digit Span Arithmetic	
CHILD	WISC-R Coding and Digit Cancellation	WCST	CPT	WISC-R Digit Span Arithmetic	
SUPPORTING SUBSTRATA	*Focus:* Inferior parietal and superior temporal cortexes *Execute:* Inferior parietal and corpus striatum	Prefrontal cortex	Rostral midbrain structures and brain stem	Hippocampus and amygdala	

Note: CPT = Continuous Performance Test (Rosvold, Mirsky, Sarason, Bransome, & Beck, 1956); Digit Cancellation (Mirsky, 1995); Stroop Test (Stroop, 1935); TMT A & B = Trail Making Test A & B (Reitan & Davidson, 1974); Letter Cancellation = Letter Cancellation Test (Talland, 1965); WAIS-R = Wechsler Adult Intelligence Scale–Revised (Wechsler, 1981); WCST = Wisconsin Card Sorting Test (Grant & Berg, 1948); WISC-R = Wechsler Intelligence Scale for Children–Revised (Wechsler, 1974).

Source: From Mirsky, A. F. (1995). *Journal of Clinical and Experimental Neuropsychology*, pp. 481–498. © Swets & Zeitlinger. Used with permission.

tention differentiated ADHD and normal children and predicted group membership, on the average, with 91% accuracy.

Posner's Model Michael Posner developed a model of attention from the perspective of cognitive psychology and neuroscience. He proposed that attention can be defined in terms of three functions: (1) orienting to events, (2) detecting signals for focal (conscious) processing, and (3) maintaining a vigilant or alert state. Separate neural networks support each attentional function, in turn. Moreover, these attentional-neural networks interact with other cortical and subcortical systems in performing cognitive operations.

In visually orienting to an event in the environment, three basic cognitive operations activate: **disengage, move,** and **engage.** Attention first disengages from the current event of focus and then moves to the new point of focus, where attentional resources engage. The operations of disengage, move, and engage link to the parietal, midbrain, and thalamic regions, respectively. Accordingly, this visual orienting system is termed the **posterior attentional system.**

The detection of stimuli, and the control of the intensity of focus to these stimuli, is linked to the anterior region (frontal lobes) of the brain. This **ante-**

rior attentional network controls and coordinates other brain regions in executing voluntary attention. A hierarchy exists in attentional processing, with the anterior system passing control to the posterior system as needed.

Finally, a **vigilance attentional system** that prepares and sustains alertness for processing high-priority targets is important to attentional functioning. Posner did not articulate the specific neural substrates undergirding this energizing system, other than to note that the generation and maintenance of arousal and alertness are the responsibility of the right hemisphere and the brain stem norepinephrine transmitter system (Posner & Petersen, 1990).

Posner hypothesized that ADHD may result from disruption of the vigilance attention system, insofar as children with ADHD are impaired in maintaining attention over time. However, applying Posner's model to the study of ADHD revealed that children with the disorder also showed deficits, relative to normal control children, on measures sensitive to the functioning of the anterior attentional system (Pearson, Yaffee, Loveland, & Norton, 1995; Swanson et al., 1991). Thus, disruption of both the vigilance and anterior attentional systems may play a role in the etiology of ADHD.

Barkley's Model   Russell Barkley (1997a, b, c) proposed a three-tiered executive model of ADHD (Figure 8.6). The first tier, behavioral inhibition, is central to the model. Behavioral inhibition involves three interrelated processes: (1) the inhibition of a **prepotent response,** (2) stopping an ongoing response, and (3) protecting an ongoing mental operation from disruption by competing external or internal events (**interference control**). These inhibitory processes are necessary for the effective operation of the four executive functions of tier 2: working memory; internalization of speech; regulation of arousal, emotions, and motivation; and reconstitution (recombining behavioral elements to create new behaviors). Tier 2 functions, in turn, affect the control, organization, and flexibility of the behavioral output of tier 3. Although the brain as a whole supports these processes, the prefrontal and frontal cortex are primarily responsible for the inhibitory and executive processes.

When inhibitory and executive processes are intact, the child develops the capacity to regulate behavior by using internal representations of events in thought and image. These internal representations enable the child to link past learning and experience with both present demands and future consequences of actions. Further, the capacity to internally manipulate and guide behavior allows for the regulation of emotion and motivation, and the generation of new behavioral patterns to augment goal-oriented behavior, particularly when something thwarts intended actions. In ADHD, impaired inhibitory control processes disrupt the operation of the executive processes. The cascading effect of this impairment results in a host of behavioral excesses and deficits, including poor impulse control, inattention, and hyperactivity.

Developmental Course

As a developmental disorder, ADHD is evident early in childhood and, with maturation, shows changing symptom manifestations. In infancy, children displaying ADHD tend to be highly active, overly responsive to stimulation, quick to anger, and show low adaptability to change. During the toddler and preschooler years, children with ADHD are constantly "on the go," seem "driven by a motor," continually manipulate objects, and shift across activi-ties. Moreover, they constantly run and climb, often without apparent consideration for the consequences of their actions. Preschoolers exhibiting ADHD are at risk for accidental injury due to their inattention, impulsivity, and high activity levels. One three-year-old, for example, was so inattentive and hyperactive that he ran into walls, doors, and other stationary objects on a daily basis!

In a preschool setting, children with ADHD often find it difficult to remain seated, fail to listen to or follow directions, become too excited when stimulated, and talk loudly and incessantly. Peers describe classmates with ADHD as bossy, uncooperative, and intrusive into their activities and games. The parents may be asked to remove their child from the preschool program if the child is also highly oppositional or aggressive. The traditional elementary school environment is referred to as the "showplace" for ADHD. The demands of school highlight the regulatory deficits of children with ADHD. Specifically, the school requirements for (1) attention to work that can be boring, tedious, and effortful; (2) organization of assignments and belongings; (3) completion of work without rushing; (4) remaining seated for long periods of time; (5) adherence to multiple classroom rules; (6) reflection before responding; (7) refraining from talking unless permitted; and (8) cooperation with others—all tax the controlling efforts of children displaying ADHD. It is during the elementary school years that children with ADHD begin to avoid homework assignments, which inevitably leads to significant conflict with teachers and parents. Further, peers often begin to move away from these children, finding their impulsivity, hyperactivity, and inattention to rules of behavior difficult to tolerate.

As children with ADHD enter middle and high school, their inability to meet the expectations for greater independence in managing the academic demands of multiple teachers leads to an ever increasing sense of failure and frustration. Perplexed, if not angry, teachers and parents continually confront these adolescents over failures to live up to expected levels of academic performance. The normal adolescent striving for independence and self-direction fuels resistance to parental offers of assistance or attempts to provide structure to the teenager's studying and home-

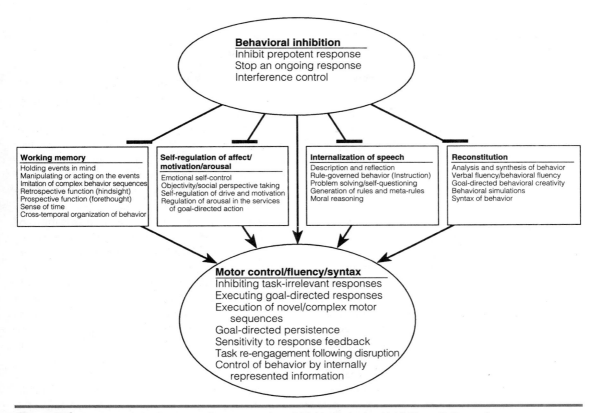

Figure 8.6 A schematic configuration of a conceptual model linking behavioral inhibition with the performance of the four executive functions that bring motor control, fluency, and syntax under the control of internally represented information. (From R. A. Barkley, "Behavioral Inhibition, Sustained Attention, and Executive Functions: Constructing a Unifying Theory of ADHD," *Psychological Bulletin, 121,* 1997b, p. 73, Figure 1. Copyright © 1997 by the American Psychological Association. Reprinted with permission)

work habits. Ongoing rejection by peers, particularly if the adolescent is aggressive, often results in the teenager gravitating toward peers who are experiencing similar difficulties. Cumulatively, these negative experiences diminish the adolescent's self-esteem and contribute to a growing realization that future educational and vocational aspirations may be unattainable.

As adolescents exhibiting ADHD move into adulthood, some show greater regulatory control and a related reduction or resolution of core symptoms of inattention, impulsivity, and hyperactivity. Unfortunately, 50% to 65% of the adolescents (Weiss & Hechtman, 1993) continue to manifest the core or

residual symptoms as they enter adulthood. Early failings in school, rejection by peers, and disappointed family members evolve into problems in achieving success in work, marriage, and family life. Not surprisingly, investigators report high rates of mood disorders, alcoholism, substance abuse, and antisocial personality disorders among adults with ADHD (Barkley, 1998). Adults with ADHD are generally gainfully employed and self-sufficient, although they tend to have poorer work records and lower vocational status than normal adult peers. Clearly, many children and adolescents manifesting ADHD continue to encounter adjustment difficulties in adulthood.

Treatment

The treatment of children with ADHD warrants a comprehensive, multimodal approach due to the multiplicity of deficits and difficulties that these children present. Each child presents a unique set of strengths and weaknesses and, accordingly, warrants an individual treatment plan tailored to his or her individual needs. In targeting the ADHD child's needs, the core symptoms of inattention, impulsivity, and hyperactivity serve as the primary point of intervention. These core symptoms, as they are manifested across contexts (family, educational, and social), expand and alter the specific treatment components. The presence of comorbid conditions (such as depression) further modifies the treatment interventions appropriate for the child. Typically, caretakers and teachers are involved in implementing treatment interventions due to their key role in engendering, exacerbating, or attenuating the child's presenting symptoms.

The two primary, and most successful interventions with ADHD are behavioral management and psychopharmacology. Behavioral management involves using learning principles to develop interventions to facilitate or inhibit behavior. Externally imposed interventions, such as token systems or response costs, appear more effective for managing the child's impulsivity, inattention, or overactivity than cognitive-behavioral interventions that focus on the child developing internal verbal self-control (Barkley, 1998).

Psychologists mold behavioral interventions to the specific needs of the child in the home, school, and community. Such interventions frequently lead to significant positive change in targeted ADHD core symptoms and coexisting emotional-behavioral difficulties. Unfortunately, this improvement in behavioral control does not often generalize beyond the specific context for which the interventions were developed. For example, the improvement in impulse control brought about by behavioral interventions in a classroom may not transfer to the home and community, unless psychologists develop additional behavioral interventions for these contexts. A serious limitation of behavioral management interventions is the rapid reappearance of the child's core ADHD symptoms when the behavioral systems are faded out. In addition, it is difficult to implement behavioral management systems for older children and adolescents because they naturally resist external structuring and control.

A variety of psychopharmacological interventions are currently available for treating ADHD. The stimulant medications (namely, Ritalin, Adderall, Dexedrine, and Cylert) are the most frequently prescribed medications for ADHD. If the child is presenting other comorbid disorders, the physician may introduce additional medications in combination with the stimulants. For example, a depressed child with ADHD may need an antidepressant medication in conjunction with a stimulant medication.

Several factors prompt the use of medication. As previously noted, behavioral improvement often does not generalize beyond the setting in which the behavioral interventions are employed. Further, behavioral interventions may not fully manage the more seriously involved children who exhibit moderate to high levels of core symptoms. Finally, parents and educators often find it difficult to employ and maintain behavioral interventions unless the psychologist who develops the interventions closely supervises and supports them.

The behavioral improvements exhibited by children treated with stimulant medications can range from slight to dramatic. Stimulant medications have enabled children with ADHD to remain in the regular classroom because their behavioral control and academic achievement has so improved. Negative parent–child interactions frequently decline, as a consequence of the child's new ability to complete homework, follow home rules, and behave appropriately in public settings. Peers can often identify when a child is medicated due to improved behavioral control, although it is unclear whether the medications contribute to increased peer acceptance. Interestingly, despite the widespread use and effectiveness of stimulant medications, neuroscientists do not completely understand the neurochemical actions of the drugs. Researchers have proposed a number of hypothesized actions, most implicating the impact of stimulant medication on the brain's neurotransmitters, specifically dopamine and norepinephrine, resulting in increased inhibitory control across cognitive and behavioral systems.

Despite the positive effects of stimulant medications, there are also several limitations: (1) side effects are common, such as appetite suppression; (2) the effects of the medications are relatively short lived (often only four hours), necessitating frequent dosing; (3) the child may show a brief intensification of core symptoms at the end of the last daily dose ("rebound effect"); (4) children often resist compliance with the medication; (5) the medications have minimal effect on certain problems (such as learning disabilities); and (6) the medications do not "cure" the disorder. Regarding the latter limitation, the core symptoms reemerge when the child is unmedicated.

Conclusion

Several developmental disorders are currently the focus of extensive research by neuropsychology and other disciplines. The neuropsychological identification of the potential brain and behavior correlates of dyslexia and the NVLD syndrome have enhanced our understanding of learning disabilities. Although much recent theorization and research has focused on disorders of reading and mathematics, other forms of learning disabilities, such as dysgraphia, await investigation. Autism has a profound and often global impact on the cognitive and behavioral development of a child. Advances have been made in the understanding of the neuropathogenesis, neuropsychological assessment, neuropsychological models, developmental course, and treatment of autism. However, the etiology of autism remains elusive, and treatment interventions often fail to significantly alter the symptoms of the disorder. Finally, ADHD is one of the most studied childhood disorders of our time. Researchers have redefined and relabeled the disorder, spawned numerous hypotheses and theories, and generated multiple interventions. Unfortunately, the etiology remains unknown; the interplay of mediating variables such as the child's personality, environmental effects, and presence of comorbid disorders remains poorly understood; and the current treatment options are limited and often ineffective. Although the entrance of neuropsychology into the study of ADHD is relatively recent, optimism remains high that its contribution will provide new and much needed direction to the study and understanding of the disorder.

Critical Thinking Questions

- Why are the symptoms of the NVLD syndrome and ADHD so often displayed by children exhibiting a wide range of developmental disorders?

- Can an autistic or Asperger's syndrome child develop normal social awareness and attachment? If so, how would this be accomplished?

- How would you respond to the comment "ADHD does not exist, it is merely a diagnosis to excuse lazy and undisciplined children?"

- As our understanding of the neural correlates of learning and neuropsychiatric disorders expands, what impact will this have on traditional psychological and educational treatment?

Key Terms

Dyslexia	Social emotional learning	Magnocellular visual system	Phonological processing
Dyscalculia	disability	Parvocellular visual system	Planum temporale
Dysgraphia	Flicker fusion rate	Saccadic eye movements	Ectopias

Cytoarchitectonic dysplasia
Working memory
Lexicon store
Metacognition
Pragmatics of language
Autism
Asperger's syndrome
Autistic aloneness
Joint attention
Echolalia
Neologism

Hyperlexia
Savant skills
Emotional perception
Theory of mind
"Stuck in set" perseveration
Fragile X
Executive planning
Response inhibition
Canalesthesia
Impaired affective
   assignment

Asociality
Extended selective attention
Response cost
Overcorrection
Attention-deficit/hyperactivity
   disorder (ADHD)
Phenylketonuria (PKU)
Gilles la Tourette syndrome
Focus-execute attention
Shift attention
Sustained attention

Encode attention
Stable attention
Disengage attention
Move attention
Engage attention
Posterior attention system
Anterior attention system
Vigilance attention system
Prepotent response
Interference control

Web Connections

http://www.cognitivedesigns.com
Cognitive Designs
Provides educational and clinical tools to teach and treat children with autism or other developmental learning disorders.

http://www.mentalhealth.com/dis/p20-ch06.html
Autistic Disorder
Very comprehensive site that provides descriptions, treatments, research references, books, magazine articles, and various links concerning autism.

http://www.mentalhealth.com/fr20.html
Attention-Deficit Hyperactivity Disorder (ADHD)
Provides a comprehensive overview of ADHD. A review of descriptions, treatment options, books, and magazine articles.

http://www.mentalhealth.com/dis/p20-ch02.html
Conduct Disorder
Provides a complete listing of materials on conduct disorder. There are links provided, review of treatments, books, and magazine articles.

http://www.mentalhealth.com/dis/p20-ch05.html
Oppositional Defiant Disorder
Provides a complete listing of materials on oppositional defiant disorder. There are links provided, review of treatments, books, and magazine articles.

http://www.bda-dyslexia.org.uk
Dyslexia
Provides a large collection of references on dyslexia.

Part Four

DISORDERS OF THE BRAIN

Chapter 9

CEREBROVASCULAR DISORDERS

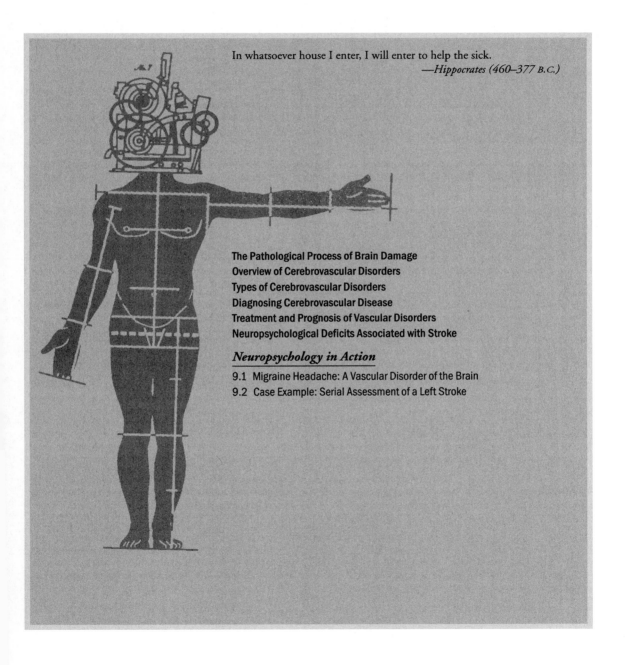

In whatsoever house I enter, I will enter to help the sick.
—*Hippocrates (460–377 B.C.)*

The Pathological Process of Brain Damage
Overview of Cerebrovascular Disorders
Types of Cerebrovascular Disorders
Diagnosing Cerebrovascular Disease
Treatment and Prognosis of Vascular Disorders
Neuropsychological Deficits Associated with Stroke

Neuropsychology in Action

9.1 Migraine Headache: A Vascular Disorder of the Brain
9.2 Case Example: Serial Assessment of a Left Stroke

Keep in Mind

■ What is a stroke?

■ How long can human brains function without oxygen?

■ How is the brain supplied with blood?

■ What are the lasting neuropsychological deficits after stroke?

Overview

The normal functioning central nervous system can be affected by a number of neurologic disorders and diseases. Some will result in similar types of damage, and some will be vastly different. Some result in focal effects, others result in diffuse damage. Physicians expect some, if not complete recovery, following many types of brain damage such as mild head injuries. Other types of brain diseases are more severe and may show lasting impairment, as is often the case in stroke, or may be even fatal, as is Alzheimer's disease, in which there is an inevitable decline culminating in death. Thus brain disorders may have a wide-ranging impact on a person's well-being. Often there are significant neuropsychological deficits that result in marked disabilities, alterations in personality, and a decline in quality of life.

The current chapter discusses the most common neurological problems and neuropsychological sequelae that are associated with cerebrovascular accidents. We discuss disorders of the brain related to tumors and head injury in the next chapter. Chapter 11 and 12 present degenerative disorders, which are good examples of diffuse and generalized involvement of brain pathology. Chapter 13 reviews disorders of consciousness, in which the typical clinical picture is also more generalized, with many behavioral adaptive skills possibly affected.

For each disorder, we examine neuropathology, neuropsychological sequelae, appropriate treatments, and case examples of patients we have treated. We present the information within a neuropsychological perspective, that is, describing the disorders with particular relevance to the relationships between brain anatomy, biological processes of the brain, and their behavioral product.

Bubbeh had to die, as you and I will one day have to die. Just as I had witnessed the decline of my grandmother's life force, I was present when it gave the first signal of its finality. It was early on an ordinary morning; Bubbeh and I were doing ordinary things. Having finished breakfast a few minutes before, I was still hunched over the sports section of the *Daily News* when I became aware that there was something very strange in the way Bubbeh was trying to wipe clean the surface of the kitchen table.

Even though we had long since realized that such household tasks were beyond her, she had never quite given up trying, and seemed oblivious to the fact that one or another of us always repeated the work after she laboriously shuffled out of the room. But when I looked up from the tabloid, I saw that her wide circular strokes were even more ineffectual than usual. Her sweeping hand had become aimless, as though acting on its own with no plan or direction. The circles ceased to be circles and soon became mere languid, useless drags of the moist cloth that was barely held in her flaccid hand, adrift on the table without purpose or weight. Her face was turned straight ahead. She seemed to be looking at something outside the window behind my chair instead of at the table in front of her. Her unseeing eyes had the dullness of oblivion; her face was expressionless. Even the most impassive of faces betrays something, but I knew at that instant of absolute blankness that I had lost my grandmother. I shouted, "Bubbeh, Bubbeh!" but it made no difference. She was beyond hearing me. The cloth slipped from her hand and she crumpled soundlessly to the floor.

I bounded to her side and called her name again, but my shouting was as futile as my attempts to comprehend what was happening. Somehow, and I remember not a moment of it, I gathered her up and staggered to the room we shared. I laid her down in my bed. Her breathing was stertorous and loud. It blew in long, forceful blasts from only one corner of her mouth, and it flapped her cheek out like a buffeted wet sail each time she exhaled from that noisy bellows somewhere down deep in her throat. I can't recall which side it was, but one entire half of her face seemed toneless and flaccid. I rushed to the phone and called a doctor whose office was not far away. Then I contacted my aunt Rose at the Seventh Avenue dress factory where she worked. Rose got there before the doctor could free himself from a waiting room filled with early-morning patients, but we knew there was nothing he could do anyway. When he arrived, he told us Bubbeh had suffered a stroke, and wouldn't live more than a few days. She outsmarted the doctor and hung on for the next 14 nights. (Nuland, 1993, p. 58–59)

The Pathological Process of Brain Damage

In this section we review examples of brain damage and their mechanisms of action within the brain. These examples are not necessarily mutually exclusive, and many conditions may result in more than one problem. They also are not totally inclusive, but are meant to provide an overview of some of the more common terms and conditions you will encounter as you read about various pathologies throughout this book. Although some examples result in specific behavioral effects, many terms, such as "lesion," are more generic and their behavioral effects often depend on the specific location and extent of damage within the brain.

BRAIN LESIONS

What are lesions, and what effects do they have on the brain? Brain **lesions** (Latin *laesio*, "to hurt") are any pathologic or traumatic discontinuity of brain tissue.

Lesions result in "holes" or "cavities" in the brain and almost always entail loss of function. Depending on their size and location, lesions result in minor or major behavioral effects. Lesions may be caused by traumas, such as punctures from bullet wounds, fragments of skull fractures, or other foreign objects entering the brain. Other events that cause lesions include cerebrovascular accidents (CVAs), surgical removal of tumors, or diseases such as multiple sclerosis or Creutzfeldt-Jacob disease ("mad cow disease").

Neurons that are completely severed often degenerate. The tissue surrounding the lesion shrinks and dies within hours. Cerebrospinal fluid then fills the cavity. With time, surrounding brain tissue may collapse the cavity, which may concomitantly distort other areas of the brain or ventricles, depending on the size of the lesion (see Exhibit 9). Any dead neuronal debris is engulfed by the brain's micro "cleaning machines," the phagocytes, which are forms of glia cells (see Chapter 2). As a result, glia cells may be all that remains in the cavity of the lesion where neurons were once active. This obviously results in a blockage or interruption of neural transmission.

ANOXIA AND HYPOXIA: OXYGEN DEPRIVATION TO THE BRAIN

Most readers will know that reduced flow of oxygen to the brain is dangerous. Cerebrovascular accidents or strokes imply by definition a disruption or stoppage of blood to the brain. Strokes almost always result in neuronal loss or degeneration. Neurons need oxygen to break down glucose into carbon dioxide and water. Furthermore, the brain has no reservoir of glucose or oxygen. Thus the brain depends on a constant and immediate supply. An elaborate blood system carries oxygen and important nutrients to the brain. Although weighing less than 3 pounds, the brain is rather demanding, requiring more than 20% of the body's oxygen to keep functioning effectively. As a result the brain is particularly vulnerable to oxygen depletion (Barnett, Mohr, Stein, & Yatsu, 1986).

If a neuron lacks oxygen for some time, the neuron will die. This **necrosis,** or *neuronal cell death,* is a direct result of a crucial interference with the cellular metabolism of the neuron. A complete absence of oxygen supply to the brain is **anoxia.** The most common causes of anoxia are cardiopulmonary failures associated with heart attacks, complications of anesthesia, accidents such as near-drowning episodes, or other severe traumas to the brain, such as are often seen in gunshot wounds to the head. In these cases, where there may be respiratory or cardiac arrest, permanent brain damage follows unless oxygen is quickly restored. Most anoxic episodes seem to result in damage to subcortical and limbic areas, the frontal lobes, and the cerebellum (Golden, Zillmer, & Spiers, 1992).

In contrast, **hypoxia** describes a reduced, but not complete, oxygenation of brain. Hypoxia typically entails not cell death, but some possible interference in the functioning of the neuron. In general, four to six minutes of anoxia may cause necrosis, although this is highly variable and depends on individual and environmental characteristics. Hypoxia can occur at high altitude, during acute cardiac crisis, during the aftermath of open-heart surgery, and during exertion in deep-sea divers. It may also be seen in carbon monoxide poisoning, may accompany sleep in the aging brain, and is present in people with chronic obstructive pulmonary disease related to chronic, intermittent lowered oxygen saturation in the blood.

A growing body of literature suggests that individuals who are otherwise healthy and who experience mild to moderate hypoxia, may demonstrate significant difficulties in concentration, short-term memory, new learning, and judgment (Barth, Findley, Zillmer, Gideon, & Surrat, 1993). At extreme altitude—that is, over 22,000 feet—hypoxia can impair a human's cognitive function, including motor speed, judgment, verbal fluency, learning, and short-term memory. Severe hypoxia produces more dramatic deficits, often resulting in irreversible brain damage. However, under specific environmental conditions (such as cold water submersion), children may recover completely from acute hypoxia, even if it has lasted as long as 20 minutes. The reasons for this are unclear, but are probably related to young age and the poorly understood effects of cold water submersion on brain metabolism.

Hypoxia can occur at high altitudes. For example, climbers refer to elevations above 25,000 feet as the "death zone," because of the low oxygen level in the air (Krakauer, 1997). The air is so thin that even con-

ditioned climbers may become hypoxic. In fact, if one were to "pluck" a person from sea level and drop him or her on Mount Everest with an elevation of 29,028 feet, death by anoxia would occur within minutes. Even when adapted to extreme elevations, many climbers must use supplemental oxygen. Nevertheless, at such high altitudes one becomes careless, sluggish, and fatigued. To conserve oxygen, the brain may diminish oxygen supply to more distal parts of the body increasing the risk of frostbite and hypothermia, and sometimes edema of the brain and death. Recent neuropsychological studies conducted on the ascent and the summit of Mount Everest clearly indicated hypoxia in climbers and a related dysfunction in memory and concentration.

Medical conditions can also affect oxygen uptake. For example, chronic obstructive pulmonary disease (COPD) is a disorder in which the lung has lost its capacity to efficiently exchange oxygen with white blood cells. **Sleep apnea** (Greek *apnoia,* "negative breathing") is a good example of chronic hypoxia during sleep. Breathing is disturbed throughout the night and often completely stops for periods as long as a minute. These hypoxic episodes often occur with more severity during REM sleep, because the voluntary muscles that assist in breathing are paralyzed during dream sleep. Under normal circumstances blood is 95% oxygenated, but in sleep apnea patients this can decrease to 50% and below. It is no wonder that people with sleep apnea complain of morning headaches, poor attention and concentration, and of course sleepiness during the day (Zillmer, Ware, Rose, & Maximin, 1988). It is not clear if the effects of hypoxia reverse with increased oxygen saturation in the blood. To some extent they seem to, because patients often completely recover. Reversibility is likely related to the length of deprivation.

HYDROCEPHALUS

Hydrocephalus is a condition in which the ventricles enlarge abnormally, because of increased CSF production, decreased CSF absorption, or a blockage of CSF flow through the ventricles. There are several medical reasons why this occurs. You may recall from Chapter 3 that the ventricles produce and circulate cerebrospinal fluid (CSF) through and around the brain and spinal cord. Spinal fluid and waste products are then reabsorbed, in part by the ventricles. The presence of blood or blood products mixing with the CSF, perhaps as a result of hemorrhage or infection, may interfere with reabsorption. This condition is called **communicating hydrocephalus.** Finally, blockage of the circulation of CSF is termed **obstructive hydrocephalus.** In young children, obstructive hydrocephalus is often caused by a congenital narrowing or stenosis of the aqueduct of Sylvius between the third and fourth ventricles. In adults obstructive hydrocephalus is most likely caused by brain tumors protruding into the ventricles.

Damage to the brain caused by hydrocephalus results from the pressure of squeezing parts of the brain against an immovable skull. If not corrected quickly, intense pressure can cut off the blood supply and result in cell death. Behaviorally, hydrocephalus results in symptoms of increased cranial pressure, such as sleepiness, severe headache, and nausea. Hydrocephalus is usually an acute condition, but physicians can reverse it by releasing the pressure; they surgically insert a tube to shunt the CSF into the peritoneal cavity of the body—the potential space around the lining of the abdominal and pelvic walls. If not treated quickly, progressive hydrocephalus can be life threatening, because it impinges on vital brain stem functions such as respiration and arousal.

Overview of Cerebrovascular Disorders

Cerebrovascular disease is reported to be the most common cause of neurologic disability in the Western world, the second leading cause of death among the oldest old (age over 85), and the third most common cause of death in the developed countries of the world. Only cancer and heart attacks affect more people. Strokes are a major health concern in the United States and can significantly affect the quality of life of those afflicted as well as their families (Zillmer et al., 1992).

In the United States, stroke affects approximately 500,000 each year, and is the major cause of disability among adults. The death rate associated with strokes is approximately 5%, corresponding to approximately 150,000 deaths each year in the United States. Another 150,000 people are left with permanent severe disability. Individuals suffering from cerebrovascular disorder place a significant financial and emotional burden on the families who take care of their loved ones. The estimated public health costs related to stroke amount to approximately $30 billion per year and are expected to accelerate steadily as advances in emergency medicine allow more stroke victims to survive (Toole, 1990).

The average age of a stroke victim is approximately 69 years (Zillmer et al., 1992). As the population of the United States is increasing, life expectancy is likewise rising. Today people are living longer and into the age groups that are more at risk from CVAs. In fact, gerontologists have called the over-65 age group the fastest-growing segment of the U.S. population (Zillmer & Ball, 1989). This rise in numbers of elderly greatly swell those at risk for strokes, creating a situation where more people in the population will actually be suffering from CVAs.

DEFINITION OF A STROKE

The term **stroke** itself is not very clearly defined and is not a precise medical term. A more technical term for stroke is **cerebrovascular accident,** or **CVA,** which describes a heterogeneous group of vascular disorders that result in brain injury. The brain's blood vessels are damaged, which can decrease blood flow within and to the brain. Simply put, stroke "suffocates" brain tissue and often produces an area of dead or dying brain tissue. A stroke always occurs in the brain and is the most common type of cerebrovascular disease. Thus, CVA or stroke is a common label assigned to clinical syndromes that are caused by blockage in blood supply or by bleeding in the brain. Stroke can result from a wide variety of different vascular diseases, but not all vascular disorders produce stroke. Although the onset of symptoms is rapid—hence the term "stroke"—the full development of the clinical picture may take an appreciable time, sometimes hours, depending on the rate of the bleed and its final cessation (Bannister, 1992).

In the past, people have conceptualized stroke as a "fait accompli." That is, once it occurred little could be done. Recent medical technology, however, has made advances in treating the stroke patient immediately, so early diagnosis and intervention have become a high priority. Physicians now treat stroke as a "brain attack," a medical emergency similar to a heart attack. Stroke can produce an array of disorders of great complexity. Most strokes occur, or are localized, in only one of the cerebral hemispheres, although in some instances there are multiple strokes or one major subcortical stroke affecting the entire brain. In general, the deficits directly relate to the location or the hemisphere where the stroke occurs.

Neuropsychologists play a crucial role in CVA diagnosis and rehabilitation. They are at the forefront in many significant advances in long-term treatment and rehabilitation of stroke patients. In addition, neuropsychologists conduct research on CVA survivors because it provides them with clinical data by which to examine localized lesions, propose strategies for intervention and rehabilitation, and indirectly, develop knowledge of the functioning intact brain (Naugle et al., 1998).

IMPAIRMENT OF BLOOD SUPPLY TO THE BRAIN

The clinical presentation of a patient after stroke reflects the damage to the anatomic structures of the brain. Disruption of major arteries can cause characteristic symptoms according to the area of the brain that artery serves (the vascular system of the brain is reviewed in Chapter 3). For example, the symptoms of a right hemisphere stroke are very much different from those of a left hemisphere CVA. Almost always behavior is disrupted, and thus physicians often consult neuropsychologists to evaluate stroke patients. The following three related neuropsychological events often occur after a stroke, all of which interfere with normal brain functioning. Victims may have to contend with these three serious consequences of stroke:

1. Disrupted blood supply decreases oxygenation, as in hypoxia or anoxia, of the involved brain tissue.
2. Related to bleeding (or hemorrhage), a space-occupying mass or pocket of blood often develops, which may press on nearby brain structures,

affecting their integrity. As a result, **intracranial pressure** or **ICP** may suddenly increase.
3. When blood spills out of the artery and into brain plasma, many toxins in the blood can interfere with normal brain metabolism. In an intact vascular system, the blood–brain barrier (see Chapter 2) protects the surrounding tissue from any toxic properties contained in blood, but exposed blood outside of the artery irritates brain tissue.

■ Types of Cerebrovascular Disorders

To effectively rehabilitate the patient and provide appropriate guidance to the family and patient, neuropsychologists differentiate between three different types and mechanisms of stroke:

1. "Temporary" strokes arise from insufficient blood supply to an area of the brain. These events, collectively called **ischemia,** often manifest in short-lasting attacks causing only transient deficits.
2. Blockage of an artery causes a more severe loss of blood supply. This **infarction** often results in more lasting neuropsychological deficits.
3. The third type of stroke is related to bleeding and to displacement of the brain that arises from a **hemorrhage.** Hemorrhages are the most severe form of stroke and often cause permanent brain damage or death.

Each cerebrovascular event is described in more detail next.

TRANSIENT ISCHEMIC ATTACKS (TIAs)

Neuropsychologists call an acute focal (localized) neurologic deficit, evidenced by a transient loss of function, a **transient ischemic attack,** or **TIA.** Recovery should take place within 24 hours, but is often complete within a much shorter time, often minutes. The attacks vary from infrequent (that is, less than one a month) to very frequent (that is, several times a day).

Rudolf Virchow, a German physician and the founder of German medicine coined the term *ischemia* (from Greek *ischein,* "to hold in check," *haima,* "blood"); literally, "a holding in check of the flow of blood," or ischemia. Deficits from TIAs clear gradually, and the patient most often returns to normal neurologic and neuropsychological functioning. An important assumption in a transient ischemic attack is that no actual damage to any neurons has occurred, just a temporary insufficiency of oxygen supply (Powers, 1990).

TIAs most commonly involve the internal carotid, middle cerebral, or the vertebral-basilar arteries. Clinically, neuropsychologists divide the deficits into the anterior circulation involving the carotid system and those affecting the posterior circulation involving the vertebral-basilar system. If the ischemic attack affects those anterior circulation, the deficits manifested will most likely relate to brief clumsiness or weakness of a limb, dysarthria, or aphasia. If the attack affects the posterior circulation, deficits may include dizziness, neglect, double vision, and numbness or weakness of the extremities. Individuals suffering from TIAs rarely lose consciousness completely, and, as already mentioned, cognitive and physical functioning usually returns to normal once the attack has ceased.

Because one of the first "signs" of stroke are TIAs, their occurrence should be taken seriously. People suffering from TIAs have a 20% to 35% higher risk of having a stroke than do normals, and go on to suffer obvious infarction, described later. There has been little research, however, to determine which individuals suffering from TIAs go on to develop the more severe infarctions. Another third continue to have TIAs without any permanent disability, and the remainder have attacks that cease spontaneously. Two-thirds of those suffering from TIAs are male or hypertensive, or both (Powers, 1990). A neurologist or neuropsychologist easily recognizes symptoms of a TIA (see Table 9.1). Unfortunately, the person suffering the TIA, because of confusion or an impaired capacity to use judgment, often does not recognize the symptoms resulting from a TIA. In other cases, the TIA symptoms are so peculiar and vague that clinicians find them difficult to establish, because of their wax-and-wane, transient nature. This is particularly frustrating to the patient, who may be inadvertently referred to a psychiatrist or psychologist, because his or her presentation does not seem to fit

Table 9.1	*Symptoms of a Transient Ischemic Attack*

Sudden tingling or numbness on one-half of the face

Confusion as to time, place, or person

Loss or impairment of speech in terms of understanding and/or communicating

Sudden slurring of speech, dizziness

Visual disturbances such as blurring or double vision

Other cognitive changes such as difficulty reading, writing, or thinking

Weakness on one side of the body (arm or leg)

any established medical categories or because physicians can find nothing physically wrong.

INFARCTIONS

When ischemia is severe enough to kill the nerve cell, neurologists consider the neuron infarcted. Infarctions result from an inadequate blood supply to an area of the brain, causing tissue death or necrosis from the lack of oxygen. This event most often relates to obstruction of the local vascular circulation by blockage or occlusion of a vessel, stopping blood flow. Occlusions are typically caused by either a blood clot or a fatty deposit lodged in a vessel. The area of the brain in which this occlusion occurs depends on clot size. Occlusion can happen to the brain as a whole, as in severe heart failure; in one of the major arteries or their branches supplying blood to the brain; or in a small capillary. Cerebral infarction is most likely the result of a thrombotic or an embolic vascular occlusion in blood flow. We discuss both ischemic events next in more detail.

Thrombosis

Thrombosis is the formation of a blood clot or *thrombus* (Greek for "clot") within the blood vessel. A thrombosis at the heart is a heart attack. A thrombosis in the brain is a stroke. The most common basic neuropathological process in infarction is that of **atherosclerosis.** In atherosclerosis irregularly distributed yellow, fatty plaques are present in large and medium-sized arteries. Fat deposits build up along blood vessel walls, reducing the size of the cerebral artery. In atherosclerosis the blood clot lodging in the vessel reduces or completely blocks blood flow through the vessel. Thus, atherosclerosis often precipitates infarction due to occlusion. Atherosclerosis is not a uniform process throughout the cardiovascular system; it can affect certain parts of the arterial system more than others. The most common location for atherosclerosis is at the bifurcation of arteries (the point where the division occurs), specifically at the common carotid artery. This condition is progressive, variable, and difficult to predict, although it tends to become worse as a person grows older. Atherosclerosis restricts blood supply to the brain and results in inadequate oxygenation of brain tissue. This produces a general decline in neuropsychological abilities of a diffuse nature. TIAs often, but not always, precede stroke that results from cerebral thrombosis.

The pathologic process underlying a thrombosis involves **platelets.** Platelets are disk-shaped cells found in the blood of all mammals. They are important for their role in blood coagulation and are produced in large numbers in the bone marrow. From there they are released into the bloodstream, where they circulate for approximately 10 days. While circulating, these cells do not adhere to each other or to the wall of a blood vessel. When the **endothelium,** the layer of epithelial cells that line the blood vessels, is breached, however, the blood-clotting properties of the platelets activate. That is, they change shape and stick to the vessel wall, each other, and red blood cells. If this occurs pathologically—that is, in a normal vessel—it leads to a thrombosis, ultimately occluding the vessel. Aspirin is an important antithrombotic agent.

The middle cerebral artery on the left side is the most commonly reported site for an occlusion. Research has shown that blood clot formation most frequently stems from abnormality within the vessel wall, and less frequently from an abnormality of the blood itself (Brown, Baird, & Shatz, 1986). If a thrombus forms and blocks the flow of blood to the brain, a cerebral infarction occurs. The area of the brain in

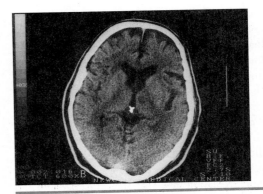

Figure 9.1   Lacunar infarcts of the thalamus as seen on CT scan. (Eric Zillmer)

which this occlusion occurs depends on the size of the blood clot. If it is large, it may lodge in one of the major arteries; if smaller, it will lodge in a branch of the major arteries. The effects of occlusions in small and large vessels differ. People with long-standing hypertension and diabetes often have occlusions of small vessels, called *lacunar infarctions* (Latin *lacuna,* "hole"), because the infarctions are generally small and round. Patients with lacunar infarctions frequently have multiple small lesions and a history of elevated blood pressure. Because the lesions are small and typically deep in the brain (see Figure 9.1), they produce, not disturbed alertness, headache, or EEG changes, but usually pure motor and sensory deficits. The disease course is often fluctuating or stepwise (Barnett et al., 1986).

Embolism

The term **embolism** (Greek *embolos,* "plug" or "wedge") refers to a blood clot that has traveled from one part of the body to another. Sometimes a piece of plaque originally formed in the heart can "break" off into the blood circulation and travel to the brain. If the blockage is not relieved rapidly, the brain area served by that artery dies of infarction. Embolism are often (up to 33%) associated with a condition known as **atrial fibrillation,** an arrhythmia of the heart. Research has recently established that cardiac surgery (such as valve replacement) may potentially contribute to cerebral emboli. When a traveling blood clot or embolism lodges in a distal intracranial branch of a blood vessel, it may block blood flow to specific parts of the brain, so a cerebral infarction occurs. At younger ages, embolic strokes are more prevalent than thrombotic strokes and are more likely to involve the anterior areas of the brain. Embolisms develop suddenly, often without immediate warning. Most often the patient is awake and active (Toole, 1990).

HEMORRHAGE

Hemorrhage (Greek *haima,* "blood," *regnynai,* "to burst forth") results from rupture of a blood vessel causing heavy spilling of blood into cerebral tissue. The large accumulation of blood within tissue is called a **hematoma.** Onset of cerebral hemorrhage is abrupt and usually occurs during waking hours, presumably because the person is more active and thus has a higher blood pressure. Although the severity may vary from a small, symptomless bleed to massive hemorrhage leading to sudden death, prognosis for cerebral hemorrhage is usually poor, especially if the patient is unconscious for more than 48 hours. A hemorrhage usually occurs when a weak spot in a blood vessel, called an *aneurysm,* ruptures. Such hemorrhages are usually massive, cause the most severe damage structurally, and often result in death. A large space-occupying bleed may discharge itself through the ventricles and can be detected using a spinal tap. Often alterations in consciousness accompany hemorrhages, ranging from disorientation to coma. Severe motor and sensory deficits are also usually present, although the degree of deficits depends on the speed and extent of the bleed. Hemorrhages occur most commonly in brain regions that are susceptible to the presence of aneurysms. Those include the putamen (50%), cerebral white matter (16%), thalamus (12%), pons (8%), cerebellum (8%), and caudate nucleus (6%; Barnett et al., 1986). There are two kinds of hemorrhagic strokes; intracerebral and subarachnoid.

Intracerebral Hemorrhage

Intracerebral means "within the cerebrum," or within the brain. In this kind of hemorrhage, a defective artery bursts and floods the surrounding brain tissue with blood. Intracerebral hemorrhages most often accompany hypertension and result in deficits localized to either left or right hemisphere. Medical and neuropsychological problems resulting from an intracerebral hemorrhage occur not only because of the disruption of blood flow that would normally reach the brain tissue from the intact artery, but also because of increased intracranial pressure on the brain tissue from the increased amount of blood flow into the skull. Large hemorrhages not only destroy brain tissue, particularly if the bleed continues, but also displace vital brain centers, which may prove fatal. Less serious hemorrhages may disrupt the integrity of adjacent brain tissue without destroying it and produce highly localized symptoms. When the bleeding does cease, there is usually no recurrence from the same site, a situation unlike that of a bleed resulting from an aneurysm.

Subarachnoid Hemorrhage

A **subarachnoid hemorrhage** occurs when a blood vessel on the surface of the brain bursts and blood flows into the subarachnoid space, the small cavity that surrounds the brain. As with intracerebral hemorrhages, a major problem that can occur from this kind of stroke is increased pressure on the brain. The extent of dysfunction seen with subarachnoid hemorrhages depends in part on how much pressure is exerted on the brain. Acute symptoms include sudden headache, vomiting, and a possible interruption of consciousness. Because of the diffuse effects on the brain, localized symptoms, such as paralysis, are typically not present during a subarachnoid hemorrhage.

Aneurysms

Aneurysms represent weak areas in the walls of an artery that cause the vessel to balloon. These localized dilations of blood vessels may be of congenital origin, but are also present after trauma, infection, and arteriosclerosis. Aneurysms can produce more significant disorders when they begin to hemorrhage and are a major cause of stroke-related mortality and disability. Aneurysm bleeds range from minor to a complete rupture resulting in a hemorrhage, as just

Although the primary symptom of migraine is a seemingly subjective and excruciating headache, migraine is, in fact, a neurological disorder of the brain's vascular structure. Symptoms consist of a moderate to severe lateralized "throbbing" headache, typically behind the eye, associated nausea, and an increased sensitivity to light, odors, and sounds. Often a family history shows similar headaches, but the diagnosis is only indicated if no evidence of other organic disease, such as tumor or stroke, could account for the symptoms. Migraines are very common: 24 million or 1 out of every 11 Americans suffer from migraine (Lezak, 1995). Migraine is more prevalent among women than men (by a 3 to 1 ratio) and occur most often between ages 30 and 45. The typical frequency of migraine is intermittent (about 2 to 5 per month), and an attack lasts between 4 and 72 hours. A migraine attack can incapacitate the victim, so high labor costs arise from decreased work productivity and increased absenteeism. About 20% of migraine sufferers experience an **aura,** a neurologic event that occurs prior to the onset of pain and is most likely caused by a TIA. The aura presents usually as a visual symptom including flashing lights, zigzag lines, or blurred or partial loss of vision. Other neurologic symptoms may also be present during an aura, including increased numbness of the skin (especially in the arms), difficulties in motor coordination, and symptoms of aphasia.

The trigeminal nerve, a large cranial nerve with three branches, has been implicated in migraine. The trigeminal nerve conveys sensory information including pain, touch, and temperature from most of the face and the scalp. A proposed mechanism for migraine implicates the sensory "pain" fibers of the trigeminal nerve that surround the cranial arteries supplying blood to the meninges. In people with migraine, these nerve fibers sometimes release chemicals known as *peptides.* As a result, blood vessels become inflamed and cranial blood flow changes, first abnormally constricting and then dilating.

Migraine auras occur during the constriction phase. This is such a common event among migraine sufferers that

---

described. Approximately 50% of aneurysms occur in the middle cerebral artery and are most likely inherited or related to a pathologic process that weakens arterial walls. Many vascular anomalies remain undetected only to begin causing problems when they rupture because of such factors as high blood pressure. The base rate for adults is 4%; and among those who have aneurysms, 20% have multiple ones. Aneurysms, which expand with time, are most often less than 6 to 7 mm in diameter, with giant aneurysms expanding to 2.5 cm. It is relatively rare that small aneurysms rupture (Bannister, 1992).

Arteriovenous Malformations (AVMs)

Arteriovenous malformations, or **AVMs,** represent direct and essentially useless communications between arteries and veins without an intervening cap-illary network. AVMs are typically congenital collections of abnormal vessels that result in abnormal blood flow. Because they are inherently weak, AVMs may lead to stroke or to inadequate distribution of blood in the regions surrounding the vessels. Rupture of AVMs may produce intracerebral as well as subarachnoid bleeding. Like aneurysms, AVMs have a tendency for recurrent bleeding. The clinical symptoms of AVMs can include headache, which is similar to migraine in that it is related to the dilation of vessels, or other more vague cognitive complaints (see Neuropsychology in Action 9.1). Often AVMs have no identifiable clinical consequence and many individuals are not aware of having the condition. The most serious complication of AVMs is bleeding, typically at a very slow rate. Table 9.2 summarizes the various types of cerebrovascular disorders reviewed in this chapter.

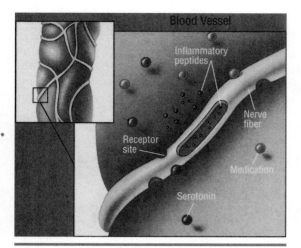

Figure 9.2 The role of serotonin in migraine (© 2000 Beth Willert. Reprinted with permission of the artist. From packaging display for GlaxoWellcome, Inc.)

naturally present in the blood to enter into brain tissue. The neurotransmitter serotonin plays a major role in migraine (see Figure 9.2). During migraine attacks, serotonin levels decrease and medications or substances that deplete serotonin (such as chocolate or the food additive MSG) often trigger a migraine. Conversely, administering serotonin (such as Imitrex) often relieves the headache.

Although many individuals experiencing migraines develop TIAs, very few go on to suffer from a CVA. Although very rare, **migraine strokes** do occur and seem to account for a small proportion of CVAs in young people, particularly females, under the age of 40 years. Medical research has demonstrated that individuals suffering from migraines are actually at less risk of suffering strokes than the general population (Bannister, 1992). This is because the migraine patient's cardiovascular system is inherently flexible, which allows the constriction and dilation of arteries in the first place (Walton, 1994).

many patients notice this as a first sign of the oncoming migraine. During the subsequent dilation, patients experience the symptoms of the migraine attack. Swollen blood vessels stimulate surrounding nerve fibers to relay impulses to the brain, where they are perceived as pain. The accompanying severe nausea perhaps relates to a compromise in the blood–brain barrier, which in turn allows toxins

Table 9.2	*Summary of Different Types of Vascular Disorders*

Arteriovenous Malformation (AVM)   Arteriovenous malformations represent abnormal, often redundant vessels that cause abnormal blood flow. Because they have inherently weak vessel walls, AVMs may lead to slow bleeding or to inadequate distribution of blood in the regions surrounding the vessels.

Embolism   A type of artery occlusion in which the clot forms in one area of the body and travels through the arterial system to another area, in this case the brain, where the clot becomes lodged and obstructs cranial blood flow. Approximately 14 percent of all CVAs are caused by an embolus.

Hemorrhage   Bleeding; literally, the escape of blood from the vessels. The most severe form of cerebrovascular accident, characterized by the rupturing of a blood vessel. Hemorrhages account for approximately 10 percent of all strokes. Most hemorrhages stem from increased blood pressure and the presence of abnormal formations of blood vessels, including aneurysms.

Migraine stroke   A rare type of stroke caused by severe TIAs, typically associated with classic migraine.

Thrombosis   A type of occlusion in which a clot or thrombus forms in an artery and obstructs blood flow at the site of its formation. This is the most common form of stroke and accounts for approximately 65 percent of all CVAs.

Transient ischemic attack (TIA)   A temporary (transient) lack of oxygen (ischemia) to the brain. This temporary lack of oxygen can cause a time-limited set of neuropsychological deficits. TIAs are technically not considered a stroke, because neuronal death does not occur.

Diagnosing Cerebrovascular Disease

Because of their sudden onset, infarctions are relatively easy to differentiate from other focal neurologic disorders such as tumors. Gradual obstruction of one vessel, however, may not produce an infarction at all. Because the occlusion develops over a long period of time, its eventual course into full occlusion may have few or mild effects, because alternate blood sources for the affected brain tissues may have formed over time. The major diagnostic task in differentiating stroke from other neurological conditions is to exclude other etiologies of lesions that produce similar clinical pictures or cause a bleed. A precise diagnosis is important to the medical team as well as the neuropsychologist in order to plan an appropriate rehabilitation program for the stroke patient. Next we review diagnostic procedures that are used to document stroke.

COMPUTED TRANSAXIAL TOMOGRAPHY (CT)

Computed transaxial tomography (CT) is a powerful, almost risk-free, technique for imaging the structure of the brain (see Chapter 6). The CT scan often provides the first evaluation in diagnosing stroke, particularly in differentiating between hemorrhagic and nonhemorrhagic stroke. On CT scans, hemorrhages appear initially as round, well-circumscribed lesions of uniform high density. Over time, the circumference of the lesions becomes more irregular and the lesion less dense. CT scans provide information not only about the location of a hemorrhage, but also size, possible edema (swelling), displacement of other brain structures, and presence of blood in the ventricular system. Tumors, which show up on CT with a different density, are easily differentiated. Contrast-enhanced CT typically does not increase detection of hemorrhages. Transient ischemic attacks (TIAs) are less easily monitored on CT because of their small size.

ANGIOGRAPHY

Angiography represents the most accurate diagnostic procedure for vascular disorders. Angiography can also provide an evaluation of collateral vessel potential and a diagnosis of coexisting neurological problems. Angiography is an invasive diagnostic procedure that entails some risk (see Chapter 6). Therefore it is usually reserved as the final diagnostic test for stroke, and CT typically precedes angiography. As reviewed in Chapter 6, the two most common routes for angiography are via the venous system and via the arterial system. Arterial angiography is the more popular one in diagnosing stroke, because it provides precise images of cerebral arteries. This is because the specialist can pass the catheter, which injects the contrast medium, up the aortic arch and selectively place it into the carotid or vertebral arteries. Angiography can also show whether the obstructing lesion is significantly impairing carotid blood flow and whether the lesion can be removed surgically. Precise diagnosis of cerebral aneurysms, AVM, artery occlusion, and **stenosis** (narrowing of an artery) are all possible using angiography.

OTHER TESTS

An alternative to angiography and imaging are noninvasive tests, typically targeted at detecting anatomic and physiologic information of the common and internal arteries. These devices, which use ultrasonic waves, function on the principle that extensive lesions to the carotid arteries may produce distorted sound wave feedback. In addition, pulse-wave Doppler imaging systems may be sensitive to blood flow velocity. In most cases, a conclusive diagnosis is not made; rather, noninvasive devices for carotid blood flow serve to screen for subsequent referral to the more invasive angiogram. Cerebrospinal fluid analysis using a lumbar puncture is also of value in ruling out or confirming a subarachnoid hemorrhage not seen on CT.

Treatment and Prognosis of Vascular Disorders

FACTORS INVOLVED IN STROKE RECOVERY

Once an individual has suffered a stroke, the type of damage or lesion and associated neuropsychological symptoms, depend on a number of medical and neuroanatomic factors. These include the extent of the lesion, the general health of the cerebrovascular system, the presence of collateral circulation in the brain, and the location of the lesion. These factors influence the extent and nature of associated cognitive symptoms, and the possibility and prognosis for recovery and extent of rehabilitation.

Size of Blood Vessel

If a small blood vessel (such as a capillary) is interrupted, the effects are more limited than the often devastating consequences of damage to a large vessel, such as the internal carotid artery or other cerebral arteries. Strokes of these large arteries can result in lesions that include large portions of the brain and produce serious behavioral deficits, coma, and even death.

Remaining Intact Vessels

If a CVA occurs in one restricted portion of the brain, the prognosis may be rather good, because healthy blood vessels in surrounding brain tissue often can supply blood to at least some of the deprived areas. In addition, the presence of **collateral blood vessels** allows redundant blood supply to take more than one route to a given region. The term *collateral* is used to describe redundant blood flow present in the vascular network following occlusion of an artery. If one vessel is blocked, a given region might be spared an infarct because the blood has an alternative route to the affected brain area. Conversely, if a stroke occurs in a region surrounded by weak or diseased vessels (as in arteriosclerosis), the effects may be much more serious, because there is no possibility of compensating. The surrounding weak zones may be at an increased risk of stroke themselves.

This communication between blood vessels by collateral channels is also known as **anastomosis** and provides an important defense against stroke. The properties of collateral communication that provides a sufficient blood supply to obstructed areas vary considerably among individuals. Thus, damage to the same vessel in different people can produce symptoms that vary considerably. Anastomosis can provide some relief to blood-depleted brain areas, particularly if the primary vessel affected is gradually blocked, rather than rapidly occluded.

Premorbid Factors

The presence of previous strokes is a strong predictor of disability. A small stroke in an otherwise healthy brain will, in the long run, have a good prognosis for substantial recovery of function. However, the effects of an additional lesion most often are cumulative. As a result, destruction of a functional zone of brain tissue may produce serious consequences for the patient.

Location

The location of brain tissue involved has neuropsychological significance. A lesion in the temporal lobe can produce a deficit in understanding speech; a stroke in the hippocampus, memory deficits; and a lesion in the brain stem, a heart failure resulting in death. Thus behavioral symptoms of vascular disorder are important clues to the neuropsychologist for locating the area of brain damage and assessing the extent of damage.

MEDICAL TREATMENT

The initial treatment of the stroke patient involves medical stabilization and control of bleeding, if necessary through surgery. Common medications include anticoagulants to dissolve blood clots or prevent clotting, vasodilators to dilate or expand vessels, and blood pressure medication and steroids to control cerebral edema. Surgeons have developed interventions over the last decades to reduce the risk of bleeding for some aneurysms by "clipping" them (see Figure 9.3). Other surgical procedures are used in the case of hemorrhages when it may be necessary to operate to relieve the pressure of the blood from the ruptured vessel on the rest of the brain. Small hemorrhages are typically not treated surgically, but are controlled by altering the patient's blood pressure.

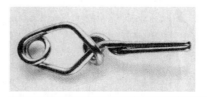

Figure 9.3 Aneurysm clip (approximate size = 6 mm).
(Eric Zillmer)

Physicians typically treat infarctions intravenously administering heparin (a potent anticoagulant agent), but only if diagnosis rules out a mass lesion from a trauma or hemorrhage (either intracerebral or subarachnoid). Administering an anticoagulant agent to a patient with a hemorrhage can be fatal, so establishing a precise differential diagnosis is very important. In medium-size bleeds surgical draining is often very effective, although this technique may leave a surgical hole in the brain that may later entail neuropsychological deficits. Other ways to decompress the brain include artificial hyperventilation, corticosteroids, and diuretics. In most cases, physicians artificially lower the blood pressure. Treatment for TIA symptoms, which is more difficult because the symptoms are ambiguous, is often restricted to pharmacological intervention with anticoagulants. An obvious danger in using anticoagulants is the inherent risk of an uncontrolled bleed.

AVMs are often surgically removed or are embolized artificially. In the later technique the surgeon delivers an agent that blocks the blood vessel close to the lesion, in some cases permanently. The embolization agent is a sponge, ball, coil, or balloon and entails certain risks. This delicate technique uses highly selective catherization procedures and close radiographic monitoring. The reason for this care is that the delivery system must advance as close to the lesion as is possible, otherwise healthy arteries may be embolized or the embolus may migrate to the lung or heart.

PREVENTING STROKE

Many people who have had a stroke say that it "struck out of nowhere"—there seemed to be no obvious warning. Typically, a stroke that occurs spontaneously results from an embolism or a hemorrhage. The fact that one can have a stroke with little or no warning testifies to the importance of identifying the many risk factors associated with stroke. The most prominent risk factor is a past history of stroke. In fact, as mentioned earlier, stroke recurrence is an important contributor to disability. In addition, common demographic factors predispose an individual to cerebrovascular disease, including:

Heredity (cardiovascular disease in one's family)

Gender (men are more at risk for stroke than women, a risk related to their higher incidence of heart disease and hypertension)

Ethnicity (African-Americans have one of the highest stroke rates, 40% higher among women and 10% higher among men)

Lifestyle indices also affect the probability of cardiovascular disease. A well-known risk factor of CVA is hypertension. Elevated blood pressure means that the force of the blood against the walls of the arteries is too high. As a result, over time the arteries become weakened and can burst. If this happens in the brain, it results in a cerebral hemorrhage. High blood pressure can also increase the force of the blood against the artery walls and break off some plaque along those walls, which then travels as an embolus through the bloodstream until it clogs a narrower vessel. The dangerous part of hypertension is that most people do not feel it and thus do not seek medical help.

Other risk factors for stroke are diabetes and high cholesterol. Individuals with diabetes run a greater risk of developing stroke. Vascular diseases are most often related to problems in artery linings, which become hardened by deposits of cholesterol, fat, calcium, and other materials such as fibrin, a substance that encourages clot formation. Fat causes plaque to build up along the lining of blood vessels, which can break off and lead to embolic stroke, or can become so built up that thrombotic stroke can occur. Because smoking is a vasoconstrictor, it is an additional risk factor for stroke. Smoking a cigarette constricts an already too narrow blood vessel.

Small amounts of alcohol may actually thin blood and can serve the same purpose as one aspirin per day. There is also some evidence to suggest that a glass of wine with dinner lowers cholesterol. Alcohol becomes a risk factor when consumed in large quantities. Excessive consumption contributes to high blood pressure and may result in ataxia (poor balance), which is often already a problem after a stroke. Also, alcohol is a sedating drug and may not interact well with other drugs. Finally, obesity contributes to the onset and maintenance of diabetes, hypertension, heart disease, and high cholesterol. Obesity is medically defined as being 25% over your ideal weight. Approximately 26% of American men and 30% of American women are overweight. Cardiovascular complications in obesity are related to the high correlation between being overweight and hypertension, a precursor of coronary heart disease.

Neuropsychological Deficits Associated with Stroke

Significant functional and cognitive impairments are often the result of stroke. These deficits can seriously impair the patient's ability to function independently, and are often incapacitating and serious enough to lead to hospitalization in a rehabilitation facility. Typically, long-term hospitalization occurs because the patient is exhibiting symptoms of inattentiveness, apraxia, communication difficulties, apathy, or general intellectual impairment.

Many factors influence cognitive changes as a result of stroke. Those include the patient's age, interval between the stroke onset and time of rehabilitation, nature of the stroke (infarction or hemorrhage), and size and location of lesion (such as right or left brain, anterior or posterior). The patient's past medical history is important, particularly as it relates to the presence of previous strokes (such as lacunar strokes), prior central nervous system trauma or disease, and premorbid level of functioning. Many stroke-related cognitive deficits may resolve over time, sometimes immediately after the stroke. For example, the more localized the effects, the more positive the prognosis. But residual deficits may remain that require an evaluation of cognitive abilities and subsequent rehabilitation (Brown et al., 1986).

Because of their complexity and variability from patient to patient, the cognitive deficits associated with stroke are not easily classified into simple categories. For didactic purposes, neuropsychologists correlate cognitive deficits with the specific type of stroke. Correlating the location of an anatomic lesion with the stroke patient's cognitive impairments has been only modestly successful. Thus the neuropsychology student should be careful not to rigidly adhere to specific patterns of deficits and recovery but instead

should realize that the disease course in individual patients varies greatly.

NEUROPSYCHOLOGICAL RISK FACTORS

Several important principles govern the properties of neuronal processes that are particular relevant to understanding the neuropsychology of cerebrovascular disorders.

Necrosis

First, neurons that have died as a result of necrosis do not spontaneously regenerate. In most instances, lost neurons in the CNS are not capable of healing after the developmental period (see Chapter 2). Thus, there is no cellular regeneration of the neuron or regrowth of damaged neurons to their normal target. Neurons lost as a result of stroke are not replaced. Fortunately, functional losses entailed by these structural losses are not necessarily permanent, because the brain has redundant pathways for supplying blood to various areas. Specifically, redundant blood supply in the brain may minimize neuronal death because there is sufficient blood supply to brain areas that have been damaged. Also, the process of rehabilitation allows some compensation of functional losses with behaviors that have been left relatively intact. Rehabilitation may alleviate enough disruption caused by stroke that the victim regains some or nearly all of his or her premorbid level of functioning. In fact, neuropsychologists have made significant headway within the last decade in developing assessment, prosthesis, and cognitive rehabilitation techniques to compensate for disrupted functional brain systems. In addition, neuroscientists are making some progress in designing drugs that facilitate the regrowth of injured neurons.

Disinhibition

An important principle of neuronal processes relevant to understanding the neuropathology of stroke relates to the capacity for inhibiting behavior after a stroke. As already discussed in previous chapters, many of the neuronal collections, particularly in the frontal lobe, serve to inhibit rather than initiate behavior.

This is important because losing inhibitory neurons to stroke may actually result in an increase in behavior or disinhibition, and often causes striking behavioral and personality changes in stroke victims. Damage to an excitatory collection of fibers, of course, results in losing some function. This is why many traumas to the brain, including stroke, often show both loss of function (such as aphasia and the inability to speak) as well as disinhibition (increased likelihood of inappropriate behavior) including impulsiveness, hypersexuality, and inappropriate feelings. This was made painfully clear to us when one of us, Eric Zillmer, was leading a stroke support group. All members of the support group had sustained a stroke, and many had significant related cognitive deficits. Almost all members demonstrated poor judgment and disinhibition when it came to operating an automobile, and they spent much time in the group discussing this. Nevertheless, they insisted on continuing to drive and drive poorly; in fact, many accidents happened in the parking lot before and after group meetings. When group participants returned from trips, they would discuss and bring along pictures of their recent accidents. They described these crashes with some bravado, reflecting very poor insight and a general lack of awareness of the dangers. This is a typical example of disinhibition because victims do not inhibit high-risk behavior, as they may have done premorbidly, that is, before the stroke. The incapacity to drive after a stroke is one of the most sensitive issues facing health care workers, and stroke victims and their families.

Disconnection Syndrome

Because the brain's substructures connect so intricately, observed deficits in a stroke patient may not necessarily correspond to the lobe or site where the stroke occurred. For example, a stroke in the visual area of the cortex (occipital lobe) ordinarily results in some form of visual impairment. In addition, however, these visual deficits may also disturb motor behavior or gait. Furthermore, a stroke may disrupt important pathways of neurons that project to other centers of the brain. This is a common problem when strokes occur near subcortical structures such as the striatum, a common stroke site. Such a stroke commonly results in higher-order cognitive deficits, because injury has severed projections to the cortex. This problem is called *disconnection syndrome*, because important pathways in the brain have been "disconnected."

ATTENTION DEFICITS

Many types of brain dysfunction typically reduce efficiency of the brain in processing information. This is certainly true for CVA. In milder cases, stroke victims cannot sustain their attention to one particular stimulus for long periods of time or select information from competing sources (selective attention). This impairment may be minimally present, and only detectable with formal neuropsychological testing, or it may be profound and easily noticeable by any observer. Sometimes cognitive changes in stroke patients are so pervasive that the patient is considerably confused and disoriented as to time, place, and person. Deficits of arousal typically relate to damage of the patient's frontal lobe circuitry or the brain stem region. In contrast, deficits in attention may relate to local or global brain damage.

MOTOR AND SENSORY IMPAIRMENT

General behavioral slowing and a reduction of psychomotor activity can be dominant characteristics of stroke. Both the right and left hemispheres are associated with changes in motor and sensory functioning from stroke. Such changes can be as benign as mild motor slowing or as debilitating as complete paralysis, particularly if the lesions are in the thalamic area or the motor and premotor area of the frontal lobes. Motor deficits of the right brain resemble those of the left brain. Right hemisphere stroke motor deficiencies, however, are generally less severe, because the nondominant left hand is not as important for skilled tasks.

Severe motor deficits are often apparent without formal testing and may involve impairment in motor speed, strength, steadiness, and fine motor coordination. Even mild deficits may significantly reduce the efficiency on highly demanding manual tasks, interfere with self-care or light housework, deteriorate handwriting skills, and slow reaction times, which may require the victim to give up driving. Diminished sensory functioning is most likely in areas of visual acuity, visual field perception, and hearing.

MEMORY PROBLEMS

Stroke victims commonly report that their memory is not as good as it used to be, and on occasion they may not recall a person's name, even when they know that person well. Many stroke patients exhibit intact memory for old learning, but not always for new learning. That is, they can remember events that happened years ago, but may be unable to remember what they had for lunch today. Unless the lesion is extensive, CVAs do not typically cause loss of primary, immediate, or long-term memory, but are most pronounced in the area of short-term memory. This most likely relates to the stroke patient's decreased capacity to organize and process large amounts of information ("chunking") in a fashion that lends itself to easier memory storage or retrieval. Not uncommonly these patients recall only a small amount of new material 30 minutes after it is presented to them.

Patients that have stroke-related hippocampal damage experience significant memory difficulties, may require repetition of new information, and may show significant problems with forgetfulness associated with a variety of everyday tasks. Such patients have frequent difficulty recalling details of recent experiences, tend to misplace things, fail to follow through on new obligations, and tend to get lost more easily in unfamiliar areas.

Stroke patients with the most severe memory deficits are virtually unable to retain any information, particularly if their attention has been directed elsewhere. Such individuals also cannot profit from repeated exposures to stimuli. They need substantial assistance in daily living and characteristically cannot take care of themselves, because they may create fire hazards at home and cannot manage financial affairs or keep track of scheduled activities. For such patients it helps to create an environment in which important objects are kept in the same place, to maintain the same daily routines, and to verbalize instructions in the same sequence. A major concern related to memory impairment is the stroke patient's ability to manage his or her own medication schedule.

DEFICITS IN ABSTRACT REASONING

Impaired judgment, loss of insight, and diminished capacity for abstract and complex thinking are common cognitive changes among stroke victims, particularly if anterior aspects of cortical areas are involved. People with mildly impaired abstract reasoning and new concept formation can often use their past accumulated knowledge to exercise reasonable judgment for routine daily activities. Those who show more serious cognitive decline often encounter difficulties with tasks requiring complex planning or organization, and with novel situations. Such patients cannot assess new situations accurately and demonstrate poor judgment, with serious consequences to themselves or others.

COGNITIVE DEFICITS ASSOCIATED WITH RIGHT BRAIN STROKES

Researchers have directed much research attention toward distinguishing the cognitive deficits between left versus right hemisphere brain damage. In general, left brain–damaged patients show markedly impaired language comprehension and communication, and right hemisphere stroke victims exhibit significantly more impairment in ability to process and execute behaviors requiring visual-perceptual ability (Lezak, 1995; Reitan & Wolfson, 1993).

Deficits affecting the right cerebral artery involve areas responsible for spatial, rhythmic, and nonverbal processing. Right hemisphere symptoms, although serious in the patient's overall functioning, can be less striking in the acute phase, particularly if they do not involve motor dysfunction. Right brain damage occurs as a consequence of right sided cerebrovascular accidents and is often associated with contralateral motor and sensory impairment. Right brain–injured patients present a variety of symptoms that pose a particular challenge to the neuropsychologist. First, the deficits often found among patients with right brain damage are not as striking initially as the deficits observed among patients with left brain damage, where the patient is often aphasic. Secondly, many right brain–damaged patients display a range of emotions from indifference to euphoria. This is in contrast to the depression often observed among patients with left brain damage. Therefore it is easy to assume that the deficits from right brain damage are not as serious as those from left brain damage. This is not true, as both types of problems can be highly disruptive to patient and family alike, often even exceeding the problems associated with left hemisphere CVAs.

For example, research has shown consistently that patients with right hemisphere stroke remain longer in rehabilitation facilities than do patients with left hemisphere strokes (Zillmer et al., 1992). This difference is related to the pervasive deficits that right hemisphere patients present in visual-spatial abilities and the extended rehabilitation required for dressing, ambulating, and other self-care behaviors.

Right hemisphere stroke victims are also diagnosed not as rapidly as are left hemisphere stroke patients. This is probably related to the difficulty that left hemisphere stroke patients display in using language—an obvious symptom that helps a family member identify that something is "wrong" with their loved one. In contrast, right brain–damaged patients often use language fluently. Thus on the surface they "sound" okay. Furthermore, right brain–damaged individuals tend to be unaware of their problems. Such patients often deny that there is anything wrong with them. As a result, patients may be blamed for being "rude," "disruptive," or "inappropriate" when they are actually exhibiting symptoms of right brain injury, including impulsivity, verbosity, inattention, and poor judgment. Thus, although neuropsychological deficits in right hemisphere stroke patients may be more subtle, they are equally and sometimes more functionally disabling than the more obvious language impairments typically associated with left hemisphere stroke.

Visual-Spatial Deficits

Deficits in right hemisphere stroke patients almost always include visual-spatial deficits, that is, the pa-

tient's capacity to accurately perceive his or her surrounding world in its completeness. Neuropsychologists report that visual-spatial deficits occur particularly after right hemisphere stroke and include both visual-perceptual as well as visual-constructional abilities. Patients with problems in spatial relationships have difficulty estimating the distance between different objects, as well as between themselves and other people or things. Common examples of mistakes that patients make with this kind of disturbance include knocking items off a table when dusting, misplacing items on tables so that they are no longer centered, or are in danger of falling off, and misjudging steps or thresholds, which puts them in danger of falling.

Obviously, a patient with spatial relations disturbance may have difficulty driving a car, and may often need help in other areas of their lives such as stair climbing, and activities of daily life such as dressing, bathing, toileting, and eating. It is in unfamiliar environments and in novel situations that driving is difficult for these patients. In case of marginal impairment, it may be helpful to limit patients to driving only in their own neighborhoods. In difficult cases a neuropsychological evaluation can aid in making this decision. Motor impersistence is also a common sign—the stroke patient cannot persist with a motor response for any length of time (such as keeping eyes closed or holding arms over the head). Often, others may perceive the patient as being oppositional or stubborn, when in fact he or she is not in control of the skills required to perform the action.

COGNITIVE DEFICITS ASSOCIATED WITH LEFT BRAIN DAMAGE

In general, cognitive profiles are most robust when associated with damage of the left versus the right brain hemisphere. For example, the middle cerebral arteries serve major sensory and motor areas, and thus significant motor and sensory deficits often affect the side contralateral to the stroke. One of the most common infarctions is that of the left middle cerebral artery in which deposits have traveled up from the heart and then blocked the middle cerebral artery. Disorders of the left middle cerebral artery most often involve cortical areas of the brain responsible for both expressive and receptive speech. Thus, one of the most dramatic symptoms of a left middle cerebral artery stroke is the impairment in speaking and/or in understanding speech. Deficits also include severe motor and tactile symptoms on the contralateral right body side in addition to expressive aphasia (see Neuropsychology in Action 9.2).

Understanding and being understood by others is the goal of most human interactions. When a stroke damages that part of the brain that controls language and communication, the effects can devastate both patient and family. Several types of communication problems can occur with stroke, and neuropsychologists play an important role in diagnosing and rehabilitating specific forms of communication problems in stroke survivors. Many patients also have apraxia, a loss of voluntary movement that makes it difficult or impossible for patients to use gestures to communicate their needs. The presence of apraxia is the main reason why speech pathologists don't routinely attempt to teach aphasic patients sign language to compensate for spoken language difficulties.

Often patients lose not only spoken language, but written language as well. Writing is one of the most complex of language abilities. If writing is disturbed by impairment to the limb that produces letters and words, neuropsychologists do not consider that a disorder of language. Rather, in written language deficits words, letters, or numbers may appear foreign or incomprehensible because the person cannot recall the form of letters. His or her attempts to write may be filled with real or imagined letters that make no sense to others. With time and training, the person may be able to understand simple written language—for example, single words such as bath or food—but still be unable to comprehend more complex written language such as sentences or paragraphs.

Many so-called behavior problems seen with stroke patients with aphasia occur because of receptive aphasia. In moderate cases, the patient can understand part, but not all of the communication. Sometimes patients' apparent noncompliance is actually caused by their misunderstanding the communication. Thus a patient may act as though he or she had not heard a word at all (so-called word deafness) or as though he or she had heard only fragments of the word. The most common defect lies not in failing to recognize that someone spoke a word, but in failing to attach meaning to the word. Some aphasics comprehend individual words, but not certain grammatical constructions.

Often stroke patients with visual disorders have considerable difficulty reading because they are blind to certain visual fields. This problem is not related to receptive aphasia; rather, the patients can't see the word—if they could, they would read it correctly—or are unaware of additional words that need to be read, as in unilateral inattention. The classification of aphasias into receptive and expressive is a useful didactic tool, but in reality most left hemisphere stroke patients have a combination of both aphasia types, because the left middle cerebral artery serves both expressive and receptive areas.

ANTERIOR VERSUS POSTERIOR STROKES

Disorders of the anterior cerebral artery may cause motor or sensory impairment involving the leg. Because the anterior cerebral arteries serve the prefrontal lobes, deficits consistent with a prefrontal syndrome, including disinhibition and dysfunction of executive skills, are also characteristic. Strokes in the posterior cerebral artery are less common and typically cause visual field loss and sensory loss of one side. Basilar artery disorders may have a similar effect as posterior cerebral arteries stroke if the posterior communicating artery provides insufficient blood supply. Those include blood flow disruption of the brain stem, including cranial nerve involvement, the cerebellum (see Exhibit 9 for example of a cerebellar stroke), and the occipital lobes.

EMOTIONAL AND BEHAVIORAL CHANGES AFTER A STROKE

After a stroke, it is common for patients to respond differently to people and events in terms of their emotional reactions. This relates in part to the experience of significant stress in the patient's life, but also to the fact that the integrity of the brain has been compromised.

Neuropsychology in Action 9.2

Case Example: Serial Assessment of a Left Stroke

by Eric A. Zillmer

The client is a 32-year-old, married, right-handed, female with 12 years of education. She worked as a manager for a fast food restaurant and lived with her husband and two young children in a two-story house. One month prior to my evaluation, she sustained a sudden onset of aphasia, right-sided weakness, and headache. CT scan showed an infarction in the area of the left cerebral hemisphere. A carotid angiogram showed an occluded internal carotid artery. Past medical history was unremarkable. There was no history of drug or alcohol use. The client was tested using the Assessment of Impairment Measure, or AIM (Zillmer, Chelder, & Efthimiou, 1995; see Chapter 14) at the start (administration 1) and one month later, at the end of her inpatient rehabilitation program (administration 2). Briefly, the AIM measures eight areas of cognitive abilities and two areas of behavioral competence. For the neuropsychology student, it is easiest to evaluate the percentage correct score. Healthy individuals are able to complete at least 90 percent of the items on each scale. Less than 80 percent correct corresponds to an impairment for that cognitive area and is highlighted by an asterisk related to the severity of impairment; * = mild, ** = moderate, *** = severe. For neuropsychologists it is important to assess the stroke victim as early as medically possible after stroke, to establish a baseline and to document improvements on subsequent testing. The administration one month after the stroke was as follows:

Subtest	Raw Score	% Correct	Impairment
I. Orientation	13	62**	Moderate
II. Sensation/perception	25	86	
III. Attention/concentration	42	74*	Mild
IV. Motor	27	76*	Mild
V. Verbal functions	18	52***	Severe
VI. Visual-spatial organization	33	94	
VII. Memory	18	44***	Severe
VIII. Judgment/problem solving	18	60**	Moderate
TOTAL SCORE	194	68**	**Moderate**
IX. Psychological distress scale	9	66**	Moderate
X. Activities of daily living (ADLs)	10	52***	Severe

* Denotes impairment associated with scores < 80% correct: * = mild, ** = moderate, *** = severe.

At the time of the initial evaluation, the client's speech was marked by paraphasias (the substitution of wrong words or phrases) and verbal perseverative tendencies (unnecessary repeating). On the orientation scale (Scale I) she was oriented to person and could state her name, age, and date of birth. She was somewhat oriented to place: She knew she was in a rehabilitation hospital, but could not give its name or location. She could write the correct date, but could not recall the current or last president. The sensation and perception scale (Scale II) showed a significant sensory and motor deficit on her dominant right side. She could not feel light touch on her right hand with single or double simultaneous stimulation. The examiner could

not accurately assess her visual acuity because of her expressive aphasia and inability to read numbers and letters.

Her attention/concentration (Scale III) was within normal limits for visually based items such as the cancelation tasks and mental control tasks requiring her to inhibit and initiate a motor response to a verbal cue. On verbal tasks, she was able to perform automatic tasks such as counting from 1 to 20 and reciting the alphabet, but could not perform any other tasks that required voluntary and purposeful speech (such as counting by serial threes and reciting the days of the week backward).

The client's gross and fine motor ability (Scale IV) and speed were intact on her nonaffected left side. However, on her dominant right side she showed a marked hemiparalysis and could not voluntarily move her right shoulder, arm, hand, or fingers. She did not show any evidence of motor apraxia and could copy simple designs adequately with her nondominant hand.

Her verbal functions (Scale V) were severely impaired, consistent with the location of her CVA in the distribution of the left middle cerebral artery. Receptive language skills were moderately impaired, as she could only follow one-step commands without difficulty. With two-step commands she became easily confused. Expressive speech was severely impaired. On the word fluency item, which requires the individual to name as many animals as possible in 30 seconds, she was only able to name one and perseverated with the word "baseball," which was an incorrect response to a previous item. She was able to correctly repeat words and phrases after the examiner, but was unable to initiate a correct response on her own. She also demonstrated alexia and agraphia for written language.

The client's visual-spatial functions were basically intact (Scale VI). She made only one minor error on this scale, which requires analysis and synthesis of the line configuration of a simple design. Figure–ground distinctions, spatial manipulation, visual sequencing, facial recognition, and spatial orientation, all tested within normal limits.

Her visual memory appeared to be within normal limits for both immediate and delayed recall procedures. However, verbal memory was severely impaired (Scale VII) secondary to her receptive and expressive aphasia. She was able to correctly repeat a list of five words for four separate trials. However, on the recognition task (two minutes later), she could identify only two words and made five false positive responses.

Her judgment/problem solving (Scale VIII) appeared moderately impaired secondary to her receptive and expressive aphasia. Yet she did demonstrate some reasoning skills on the purely visual problem-solving items such as the visual analogies. On the psychological distress scale (Scale IX), she showed a moderate degree of psychological distress. She could perform on her own about 50% of the ADLs (activities of daily living) listed (Scale X).

The client's overall neuropsychological picture based on the initial AIM showed a moderate degree of cognitive impairment for left hemisphere functions. This was consistent with the site of her CVA (Zillmer, Efthimiou, McClain, Harris, Resh, & Chelder, 1994). Cognitive areas that were relatively unimpaired included sensation, perception, and visual-spatial organization. An examiner retested the client one month later, after she had completed her inpatient rehabilitation program. The results were as follows:

Overall, scores improved by 17 percent on the posttest administration of the AIM. The most significant improvement occurred in orientation, verbal functions, memory, judgment/problem solving, psychological distress, and activities of daily living skills. The client correctly responded verbally to all the orientation questions except for one, which asked what town the hospital was located in. Verbal functions improved dramatically. The client showed good receptive speech in that she was now able to follow two-step commands easily. Verbal fluency remained limited but still showed a dramatic improvement. On the animal fluency item, she went from 0 words to 5 words and could now read and write sentences to dictation. Memory functions showed a significant improvement in her verbal memory, as she could now encode verbal information and retrieve it spontaneously. Judgment/problem solving showed some problems with concrete

Continued

Subtest	Raw Score %	Correct %	Change	Residual Impairment
I. Orientation	18	86	+24	
II. Sensation/perception	29	100	+14	
III. Attention/concentration	41	94	+20	
IV. Motor	32	90	+14	
V. Verbal functions	25	72*	+20	Mild
VI. Visual-spatial organization	32	92	0	
VII. Memory	28	68**	+24	Moderate
VIII. Judgment/problem solving	25	84	+24	
TOTAL SCORE	**230**	**85**	**+17**	
IX. Psychological distress scale	4	86	+20	
X. Activities of daily living (ADLs)	18	90	+38	

* Denotes impairment associated with scores < 80% correct: * = mild, ** = moderate, *** = severe.

Continued

thinking, but generally good common sense, reasoning, and judgment. The reported amount of psychological distress experienced by this young woman decreased by 20%, and she showed a 38% increase in her level of independent functioning in her ADLs.

Neuropsychological testing proved a very valuable technique in tracking this young woman's recovery from stroke. It was also effective in demonstrating the breadth of improvement this client made in cognitive, psychological, and physical skills, as well as documenting the residual areas of impairment in verbal functioning and verbal memory. The neuropsychology student should note that the precise extent of this patient's deficits and partial recovery is not obvious even to health care workers and the immediate family. That is why neuropsychological testing can be so important, not only in quantifying cognitive abilities, but also in setting realistic expectations for recovery and rehabilitation. In this case, the family was focusing mostly on the patient's residual impairment in memory and language. In charting the patient's remarkable recovery, I was able to help the family reframe their perceptions of the perceived strengths and weaknesses, thus helping them also cope with this potentially devastating disease.

Depression

Depression is a common and not very surprising reaction to stroke. Depression may be indicated if patients feel overwhelmed with sadness, believe they have failed completely, blame themselves for their problems, and often feel like crying. Poor sleep, decreased appetite, low self-esteem, and reduced efficiency are present as well. Whenever people experience loss, depression is a natural response. Depression is most likely to occur among patients with right-sided weakness and corresponding left hemisphere stroke. Often a patient does not show signs of depression until 6 to 12 months after a stroke when the scope of the loss has sunk in and there is time to think about how life has changed. Research and experience tells us that depression is best treated with a combination of psychotherapy and antidepressant medication (Freedman et al., 1978).

Apathy

Apathy or indifference involves lack of emotions. The person isn't sad or happy. In fact, the person may not seem to have any emotions. The voice sounds monotone, the face lacks expression, and if you ask the patient what he or she feels, the answer will be neutral, or without affective tone. On occasion patients who lack vocal and facial expression nevertheless report that they feel depressed, afraid, or angry. Both depression and apathy are quite common after a stroke, in part related to the loss of function that can accompany stroke, but also related to reduced brain efficiency after such trauma. Thus, part of the depression or apathy in a stroke patient is related to the stroke itself. In this sense the depression is more biological than psychological.

Euphoria

Euphoria is an overriding positive emotional response that is "too happy," given the circumstances. Euphoric people are not sad, indifferent, or apathetic; in fact, they are full of ideas and energy. Patients with euphoria seem positively happy about or despite their condition. Euphoria goes beyond a capacity to overcome obstacles—it is as if no obstacles existed. Apathy and euphoria are especially common among patients with left-sided weakness—that is, those suffering from right hemisphere stroke.

Impulsive Behavior

An impulsive emotional response is one that seems to come without warning. Patients who have labile emotions will cry or laugh in response to events or phrases that others around them might find only mildly arousing. For example, most people respond to the National Anthem before a baseball game with a smile. The stroke patient may respond with seemingly uncontrolled tearfulness or laughter. Labile emotional responses usually embarrass the patient and upset the family members. As a consequence, family members often avoid talking about important family topics, lest the discussion "upset" the patient. It is important to remember that labile emotional responses are a physiological and not an emotional response to a stroke. In fact, patients often cry in response to happy events—as when a therapist compliments them.

Impulsivity of behavior also affects a person's ability to stop motor actions. For example, a stroke survivor may automatically stand up and begin to walk on legs that cannot support him or her. This is dangerous to the well-being of the stroke patient, and therapists spend much time in rehabilitation helping the person to inhibit dangerous or inappropriate behaviors.

Lack of Initiation

On the other end of the spectrum, strokes can also impair a person's ability to initiate (or start) a behavior (akinesia). For example, the person may be hungry, and food may be sitting there ready to be consumed, but the person fails to bring the food to his or her mouth. In the extreme, the person may fail to chew once food has been placed in his or her mouth. The inability to initiate behavior may appear in the person's verbal responses. For example, it may take a very long time to answer questions. A difficulty related to problems initiating actions is the perseveration of behavior. Perseveration is the inability to stop behaviors once they have started. A patient may perform a motor movement over and over again, unable to stop it. Motor rigidity, perseveration, motor impersistence, and disinhibition are common problems in stroke patients and generally improve with rehabilitation.

Poor Judgment

Many stroke victims demonstrate poor judgment. Ironically, many such patients often can verbalize the appropriate actions they "should take," but can't follow through with those actions. For example, individuals with a spatial problem may be able to verbalize the steps in preparing a cup of coffee, but nevertheless continue to let coffee overflow when pouring a cup. It is as if their words and actions were not related. The brain trauma has impaired their ability to monitor their own behaviors and to understand the consequences of their own actions.

Conclusion

In general, damage to the brain may result from either primary or secondary damage, and may have either acute or long-term effects. In addition to damage within the immediate area, there may also be damage to more distal areas because of disconnected neuronal pathways. The diagnosis of primary damage relates to the initial injury or insult to the brain. If axons are completely severed or destroyed, the damage is often permanent and that tissue is lost. Secondary brain damage, in contrast, may result in either permanent or temporary damage. Secondary damage is caused by the aftereffects of the primary injury. Hemorrhage or bleeding causes oxygen deprivation and can lead to cell death known as necrosis. Edema, or "brain swelling"; hemorrhage; and infection may all cause increased cranial pressure. This pressure in the nonexpanding skull may effectively "squeeze off" areas of brain functions. If these secondary effects can be controlled quickly, the damage and functional effects may reverse in the acute stages of recovery. What is considered primary damage in one situation may be secondary damage in another. For example, a head injury, discussed in the next chapter, may cause primary axonal severing, destruction of brain tissue, and secondary swelling and hemorrhaging. A stroke's primary damage may be caused by a hemorrhage, but there may still be secondary swelling and intercranial pressure. Sudden traumas such as stroke tend to have more striking and noticeable behavioral effects than slowly emerging processes.

The most frequently encountered cerebrovascular disorders may at times produce multiple cognitive disabilities, yet often such dysfunction is relatively localized in terms of the anatomic area involved as well as the corresponding neuropsychological sequelae. However, more general neuropsychological disabilities are possible when, for example, larger areas of the brain are infarcted. In Chapter 10 we discuss other neurologic disorders of the brain, specifically tumors and traumatic head injuries.

Critical Thinking Questions

- What are the neurological, behavioral, and emotional symptoms of a stroke?
- What are the major forms of treatment for stroke?
- Why do some stroke victims downplay their illness, whereas others go into a deep depression?
- Describe the most common neuropsychological deficits associated with stroke.

Key Terms

Lesions
Necrosis
Anoxia
Hypoxia
Sleep apnea
Hydrocephalus
Communicating
  hydrocephalus
Obstructive hydrocephalus

Stroke
Cerebrovascular accident
  (CVA)
Intracranial pressure (ICP)
Ischemia
Infarction
Hemorrhage
Transient ischemic attack
  (TIA)

Thrombosis
Atherosclerosis
Platelets
Endothelium
Embolism
Atrial fibrillation
Hemorrhage
Hematoma
Intracerebral

Subarachnoid hemorrhage
Aneurysms
Arteriovenous malformations
  (AVM)
Aura
Migraine stroke
Stenosis
Collateral blood vessel
Anastomosis

Web Connections

http://www.med.harvard.edu/AANLIB/home.html
Harvard Medical School—CVA Facts
This site for the Whole Brain Atlas has an excellent section of images demonstrating various types of CVAs discussed in our text. A great way to visualize the extent of damage different types of cerebrovascular accidents may manifest.

http://neurosurgery.mgh.harvard.edu/vaschome.htm
Brain Aneurysm and AVM Center
Links you to the Harvard Brain Aneurysm and AVM Center at Mass General, where you can find discussions of the latest treatment for these and other cerebrovascular disorders.

http://www.stanford.edu/group/neurology/stroke
Stroke Awareness
Stanford Medical Center's site for stroke awareness and treatment information.

http://www.ninds.nih.gov
National Institute on Neurological Disorders and Stroke
An excellent site for the most up-to-date information on CVAs and related disorders. Internal search engines allow you to be as specific as you would like in obtaining information.

Chapter 10

TUMORS AND TRAUMATIC HEAD INJURY

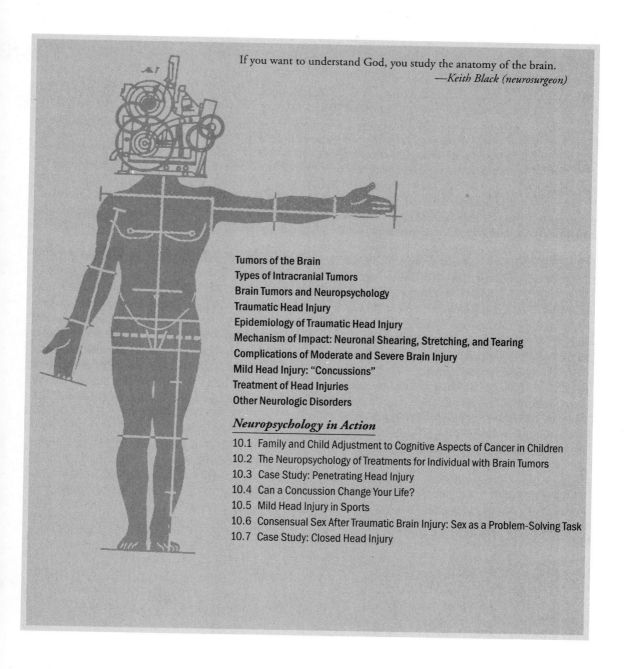

If you want to understand God, you study the anatomy of the brain.
—*Keith Black (neurosurgeon)*

Tumors of the Brain
Types of Intracranial Tumors
Brain Tumors and Neuropsychology
Traumatic Head Injury
Epidemiology of Traumatic Head Injury
Mechanism of Impact: Neuronal Shearing, Stretching, and Tearing
Complications of Moderate and Severe Brain Injury
Mild Head Injury: "Concussions"
Treatment of Head Injuries
Other Neurologic Disorders

Neuropsychology in Action

10.1 Family and Child Adjustment to Cognitive Aspects of Cancer in Children
10.2 The Neuropsychology of Treatments for Individual with Brain Tumors
10.3 Case Study: Penetrating Head Injury
10.4 Can a Concussion Change Your Life?
10.5 Mild Head Injury in Sports
10.6 Consensual Sex After Traumatic Brain Injury: Sex as a Problem-Solving Task
10.7 Case Study: Closed Head Injury

Keep in Mind

■ What happens when a tumor grows in the brain?

■ Do different injuries to the brain have similar effects on the brain, or should we expect a variety of effects?

■ What is the difference between a penetrating and a closed head injury?

■ What role do neuropsychologists play in the diagnosis and treatment of head injuries?

Overview

Neurologists commonly differentiate neurologic disorders of the brain by whether they have a particular focus or site, or are more generalized, affecting the brain as a whole. There are, however, many exceptions to this simple classification paradigm. As discussed in Chapter 9, a stroke or a bleed in the brain is a focal disorder because the damage occurred at a specific location. In contrast, many small bleeds or very large hemorrhages often present a diffuse clinical picture. Similarly, a single brain tumor may represent a very precise focal deficit, whereas a large tumor or multiple small tumors of the brain may leave the patient with more wide-reaching deficits, which typically entail diffuse neuropsychological deficits. For the most part, neuropsychologists consider tumors focal disorders of the brain, because most often they entail more or less circumscribed brain damage.

In contrast, diffuse disorders most often involve dysfunction of the entire brain and most frequently appear in closed head injuries, toxic conditions, and degenerative disorders. As mentioned, this classification paradigm is not entirely accurate, but it helps the neuropsychologist make an overall determination of the severity and extent of possible dysfunction. In a car accident, the rotational forces on the head often result in blunt trauma to the brain, and thus cause diffuse damage. In contrast, a gunshot wound to the head may present a relatively localized, but devastating trauma to the brain and may have more localized deficits. So keep in mind that this categorization is not a hard-and-fast rule. In principle, focal disorders may interrupt a very small area of brain functioning, whereas other areas of the brain remain relatively intact. Sometimes the loss of brain tissue is so small that it may not be noticeable except with sophisticated neuropsychological testing or advanced imaging techniques.

In this chapter, we first discuss the more focal disorder of brain tumors. Later we discuss the more diffuse traumas of the brain related to head injury. Finally, we discuss other, less frequently encountered neurologic disorders, including brain abscesses, infections, and neurotoxins.

Tumors of the Brain

If her brain tumor had shown up 10 years ago, Melinda Schuler would not have had much of a chance. Few doctors would even have tried to remove the malignant growth, located within her right frontal lobe. The tumor had already taken over one-sixth of her cranium, pushing her brain down and to the left. Had it been left alone, the cancer would have kept inexorably compressing useful tissue, robbing the patient of speech, movement, consciousness, life itself—all within months. If surgeons had tried to cut it out, there would have been a risk of taking too little, leaving cancerous tissue to grow again, or taking too much, causing profound and irreparable brain damage. Fortunately for Schuler, the tumor was discovered in 1997 rather than in 1987. In the intervening decade, brain surgery advanced dramatically, enabling surgeons to refine their operating techniques enormously with more sophisticated medical technology. Today they can chart a far safer passage to tumors hidden deep in the brain.

To reach such a tumor, a team of specialists first drill a series of holes into the patient's skull, not unlike the burr holes used in trephination discussed in Chapter 1. Then the surgeon connects the holes with a surgical jigsaw. After he or she lifts the oval-shaped piece of skull, the dura mater is exposed, a thick membrane that protects the brain and spinal cord. Melinda's tumor was sitting right in the middle of her motor area. To operate on the tumor, and not leave her paralyzed, the neurosurgeon had to navigate carefully, dividing the tumor from the normal brain, cauterizing severed blood vessels along the way. Gradually the tumor was cut away from Melinda's brain and extracted. A lab autopsy verified the diagnosis of the initial biopsy: a malignant astrocytoma, a slow-growing but dangerous tumor (discussed later). Schuler's death sentence had been postponed, perhaps by years. By the following day, she would be walking the halls. Textbooks would project that she would live three to five years more, even after her successful operation. No matter how careful the surgeon cuts out the malignant tumor, the few stray cancer cells that are inevitably left behind will begin to grow again.

The term **tumor** refers to a morbid enlargement or new growth of tissue in which cell multiplication is uncontrolled and progressive. Tumors are also called **neoplasms,** which means "new tissue." The new cell growth resembles cells already normally present in the body. This growth is, however, often arranged in disorganized ways, does not serve any functional purpose, and often grows at the expense of surrounding intact tissue. Brain tumors make up approximately 5% of all cancers and appear in approximately 2% of all autopsies. Because cancer is the second most frequent cause of death, the actual number of victims suffering

from brain tumors is actually quite high. Brain tumors can occur at any age, but are most common in early and middle adulthood (Golden et al., 1992).

Brain tumors can be conceptualized according to two principal forms:

1. **Infiltrative tumors,** which take over (or infiltrate) neighboring areas of the brain and destroy its tissue
2. **Noninfiltrative tumors,** which are encapsulated and differentiated (easily distinguished from brain tissue), but cause dysfunction by compressing surrounding brain tissue

Tumors can further be classified according to two additional descriptors:

1. **Malignant,** which indicates that the properties of the tumor cells invades other tissue and are likely to regrow or spread
2. **Benign,** which describes cell growth that is usually surrounded by a fibrous capsule, is typically noninfiltrative (noninvasive), and will not spread

The primary feature of malignant tumors is that they are much more likely to reappear after surgical intervention. Because they are infiltrative, it is difficult to completely remove malignant tumors surgically. Malignant tumors may also "travel" to other organs in the body through the bloodstream. This form of spreading is called **metastasis.** Metastatic brain tumors typically originate from primary sites other than the brain, most frequently the lung or the breast. Even benign tumors, however, are troublesome if they occur in the brain. This is because the skull completely encloses the brain and any mass-producing lesion displaces healthy brain tissue. You may already realize that nerve cells are not likely to cause brain tumors, because neurons do not grow or heal spontaneously. This is correct. Tumors of the brain arise mostly from the supporting cells of the brain. As a result neurons are only indirectly affected. **Neuromas** are tumors or new growths that are largely made up of nerve cells and nerve fibers.

One method of evaluating the malignant features of a brain tumor is to **grade** them from slow-growing neoplasms to rapidly growing tumors. The grade of a tumor is determined by its malignancy, the tendency of a tumor to grow at a fast rate, causing severe destruction of brain tissue and eventually death. Grading is from 1 to 4, with a Grade 1 tumor representing a slow-growing tumor accompanied by few neuropsychological deficits. Grades 2 and 3 represent intermediate rates of growth and neuropsychological dysfunction. Grade 4 tumors grow fast and typically have a poor prognosis for recovery. Table 10.1 reviews the different characteristics of brain tumors. Neurological and neuropsychological dysfunction results from the invasion and destruction of brain tissue by the tumor. Secondary effects include increased intracranial pressure (ICP) and cerebral swelling (edema), which displace and compress brain tissue, cranial nerves, the cerebral vascular structure, and the cerebrospinal fluid system.

 ## Types of Intracranial Tumors

INFILTRATING TUMORS

As already mentioned, infiltrative tumors are not clearly differentiated from surrounding brain tissue. The most common infiltrative tumors are **gliomas,** which make up approximately 40 to 50% of all brain tumors. Gliomas are relatively fast-growing tumors that arise from supporting glia cells (see Figure 10.1 and Exhibit 9). Any type of glia cells can form a tumor, including gliomas (arising from neuroglia-cells), astrocytomas (which are formed from astrocyte cells), and oligodendrogliomas (composed of oligodendrocyte cells). A particularly destructive and fatal glioma is the **glioblastoma multiforme (GBM),** which generally arises after middle age and is most often confined to one hemisphere. A GBM is typically a large, Grade 4 tumor, growing very rapidly, with symptoms arising within several weeks. Surgical removal is often incomplete because of the highly infiltrative and malignant characteristics of these tumors. Thus, regrowth and eventual death are common within 6 to 12 months after surgery, even after aggressive radiation therapy. **Astrocytomas** are infiltrative tumors of astrocytes, a type of glia cell. Astrocytomas grow more slowly than GBMs, thus they have a somewhat better prognosis. Gliomas of the

Table 10.1 *Characteristics of Intracranial Tumors*

1. Characteristics of brain tumors
   - Atypical, uncontrolled growth of cells
   - Cells do not serve functional purpose
   - Tumor grows at the expense of healthy cells

2. Infiltrating tumors
   - Take over and "invade" neighboring areas of the brain and destroy surrounding tissue

3. Noninfiltrating tumors
   - Are encapsulated, well differentiated, and noninvasive

4. Malignant
   - Indicates that the properties of the tumor cells invade other tissue and that there is a propensity for regrowth

5. Benign
   - Describes abnormal cell growth that is usually surrounded by a fibrous capsule and is noninfiltrative; a much smaller probability for regrowth

6. Grading
   - A classification system of tumor growth. Grading is in order of increasing malignancy from Grade 1 to Grade 4, depending on cell type

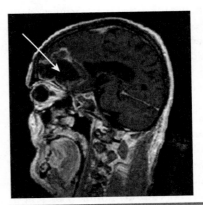

Figure 10.1 MRI examination of a patient with a cerebral glioma. The patient had suffered from increasing headaches for six weeks, memory impairment, and increasing paresis of the left side. Walking remained undamaged. MRI examination indicated a tumor 65 x 56 x 69 mm in size in the right frontal lobe. The tumor displaced the anterior part of the right lateral ventricle and moved a part of the corpus callosum to the left. (Dorota Kozinska, University of Warsaw, Poland)

brain stem are typically astrocytomas and often affect cranial nerves V, VI, VII, and X. Finally, an **oligodendroglioma** is a rare, slowly growing tumor that mostly affects young adults.

NONINFILTRATING TUMORS

Meningiomas

The most common noninfiltrative tumors are the **meningiomas,** which represent approximately 15% of all brain tumors. Meningiomas are highly encapsulated benign tumors that arise from the arachnoid layer of the meninges. Their incidence increases with age and they are more frequent in women than in men (by a 2 to 1 ratio). Meningiomas grow very slowly and can become rather large before the gradually increasing pressure on the brain and displacement of surrounding healthy brain tissue cause symptoms. Technically, a meningioma is not a brain tumor, because the growth is in the brain's covering, outside the brain. This is why we refer to all tumors discussed in this chapter as *intracranial* (within the skull), rather than as *brain* tumors. With meningiomas, brain tissue is not destroyed, but neuropsychological impairments may appear because the space-occupying mass puts physical pressure on the cortex, especially in large meningiomas. Because meningiomas grow over many years, the brain can often accommodate the size of the tumor. Thus focal or severe deficits usually do not accompany this type of tumor. Because the brain adapts to the slowly growing meningiomas, tumors in the frontal area may grow relatively large before intracranial pressure produces behavioral symptoms. Therefore meningiomas often cause no symptoms and remain undiagnosed, only to be discovered later on autopsy.

The neurosurgeon finds meningiomas relatively easy to remove because they are encapsulated outside the brain. Removal can, however, become complicated if the tumor is difficult to access, as when the lesion is in the intrahemispheric fissure or the inferior parts of the brain. Meningiomas arising from the optic nerve sheath may be particularly difficult or impossible to remove, because they almost envelop the optic nerve. Nevertheless, because they are encapsulated and benign, meningiomas offer the best prognosis for complete recovery of any of the brain tumors.

Metastatic Tumor

A malignant but encapsulated tumor is a **metastatic tumor.** *Metastasis* is a medical term for the transfer of disease from one organ or part not directly connected with it. The capacity to metastasize is a characteristic of all malignant tumors. Metastatic tumors arise secondarily to cancerous tumors, which have their primary site in other parts of the body, such as the lungs, breasts, or lymph system (Earle, 1955). The secondary growths arise because cancer cells from the primary neoplasm detach. The blood stream can carry the cells to the brain, where they multiply. This is why early diagnosis in cancer is so important: to keep tumor tissue from "metastasizing." Metastatic brain tumors typically have multiple sites and represent up to 40% of all brain tumors seen in the elderly. They generally grow fast and typically occur at the junction of gray and white matter, close to the cortex surface, although they can grow at any location in the brain. Metastatic brain tumors in adults arise most frequently from bronchogenic carcinoma (lung cancer), adenocarcinoma of the breast (breast cancer), and malignant melanoma (skin cancer).

A typical clinical picture in metastatic tumor is the diagnosis of an elderly man with lung cancer related to a long history of cigarette smoking. Examination of the patient's lymph nodes reveals evidence of a tumor. Twelve weeks later the patient develops a gait disturbance. Neuropsychological evaluation reveals that the patient is cognitively intact, but has motor slowing on the left side, an intention tremor, and difficulty walking in a straight line. Diagnostic imaging shows a metastatic tumor in the left hemisphere of the cerebellum (recall that cerebellar deficits involve the ipsilateral arm and leg). Despite intensive chemo- and radiation therapy, the patient dies. The prognosis in metastatic brain cancer is typically poor because cancer invades multiple organs and produces multiple growths in the brain. Neurosurgeons usually do not consider extracting metastatic tumors if multiple sites are present. But as with any disease there are exceptions, and the disease progress is often difficult to predict. For example, U.S. cyclist Lance Armstrong was diagnosed with testicular cancer. His cancer metastasized to his lungs and his brain, spawning multiple tumors. After surgery Armstrong made a remarkable recovery and has not only stayed cancer free, but went on to win the month-long 1999 and 2000 Tour de France, the most grueling bicycle race in the world.

Acoustic Neuroma

Acoustic neuromas are progressively enlarging, benign tumors within the auditory canal arising from Schwann cells of the VIIIth cranial nerve, the auditory vestibular nerve, which sends sensory hearing and equilibrium information to the brain. Initial symptoms include ringing in the ears (tinnitus), followed by partial deafness, such as in distinguishing speech sounds and rhythmic patterns. Acoustic neuromas typically begin to grow in the internal auditory canal and then grow medially. They affect the Vth (the trigeminal nerve, which provides sensory information of the face and motor control for chewing and swallowing) and the VIIth cranial nerves (the facial nerve, which provides sensory information from the tongue and motor control of facial expressions and crying). As a result, the patient may lose his or her sense of hearing, followed by complaints of a loss of taste on one side. Physicians often consult audiologists in diagnosing acoustic neuromas.

Pituitary Tumors

The classification and neuropathology of **pituitary tumors** is complex because of the pituitary gland's relationship to the chemistry of the nervous and endocrine systems. Scientists traditionally divide pituitary tumors into **functioning** and **nonfunctioning adenomas.** Pituitary adenomas are benign neoplasms of the pituitary gland. Nonfunctioning adenomas produce symptoms caused by pressure on the pituitary and adjacent structures. As the tumor grows out of the sella—the bony capsule that holds the pituitary—headaches are common. Visual field deficits may also occur due to compression of the optic chiasm (bitemporal hemianopsia). Hypothalamic compression usually causes diabetes insipidus.

Functioning pituitary tumors play an "uninvited" role in the operation of the pituitary gland, often affecting the release of the gland's hormones. Function-

ing tumors of the pituitary include the **acidophilic adenoma,** a tumor usually found in the anterior lobe of the gland. The acidophilic adenoma provokes excessive secretion of growth hormones, often resulting in giantism, a condition featuring enlarged jaw, nose, tongue, hands, and feet. The **chromophobic adenoma** also appears in the anterior aspects of the pituitary gland and often produces hyper- or hypopituitarism. **Basophilic adenomas** also occur in the anterior lobe of the pituitary gland, but give rise to excessive secretion of ACTH, which can cause **Cushing's syndrome.** This syndrome, named after Boston surgeon Harvey Cushing (1869–1939), is a severe systemic illness most often seen in females, which includes neurological symptoms and changes in bone structure, hypertension, and diabetes. The ACTH-secreting tumor is the most serious condition encountered by any of the pituitary tumors and can necessitate complete removal of the tumor, including the pituitary gland.

CHILDHOOD TUMORS

Childhood tumors are less frequent than brain tumors in adults. The most frequent is the **medulloblastoma,** a rapidly growing and very malignant tumor located in the inferior vermis close to the exit of cerebrospinal fluid from the fourth ventricle. This type of tumor accounts for about two-thirds of all tumors in children and causes increased intracranial pressure due to obstructive hydrocephalus. Early symptoms include vomiting and headache. Other common childhood tumors are cerebellar astrocytomas, gliomas of the brainstem and optic nerve, and pinealomas. Pineal tumors are most common in prepubescent boys. The tumor often compresses the aqueduct of Sylvius, causing hydrocephalus, papilledema, and other signs of intracranial pressure. Table 10.2 summarizes the different types and features of brain tumors.

DIAGNOSIS OF BRAIN TUMORS

The overall incidence of brain tumors for males and females is about equal, but cerebellar medulloblastomas and glioblastoma multiforme are more common in males, and meningiomas are more frequent in

Table 10.2	*Types of Brain Tumors*

Acoustic neuroma   A benign tumor growing from the sheath of the acoustic nerve at the cerebellopontine angle

Gliomas   A tumor composed of tissue representing neuroglia; the term *glioma* is often used to describe all primary, intrinsic neoplasms of the brain and the spinal cord

Glioblastoma   Malignant forms of astrocytoma

Glioblastoma multiforme   An astrocytoma of Grade 3 or 4, a rapidly growing tumor usually confined to one cerebral hemisphere and composed of a mixture of spongioblasts, astroblasts, and astrocytes

Astrocytoma   A malignant tumor composed primarily of astrocytes

Ependymal glioma   A bulky, solid, firm vascular tumor of the fourth ventricle

Oligodendroglioma   A neoplasm derived from and composed of oligodendrogliocytes

Optic glioma   A slowly growing glioma of the optic nerve or optic chiasm, associated with visual loss and loss of ocular movement

Meningioma   A typically benign tumor arising from arachnoid cells; produces neuropsychological deficits by exerting pressure on surrounding brain substances or cranial nerves

Metastatic tumor   A growth of a tumor, often multiple, distant from the site primarily involved in the morbid process

Pituitary adenoma   A tumor of the pituitary gland; pituitary adenomas are often classified as functioning (changing the secretion of the pituitary gland) and nonfunctioning (benign)

Pinealoma   A tumor of the pineal body

females. The overall frequency of various types of intracranial tumors is approximately 45% for gliomas, 15% for pituitary adenomas, 15% for meningiomas, 15% for metastatic brain tumors, and 10% for other types.

Early behavioral symptoms in the diagnosis of tumor include a sudden onset of headaches, nausea, loss of cognitive function, or seizures. The intracranial pressure triad often accompanies the growth of brain tumors and includes

1. Headache
2. Nausea and vomiting
3. A positive papilledema, a swelling of the optic disk in the eye

Of course, not every patient complaining of a headache has a brain tumor, but headache often accompanies brain tumor because of the enlarging tumor mass.

The introduction of the CT scan and the more recent MRI has literally revolutionized diagnosis of tumors. High-resolution CT can visualize even tiny tumors. Three-dimensional reconstruction can often demonstrate the intimate relationships of the tumor to its surrounding brain structure, facilitating precise removal of the tumor by surgeons. Today, neurologists most efficiently diagnose brain tumor using CT or MRI, which often provides the definitive diagnosis (see Chapter 6 for a comprehensive review of medical diagnostic procedures). Neurologists have used functional MRI (fMRI) to differentiate brain tissue from tumor tissue as well as to identify areas of the brain that are particularly vital for cognitive functions. This is often important, because using fMRI neurologists can identify a safe corridor through the brain into the tumor, which the surgeon can then use. In addition, fMRI can help differentiate whether or not the cancer itself contains vital brain tissue. Somatosensory evoked responses and direct stimulation of the brain can also help separate important brain tissue from brain tumor tissue. Neurologists often use plain x-ray films in diagnosing and planning surgery to remove meningiomas, because this type of tumor can erode the skull in a high percentage of patients, as shown in radiographic changes on skull x-ray films.

Angiography can occasionally be useful in tumor diagnosis to identify which primary branches of the cardiovascular system supply the tumor with its blood supply. Modern imaging is most effective in diagnosing the presence of a tumor, but not in diagnosing its type. Histological examination via brain biopsy is necessary to precisely diagnose the type of tumor and to select the most appropriate intervention. Neurologists most frequently do this using CT-guided stereotaxic biopsy, which interfaces stereotactic frames that fasten to the patient's head with steel pins. A biopsy needle is affixed to the frame, which the neurosurgeon can move with precision in all three dimensions. Using this procedure and with the patient under local anesthesia, the neurosurgeon can take a brain specimen through a burr hole. Subsequent laboratory examination can then provide the exact diagnosis of the tumor.

TREATMENT OF BRAIN TUMORS

The preferred treatment for brain tumors is total surgical excision of the tumor whenever possible. The prognosis for recovery after removing a brain tumor depends on two primary factors, the location and type of tumor. For example, a relatively simple surgical excision might involve a well-differentiated tumor, such as a meningioma, particularly if the tumor is in an easily accessible location (as in superior aspects of the cortex). If the tumor is malignant, local radiation therapy typically follows surgical removal to prevent regrowth. If the tumor is inaccessible, for example, in the region of the thalamus or brain stem, radiation therapy is the primary intervention. A fast-growing glioblastoma in a nonresectable location is often fatal within 12 months. Thus, the prognosis for GBMs is not good, but combined treatments have a small success rate. For difficult-to-access tumors, located at the base of the skull or covering the superior sagittal sinus, the neurosurgeon often uses a sophisticated operating microscope or a laser.

Chemotherapy for brain tumors is playing an increasing important role in the battle against cancer. Chemotherapy is most effective in tumors that have a high growth fraction, that is, that are actively dividing and producing DNA. When a tumor is young, most of its cells are making DNA. When antitumor drugs reach tumor cells in the phases of cell cycling, the cells die. As the tumor ages, growth fraction decreases and drug sensitivity declines. Thus the most effective form of chemotherapy is when the tumor is young and 100% of its cells are in the growth fraction—this again emphasizes the importance of early diagnosis. However, the blood–brain barrier (BBB), which protects the brain from foreign substances, complicates chemotherapy for brain tumors. The blood–brain barrier prevents cancer-killing drugs from entering brain tissue via the bloodstream. Thus antitumor drugs targeting brain tumors are limited to agents easily transported across the BBB—typically, very lipid-soluble substances. In recent years, however, researchers have discovered that some chemicals (such as RMP-7) are highly effective in opening the blood–brain barrier by making capillary walls "leaky."

As a result, chemotherapy drugs can act directly on the tumors, increasing their effectiveness as much as tenfold.

Medicine will only achieve a cure in the fight against brain tumors, however, when it can enlist the patient's own immune system to attack the cancer. Tumors produce a chemical that tricks the immune system into ignoring them. Recent genetic engineering research in animals has shown some promise in discovering substances that turn off the tumor cells' ability to produce their own vaccine. The tumor cells then become immediate targets of the immune system, which destroys them.

Treating brain tumors is not only complicated from a scientific perspective, but it also takes a psychological toll on the patient as well as the family (see Neuropsychology in Action 10.1). As a result, psychologists also play an important role in counseling patients undergoing cancer treatment or in hospice centers—health care centers that provide medical and emotional support for the terminal ill and their families.

Brain Tumors and Neuropsychology

The neuropsychological manifestations of brain tumors depend on the location, size, and grade of the tumor, rather than on its histological type. Smaller tumors near primary motor areas may cause seizures and loss of motor function, whereas deeper intracranial tumors may grow rather large before focal clinical symptoms appear. Evaluations also find a general decline in adaptive areas as well as in overall cognitive functioning, because the tumor displaces neighboring areas. The neuropsychological deficits of a GBM (glioblastoma multiforme) are profound (Smith, 1966). The destruction of whichever cerebral hemisphere is involved is severe and nearly complete. In the acute stages of GBM, neuropsychological evaluation is typically not undertaken, because the deficits are so severe and the overall medical condition of the patient is of most concern. Patients with astrocytomas may have longer histories of increasing problems, because of the slow growth of these neoplasms.

Oligodendrogliomas typically produce few neuropsychological effects because they grow so slowly.

Focal neuropsychological symptoms of brain tumors stem from localized destruction, compression of nervous tissue, or altered endocrine function. Tumors in the frontal lobes are most commonly meningiomas and gliomas. They can produce both localized and generalized cognitive deficits, including expressive aphasia (if located in the dominant hemisphere) or difficulties smelling (anosmia) related to a meningioma at the base of the frontal lobe. Inattention and changes in motivation commonly accompany tumors affecting both frontal hemispheres. Parietal lobe tumors may contralaterally impair sensory modalities, stereognosis, contralateral homonymous hemianopsia, and apraxia. Speech disturbances, agraphia, and finger agnosia may appear if the left hemisphere is involved, and neglect is characteristic of patents whose right hemisphere is affected.

Temporal lobe tumors may produce mixed expressive and receptive aphasia of the dominant temporal lobe. Nondominant temporal tumors often do not have "obvious" cognitive signs. Tumors deep in the temporal lobe may cause contralateral hemianopsia. Occipital lobe tumors most often entail visual deficits, typically a contralateral quadrant defect in the visual field or a hemaniopia with sparing of the macula. Subcortical tumors involving the internal capsule produce contralateral hemiplegia. Thalamic tumors produce contralateral sensory impairment. Basal ganglia tumors often result in tremors. All brain tumors may produce seizures, which may be preceded by an aura that may indicate the location of the tumor.

Metastatic tumors are often associated with neuropsychological test results indicating focal areas of deficits. Skills that the tumor does not affect may be relatively intact. Later stages of metastatic tumors with numerous sites and sizes may produce a diffuse loss of most neuropsychological abilities. Acoustic neuromas typically do not entail severe cognitive loss, but rather, a hearing impairment. A meningioma produces its behavioral effects by compressing the brain. Meningiomas near the optic nerve result in visual disturbances and are difficult to remove because of their location. Pituitary tumors also produce visual field defects because of the close relationship between the optic chiasm and the pituitary gland.

Neuropsychological evaluations have proven most useful in establishing a cognitive baseline before neurosurgery and in evaluating outcomes of patients after surgery. As already mentioned, neuropsychologists also provide counseling and education to brain tumor patients and their families. More recent research has focused on the neuropsychological implications of radiation therapy (see Neuropsychology in Action 10.2).

Traumatic Head Injury

The Kennedy clan (of John F. Kennedy fame, among others) engage in an annual family ritual during their skiing vacation in Aspen, Colorado. The Kennedy clan and friends gather at a mountaintop bar, waiting until the lifts shut down at about 4 P.M. Then, with few other skiers on the trails, they play football down the slope, with skis but no poles. A cross between Frisbee and touch football, "ski football" is an old Kennedy pastime. They divide into two teams and start tossing a makeshift football through the thin mountain air toward a goal, typically a trail marker. The rules of the game demand that a player must pass the ball to a teammate within 10 seconds or turn the ball over. This seems like a lot of fun, but inherent in skiing, as is true for most sports, is risk in the form of speed. Sports, in fact, account for 17% of all head injuries, second only to motor vehicle accidents. The most dangerous sports are equestrian events, gymnastics, and cheerleading. Among intercollegiate sports, gymnastics, football, lacrosse, and ice hockey are the most likely to lead to head injuries. Skiing is actually a relatively safe sport—there is less than one death per one million skied days. But that New Year's Eve afternoon the conditions were getting worse, the slopes were slick and icy, and the sun was setting behind the mountains, making it hard to see in the shadows and flat light. On the quintessential "last run" on the last day of the year, Michael L. Kennedy, the 39-year-old son of Ethel and the late Senator Robert, turned his head to catch the ball. He hit a fir tree head first on the left side of the trail.

N e u r o p s y c h o l o g y   i n   A c t i o n   1 0 . 1

Family and Child Adjustment to Cognitive Aspects of Cancer in Children

by Lamia P. Barakat Ph.D., Assistant Professor of Psychology, Department of Psychology, Drexel University.

Lisa is a 21-year-old woman referred to me by her pediatric oncologist. She was experiencing depressed mood, the possibility of pseudoseizures (behavioral manifestations of seizures with no associated neurologic changes), and family conflict. When she was 10 years old, Lisa had been treated for acute nonlymphoblastic leukemia through bone marrow transplant. Her bone marrow transplant included high-dose, whole-body radiation. Sequelae included apparent seizures (particularly when stressed); cognitive deficits, specifically limitations in short-term memory and attention span; cataracts; and infertility. After medical treatment, Lisa's school performance declined, although she graduated from high school, and she became socially isolated. At the time of referral, Lisa lived with her parents, who worked full time, and her younger brother, who was in college. She spent most of her time alone at home engaged in few activities. Her parents were caring and protective. They did not encourage Lisa to branch out of the home, fearing she would have a seizure in a public place. They were

uncertain of her capabilities and viewed the cancer and its consequences as severe and insurmountable. The family had experienced the death of another daughter from epilepsy and congenital abnormalities. In spite of her current situation, Lisa hoped to go to college, get married, and have children. Although Lisa's parents can be described as supportive and caring, the complexities of Lisa's medical condition, including her cognitive limitations and her unrealistic expectations, have placed a considerable burden on the family as a whole. As a result, the family was not coping and adapting well.

The role of the patient's cognitive factors in family functioning is complex; some detrimental effects may appear, but some families can cope with these problems. In addition, adequate family functioning accompanies higher intellectual functioning in children treated for cancer (Carlson-Green, Morris, & Krawiecki, 1995). The key to understanding the relationships among cognitive aspects of childhood cancer, child adjust-

ment, and family functioning may be to look at child and parent perceptions or appraisals of the illness's impact. A series of studies on childhood cancer survivors and their parents consistently relate perception of life threat associated with cancer and its treatment in the past and present, and appraisals of treatment intensity, to child, parent, and family adjustment (Barakat et al., 1997). However, objectively rated intensity of the treatment, severity of medical late effects (including cognitive impairments and special education placement), and history of cranial radiation treatment did not correlate with adjustment. Similar results characterize children treated for hypothalamic brain tumors. Perceived change in the child's academic, social, and behavioral functioning, as rated by parents following diagnosis and treatment, strongly correlate with child adjustment and general family functioning, whereas aspects of treatment and objective ratings of medical late effects did not (Foley et al., in press).

These findings provide strong evidence for the importance of child and

---

Yes, it was reckless to ski while playing a daring game of mountainside football. The ski patrol had warned against it. Tossing a makeshift football back and forth may have distracted Kennedy just enough that he was not able to stop or swerve before striking the tree. According to eyewitnesses, Kennedy—a good skier—first struck the tree with a tip of his ski, which caused him to catapult slightly and slam his head directly into its trunk without slowing down. With his

three youngest children watching in horror, Michael Kennedy died of a severe head injury to the back of his fractured skull. His injury must have damaged his brain stem, because his sister Rory, who was the first to his side, noticed no pulse or breathing. The medulla oblongata, a part of the lower brain stem, mediates vital functions necessary for life such as respiration, blood pressure, heart rate, and basic muscle tone. Damage to the medulla can interrupt motor and sen-

parent subjective appraisals or perceptions of cognitive limitations in understanding child and family functioning following cancer diagnosis and treatment. Importantly, preventive interventions can modify child and parent appraisals of cognitive limitations and the impact of the illness, to improve long-term family adaptation. It is essential to work with families from the point of cancer diagnosis to provide a realistic but optimistic framework for understanding children's capabilities and needs. The intervention must consider the child's ability to comprehend this information, given cognitive limitations.

Such interventions must also take into account developmental process in families. As the children grow older, families must be able to reassess and then reintegrate the meaning of the cognitive limitations for their children and their families. For example, as children enter formal schooling, families must balance the need to address potential learning problems with the need for children to engage in routine activities with peers. As children reach adolescence and plan to leave home, families must be able to set realistic academic and vocational goals with their children while allowing them to achieve independence in functioning. On the flip side, counselors must guide children and adolescents in choosing academic, vocational, and social goals that they can attain and that will bring some success.

In addition to addressing perceptions, it is necessary to develop positive changes in family interactions (such as interactions around homework, rules in the home, and peer relationships) to promote children's competencies and in turn improve functioning. In relation to this, planning must address the role of other systems, such as the school, church, and medical treatment team. Frequent communication among these systems decreases conflicting information provided to families and improves coordination of interactions. For instance, the child, parents, and teachers may cooperatively develop and implement a plan aimed at homework completion, that provides structure and motivation and builds on the child's cognitive strengths.

Finally, improving parent resources and coping helps improve the functioning of families dealing with the long-term strains of treatment for cancer and of cognitive changes. Family-to-family contact and support through multiple-family groups is an integral part of bolstering children and their parents' resources. Families learn from one another which coping strategies most facilitate healthy family development as the childhood cancer survivor moves into adulthood.

After a complete neurological and psychological evaluation, neuropsychologists diagnosed Lisa with grand mal

seizures, pseudoseizures, and major depression with dissociative features. Treatment entailed achieving a therapeutic dosage of medication for her seizures, and individual and family therapy. The goal of family therapy was to help Lisa and her parents realistically assess her skills and recognize her potential. Initially, through increasing her responsibility in the home, trips to the mall (where she was free to shop on her own), and engagement in hobbies, Lisa's sense of competence improved. Her parents' perceptions of her abilities became more optimistic, and their appraisals of her illness's severity lightened. Lisa and her parents began to focus on increasing Lisa's independent functioning. She successfully entered a vocational rehabilitation program and made plans for a clerical position in the future. She began to make friends and to attend social functions through her rehabilitation program. Lisa made a number of overnight visits with siblings, and her parents took a long-needed vacation without their daughter. Concurrently, counselors gently guided Lisa through cognitive interventions to understand and come to terms with her limitations, particularly those relevant to her hopes for a college education and children. Lisa's pseudoseizures and depression remitted.

---

sory pathways as well as threaten life itself. The death, ruled accidental, adds yet another tragedy to America's most famous clan.

Would a helmet have saved his life? Those who survive head injuries often sustain significant brain damage, which can change them for a lifetime, both physically and emotionally. This can result in a markedly altered lifestyle for the survivor and those who take care of him or her, the family, and loved ones.

 Epidemiology of Traumatic Head Injury

Human brains have evolved over hundreds of thousands of years, but only recently have people invented technology, both recreational and occupational, that has put brains in motion, often at high speeds. The skull and the dura mater protect the brain well, but are no match for the physical forces unleashed

Neuropsychology in Action 10.2

The Neuropsychology of Treatments for Individuals with Brain Tumors

by Carol L. Armstrong Ph.D., Department of Neurology, University of Pennsylvania and the Joseph Stokes Research Institute, Children's Hospital of Philadelphia.

Effective brain tumor treatment is always a compromise, involving the protection of healthy cells and the destruction of aggressive cancer cells that have infiltrated healthy tissue. Treatment choices are complex and should involve input from a team of oncological professionals, including neurosurgeon, oncologist-hematologist, radiation therapist, neuroradiologist, neurologist, and neuropsychologist. Surgical interventions range from biopsy, or the removal of enough tissue for microscopic determination of histologic type and pathologic grade of tumor cells, to the resection of 100% of tumor tissue as a method of preventing tumor regrowth. Brain surgery may also involve Wada testing or fMRI (see Chapter 6), with the aid of the neuropsychologist in determining hemispheric dominance of movement and language, and help from the neuroradiologist in outlining blood flow patterns in the brain. Specialists also may use brain mapping to localize function and preclude resection of brain tissue crucial for language or memory.

Besides surgical treatments for brain tumors, medical professionals often give radiation therapy and chemotherapy, either alone or in combination. The most common method of radiotherapy involves external photon beam radiation, which technicians administer a total dose of radiation in fractions over a period of about six weeks, five days a week. If the treatment is to prevent metastasis or the seeding of tumor cells by blood- or lymph-based cancer, then radiation may include the whole brain. However, to shrink or prevent the spread of a primary tumor, radiation is focused on just parts of the brain. The best current alternative therapies include conformal and stereotactic radiotherapy, surgical placement of chemotherapy wafers in the tumor bed, and gene therapy.

The natural history of radiotherapy effects is not well understood. Experimental animal studies demonstrate brain damage or decreased cell density from radiotherapy. Several studies in humans have associated damage to the brain's white matter with delayed radiation effects (Corn et al., 1994). In addition, chemotherapy interacts with radiotherapy to exacerbate radiation damage. Although studies of children and several retrospective studies have found alarming effects of radiation injury, some studies of adults have not. The methodology used is often the source of the discrepancies. For example, retrospective studies find abnormally high rates of white matter damage, low IQ, memory impairment, and even dementia in both adults and children from 3 months to many years after irradiation (DeAngelis, Delattre, & Posner, 1989). A late effect, up to 20 years post treatment, may result in an atherosclerotic-like disorder if carotid arteries were irradiated. Conclusions are confounded when patients are tested at irregular time periods, only brief neuropsychological evaluations are conducted, or no baseline neuropsychological testing (before treatment) is ordered.

Memory deficits have been implicated as the most frequent and severe delayed effect of radiation therapy. Researchers consider the early delayed effects, occurring two to three months after completion of radiation treatment, to be mild and temporary. The late delayed effects of radiation therapy, are more severe, may progress, and are irreversible. We compared longitudinal research on patients who received radiation therapy to patients with similar tumor types but who did not have radiotherapy. Patients with low-grade cortical, primary brain tumors often have long life expectancies and relatively few cognitive deficits. Neuropsychologists give these patients a repeatable, comprehensive battery of tests that includes many sen-

---

on the brain during a head injury, which often can result in brain damage. Head injuries do not occur in isolation; additional injuries are common, and thus most cases require additional medical attention to other seriously traumatized parts of the body, complicating the overall prognosis and intervention.

Accidents are the leading cause of death in people ages 1 to 30. In the 1970s the medical profession first recognized head injuries, and in particular those related to motor vehicle accidents (MVAs), as a national epidemic. Researchers estimate that 500,000 people suffer brain injury every year. Ten percent of all head

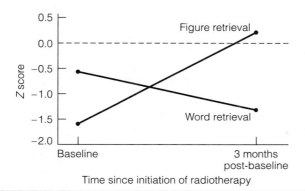

Figure 10.2 Double dissociation of patients' word and figure retrieval after delay at baseline and at point of early delayed phase of radiotherapy. (From C. Armstrong, B. Corn, J. Ruffer, A. Pruitt, J. Mollman, and P. Phillips, "Radiotherapeutic Effects on Brain Function: Double Dissociation of Memory Systems," *Neuropsychiatry, Neuropsychology, and Behavioral Neurology,* Philadelphia: Lippincott-Ravens Publishers, 2000, *13,* 100–111. Reprinted with permission)

sitive measures of attention and memory processes. Evaluations occur just prior to irradiation, and then at 3-, 6-, and 12-month intervals. Thus far we have learned that robust patterns of neuro-cognitive change appear during the first year after radiotherapy (see Figure 10.2). Visual-perceptual memory learning and recall are impaired at baseline but improve steadily over one year. Verbal-semantic retrieval is often not affected at baseline, but declines at the early delayed phase. Researchers think the early delayed phase of radiation damage is due to interruption of myelin synthesis, which stems from inhibition of glial mitosis. Thus, verbal-semantic retrieval appears sensitive to the damaging effects of radiotherapy, and may be sensitive

to the more crucial late delayed phase of irradiation. The initial impairment and improvement in visual memory may represent recovery from surgical injury to the hippocampal memory system.

We discovered that radiation selectively impairs verbal-semantic memory significantly more than motor control, visual and auditory attention, visual and auditory working memory, visual long-term memory, language, visual-spatial perception, processing speed, and reasoning. Why would retrieval be so sensitive to radiation? Retrieval, the endpoint of remembering, depends on reconstructive processes in which the system associates the contents of current consciousness with information stored in permanent memory. Several

other cognitive processes could theoretically account for the patients' failure to retrieve words from long-term memory, including failure of selective attention, working memory deficit, slowed processing speed, and failure to regenerate the attributes of the target. However, we found that none of these related cognitive processes explained the retrieval impairment. We are pursuing the questions of whether the rate of reconstruction of current memory or the recall of novel arrangements of memory attributes predicts the retrieval deficit, and how these processes correspond with regions of the brain's white matter.

Neuropsychological findings have influenced the treatment of brain tumors. Neuro-oncologists have become more selective about the doses and timing of radiotherapy. Radiation oncologists may advise patients about the early delayed effects on memory. Patients are more likely to receive referrals for rehabilitative therapies, and neuropsychologists are more cautious when recommending return to work. Neuro-oncology researchers are investigating other potential damaging effects on the brain, such as the possible association with Alzheimer-like neural changes in gray matter. Researchers are also aiming studies at developing pharmacologic treatments to block the damaging effects of radiotherapy, and at identifying chromosomal markers of beneficial sensitivity to cancer treatments. Neuropsychologists can play an important role in helping to understanding the cognitive changes associated with brain tumor treatment.

injuries are in the moderate to severe range (Levin, Benton, & Grossman, 1982). An estimated 1 to 2 million living Americans have sustained moderate to severe brain trauma (Bond, 1986). After MVAs, the causes of head injuries are, in order, sports injuries, falls, violence, and industrial accidents. In individu-

als younger than 45 years, head injuries cause more deaths and disability every year than any other neurologic illness. Those most at risk are young, under age 30, single, and male. The male–female ratio may be as high as 4 to 1. Young adults between ages 15 and 24, followed by children and adolescents ages 5 to 14, are at highest risk for traumatic brain injury. But no one is immune. Studies implicate alcohol in one-third to one-half of all traumatic head injuries. In fact, head injuries are such a significant health problem among developed countries that they play a role in approximately half of all deaths related to trauma (Rimel, Giordani, Barth, Boll, & Jane, 1981).

Most often head injuries show no visible physical "scars." However, significant changes in behavior and emotion follow head injuries, often most noticeable by people close to the victim. Only 20 years ago, hospitals typically discharged survivors of head injuries, after recovering medically, without consideration of whether they had recovered cognitively or emotionally. Neuropsychologists now know that even mild head injuries may entail a variety of learning and mood disorders (Diamond, Barth, & Zillmer, 1988). Head injuries also place a financial burden on society. On average, each brain injury costs over $100,000 in acute medical care and rehabilitation. Neuropsychologists play an important role in assessing survivors and in providing rehabilitation. Because of the complexities of brain functions and the sequelae of traumatic brain injury, the neuropsychology student must understand the pathophysiologic aspects of head trauma as well as their neuropsychological correlates.

Mechanism of Impact: Neuronal Shearing, Stretching, and Tearing

Bumps to the head are something everyone has endured. But when does a "bump" become a traumatic brain injury, or TBI? The pathomechanism of head injuries relates to the physical forces placed on the neuron, specifically the axon and cell body. Neurologists have described these forces as shear and straining effects at the neuron level. The axon in particular can only take a certain amount of physical stress; the axon's **tensile strength** is its resistance to longitudinal stress, measured by the minimal amount of stress required to rupture the axon. Brain trauma may deform, stretch, and compress the brain and its tissue, exceeding normal tissue's extendability, particularly

along the axon (Levin, Benton, & Grossman, 1982). These forces may tear the axon, and once damaged, the axon may degenerate back to the cell body, which may lead to cell death. This process is called **retrograde degeneration.** Conversely, the tear or rupture of a cell body can lead to the axon fiber degenerating: **anterograde degeneration.** Because the neuron dies, the now-damaged axon is not activated by the postsynaptic axon. This may lead to a "domino effect;" that is, metabolic changes in the postsynaptic neuron and possible cell death. The shearing effect on axons is most noticeable at the junction of gray and white matter regions of the brain (Naugle et al., 1998). Recent advances in understanding of neuronal changes in the brain have improved knowledge of the microanatomic changes related to TBI. This knowledge has confirmed the long-assumed idea that during brain trauma, real physical changes at the cellular level may have associated cognitive deficits.

These types of degeneration most likely result from rapid acceleration and deceleration that shake the "Jello-like" brain within the cranial cavity. The types of traumas most likely to cause such shaking are closed head injuries, in which the head impacts another object or is suddenly thrown back in whiplash. Only neurons that are not completely severed may "resprout" axonal projections. Shearing, tearing, and stretching may result in axonal sprouting, or new growth from the damaged neurons. Perhaps these new connections will bypass damaged areas and restore function. New axonal sprouting, however, is not always beneficial. Neurons may also form unwanted connections, resulting in behavioral disturbances. Apparently much axonal activity takes place in the area of the neuronal injury. There may be not only axonal sprouting from damaged neurons, but also collateral sprouting from nearby intact neurons.

Damage to the brain itself results either from an object penetrating the skull, or from rapid acceleration or deceleration of the brain. Thus it is useful to divide the mechanisms of impact according to two major classifications of head injuries:

1. Head injuries associated with a penetrating mechanism, called **penetrating head injury**

2. **Closed head injuries,** associated with a blow to the head, but not penetrating the skull

PENETRATING HEAD INJURY

A penetrating head injury occurs when a small object has lodged in the brain, such as a knife, scissors, or a bullet from a gun. Penetrating head injuries are very dangerous to the cortical integrity of the brain, because of two factors. The first factor is the location and extent of the damage. For example, a gunshot wound to the brain stem is almost always fatal. Conversely damage to a cortical association area may entail "less" damage. The second factor is the complications typically associated with penetrating head injuries, which include infection and hemorrhaging.

Although most gunshot wounds to the head result in fatal brain damage, survivors almost always receive a neuropsychological evaluation to outline the deficits and residual strengths associated with the injury. We have consulted on many cases in which patients with seemingly fatal penetrating head injuries have survived, although with neuropsychological deficits (see Neuropsychology in Action 10.3).

Another account of penetrating gunshot wound from our clinical experience concerns a depressed man who tried to kill himself by using a shotgun. He placed the shotgun underneath his chin, pointing the gun straight up, and pulled the trigger. The blast removed his chin, nose, mouth, and most of the prefrontal cortex. The suicide attempt also left him blind. But vital areas of the brain including the brain stem, hypothalamus, and subcortical structures, remained intact, and the patient survived. Interestingly, the patient had inadvertently given himself a prefrontal lobotomy. His depression was not present any more, but he had many cognitive deficits and a very bad temper. In another, final example, during a prison fight one inmate plunged a pair of scissors in another inmate's brain, straight down the parietal cortex. The scissors missed the superior sagittal sinus and must have been short enough to avoid penetrating subcortical areas. The prisoner walked into the emergency room with the scissors still implanted in the skull—only the handles showed!

Penetrating head injuries can greatly damage the brain, which is often incompatible with sustaining life. A large-caliber gunshot wound to the brain usually causes death, because there is significant tearing of blood vessels and destruction of brain tissue along the bullet's path through the brain. Small-caliber gunshot wounds can also be fatal, because they can "bounce" within the skull, fatally damaging a strategic area of the brain.

Self-inflicted gunshot wounds to the head are the primary way men commit suicide, followed by jumping off high buildings and hanging. There are over 25,000 suicides in the United States every year, a majority from gunshot wounds.

People who survive penetrating head injuries are often disabled for life. A well-documented case is James Brady, who was President Ronald Reagan's press attaché. During an assassination attempt by John Hinckley, Jr., Brady was struck by bullets to his right frontal lobe. Hinckley used "killer bullets," which, on impact, explode into hundreds of fragments. Surgeons completely removed Brady's right frontal lobe, which was seriously damaged. Hinckley, a paranoid schizophrenic, later used the insanity defense to avoid prison; he is currently hospitalized in St. Elizabeth's Hospital in Washington, D.C. Brady was left hemiplegic on the left side of his body and has many other, more subtle, neuropsychological symptoms. He and his wife have been the primary political forces behind the Brady Bill, which seeks to control handgun purchases by former mental patients and people with a criminal record. Countries that monitor gun purchases have shown dramatic success in reducing gun-related deaths and injuries. For example, in Norway, a small, northern European country of approximately five million, only seven deaths were attributed to gunshot wounds to the head in 1993. The latest statistics from the U.S. Department of Justice report that of all homicides perpetrated in 1998, 52% or 14,000 were committed with handguns.

CLOSED HEAD INJURY

There are many different causes of closed head traumas, but common to all is the fact that the brain

Neuropsychology in Action 10.3

Case Study: Penetrating Head Injury

by Eric A. Zillmer

This case concerns a patient I saw on a trauma intensive care unit (ICU). The client was a 25-year-old, right-handed, unemployed, single mother with a 12th-grade education. She was suffering from severe depression when she shot herself in the forehead with a small .32-caliber pistol. She was right-handed and held the pistol to her right temple, an inch above her right eye. With her two young children in the home, she then pulled the trigger. The bullet pierced her right frontal skull, sending fragments of bone into her right frontal and parietal lobe. The bullet itself, sterilized by the heat from the acceleration from the gun barrel, came to rest in the left frontal lobe (see Figure 10.3). Damage to her brain was confined to her frontal lobes. She did not injure subcortical structures and motor areas of the frontal lobes, and no vital arteries or veins were severed. In a way she lobotomized herself, and surprisingly, she was actually conscious and responsive when she arrived in the emergency room!

She underwent a right frontal craniotomy for debridement of the gunshot because the bone and skin fragments presented a risk for infection. Surgeons inserted a metal plate in her right skull to repair the damage where the bullet had entered. The bullet itself was too deeply lodged in the brain to be removed. The neurosurgeon decided not to extract the bullet, because doing so would have required cutting through intact brain tissue to reach the bullet. The bullet remained in her brain.

I conducted a neuropsychological evaluation while the client was still in the trauma intensive care unit, three days post trauma. I decided to administer a short neuropsychology screen to the patient, that is, the Assessment of

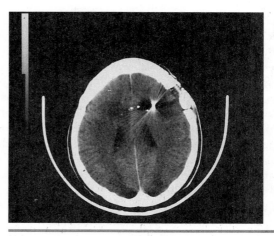

Figure 10.3   CT scan of .32-caliber bullet gunshot wound. CT scan shows that the gunshot was to the right frontal area with bone fragments in the right frontal lobe. (Eric Zillmer)

undergoes either marked **acceleration** and/or **deceleration.** In acceleration, the brain experiences a significant physical force that propels it quickly from stationary to moving. Examples are the brain being hit by a moving object such as a baseball bat or a car, or a passenger in a rocket accelerating very fast. In deceleration the brain is already in motion, traveling at a certain speed, and then stops abruptly, sometimes instantaneously. Examples include most motor vehicle accidents and the skiing accident described earlier. The kinetic potential—that is, the physical forces acting on the brain—can be expressed mathematically for both types of injuries.

Let's start first with acceleration injuries. You can measure acceleration by noting the time elapsed from the start of acceleration and multiplying it by the ac-

Impairment Measure or AIM (Zillmer et al., 1995; see Chapter 14). Briefly, the AIM measures eight areas of cognitive abilities and two areas of behavioral competence. For the neuropsychology student, it is easiest to evaluate the percentage correct score. Healthy individuals can complete at least 90% of the items on each scale. Less than 80% correct corresponds to an impairment for that cognitive area, which is highlighted by an asterisk related to the severity of impairment: * = mild, ** = moderate, *** = severe. The results from the evaluation were as follows:

I could not administer the full AIM because of the patients level of fatigue and poor endurance. The results showed that she was alert and oriented to person, place, and time. She was aware that her speed of processing was extremely slow and kept asking, "Why am I taking so long to respond to these questions?" Attention was mildly impaired. She could repeat up to five digits forward and could do automatism, such as counting from 1 to 20 and reciting the alphabet. On tasks requiring more sustained attention/concentration, however, she showed moderate problems, as she could only repeat

up to two digits backward and made errors adding serial threes.

Her motor functions showed decreased motor speed and motor-sequencing problems on the nondominant left hand. Visual-spatial functions showed mild problems in spatial orientation and a left visual neglect syndrome. Copying of designs showed a neglect of the left visual space. For example, her drawing of a clock was missing the numbers from 6 to 10 on the left side. Receptive speech was adequate—she could follow two-step commands, but her processing speed was very slow. Expressive speech showed markedly decreased fluency. Immediate visual and verbal memory were adequate. On delayed recall, however, she showed mild to moderate short-term memory problems. Her overall abstract reasoning and planning were significantly impaired.

I include this evaluation using the AIM here to demonstrate the neuropsychologist's role in a critical care setting as well as document the neuropsychological functioning of a gunshot victim. In making this neuropsychological evaluation, I established some cognitive impairment and identified this client as a potential rehabilitation patient. The relatively mild degree of impairment, given the nature of the trauma, suggests that the integration centers of the brain were spared from damage. It could have been a lot worse neuropsychologically and medically, although the patient continued to struggle with depression.

Subtest	Raw Score	% Correct	Impairment
I. Orientation	18	86	
II. Sensation/perception*	21	72*	Mild
III. Attention/concentration	31	70*	mild
IV. Motor	30	84	
V. Verbal functions	29	84	
VI. Visual-spatial organization	27	78*	Mild
VII. Memory	29	70*	Mild
VIII. Judgment/problem solving	9	50***	Severe
TOTAL SCORE	**194**	**76***	Mild
IX. Psychological distress scale	N/A		
X. Activities of daily living	N/A		

Note: N/A = incomplete administration of the scale. * indicates impairment associated with scores < 80% correct: * = mild, ** = moderate, *** = severe.

celeration of gravity, or $g = 9.8$ m/sec^2 and time, according to the following formula: velocity (v) = the product of acceleration (g) and time (t) or $v = gt$. For example, think of yourself jumping off a 3-meter-high diving board. There are two ways you could get hurt. The first is related to acceleration from the forces (in this case from gravity) that your brain is experiencing during the period of free fall. In mathematical terms,

you can calculate this using the preceding formula. Thus maximum impact velocity (v) for a 3-meter board would be 12.94 m/sec, corresponding to approximately 29 mph maximum impact speed (depending how high you jump off the board).

The second type of injury you could receive is related to how fast your kinetic energy that you have acquired (29 mph), as a result of the free fall deceleration, is absorbed by your body and brain. For example, you may have performed a jump in which you landed flat on your stomach. In this case you decelerate much more quickly than you would if you entered the water with your feet first. You can calculate deceleration (a) by dividing velocity over time ($a = v/t$). You have already calculated the velocity, so all you need to establish is the time it takes to decelerate. If that time period is instantaneous—if you were to hit the asphalt rather than the water—the deceleration would be very high and injury very likely. If, however, it takes the diver one or two seconds to decelerate, then the forces are much less. The time of deceleration is an important variable in the deceleration equation. If very short, it corresponds to higher deceleration. This is why downhill skiing crashes or race car crashes that take a "considerable" amount of time, although looking horrific to the observer, are actually safer, because the brain is decelerating more slowly.

Using the preceding formula, a springboard diver experiences approximately a corresponding deceleration of 16.28 m/sec^2 or approximately 2 g when jumping off a 3-meter board. If you were to hit asphalt from the same height, the approximate deceleration expressed in mathematical terms would be over 50 g! In their cars, racecar drivers at the Indy 500 carry g-meters, which can corroborate the amount of gravity forces the driver experiences during a crash. In one crash during practice, a driver hit the retaining wall almost head on. The g-meter indicated a force of 87g, incompatible with sustaining life. Because car racing is very dangerous and drivers are at risk for closed head injuries, Indy racecar drivers undergo preseason neuropsychological testing, to establish a baseline in cognitive abilities if injuries occur during the season. This is also the case for the National Hockey League (NHL), which has started baseline neuropsychological testing for all its players, to evaluate the effects of mild closed head injuries (also called *concussions*), which have cut short some of the players' careers.

In closed head injuries, the physical forces acting on the brain tissue may occur at the point of impact (an **impact injury**) or its opposite pole, because the brain "tears" away from the skull (**countercoup injury**). Diffuse injury is also common and most likely to occur at the frontal lobes and temporal poles, be-

cause of the uneven, "sandpaperlike" surface of the tentorial plates that hold those brain structures in place. The physical forces may shear, tear, and rupture nerves, blood vessels, and the covering of the brain. In severe head injury, those forces are so strong that they reduce the brain to a bloody, swollen pulp. As a result, there may be severe complications associated with neuronal disruption, ischemia, hemorrhaging, and edema.

ASSESSING THE SEVERITY OF BRAIN INJURY

The severity of a traumatic head injury has been most often associated with corresponding scores on the **Glasgow Coma Scale,** or **GCS** (Teasdale & Jennett, 1974). This measure gives the head injury trauma team a rapid, reliable measure of coma depth by assessing separate symptoms, including language, consciousness, and motor domains. Neuropsychologists generally accept the GCS as the standard measure for determining severity of injury in patients with compromised consciousness, from the mildest confusional state (scores over 13) to deep coma (scores below 5; see Table 10.3). Medically, coma is defined as a score of 8 or less, which corresponds to a severe head injury. Thus the standard definition of coma is that a patient cannot open his or her eyes, make any recognizable sounds, and follow any commands (Levin et al., 1982). Depth of coma, along with posttraumatic amnesia (described later in this chapter), is a reliable measure of the overall level of brain damage and prognosis. The Glasgow Coma Scale has proven a good outcome measure following coma, with scores greater than 8 indicating a good recovery. Greater mortality is typically associated with scores below 7.

Coma is not the same as "being asleep." In fact, EEG monitoring shows that a comatose patient has sleep–awake cycles even while in coma. Coma is directly associated with an injury to those areas of the brain, typically the lower brain stem and reticular activating system (RAS), that are involved in brain arousal. Although it is not clear what precisely causes coma, researchers believe it is related to RAS damage. In animal experiments, researchers found that a linear acceleration blow did not result in coma, but

Table 10.3	*Glasgow Coma Scale*	
Dimension	**Score**	**Description**
Eye opening (E)		
Spontaneously	4	Eyes are open; scored without reference to awareness
To speech ("Open eyes")	3	Eyes are open to speech or shut without implying a response to a direct command
To pain	2	Eyes are open with painful stimulus to limbs or chest
Not at all	1	No eye opening, not attributed to ocular swelling
Best Verbal Response (V) ("What year is it?")		
Oriented	5	Aware of self, environment, time, and situation
Confused	4	Attention is adequate and patient is responsive, but responses suggest disorientation and confusion
Inappropriate	3	Understandable articulation, but speech is used in a non-conversational manner or conversation is not sustained
Incomprehensible	2	Verbal responses (moaning), but without recognizable words
None	1	
Best Motor Response (M) ("Show me two fingers.")		
Obeys commands	6	Follows simple verbal directions
Localizes pain (by touch)	5	Moves limbs to attempt to escape painful stimuli
Withdraws from pain	4	Normal flexor response
Abnormal flexor response	3	"Decorticate": abnormal adduction of shoulder
Extensor response	2	"Decerebrate": internal rotation of shoulder
None	1	Flaccid
Glasgow Coma Score (E + V + M) = 3 to 15		

Source: Adapted from "Assessment of Coma and Impaired Consciousness," by G. Teasdale and B. Jennett (1974).

when the head was free to move in a rotational plane, as in injuries from motor vehicle accidents, coma did appear. Coma is also not a binary phenomenon: It is incorrect to conceptualize the patient as either in a coma or not. Rather, coma falls along a continuum. That is, patients can be in a deep coma or in a light, shallow coma, or somewhere in between. (Alternatively, head injury survivors may not be in a coma at all, but may be confused and disoriented.) When patients recover from coma, they do not "suddenly awake" from it. Rather, they slowly progress from deeper stages to more shallow stages of coma. In this respect the GCS has been a very useful tool for monitoring recovery of comatose patients. Limitations of the GCS are twofold: First, incorrect assessment is possible because of confounding factors including eye swelling that prohibits assessment of eye opening, and the presence of an endotracheal tube and the use of drugs (such as barbiturates or anticonvulsants), both of which can prevent verbal response. The second limitation relates to the fact that a very small lesion to the brain stem can cause coma, although most of the brain is not injured. In such a case the coma, while serious and potentially life threatening, is not a good overall indicator of overall brain damage, because the cortex, for example, may be entirely intact.

Research has demonstrated a relationship between the severity of a head injury, defined by the GCS, and neuropsychological outcome. The most severe injuries entail the most substantial neuropsychological deficits (Levin et al., 1982). Although initial severity of GCS is an important prognostic indicator for the patient's survival, other indicators, such as number of days to reach a GCS of 15, have also been associated with long-term neuropsychological outcome.

Complications of Moderate and Severe Brain Injury

The major complications of moderate and severe closed head injuries are edema of the brain and associated brain herniation, intracranial bleeding, and skull fractures. We describe each of these processes next because they are important variables for a positive neuropsychological outcome:

EDEMA

Edema of the brain refers to swelling. Just as swelling follows a bruise to a leg, the brain swells as a result of trauma. The problem with brain edema is that there is no space for the brain to swell into. As a result, internal pressure of the brain increases, often dramatically. Therefore the trauma team almost routinely places an intracranial monitoring catheter into the ventricles or the subarachnoid space to monitor **intracranial pressure,** or **ICP.** Intracranial pressure can cause diffuse damage to the brain. In fact, in moderate and severe head injuries, severe and uncontrollable ICP is the main cause of death.

BRAIN HERNIATION

Besides head injury, other pathological processes occur in the brain, including hemorrhages, tumors, or infections, which may displace and deform the brain. This process, called **brain herniation,** is associated with increasing intracranial pressure often related to the presence of a large pocket of blood (also called a *hematoma*). In more than 75% of severe closed head injury (CHI) cases, there is an associated ICP of greater than 20 mm Hg (or Torr; normal is 0 to 15). Such a high ICP often results from an intracranial hematoma and a generalized swelling of the brain. These displace the brain downward. This **transtentorial herniation** is characterized by downward displacement of the parahippocampal gyrus and uncus of one or both temporal lobes through the tentorial hiatus. There is only one large opening in the skull, the foramen magnum, which is the normal anatomic site of the lower brain stem. Brain herniation can place extreme pressure on the lower brain stem, typically cutting off the cranial nerve III (the oculomotor nerve) and compromising the integrity of the brain stem. The cranial nerve symptom causes initial constriction, followed by dilation of the pupil on the herniation side. Furthermore, the patient may lose motor functions on the same side as the herniation. Compression of the posterior cerebral artery may obstruct blood circulation and eventually cause necrosis. In the herniation syndrome, consciousness deteriorates

to a state of deep coma within minutes to hours. If left untreated, the patient goes into a coma and dies of respiratory failure because the brain centers, among them the medulla oblongata, have been damaged and life-sustaining functions cease to operate.

Because edema thus progresses to brain herniation, controlling ICP is the main medical issue in acute closed head injury. Medical trauma personnel carefully monitor ICP, and if it is elevated they treat it, often aggressively. Lowering the patient's blood pressure medically or by hyperventilation is often enough to stabilize ICP. In extreme cases the trauma staff artificially places the patient in a coma. Of course, he or she is already in a coma related to the brain injury, but a pharmacologically induced coma additionally reduces brain metabolism and hence swelling. A last resort in controlling ICP is evacuation (surgical removal) of a lobe, such as the right frontal one, to make room for the brain to swell into. This happened to one of our patients, Frank, a 22-year-old college student. One night he joined a friend to travel by car to a questionable location of the city to buy marijuana. Similar drug transactions usually end without incident, but the drug dealers mistook Frank for someone else who, the night before, either did not pay for drugs or started an altercation. Whatever the reasons, his attackers were never caught. They pulled Frank from the car, beat him up with a baseball bat, and left him for dead. Miraculously, he survived, but with a severe closed head injury and in a coma. His ICP was so severe that he would have not lived had not the neurosurgeons removed his right frontal lobe, although there was no specific injury to that lobe. They simply removed it because Frank's brain needed the additional space to expand. Frank has now been through 10 years of rehabilitation. He has severe cognitive deficits and needs supervision 24 hours a day. His life has changed dramatically. He has had to learn all over again how to walk and talk. The rehabilitation hospital where Frank now lives has built a special room for him with soft padded walls, because of his uncontrollable temper. To his parents he is a completely different person from who he was before the assault. His parents deal with the situation as if their son had died that night and as if the new Frank were their new son.

EXTRADURAL AND SUBDURAL HEMORRHAGE

As a result of a head injury, cerebral blood vessels may tear, producing pools of blood within and between the meninges. Subdural and extradural bleeding frequently complicate head injuries and are medically significant. A **subdural hematoma,** particularly, may be associated with trivial bleeding only to cause problems weeks later after the injury. Acute subdural or intracerebral bleeds most often appear in severe head injury. Together with brain edema, they are present in most fatal cases. The classic symptom in the subdural is an initial period of unconsciousness, but because the dura adheres tightly to the skull the bleeding delays, and a prolonged interval occurs during which the patient is conscious and functioning more or less normally. Once the bleed enlarges, it pushes the brain laterally and downward, causing brain herniation. As the hematoma enlarges, level of consciousness deteriorates quickly. This sequence of events is very dangerous, because the patient seems to have recovered from the trauma to the head, only to deteriorate once more quickly—and often fatally.

The frequent subdural hematoma corresponds to a bleed between the dura and the arachnoid space. A subdural hematoma is most likely caused by an acute venous hemorrhage related to rupture of a cortical vein, such as the superior sagittal sinus. Subdural bleeding typically occurs over the outward surfaces of the frontal and parietal lobes. Subdural hematomas are medical emergencies and typically develop within one week after the injury (if the bleed is slow) to as quickly as within one hour. Skull fractures (of which motor vehicle accidents are the most frequent cause) cause over half of all subdurals. Alcohol is a major catalyst, because of its anticoagulant properties in blood. Left untreated, the brain pressure increases to such a degree that the brain herniates, ultimately resulting in death. Symptoms of subdural hematoma include contralateral hemiparesis, ipsilateral pupil dilation, and changes in level of consciousness. Radiologists can easily make the diagnosis using CT imaging.

The less frequent **extradural hematoma** is a bleed that occurs between the skull and the dura. Bleeding of the large middle meningeal artery most often causes an extradural hematoma. An **epidural hematoma** represents a bleed between the meninges and the skull and is less common only occurring in 1% to 3% of major closed head injuries. The cause of an epidural is most often related to the rupture of an artery, but in some cases an epidural develops as a result of injury to a meningeal vein or to the dural sinus.

Surgeons treat an epidural or subdural hematoma by drilling one or more burr holes over the parieto-occipital and temporal regions. This drains the pocket of blood and is the most rapid and effective intervention. In essence, the hematoma drains through a shunt placed within the bleed. Drainage needs to occur as quickly as possible once the hematoma has been diagnosed, and before the blood coagulates, which would have to be removed by neurosurgery. If such intervention occurs in a timely manner, the outcome of the subdural or epidural hematoma is generally good, with few if any cognitive deficits.

INTRACRANIAL BLEEDING

"Space-occupying clots" appear in about 15% of fatal head injuries. Most frequent are microscopic hemorrhages, commonly formed by shearing forces that tear blood vessels in subcortical white matter, the corpus callosum, and the orbital surfaces of the frontal and temporal lobes. Focal lesions do not occur as frequently, but appear as contusions and intracranial hematoma (a collection of blood, typically clotted). Technically, epidural and subdural hematomas are not intracerebral hematomas, in which the bleed is intracranial—that is, within the brain. Epidural and subdural bleeds are actually outside the brain. Intracerebral hematomas are more difficult to treat than epidural and subdural hematomas and may require emergency neurosurgery.

SKULL FRACTURES

Examiners find skull fractures in approximately 75% to 90% of all patients with intracranial or epidural hematoma. There are two different types of skull fractures. The first is the relatively benign linear fracture, which results in a rather distinct, straight line. The second is the more complicated depressed skull fracture, in which the impact has often driven fragments of the skull into the underlying dura and brain. Location is another important variable. Fractures to the base of the skull are difficult to detect in x-ray films and often entail more damage than do the simple linear fractures. Although the brain can be severely damaged without any skull damage, the presence of a skull fracture always gives rise to the possibility of infection, CSF leaks, and bleeding. Skull fractures may also rupture meningeal arteries or large venous sinuses, resulting in epidural and subdural hematomas.

The relationship between skull fractures and neuropsychological functioning has been debated. Clearly, for the skull to fracture a significant force must have acted on the cranial plates. This force may have transferred to the brain, making actual brain damage more likely. The physics of skull fractures are complicated. In a skull fracture, the skull itself may have absorbed much if not most of the kinetic energy, thereby protecting the brain from damage. This is analogous to falling off a bicycle while wearing a helmet. The helmet absorbs much of the physical force, which transferred to the physical structure of the helmet (often destroying it), thereby protecting the head and the brain. For these reasons, skull fractures may not be directly related to specific levels of neuropsychological dysfunction. However, brain damage is more likely in skull fractures because the initial forces that fractured the skull must have been high, increasing the likelihood of brain damage.

POSTTRAUMATIC EPILEPSY

Seizures are a major complication after head injury. Posttraumatic epilepsy follows about 10% of severe closed head wounds and 40% of penetrating head injuries. The causes of the seizures relate to the presence of scar tissue, specifically alterations in neuronal membrane function and its structure. Neurologists consider seizures stemming from a head injury secondary, because they result from a known pathologic lesion. It is difficult to predict which head injury survivor may develop seizures, because onset can delay as much as two years after the trauma. Risk factors that increase the likelihood of developing posttraumatic seizures include penetrating type head injury, severity of brain damage, prolonged periods of coma, posttraumatic amnesia (described later in this chapter), inflammation associated with the wound, and residual neurologic symptoms. Seizures are such a frequent complication of head injury that patients receive anticonvulsant medication prophylactically (routinely) to control even the possibility of seizures.

Mild Head Injury: "Concussion"

The concept of a mild head injury is relatively recent. In the early 1980s, one of our mentors, Jeffrey T. Barth from the University of Virginia Medical School, was curious about what happens to patients who report to the emergency room for a head injury complaining of a concussion. These patients typically have had no or a very short loss of consciousness, followed by prompt recovery without any localizing neurologic signs. They exhibit few immediate cognitive or physical complaints beyond a headache, feeling dizzy, and vague memory problems. Together with a team of neurosurgeons and neurologists, Barth examined hundreds of patients who were turned away from the emergency room, usually with no referral followup, because their injury was not thought to be severe enough to hospitalize the patient. The assumption was that there were no long-term problems. In the early 1980s, concussions were not considered a medical emergency.

Perhaps this indifference relates to how society deals with mild head trauma. For example, in athletics, concussions are often tolerated with some bravado: "I was hit in the head and didn't know the score of the football game." In fact, TV football announcers recount how "amusing" it was to have someone knocked out, only to return to the opponent's sideline rather than his own. They recall with great humor how a teammate, after being knocked out, proceeded to run with the football in the wrong direction. Similarly, the symptoms of "seeing stars" has not been thought of as a neurologic symptom in this society, although it clearly is, but as a relatively benign, perhaps comic, event. In fact, many comic strips use "stars" to characterize transient confusion (see Figure 10.4).

Until very recently, researchers have not studied and understood the medical, neurologic, and psychological manifestations of mild head injuries. Over the last 15 years, an appreciation for milder forms of injuries to the head has appeared in the scientific literature. Mild head injuries often entail dizziness, fatigue, or headaches, with no loss or only brief loss of consciousness (Levin, Eisenberg, & Benton, 1989). The traditional literature often calls this type of head injury a "concussion." But neuropsychologists now treat mild head injury as a significant medical event that has real, even long-term, consequences (see Neuropsychology in Action 10.4). This finding is related not only to clinical evidence, in which patients have complained of physical and cognitive symptoms, but also to experimental evidence. Research studies have demonstrated that earlier studies using only the light microscope were incorrect in finding no reliable association between mild head injury and pathologic lesions in the brain. Recent animal research, using

histologic staining techniques, shows that neurons exposed to forces consistent with a mild head injury are damaged and die (Barth et al., 1983).

There are three important findings that have emerged from this body of research that are important to mild head injuries:

1. Mild head injuries usually go medically unnoticed. The medical community does not widely recognize the often debilitating sequelae of such injuries (Diamond et al., 1988).
2. During mild head injury, the physical energy transferred to the brain is related to linear and rotational mechanical forces associated with the sudden acceleration and/or deceleration. These forces can result in shearing or stretching, and even in necrosis (cell death) of neurons, which are the central building blocks of the central nervous system (for example, see Levin et al., 1982).
3. Head injuries, including the mild variety, are cumulative in effect. For example, Gronwall and Wrightson (1975) conducted one of the first investigations to establish that after a second concussion the capacity of adults to process information declined significantly. Thus, repeated blows to the head, such as those occurring in boxing and

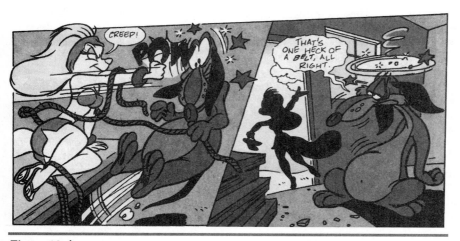

Figure 10.4 Animaniacs. (From DC Comics, *Animaniacs*, September 17, 1996. Copyright © 1996–2000 by Warner Bros. All rights reserved. Reproduced by permission)

Neuropsychology in Action 10.4

Can a Concussion Change Your Life?

by Ronald M. Ruff Ph.D., *Director of Neurobehavioral Rehabilitation, St. Mary's Medical Center, Associate Adjunct Professor, Department of Neurosurgery and Psychiatry, University of California at San Francisco.*

After attending a research meeting in Vail, Colorado, on traumatic brain injuries, my colleague, a 42-year-old neurosurgeon, decided to hit the ski slopes. While descending a modest incline, he lost his balance and fell, striking his head. He was immediately knocked unconscious for a period of only 10 to 15 seconds. On awakening, he experienced confusion that cleared in minutes, with the exception of a very modest vertigo that persisted but did not interfere with his ability to ski down the mountain. Because my mentor and friend, who is a renowned specialist in brain trauma, continued to ski that day, I thought this concussion had had no effect on him. However, on returning home he did report that he was a bit more distractible and that his memory was flawed, for example, when remembering the location of his Dictaphone, briefcase, and keys. He also noticed that when talking with colleagues and residents, he could no longer quickly recall references to articles. His speed of information processing was not affected, nor was his skill and judgment as a neurosurgeon; however, he did fatigue more quickly than before.

What exactly is a concussion? The term *concussion* refers to an injury to the brain, resulting either from a collision between the head and an object or from a rapid, forceful acceleration and deceleration. Neuropsychologists typically diagnose a brain injury when the consequences include one or more of the following: (1) an alteration or loss of consciousness; (2) a loss of memory for the events immediately before and after the injury; and (3) neurologic symptoms. The degree of injury can vary significantly, from a very mild concussion to death. The term "concussion" and "mild traumatic brain injury" are frequently used as synonyms, although I focus here on mild traumatic brain injury. What features separate a mild from a moderate brain injury? Medical professionals generally accept that a "mild" rating should not involve a loss of consciousness that exceeds 30 minutes; in addition, memory loss for events following the trauma should not exceed 24 hours, and the neurologic symptoms should not lead to a deterioration of the patient's GCS score below 13.

How many of us sustain a mild traumatic brain injury? Neurologists classify approximately two-thirds of all brain injuries as mild. In the United States alone, researchers estimate that approximately 1,300,000 individuals sustain a mild traumatic brain injury each year. Approximately half are the result of motor vehicle accidents, and the rest involve assaults, falls, or sports-related injuries (such as in skiing, boxing, football, horseback riding, and ice hockey). What happens to the brain during mild traumatic brain injury? At present, the best data is derived from studies of concussed animals or from humans who, in addition to having concussions, died of other medical complications such as chest wounds. Particularly because of rotational forces, brain cells tear, and this shearing of axons most often occurs in subcortical and frontotemporal regions. Because impact to the brain from the outside can vary so significantly, tearing and shearing of cells can also vary among individuals. However, postmortem examinations of concussed brains have provided evidence of microscopic changes, which can no doubt lead to neurophysiological and neurochemical alterations.

What typical difficulties do patients encounter? By evaluating patients in the first phases following a mild traumatic brain injury (TBI), researchers have documented frequent impairments on neuropsychological tests of sustained attention, memory and learning, and measures that capture speed of information processing. Most mild TBI survivors enjoy a favorable recovery in three to six months after the injury. That is, these patients improve up to a level that is not statistically below that of a control group. One study even found a way to test patients before and after a mild TBI. Before the playing season, researchers tested college football players who had never sustained a brain injury and did followup testing on those who later sustained a mild TBI. This retesting revealed an initial drop on neuropsychological testing, with a positive recovery in the following weeks. However, a large body of literature has unequivocally demonstrated that not all mild TBI patients enjoy a favorable recovery. A minority continue to have not only persistent cognitive problems, but also physical problems, which typically include headache, vertigo, dizziness, energy loss, and in some cases a heightened sensitivity to noise, light, alcohol, or medications. Emotional reactions commonly include irritability, elevated anxiety, or depressive symptoms. These cognitive and physical problems can in turn lead to emotional, psychosocial, and vocational changes. Neuropsychologists use the term "postconcussive disorder" for such cases. In the literature, researchers have estimated that postconcussive disorders occur in 10–20% of all mild TBI cases (130,000 to 260,000 cases each year in the United States). Over the years, the importance of a careful neuropsychological evaluation of patients with mild TBI has become more and more recognized.

What is the neuropsychologist's role in evaluating mild TBI? The objective tools that physicians tend to rely on for diagnosing brain injuries include computed transaxial tomography (CT), and magnetic resonance imaging (MRI). However, for mild TBI, these neuroimaging techniques lack sufficient sensitivity to visualize microscopic changes. Thus CT and MRI scans are, as a rule, "normal" in most mild TBI cases. Although the newer dynamic neuroimaging techniques such as positron emission tomography (PET) and single-photon emission computed tomography (SPECT) scans have demonstrated greater sensitivity in case studies, more research is required to

determine whether these newer techniques can objectify mild TBI conclusively. Because objective tools cannot yet reliably evaluate the potential brain damage involved in mild TBI, medical teams frequently assign to neuropsychologists, using subjective tools, the task of providing answers. Using psychometric tests, neuropsychologists are uniquely qualified to delineate the upper thresholds of cognitive functioning. Based on a pattern analysis across a neurocognitive test battery along with a psychodiagnostic evaluation, neuropsychologists can reach a diagnosis to determine the extent to which brain damage has contributed to the postconcussive disorder. The three key challenges for making a differential diagnosis are (1) estimating preinjury functioning levels, (2) evaluating comorbid factors, and (3) exploring interactions among the postinjury problems. Estimating preinjury functioning is paramount for capturing not only "deficits" but also any decline in functioning.

To illustrate, let's return to the earlier-mentioned neurosurgeon who struck his head while skiing. Many neuropsychologists use an impairment index that largely represents a common notion that a deficit is defined by a score that falls two standard deviations below the mean. However, this notion may lead to false negatives. For example, a 50% drop in performance in an individual whose preinjury functioning levels were at the 95th percentile will result in a postinjury performance at the 45th percentile. This neurosurgeon commented, with respect to the challenges neuropsychologists face:

> [P]erceptions of a disease by one who has not had the disease as a patient tend to

be modestly inaccurate. Recovery from a head injury appears to be a long process, one requiring innumerable strategies for compensation. Neurocognitive testing will indicate part of the story, only if the results are abnormal; it leaves something to be desired in predicting levels of performance for those who are adequate competitors in a modern society. (Marshall & Ruff, 1989, p. 278)

In addition to capturing a relative loss based on a comparison with the patient's estimated preinjury functioning levels, it is also crucial that the neuropsychologist become aware of pre-existing medical risk factors (history of alcohol or substance abuse; prior concussion), as well as cognitive risk factors (pre-existing learning disabilities), and emotional risk factors (such as hysteria, somatization, and secondary gain). Concurrent medical injuries are common in mild TBI cases, including neck, shoulder, and rib fractures, which can result in a pain syndrome. Excessive pain can interfere with sleep, and always results in emotional reactions that can in turn affect neurocognitive functioning. More systematic research is called for to evaluate mild TBI cases with and without comorbid medical injuries. Finally, the interactions among postinjury problems require careful analysis. Postconcussive syndromes derail some patients from their vocations as a result of a combination of factors (such as headaches, vertigo, attentional difficulties, and mood changes). All of us who work in this field believe that we must stress prevention. The mandatory introduction of helmets, safety belts, and airbags has reduced TBI rates. Be careful: A concussion has the potential to change your life!

football, are especially dangerous to the athlete's health.

POSTCONCUSSIONAL SYNDROME

Medical personnel often call the behavioral and cognitive sequelae of mild head injury "postconcussional syndrome." These sequelae range over a variety of somatic and neuropsychological symptoms, including headache, irritability, dizziness, lack of concentration, and impaired memory. Researchers have documented the symptoms of mild head injury most frequently with motor vehicle accidents. However, analogous situations with acceleration/deceleration of the head arise in the context of competitive sports. Many sports involve speed and the potential for collision. In fact, as already mentioned, 17% of all head injuries are sports related.

For example, research with football players suggests that many effects of sports-related collisions (such as tackling) that were originally thought to be relatively benign, actually have measurable neuropsychological consequences in college athletes. These collisions may not only diminish the performance of players on the field, but can also compromise their health off the field. Full appreciation of impact injuries has only recently developed as many National Football League quarterbacks have complained of the effects of repeatedly being hit in the head. Frequent head impact places them at risk for losing consciousness even when experiencing relatively minor concussive forces to the head. In some cases this has resulted in cognitive changes, including excessive dizziness and difficulty in concentrating. Several players were forced to retire, and rules were changed, disallowing tackling with the helmet or "spearing" to the opposing player's head.

Researchers have studied the neurologic aspects of professional boxing in more detail; these aspects are easily appreciated by the public because of the knockout (KO), which is a neurologic event synonymous with cerebral contusion. Only recently have researchers examined the neurologic aspects of amateur boxing, where duration of fights, rules, and protective devices differ from professional boxing (for example,

see Jordan, 1987). Other less obvious sports-related neurologic effects appear in soccer players who frequently head the ball. Findings indicate more electroencephalographic (EEG) abnormalities among national team players (Tysvaer, Storli, & Bachen, 1989) and more neuropsychological dysfunction among college players (Witol & Webbe, 1993). That football and soccer can involve potential mechanical forces to the head that can cause injury seems disturbing, particularly at the nonprofessional, "recreational" level. At that level many elementary school, high school, and college players (see Neuropsychology in Action 10.5, p. 348) are particularly vulnerable to the developmental delays related to such head injuries (Levin et al., 1982; Levin & Eisenberg, 1979).

Treatment of Head Injuries

An acute traumatic brain injury often entails severe neurologic impairment. In severe head injuries the patient is comatose when the medical emergency unit arrives. The initial management of severe head injury follows the ABC assessment, in which A = airway; the medics establish a respiratory airway, often freeing the pharynx from blood and other obstructions. If they do not establish an airway, anoxia will result, adding to the physical injuries of the brain. B = breathing; after a clear airway has been established, medics assess the patient's breathing. Then the team establishes regular breathing, if necessary artificially, with sufficient oxygen, because hypoxia is common in head injuries. Alterations in breathing may be related to brain stem dysfunction. Medics then evaluate circulatory status (C) by examining blood gases and blood pressure. They initiate intravenous infusion, including blood replacement. Then, once the patient has been medically stabilized, they obtain diagnostic imaging using CT and MRI. Next a neurologist conducts an evaluation to ascertain the level of consciousness and presence of neurologic symptoms. If the patient remains in a coma, the team may hospitalize him or her in a neuro-intensive care unit, which has a specialized environment that facilitates care of comatose patients.

As already mentioned, intracranial monitoring is the cornerstone of medical therapy. If ICP remains normal, the patient undergoes intensive supportive care. If ICP is elevated, medical personnel use aggressive measures to reduce it. These include controlled ventilation, which decreases cerebral blood volume and constricts cerebral vessels thus lowering ICP. Steroid therapy may prevent intracerebral edema. Patients are typically temperature controlled with heating/cooling blankets, because elevated body temperature increases metabolic rate and hypothermia leads to other medical complications. Sometimes medical personnel administer diuretics to reduce the ICP. If these measures do not control ICP, the prognosis is typically poor, and more aggressive measures are taken, such as inducing barbiturate coma and doing surgery. Administering a large dosage of barbiturates decreases the cerebral metabolic rate and constricts cerebral vessels. Inducing barbiturate coma is controversial, because it may contribute to additional neuropsychological sequelae. A final measure is to remove part of the brain to make space available.

NEUROPSYCHOLOGICAL MANIFESTATIONS

Neuropsychological sequelae, of course, are very prominently associated with traumatic brain injury. They range from complaints of memory difficulty to problems with attention and concentration, as well as alterations in mood. Neuropsychologists play an important role in objectively assessing residual ability after mild, moderate, and even severe head injuries, once the patient has been medically stabilized and is no longer in a coma or in acute medical care. Besides the cognitive effects of brain injury, personality changes from frontal lobe damage may affect the patient's well-being and quality of life (see Neuropsychology in Action 10.6, p. 350). Neuropsychologists routinely test head injury survivors, because unless tested, cognitive deficits, especially memory, may at first go unnoticed, but cause problems later when the patient returns home or to work. Most recovery after severe head injury occurs within the first six months, with smaller adjustments continuing for

perhaps as long as two years. In the past, rehabilitation experts have waited until the "natural" healing cycle has finished before initiating rehabilitation. More recent thinking has proven that rehabilitation is most effective when started as early as medically possible (Levin et al., 1989).

ANTEROGRADE AND RETROGRADE AMNESIA

Memory problems constitute a major deficit for people who have sustained traumatic head injuries and are of special interest to neuropsychologists. In fact, head injury experts grade the severity of a head injury in part on the patient's memory surrounding the accident. Such memory problems are called **posttraumatic amnesia,** or **PTA. Retrograde amnesia** is the loss of memory for the interval preceding the injury. Conversely, **anterograde amnesia** is the loss of memory for events after trauma or disease onset. Although the patient may also have residual short-term memory impairment from the head injury as well as other cognitive deficits, neuropsychologists have established retrograde and anterograde amnesia as a relative robust measure of the severity of trauma and its associated cognitive symptoms. Because cortical and subcortical structures mediate memory, PTA has proven a better overall indicator of brain damage than length and depth of coma, which may relate to isolated damage of the brain stem. Neuropsychologists consider these types of amnesia to relate mostly to anterior temporal lesions, an anatomic area particular vulnerable to head injuries, because of the bony features surrounding this area of the brain (Golden, Zillmer, & Spiers, 1992).

Neuropsychological Evaluation

Often other medical personnel ask neuropsychologists to evaluate head-injured patients at their bedside, close to the time of their accident, while they are still hospitalized (see Neuropsychology in Action 10.3). This exam is typically brief and serves to assess if the patient can tolerate more formal, longer testing. It also establishes a baseline of overall cognitive abilities

Neuropsychology in Action 10.5

Mild Head Injury in Sports

by Jeffrey T. Barth Ph.D., Raymond Fowler Professor of Psychology, University of Virginia Medical School.

Interest in sports mild head injury evolved from two sources: (1) broad, clinical public health concerns regarding mild head trauma, usually associated with motor vehicle accidents and sometimes resulting in controversial long-term disability and costly litigation; and (2) media attention to multiple concussions in high-profile athletes such as National Football League quarterbacks. Before the late 1970s and early 1980s, neurologists believed that mild head trauma resulted in no clinically significant impairment or neuropathology, and that any lasting deficits in cognitive functions after such injuries was purely psychiatric in nature (depression, hysteria, or malingering). Athletes incurring mild head injuries or concussions usually suffered in silence because of their "macho" images, financial incentives to play, and internal need to succeed in competition ("You can't make the club if you're in the tub").

Early clinical/epidemiological studies (Barth et al, 1983; Rimel, Eisenberg, & Benton, 1989) revealed neuropsychological deficits in new and rapid problem solving, attention and concentration, and memory that lasted at least three months post trauma. The research definition of mild head injury for these studies was a Glasgow Coma Scale score of 13 to 15, less than 20 minutes loss of consciousness, and less than 48 hours hospitalization (later studies added a fourth criteria of no neuroimaging evidence of lesion). At about this same time, Gennarelli (1983, 1984) and Ommaya (Ommaya & Gennerelli, 1974) were performing primate studies to evaluate the histologic effects of mild acceleration-deceleration head trauma. They discovered axonal shear strain in the brain stem in this experimental model, similar to the diffuse axonal injury noted in more severe cerebral trauma. A few years later, in the mid-1980s, controlled and prospective clinical studies of mildly head-injured patients revealed neurocognitive deficits one month post trauma. Yet little, if any, impairment appeared two months later, suggesting a rapid recovery curve if there were no complicating factors.

This flurry of research, as is often the case, created more questions than it actually answered. Although there appeared to be a growing consensus that mild head injury was not as innocuous as previously thought, recovery curves lacked definition and individual vulnerability, and neuropsychologists did not fully understand complications of mild head injuries. The field needed research that would truly control for individual vulnerability or pre-existing factors, which would influence outcome in this population. The most precise method for controlling these pre-existing factors would be to assess neurocognitive functions in a laboratory setting before and after administering a controlled mild head injury to a human subject. In this way the individual would act as his or her own control. However, ethical considerations certainly preclude such experimentation. To follow such a research course in the natural environment, it is necessary to accurately predict who is most likely to suffer a low grade or mild head injury (concussion), assess that popula-

for future comparisons. An example of such a neuropsychology consult follows:

Neuropsychology Note. Results from brief neuropsychological procedure, post-MVA with LOC (loss of consciousness) 30 min, revealed a 33 yowm (year-old white male) who was oriented ×3 (to self, time, and place) and attentive/cooperative with the exam. The patient was able to follow simple commands involving two-step learning. Memory appeared WNL (within normal limits) for immediate and short-term verbal/visual material. Expressive/receptive speech also WNL. No sensory deficits including astereognosis, finger agnosia, neglect, right–left confusion, or hemianopsia, were observed. The patient did manifest a bilateral resting hand tremor as well as motor incoordination, and difficulty in initiating specific motor movements. Perseveration of motor behavior was also apparent. Additional frontal lobe signs included poor reasoning ability and judgment.

Results are consistent with mild to moderate head injury and bilateral frontal lesions as seen on MRI from 1/11/97 revealing contusions in the inferior frontal re-

tion, wait for such an event to occur, and then do a followup neuropsychological evaluation.

The practical solution to this research problem was to determine who was at high risk of experiencing an acceleration–deceleration mild head injury (similar to the type of linear rotational brain trauma experienced in motor vehicle accidents) within a natural, yet controlled environment. Barth and his colleagues at the University of Virginia (Barth et al., 1983) identified college football players for this purpose and used a brief battery of neuropsychological tests to assess 2300 athletes at 10 universities in the Northeast during preseason practices over a four-year period. The researchers reassessed players sustaining head trauma with confusion or alteration in consciousness (no loss of consciousness), and a control group, at 24 hours, 5 days, and 10 days post trauma, as well as at post season. One hundred and ninety-five mildly concussed athletes exhibited statistically significant neurocognitive decline within 24 hours and at 5 days post injury, compared to red-shirted players, who were used as a control group. These mildly head-injured athletes took advantage of the practice effect and reached the performance level of the control group by 10 days post trauma. This study

suggested that young, bright, healthy, well-motivated individuals who experience very mild, uncomplicated head trauma without loss of consciousness will likely follow a very rapid recovery curve and will have no lasting disability.

While this clinical and laboratory research was underway, the sports medicine community was also struggling with the potentially serious consequences of cerebral concussion in athletes. The earliest research in this area focused on professional boxing, where the purpose of the sport is to render an opponent unconscious through successive blows to the head. Severe, acute, traumatic brain injury and chronic boxer's encephalopathy can result from single impacts and multiple (cumulative) mild head injuries, respectively. Clearly, head trauma in boxing represents the more severe end of the sports head injury continuum.

Concussion in American football, soccer, ice hockey, and rugby has become a major focus of attention in high school, college, and professional sports. The most salient concerns for team physicians and athletic trainers are (1) reliably determining the severity of concussion, (2) evaluating the immediate and long-term effects of multiple head injuries, and (3) developing valid return-to-play criteria to avoid catastrophic neurologic injury such as second impact

syndrome. Second impact syndrome involves an unusual quick and often fatal swelling of the brain when a second impact to the head occurs and the effects of the initial injury have not completely healed. Sports medicine scientists and clinicians such as Torg (1982) and Cantu (1996) have developed severity classification scales, most of which use level of consciousness/confusion and amnesia as the primary criteria for characterizing a concussion as mild, moderate, or severe (grades I, II, and III). Severity level and number of concussions experienced have direct implications for treatment and return-to-play decisions. Unfortunately, with the exception of the data from the University of Virginia football study, there exist few scientific data on which to base such decisions, so physicians and trainers must rely on anecdotal evidence and clinical experience to assure athlete safety.

The future of research on sports-related mild head injury is expanding and will be best served by prospective neuropsychological study of athletes at high risk for multiple concussions. The focus of sports medicine in the new millennium should be on better protective equipment and devices, rule changes, and pooling of information into a comprehensive concussion data bank to better define safe return-to-play criteria.

---

gions. Psychologically, the patient appears very distressed and depressed about his hospitalization and MVA, with suicidal thoughts present (but no specific plan). No other psychiatric symptoms were noted (hallucinations, delusions). Patient should be placed on suicide watch. Psychiatric consult should be ordered, and relocation to psychiatric ward should be considered to better manage suicide threats when the patient is medically stable. Other recommendations include comprehensive neuropsychological and psychological evaluation within the next four weeks to identify functional strengths and weaknesses. Cognitive

residual effects that may hinder this patient's ability to return to his previous employment as a manager include his ability to function independently in life, and his need for outpatient psychotherapy. This testing can be done on an in- or outpatient basis and should be repeated over a 6- to 9-month period to monitor his recovery. Once he is discharged I also recommend him joining our head injury group meetings, designed for individuals and families with histories of head injuries.

Signed: *Dr. Eric A. Zillmer,*
Neuropsychologist

Neuropsychology in Action 10.6

Consensual Sex After Traumatic Brain Injury: Sex as a Problem-Solving Task

by Carrie Hill Kennedy Lieutenant, Medical Service Corps, United States Naval Reserve, Naval Medical Center Portsmouth, Virginia.

John, age 24, and Theresa, age 22, are two traumatically brain-injured adults. John suffered a head injury at age 17 in a motorcycle accident. At age 20, Theresa suffered a head injury when a drunk driver struck her car as she waited at a red light. As a result of their injuries, John and Theresa currently live in a community-based rehabilitation facility.

John experiences hemiplegia, difficulty in planning for future events, and memory and attention deficits. Theresa experiences seizures, as well as severe speech and memory deficits. John and Theresa enjoy each other's company and often attend community events together. More recently, John and Theresa have become interested in a physically intimate relationship.

The last issue is a concern for the agency that provides their rehabilitative services. With their specific cognitive deficits, can John and Theresa *consent* to have sex? Can they each make an informed decision using information on sexual conduct, diseases, and pregnancy? Is either at a high risk of being victimized because of an inability to adequately protect him- or herself from unwanted sexual advances? To explore the answers to these questions, let's consider the issues of TBI (traumatic brain injury) and sexuality.

A common problem for people who have suffered a TBI is that of impaired sexuality. Because the incidence of TBI is high, particularly in young men ages 15 to 24, neurologists, psychologists, and neuropsychologists frequently address the issue of impaired sexuality. In fact, each year approximately two million Americans suffer a TBI. Of these, an estimated 300,000 cases are severe enough to require hospitalization, and of these 85,000 will experience permanent neurologic deficits (Silver et al., 1994).

After a head injury, the often ambiguous rules and rituals pertaining to sex can become even more difficult. Adverse effects of TBI on sexuality range from sensorimotor deficits and bowel and bladder dysfunction, to changes in sex drive and various male and female genital sexual dysfunctions. In addition to the neurologic, physical, and emotional effects on sexuality are cognitive changes associated with TBI. Cognitive changes can affect sexuality in a variety of ways, including impairment of the ability to make safe choices regarding sexual behavior. The individual can be physically able to engage in a sexual relationship, and even be interested in pursuing one, but at the same time be cognitively incapable of consenting. An inability to make decisions can result in victimization, unwanted pregnancies, and diseases.

One hallmark of a moderate to severe TBI can be the loss of the ability to make complex decisions requiring judgment, insight, preplanning, reasoning, organization, and impulse control. Clearly, such cognitive deficits can impair the ability to consent to sex. When this issue arises, the neuropsychologist serves two main roles. First, the neuropsychologist can assess an individual's capacity to consent to sex along with formal testing of his or her cognitive and functional strengths and weaknesses. Second, the neuropsychologist can recommend rehabilitative and educational strategies that are specially geared to a person's functioning level and cognitive abilities. In this way, neuropsychologists can

---

In general, the long-term neuropsychological effects of head trauma may vary considerably, and depend on the strength of the trauma and the medical condition of the head injured. Not all head traumas produce significant neuropsychological deficits. Others cause permanent and severe deficits. In general, neuropsychologists consider closed head injuries a diffuse disorder of the brain, because they may affect many different areas of the brain. Thus, differences in neuropsychological presentation in a head-injured protocol typically relate to the patient's level of overall deficits. Neuropsychology in Action 10.7 gives a good example of the neuropsychological profile of a head injury survivor.

optimize the decision making and safety of TBI survivors, while facilitating the return of an important aspect of quality of life, that of sexual intimacy.

Using an instrument such as the Sexual Consent and Education Assessment (SCEA—see Kennedy, 1999), neuropsychologists make a capacity determination based on prescribed legal criteria for consent. Legal criteria for sexual consent vary from state to state. In fact, a person may be deemed capable to consent in one state and not in another. Generally, however, the three criteria are knowledge of sexual conduct, knowledge of the consequences of sexual activity, and the ability to protect oneself by saying no. Although, taken together, these criteria determine the capacity of any given individual, each criterion is also a separate entity directly related to cognitive abilities that neuropsychologists can measure.

The first two criteria for capacity for sexual consent, regarding the nature of sexual conduct and consequences of sexual activity, are a function of crystallized intelligence (knowledge that has been acquired over the years) in most adults. That is, individuals who have had previous sexuality education and/ or sexual experience are more likely to retain general knowledge and information regarding sexuality. Later, such adults who have suffered a TBI typically have little difficulty communicating their understanding of the nature of sexual conduct and the various consequences

of sexual activity. However, individuals who have not yet obtained general knowledge about sexuality, must learn it for the first time. After TBI, attentional, memory, and executive function deficits significantly hinder new learning and can make a task such as learning basic sexual knowledge daunting. Individuals who suffered a TBI prior to AIDS education readily show this difficulty. Many moderate to severely head-injured residents in rehabilitation facilities still cannot recount the basic facts regarding HIV, AIDS, and their relationship to sex.

The third criterion, however, protecting oneself by saying no, seems to be the most significant hurdle for moderate to severely head-injured individuals. This particular neuropsychological task appears to be an executive decision involving a complex string of decision making, reasoning, judgment, and planning. This third criterion is an interesting issue. According to Lezak (1995), "executive functions consist of those capacities that enable a person to engage successfully in independent, purposive, self-serving behavior" (p. 42) and are described as having four components: (1) volition, (2) planning, (3) purposive action, and (4) effective performance (p. 650).

To date, little research has explored the area of consent and executive functions. Preliminary findings suggest that neuropsychological tasks such as the Tower of London–Drexel University (Culbertson & Zillmer, 1998c), the Modified Wisconsin Card Sorting Test, and word

fluency (Lezak, 1995) may be able to identify those who can consent to sexual activity (Kennedy & Zillmer, 1999). These neuropsychological tests seem to tap the frontal lobe functions, particularly the ability to preplan and inhibit. Additional research will provide further information regarding sexual consent and related neuropsychological requirements. In turn, investigation of these questions will also provide the basis for developing more effective rehabilitative strategies to help people suffering neurologic damage in regaining important parts of their lives, not least of which will be sexual intimacy. This leads us back to our original questions about John and Theresa.

John and Theresa were both tested using the SCEA and a neuropsychological battery. Theresa easily passed all aspects of the assessment, whereas John showed significant difficulty with the concepts of sexually transmitted diseases (STDs) and protection against them. John was declared not capable of giving consent until he could successfully complete an educational program dealing specifically with diseases and methods of protection. The educational program, which John completed, included methods of learning that were optimal for John given his neuropsychological test findings. Subsequently, the rehabilitation facility worked with John and Theresa with regards to establishing privacy, and their subjective quality of life is vastly improved.

Other Neurological Disorders

BRAIN ABSCESS

Brain abscesses are similar to tumors, both in appearance and on visualization using imaging. Compared to a tumor, however, a brain abscess arises from an infection spreading to the brain or originating in the brain. Abscesses begin as an area of generalized inflammation and progress to a "walled off," localized pocket of pus within the brain. The abscess can gradually expand, destroying and compressing brain tissue as it grows. Compared to brain tumors, however, imaging typically reveals a hollow

Neuropsychology in Action 10.7

Case Study: Closed Head Injury

by Eric A. Zillmer

The client is a 39-year-old, right-handed, male with a 12th-grade education. He sustained a closed head injury in a motor vehicle accident in which he was an unrestrained driver. His Glasgow Coma Scale score on admission to the emergency room was 4, severe. He was unconscious and had alcohol on his breath (BAL, blood alcohol level, of .32, legal limit ≤ .10). Within days of admission, medical personnel noted decerebrate posturing, which is characterized by an absence of muscle tone. Initial CT scan showed multiple hemorrhagic contusions of the frontal lobes, right corpus callosum, bilateral temporal right brain stem injury, and a fractured right frontal bone. When discharged from the trauma unit, he had a GSC score of 9. His eyes were open, and he could occasionally follow one-step commands.

The client was evaluated using the Assessment of Impairment Measure (AIM—Zillmer et al., 1995; see Chapter 14) two months after his trauma and as he was just beginning his inpatient brain injury rehabilitation program. On the AIM less than 80% correct indicates an impairment for that cognitive area and is highlighted by an asterisk related to the severity of impairment; * = mild, ** = moderate, *** = severe. The results from the evaluation were as follows:

Subtest	Raw Score	% Correct	Impairment
I. Orientation	17	82	
II. Sensation/perception	20	70*	Mild
III. Attention/concentration	33	74*	Mild
IV. Motor	25	70*	Mild
V. Verbal functions	26	74*	Mild
VI. Visual-spatial organization	23	66**	Moderate
VII. Memory	26	64**	Moderate
VIII. Judgment/problem solving	18	60**	Moderate
TOTAL SCORE	188	69**	Moderate
IX. Psychological distress scale	11	58***	Severe
X. Activities of Daily Living	19	96	

* indicates impairment associated with scores < 80% correct: * = mild, ** = moderate, *** = severe.

center within the abscess differentiating it from a tumor, which appears more "solid." In addition, the patient typically presents with a history of a prior infection.

INFECTIONS

Infections and infectious diseases tend to attack specific brain structures depending on the type. At least 20 different types of infections affect the brain. Many are obscure and rare. Among the well studied are **meningitis, herpes encephalitis,** and the **human immunodeficiency virus (HIV).** Meningitis is a bacterial or viral infection of the meninges that pro-

vide the protective covering of the brain. Meningitis can also be a result of brain surgery (there is an up to 5% incidence rate), and physicians routinely administer antibiotics to patients who have undergone intracranial procedures, to prevent such infections. Interestingly, such infections acquired during brain surgery vary, not only from hospital to hospital depending on the thoroughness of sterilization of the operating room, but also among operating rooms within a single hospital. Such data are, however, not commonly published for the consumer, for obvious reasons. Herpes encephalitis (not to be confused with genital herpes) aggressively attacks the medial temporal and orbital frontal areas. This appears to de-

The patient was alert and oriented to person and place and somewhat to time. He did know the exact date, but did not recall the current or last president. Sensation/perception showed mildly impaired visual acuity (vision tested at 20/50 for both eyes together), and stereognosis was markedly impaired bilaterally. Motor functions were moderately impaired on the dominant (right) hand for fine motor speed. He showed motor perseverative responses and had difficulty with motor inhibition. Graphomotor skills were severely impaired with marked tremors, which distorted the overall gestalt of the figures and made his handwriting completely illegible. These significant sensory and motor deficits could have been caused by the brain stem injury.

Immediate verbal attention was moderately impaired, as the patient could only repeat four digits forward. He was able to do automatic tasks such as reciting the alphabet and counting from 1 to 20. However, on sustained attention tasks, he showed significant problems. He was unable to add serial threes, and could only repeat two digits backward.

Receptive speech was adequate for following two-step commands. Expressive speech showed markedly decreased verbal fluency. Visual-spatial functions showed moderately impaired spatial orientation but good figure/ground perception, visual sequencing, and facial recognition.

Overall memory functions were severely impaired for immediate and short-term memory. Recognition did not help with information retrieval, suggesting a problem with initial coding and storage of information. Judgment/problem solving was moderately to severely impaired. Thought processes were very concrete. When asked to interpret the saying "You can't judge a book by its cover," he replied, "Can't see the words in there." Also his capacity to find similarities and differences between objects was grossly impaired. He said an apple and an orange were alike in that they were both vegetables and the way they were different was that they were vegetables too. Difficulties in these areas suggest problems with integrative functions of the brain such as the frontal lobes and the corpus callosum (both of which appeared as contusions on CT scans).

The AIM in this case helped establish a baseline screening for a severely impaired closed head injury client. His deficits are global in nature with pronounced impairment in the brain stem area affecting his general level of arousal and impaired motor capacity. The AIM also illustrated that integration centers of the brain were markedly impaired, consistent with damage to the frontal lobes and the corpus callosum.

---

stroy much of the limbic system, especially the hippocampus. The result is a near total inability to learn new information (anterograde amnesia). The HIV/AIDS virus has wider effects on the brain, because it progressively destroys the immune system. The virus itself may have direct consequences for the brain, but it also opens the brain to opportunistic infections and other diseases that can attack the brain.

NEUROTOXINS

Neurotoxins include any substances that are poisonous to the brain (Lezak, 1995). These may include drugs, alcohol, solvents, fuels, pesticides, and metals such as lead or mercury. Many substances can be toxic to the brain in high doses, whereas they may not be toxic in low doses. Many prescription drugs fall into this category; for example, lithium, which is used to treat bipolar affective disorder (manic depression).

Many heavy metals, such as lead or mercury, can be extremely damaging to the body and the central nervous system, even in low dosages (Zillmer, Lucci, Barth, Peake, & Spyker, 1986; Zillmer, 1995). Although not many people come in contact with heavy metals, the general population may be exposed to some toxins routinely or by accident. For example, more than half a million accidental poisonings from pesticides are reported each year worldwide (Ecobichon &

Joy, 1982). One common group of pesticides are chlorinated hydrocarbon insecticides (for example, chlordane, heptachlor, and lindane) which people use extensively to combat household pests such as flies, cockroaches, fleas, termites, and mosquitoes as well as agricultural crop enemies. Because chlordane maintains its effects for approximately 15 or more years after application, it offers an economically appealing long-term treatment against termites. Chlordane is readily absorbed through the gastrointestinal tract, respiratory tract, or unbroken skin, and is stored in body fat. Once absorbed, chlordane is an axon poison, which disturbs the normal action of the sodium-potassium adenosinetriphosphatase (ATPase) pump, interfering with the transmission of nerve impulses. Because of its chemical stability, chlordane can be detected in approximately 70% of U.S. homes today, and ranks among the most ubiquitous neurotoxic materials being released into the ecosystem (Zillmer, Montenegro, Wiser, Barth, & Spyker, 1996).

In general, toxic effects on the brain cannot be described in simple terms, because the mechanisms of action are so varied. Most common are cognitive deficits ranging from mild to severe on tasks requiring speeded processing, problem solving, and delayed memory. Somatization, hysterical features, and depression often dominate the clinical picture. Thus, the medical profession increasingly recognizes that chemicals can have significant neuropsychological effects (Hartman, 1988) and that neuropsychology offers promise in increasing knowledge of the effects of toxins on the human CNS, describing specific patterns of performance, and monitoring the course of treatment.

Conclusion

Brain tumors and head injuries affect a significant proportion of the population and may lead to many debilitating conditions. Neuropsychologists play an important role in evaluating the cognitive profile of those patients and in actively rehabilitating for these conditions. Furthermore, neuropsychologists are at the forefront in researching tumor treatment and TBI rehabilitation. Neuropsychologists are most interested in how such conditions result in specific neuropsychological deficits and disabilities in adaptive behaviors. Such research not only improves the patient's care but also provides new knowledge on the normal functioning brain. The next three chapters focus on the relationship between diffuse neuropsychological deficits and dementing conditions such as encountered in Alzheimer's disease and disorders of consciousness.

Critical Thinking Questions

■ Would you want to know what type of cell a tumor arises from, if a family member of yours had brain cancer? Why? Should physicians routinely inform their patients of such medical details?

■ How do children who suffer from brain tumors react differently to their disease from the way adults do? How do their families react?

■ Can a head injury change a person's life?

■ What is the neuropsychologist's role in diagnosing and treating the victims and their families who suffer from brain tumors?

Key Terms

Tumor
Neoplasm
Infiltrative tumors
Noninfiltrative tumors
Malignant tumors
Benign tumors
Metastasis
Neuromas
Grade of tumor
Gliomas
Glioblastoma multiforme (GBM)
Astrocytomas
Oligodendroglioma

Meningiomas
Metastatic tumors
Acoustic neuromas
Pituitary tumors
Functioning adenomas
Nonfunctioning adenomas
Acidophilic adenoma
Chromophobic adenoma
Basophilic adenoma
Cushing's syndrome
Medulloblastoma
Ependymal glioma
Optic glioma
Pituitary adenoma

Pinealoma
Tensile strength
Retrograde degeneration
Anterograde degeneration
Penetrating head injury
Closed head injury
Acceleration
Deceleration
Impact injury
Countercoup injury
Glasgow Coma Scale (GCS)
Edema
Intracranial pressure (ICP)
Brain herniation

Transtentorial herniation
Subdural hematoma
Extradural hematoma
Epidural hematoma
Posttraumatic amnesia (PTA)
Retrograde amnesia
Anterograde amnesia
Brain abscesses
Meningitis
Herpes encephalitis
Human immunodeficiency virus (HIV)

Web Connections

http://www.med.harvard.edu/AANLIB/home.html
The Whole Brain Atlas (Brain Tumors)
Shows MRI and SPECT images of various neoplastic diseases, including glioma, metastatic tumors, and meningioma.

http://www.tbilaw.com
Brain Injury Information Page
Provides information about brain injury, concussion, and head injury.

http://health.yahoo.com/health/Diseases_and_Conditions/Disease_Feed_Data/concussion
Concussion Health Page
Page on causes, prevention, incidence, and risk factors of concussions.

Chapter 11

NORMAL AGING AND DEMENTIA: ALZHEIMER'S DISEASE

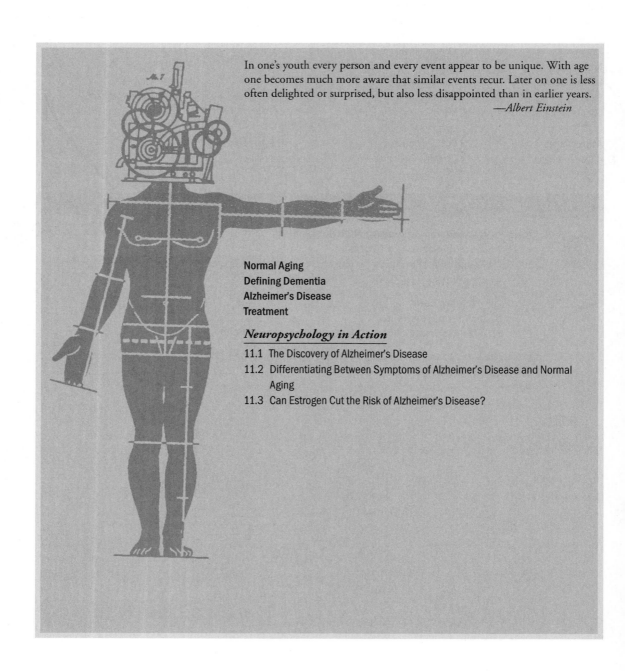

In one's youth every person and every event appear to be unique. With age one becomes much more aware that similar events recur. Later on one is less often delighted or surprised, but also less disappointed than in earlier years.
—*Albert Einstein*

Normal Aging
Defining Dementia
Alzheimer's Disease
Treatment

Neuropsychology in Action

11.1 The Discovery of Alzheimer's Disease
11.2 Differentiating Between Symptoms of Alzheimer's Disease and Normal Aging
11.3 Can Estrogen Cut the Risk of Alzheimer's Disease?

Keep in Mind

- Is dementia inevitable? How does healthy "normal" aging differ from dementia?
- Are dementia and Alzheimer's disease synonymous?
- Does Alzheimer's disease selectively affect "memory" structures of the brain?
- Why is Alzheimer's disease so difficult to diagnose?

Overview

The elderly are the fastest growing segment of the U.S. population. More than 11% of the population, nearly 26 million, is older than 65. This compares to only 4% at the turn of the century. In 1900 about 1% of the population in Western industrialized countries was over 75 years old. Today that number has mushroomed to about 7% and has not yet peaked. Life expectancy has increased to an average of 71 years for men and 77 years for women. In the year 2030 there will be 55 million people over 65, constituting approximately 20% of U.S. citizens. The 85-and-older group is expected to double its present size.

Because of this change in demographics, tremendous research interest has focused on understanding the neurologic conditions that target the elderly. Among these conditions are a group of disorders that cause global declines in cognitive and behavioral functioning. These syndromes are collectively known as the *dementias*. They have no one cause, and most etiologies are still a mystery. Many dementias have no known cure. Dementia is often progressive, eventually affecting numerous higher mental facilities. In short, dementia may be thought of as the "thief of the mind," sometimes first robbing memory, communication ability, or visual-spatial skills, but then returning to steal other aspects of mental functioning.

Although epidemiologic studies estimate that 1–5% of the population between 60 and 70 years old suffer from dementia, the incidence increases exponentially with age, so that by age 85 the prevalence of dementia in the population is estimated at between 18% and 85% (Kay, 1995; Johansson, 1991). With a top-heavy population of aging baby-boomers, the problem of identifying dementia and providing medical and psychological services to patients and families is becoming increasingly important. About 10% of Americans over age 65 live in specialized settings (such as residential care facilities or assisted living), and over a million live in nursing homes. Although the elderly only constitute 11% of the American population, they account for over 40% of hospitalization days in acute care hospitals. They buy 25% of all prescription drugs and use 30% of the total health budget. Clinical neuropsychologists contribute valuable assessment skills to distinguish normal aging from dementia. They also play an important role in health care decision making, helping match level of care to an elderly patient's actual needs.

In this chapter, we examine the differences between normal aging and dementia and address questions regarding the aging brain and neuropsychological functioning. For example, is there an inevitable cognitive decline with age? These differentiations can be made by considering the neuropsychological profiles of both healthy older individuals and those with **dementia**. We examine dementias in both this chapter and the next. This chapter presents an in-depth look at the most common dementia syndrome: Alzheimer's disease, or AD. This cortical dementia is examined from a neuropathological, neuropsychological, and behavioral perspective. In the next chapter, the subcortical dementias of Parkinson's disease, Huntington's disease and Creutzfeldt-Jakob's disease are presented.

Normal Aging

What determines whether getting older brings wisdom, contentment, and a sense of fulfillment, or despair and sadness, regret, and a feeling of loss? The well-known psychologist and developmental theorist Erik Erickson has described this as a conflict between achieving "integrity" versus "acknowledging despair." To achieve integrity, the person must accept his or her own life. According to this theory, people who achieve integrity use past experiences, accumulated knowledge, and mature judgment, and seek to improve the path for younger generations. The state of wholeness or completeness that may accompany a sense of fulfillment allows the older person to remain productive and creative, and adds a sense of purpose and closure to life. The negative alternative to achieving integrity is despair and futility—a sense that a lifetime has been wasted, leaving no energy for making constructive use of accumulated experience.

Old age presents many challenges. Socially, older people may feel increasingly isolated with adjustment to retirement and death of friends or a spouse. Physically, age brings the threat of increased ailments and chronic illness. Cognitively, older people are often concerned with the possibility of memory problems and mental slowing. But despite these challenges, many older people find their happiness increases with age. A large study of 2727 participants aged 25–74 found, on average, that younger adults harbored more negative emotions of sadness, anxiety, and worthlessness than did older survey respondents (Mroczek & Kolarz, 1998). The happiest elders were those who maintained significant relationships and were more extraverted. The authors also speculated that increased self-knowledge with age helped older people know and thus minimize the impact of negative external forces on their moods.

COGNITIVE CHANGES ASSOCIATED WITH AGING

The extent of functional cognitive impairment from aging is the subject of some controversy. Does aging entail inevitable cognitive decline? And if so, in what areas? Some individuals deteriorate appreciably before reaching age 60, whereas others who are much older retain much of their cognitive ability. Can "normal aging" result in such variation?

Cross-sectional studies comparing older to younger age groups generally indicate that stored knowledge in memory (long-term memory) and habitual ways of solving problems (**crystallized intelligence**) resist the effects of aging. However, novel reasoning and the efficiency of solving new problems or responding to abstract ideas (**fluid intelligence**) decline with advanced age. Fluid intelligence is most directly related to the influences of changing biological factors and is relatively unaffected by higher levels of experience or education. In contrast, crystallized intelligence represents an accumulation of acquired skills and general information, and is more related to formal education or diverse social experiences and less sensitive to biological processes. The most reliable decline in age group comparison studies shows up in three areas of intellectual activity, all of which are considered fluid markers of intelligence: (1) new learning, (2) abstract and complex new problem solving, and (3) behavioral speed. Because these declines are also present in dementias such as Alzheimer's disease, it is important to differentiate whether these changes herald the start of a progressive dementia or are qualitatively different.

Because much individual variation in cognitive functioning is possible, longitudinal studies are providing clues to the question of "inevitable" cognitive decline and the factors that contribute to successful aging. A series of interesting studies conducted in Sweden document the neuropsychological performance of the oldest segment of the population. In one study, researchers gave neuropsychological tests, twice, two years apart, to over 300 people between the ages of 84 and 90 (Johansson, 1991). This study of the oldest old (84–90 years old) found surprising stability in neuropsychological functioning between the first and second test sessions. Researchers expected that people at this advanced age would decline over two years. However, two-thirds of the sample (66%) remained at the same cognitive level, whereas 31% declined (Johansson, Zarit, & Berg, 1992). Almost half (42%) remained in the normal range of functioning during the two-year time period. This finding was surprising not only in that a large portion of the sample showed stability of cognitive function over time, but also that a significant portion of quite elderly adults still had "normal" cognitive function.

Johansson and his colleagues (Johansson, 1991) suggest that terminal decline, or proximity to death, may relate more to cognitive functioning than to chronological age. Among other neuropsychological tests, these examiners administered the digit span task, at regular intervals, to normally aging Swedes over age 70. This requires repeating increasingly longer series of digits either in sequential or reverse order, respectively, until the testee misses them. For the 70- to 88-year-olds studied over time, Johansson examined two groups: those who died before age 85, and those still living. Those alive at age 85 showed a consistent performance as they aged; those who died before age 85 started showing a drop in backward digit span by age 75 and marked drops in both forward and backward span lengths by age 79.

Thus one cannot assume that cognitive decline is a marked and inevitable result of advancing age. Many factors contribute to loss of intellectual functioning. Progressive dementia and other degenerative neurological disease are obvious factors. The person's medical condition and degree of physical frailty certainly contribute. Older people have a higher probability of cardiovascular problems and chronic physical ailments. Also, older people may suffer more cognitive problems secondary to depression or medication regimen. People who are healthy and active appear to have more "functional reserve" or capacity and may be less susceptible to the effects of the aging process or to the effects of acute illness. In other words, they may bounce back more easily.

An example of functional cognitive reserve is evident in the longitudinal study of aging and Alzheimer's disease called the Nun Study. David Snowdon of the University of Kentucky is following 678 Roman Catholic sisters who have agreed to regular cognitive and medical assessments and brain donation at death. Snowden and his colleagues are seeking to shed light on the factors that lead to increased longevity as well as on the determinants of Alzheimer's disease and other brain disorders such as stroke. What is unique about this research is the availability of records from young adulthood and throughout the time each nun resided in the convent. An examination of linguistic complexity, gleaned from autobiographies written between ages 18 and 32, indicated that poorer linguistic ability early in life strongly related to lower cognitive functioning, dementia, and markers of Alzheimer's disease in the brain later in life (Snowdon, Greiner, Kemper, Nanayakkara, & Mortimer, 1999).

BRAIN CHANGES ASSOCIATED WITH AGING

Throughout this book we have reiterated that the goal of neuropsychology is to understand the relationships of brain structure and function to behavior. How does aging affect these relationships? The aging brain undergoes visually apparent structural changes such as diminution in size, flattening of the cortical surface, and increasing amounts of intracranial space. Concomitant changes take place at the neuroanatomical and biochemical levels. Reseachers have reported some loss of neurons, changes in neuronal size, altered dendritic processes, and an increased frequency of **neurofibrillary tangles** and **senile plaques** with normal aging.

However, the brain does not age uniformly. Neuron loss and cortical thinning may have led to one of the myths of human neurobiology, namely, that throughout adulthood people lose an enormous number of neurons from the brain each day. Quantitative studies, using automated equipment and correcting for total tissue volume, suggest that many areas of the brain such as the **striate cortex** and parietal cortex do not lose an appreciable number of neurons over the life span. By contrast, the **neostriatum** and the frontal cortex lose 15–20% of their neurons between young adulthood and old age. The most likely set of age-related neuronal changes specifically affects the prefrontal cortex. Neuronal loss in this area could account directly for some of the fluid intelligence changes in cognitive functions reported to occur with aging. Also, neurotransmitter changes can occur as the result of structural changes and may predispose older people to problems such as depression, memory problems, and brain disorders. For example, when dopamine levels drop past a critical threshold, Parkinsonism is the result.

Because cognitive functioning varies widely among older people, one might also expect a range of individual variability in physical brain changes. When assessing the degree of cortical **atrophy,** gross inspection of the brain reveals wide variation (see Figure 11.1). In the Swedish study (Johansson, 1991), 85% of elderly persons' brains seemed to have little to no evidence of cerebral atrophy. However, all did show some neuropathologic markers usually associated with dementia, including signs of ischemia, neurofibrillary tangles, and plaque formations. In individuals over age 85, gray matter atrophy is often apparent on CT in both demented and nondemented people. White matter attenuation (thinning of the white matter) relates to cognitive changes associated with fluid intelligence, such as slowed speed of behavior, poorer spatial ability, poorer arithmetic, and memory recognition skills (Johansson, 1991). As imaging methods become more specific, it will be interesting to see if specific brain areas show more atrophy than others and if these areas correlate with neuropsychological functioning.

Summary

The findings from various researchers in aging and cognition suggest that both crystallized and fluid intelligence are important for successful functioning in advanced age. Ability, level of education, and knowledge gained early in life seem to provide some buffer against later brain disorders. Not everyone ages cognitively at the same rate, and many retain high abilities into advanced age. Some individuals may suffer devastating effects, both physical and cognitive, whereas others suffer relatively few effects. Therefore, among groups of older people age is not the only, or best, predictor of cognitive decline or mortality. The process of aging increases the probability of cognitive problems. Aging also results in a loss of neurons, but this by itself does not seem to differentiate between normal aging and dementia. Different measures of functional capacity may well be the key to identifying those at greatest risk. Advanced imaging methods correlated with neuropsychological functioning hold promise for more precisely relating structure to func-

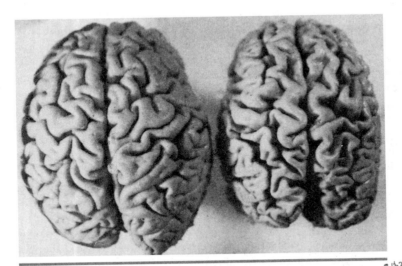

Figure 11.1 Normal brain (left) and brain showing widespread cortical atrophy (right). Note the thinner gyri, wider sulci, and widening of the interhemispheric fissure on the right. Cortical atrophy indicates loss of neuronal connections but not necessarily clinical dementia. (From Erin D. Bigler, "The Clinical Significance of Cerebral Atrophy in Dementia," *Archives of Clinical Neuropsychology, 2,* 1987, Figure 1, p. 178. Copyright © 2000 Elsevier Science, Ltd. Reprinted with permission of the authors and publisher)

tion. This will also aid in identifying people at greatest risk for developing dementia and in ultimately answering the question, What is the difference between normal aging and dementia?

Defining Dementia

With public and scientific attention focused on progressive dementia, one might expect general agreement among health professionals when referring to dementia and subtypes of dementia such as Alzheimer's disease. Surprisingly, there is no such agreement. Given the cornucopia of terms used to refer to dementia and subtypes of dementia (see Table 11.1), no wonder people get confused. Professionals and laypeople alike may confuse dementia—the behavioral syndrome—with one particular condition, such as Alzheimer's disease. Patients and families often understand dementing conditions as "hardening of the arteries," "senility," or "old-timers' disease," which often reflects a perception that the problem is inevitable in aging. In the most generic sense, dementia refers to a behavioral syndrome and not one disease or cause. It denotes conditions that may have a variety of causes or etiologies. Some dementias may be treatable, some may not. Some stem from disease processes that inevitably become worse, and some from toxic exposure or injury, resulting in a behavioral decline that plateaus.

The dementia syndrome is a cluster of behavioral symptoms that may or may not point to a disease, but dementia is not a disease entity in and of itself. The various subcategories of dementia usually relate to the suspected disease, cause, or primary site of damage (for example, cortical versus subcortical). Researchers have found well over 50 causes of dementia; Table 11.1 lists a sampling. Among the most well known are the degenerative dementias caused by a progressive and unrelenting disease process such as Alzheimer's or Parkinson's disease. Neurologists have traditionally categorized these disease processes as cortical, subcortical, or mixed, depending on the degree to which they affect gray or white matter areas of the brain. Vascular, infectious, and toxic conditions, as well as a variety of other brain conditions may also result in dementia.

Table 11.1 *Representative Causes of Dementia*

Progressive Dementias	**Potentially Static Dementias**
Cortical Dementias	**(continued)**
Alzheimer's disease	*Infectious Conditions*
	Herpes encephalitis
Motor neuron disease	
	Miscellaneous Conditions
Pick's disease	Tumor
Progressive aphasia	
	Normal pressure hydro-
Wilson's disease	cephalus
Subcortical Dementias	
Huntington's disease	Trauma
Parkinson's disease	**Potentially Reversible**
	Dementias
Progressive supranuclear	*Systemic Illness*
palsy	Severe anemia
AIDS dementia	Uremia
Creutzfeldt-Jakob disease	*Deficiency States*
	B_{12} deficiency
Mixed Dementias	
Lewy body dementia	*Endocrine Disorders*
	Addison's disease
Vascular dementias (such	
as multi-infarct dementia,	Thyroid disorders
or MID)	*Drug Toxicity*
	Anticholinergics
Binswanger's disease	
	Antipsychotics
Potentially Static Dementias	
Toxic Conditions	**Pseudodementia**
Alcoholic dementia	Depression
Heavy metal poisoning (such	
as lead and mercury)	

Multi-infarct dementia results from progressive small strokes. Some of these conditions are progressive, whereas others, such as the dementia resulting from herpes encephalitis, may be static, rarely worsening over time. Although most dementing conditions encountered by neuropsychologists represent persistent and/or progressive states, researchers have also documented "reversible" or temporary dementias. Reduced metabolic efficiency accompanies aging, making older individuals especially susceptible to conditions and substances that they might have tolerated when younger. For example, symptoms of dementia can stem from adverse reactions to medications (such as sedative-hypnotics and anticholinergic drugs), nutritional disorders (such as thiamine deficiency and pernicious anemia), metabolic disorders (hypoglycemia, hypercalcemia, kidney failure), psychiatric disorders (severe mood disorders, psychosis), and other conditions such as anesthesia or surgery. However, when these conditions are treated, the dementia is usually reversible and the patient returns to baseline.

DIAGNOSTIC CRITERIA FOR DEMENTIA

No one set of criteria represents definitive agreement regarding the diagnosis of dementia. Somewhat varying diagnostic standards are described in the *Diagnostic and Statistical Manual*, vol. 4 (*DSM-IV*) and by the National Institute of Neurological and Communicative Disorders and Stroke-Alzheimer's disease and Related Disorders Association (NINCDS-ADRDA; McKhann et al., 1984). However, experts agree about some of the major features of dementia. The first is that dementia results in a *loss of cognitive or intellectual function.* This feature implies a decline that is acquired and unusual. It is acquired, because people born with impaired intellectual function, having developmental disorders such as mental retardation, do not have dementia simply by virtue of poor intellect, although they too can develop dementia. The loss of cognitive or intellectual functioning must also be unusual or outside of the realm of what would be expected with normal aging. As we discussed, aging may bring about mild cognitive decline, particularly in memory and cognitive processing speed. But the decline associated with dementia represents a marked change from previous levels of intellectual and memory ability. Although the most well known subtypes of dementia have a predilection for the elderly and result in inevitable deterioration, this broad definition of dementia could hypothetically refer to the sudden loss of intellectual function from head injury in a 17-year-old.

Although patterns of impairment may differ, the second area of diagnostic agreement in dementia involves *multiple areas of cognitive impairment.* The abilities impaired in dementia may represent all cognitive functions or may present different patterns of neuropsychological disability. Both sets of criteria for dementia identify memory impairment as a promi-

| Table 11.2 | *Diagnostic Criteria for Dementia* |

Criterion	DSM-IV	NINCDS/ADRDA
Memory impairment	R	R
Impairment of additional area of cognition (such as language, construction, praxis, or executive functioning)	R	D
Confirmed on mental status tests	NS	R
Impaired/decline in social or occupational function	R	NS
State of consciousness unclouded	R	R
Evidence of specific organic factor etiologically related to the disorder or absence of conditions other than organic mental syndrome	R	NS

Note: R = Required, D = Desirable but not required, NS = Not specified.

Source: Adapted from Rebok and Folstein (1993) and Katzman, Lasker, and Bernstein (1988).

nent and necessary feature. However, it is the multiple, and often diffuse cognitive decline that characterizes dementia.

In summary, the term *dementia* in its broadest sense refers to a group of conditions and diseases that share some similar neuropsychological and behavioral symptoms, although the underlying causes may vary widely. The prime identifying feature is a decline in multiple areas of cognitive functioning, including memory. Beyond this initial definition of dementia, however, lies what is probably most important in working with patients suffering from dementia—an understanding of the different neuropsychological presentations of dementia subtypes.

SUBTYPES AND CLASSIFICATIONS OF DEMENTIA

Cortical versus Subcortical

Traditionally, the primary demarcation among subtypes of dementia has followed the attempt to distinguish between cortical and subcortical dementias. **Cortical dementias** primarily affect the cerebral cortex, or gray matter. Alzheimer's disease is typically included within this category. In **subcortical dementias,** the disease state predominantly affects the white matter, or neuronal connections between cortical areas and gray matter structures below the cortex. The term *subcortical* was first used to describe the neuropathology and accompanying pattern of cognitive deficits associated with progressive supranuclear palsy (Albert, Feldman, & Willis, 1974). Since that time, it has expanded to include Huntington's disease and Parkinson's disease and may also refer to diseases such as AIDS-related dementia and some depressions. The difficulty with this differentiation, both neuroanatomically and behaviorally, is that these disorders do not conform to strict cortical–subcortical boundaries in the brain. For example, Alzheimer's disease typically causes significant cortical neuronal loss and atrophy, but also specifically attacks the hippocampus, a subcortical limbic system structure. In contrast, diagnosticians usually identify Parkinson's disease by the subcortical structure that it targets, the substantia nigra, although evidence suggests that it also affects some higher cortical functions such as executive functioning. Even when evidence indicates that a disease only targets subcortical structures, "cortical" effects may appear because of the disconnection of neural pathways in the white matter that connect the gray matter areas. Although we use the terms "cortical" and "subcortical" dementia as general categories, you must loosely interpret them to imply a major or primary area of damage rather than an exclusive area of damage.

Static versus Progressive

All dementias that result from a disease process are progressive. Diseases such as Alzheimer's, Pick's, Huntington's, or Creutzfeldt-Jakob inevitably follow a continuous cognitive and behavioral decline. Other conditions, however, may cause a static, or steady-state cognitive disorder. A neurotoxic substance (such as lead or alcohol) or infection (such as herpes encephalitis) continues to cause brain damage as long as it is present. But when the condition is arrested, the resultant dementia usually plateaus.

Both static and progressive dementias can begin with a sudden change of functioning, over days or weeks, or a more insidious or gradual onset, over the course of months or years. Lead may poison the brain for a period of years before impairment appears. Herpes encephalitis, in contrast, is an acute infectious condition with sudden and dramatic effects on the brain. Progressive dementias can also vary in their course. The progression, as in the case of Alzheimer's disease, is gradual. However, there may be long periods during which the decline plateaus. Vascular dementias often produce a stepwise progression, as multiple infarcts or strokes occur at different times. Only repeated neuropsychological testing and keen observation by the neuropsychologist, patient, or family can reveal the progression of the dementia.

Reversible versus Irreversible

Researchers have focused primarily on irreversible and progressive dementias. However, clinicians are likely to see a variety of patients with dementia-like symptoms that may remit with time. Part of the diagnostic problem with the so-called reversible dementias is that these people may actually have **delirium** rather than dementia. Delirium does not signal dementia, but is a transient cognitive problem associated with an acute confusional state. Typically, individuals with delirium have poor attention, disorganized thinking, perceptual disruption, disorientation, memory impairment, and an altered state of consciousness. Because delirium and dementia share memory impairment and disorientation, they can be easily confused. However, with delirium, the symptoms develop over a period of days or hours and are caused by specific organic problems such as overmedication or an acute or worsening medical condition. Many medical problems listed as potentially reversible dementias in Table 11.1 cause delirium. Moreover, it is not uncommon for patients with dementia to develop delirium. For example, they might go into the hospital to have surgery or to be treated for an acute medical condition. Perhaps their already lowered cognitive capacity causes vulnerability to the cognitive effects of general metabolic dysfunction. People who become delirious for short periods of time and then

Neuropsychology in Action 11.1

The Discovery of Alzheimer's Disease

by Mary V. Spiers

A piece of recently uncovered neuropsychology history puts to rest doubts about Auguste D., the first case of Alzheimer's disease ever described. After having gone missing for nearly 90 years, Alois Alzheimer's blue cardboard file was found by psychiatrists in the archives of the University of Frankfurt, Germany, in 1996. Among the 32 sheets were Alzheimer's handwritten interview notes, samples of Auguste D.'s "amnestic writing disorder," and a report of the course of the disease. Alzheimer's first notes are as follows:

> Nov. 26, 1901
>
> She sits on the bed with a helpless expression. What is your name? *Auguste.* Last name? *Auguste.* What is your hus-

band's name? *Auguste, I think.* Your husband? *Ah, my husband.* She looks as if she didn't understand the question. . . .

> What is this? I show her a pencil. *A pen.* A purse and a key, diary, cigar are identified correctly. At lunch she eats cauliflower and pork. Asked what she is eating, she answers *spinach.* . . .

> When objects are shown to her, she does not remember after a short time which objects have been shown. In between she always speaks about twins. When she is asked to write, she holds the book in such a way that one has the impression that she has a loss in the right visual field. Asked to write *Auguste D,* she tries to write *Mrs.* and forgets the rest. It is

necessary to repeat every word. (Maurer, Volk, & Gerbaldo, 1997, p. 1547)

Dementia had been described before, with terms such as "paralytic dementia," "atherosclerotic dementia," and "senile dementia." What made Auguste so unusual was that she was so young, only 51. After 4½ years Auguste died. When Alzheimer published his description of this case (1907/1987), he had examined her brain and could describe the unique histologic findings of neurofibrillary tangles: "The nucleus and the cell have fallen apart and only a tangled bundle of fibrils points to the place in which there was once a ganglion cell" (Alzheimer, 1907/1987). He had even

recover do not have a dementia, even a reversible one. One difference in presentation is that people with dementia, other than in the late stages, are alert and can respond to what is going on around them. People with delirium are grossly confused and disoriented to their surroundings. A true "reversible dementia" should meet the behavioral criteria for dementia discussed earlier. In other words, the individual must show dementia in the absence of a delusional state.

The rest of this chapter focuses on Alzheimer's disease. This represents the most clearly understood dementia. Research continues on the question of reversibility. Several possibilities exist. For example, anticholinergic drugs impair memory functioning. Maybe lowered cognitive functioning caused by large doses of a medication can indeed permanently reverse when the person stops taking it. Or perhaps dementia symptoms stemming from overmedication indicate the early stages of dementia in an already compromised brain, so that discontinuing the drug only temporarily raises cognitive functioning.

Alzheimer's Disease

Alzheimer's disease (AD), named after its discoverer, Alois Alzheimer (see Neuropsychology in Action 11.1), is a cortical dementia that is irreversible and results in an inevitable decline. It is the most devastating and prevalent of the dementias, representing more than 50% of diagnosed dementia cases (Kay, 1995). Researchers estimate that Alzheimer's disease affects between 1.5 to 3 million people in the United States over age 65, with an incidence of new cases increasing exponentially between ages 65 and 85 (Terry & Katzman, 1992).

There appears to be no single cause for Alzheimer's disease, and in most cases the etiology remains unknown. AD is linked to increased age, which has led

drawn pictures of Auguste D.'s neuro-fibrillary tangles (see Figure 11.2). To Alzheimer, this represented a new entity of "presenile dementia." In 1910, Krae-pelin included the new syndrome of Alzheimerische Krankheit (Alzheimer's disease) in his famous textbook of psychiatry.

A controversy erupted after their discovery of Alzheimer's file because the original autopsy findings also indicated that Auguste D. had arteriosclerosis in smaller blood vessels, a fact that today is a criterion excluding pure Alzheimer's disease. Other scientists argued that she may have had a metabolic disorder. Finding Auguste D.'s brain would be the only way to resolve the question of whether she had what we now recognize as Alzheimer's disease. After a two-year search yet another group of German researchers found more than 250 slides of Auguste's brain in the basement of the University of Munich. German researchers have been able to confirm the two classic signs

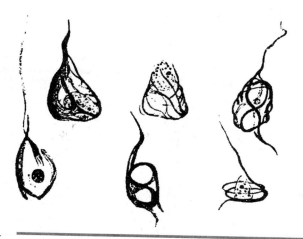

Figure 11.2 Alzheimer's drawings of neurofibrillary tangles from the brain of Auguste D. (From K. Maurer, S. Volk, and H. Gerbaldo, "August D. and Alzheimer's Disease," *The Lancet*, 1997, *349*, Figure 5, p. 1549. Reprinted with permission)

of Alzheimer's disease in the brain of Auguste D.: neurofibrillary tangles and amyloid, or senile, plaques. This puts to rest the notion that Auguste D. may have had a disease process other than Alzheimer's. However, the question of whether she had a coexisting vascular problem is likely to fuel debates for some time.

some to speculate that it is a disease of "accelerated aging"—implying that if we all lived long enough, Alzheimer's disease would be inevitable. About twice as many women as men in the older population have AD. It is not clear if this represents a sex difference or a predominantly female elderly population. People with more education seem less likely to develop Alzheimer's, but again, this is probably more a marker of larger cognitive reserves acting as a buffer between neuropathology and disease manifestation than a suggestion that graduate degrees will ward off the disease.

Alzheimer's disease does not have a strong genetic component in most cases. It does seem to run in a few families, but probably fewer than 150 families worldwide. In these families, the pattern of the disease is autosomal dominant, meaning the family pedigree shows about 50% of the family members as having Alzheimer's. The most likely chromosonal culprits in genetically established Alzheimer's appear to be chromosomes, 1, 14, and 21. Interestingly, people born

with Down's syndrome or trisomy 21 (named because the disorder results from an abnormality on chromosome 21) inevitably develop a dementia, usually by age 40. The associated brain changes corresponding to Alzheimer's (neurofibrillary tangles and senile plaques) appear years before clinical diagnosis. Recent genetic research has focused on a genetic protein called ApoE4, which seems associated with Alzheimer's and which may eventually assist in the diagnosis of patients with the disorder. In sum, although the biomedical research searching for causes and markers of the disease appears promising, scientists still know very little about the actual causes of Alzheimer's disease.

THE DIAGNOSTIC PROBLEM OF ALZHEIMER'S DISEASE

A definitive diagnosis of Alzheimer's disease requires the behavioral presence of dementia and the identification of neuropathological markers of Alzheimer's.

No single medical test can identify AD, short of a brain biopsy revealing the characteristic neurofibrillary tangles and neuritic plaques, which are most predominant in the hippocampus and cortical association areas. Because biopsy is not a procedure to which most people would submit, a definitive diagnosis cannot be made until autopsy. The clinical diagnosis of AD largely depends on evidence related to behavioral and neuropsychological profiles and on ruling out all other identifiable causes of dementia, such as those listed in Table 11.1. The clinical diagnoses of "probable" and "possible" AD reflect, in large measure, the certainty with which other causes of dementia can be excluded. In this chapter we also refer to probable Alzheimer's disease as "senile dementia of the Alzheimer's type" (SDAT), to reflect the probable nature of the diagnosis.

THE NEUROPATHOLOGY OF ALZHEIMER'S DISEASE

Major Brain Structures Affected by Alzheimer's Disease

There are two very interesting facts regarding the neuropathology and pathophysiology of Alzheimer's disease. First, the disease targets specific regions of the brain. Second, disease-targeted structures sustain massive cell loss. Although AD is a "cortical dementia," because major areas of the cerebral cortex show massive cell loss and brain shrinkage, this disease does not respect cortical boundaries. It greatly affects major subcortical limbic system structures such as the hippocampus and amygdala. Most pathologic changes occur in the cortical temporal-parietal association areas and the *subcortical limbic cortexes*. Specifically, the disease destroys the major pathways to and from the hippocampus, cutting off direct connections to association cortexes.

Gross postmortem inspection of the brain often finds cortical atrophy. In Figure 11.3 the most marked atrophy is in the frontal, temporal, and parietal areas. The gyri are thinned, and the sulci are noticeably widened. Researchers estimate that in AD about half of the large neurons deteriorate (Terry, Peck, de Teresa, Schecter, & Horoupian, 1981), resulting in a loss of volume. Specifically, these neurons lose dendritic arborization, or branching. The ventricles also enlarge, because of cortical thinning (see Figure 11.4). Although dementia severity increases with increased cell death, longitudinal comparisons of global cerebral atrophy to dementia severity do not reliably indicate dementia (Bigler, 1987; Johansson, 1991).

A closer look at specific structures reveals that they sustain massive cell loss. In fact, SDAT appears to follow structural borders. Chief among these are the parietal and temporal cortexes, the hippocampus and the

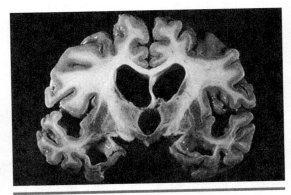

Figure 11.4 Coronal view of an Alzheimer's disease brain, showing widened ventricles. In particular, note also the thinning of the temporal lobes at the bottom of the picture. (From WebPath, courtesy of Edward C. Klatt, M.D., Department of Pathology, University of Utah, Salt Lake City, Utah, USA)

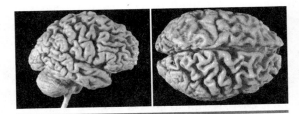

Figure 11.3 Lateral and superior views of cortical atrophy in the postmortem brain of an Alzheimer's disease patient. (From WebPath, courtesy of Edward C. Klatt, M.D., Department of Pathology, University of Utah, Salt Lake City, Utah, USA)

structures leading to it (entorhinal cortex and the perforant neural path), the amygdala, and specific nuclei of the thalamus (VanHoesn & Damasio, 1987). In addition, certain subcortical frontal areas are implicated, such as the nucleus basalis of Meynert and the olfactory areas. Noticeably spared are the primary motor and sensory areas (tactile, auditory, visual) and the basal ganglia. The affected structures correspond to areas of higher cognitive functioning and memory, leaving relatively untouched more basic sensory and motor abilities.

Histologic Markers

The two neuropathological findings Alzheimer (1907/1987) identified, still considered the primary markers of the disease, are neurofibrillary tangles and neuritic, or senile, plaques. These are evident by microscope inspection after brain biopsy at autopsy. Neurofibrillary tangles resemble entwined and twisted pairs of rope within the cytoplasm of swollen cell bodies (see Figures 11.2 and 11.5). Tangles consist of proteins, termed tau proteins, that are believed to accumulate as a result of abnormal phosphorylation. The excessive collection creates tangles that are dispersed throughout the brain but disproportionately in the areas just listed, including the temporal-parietal areas and the hippocampal complex. The specificity of structural deterioration in Alzheimer's extends to the cellular lay-

ers of the cortex. For example, within the six-layered isocortex of the cortical association areas, tangles and plaques devastate layers 3 and 5, whereas other layers are relatively spared (VanHoesn & Damasio, 1986).

Alzheimer described neuritic plaques as "clump-like deposits in the neuropil." They are round aggregates of "cellular trash" that have a particular affinity for the regions where the majority of synapses lie (the neuropil). The synapses eventually disintegrate, leaving holes and misshapen neurons where there were once active connections (see Figure 11.6). Plaques are likely to concentrate in the frontal and temporal regions (Zubenko, Moossy, Martinez, Rao, Kopp, & Hanin, 1989) and are numerous around the hippocampal formation. Note that tangles and plaques are not specific to Alzheimer's disease. They also appear in normally aging individuals without evidence of dementia, as well as in other degenerative diseases. It is the pattern and quantity of these markers that defines Alzheimer's.

An exciting recent discovery is that the substance of neuritic plaques and tangles may lead to hypotheses regarding possible causes of and treatments for Alzheimer's disease. The neuritic plaques found in AD contain an amino acid peptide protein core termed **beta-amyloid (β-amyloid)**. As a result, these neuritic plaques are also called *amyloid plaques*. Bradshaw and Mattingly (1995) review several possibilities

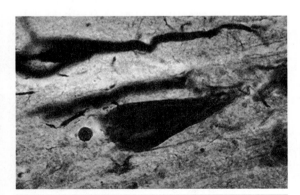

Figure 11.5 Twisted neurofibrillary tangles are a major histologic marker of Alzheimer's disease. (From WebPath, courtesy of Edward C. Klatt, M.D., Department of Pathology, University of Utah, Salt Lake City, Utah, USA)

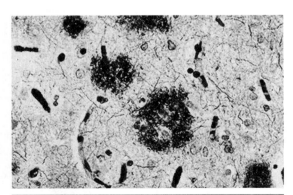

Figure 11.6 The round clumps of "cellular trash" form the neuritic plaques of Alzheimer's disease. (From WebPath, courtesy of Edward C. Klatt, M.D., Department of Pathology, University of Utah, Salt Lake City, Utah, USA)

for how β-amyloid may operate. First, it is coded on chromosome 21, the same chromosome responsible for Down's syndrome. The behavioral significance of this is that if they live past 30 people with Down's syndrome often show Alzheimer-like dementia symptoms. Therefore, chromosome 21 may be responsible for both problems. Second, there is debate on the function of β-amyloid. Is it a cause of the disease, a by-product of the disease, a "protective reactant," or an autoimmune response?

A team of neuroscientists from Duke University have discovered an additional protein in plaques and tangles that may also be a link to SDAT. It is *apolipoprotein E4* (ApoE4), one of four possible variants, or alleles, of the protein ApoE. Seventy-five percent of people have the ApoE3 variant (Corder et al., 1993), but risk for developing Alzheimer's disease increases to 90% if a person inherits the ApoE4 variant from both parents. In addition, a double set of ApoE4 alleles also lowers the mean age of onset. ApoE4 is responsible for ferrying cholesterol into the brain; however, researchers are currently investigating how this protein may operate in SDAT. It appears on yet another chromosome, chromosome 19, which binds with β-amyloid in cerebrospinal fluid. The exact mechanism for this binding process is not yet known; however, researchers hypothesize that ApoE4 may not be the direct or sole cause of the disease (see Bradshaw & Mattingly, 1995); rather, the protective factors that ApoE2 or E3 provide may be lost.

Neurotransmitter Systems Altered by Alzheimer's Disease

Of the many neurotransmitter systems in the brain, researchers are now finding that SDAT may touch multiple systems. However, the most consistent evidence of a neurotransmitter with a direct effect on memory processes in Alzheimer's disease is **acetylcholine (ACh).**

In the brain, acetylcholine is synthesized in a group of neurons called the *basal forebrain cholinergic complex (BFCC).* The cell bodies of these neurons lie in the basal forebrain structures of the nucleus basalis of Meynert, the diagonal band of Broca's area, and the globus pallidus. These axons project to the hippocampus and the cerebral cortex, primarily the frontal and temporal cortexes. The BFCC is a subcortical component of the limbic system and the major source of choline for the hippocampus and cortex (Coyle, 1985). Researchers have long known that acetylcholine plays a role in memory. Drachman (1977) demonstrated that blockage of receptors causes memory loss even in young adults. In Alzheimer's disease, the devastation of the BFCC neurons profoundly depresses brain levels of acetylcholine, perhaps as much as 60–90% (Terry & Davies, 1980; Bowen, Benton, Spillane, Smith, & Allen, 1982).

Some of the other neurotransmitters implicated in Alzheimer's disease are the catecholamines, the amino acid glutamate, and the neuropeptides somatostatin and corticotrophin. However, at this juncture, none of these neurotransmitters seem to play a clear role in SDAT. Researchers have reported that all are reduced in AD, but their reduction may be secondary to the disease process. For example, general stress also reduces somatostatin. As you might imagine, research in this area is progressing quickly, because of the push to find appropriate pharmacological treatments.

Neuroimaging in Alzheimer's Disease

Gross neuroimaging of the brain in patients with Alzheimer's disease may indicate cerebral atrophy on CT or MRI. The EEGs of Alzheimer's patients are likely to show generalized slowing (LaRue, 1992). Degree of atrophy or slowing taken in isolation are not reliably associated with degree of neuropsychological impairment (for example, see Bigler, 1987) but the degree of ventricular enlargement seen over time as the cortex atrophies accompanies increasing cognitive impairment (Burns, Jacoby, & Levy, 1991). Special imaging procedures demonstrate the enlarged hippocampal fissure that results from neuronal loss, tangles, and plaques that begin early in the disease process. Although researchers can only visualize this fissure by using an angled CT or MRI, it may be one of the best early Alzheimer's markers accomplished through noninvasive neuroimaging procedures. Also characteristic of AD is a pattern of metabolic and/or vascular insufficiency seen in the temporal-parietal area, which shows up on PET and SPECT scans. This hypometabolism can be either unilateral or bilateral and depends on factors such as severity of illness, gender, and age at onset (for review, see Forstl & Hentschel, 1994).

CTs and MRIs are primarily useful, not to confirm a diagnosis of Alzheimer's disease, but to rule out other conditions such as tumor or **multi-infarct dementia** caused by multiple small strokes or ischemic attacks. However, promising new methods of analyzing volume and ratio of specific structures through structural imaging may help confirm diagnosis of AD. PET and SPECT scans appear most sensitive for detecting the characteristic patterns of SDAT. These imaging measures are then correlated with neuropsychological measures to provide a dynamic picture of the disease process.

CLINICAL PRESENTATION AND NEUROPSYCHOLOGICAL PROFILE OF ALZHEIMER'S DISEASE

The clinical presentation of Alzheimer's patients can vary but many share characteristic patterns (see Neuropsychology in Action 11.2). The most consistent deficits across patients with autopsy-documented AD are memory and fluent anomic aphasia (for example, see Price, Gurvit, Weintrub, Geula, Leimkuhler, & Mesulam, 1993). Visual-spatial difficulties are also characteristic. These deficits correspond with neuroimaging studies showing patterns of hypometabolism in limbic and association areas in early stages of the disease. In this classic presentation, some frontal areas of the brain appear relatively spared. This also corresponds with neuropsychological testing and clinical observation indicating that despite severe memory impairment, many Alzheimer's patients retain an appropriate "social facade," do not have a Broca-type (nonfluent) aphasia, and retain normal strength and simple motor speed until the end stages of the disease. However, the impairments progress over time, gradually affecting all higher mental functions of the brain. What follows is a description of the neuropsychological and behavioral performance, according to

functional area, typical of those with SDAT. Because memory dysfunction is the hallmark of AD, we devote more discussion to this problem than to the other functional areas.

Memory

Alzheimer's globally and profoundly impairs memory. New declarative learning problems at all levels (encoding, storage, and retrieval), and retention over time are usually noticed first. In addition, structures of the brain that hold previously well-learned semantic knowledge information in organized associational frameworks, begin to deteriorate. Finally, short-term memory span, names of family members, and familiar stories fragment. The only type of learning that appears to persist lies outside the corticolimbic system, with certain types of nondeclarative learning.

Long-Term Declarative Memory   As in other conditions that produce "amnesia," SDAT results in profound difficulties in learning new declarative information. As discussed in Chapter 5, declarative memory can be loosely divided into episodic and semantic memory. People with SDAT have deficits in both. One of the first and most prominent symptoms of Alzheimer's disease is a deficit in new declarative learning, often called *anterograde amnesia* to differentiate it from retrograde amnesia (deficit in remote recall). On neuropsychological testing, SDAT patients in the mild to moderate stages of the disease typically show marked impairment on both verbal and visual learning tasks, although the progression may begin with one area being of greater deficit. Performance on list learning over trials usually does not progress much beyond an immediate memory span length. In other words, if a person has a memory span of four or five items, five attempts to learn a nine–word list often reveals a flat learning curve beginning with recall of four to five items and ending with recall of four to five items. Verbal recall of stories and word lists shows a large number of perseveration and intrusion errors (among others, see Butters et al., 1988). For example, the person may repeat words from the same list as if recalling them for the first time or may recall one aspect of a design that is presented, such as a dot in a box, as

Neuropsychology in Action 11.2

Differentiating Between Symptoms of Alzheimer's Disease and Normal Aging

by Mary V. Spiers

Although memory impairment is the hallmark of Alzheimer's disease, those over age 65 (the time of life when Alzheimer's is most likely to manifest) often decline in memory ability. The key is to differentiate between general complaints of forgetfulness and lowered cognitive functioning that accompany normal aging, and cognitive indicators of incipient dementia. Consider the following two scenarios, which are compilations of cases seen by the authors:

Case 1: Mrs. C. Mrs. C is a 90-year-old woman from a small midwestern town who has lived by herself for the last 10 years since her husband died. She is active in her church and volunteers at a local thrift shop. At home she spends most of her time reading, keeping up with correspondence to family and friends, and talking with neighbors on the phone. She

drove her car until a year ago, when after increasing restrictions on night driving due to failing eyesight, she agreed with her physician that she should give it up. She tells her family that her memory is quite poor. She can read through a whole book but says if she picked it up again it would be "just like reading a new book." She watches the news daily, and is interested in following the elections and candidates for office. Mrs. C has a definite opinion regarding who she likes, although she doesn't remember many of the details of current events, and says the news "goes in one ear and out the other." However, she does remember major life events, if asked about them by her children. She can recount episodes from her teens and twenties quite well and tells old family stories from her childhood with incredible detail and animation. For the first time in

her life she has had to start taking several prescription medicines for heart problems. At first she needed nearly constant prompting to remember to take her three daily doses at the right times. However, over the course of two to three months she learned her medication routine. She always remembered to take her pills when she got up and before bed but frequently forgot the 11 A.M. pill.

Case 2: Mrs. R. Mrs. R is a 75-year-old woman who is married and lives with her husband. Mr. and Mrs. R have always had an active social life, getting together with friends quite often to go dancing or play bridge in their retirement community. Within the last several years, Mr. R has noticed that his wife doesn't seem to be paying attention when they play bridge anymore. She has made wrong bids, and makes mistakes keeping score. She

---

five or six dots in a box. The person may recall specific events or stimuli across situations, intruding elements from one story into another story or remembering elements of one design as part of another. Although all people with classical amnesia show profound difficulties in new learning, this repeating and confusion of memory differs from most other amnestic dysfunctions that the corticolimbic circuit causes. Intrusions and perseverations are most common in two conditions, Alzheimer's disease and Korsakoff's amnesia, which also involve similar patterns of frontal lobe involvement. Butters (for example, see Butters et al., 1988) hypothesized that the similar pattern of intrusion and perseveration errors in SDAT and alcoholic Korsakoff's amnesia may be caused by a significant loss of cholinergic neurons in the basal forebrain area.

Although many normal elderly people may forget, they can often remember lost thoughts with the help of retrieval cues. This facilitation of memory by retrieval cues also characterizes Huntington's disease, but the memory problem in Alzheimer's is more global and profound. People with AD show impairment in encoding, consolidation, and retrieval. The constellation of memory deficits in AD greatly hinders retrieval because it depends on proper encoding, organization, and consolidation of material to be remembered. Thus retrieval cues will not aid Alzheimer's patients' recall of information, suggesting that encoding and consolidation have not taken place. Besides the fact that SDAT patients show flat learning curves, demonstrating little to no ability to profit from practice, any information that the patient may

usually makes a joke about these things, saying to her friend, "Lucy, you're just trying to distract me so you'll win." Everyone has a big laugh, which seems to just egg her on. Mrs. R particularly likes to tell stories of when they were young, and she has a lot of them to entertain everyone. When the conversation turns to the day's news, Mrs. R seems to have little comment on current events, although she and her husband have always watched the news together every night. She seems to get news stories mixed up. Mrs. R says she just doesn't have too much use for the news, "it goes in one ear and out the other." A new couple has joined their dancing club, and much to Mr. R's embarrassment Mrs. R keeps reintroducing herself to them even after four months. After a while it became comical, and Mrs. R says she does it on purpose for a joke. Mrs. R has taken medication for the past 15 years, and has always managed well. But now her husband feels like he must remind her to take her pills because he noticed she often doesn't put it out by her plate as she used to. She resents being reminded and says accusingly, "I put it out. Are you sure you didn't just take it and put it away when you cleared the table?" This behavior is upsetting to Mr. R, but the thing that bothers him most is that his wife, who had been a good cook, is now very disorganized in the kitchen. After he noticed that a cake tasted salty, he watched her as she prepared other things. She often added ingredients twice or totally left out essentials of her recipes.

Both Mrs. C and Mrs. R have trouble remembering in areas in which they were previously more able, and seem to have declined from their own former levels of ability. In some respects, both show a similar pattern of memory loss in that remote memory, or information learned many years ago, such as stories from childhood or facts related to work or home persist remarkably well in comparison to new learning. Difficulty remembering what the news commentator said, or learning a new medication routine or new names, presents more of a problem in both cases. These similarities between normal aging and dementia can prompt dread in people who see themselves as less able to rely on their powers of memory. However, there are several notable differences between the two cases. First, Mrs. C seems to have some insight into her memory difficulties, whereas Mrs. R rationalizes, jokes, and blames others for her poor memory. Second, Mrs. C learns and retains some new things, even though the learning may take longer. Mrs. R, in contrast, not only is showing difficulty learning new things but appears to be losing her ability to perform previously well-learned tasks, such as cueing herself to take her own medication or to cook. Finally, there is a suggestion that Mrs. R's problems seem more pervasive, in that she may also have problems in concentration, attention, calculation skills, and name finding. Mrs. R's memory difficulties are characteristic of dementia, possibly Alzheimer's disease, and may appear paradoxical to patients' families, who can see that their family member is socially appropriate and retains remote and overlearned information quite well. It is easy to discount the importance of cognitive problems. A comprehensive neuropsychological evaluation can help answer these questions.

---

have remembered immediately after presentation quickly disappears. As the disease progresses, information is lost faster and faster. Although many people benefit from practice over days and weeks, SDAT patients do not seem to show this consolidation of declarative learning.

Breakdown of Semantic Knowledge   People afflicted with this disease have another fundamental problem of memory, which pervades the entire organization of knowledge. As we discussed in Chapter 5, the brain stores information at the site where it was first processed. In other words, most visual-spatial information is stored in the posterior areas of the cortex, primarily the parietal and posterior temporal lobes. Auditory information is stored in the temporal lobes, and so on. The dominant theory of memory consolidation, simply put, is that the hippocampus, which has afferent and efferent projections to most areas of the cortex receives to-be-remembered information, codes it for storage, and sends it back to the original processing site (Squire, 1987). Researchers believe memory for information and facts is not stored as separate and complete units (for example, all information about robins stored in one node). Rather, they hypothesize that the brain contains associations of meaning, "semantic networks," whose individual nodes may contain pieces of information or attributes, such as "bird," "wings," "small," and "red breast," which when activated as a pattern lead to the recognition of "robin."

Most amnestic patients, although they cannot encode new information, have an intact semantic organizational network for information. In Alzheimer's disease, the memory disorder is much more pervasive, involving a progressive disintegration of this associational network, eventually even for old learned information. The evidence for this loss of knowledge through semantic degradation rests on several findings. First, neuropsychologists noticed that AD patients do not organize new information semantically as they are attempting to learn it. Thus, if presented with word lists that have inherent semantic categories, such as fruits, vegetables, and items of clothing, most people learn and recall information within semantic categories, clustering the information together. This "semantic clustering" is deficient or nonexistent among AD patients, who instead show a serial ordering or primacy/recency effect. Secondly, AD patients appear to lose conceptual knowledge. Fluency tasks often reveal an interesting pattern. Asked to name as many animals as possible in 60 seconds, people with AD often can retrieve superordinate and high-frequency category exemplars such as cat or bird, but show difficulty retrieving subordinate category exemplars such as leopard or robin. This degradation seems to be more than just a problem in retrieving semantic information from long-term memory. This degradation has been shown to be consistent across tasks, so that the patient may also have difficulty in defining "robin" or naming a picture of a robin (Hodges, Salmon, & Butters, 1992). These difficulties represent neuropathological changes of higher-order intermodal association cortexes strongly involved in semantic networking (for example, posterior-temporal, inferior parietal) rather than classical language problems associated with the frontal operculum (Broca's area), superior temporal gyrus, or supramarginal gyrus. As the disease progresses, these connected memories or knowledge structures seem to break down to such a degree that even the identity and association of family members eventually become confused in the patient's mind.

In this discussion of memory in AD, we have focused primarily on the encoding, storage, and retrieval processes of declarative long-term memory. These are undoubtedly the areas of the most recognizable and profound memory difficulty. Two areas of memory that appear less affected by Alzheimer's are short-term memory span and nondeclarative long-term memory.

Relatively Spared Memory Systems   On short-term memory tasks such as length of digit span forward, AD patients perform relatively well in the early stages of the disease. In later stages, short-term memory retention declines. However, if the examiner looks closely at short-term memory capacity, or working memory, it is typically compromised.

Alzheimer's patients do relatively well on some nondeclarative memory tasks. Separate nondeclarative memory systems exist outside of the subcortical limbic system. The workings of these systems for the most part seem implicit, or outside consciousness. Learning skills with a large motor and practice component such as riding a bike or typing, or learning psychomotor tests such as pursuit rotor or mirror tracing seem to be part of a motor skills learning system. It is not yet clear whether other systems controlling classically conditioned responses, and priming represent yet other nondeclarative memory networks, or if they are subcomponents of a single nondeclarative network.

People with AD show normal performance on some nondeclarative tasks and impairment on others. Soliveri (Soliveri, Brown, Jahanshahi, & Marsden, 1992) describes the pattern of nondeclarative memory performance in various neurologically impaired groups. Most people with Alzheimer's disease perform well on motor learning tasks that researchers think represent an unimpaired striatal system. However, the picture is different with priming tasks. The methodology of priming, discussed in Chapter 5, assumes that previous exposure to an item will facilitate its future processing. Word stem completion priming tasks typically first present a list of words, such as *there, church,* and *leaf.* Later they present three-letter stems such as *the___, chu___* and *lea__.* Typically amnestics—even though they have not been able to demonstrate learning of the words through declarative means, namely spontaneous recall—are likely to produce the targeted words on word stem completion tasks. People with AD usually cannot perform these tasks well. Interestingly, on perceptual priming tasks that present complete and incomplete figures, AD patients seem to do better in some instances. Because of this pattern, researchers suggest that Alzheimer's patients confront a specific difficulty in implicit verbal priming while maintaining nondeclarative learning abilities in perceptual priming and in attaining motor skills. Why would this be so? Verbal implicit priming tasks are probably another pointer to the AD breakdown of the semantic network. Motor skill learning is intact because it is controlled by the striatum, which is relatively unaffected in AD. Perceptual priming seems to point to a relatively more intact visual object recognition system, which may not be affected until late in the disease process.

Language/Speech

Patients with Alzheimer's disease do show language problems, but these cannot be neatly characterized with other classic aphasias. In fact, the aphasia progressively worsens both in degree and type. Early in the disease process, AD patients show an anomic aphasia, characterized chiefly by word-finding and -naming difficulties (Cummings, Benson, Hill, & Read, 1985). A confrontation naming test (such as the Boston Naming Test), in which the person must retrieve the exact name of an item from line drawings, often results in semantic and circumlocution (talking around) errors. An AD patient is more likely to say "tool" for "hammer" or "some type of musical instrument" for "harmonica," indicating that he or she recognizes the semantic category but can only retrieve the general category or the wrong exemplar from the same category (for example, see Hodges, Salmon, & Butters, 1991). This type of anomia, along with the difficulty in semantic fluency tasks discussed earlier, suggests a semantic anomic aphasia. As the dementia progresses, language problems become more profound. Comprehension problems begin to appear, followed by problems in repeating information, and last, declines in fluent conversational output may appear that resemble a global aphasia (Zec, 1993; Cummings et al., 1985).

Visual-Spatial Functioning

Visual-spatial problems crop up by the middle stages of Alzheimer's disease, if not before. Mr. T, a 70-year-old retired salesman and a patient of ours, came in for neuropsychological evaluation at the request of his wife and neurologist. When they moved to a new retirement community in Florida, Mr. T's wife noticed a change. He started getting lost while driving in the neighborhood, sometimes ending up at the other end of town; embarrassed and angry, he would have to call his wife. Even though they had been there for nearly a month, he kept losing his way, and blamed it on the fact that "all those tract houses built in the 60s look alike." Accompanied by his wife, Mr. T could follow the correct route; however, Mrs. T was a bit nervous about riding with her husband. She reported he had a tendency to drift to the left, and on several occasions she had to shout at him to avoid hitting another car. What was most disconcerting to Mrs. T, however, was the fact that Mr. T seemed disoriented in his own home, often heading out to the kitchen to use the bathroom.

The problems Mr. T is showing reveal two things. First, he has marked visual-spatial impairments in his daily life. Most obviously, he cannot orient himself in his environment, either in the neighborhood or at home. He does not have good spatial sense when he is driving. He veers to the left and seems to have lost his "inner compass." Second, moving to a new residence may unmask a condition that was not evident in a more familiar environment. Mr. T did not have a stroke or some other neurologic event that occurred suddenly. His wife discovered his spatial problems when they moved. Although Mr. T would still have been able to function in his old home, as his dementia progressed it would have only been a matter of time before he was getting lost in his old, familiar neighborhood and becoming disoriented in his home of 15 years.

On neuropsychological examination, AD patients usually show poor performance on a number of visual-spatial measures. As in the other functional domains, the degree of impairment corresponds to the stage of dementia. Tests of line orientation (for example, the Benton Judgment of Line Orientation Test), spatial construction tasks (such as the WAIS-R Block Design), copying (such as the Rey-Osterreith Complex Figure Test, Bender Gestalt), drawing (such as the Clock Drawing Test) and visual integration (such as the Hooper Visual Organization Test) are

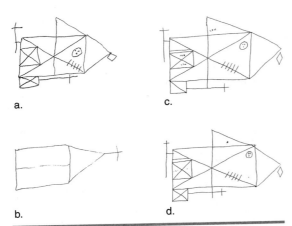

a.

c.

b.

d.

Figure 11.7 Drawing and memory performance on a modified Rey-Osterreith figure drawn by a patient with Alzheimer's disease and a normal elderly person: (a) AD copy, (b) AD immediate recall, (c) normal control copy, (d) normal control immediate recall. (Courtesy of David Libon, Ph.D. Reprinted with permission)

the most likely to be affected (for review, see Zec, 1993). Complex tasks such as the Rey-Osterreith seem more sensitive to impairment in the early stages of the disease than are simple drawing tasks. Figure 11.7 shows drawing performance in a patient with autopsy-confirmed Alzheimer's disease. The patient made these drawings in the early stages of the disease. The more complex Rey figure is somewhat impaired even on the copy. As the dementia progresses, copying designs also becomes distorted.

General Intellectual Functioning

Experts often say that Alzheimer's disease, like other dementias, results in a "decline in general cognitive functioning." However, as noted, all functions do not decline at the same rate, so it is more useful to consider the subcomponents of measures of global intellectual functioning. We focus here on verbally mediated tasks of abstract reasoning, judgment, fund of information, and speed of cognitive processing.

The ability to abstract a higher-order construct is often impaired in even mild SDAT (Zec, 1993). Verbally, the patient may be unable to say how two ob-

jects or concepts are alike, such as a phone and a radio (for example, on the WAIS-R Similarities Test). Visually, the person may be unable to state a common principle that relates multiple figures (for example, on the Category Test or the Ravens Progressive Matrices). This deficit is a problem in conceptualization and abstract reasoning. Thus people with Alzheimer's dementia do poorly on a number of tasks that require reasoning and problem solving.

We use the term "fund of information" to refer to accumulated knowledge over the life span. Often neuropsychologists measure this via tests of vocabulary knowledge (for example, WAIS-R Vocabulary) or overlearned information. For example, someone who has lived in the United States for several years should know in what month Memorial Day falls. However, few formal tests measure specific areas of expertise that may accumulate from a person's line of employment. This knowledge store is one of the few areas that remain preserved until the later stages of the disease.

Although SDAT patients are slower on speeded complex tasks (for review, see Zec, 1993), they do not exhibit the **bradyphrenia,** or extremely slow information processing speed characteristic of patients with subcortical dementias.

Executive Functioning

Although deficits are subtle early on, difficulties in executive control are evident to caregivers. For example, in an attempt to compensate for memory loss, a person may keep notes. But without an adequate executive strategy, increased disorganization may show up in notes found in various places around the house, and tasks started but left unfinished. Family members often notice perseveration of thought because the person tells stories over and over, or asks questions repeatedly. The person may be less flexible than before. Many apparent "personality" changes may actually stem from frontal impairment. Repeated behaviors, such as checking and rechecking, may emerge from the combined effect of a poor memory and increased perseveration.

An interesting aspect of dysfunctional executive ability is that many Alzheimer's patients seem to lose **metacognitive awareness,** or the inability to self-monitor their own behavior and performance. Many clinicians describe AD patients as having little insight into their own deficits. Often they appear generally unaware or unconcerned about the magnitude or consequences of their deficits. Is this psychological response understandable as a defense mechanism against the devastating effects of the disease? Not in the typical sense. Many AD patients seem truly unaware of their difficulties, and consistently overestimate their abilities to accomplish things.

Problems in the ability to organize, plan, and use appropriate strategies for problem solving in patients with Alzheimer's disease often appear on tests designed for evaluating strategic processing (such as Tower of London or Tower of Hanoi) and qualitatively on tests designed for other purposes such as visual-spatial problem solving (such as the Block Design Test of WAIS-R). Intrusions and perseverations often show up on memory tests. Perseveration is evident as an inability to shift sets on tests that require flexible problem solving (for example, Wisconsin Card Sorting Test or Trails Making Text–B).

Orientation, Attention, and Level of Consciousness

Alzheimer's disease is not an altered state of consciousness, such as delirium. General orientation and selective attention persist until late in the course of the disease. However, more complex forms of attention such as divided and alternating attention decline from the early stages. Orientation for person, time, and place is generally intact until the moderate to severe stages of AD.

Motor and Sensory Function

In relation to other areas of functioning, motor and sensory abilities are relatively preserved throughout the course of Alzheimer's disease. Simple motor speed and strength persist until late in the course of the dementia. However, more complex motor behavior, which may involve coordination or skilled movement, declines earlier.

The disease process seems to spare sensory functioning—that is, visual, auditory, and tactile acuity. Olfaction is the only primary sensory area affected:

Sense of smell is compromised even in the mild stages of the disease (Jones & Richardson, 1990). Many AD patients complain of visual disturbances such as difficulty in reading, interpreting pictures, and recognizing familiar people. Although opthamologists often find good acuity and full visual fields, neuropsychological testing often reveals visual-perceptual and visual-spatial deficits, which may cause the self-reported visual disturbances.

Mood, Emotion, Personality, and Insight

As with Alzheimer's (1907/1987) famous patient, clinicians may first refer people for psychiatric symptoms. In some cases these symptoms stem from the cognitive difficulties accompanying Alzheimer's disease, but in other cases the symptoms, such as depression, may represent an additional disorder. Suspiciousness of others and frank paranoid delusions can manifest memory dysfunction. One 70-year-old woman tearfully related that her husband had begun accusing her of stealing his glasses and other personal items. After 50 years of marriage, he also accused her of having an affair. On questioning it became apparent that he was accusing her of taking things he was misplacing. Because of his impaired time estimation, not uncommon in AD, five minutes could seem like an hour, or an hour like five minutes. So when she went to the grocery store on a quick errand, it seemed like an eternity to him. He had little insight into his memory difficulties and in trying to make sense of a frustrating situation, externalized the problem and blamed his wife.

Symptoms that herald a significant about-face in personality usually raise a red flag for family members. Such patients are most likely to be seen by mental health professionals. However, psychiatric symptoms that are exacerbations of premorbid personality styles make recognizing change extremely difficult. A woman always considered impulsive and distractible, flighty or disorganized, may at first seem simply eccentric when she begins to lose track of daily memories. When attempting to deal with memory loss, the person is likely to carry on with coping styles and defense mechanisms characteristic of earlier times. As memory becomes less reliable, a person concerned with order, timeliness, or organization may obsessively check dates, doctor's appointments, medications, memos, and lists.

Depression and Dementia A common problem in making a differential diagnosis of behavioral disturbances among the elderly is to distinguish psychological depression from global loss of intellectual function. The most effective way to make these diagnostic determinations is to obtain formal psychometric testing from a neuropsychologist, who can describe the patient's cognitive functioning in detail, recognize normal and abnormal patterns of performance, and establish a baseline of performance against which to measure any changes over time. In addition, more subjective guidelines may include the depressed patient's tendency to exaggerate memory problems when compared to the demented patient's tendency to deny or minimize them. It is important to query for information regarding any situational/environmental life crisis that might have precipitated a depressive reaction but that would not be expected to trigger a dementia process. Because some elderly patients are heavily medicated, it is also important to review all prescriptions to determine if any, alone or in combination, interfere with optimal cognitive functioning. Of course, depression may also coexist with a cognitive disorder. Approximately 40% of people with AD may also suffer from depression or symptoms of depression, although major depressive episodes are relatively rare (Cummings, 1994).

A common differential diagnostic issue with which consulting neuropsychologists deal is the referral to distinguish between depression and dementia in elderly patients. Here is a possible scenario:

When asked about her husband's behavior during an initial interview, Mrs. S related that her husband no longer appears interested in his daily activities and hobbies. He used to tinker with their cars and had a hobby of building wooden clocks. He has gradually given both of these up over the past year and a half and says he is no longer interested in them. He spends much more of his day sleeping than he used to, although he is up a lot at night. He has also lost weight and doesn't seem to have a strong interest in eating. In fact, says his wife, Mr. S doesn't seem to have a strong interest in anything. "If it wasn't for me," she says, "he'd probably spend his whole day sitting in his chair. I try to give him things to do, like crossword puzzles or little things to fix, but when I come back, he hasn't gotten anywhere. We don't see our friends anymore because he just doesn't seem to have much to say." Mr. S agreed that he had given up most of his former hobbies, saying he just wasn't interested in them anymore, although he wasn't sure why. He didn't admit to feeling particularly sad or discouraged about these or any other events. Largely, he appeared to be apathetic, not particularly moved in any direction either to be excited and motivated to accomplish things, or to be despondent about his situation. Although he didn't seem to display internal motivation, Mrs. S did say that her husband would accompany her on outings when she planned them. Recently, they had gone to New England on a four-day chartered bus trip with members of their church. Mr. S went along on all the activities and did not spend time sleeping during the day.

At first glance, Mr. S appears to suffer from symptoms suggestive of depression: He has lost interest in previously enjoyable hobbies and activities, and his eating and sleeping habits have changed. Curiously, however, he does not admit to depressed mood or show other subjective or affective signs of depression. He also will become involved in some activities. At this point, three possibilities need to be considered: (1) Mr. S may have primary depression, (2) a dementing process may explain Mr. S's depressive symptoms, or (3) Mr. S may have both progressive dementia and depression. Further discussion of depressive symptoms and testing for depression may reveal motivational and affective difficulties, perhaps a reaction to a more sedentary lifestyle after retirement, or problems related to his current life situation over the past several years. Chronic medical problems, if they exist, are likely to result in decreased energy, a loss of vitality, and depressed mood. However, it is also possible that these symptoms may be largely explained by dementia. Mr. S may have given up former hobbies such as clock building because he no longer has adequate visual-spatial functioning or the organizational and planning abilities to successfully approach novel or complex problems. He also may suffer from "cognitive inertia." If this is the case, what appears to be poor motivation may be an inability to structure and organize in such a manner as to accomplish tasks. Although at first only complex projects may be affected, later in the disease even straightforward tasks such as washing dishes or taking out the garbage may be difficult to begin, because the patient does not know where to start. Other possibilities to consider, consistent with AD, are that he may have little insight into his difficulties and so may appear vague and somewhat detached when speaking about himself. Certainly, further interviewing and testing concerning memory and other cognitive problems are warranted. The primary objective here is not to differentiate between dementia and depression based on a brief description of Mr. S's difficulties. Rather, the point is to consider that, especially when psychiatric symptoms present themselves for the first time in older patients, these may signal underlying cognitive problems. Although seeming changes in personality and mood occur with some frequency in Alzheimer's disease, they are not necessary or particular to this disease.

Treatment

No treatments currently available can reverse, halt, or slow the progression of Alzheimer's disease. We simply do not yet know enough about the neurophysiology and causes of the disease to develop medical treatments tailored to attack the underlying mechanisms. What, then, does treatment focus on? First, there is a big push for psychopharmacologic investigators to develop drugs that will enhance cognitive functioning. Many drugs are in the experimental stages, and a few have made it to market. Most target the cholinergic system, and therefore memory. Second, both pharmacologic and behavioral interventions are aimed at ameliorating psychiatric symptoms and excess disability (that is, additional cognitive and psychiatric impairment not directly attributable to the disease). With each of these treatments, the goal is to improve quality of life for both the AD sufferers and their caregivers. In this section we provide an overview of psychopharmacologic and behavioral approaches to intervention.

TREATMENTS FOR COGNITIVE ENHANCEMENT

As discussed earlier, acetylcholine (ACh) is the neurotransmitter system that holds the most promising physiological link to Alzheimer's disease. Many drugs targeting the cholinergic system seek to increase its production or action and therefore to compensate for the impaired cholinergic production in the basal forebrain, including the nucleus basalis. Researchers have tried varied approaches to augment levels of brain ACh. One approach is to increase the availability of ACh precursors such as choline. Because large quantities of choline are found in lecithin, a substance contained in foods such as egg whites and chocolate, researchers once thought that by increasing dietary choline, they might also elevate brain levels of ACh. However, no clear improvements in memory have materialized from this or other approaches. Other pharmacologic approaches have attempted to target the synaptic transmission itself. One method increases ACh by blocking its breakdown by inhibiting acetylcholinesterase. Other methods strive to directly increase the output of ACh or stimulate the postsynaptic cholinergic (muscarinic) receptors to increase firing. Physostigmine (Synapton) was one of the first cholinergic augmenting drugs that clinical trials tested with AD patients in the mid-1980s. Although some studies suggested improvement, this gain appeared minimal in light of overall declining functioning. But there is some indication that longer-term use may result in more gain (for review, see Ashford & Zec, 1993). In the mid-1990s, tacrine (Cognex), which is a long-acting acetylcholinesterase inhibitor, received a flurry of attention. It appeared to show some positive effects but also resulted in a side effect of liver toxicity. To date no fewer than 10 drugs have been designed specifically to enhance cholinergic activity in the brain. At this point, however, the search is still on to find the right combination of noticeable memory enhancement coupled with tolerable side effects.

Alternative experimental approaches aimed at understanding the pathophysiology of Alzheimer's disease hold the promise of future therapeutic benefit. Nerve growth factor (NGF) and estrogen replacement

Neuropsychology in Action 11.3

Can Estrogen Cut the Risk of Alzheimer's Disease?

by Mary V. Spiers

Estrogen may protect against the development of Alzheimer's disease in later life—this is the claim of several teams of researchers who have observed that postmenopausal women on hormone replacement therapy are less likely to develop Alzheimer's disease. One clue that originally alerted researchers to a possible link was the observation that more women than men develop AD. Of course, the average life expectancy for women is longer than for men. However, men convert some testosterone into estrogen throughout their lives, whereas older women have greatly reduced estrogen levels. The other clue was that estrogen enhances the functioning of the cholinergic nucleus basalis of Meynert, and may even encourage cell growth. A longitudinal study conducted at Columbia University followed over 1000 postmenopausal women of various socioeconomic and ethnic groups with an average age of 74, over a five-year period. Across groups, those who had used estrogen for 10 years or more were a third less likely to develop AD than those who had not. This is a very encouraging finding. But estrogen is a double-edged sword. Although some research suggests it has beneficial effects in slowing heart disease and bone deterioration, other research has also linked it to increased incidence of breast cancer and uterine endometriosis. Future research in this area with controlled studies should help to determine the risk–benefit ratio of therapeutic estrogen replacement to ward off Alzheimer's.

---

therapy (see Neuropsychology in Action 11.3) are two methods being researched to increase cholinergic neuronal functioning. NGF is part of a family of **neurotrophins,** or neuron-feeding nutrients, that researchers have long known sustain neural viability in the autonomic nervous system. The cholinergic system neurons in the basal forebrain also have specific receptors for NGF. In animals, antibodies to NGF result in neuronal shriveling and death. Also in animals, introducing NGF appears to increase ACh functioning, and learning and memory behavior in those with lesioned brains. NGF may prove therapeutic in AD if it can sustain life and promote growth of surviving cholinergic neurons. Methods suggested include intraventricular infusion of NGF through a pump (Olson, 1990), attachment of NGF to a gene that can specifically target the ACh system through a retrovirus, and direct neural implants of tissue with active NGF (Dunnet, 1991).

A pharmacologic treatment to halt or reverse the memory and cognitive loss suffered in Alzheimer's disease is likely to emerge as our understanding of the underlying pathophysiology develops. Probably this will involve a multifaceted approach to treatment, because large areas of the brain are affected. The treatments reviewed here primarily target the most common and prominent symptom of new learning. A truly effective solution will have to conquer the pervasive cognitive decline.

COGNITIVE, BEHAVIORAL, AND PSYCHIATRIC SYMPTOM CONTROL

The other avenue of treatment for Alzheimer's disease aims at symptom control. Behavioral, psychiatric, and cognitive difficulties can emerge either associated with the progression of the disease itself or attributable to processes above and beyond those symptoms, that can be explained by the disease itself—a condition termed "excess disability." Attempts to manage these symptoms use either pharmacologic or behavioral tools.

Common behavioral and affective symptoms associated with dementia include depression, insomnia, persecutory ideation, hallucinations, apathy, agitation, irritability, and purposeless or inappropriate activity patterns. Minor tranquilizers or antidepressants may aid depression and insomnia, but pharmacologic treatment of psychotic symptoms such as delusions or hallucinations may cause serious unwanted side effects. Neuroleptics may further impair cognition, increase agitation, and cause other unwanted motor symptoms.

Alzheimer's patients are also susceptible to illness and conditions associated with aging such as respiratory or urinary tract infections, and hearing and vision problems. The associated behavioral problems associated with this "excess disability" can include decreased or increased activity levels, delirium, or hallucinations. In the case of illness, when the condition resolves the behavioral problem likewise should sub-

side. Visual or hearing problems may also amplify hallucinations or sensory illusions.

Because of the severe memory deficit, behavioral management strategies based on learning and responding to reinforcement paradigms can easily prove futile. Instead, most management strategies seek to restructure the environment to ensure safety, provide appropriate stimulation, and redirect inappropriate behavior. As the disease progresses, the person needs more constant supervision. Many nursing homes have specially designated Alzheimer's units because of the difficulties of behavioral management. If a patient is living at home, the burden on caregivers can be enormous. Respite care in the form of dementia "day care" programs serves the purpose of providing appropriate activity and behavioral management, as well as a needed break for caregivers.

Conclusion

Psychological studies of the elderly have established that aging itself does not necessarily cause dementia. Instead, aging produces predictable changes in patterns of abilities in crystallized and fluid intelligence. Healthy and active individuals in their 60s, 70s and 80s do not necessarily differ substantially from their past level of functioning in the level of their cognitive skills or abilities. Relatively stable skills include well-learned verbal abilities such as reading, writing, and speaking, simple arithmetic ability, and immediate and long-term memory. In contrast, short-term memory, abstract and novel problem solving, and behavioral slowing are examples of types of functioning that normal aging may compromise. Health care costs, the aging of the American people, and a renewed concern for well-being of older people have hastened inquiries and interest in this area. Although elderly people are at high risk for diseases that impair cognitive functioning (such as Alzheimer's disease), cognitive impairment is potentially reversible in 5–20% of dementia cases (for example, in nutritional deficiencies). An understanding of precise neuropsychological deficits can improve the medical management even of patients with irreversible dementia. Neuropsychologists play an important role in comprehensive medical, functional, psychosocial, and neuropsychological assessment. Assessment of mental status and cognitive abilities yields valuable information about prognosis, and is important in monitoring a patient's health or illness, and helping the patient make further life plans (Zillmer, & Passuth, 1989; Zillmer, Fowler, Gutnick, & Becker, 1990).

Critical Thinking Questions

■ Will exercising one's mind help ward off dementia? Must one "use it or lose it"?

■ How is Alzheimer's disease best identified in life?

■ How can a neuropsychological profile aid dementia sufferers and their families?

■ How does the Alzheimer's disease patient's concept of self change with the progression of the disease?

Key Terms

Dementia	Striate cortex	Delirium	Bradyphrenia
Crystallized intelligence	Neostriatum	Alzheimer's disease	Metacognitive awareness
Fluid intelligence	Atrophy	Beta-amyloid (β-amyloid)	Neurotrophins
Neurofibrillary tangles	Cortical dementia	Acetylcholine (Ach)	
Senile plaques	Subcortical dementia	Multi-infarct dementia	

Web Connections

http://www.alzforum.org
Alzheimer's Forum
A nonprofit foundation which has established this site to serve the scientific and clinical research community.

http://www.informatik.fh-luebeck.de/icd/icdchVF-D-Index.html
ICD-10 Codes for Dementing Disorders
Provides a classification system (the ICD-10) of mental and physical disorders used by the World Health Organization. Includes a brief description and diagnostic criteria for most major brain diseases.

http://pni.med.jhu.edu
Johns Hopkins University Division of Psychiatric Neuro-Imaging
These pages describe quantitative brain analyses of neuropsychiatric disorders such as Alzheimer's disease, using MRI, fMRI, and SPECT imaging.

http://www.agelessdesign.com
Ageless Design: Smarter, Safer Living for Seniors
This is the site of the first organization to dedicate its resources, imagination, and heart to creating smarter, safer living for seniors. By recommending logical, cost-effective home modifications, unique ideas and products, homes can accommodate those dealing with age-related conditions and embrace the special needs of people as they age.

http://dementia.ion.ucl.ac.uk/
Dementia Web
This site is based at the National Hospital for Neurology and is supported by The Institute of Neurology and the Division Imperial College School of Medicine. The site provides updates on dementia research, a virtual chat room, a dementia support group, and other links.

http://www.mentalhealth.com/dis/p20-or05.html

Internet Mental Health: Dementia

This page provides diagnosis, treatment, and research reports for caregivers and specialists.

http://tv.cbc.ca/national/pgminfo/memory/index.html

The National Online—In Search of Memory

This page provides information on three forms of memory: semantic memory, procedural memory, and episodic memory. It relates these memory forms to different dementia disorders.

Chapter 12

SUBCORTICAL DEMENTIAS

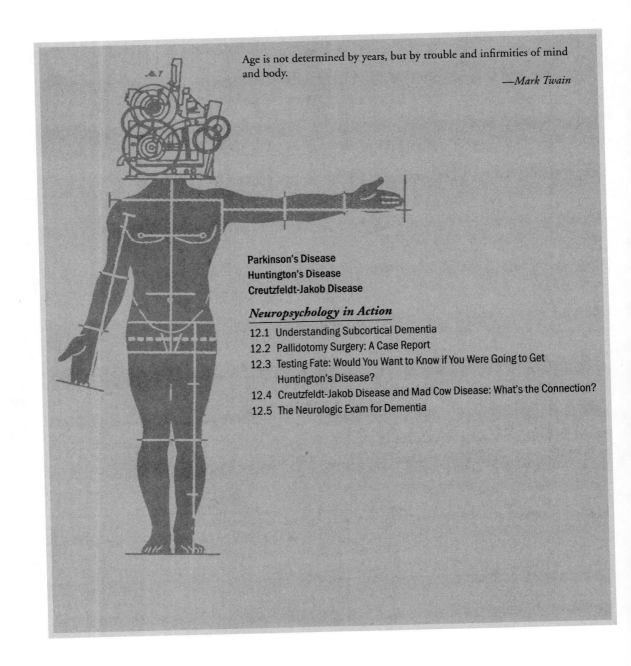

Age is not determined by years, but by trouble and infirmities of mind and body.

—*Mark Twain*

Parkinson's Disease
Huntington's Disease
Creutzfeldt-Jakob Disease

Neuropsychology in Action

12.1 Understanding Subcortical Dementia
12.2 Pallidotomy Surgery: A Case Report
12.3 Testing Fate: Would You Want to Know if You Were Going to Get Huntington's Disease?
12.4 Creutzfeldt-Jakob Disease and Mad Cow Disease: What's the Connection?
12.5 The Neurologic Exam for Dementia

Keep in Mind

■ How do the cortical and subcortical dementias differ from each other?

■ How do behavioral motor presentations differ among subcortical disorders?

■ What are the symptoms and progression of Huntington's disease and Parkinson's disease?

■ How is Creutzfeldt-Jakob disease acquired?

Overview

Subcortical dementias are so named because, although these conditions often affect cortical areas and functioning, the structures that are prominently damaged are subcortical. Parkinson's disease and Huntington's disease attack the basal ganglia; Parkinson's disease targets the substantia nigra and Huntington's, the caudate nucleus. Creutzfeldt-Jakob disease affects yet another noncortical structure, the cerebellum. The common behavioral feature characterizing these and most subcortical dementias is slowed cognitive and motor dysfunction. What is interesting is the manner in which each disease affects the motor system in a different way. You can truly appreciate the complexities of the motor system by examining these diseases. Motor problems present great physical limitations and hardship. These dementias, however, do not represent only motor system dysfunction. The dementias we present in this chapter are progressive and involve multiple functional systems. We present Parkinson's disease in greater detail than the other disorders because it is more common, and these patients are more likely to be seen by clinical neuropsychologists.

Parkinson's Disease

Parkinson's disease does not inevitably lead to dementia, but the proportion of cases is large enough to warrant inclusion in the discussion of dementia. In addition, recent evidence suggests that even those who don't meet the criteria for dementia may have neuropsychological impairments in circumscribed areas. Parkinson's disease, or idiopathic parkinsonism as it is also known, is the most common manifestation of parkinsonism. **Parkinsonism,** like *dementia,* does not refer to a particular disease but to a behavioral syndrome marked by the motor symptoms of tremor, rigidity, and slowness of movement. This cluster of motor symptoms may be caused by Parkinson's disease but also by drugs, encephalitis, toxins such as carbon monoxide and manganese and injury. Mohammed Ali, the famous boxer, developed parkinsonian symptoms (called *dementia pugilistica*) following repeated blows to the head (see Figure 12.1).

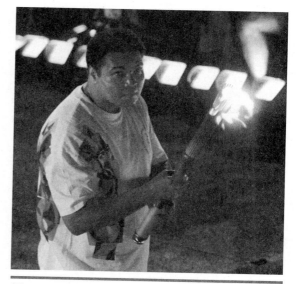

Figure 12.1 Mohammed Ali, who developed Parkinsonian symptoms from boxing, lit the flame in the 1996 Summer Olympics. (AP/Wide World Photos)

Neuropsychology in Action 12.1

Understanding Subcortical Dementia

by Jeffrey L. Cummings M.D., Professor of Neurology and Psychiatry, UCLA School of Medicine.

Subcortical dementia is a clinical syndrome characterized by slowness of cognitive processing, executive dysfunction, difficulty retrieving learned information, and abnormalities of mood and motivation. The syndrome is produced by disorders affecting frontal-subcortical circuits, including lesions of the striatum, globus pallidus, and thalamus.

Kinnier Wilson (1912), in his original description of Wilson's disease, recognized the clinical features of subcortical dementia, which von Stockert (1932) described again in the context of discussing postencephalitic **Parkinson's disease**. Martin Albert and colleagues (Albert et al., 1974) reintroduced the syndrome into clinical neurology in descriptions of the subcortical dementia of progressive supranuclear palsy at Boston

University in 1975. Substantial controversy centered on this syndrome when researchers first introduced it. Critics of the concept suggested that most dementia syndromes include both cortical and subcortical abnormalities and that the clinical phenomenology was not distinctive enough to guide differential diagnosis. Subsequent experiences have helped to remold the concept and to account for these criticisms. For example, the subcortical changes in Alzheimer's disease in the nucleus basalis of Meynert lead to a cholinergic deficiency that manifests at the cortical level. Thus, although the pathology is subcortical in location, the dysfunction primarily affects the cerebral cortex. Likewise, although there are cortical changes in Huntington's disease they are minor compared to the marked

subcortical abnormalities, and the mental status changes correlate with the subcortical rather than the cortical abnormalities. Thus, even within these mixed syndromes it is possible to identify cortical and subcortical patterns of dysfunction.

Researchers have increasingly well-documented the clinical features of subcortical dementia (Cummings, 1986). Slowing of cognition stems from the increased central processing time imposed by subcortical disorders. Patients have prolonged response latencies and slowed complex reaction times. They show executive dysfunction, including difficulty with set shifting, as measured by tests such as the Wisconsin Card Sorting Test or Trails B of the Trail Making Test; reduced verbal fluency on tests of

Although the cause of Parkinson's disease is unknown, and the disease is therefore called idiopathic, it is known to selectively affect the substantia nigra and the dopaminergic systems of the brain.

Parkinson's disease affects an estimated 1% of the population of the United States over age 50, with the incidence of new cases appearing to peak between ages 60 and 64 (Koller et al., 1987). Parkinson's rarely occurs before age 40. Some sources suggest the rate of new cases declines after age 65; others argue that it does not decline until the eighth decade (for review, see Kay, 1995). Parkinson's disease appears more common in men than women, although no differences in risk factors have been identified. Dementia in Parkinson's disease does, however, appear age related. About 40% of those with Parkinson's

meet the criteria for dementia (Kay, 1995). However, only about 12% of Parkinson's patients in their 50s have dementia, as compared to about 70% of those over 80 (Mayeux et al., 1992). Younger Parkinson's patients are likely to function well, but dementia is more likely with increased age and disease severity. People most likely to have dementia seem to be those who have either had the disease for a longer period of time, or are older at the time of diagnosis (Kay, 1995). Researchers do not yet know if Parkinson's is the direct cause of the dementia. Parkinson's patients with dementia could have a comorbid disease process such as Alzheimer's disease. In any case, the rate of dementia in those with Parkinson's disease is quite high compared to the population at large.

word list generation, such as the number of animals that can be named in one minute; impoverished motor programming, as measured by tests such as execution of serial hand sequences; and poor abstracting abilities when asked to interpret proverbs or to distinguish among similar concepts. Memory abnormalities are primarily of a retrieval deficit type. Patients store information at nearly normal rates but have difficulty retrieving the information in a timely way. Thus, on tests of recall they do poorly, but on tests of recognition memory they may perform in the normal range. This recall deficit includes both recent and remote information.

Patients with subcortical dementia show neuropsychiatric as well as neuropsychological abnormalities. Apathy and depression are particularly prominent. Less common are irritability, disinhibition, mania, and psychosis. Motor abnormalities also accompany most subcortical dementias when the disease involves striatal structures, the substantia nigra, or globus pallidus. Parkinsonism and chorea are the predominant motor manifestations in patients with subcortical dementia.

Recent advances in neuroanatomy contribute to neuropsychological understanding of subcortical dementia syndromes. Five frontal subcortical circuits link regions of the premotor cortex to areas of the striatum, globus pallidus, and thalamus. The dorsolateral prefrontal subcortical circuit mediates executive function and projects from dorsolateral prefrontal regions to the head of the caudate nucleus, globus pallidus, dorsomedial thalamus, and back to the prefrontal cortex. The anterior cingulate region in the medial prefrontal region mediates motivated behavior via a frontal subcortical circuit including the nucleus accumbens, globus pallidus, dorsomedial thalamus, and anterior cingulate. An orbitofrontal subcortical circuit mediates the social governance of behavior and includes orbitofrontal cortex, inferior caudate nucleus, globus pallidus, and dorsomedial thalamus. Dysfunction in the lateral prefrontal-subcortical circuit produces executive dysfunction; abnormalities of the anterior cingulate-subcortical circuit result in apathy; and abnormalities of the orbitofrontal-subcortical circuit produce disinhibited, tactless behavior (Cummings, 1993).

Treatment of patients with subcortical dementia depends on the specific etiology of their syndrome. Parkinsonian disorders and Parkinson's disease are treated with levodopa and other dopaminergic agents. The depression syndrome in many patients with subcortical dementia typically responds to antidepressant agents such as selective serotonin uptake inhibitors. The apathetic syndrome may respond to dopaminergic agonists or psychostimulants such as methylphenidate. Cognitive dysfunction in patients who have a cholinergic disturbance—such as those with Parkinson's disease—may respond to cholinergic therapies such as cholinesterase inhibitors.

NEUROPATHOLOGY OF PARKINSON'S DISEASE

Parkinson's disease (PD) is marked by a loss of dopaminergic cells and pigmentation in the substantia nigra (black substance) (see Figure 12.2). It is also characterized by **Lewy bodies,** which are small, tightly packed granular structures with ringlike filaments found within dying cells. Although Lewy bodies are pathognomonic markers in cells of the substantia nigra, PD patients may also have concentrations of them in other pigmented subcortical areas such as the locus ceruleus or unpigmented areas such as the nucleus basalis of Meynert, autonomic ganglia, and hypothalamus. Lewy bodies may also appear in cortical areas. Although the pattern of concentration

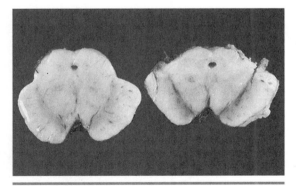

Figure 12.2 The substantia nigra of a Parkinson's patient shows a loss of dark pigmentation (left) in contrast with a normal midbrain section (right). (From WebPath, courtesy of Edward C. Klatt, M.D., Department of Pathology, University of Utah, Salt Lake City, Utah, USA)

of Lewy bodies in the substantia nigra indicates PD, the presence of Lewy bodies in the brain is not specific to PD. They may also appear in normally aging people, Alzheimer's sufferers, and those with other progressive neurodegenerative conditions. This leads to speculation that Lewy bodies are either (1) indicators of a general disease process or (2) markers of cell death.

The darkly pigmented, or melanized, substantia nigra is a midbrain structure that is part of a group of subcortical structures that collectively make up the basal ganglia. The basal ganglia, which reciprocally connect to the premotor cortex and the supplementary motor areas via the thalamus, largely function to control the fluidity of overlearned and "semiautomatic" motor programs (Bradshaw & Mattingly, 1995). The loss of dopamine from the substantia nigra is directly related to the problems of movement initiation and motor rigidity in Parkinson's (Bradshaw & Mattingly, 1995). Aging itself takes a toll on the dopamine system, and some cell loss is expected. But the dopaminergic degeneration in PD is several times that of normal aging. Perhaps the reason that noticeable parkinsonian symptoms don't appear in older individuals is because there is a "dopamine threshold," estimated to be breached at between 50 and 80% cell loss (Bradshaw & Mattingly, 1995) before symptoms appear.

CLINICAL PRESENTATION AND NEUROPSYCHOLOGICAL PROFILE OF PARKINSON'S DISEASE

When a physician refers patients with Parkinson's disease to a consulting neuropsychologist, the diagnosis has usually been well established from the characteristic **resting tremor** and allied motor symptoms. In this case, the referral is usually to help determine the presence or extent of cognitive decline. However, physicians may refer patients to either a psychotherapist or a neuropsychologist or to aid in diagnosis before the "classic" symptoms appear. Unlike stroke, which presents with sudden motor weakness, PD is insidious, slowly sneaking up on its victim. The patient may first sense vague aches and pains, and wonder if arthritis is developing. A general feeling of

tiredness or malaise may come first, which could easily be attributed to overwork or "burnout." Other PD patients may first report feeling irritable or depressed. These symptoms may be met with assurances, a suggestion to undertake medical tests, or a referral to a psychologist to investigate possible psychosomatic problems or depression. As the disease continues to progress, subtle motor symptoms begin to appear. Perhaps the person notices weakness in an arm or leg, problems in writing, holding a pen, or typing. Voice quality becomes softer and more monotone, and facial expression appears flat to others. If the symptoms are limited to one side of the body, it may appear that the person has suffered a mild stroke. It is nearly impossible to diagnose Parkinson's at this stage because the classic motor symptoms have not yet emerged. It would also be rare to even suspect Parkinson's, because these initial symptoms could herald a multitude of different problems.

The cognitive profile of those diagnosed with Parkinson's disease usually falls into two general categories: Parkinson's with dementia and nondemented Parkinson's. As previously mentioned, the incidence of dementia in PD is higher than in the general population. On testing, those with dementia may appear more like Alzheimer's patients. However, it is not known if this dementia stems from a co-occurring Alzheimer's disease process. Raskin and colleagues (Raskin et al., 1990) have suggested two possibilities for the occurrence of dementia in PD patients. First, demented PD patients may represent a qualitatively different subgroup, experiencing a later onset of symptoms and showing more subcortical and frontal atrophy. The second explanation is that this group may differ only in degree, with a more pronounced progression of cognitive decline.

This section examines the cognitive profile of nondemented Parkinson's patients. For many years researchers believed that Parkinson's entailed no significant mental status changes. Now, most researchers and clinicians do not believe that to be the case. More recently a number of authors have well documented these changes. Some have also suggested that the cognitive profile is heterogeneous, that there may be several subgroups of Parkinson's disease, possibly pointing to subgroups of neuropathology (Dubois,

Boller, Pillon, & Agid, 1991). Others have also raised questions about lateralization of cognitive deficits. Do cognitive deficits in any way parallel the type and degree of motor symptomatology?

Just as memory dysfunction is the hallmark of Alzheimer's disease, motor dysfunction is characteristic of Parkinson's. Our review of functional systems begins with the clinical presentation and neuropsychological dysfunction of the motor system.

Motor

The motor symptoms of Parkinson's disease generally fall into groups of positive and negative symptoms (see Table 12.1). Positive symptoms indicate an excess of motor behavior, or abnormal motor reactivity, whereas negative symptoms indicate a diminution or loss of motor functioning. Some experts believe that negative symptoms may manifest before the positive symptoms, although they may be frequently missed. You can think of **bradykinesia** as a poverty of movement that is not only slowed but reduced in magnitude. Semiautomatic movements such as walking, arm swinging, blinking, swallowing, and facial expressiveness may appear almost frozen, as if the person is robotlike and must consciously think to move. The description of a Parkinson's patient as having "**masked facies**"—denoting a masklike face—captures the essence of an emotionless face. The person's demeanor may seem depressed; a vacant stare may be produced by the combination of reduced facial emotion, slow speech, and decreased eye blinking. In addition to slowness, many movements decline in magnitude. Parkinson's patients do not take long steps and swing their arms high in the air, but exhibit a rapid, small, shuffling, **festinating gait.** Handwriting also gets slower and smaller (**micrographia**), and the voice becomes softer as the ability to project sound of one's voice becomes increasingly difficult. PD patients also describe difficulty in initiating movement, or **hypokinesia**, and may have to consciously think to begin walking, to turn around, or to lift a fork. During the movement, the person may also freeze, and may need to "will" the action to continue. Ironically, it may also be difficult to stop an action such a walking or writing, which has led to the suggestion that PD results in a fundamental deficit in initiating and terminat-

Table 12.1	*Motor Symptoms of Parkinson's Disease*

Positive Symptoms

Resting tremor

Rigidity (cogwheel) 경직.
  Stooped posture

Impaired righting reflex/poor balance

Negative Symptoms

Bradykinesia: slowness of movement

Hypokinesia: reduced motor initiation

Gait disturbance
  Slow
  Festinating (rapid small steps)
  Freezing

Masked facies: reduced facial expression

Slowed speech

Decreased voice amplitude

Ocular disturbances
  Decreased blink rate
  Decreased light accommodation
  Slowed saccades

ing semiautomatic motor programs (for example, see Bradshaw & Mattingly, 1995).

Despite the debilitating effect of the negative symptoms of Parkinson's disease, the positive symptoms of PD are perhaps the most noticeable, and most people recognize them as the hallmarks of the disease. Chief among these are a resting tremor and rigidity. **Resting tremor,** as opposed to a cerebellar intention tremor, is often characterized as "pill rolling." This rhythmic shaking, often first occurring in one hand or the other, looks as if the person might be rubbing or rolling a coin or pill between thumb and forefinger. The tremor stops or lessens with voluntary movements such as reaching, swinging the arm, grasping, or manipulating objects. When the person is sleeping, the tremor usually disappears.

However, with heightened states of alertness, concentration, or nervousness, the tremor is likely to increase. The degree of tremor at any one time is partly due to the voluntary–involuntary nature of the movement, the level of alertness, and the level of stress. It is not always predictable, coming in bursts, but it does increase in speed, and may become more violent as the disease progresses. In the early stages it is not uncommon for the tremor to influence only one side of the body, affecting the hand and foot first, and maybe one side of the face. Eventually it moves to the contralateral side, and affects all extremities.

Rigidity, the other major positive symptom, occurs as a tightening of muscles and joints. When a neurologist tries to move the person's wrist, elbow, or knee, there is persistent resistance to this passive movement. Sometimes this resistance appears as a ratcheting movement, as if the person's joint were a cogwheel (cogwheel rigidity). Muscles may appear tensed, and feel contracted to touch, even when the person is relaxing. This increasing rigidity may result in the characteristic stooped or hunched posture of Parkinson's disease. In addition to a more rigid posture, poor balance and the inability to adjust posture may be evident. The inability to catch oneself quickly, or impaired righting reflex, may appear if the person is pushed or missteps.

On neuropsychological testing of the motor system, Parkinson's patients are extremely slow, with poor reaction times. This is certainly evident on basic tasks that may require simple speeded movement, such as finger tapping. Poor motor performance is also evident on many other tasks that have a speeded motor component such as copying geometric designs with blocks within a specified time limit (such as WAIS-R Block Design).

Because Parkinson's disease usually begins as a lateralized motor disorder, some have speculated that the cognitive profile may also show lateralized impairment. Indeed, this may be the case. People with hemiparkinsonism often do show a neuropsychological profile consistent with what would be expected from lateralized cortical damage (Raskin et al., 1990). Exclusively left-sided motor symptoms link to more right hemisphere deficits. Raskin also suggests that this profile may reflect unilateral damage to basal-cortical pathways, resulting in disconnection, rather than unilateral lesions of the basal ganglia.

Motor symptoms may result in lateralized neuropsychological profiles—but is there a relationship between the degree of motor impairment and the severity of cognitive dysfunction? Parkinson's patients followed for up to 10 years did not show evidence of such correspondence (Portin & Rinne, 1986). Although drugs that targeted the motor symptoms, such as L-dopa, had great impact on motor performance, they had little effect on cognitive performance.

Visual-Spatial

Of nonmotor, higher cognitive functions, visual-spatial deficits in nondemented Parkinson's disease are among the most commonly reported in the literature and among the most controversial. Many studies have found that PD patients do poorly on spatial tasks that have a motor component. This is not surprising. But there is evidence for impairment on visual-spatial tasks whether or not there is a motor component (for example, see Raskin et al., 1990, for review). However, enough studies show mixed results, or no impairment on visual-spatial tasks, to throw the issue of spatial impairment into doubt (for review, see Dubois et al., 1991). To what can we attribute this discrepancy? In part, it may be caused by the heterogeneity of presentation in Parkinson's patients. Different patients may have somewhat different pathology and thus have different clinical presentations. As discussed, those with more left-sided motor impairment may show more right hemisphere damage (visual-spatial deficits). Some studies include patients in more advanced stages of the disease. Some PD patients may have a comorbid dementia. In any case, factors having to do with possible subgroups of PD patients continue to cloud the picture of visual-spatial functioning.

In nondemented Parkinson's sufferers who have visual-spatial dysfunction, does such dysfunction point to parietal impairment or some other mechanism? First, PD patients may report having difficulty orienting themselves in space. For example, when having to walk around the house in the dark without the aid of visible landmarks or outside in a fog, one person relates, "I used to walk alone in the wood, fog or no fog, but when the symptoms of Parkinson's disease appeared, I noticed that I could not orient myself any more, and in case of fog, I got lost" (Dubois et al., 1991, p. 203). Spatial abilities require the person to visualize the relative position of objects in three-dimensional space, and to make a motor response, in order to orient him- or herself or other objects in that space. Therefore the visual-spatial-motor aspects link in an overall spatial framework. Disease could theoretically disrupt this network in the parietal lobes or anywhere along the visual-motor system. Some have suggested that the basal ganglia play a role in the visual-motor aspects of visual-spatial problems in PD patients (Danta & Hilton, 1975; Dubois et al., 1991). But what about patients who have visual-perceptive difficulty but no visual-motor problems? For example, a popular test used by neuropsychologists, Benton's Judgment of Line Orientation Test (Benton et al., 1983), requires matching drawings of lines in various orientations to a template (see Figure 12.3). It does not require drawing or movement of the body. Yet many nondemented PD patients have difficulty with this task (Goldenberg, Wimmer, Auff, & Schnaberth, 1986). One explanation is that any disruption

in the visual-spatial-motor circuit may impair performance. Another suggestion is that even in tasks where a person does not use a motor response, he or she still has an internal representation of a perceptual-motor response (Villardita, Smirni, LaPira, Zappala, & Nicoletti, 1982).

In summary, although it is not clear if all Parkinson's patients experience visual-spatial dysfunction, a sizable proportion do. Certain subgroups of patients or those in more advanced stages of the disease, for example, may show the most difficulty. The parietal lobes, per se, do not appear chiefly responsible for the problem. Rather, the basal ganglia are implicated, in a larger visual-spatial network.

Executive Functioning

Many Parkinson's disease patients have executive functioning difficulties. Difficulties with specific executive functions can be evident, although most do not have difficulty with abstract thinking (Raskin et al., 1990). These deficits show up early in the disease process, and thus appear to result directly from the disease (for review, see Dubois et al., 1991).

Among executive dysfunctions reported in the literature are difficulties with changing mental sets, maintaining mental sets, and temporal structuring. The inability to switch mental set in response to environmental demands, or perseveration, shows most clearly on neuropsychological testing through measures that require strategy shifts to solve problems (such as the Wisconsin Card Sorting Test) or an alternating response between two different types of stimuli (such as the Trail Making Test B or the Stroop Test). Someone who has set-shifting problems repeatedly tries to use the same strategy, even if it is not working. Investigators have found that Parkinson's disease patients do not make more total errors on these types of tasks, but the errors they do make are perseverative (Raskin et al., 1990; Dubois et al., 1991). The perseverative problem in maintaining set occurs after the patient tries a new or different strategy. It is a tendency to revert back to a previous strategy after switching "mental set." Some have also explained the verbal fluency difficulties of this group as a problem of set maintenance (Dubois et al., 1991). Verbal fluency tasks typically require the person to list as many words as

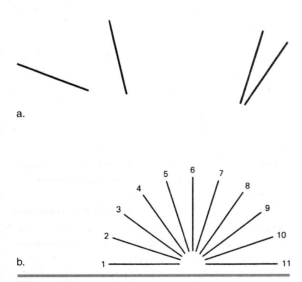

Figure 12.3 The Judgment of Line Orientation Test. Two examples of double-line stimuli (a) to be matched to the template below (b). (From A. L. Benton, K. deS. Hamsher, N. R. Varney, and O. Spreen, *Contributions to Neuropsychological Assessment,* New York: Oxford University Press, 1983. Reprinted with permission)

possible that begin with a specified letter or belong to a specified category. The problems seems most evident when the person uses several different letters. First the task is to name as many words, within a one-minute time period, that start with the letter *F,* then to name all the possibilities that begin with *A,* then with *S.* In such tasks, during the middle of the *S* sequence Parkinson's patients may revert to words that begin with *F* or *A* (Lees & Smith, 1983).

A difficulty in "time tagging" events is a problem in temporal structuring. Researchers have reported Parkinson's patients may have memory for news events without associated memory for the event order (Sagar et al., 1988). In daily life this can translate into problems remembering "when" medications have been taken, or learning the sequence of new tasks. Temporal ordering is an executive problem that interacts with memory.

Not all of the frontal lobe is involved in the dysexecutive problems of Parkinson's disease. Rather, the premotor area and the basal ganglia with its associated projections to the frontal lobes are implicated.

Language/Speech

Parkinson's disease typically does not produce classical aphasia. Also, few to no linguistic impairments appear involving grammar and sentence structure (Dubois et al., 1991). So general language processing and comprehension are intact. Some researchers indicate that more subtle problems in understanding grammatical complexity may be evident on more sophisticated neuropsychological tests (Levin, Tomer, & Rey, 1992). However, close to 70% have difficulties with articulation and the neuromechanical aspects of speech production (Levin et al., 1992). We have mentioned that PD patients lose voice amplitude and vocal emotional expression (**dysphonia**), which results in monotonous voice. Other speech irregularities may include segmented accelerated bursts of speech (**tachiphemia**) and compulsive word or phrase repetition (**palilalia**).

Tests measuring aspects of expressive or receptive aphasia reveal little impairment in Parkinson's patients. However, they may perform poorly on semantic fluency and word-finding tasks (such as the Boston Naming Test). However, as discussed previously, these tasks are better conceptualized as belonging in another domain (executive functioning). Behavioral assessment of speech is the method that will reveal the characteristic dysarticulation problems.

Memory

Compared to Alzheimer's disease, memory functioning is relatively spared in Parkinson's disease, even in demented PD patients (Sagar et al., 1988). Digit repetition and block-tapping repetition are usually preserved (for review, see Dubois et al., 1991). On tests involving episodic memory, paired associate learning, auditory verbal learning and visual reproduction of geometric designs, PD patients do show a recall deficit but demonstrate encoding and registration of declarative material through recognition tasks (for reviews, see Dubois et al., 1991; Levin et al., 1992). The implication of this pattern is that strategic memory processes for organization and retrieval of declarative information are defective.

Nondeclarative learning presents a mixed bag in Parkinson's disease. Verbal priming and perceptual motor adaptation are largely unimpaired in nondemented Parkinson's patients (Crosson, 1992; Heindel et al., 1989). However, nondelarative learning, which relies on intact motor or executive functioning, is often deficient. The ability to learn new motor skills declines as the disease progresses (Crosson, 1992). This is not surprising, considering the general dysregulation of the motor system. Procedural learning, measured by rule-learning tasks such as the Tower of Toronto, may be deficient, but results are mixed. At times PD patients perform poorly because of a problem in maintaining mental set for the rule, again pointing more to a problem in executive functioning than to a memory registration problem.

Most of the apparent memory difficulties experienced by Parkinson's patients stem from interactions among the executive system, the memory registration system, and the motor system. Parkinson's patients may show difficulty in motor skill acquisition. Non-demented Parkinson's patients can passively register declarative information in short-term and long-term memory. However, many have trouble using this information effectively. This includes effectively organizing information to be recalled, maintaining a consistent mental set when trying to learn or retrieve information, and time tagging or knowing not only that something has occurred but "knowing when" it happened.

Mood, Emotion, Personality, and Insight

A large proportion of Parkinson's disease patients suffer from depression. There is continuing debate over whether the mood disorder is a primary dysfunction of the disease or a secondary result of the medications used to treat the disease. To those suffering from depression, the debate may seem academic. Some also suggested that depression may be a natural reaction to realizing that the patients have Parkinson's disease. Although this probably occurs to some degree, it does not seem to explain enough. PD patients seem to be more depressed than patients with many other chronic diseases (Raskin et al., 1990).

Although few standardized neuropsychological tests measure expression of emotion, researchers have studied this in Parkinson's patients. The findings are somewhat equivocal, but some suggest that PD patients have a dysfunction in emotional expression associated with a right-frontal focus (for example, see Ross, 1985). They may have difficulty in showing an angry face or a surprised face but may be able to recognize emotional expression. Does this finding suggest a cortical deficit in emotional expression? Or rather a problem in the more mechanical aspects of emotional expression? Because of the "masked facies," it is hard to tell if emotional expression is lost or just diminished in frequency and intensity. Future research may help answer this question.

TREATMENTS FOR PARKINSON'S DISEASE

Without treatment, patients with Parkinson's disease are souls trapped in the cages of their bodies, unable to command or coax their mutinous muscles into action. Out of the tragedy of this disease, however, has emerged a palette of treatments that are worth examining, not only for addressing PD, but because they represent creative and forward-thinking approaches to the treatment of aging-related brain disorders in general. Interestingly, the treatment for PD appears to be traveling full circle from surgery to drugs to surgery. In addition, gene therapies, tissue implants, and various approaches to prevention are on the horizon.

The first surgical approaches to Parkinson's disease in the late 1950s were based on the idea of alleviating symptoms by interfering with what was thought to be "malfunctioning circuitry" in the basal ganglia through heat-induced surgical lesioning of the global pallidus. By 1960, a group of Swedish researchers could demonstrate motor improvement in a significant number of their patients. However, this treatment preceded the advent of CT scans, MRIs, and the precision stereotaxic and electrode recording tools needed to locate specific neurons. The imprecision of this surgery made negative side effects likely.

The discovery of L-dopa as a possible treatment for Parkinson's disease in 1961 (Birkmayer & Hornykiewicz, 1961) was revolutionary and heralded a new approach to the treatment of neurodegenerative diseases. With the advent of a seeming miracle drug, surgical approaches fell by the wayside by the late 1960s. Today, there exists a menu of drugs that act not only on the dopaminergic system, but also on related neurotransmitter systems.

In Paris in the 1860s, **anticholinergics** extracted from plant sources (such as scopolamine from jimsonweed, black henbane, or deadly nightshade) were the first treatments used for Parkinson's disease. Although the mechanism of action was not known at the time, these solanaceous alkaloids acted by blocking the action of acetylcholine, offering some symptomatic control of motor systems for tremor and rigidity. However, the side effects of "anticholinergic intoxication" limit their usefulness. Possible systemic effects, including dry mouth, blurred vision, constipation, weak bladder, and cognitive effects such as memory problems, confusion, slurred speech, and visual hallucinations, can create more than a small nuisance for patients. Physicians now prescribe synthetic anticholinergics of different types, if at all, during the early stages of the disease, and usually in combination with levodopa.

L-dopa is the left (levo) form of the dopa molecule, a simple amino acid. Prepared as a drug, it is called *levodopa*. Plants and animals manufacture it, and it appears naturally in fava beans and other legumes. Levodopa, being a dopamine precursor, directly metabolizes into dopamine. Cousins of levodopa include dopamine agonists and analogs that mimic the action of dopamine by stimulating its release, whereas reuptake blockers work by preventing reuptake at the synapse to retard metabolic removal. Drugs acting on the dopaminergic neurotransmitter system are still the best family of drugs found to alleviate tremor, bradykinesia, and rigidity. The difficulty with these orally ingested drugs, however, is that they convert to dopamine in the body and don't easily penetrate the blood–brain barrier. Probably less than 1% actually crosses over to be useful to the striatum, causing systemic buildup of dopamine in organs such as the liver and kidneys. Therefore medications usually combine levodopa with a decarboxylase inhibitor (such as Carbidopa) to prevent the conversion to dopamine until it crosses the blood–brain barrier. Because Carbidopa cannot cross the blood–brain barrier, it acts as a protector against conversion in the body until it releases the levodopa into the brain. This arrangement delivers about five times the dopamine to the targeted area, greatly enhancing the drug's effectiveness.

Physicians may also use other drugs to treat Parkinson's disease, either as adjuncts or to counteract side effects of long-term dopaminergic drug usage. Doctors may add MAO-B inhibitors, antidepressants, and agents to counteract the effect of dyskinesia to the complex menu, which must be taken at intervals as frequently as every four hours. These drugs are extending the survival of Parkinson's disease patients, but not without a price. The side effects of dopaminergic drugs, including vivid nightmares, disturbed sleep, perceptual illusions, and hypomania can be very disturbing. Also, after a long course of treatment, usually 10 years or so, the drugs lose effectiveness, dopaminergic neurons become hypersensitive, and the therapeutic window becomes shorter in duration, resulting in a severe on–off syndrome. During the on phase, the drug exerts its action but may overshoot, resulting in an effect akin to an overdose. In this phase severe dyskinesia resembling choreic movements and dystonia involving muscular posturing may result. This may cycle quickly to off symptoms, which include the disease symptoms, particularly freezing, severe tremor, and panic.

L-dopa could not live up to the hopes that pharmacologic substitution of missing dopamine would be sufficient treatment. The debilitating "on–off" drug phenomena led to the return of surgical techniques. These operations are currently intended for those for whom the drug treatments are no longer working. This time, however, high-tech precision imaging of the brain results in a greater chance of locating the offending neurons. Currently two types of operations are being conducted. The first operations focused on surgical lesioning of offending neurons. The second wave of surgeries, deep brain stimulation operations, involves nondestructive electrical interference.

Pallidotomy, the Parkinson's surgery of the late 1950s, was revived in the early 1990s. Surgeons use it in an attempt to alleviate the abnormal uncontrolled movement of dyskinesia and the frequent on–off symptoms. In pallidotomy, surgeons lesion the ventral, or internal portion, of the globus pallidus by heat-coagulating the neurons. Studies have shown that the decreased dopamine in the basal ganglia causes the motor portions of the pallidum to become overactive. This hyperfiring, in turn, inhibits the thalamus and portions of the brain stem (which causes bradykinesia and dyskinesia). Lesioning the posteroventral portion of the pallidum arrests this excessive output to the thalamus and brain stem (see Neuropsychology in Action 12.2). Surgeons use a second lesioning procedure on a portion of the thalamus, **thalotomy,** to attack tremor. Interestingly, they also use this procedure for patients with tremor caused by MS, essential tremor of old age, cerebellar tremor, and poststroke tremor. These two operations are typically unilateral and not done in combination. In fact, the lesion sites for the two operations are only millimeters apart. Bilateral lesions done at the same time seem to greatly increase the risk of cognitive deficits. In pallidotomy, the risk may be greatest for memory difficulty and confusion. For thalotomy, speech dysfunction seems to be the greatest risk.

Deep brain stimulation procedures represent the newest variation of these surgeries. The target site is the same as in thalotomy, except that instead of a destructive lesion, surgeons transmit electrical interference to the neurons via a permanently implanted lead. An implanted adjustable neurostimulator operates somewhat like a pacemaker and can be turned on and off by the patient.

Although these surgeries represent new hope for patients for whom drugs are no longer effective, they are palliative, not curative. Patients experience relief of symptoms, and around 80% of people may improve, but they must still take medication. The progression of the disease continues.

Huntington's Disease

Huntington's disease (HD), although very rare, has been well studied in the last quarter of the 20th century. Why the resurgent interest in a disease that physicians described over a century ago and then seemingly left to languish until the 1960s? From 1872, when George Huntington described this "hereditary chorea," until the 1960s, researchers paid little attention to this neurologic disease, which causes adults in the prime of their lives to seemingly "go insane," develop a tendency toward suicide, and suffer devastating motor impairment in the form of chorea. Families of Huntington's disease sufferers have spearheaded the search for the gene that controls the disease. For neuropsychology, the specificity of this disease offers a window to learn about the widespread behavioral effects of caudate nucleus deterioration.

George Huntington was not the first to describe the twisting, writhing, grimacing choreic movements, which are reminiscent of a puppet at the hands of a sinister master. In the 16th century, "peculiar" families were described but the hereditary nature of the disease did not appear to come into the medical consciousness until evolutionary theory emerged in the mid-1800s (Wexler, 1995). Other physicians before Huntington hypothesized about the hereditary nature of the disease, but it was young George Huntington, just 22 years old, who in his 1872 paper described the disorder most clearly and most completely. He emphasized the emotional and psychological aspects of the disease, describing "the tendency to insanity, and sometimes that form of insanity that leads to suicide." This became the classic account of the disorder, forever after associated with the name Huntington.

The story of the search for the "Huntington's gene" begins in the late 1960s. After years of relatively little scientific interest in this apparently incurable disorder, two families picked up the torch. Marjorie Guthrie, ex-wife of Woody Guthrie, the famous singer, who had Huntington's disease, founded an organization of Huntington's families to raise money for research. The Wexlers, whose story is told in the book *Mapping Fate* (see Neuropsychology in Action 12.3) were instrumental in pushing basic scientific research toward the search for the gene. Nancy Wexler, at risk for Huntington's disease herself, was active in the study of colonies of Huntington's families in Venezuela. Largely through the energy generated by these and other at-risk families, researchers pinpointed the offending gene in 1993. This discovery does not translate into an immediate cure or treatment. However, it does provide the first hopeful step in that direction.

Huntington's disease (HD) is a progressive subcortical dementia. This rare disease, affecting about 5–10 people out of every 100,000, is linked to the gene ITI5 on chromosome 4 and is passed on by one parent in a autosomal dominant inheritance pattern. As far as genes go, ITI5 is a big one, with over 300,000 base pairs, and is evident in all tissues with the body. People with normal versions of the gene have between 11 and 34 repeats of the trinucleotide CAG (cytosine, adenine, guanine), which codes the gene. However, those with the Huntington's positive gene have 37 to as many as 100 or more repeats. More repeats entail earlier onset and greater severity of symptoms. There is some overlap between normal and abnormal functioning, making 35–40 a borderline range. When operating normally, ITI5 produces the amino acid glutamine. It is not clear how the body uses glutamine, or the exact function of ITI5, but researchers know that expanded gene sequence repeats on other genes characterize inherited diseases such as myotonic dystrophy and spinobulbar muscular dystrophy, which affected President Kennedy.

Autosomal dominance translates into a 50% chance of developing the disease. Because this disorder runs

Neuropsychology in Action 12.2

Pallidotomy Surgery: A Case Report

by Barbara L. Malamut Ph.D.

The following case report profiles one "typical" patient who underwent right pallidotomy in an attempt to alleviate some of his adverse motor fluctuations. M.J. is a 56-year-old, right-handed man with a 16-year history of Parkinson's disease. His symptoms first began on the left side of his body with abnormal spontaneous movements of his foot, including a rhythmic tapping and an involuntary curling up of his toes. After about 10 years, his motor deficits worsened and he suffered from significant bilateral symptoms including bradykinesia, rigidity, and motor fluctuations. He had dyskinesias when his medication was "on" and freezing when "off." Other than Parkinson's disease, M.J. had no other major medical or psychiatric problems. He was forced to go on medical disability three years ago. He has few hobbies, spending his days maintaining the house, walking the dog, doing yardwork and some cooking. M.J. acknowledges a feeling of depression, which increases when he does not feel well.

When he arrived for his presurgical neuropsychological assessment, M.J. presented as an alert, oriented, pleasant, and cooperative man with a stiff, slow gait. Dystonic posturing of his head and upper torso was evident when sitting. Although his facial expression was fixed, he displayed a range of affect. A moderate tremor, which was greater on the left, was also evident. His spontaneous speech was soft in volume, with a choppy cadence, but his language was intact. No disturbance in thinking was noted during the interview. Results of neuropsychological testing indicated a few areas of mild impairment that were consistent with Parkinson's disease. These included problems with speed of mental processing, working memory for both auditory-verbal and visual-spatial information, visual scanning, graphomotor control, and retrieval of verbal and visual-spatial material. Recognition memory was intact. Consistent with his self-reported history, M.J. was depressed, socially isolated, and withdrawn.

M.J. was a good candidate for pallidotomy because he was generally in good physical and mental health, his neuropsychological profile did not indicate cognitive decline or dementia, and his medications had lost much of their effectiveness. The day of M.J.'s surgery, he was injected with a local anesthetic and fitted with a stereotactic frame necessary to locate the area to be le-sioned (see Figure 12.4). With the frame in place, a CT scan was done and compared to his previous MRI, to identify the precise placement of critical brain structures. After drilling a tiny hole through M.J.'s skull, the surgeon inserted a small canula, or tube, through the dura mater and snaked a microelectric probe through his brain toward his right pallidum. As the probe approached the area of neuronal hyperactivity, sound bursts became more frequent. The surgeon first stimulated the area to observe motor response. (M.J. was conscious so his responses to stimulation could be tested and any adverse affects on vision or speech could be noted before actual lesions were made.) Being careful not to affect the nearby optic tract, the surgeon then made a small heat-induced lesion to permanently destroy the overactive neurons of the pallidum. After this surgery, M.J. needed a few stitches and was released within 24 hours. M.J. experienced no surgical complications.

Six months later M.J. returned for a neuropsychological reevaluation to monitor his cognitive status. He reported that since surgery, his left-sided rigidity had disappeared and he no longer had pain or involuntary movements when

in families, HD is not suspect unless there is a family history. In those with a family history, a simple genetic test can determine the presence of the disease, but much to the surprise of many scientists, most at risk have chosen not to be tested (see Neuropsychology in Action 12.3).

NEUROPATHOLOGY OF HUNTINGTON'S DISEASE

Deterioration of the caudate nucleus bilaterally plays a primary role in the neuropathology of Huntington's disease, although ultimately HD affects multi-

walking. On observation, he no longer had dystonic posturing, but did continue to walk with a slow, shuffling gait. In addition, his speech was now normal in volume but he had developed a mild stammer. Overall, M.J. was pleased with the results of his surgery, although he realized this was not a cure. Improvement relative to his preoperative neuropsychological evaluation was noted in speed of mental processing, working memory for both auditory-verbal and visual-spatial information, and graphomotor control. M.J.'s problems with depression remained, and he was started on antidepressant medication and agreed to begin psychotherapy.

This case raises several critical and common issues regarding pallidotomy surgery. Although pallidotomy very effectively alleviates many motor symptoms and pain associated with later stages of Parkinson's disease, it does not cure the disease or return the patient to preinjury functioning. The long-term benefits and risks of pallidotomy are not known. Studies currently under way are examining the cognitive sequelae of the pallidotomy procedure in comparison to the natural progression of the disease. The newest procedure, approved by the FDA in July 1997, is deep thalamic stimulation, which works as a type of electronic pacemaker interfering with the ventral intermediate thalamic nucleus. The surgery, performed like pallidotomy, primarily reduces tremor but may have little effect on the other Parkinson's symptoms. This surgery, un-

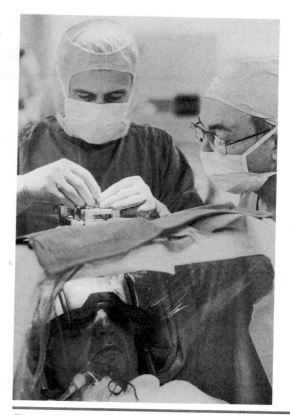

Figure 12.4 In the pallidotomy surgery for Parkinson's disease, the surgeon is using the triangulation of three coordinates of the frame to pinpoint the patient's globus pallidus. (Steve Ueckert, *Houston Chronicle*, January 22, 1996, p. 4a)

like pallidotomy, does not result in permanent lesions. Other treatment modalities currently being explored such as gene therapy and fetal implant surgery, may be promising avenues for the future. These procedures may actually arrest or reverse Parkinson's, rather than just ameliorate some of its motor symptoms.

ple brain systems. The caudate nucleus is one of the structures that comprise the striatum, along with the globus pallidus and putamen. The striatum is part of the basal ganglia, which is responsible for modulating motor activity. However, the role of the striatum is somewhat different from that of the substantia nigra, which is primarily affected in Parkinson's disease. Although the substantia nigra is responsible for proper initiation and termination of movements, the striatum controls the proper timing, ordering, and sequencing of movement patterns (Bradshaw & Mattingly, 1995). The caudate nucleus has reciprocal

Neuropsychology in Action 12.3

Testing Fate: Would You Want to Know If You Were Going to Get Huntington's Disease?

by Mary V. Spiers

Would you take a test to see whether you would develop an inherited brain disease in the future? This is the question facing family members of people with Huntington's disease, a subcortical dementia with devastating motor and cognitive consequences. Fortunately the disease is rare, but if it runs in your family, you have a 50% chance of developing this autosomal dominant genetic disease. There is no cure and there is no treatment, and if you do have it you may pass it on to your children. You are also likely to die while in your 50s. Would knowing this help you to plan? Plan not to have children, perhaps plan not to even marry, perhaps try to pack a lot of living into a short time? Would knowing lessen your worry? Or would knowing be a traumatic experience? Would you consider suicide? Would you always be on guard watching and waiting for the first symptoms to appear?

These questions face the 125,000 people at risk for the disease in the United States. In 1983 researchers discovered a genetic marker that paved the way for the first testing for Huntington's disease. Then 10 years later, in 1993, researchers located the gene ITI5 (named "Interesting Transcript") on the short arm of chromosome 4, and the test became much more accurate. Only a simple blood test is required. Scientists predicted a flood at testing centers. But there has only been a trickle of people, about 6% of those at risk. Why is this? The answers come from those at risk. Alice Wexler, author of the book *Mapping Fate,* describes the story of her own family, and of her mother, who died of HD. After her mother's diagnosis in 1968 the Wexler family, led by her father and sister, spearheaded one of the most innovative approaches to scientific investigation, bringing scientists and families together in collaborative efforts to search for the Huntington's gene. The book chronicles the scientific and per-sonal odyssey of the discovery of the gene. Alice Wexler describes her own ambivalence and the feelings of others who have struggled with the idea of getting tested. Some have taken the test, mentioning control and relief from uncertainty as major reasons. Others are concerned about confidentiality of their medical records and possible denial of insurance coverage. For those who have tested positive, the experience is often traumatic, and surprisingly, may not alleviate the anxiety because there is no certainty as to when the symptoms may develop. Even for those who test negatively, the result may come as a shock as they realize they have built their lives around the possibility that they might develop a fatal disease. Alice Wexler, like so many others, has decided against being tested. If you were at risk you could test your fate. But would you want to?

---

projections (afferent and efferent neurons) to a number of limbic and prefrontal areas. Although HD primarily affects the caudate, it may also affect the putamen, other areas of the striatum, and possibly other limbic system structures such as the hippocampus. By the end stages of the disease, the frontal lobes may also shrink by 20 to 30% (Vonsattel, 1992).

In HD patients who are showing the symptoms of the disease, structural neuroimaging techniques such as CT or MRI clearly reveal the loss of cell mass in the caudate and a widening of the ventricles. On MRI, the volume of the caudate and other basal ganglia structures are clearly reduced. The apparent structural deterioration of the caudate corresponds to a downward progression of behavioral functioning. Functional neuroimaging via PET scan is more sensitive to early changes and can reveal hypometabolism in the frontal and striatal regions before deterioration is evident structurally (Hasselbalch et al., 1992) and before a clinical diagnosis (Penny & Young, 1993).

CLINICAL PRESENTATION AND NEUROPSYCHOLOGICAL PROFILE OF HUNTINGTON'S DISEASE

How do the symptomatology and neuropsychological functioning of the HD sufferers differ from profiles of AD or Parkinson's disease? Huntington's disease results in a unique pattern of impairment in which difficulties associated with frontal lobe functioning and motor functioning are prominent. Although Parkinson's disease also results in frontal executive system and motor impairment, the presentation differs in some ways. The caudate nucleus, rather than the substantia nigra, is the main culprit in HD.

Many of the cognitive difficulties of HD patients likely stem from a breakdown in premotor frontal lobe functioning and the connectivity of the caudate-frontal system. Early in the disease process HD patients show characteristic frontal signs of rigidity, perseveration, and difficulty switching mental set in daily life, as well as on neuropsychological testing. Some dysfunctions stem from the impacts that poor executive organizational abilities and attention/concentration problems have on cognitive functioning. For example, the memory difficulties of HD patients seem largely attributable to poor executive functioning. Capacity for learning new information declines in HD, but the picture differs from the AD profile. HD patients demonstrate low levels of free recall but improve greatly if given a recognition test. Why? Apparently they encode new information, or multiple-choice recognition tests would not aid performance. Huntington's patients seem to suffer primarily from a retrieval problem caused by ineffective memory search operations. They may have a poor ability to differentiate what they know from what they don't know (for review, see Brandt & Bylsma, 1993). This problem in strategic memory processing and metamemory (knowledge of one's own memory) appears attributable largely to frontal lobe and executive functioning difficulties rather than to hippocampal involvement, although both may interact to some degree. Executive difficulties probably also interact with other cognitive processes such as verbal and spatial conceptualization and processing.

The final manner by which the striatal-frontal lobe complex may exert its effects on cognitive functioning is through multiple connections to other areas of the brain. HD patients seem to have difficulty orienting themselves in space, which may be a parietal dysfunction. For example, the old-time child's game of blind man's bluff, in which one child is spun around blindfolded and then required to tag others by sound alone as they call out, would be very difficult for HD patients. Potegal (1971) has explained this egocentric spatial disorder as a problem in readjusting, or the caudate's ineffectiveness in modulating changes in spatial position. Although research has not yet confirmed this interpretation, it appears reasonable, given the role of the striatum in modulating other motor activity.

The emotional difficulties experienced by many HD patients likely result from prefrontal and limbic system interactions. HD patients exhibit a disproportionately high degree of affective disturbance, in the form of depression and manic depression. The suicide rate of 6% (Farrer, 1986) is higher than in other degenerative disorders. Are these emotional disturbances a response to a desperate situation, or perhaps a symptom of frontal-subcortical impairment? Suicide may be an understandable response, given the severe cognitive devastation that people in the early stages of the disease can anticipate. HD sufferers are no strangers to what will befall them. They have seen a parent, a grandparent, aunts, and uncles succumb to the same horrible disease. However, the rate of emotional disturbance in Huntington's disease is higher than expected. Depression is the most common affective disturbance (Brandt & Bylsma, 1993), but the literature reports a wide range of affective and psychiatric disturbances in HD patients. These include anxiety, apathy, irritability, impulsivity, aggression, sexual disturbance, schizophreniform thought disorder, and psychosis involving hallucinations and delusions (for reviews, see Brandt & Bylsma, 1993; Bradshaw & Mattingly, 1995). Interestingly, the emotional disturbances often precede motor symptoms. At this point the affected individual may not even be aware of his or her diagnosis. These emotional symptoms can be best conceptualized as a symptom of the disease, or a predisposition toward symptoms such as depression. However, this is not to say that reactions to the illness do not contribute to the picture of emotional disturbance. A reaction to the severity of the disease can compound a predisposition to depression.

The motor difficulties of HD are characterized by **chorea:** twisting, writhing, undulating, grimacing movements of the face and body. Interestingly, over-medicated Parkinson's patients also show choreic movements. This has led to the hypothesis that the dopamine system lies at the root of both these problems. Obviously, this gross motor dysfunction seriously hinders everyday activity. Like PD patients, HD patients are slow motorically (bradykinesia). Also, as in PD, the chorea tends to disappear with sleep and increase with stress. Unlike PD, HD patients walk with a wide-based gait. Their speech is dysarthric, becoming increasingly erratic in its rate of production, and staccato with intermittent pauses. They become clumsy and uncoordinated, unable to do fine-grained work. In testing HD patients, these severe motor difficulties disrupt performance on other tests that have a motor component, even if the test is designed to measure other functions such as visual problem solving. In assessing the cognitive performance of Huntington's patients, motor-free tests provide the clearest picture.

There is currently no cure for Huntington's disease, and the treatments that exist focus primarily on the relief of emotional symptoms such as depression and hallucinations.

◼ Creutzfeldt-Jakob Disease

Creutzfeldt-Jakob Disease (CJD), a dementia long hidden in obscurity because of its rarity (one that most neuropsychologists have never seen personally in one of their patients), has suddenly leapt into the limelight because of its connection to "mad cow disease" and because of the fear that its incidence is increasing. It is a compelling disease, unlike the other dementias we have considered, because of both its speed of progression and mode of transmission. With a malignantly cascading decline over three to four months, it is the most quickly progressing dementia. Scientists have long known that humans can transmit this disease via transplants of affected neural tissue, cornea transplants, or contamination via medical procedures, but it is now also becoming clear that CJD and its variants can cross species through the consumption of tainted meat containing neural tissue. Extensive spongelike holes appear in the brains of its victims, giving it the fitting name "spongiform encephalopathy." The mechanism by which the brain

becomes infected has eluded scientists for decades because CJD does not manifest the symptoms of typical acute infections. Virologists, biologists, and chemists are joining clinicians to unravel the mysteries of this disease.

In the early 1900s, Bertha, a 23-year-old German woman was a patient of Hans Gerhard Creutzfeldt. Creutzfeldt, an assistant of Alois Alzheimer at the Munich Psychiatric Clinic, was, like Alzheimer, trying to clarify the differences and similarities between behaviors understood as "psychiatric" and "neurologic." Creutzfeldt noticed that Bertha showed many behaviors typical of other mental illnesses, such as believing she was possessed by the devil, neglecting her hygiene, and posturing strangely. However, other symptoms suggested frank brain impairment. Bertha also had an unsteady gait, twitchy eyes, a voluntary tremor, and a tendency to giggle inappropriately. These latter symptoms, which we now recognize as indicating subcortical motor and emotional dysfunction, were Creutzfeldt's clues. After Bertha died, Creutzfeldt examined her brain tissue under the microscope. What he saw were the little "stars" of astrogliosis (see Figure 12.5) dotting her brain. In 1920, he published his paper describing Bertha. With the synchronicity that often occurs in science, Dr. Jakob reported a similar case in 1921. Creutzfeldt and Jakob thus shared the distinction of discovery.

Creutzfeldt-Jakob disease (CJD) is a quickly progressive subcortical dementia estimated to affect only one person in a million per year. This is extremely rare even in comparison to Huntington's Disease which affects 5–10 per 100,000. It appears around the world with the same prevalence, and does not seem to vary across groups or cultures. Although Creutzfeldt's patient was young, most cases have been in their 50s or 60s. For the most part researchers have hypothesized that CJD spontaneously arises as a random mutation. As long as it is not passed on to others, the disease dies out with its victim. Some variants of CJD may manifest themselves differently in the behavior of those it afflicts. For example, the extremely rare familial CJD variant termed **Gerstmann-Straussler-Scheinker syndrome (GSS)**, reported in only a handful of families, results in a "fatal insomnia." This is the only reported incidence of transmis-

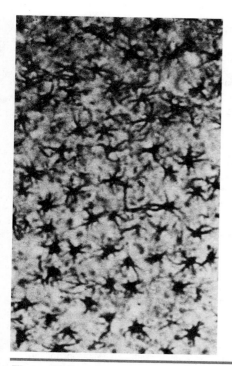

Figure 12.5 The dark stars of astrogliosis. (D. Carlton Gajdusek)

sion other than through external infection. Researchers believe that in older people CJD incubates for years before manifesting.

One of the most alarming aspects of this disease, and the reason it has been catapulted out of obscurity, is its relationship to other spongiform encephalophies (SEs). Variations of SE, as mentioned, are aptly named: Portions of the brain actually resemble a sponge, because of the microscopic pattern of holes. Researchers have identified SEs in species from minks to sheep (scrapie) to cows (bovine spongiform encephalophy or "mad cow disease") to humans (Creutzfeldt-Jakob disease and kuru). In his book *Deadly Feasts,* Richard Rhodes chronicles the history of the SEs. He describes the history and current status of research into CJD and kuru. **Kuru** is a SE that the Fore people of New Guinea contract, which presented itself when they began ritually cannibalizing their dead at the beginning of the 1900s. Rhodes

(1997) also describes the history of the research, which suggests that SEs can easily leap across species and that they are probably variations of the same disease process. In his book he predicts an alarming rise in the incidence of CJD (see Neuropsychology in Action 12.4).

NEUROPATHOLOGY OF CREUTZFELDT-JAKOB DISEASE

The cause of Creutzfeldt-Jakob disease has eluded scientists until recently because it is a transmissible or infectious agent with none of the usual symptoms of acute infection. In fact, scientists first thought that kuru could be genetic, because it occurred primarily among the women and children of the Fore people. However, only the women and children were eating the dead in a mortuary love feast. Men believed contact with women weakened them, and they did not partake in the ritual. Acute infections are easily identified by noticing the body's defensive immune system response. Inflammation, increased numbers of lymph cells in cerebrospinal fluid, and fever are typical, yet none of these symptoms occur in CJD or any of the spongiform encephalopathies.

No one knows where this infectious agent originally arose from. Perhaps from a randomly occurring mutation. This might account for the rarity in the population at large and the fact that CJD occurs with equal frequency throughout the world. However, in the last century, spongiform encephalophy has also been transmitted by eating infected neural tissue. This has happened both within species such as cows (bovine spongiform encephalopathy or mad cow disease) and across species. Mice, hamsters, and even primates injected with kuru have developed SE. Humans who have eaten infected meat have developed CJD (see Neuropsychology in Action 12.4). Many scientists now believe CJD to be a slow virus that incubates over years, perhaps in the spleen, and is camouflaged in cells so as not to be recognized as an invader. Some have also hypothesized that slow viruses are responsible for Alzheimer's, Parkinson's, and atrophic lateral sclerosis (ALS).

What exactly do SEs, specifically CJD, do to the brain? Certain areas of the brain look spongy, taking

Neuropsychology in Action 12.4

Creutzfeldt-Jakob Disease and Mad Cow Disease: What's the Connection?

by Mary V. Spiers

In his book *Deadly Feasts,* Richard Rhodes traces the history of spongiform encephalophathies in humans and other species. He reflects scientists' views that these diseases are variations of the same infectious process and that the ingestion or injection of diseased neural tissue can spread many SEs within or across species. He also forecasts an alarming rise in human encephalopathies over the next few years if people do not contain and eliminate the disease in the animal food supply.

How exactly did mad cow disease (bovine spongiform encephalopathy, or BSE) arise and become a threat to humans? Farmers routinely give cattle protein supplements: dairy cows all through their life, and beef cattle for end-stage fattening. As long as farmers fed cattle largely vegetable protein (such as soy) or fish protein along with their diet of grass or hay, and no transmission from randomly affected cattle occurred, BSE did not arise. However, during the 1980s a series of events in Great Britain triggered a BSE epidemic. One factor was that, because the pound was devalued, the price of soy and fish meal increased, so the agricultural industry began to rely more heavily on animal sources of protein. Animal protein typically comes from the by-products of slaughterhouses—bones and offal (guts, heads, tails, and blood) are processed into bonemeal pellets or powder and fed to other cattle. As long as the rendering process killed any disease, bonemeal was a good source of protein. During the 1980s in Britain, changes in the rendering process lowered the bonemeal processing temperature and abandoned fat removal, no longer destroying BSE in tissue. By the late 1980s, BSE had spread throughout Great Britain and had infected over 2000 cattle. Farmers noticed that their cattle were "becoming aggressive, rather nervous, knocking other cows . . . and becoming dangerous to handle. . . . If you shooed her, she would stumble, particularly on the back legs, and go down, and then scrabble along" (p. 172). In 1988 the British government ordered milk from affected cows destroyed. However, not until an outbreak in humans occurred, in 1996, were massive number of beef cattle destroyed. The base rate for CJD is one in a million in people over the age of 50. CJD cases developing under that age are extremely rare. In the world, there had been only 10 known adolescent cases. Only with kuru-associated cannibalism did researchers notice that young people developed spongiform encephalophathy with a shortened incubation period. Between 1991 and 1996, 10 cases of a CJD variant of people under age 40 emerged in Great Britain. According to statistical probability, this is an epidemic. Only time will tell if awareness has stopped the spread.

on a characteristic spongiform pattern. CJD, like kuru, attacks the cerebellum, but it also damages the cerebrum. Microscopically, the "stars" of astrogliosis that Creutzfeldt found were the result of the glial cells, or the "cleanup machines" of the brain, filling in after neuronal tissue had died. Astrogliosis is the aftereffect, not the cause of the disease. Amyloid plaques are also numerous, but as already discussed, these are not specific to CJD but are also found in other diseases such as AD.

Patricia Merz, with the aid of her electron microscope, first found small, twisted sticklike fibers in the cells of tissue samples of sheep with the sheep version of spongiform encephalophy, called "scrapie" (Merz, Sommerville, Wisneiwski, & Iqbal, 1981). Interestingly, she could then correctly distinguish between healthy controls and affected victims with CJD on the basis of these scrapie-associated fibrils (SAFs) in spleen and neural tissue samples. Merz hypothesized that SAFs may be the disease agent, which incubates in the spleen over years before affecting the brain. SAFs have been found in kuru as well as CJD brains, but not in AD, Parkinson's, or ALS brains. This was the first indication of a disease agent specific to spongiform encephalopathies such as CJD.

The name that has become popular in referring to SAFs is *prions* (Pruisiner, 1982). Currently, several different variations or strains have been identified. Prion proteins (PrPs), the protein components of prions, which are present in both normal and afflicted individuals, have been the target of research interest in CJD. However, infected PrP resists normal protein digestion via enzymes. Interestingly, both diseased and normal PrP have the same DNA specifications. This helps explain the riddle of why the body's immune system does not attack the infected protein. It doesn't recognize the protein as foreign! However, one of the unsolved mysteries of this disease is to understand how a normal protein changes to an abnormal protein with the same structural DNA. Several hypotheses exist to explain the mechanism of action. One is that there may be a very small virus, termed a *virino,* that has not yet been identified. Proteins are not known to mutate on their own, but perhaps small bits of "naked" nucleic acid infected with the virino, divorced from their cells, attach themselves to proteins and force the mutation. Another explanation involves a very interesting nonbiological form of replication. Nobel prize winner Carleton Gajdusek (1988) has postulated that something else must be transporting the infectious agent, because even when the nucleic acid is destroyed by radiation, the "infection" persists. He explains this as a crystal nucleation process. Similar to how crystals such as diamonds form in nature, the infection provides the pattern that is the nucleus, or catalyst, for the reaction. Successive proteins then mutate by patterning themselves after the original. If this sounds like science fiction, scientists have already dubbed this the "Ice 9" metaphor after a Kurt Vonnegut novel in which all the water on earth turns to ice, in a crystallization process.

Whether a yet undiscovered virino, nuclear crystallization, or some other process is causing CJD, scientists are pursuing this disease with renewed vigor because of its unfortunate recent resurgence. We now turn to the clinical aspects of CJD.

CLINICAL PRESENTATION AND NEUROPSYCHOLOGICAL PROFILE OF CREUTZFELDT-JAKOB DISEASE

Even though emotional symptoms may be first evident, the hallmark of CJD, as well as other spongi-form encephalopathies such as kuru, is motor symptomatology. The motor symptoms are those expected of cerebellar and subcortical dysfunction. Movements become uncoordinated, walking resembles a drunken stagger, and speech is slurred and inarticulate. Involuntary tremors and choreiform grimaces emerge, and finally victims can't swallow and so may die of starvation. Visual function alters, eventually leading to blindness in some people. These cerebellar and subcortical motor problems may follow initial, emotionally related complaints of mood disorders such as anxiety, depression or hypomania, fatigue, difficulty sleeping, and attention/concentration problems. As with the confusion over Creutzfeldt's patient Bertha, these symptoms may lead one to first believe that a pure mood disorder is present, or, in Bertha's case, which was more advanced, a delusional or psychotic disorder. However, the classic motor symptoms quickly reveal themselves.

The dementia of CJD and its variants has a very rapid progression, typically less than a year and usually within three to four months. Kuru has a similar progression. The Fore people of New Guinea categorized the disease (using pidgin) in five stages: (1) *kuru laik i-kamap now* ("kuru like he come up now") the first stage before motor symptoms are present, (2) *wokabout yet* ("walk-about yet") motor and gait problems apparent, (3) *sindaun pinis* ("sit down finish") inability to walk, (4) *slip pinis* ("sleep finish") stuporous state, and (5) *klostu dai nau* ("close to die now") final stage, swallowing lost (Rhodes, 1997). Some have likened the progression to classic advanced parkinsonism, but it certainly has features of Huntington's disease, too.

Neuropsychological testing of CJD patients is rarely done, not only because of the rarity of the disease, but also because of its circumstances. By the time the disorder is identified, patients are untestable. Unfortunately, at this time, there are no treatments and no cure. Perhaps the only fortunate aspect is that the disease dies out if it is not passed along. The level of kuru in the Fore people has dropped dramatically since they have stopped eating infected tissue.

Neuropsychology in Action 12.5

The Neurologic Exam for Dementia

by Allen J. Rubin M.D.

Watching a neurologist at bedside can be perplexing. A process of inference is at work that is not apparent to the onlooker. It begins with history taking, which incorporates as data every symptom the patient describes, and the form and pattern of the descriptive process. The physical aspects of examination are selective in some respects, and elaborated in others, to serve an incipient process of hypothesis testing at work during the examination. An active set of principles working inwardly guides the conduct of the neurologist. I undertake here to make those inferential processes and those principles explicit, in a general form.

The neurologist examines the central nervous system with an attitude that differs from the common attitude toward the body and its symptoms. The neurologist applies an invisible reference "map" derived from neuroanatomy and neurophysiology, and from encounters with past patients and syndromes. She or he seeks to define and localize a symptom as an epiphenomenon of unwitnessed internal mechanisms, respecting the rules of nervous tissue function rather than the culturally validated rules of somatic experience. In the examination of aging and dementia, the neurologist is, in addition, sensitized to a number of pivotal issues in history taking, and pivotal physical signs that narrow the selection of possible causes. A set of diagnostic hypotheses, ranked by priority, is the goal of the examination, then (most often) to be explored by laboratory and neuroimaging investigations, before the neurologist recommends treatments.

The neurologist's attitude is "phenomenological" in the sense that he or she must "bracket" or hold uninterpreted the symptom as the patient presents until a precise neurologic meaning can be attributed to the symptom (we will call these "*symptom hypotheses*"). Therefore, most of the examination effort focuses on the adept taking of a history, often from observers and family as well as the patient. The neurologist applies the tools of physical examination to clarify symptoms, achieve more precise localization, and select a favored hypothesis.

The model yielding symptom hypotheses always includes attention to these seven issues:

1. Clinical Course

Sudden onset (suggesting vascular or pharmacologic causes)

Insidious progression (suggesting metabolic, neoplastic, inflammatory, infectious, or degenerative causes)

Episodic or paroxysmal occurrence (suggesting epileptic or vascular causes)

Exacerbating-remitting course (suggesting inflammatory or demyelinating causes, or disorders deriving from variable systemic illness, or related to neuromuscular junction fatigue)

2. Hierarchical Level of Advancement

Within the nervous system as a whole, symptoms localize to a "level of organization": muscle, neuromuscular junction, peripheral nerve, spinal root, spinal cord, brain stem, or brain. Within the brain "level," symptoms will vary from simple (for example, segmental loss of light

perception) to complex (smelling colors, misattributing meaning to objects), from unimodal (for example, primary motor outputs or primary sensory inputs), to heteromodal (for example, converging complex functions, personality, or the flexibility, anticipation, and organizing executive functions of the frontal lobe). The "level" and "complexity" of the symptom lead the inferential process selectively to parts of the nervous system in which these qualities must necessarily be generated.

Within the *central nervous system, where neuropsychological dysfunction will arise,* elicited history amplifies these issues:

3. "Central Quality" of Symptoms

The presentation of a system may direct the inferential process away from the peripheral nerves to the central nervous system (CNS), the spinal cord and brain. A patient may describe a limb as disobedient or clumsy rather than weak or limp, may describe a limb sensory deficit as a regional perversion of normal sensation rather than numbness. In the visual system, lateralized inattention or distortions (metamorphosis, color alteration, movement or space misperception, or apparitions, for example) are central in origin. Paroxysmal intrusive experiences, seizures, unrealistic experiences, failure of reality testing, or any symptom reporting the disruption of the individual's normal connection to the social or sensory environment raise the specter of brain disease.

4. Lateralization

Co-occurrence of dysfunction in the same-side arm and face may place a suspect lesion contralaterally above the pons, and dysfunction in the same-side leg and arm may place a suspect lesion above the level of synapse within the cervical spinal cord. The presence of "crossed symptoms" (such as right face with left arm) invites exploration of localization within regions of anatomic crossing of specific projections, such as the crossing of paths in the brain stem. Coincidence of multiple lesions may imitate, in some cases, a single lesion in a complex region. Therefore neuropsychologists must rewrite the logic of inference to entertain all possibilities. Neuroimaging and electrophysiological tests can corroborate the inference of a focal lateralized hemispheric syndrome, and lateralized neuropsychological findings can substantiate and clarify the diagnosis.

5. Heritable Factors and Risk Factors

Past nervous system insults (such as trauma), vascular disease outside the nervous system (such as coronary disease and cardiac arrhythmia), systemic illnesses (such as immune system compromise, hyperlipidemia, diabetes mellitus, and autoimmune diseases) all narrow the guesswork in selecting a specific pathologic process in brain. Occurrence of CNS diseases in preceding generations (such as dementias, Huntington's disease) renders certain diagnoses more likely.

6. Confluence, Association, Dissociation, Disconnection

Confluence of symptoms (such as ipsilateral motor and sensory findings), association (such as right-sided weakness with aphasia, chronic vertigo with loss of facial sensation, right–left confu-

sion with agraphia), or dissociation (such as preservation of pain sensation only on the right and preservation of vibratory sensation only on the left; loss of voluntary facial movement but preservation of automatic emotional facial mimicry) all point to a CNS localization. Lastly, history or examination can identify disconnection of cerebral processes, which may be identified by history or examination (for example, alexia without agraphia, conduction aphasia with isolated loss of language repetition) and can place lesions in the interconnecting brain white matter connections.

7. Syndrome Recognition, Including Neurobehavioral Profiles

A neuropsychologist may advance a "diagnostic hypothesis" of a distinct disease syndrome, subject to confirmation with selected laboratory tests (genetic DNA studies, metabolic-hematologic studies, CT or MRI neuroimaging, Doppler or contrast angiography, electroencephalography, sensory evoked responses, cerebral fluid examination, quantitative visual perimetry, and brain biopsy) and neuropsychological consultation.

The following three cases of progressive diseases among the elderly illustrate how the symptoms and findings converge to allow diagnostic hypotheses:

Case 1

At 62 a woman patient retired from her work as an effective office manager; at that time she was involved in dancing and was a competitive bridge player as recreation. At 75 she presented with an insidious course of handwriting shrinkage, tremor at rest, stooping, and shuffling in gait. At 79 she had the onset of tiredness and discouragement with lack of motivation and failure of initiative, dysphoric mood and agoraphobia.

Pertinent examination: Her mental state was normal, with the exception of verbal memory, which benefited by cuing. Orthostatic hypotension was present. She exhibited masked facies and bradykinesia. A resting tremor was observed. Rigidity was present in passive movements. She required the aid of her arms to rise from a chair, and walked with diminished arm swing and shortened steps. Coordinated movements were slow but accurate. Reflexes were normal.

Summary: An insidious CNS disorder with predominantly motor impairment respecting a specific degenerative pattern. A disorder of memory retrieval may be emerging.

Principal diagnostic hypothesis: Parkinson's disease with secondary depression and anxiety disorder. Possible early subcortical dementia.

Case 2

At 58 a financial planner found himself taking additional time to perform routine tasks, and found that he could not manage phone transactions. His personality became irritable, obsessive, with reduced frustration tolerance and temperamental flares over trivial matters. He found he could not plan or organize as before, and he had several "near misses" in driving over a short period.

His examination showed slowed velocity of ocular refixation movements (saccades), motor impersistence of tongue protrusion, and poorly sustained grip. His speech was grammatic and expressive, but dysrhythmic. With mental effort he showed choreic movement in the face and all extremities. His gait was slightly widened in base. His muscle stretch reflexes were hyperactive.

Summary: An insidious progressive brain disorder with frontal executive functional impairment and evolving irritable

Continued

Continued

personality, accompanied by an adult-onset choreic movement disorder. Frontal-subcortical localization is suspected.

Principal diagnostic hypothesis: Huntington's disease. If the family history is negative for this genetic disorder, confirmation of the diagnosis can be sought through DNA testing.

Case 3

A 65-year-old retired judge experiences slowly progressive impairment. He has difficulty in word finding and adopts a "circumlocutory" speech. He misplaces objects and cannot retain the content of his reading. He loses direction when he walks in unfamiliar places, and he finds that he cannot continue his hobby of constructing models. After several years, he loses insight that he is impaired, and accuses his wife of being a malevolent impostor. His memory impairment is not helped by cues or reminders.

The neurologic examination, other than the mental status, is entirely normal, although he has difficulty cooperating with the examiner.

Summary: A progressive disorder manifesting anomic aphasia, visual-spatial impairment, and apraxia, all cortical dysfunctions. memory encoding is impaired, and not benefited by recognition. The absence of any motor impairment is striking.

Principal diagnostic hypothesis: A cortical degenerative dementia such as Alzheimer's disease is likely. The medical team will undertake a search for treatable and reversible conditions that imitate this pattern.

Conclusion

Subcortical dementias primarily target subcortical structures in the brain. The hallmark of these dementias is motor system disorder, but the behavioral impairment also targets many higher cognitive functions. Parkinson's disease patients are more likely to develop dementia as they age, although dementia is not inevitable. This chapter has examined the neuropsychological profile of nondemented PD patients. In addition to the characteristic motor symptoms, Parkinson's patients often show lateralized motor dysfunction. There is also often visual-spatial and executive dysfunction. Language difficulties are typically minor, and memory difficulties, in comparison to Alzheimer's disease, primarily involve executive aspects of memory. Parkinson's patients also frequently suffer from a concomitant mood disorder. The pharmacological and surgical treatments for Parkinson's disease are among the most promising treatments for any of the dementias.

Huntington's disease, is a good example of a contrasting subcortical dementia with motor difficulties different from those of Parkinson's disease. It is also a good example of a progressive hereditary disease. The neuropsychological profile of HD illustrates the executive functioning problems caused by compromise of the striatal-frontal lobe complex. Interestingly, HD patients also show a significant affective disturbance. Finally, Creutzfeldt-Jakob disease, although quite rare, is a good example of a fast-acting dementia that is transmissible via infected neural tissue.

Differential diagnosis among dementia subtypes can be quite complex. In this chapter and the last we have discussed only some of the major exemplars of dementia. There are many more subtypes that practicing neuropsychologists must come to recognize and differentiate. The study and recognition of dementias requires much experience with a number of dementia subtypes, and careful assessment and observation of behavioral differences. In this endeavor, neuropsychologists work in close conjunction with neurologists specializing in geriatrics. We end this chapter with a look at how neurologists approach evaluation and diagnosis in differentiating dementia subtypes (see Neuropsychology in Action 12.5).

Critical Thinking Questions

- ■ It may soon be possible to test for many neurologic diseases. Would you want to be tested for the possibility of future dementia?

- ■ How is the behavioral quality of subcortical motor disorders presented in this chapter similar or different from the cortical motor disorders such as apraxia presented in Chapter 4?

- ■ How do the subcortical and cortical motor systems work together?

- ■ What are the ethical and scientific issues in the treatment of dementias?

Key Terms

Parkinsonism	Festinating gait	Palilalia	Creutzfeldt-Jakob disease
Subcortical dementia	Micrographia	Anticholinergics	(CJD)
Parkinson's disease	Hypokinesia	Pallidotomy	Gerstmann-Straussler-
Lewy bodies	Resting tremor	Thalotomy	Scheinker syndrome (GSS)
Resting tremor	Rigidity	Huntington's disease	Kuru
Bradykinesia	Dysphonia	(HD)	
Masked facies	Tachiphemia	Chorea	

Web Connections

http://www.mentalhealth.com/dis/p20-or05.html
Internet Mental Health: Dementia
This site offers descriptions, information on treatment, recent research links, and publication listings.

http://www.nimh.nih.gov
National Institute of Mental Health (NIMH)
Home page of NIMH provides links to research activities and news.

http://www.mentalhealth.com
Internet Mental Health
This site provides information on a number of psychological disorders, medications, research, and reprints of articles.

Chapter 13

ALTERATIONS OF CONSCIOUSNESS

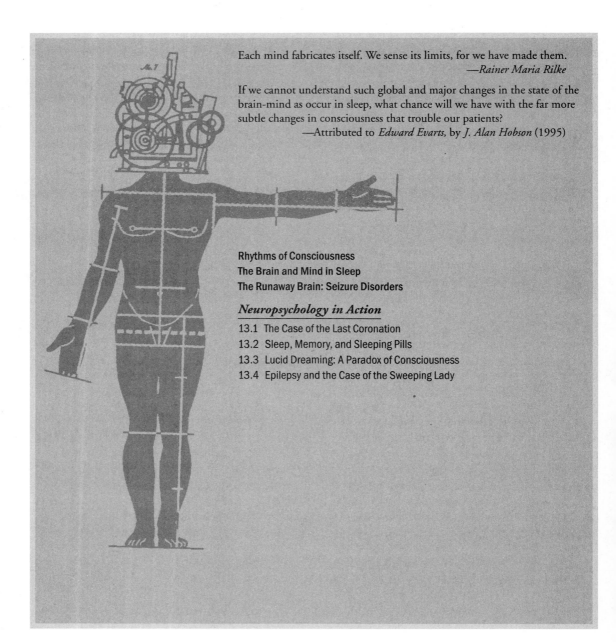

Each mind fabricates itself. We sense its limits, for we have made them.
—*Rainer Maria Rilke*

If we cannot understand such global and major changes in the state of the brain-mind as occur in sleep, what chance will we have with the far more subtle changes in consciousness that trouble our patients?
—Attributed to *Edward Evarts*, by *J. Alan Hobson* (1995)

Rhythms of Consciousness
The Brain and Mind in Sleep
The Runaway Brain: Seizure Disorders

Neuropsychology in Action

13.1 The Case of the Last Coronation
13.2 Sleep, Memory, and Sleeping Pills
13.3 Lucid Dreaming: A Paradox of Consciousness
13.4 Epilepsy and the Case of the Sweeping Lady

Keep in Mind

- Can "brain" states differ from "mind" states?
- What brain mechanisms are responsible for the "paradox" of REM sleep?
- What alterations of consciousness are represented by different seizure types?
- Do alterations in conscious alertness result from similar biological mechanisms?

Overview

You can conceptualize **consciousness** in a number of ways. Awareness, level of mental alertness, and level of attention are common representations. Consciousness can also imply the mind's subjective experience of brain states and processes that are available to perception. These various definitions (reviewed in Chapter 5) point to a number of different functional anatomic areas depending on the aspect of consciousness under consideration. Disorders of these disparate functional systems also result in a variety of disorders of consciousness. For example, we have discussed alterations in conscious "knowing, or agnosias of the visual system. The total unawareness of one side of the body, or neglect, is a very dramatic dysfunction of normal conscious awareness. These disorders of lowered, distorted, or piecemeal awareness can occur in any sensory modality. Synesthesia, or the abnormal melding of sensory-perceptual experiences, represents yet another alteration of consciousness that we have covered. Studying these disorders provides fascinating glimpses into the altered workings of normal waking consciousness.

In this chapter, the focus turns to alterations in levels of alertness and arousal. These alterations fluctuate throughout day and night according to preset circadian rhythms. Studying these daily rhythms, as people move from waking to sleeping and dreaming, offers lessons in the limits of normal brain alterations of consciousness. Disrupted flow of these rhythms can result in a variety of sleep disorders. Some, such as the rare circadian rhythm disorder (see Neuropsychology in Action 13.1) can threaten life itself. Others, like narcolepsy, show major disruptions of the REM cycle and result in sleep intrusions into wakefulness. Most sleep disorders disrupt cognition in some way. In sleep apnea, for example, memory and concentration difficulties are prevalent.

Seizures represent another set of consciousness disorders. Seizure events of various types represent alterations of daytime alertness. These internally generated brainstorms of activity manifest differently, largely according to the location of the seizure focus in the brain. Typically neurologists categorize them as either generalized or partial seizures, depending on the extent of brain involvement during the seizure episode. In the section on seizures, we discuss the general classification scheme. Seizures can occur as a result of a variety of causes. Neurologists consider most people with repeat seizures to have an **epileptic syndrome.** This of course is potentially more threatening to brain function than is an isolated seizure event. We discuss the neuroanatomy and neurophysiology of epilepsy as well as the neuropsychological consequences and types of treatments available.

Neuropsychology in Action 13.1

The Case of the Last Coronation

He was Italian, 53 years old, and an industrial manager whose health had been fine except for some problems with high blood pressure. Much to his misfortune, he was destined to show researchers how dire things can get, when the body's internal clock runs amok.

In 1985, the man developed insomnia. His sleep fell to only two or three hours a night, he became impotent, and he began to have difficulties with his digestion and developed a high temperature. Within two months, he could sleep for only an hour a night and was often observed rising from his bed, standing and giving a military salute. He told his family that he was dreaming of a coronation. By the time the man was admitted to the hospital in Bologna, he had ceased to sleep normally at all. He was alert when spoken to, but when left alone would drift into a stupor in which he would gesture as if communicating in a dream. His doctors tried to treat him with a variety of strong drugs, none of which had a lasting effect. In the eighth month of his illness, the man's stupor was relieved only by episodes in which he screamed and thrashed about. In the ninth month he died.

Examining his otherwise normal brain, doctors found that certain regions of the thalamus had degenerated. The man's rare disease supported suspicions that sleep, at least non-dreaming NREM sleep, is affected by chemical processes in the thalamus. Just below that structure, near the base of the brain, is a bean-sized region known as the *hypothalamus*. The hypothalamus sends out signals that regulate basic processes such as hunger and sex, and affect emotions such as anger. It is also a central control for the biological clock that controls sleep; when the hypothalami of mice are damaged, the mice lose any semblance of orderly or regular sleep.

This man's misfortune also displayed the genetic nature of this sleep disorder. The doctors learned from one of the man's relatives, also a doctor, that in the last six generations of the man's family at least 14 relatives, including his sisters, had died of the same bizarre condition.

Source: "The Case of the Last Coronation," reprinted/adapted from *Hippocrates*, March–April 1988.

Rhythms of Consciousness

Cyclic changes are inherent in the passing of seasons, in weather patterns, in tidal ebbs and flows, and in the rising and setting of the sun. In humans, mood and energy level respond to seasonal shifts, menstruation cycles follow monthly rhythms, and sleep and wakefulness cycles oscillate daily in a **circadian** (Latin for "about a day") **rhythm.** Humans also respond to shorter **ultradian** 90-minute cycles of heightened and lowered brain arousal. The autonomic system of the brain controls the rhythms of heart rate and respiration. The brain itself is a web of neuronal circuitry with a frequency measured in cycles per second (cps) on an EEG (see Chapter 6 for a detailed discussion of EEG). It alternates between periods of brain asynchronicity, usually indicative of an alert brain state, and periods of "altered consciousness" synchronicity, in which groups of neurons oscillate rhythmically. Some of these synchronous oscillations, such as those occurring during sleep, represent normal variations. Others, which occur during seizures and coma, may suggest pathology. Many of the normal internal rhythms of the body and brain—such as sleep, for example—are calibrated in response to external environmental changes such as the light–dark cycle. Scientists do not yet understand a great deal about the complex interplay between the many human rhythms and external environmental rhythms affecting human functioning.

In addition to these questions, neuropsychology is interested in how brain states, measurable via dynamic imaging means such as EEG and PET, correspond to mind states in both ordinary and pathological functioning. In absence seizures, slow-wave synchronous activity abruptly interrupts the normally asynchronous waking state. It would appear, then, that slow synchronous brain activity heralds pathology. But absence seizures in children, which are marked by brief lapses in consciousness, show the same 3 cps synchronous brain waves characteristic of normal delta-stage sleep. The EEGs of people in coma also show this slow synchronous wave. Masters of meditation, however, can produce delta waves and remain seemingly "conscious." Although the EEG can record similar brain states in two different people, mind states and awareness can range considerably. Therefore, similar brain wave frequencies can imply pathologic "unconscious" mind states, normal sleeping mind states, or fully conscious mind states. Although the EEG provides clues as to *whether* one is thinking or not, it does not capture the subjective experience of the mind.

Many interesting questions of consciousness revolve around alertness and level of arousal. We examine sleep in some depth in this chapter because of its rhythmic brain activity and the paradoxical and fascinating nature of the dreaming REM stage. Deep within the hypothalamus, a biological clock—in conjunction with the visual system— calibrates the sleep–wake cycle. A case example illustrates how chaotic sleep and health can become without this clock (see Neuropsychology in Action 13.1). Sleep disorders such as narcolepsy also illustrate the manner in which sleep–wake rhythms may become confused, resulting in daytime sleep intrusions and fragmented nighttime sleep.

Scientists are just beginning to understand the brain mechanisms underlying neuronal rhythm in sleep as well as in seizures. At a neuronal level, neurons and neuronal systems maintain a fine balance between excitatory and inhibitory balance. An individual neuron may receive both excitatory and inhibitory messages from the neurons that synapse on it. The neuron fires or not, depending on how these messages add up. Excitatory and inhibitory neurons may also synapse with each other in a loop and oscillate in their intercommunication. The thalamus, a powerful pacemaker, has afferent and efferent neural connections reaching throughout the cortex. At a cell assembly level, the same sort of oscillation, the *thalamocortical loop,* operates between the thalamus and the cortex. Interestingly, the thalamus appears able

to initiate thalamocortical synchronous oscillations without external input. Although researchers know that peculiarities in the ion channels of thalamic cell membranes allow these cells to generate and sustain a rhythm, it is not clear what triggers this behavior. In general, scientists can describe how certain local groups of cells begin to oscillate, and how certain widespread cortical brain-controlling mechanisms, such as the thalamus, generate rhythm, but why this occurs is a matter of speculation. Studying rhythmic brain activity in behaviors such as sleep and seizures may help elucidate these mechanisms.

The Brain and Mind in Sleep

Is sleep unconscious? As a laptop computer goes "to sleep," it shuts down—it is unresponsive and the hard disk spins down until it is "awakened" again with a touch. But the machine analogy of a steady state does not do justice to the complex ebbs and flows of the sleeping human brain. Sleep is a drifting down into deeper levels of unawareness of the world which then lighten and deepen in a rhythmic pattern during the night. Seemingly unresponsive to the majority of external sensory stimuli, intense emotions, and hallucinations arise created by the spontaneous firings of the brain itself. How conscious are we, or can we be, during sleep? Delta waves at a frequency of 1/2 to 4 cycles per second represent the deepest stage of sleep. Yet what of expert mediators who can produce delta waves and remain conscious? They describe their change in awareness of themselves as progressing from the experience of "self" to a "point of still awareness" (Kenyon, 1994). During REM sleep dreams occur, but people are usually quite oblivious to the fact that they are in a dream state and usually forget the dream. Some people, however, are "lucid" dreamers, knowing they are dreaming during their dream, and able to influence theme and outcome, thoughts and emotions. There is much to learn in the emerging area of brain function during sleep. This section explores how consciousness, awareness, and arousal operate through the window of sleep and dreaming. We discuss the known brain mechanisms that govern levels of arousal through the neurology and physiology of normal sleep, and finally, sleep disorders of particular interest to neuropsychology.

SLEEP ARCHITECTURE

The cycle of brain activity during sleep is embedded within the larger circadian rhythm of wakefulness and sleep. The sleep rhythm is a 90-minute cycle of descending and ascending states of cortical arousal. It is punctuated at the end of each cycle by periods of such intense brain activity that the sleeping brain appears active, almost in a waking state. This general pattern is highly stable across people, although there is much variability in the amount of time spent in each phase, depending on such factors as age, physical condition, and other individual variables.

The two general stages of sleep are known as **REM** (rapid eye movement sleep) and **NREM** (non-REM sleep). Both have characteristic EEG patterns and physiological correlates (see Table 13.1). As discussed in Chapter 6, scientists describe EEG waves in terms of their amplitude, which is a measure of microvoltage, and their frequency or speed, measured as the cycles per second (cps) of a complete wave. Scientists may also describe the overall characterization, or pattern of waves as synchronous or asynchronous (arhythmic), according to the degree or tendency of neural circuits to fire together in rhythm. The EEG provides a dynamic view of activity in the sleeping brain. Figure 13.1 portrays the characteristic EEG

waves and patterns of each stage of sleep. Notice that as EEG slows, wave amplitude correspondingly increases. For each stage of sleep there are characteristic waveforms, such as alpha, theta, and delta, and for REM a form that looks like a sawtooth. In addition, certain forms may be superimposed, such as sleep spindles and K complexes in stage 2 sleep. During the waking state, the neural circuits fire in a characteristic 40 cps, low-voltage desynchronized pattern. Merely closing the eyes starts a shift toward coordinated rhythmic neural circuit oscillation. Synchronized bursts of alpha waves (8–12 cps) appear superimposed on the background of the faster brain rhythm. The person literally descends into sleep as the EEG waves become slower, higher, and more rhythmic with each stage. Finally, in the deepest (stage 4) sleep, EEGs show 50% or more delta waves. This high-amplitude (100–200 microvolts) slow-wave (0.5–2 cps) rhythm indicates that the cortical circuits are oscillating at the slowest periodicity. It is not surprising that if one is awakened from stage 4 sleep, which is likely to occur around 60 minutes after sleep onset, one takes several minutes to recover from deep-sleep grogginess.

NREM and REM sleep represent different states of consciousness. Progressing through the stages of NREM sleep, the person becomes increasingly difficult to arouse. It takes a bit of commotion to wake someone from stage 4 NREM sleep. The brain is less active and becomes less capable of organized activity. Some individuals may vocalize, but this speech usually does not seem logical. Some motor behavior may occur as well, and sleepwalking sometimes accompanies NREM sleep. Although NREM sleep is associated with a sleeping brain, curiously the body is "awake," twitching and turning. Sometimes the twitching is so strong that the person may kick. This is called **nocturnal myoclonus** (restless leg syndrome) and can be so strong that it may wake the person up.

After the first descent into deep sleep, there is a progressive lightening that culminates at 90 minutes after sleep onset in the first REM period (named for the prominence of rapid eye movements). REM sleep shows many contrasts with NREM sleep (see Table 13.2 on p. 412). The most striking feature is REM sleep's relatively high level of alertness, much like stage 1 sleep. In fact, the first time sleep researchers measured REM sleep via EEG they thought the subject had awakened.

Table 13.1	**EEG Sleep Stage Characteristics in Adults**			
Stage	Frequency (cps)	Amplitude (microvolts)	Waveform	% Time
NREM				
1	4–8	50–100	Alpha, theta	5
2	8–15	50–150	Theta, sleep spindle, K complex	45
3	2–4	100–150	20–50% delta	12
4	0.5–2	100–200	>50% delta	13
REM	Mixed	50–100	"sawtooth"	25

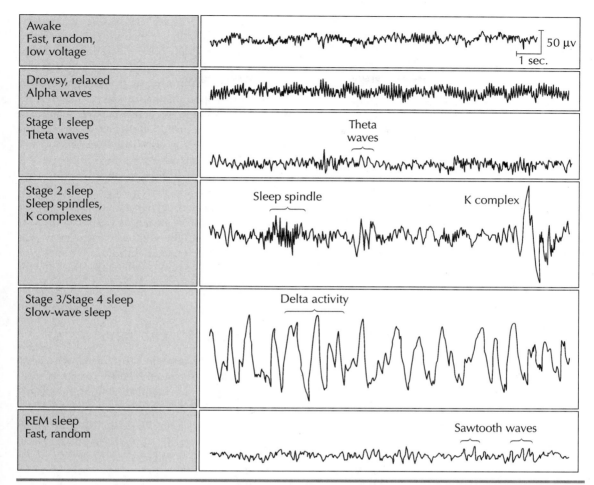

Awake Fast, random, low voltage	
Drowsy, relaxed Alpha waves	
Stage 1 sleep Theta waves	Theta waves
Stage 2 sleep Sleep spindles, K complexes	Sleep spindle K complex
Stage 3/Stage 4 sleep Slow-wave sleep	Delta activity
REM sleep Fast, random	Sawtooth waves

Figure 13.1 EEG patterns representative of stages of sleep. As a person moves into deeper stages of sleep, the characteristic EEG pattern moves from low-amplitude fast waves to high-amplitude slow waves. REM sleep more closely resembles waking. (From James S. Nairne, *The Adaptive Mind*, Pacific Grove, CA: Brooks/Cole, 1997, p. 216, Figure 6.5. Adapted from P. Hauri, *Current Concepts: The Sleep Disorders*, Peapack, NJ: Pharmacia & Upjohn, Inc. 1982. Reprinted by permission of the author and publisher)

The characteristic REM EEG pattern of low-voltage, random, fast "sawtooth" waves is a dynamic representation of the sleeper's internally generated heightened cortical arousal is associated with intensive processing of the internal mind state of dreaming. The first REM period may be quite short, lasting less than five minutes. Thus in REM sleep the brain is active and seemingly awake. A person awakened during REM sleep often reports dreams. However, the body is immobile during REM sleep. In fact, all voluntary muscles are temporarily "paralyzed" from the neck down. Both females and males show sexual response (lubrication or erection). As the night progresses, Figure 13.2 (p. 412) illustrates how REM periods lengthen at the end of each 90-minute cycle. Correspondingly, stages 3 and 4 sleep taper off in the early morning hours. In general, normal sleepers spend 75% in NREM sleep and 25% in REM sleep over a night's sleep.

What we have just described is normal adult sleep. Variability in this cycle depends on age and several

Table 13.2 *Comparison of NREM and REM Sleep Events*

Event	NREM	REM
Occurrence	> in first half of night	> in second half of night
Eye movement	Slow, rolling	Rapid, conjugate
Mentation	Short, ordinary, Fragmented	Dreams Vivid, emotional
Sensory processing	Lowered	Inhibited
Motor response	Relaxed	Atonic Benign paralysis
Autonomic nervous system variability	Low	High
GSR variability	High	Low
CNS temperature	Decreases	Increases
Sexual response	Low	High
Neurotransmitter activity		
Aminergic	High	Low
Cholinergic acetylcholine	Low	High
Hormonal secretion rate		
Growth hormone	High	Low
Parathyroid hormone	High	Low
Lutenizing hormone	Low	High

other factors (see Figure 13.3). Infants, in contrast, spend 50% of their sleep time in REM sleep, and a large proportion of their NREM sleep in stage 4 sleep. By late middle age most people have lost all of this physiologically restorative Stage 4 sleep and retain only a small proportion of REM sleep. Why this tremendous variation in the developmental qualities of sleep? The answer may lie in the functions various types of sleep serve in growth and development.

Among other phasic events, the pituitary, under control of the hypothalamus, releases somatotrophin (growth hormone) during Stage 4 sleep, and the immune system is particularly active. During rapid growth and development, stage 4 sleep may be more necessary. Stage 4 sleep is often termed *restorative sleep* because it also increases in adults in response to intense physical exertion. At older ages this growth-and-tissue-repair function of growth hormone becomes less available.

SLEEP ANATOMY AND PHYSIOLOGY

Circadian clocks (from the Latin for "about a day," as noted earlier), which set the daily pattern of sleep and wakefulness, are intrinsic to most living organisms. This clock may have been patterned in ancient times and embedded in DNA as all life on earth

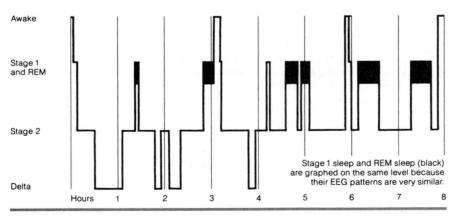

Figure 13.2 Polysomnograph of a typical night of adult sleep. At the beginning of the night, REM periods (in black) are short, and delta sleep (stages 3 and 4) is longer. As the night progresses, delta periods become shorter and REM periods become longer. (From P. Hauri, *Current Concepts: The Sleep Disorders,* Peapack, NJ: Pharmacia & Upjohn, Inc. 1977, p. 8, Figure 2. Reprinted by permission of the author and publisher)

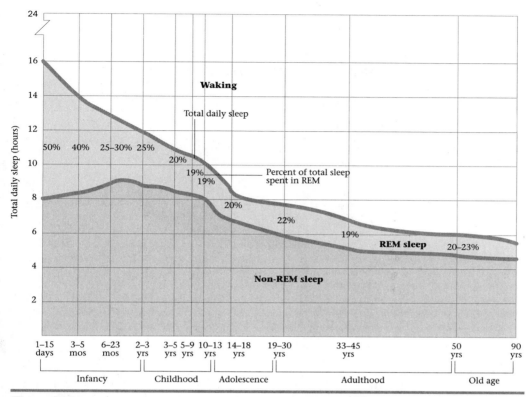

Figure 13.3 Average changes in sleep stage percentages over the life span. Average daily sleep stage percentages are highest in infancy, decline during childhood, and then are fairly stable throughout middle adulthood. (From W. Weiten, *Psychology: Themes and Variations,* 4th ed., Pacific Grove, CA: Brooks/Cole, 1998, Figure 5.8, p. 187. Originally from H. P. Roffwarg, J. N. Muzio, W. C. Dement, Ontogenetic development of human sleep–dream cycle. *Science, 152,* 604–619. Adapted with permission of the authors)

learned to respond to the rhythms of the cycles of days, months, seasons, and years. Even plants have a rudimentary circadian triggering mechanism. The heliotrope folds its leaves at night and opens them in the morning, but it is not directly guided by the light of the sun. Even in a dark room it continues opening and closing, according to daily cycles, according to some internal timing mechanism.

In humans, and all mammals, a more specialized circadian clock nestles in the **suprachiasmic nucleus (SCN)** of the hypothalamus. If the SCN is removed from the brain, the neurons continue to fire according to the programmed daily rhythms. However, if the SCN were totally dependent on genetic program-

ming, what would happen when traveling to the other side of the world? The daily internal clock must have a way to resynchronize according to the light–dark cycle. That indeed is the case. In fact, if left without any natural light cues, humans will revert to about 25-hour-per-day cycles of waking and sleeping. Natural light, or in some cases an alarm clock, apparently resynchronizes the human circadian clock each day for functioning in accord with a 24-hour day. The two halves of the SCN lie just above the optic chiasm and receive light via neural input from the two visual fields as they cross hemispheres to the opposite sides of the brain (see Figure 13.4). When this internal clock runs amok, sleep patterns can be greatly,

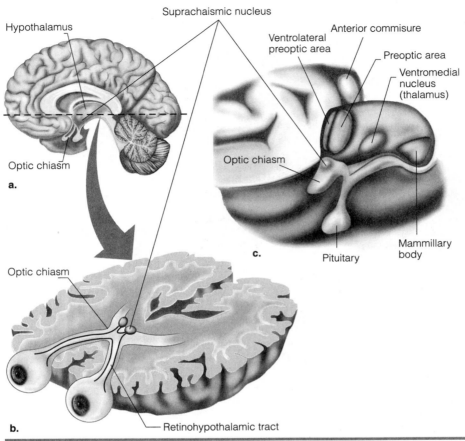

Figure 13.4 The suprachiasmic nucleus (SCN) of the hypothalamus. A (a) sagittal and (b) horizontal section of the human brain showing the SCN in relationship to the optic chiasm; (c) exploded view of the hypothalamus showing the SCN in relation to other nuclei. (Adapted from [a] James W. Kalat, *Biological Psychology*, 6th ed., Pacific Grove, CA: Brooks/Cole, 1998, Figure 9.6c; [b, c] modified from P. J. Pinel and M. Edwards, *A Colorful Introduction to the Anatomy of the Human Brain*, p. 195, Figure 11.6. Copyright © 1998 by Allyn & Bacon. Reprinted by permission)

even fatally disrupted (see Neuropsychology in Action 13.1).

Scientists do not yet know how the human circadian clocks signal sleep onset each night and awakening each morning—perhaps through qualitatively different signals, or via a gradual change in the release of neurotransmitter molecules. Clifford Saper, of Harvard, and his colleagues (Sheim, Shiromani, McCarley, & Saper, 1996) have suggested that the ventrolateral preoptic (VLPO) area of the hypothalamus may be the "master switch" to arousal (see Figure 13.3). Researchers have observed this somnolence center to be the only brain center that is more active during sleep than wakefulness. Other researchers have identified a peptide molecule named "factor S" and claim it may be one of the neurotransmitters most directly responsible for setting off the downward drift into sleepiness. Injected into the hypothalamus, factor S induces sleep and raises body temperature. It also appears to trigger the release of "interleukin 1," which raises many interesting questions about the immunoprotective function of sleep. This collective evidence points to a strong role for the hypothalamus as the "biological sandman."

When activated, the hypothalamus sends its molecular message to the thalamus and the reticular activating system of the lower brain stem. Gradually, the brain moves from a state of processing external sensory information to a closing off of inputs from vision, hearing, and touch. During alertness, the thalamus relays inputs from most sensory systems, except for smell. The thalamus constantly communicates with the cortex through a feedback system of millions of thalamocortical loops. With high alertness, neuronal firing is frequent and finely tuned. Any external sensory "noise" against this background is easily picked up because the brain discriminates it from the high-frequency background rhythm by its irregularity or novelty. As alertness drops, at a certain point the thalamocortical loops start oscillating to their own rhythm, in a sort of internal dance between the thalamus and the cortex.

On an EEG, this is also when the sleep spindles (12–14 cycles per second) emerge, typical of stage 2 sleep. With the slowed frequency of thalamocortical firing, orientation to and processing of external stimuli is less likely. The brain turns inward, attention drifts, and the sleeper becomes oblivious to his or her surroundings. Currently, the thalamocortical loop stands as the primary mechanism in sleep onset and in maintenance of lowered attention to external stimuli. As sleep continues to deepen, responsiveness to the outward environment lessens even further. Yet many parents of newborns apparently maintain vigilance to their baby's stirrings while sleeping. Perhaps future research will reveal if another mechanism monitors the environment during sleep, or if sleep remains lighter for those who must remain alert. Animals in the wild, who must retain more alertness to danger, show lighter and more fragmented sleep than zoo and domestic animals. Perhaps this is also the case with humans.

THE RETICULAR ACTIVATING SYSTEM AND REM SLEEP

Approximately every 90 minutes, and lengthening throughout the night, a sleeper enters stage REM sleep. The cortical activity of high-frequency sawtooth EEG waves in the theta range nearly resembles a waking brain state, yet the sleeper is turned inward. The view is an internal movie as scenes and images flash by and fall away. Willful movement is impossible, because the motor neurons have temporarily lost communication with the spinal cord. Sensation from the outside world is turned down to its lowest point. For all practical purposes, more than any other stage of sleep, the sleeper is in a cocoon, insulated from the outside world and unable to act on it, yet with a very active mind. What are the brain mechanisms responsible for this paradox? Although science does not yet understand the complete workings of REM sleep, it is evident that the **reticular activating system (RAS)** is the primary mechanism for turning REM sleep on and off. In this section we discuss both the mechanical aspects and the chemical transmitters that play a role in REM sleep.

The RAS maintains cortical arousal. It arises from deep within the brain stem (see Figure 13.5). During wakefulness, the high activity in the ascending RAS stimulates the brain via projections into many different neurologic systems in the cortex. The nuclei of the gigantocellular tegmental field (GTF) located in the higher pons appear to generate these brain waves. Left unchecked, they fire spontaneously producing a

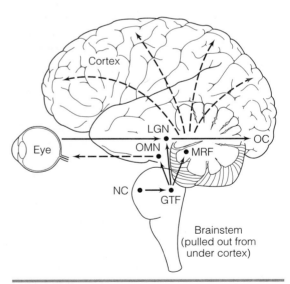

Figure 13.5 Schematic diagram of the REM system. OMN = oculomotor nuclei; MRF = midbrain reticular formation. (From P. Hauri, *Current Concepts: The Sleep Disorders*, Peapack, NJ: Pharmacia & Upjohn, Inc. 1977, p. 15, Figure 5. Reprinted by permission of the author and publisher)

high level of activity. During stages 1 and 2 the nucleus cereleus (NC) becomes active and acts as an inhibitory control on the GTF, dampening the firing. Cortical activation continues to slow through stages 3 and 4. Then, during REM sleep the NC releases its inhibition of the GTF, leaving it free to activate again, sending spikes through the cortex and activating the cortex into a higher level of arousal. One particular set of discharges are termed PGO spikes because they travel from the pons (P) to the lateral geniculate nucleus (LGN) of the thalamus to the occipital cortex (OC). The lateral geniculate nucleus is part of the visual pathway from the retina to the occipital cortex. The internally generated PGO spikes intercept this pathway midway. Interestingly, the PGO spikes fire in pulsating bursts. This is an additional indication that the thalamus may be synchronizing brain rhythms. Although it also happens during waking hours, PGO bursts are more active in REM sleep. The stimulation that finally reaches the occipital cortex gives rise to dream images and the corresponding rapid REM characteristic of this stage. The occipital lobes are therefore excited without external visual input. Given this scenario, it is curious that eyes move. But they appear somehow calibrated to move in conjunction with scene changes of dreams. Researchers think that bursts from the pons also stimulate nearby oculomotor neurons, resulting in corresponding eye movements (Hobson, 1995).

Areas other than the occipital lobes also activate during REM sleep. In rats, rabbits, and cats, single-neuron recording has demonstrated that the theta rhythm emanates from the hippocampus; specifically in the dentate gyrus and the entorhinal cortex (Winson, 1972). However, the signal to activate the theta rhythm has its trigger in the brain stem within the RAS. This hippocampal activation during REM sleep has ramifications for proposing a role for memory within REM sleep. We discuss this issue further in considering the functions of REM sleep.

Many of the REM sleep occurrences listed in Table 13.2 have brain stem mechanisms. "Sleep paralysis" occurs because it is simply too dangerous to act out dreams. Although we may see or sense movement in dreams, through active central motor neuronal activity, the motor neurons responsible for actually carrying out the action are "turned off" at the level of the spinal cord. The active reticular firing in the medulla during REM sleep inhibits the spinal motor pathways. This greatly reduces muscle tone *(atonia),* and for all practical purposes paralyzes the sleeper. When researchers surgically turned off cats' medullar inhibitory mechanism, the cats actually became physically active during REM. They stalked, attacked, hissed, and otherwise acted out the drama of their dreams.

REM sleep dampens external sensory stimulation. The pontine excitement also inhibits peripheral nerve pathways where they synapse with the spinal cord. During all stages of sleep, after an initial rise in the first two hours, respiration rate and body temperature gradually diminish. Body movement and systolic blood pressure also increase during the night. These changes continue during REM but tend to fluctuate more than during NREM sleep. As the night progresses and REM periods lengthen, fluctuations become more variable from REM period to REM period.

As with all behavior, REM sleep combines structural and functional processes. The neurophysiological processes provide the fuel for the mechanical processes we have just discussed. Many brain neurotransmitters decline only slightly during REM sleep. The question is, Do certain neurotransmitters operate differently during REM sleep? Apparently so. Within the locus ceruleus researchers have observed a cluster of neurons, which they labeled "REM off" cells, which completely stop firing during REM sleep (Hobson, 1995). Because these cells otherwise release norepinephrine and serotonin, the consequence is a relative unavailability of these substances to the brain during REM. J. Alan Hobson (1995) hypothesizes that the lowering of these aminergic transmitters plays a role in the "lack of self-reflective awareness, disorientation, and logical fallacy" in verbal reports of dreaming during REM sleep. Hobson also postulates that serotonin and norepinephrine act as long-term neuromodulators on the brain. As NREM sleep commences, "REM off" cells begin to slow their firing rate, with the functional result of slowly releasing their hold on the "rational" cortex. The mind becomes more disinhibited during sleep, but is especially free to wander during REM owing to a now complete lack of aminergic transmission. At the end of the REM cycle, the cells "turn on," activating at a higher level of serotonin and nor-epinephrine. This level then tapers off, leading to the next REM period. From this information, it is possible to speculate that lengthening REM periods during the night may result from progressively lower levels of aminergic neurotransmitter release during the night.

Another neurotransmitter of interest in REM sleep is acetylcholine (ACh). Interestingly, ACh increases during REM sleep in animals and can trigger "spectacularly long and intense" REM periods when administered in high doses. As we discussed in previous chapters, ACh is important in facilitating memory processing. We take up REM's role in memory consolidation in the next section.

FUNCTIONS OF REM SLEEP

Scientists know that slow-wave delta sleep is physically restorative, but the debate over the purpose of REM sleep has ranged from postulations that it serves as a type of mental "garbage dump," to Freud's assertion that dreams are the "royal road to the unconscious." Science is now aware of at least two behavioral functions that REM sleep may serve. The first is memory consolidation. The second is the intrapsychic function of dreaming. With a nod to Freud, neuropsychologists now conceptualize the psychological function of dreaming somewhat differently from Freud. Because scientists have again blessed the study of personal internal conscious processes, the study of dream function is once more opening up. Next we introduce an area of study that is likely to provide many insights into the functioning of the conscious and subconscious minds.

Memory Consolidation and REM Sleep

The physiological means by which long-term memory storage occurs is most likely through long-term potentiation (LTP) of special glutamate neurotransmitter receptors (NMDA receptors) in the hippocampus. Memory consolidation may also be inhibited by GABA (see Neuropsychology in Action 13.2). The hippocampus actively produces theta waves during REM sleep, as well as during stage 1 and 2 sleep. The important link between sleep and memory is

that LTP in the hippocampus occurs during the production of theta rhythms (Larson & Lynch, 1986). Researchers have long thought that memory consolidates during sleep, because people can remember more after sleep. Sleeping pills may interfere with this process. However, it has been difficult to know if sleep or REM itself accounts for the memory boost, or if people just remember better when other information doesn't interfere. Now animal and human experiments have provided more evidence that memory is processed during sleep. Using rats, a team of researchers have recorded from individual neurons of the hippocampus (Pavlides & Winson, 1989). While the rats were awake, and moving about learning their position, only specific spatial coding neurons fired. Later during sleep, and particularly during production of the theta rhythm, these same neurons, and *only* these same neurons, fired at an even higher rate than during waking learning. This finding suggests that rats were reprocessing and strengthening the information during sleep.

In another experiment, a group of Israeli researchers studied memory consolidation and sleep under three different conditions. The task involved having to identify perceptual targets embedded in a visually noisy background. With learning and practice, people can usually improve their speed in picking out targets. In the first condition, researchers let people sleep normally after their initial practice session. In the second condition, researchers awakened people each time they entered REM sleep, effectively depriving them of REM sleep. In the same manner, in the third condition researchers deprived people of delta sleep within stages 3 and 4. The two groups that were allowed REM sleep showed enhanced task learning on awakening. All those who underwent REM sleep deprivation, in contrast, showed either less improvement or an actual decrement in performance (Karni, Tanne, Rubenstein, Askenasy, & Sagi, 1994). Together, the findings from both animal and human research suggest that stage REM sleep plays a role in memory consolidation. However, whether REM plays a unique role in memory consolidation is still a matter of debate. This is a promising area of research for neuropsychologists and neuroscientists interested in the relationships among REM, ACh, and hippocampal consolidation through LTP.

Neuropsychology in Action 13.2

Sleep, Memory, and Sleeping Pills

by J. Catesby Ware Ph.D., Professor, Departments of Medicine and Psychiatry, Eastern Virginia Medical School, Director, Sleep Disorders Center for Adults and Children, Sentara Norfolk General Hospital, Norfolk, Virginia.

Several years ago, a friend from California flew to New York to give an invited talk. He was anxious because at least one big name in his field was to be present with data that did not support his work. He arrived in New York at 5 P.M.; made it to the hotel by 6 P.M.; returned from dinner at 9 P.M.; reviewed his presentation scheduled for the next morning, and was in bed by 11 P.M. After tossing and turning for 45 minutes, he took the then recommended dose of a short-acting sleeping pill, 0.5 mg of triazolam (Halcion). After a half an hour of continuing wakefulness and becoming more worried that he would not give a good presentation if he got no sleep, he took an additional 0.25 mg of triazolam. He dosed briefly but woke up at 1 A.M. and took a third dose of triazolam, 0.25 mg. Soon thereafter he fell asleep and slept soundly the rest of the night.

The next day as he was leaving the conference in the late afternoon, a graduate student stopped him with a question about his presentation. My friend was alarmed to realize that not only did he not remember giving his presentation, he remembered little about his day at the conference. He then surprised the gradu-ate student by asking her about what he had said. According to her, he had given a well-reasoned and well-received presentation. He had responded to questions appropriately and acted normally.

My friend had experienced anterograde amnesia. Anterograde amnesia is the inability to remember what happens after a particular event, in this case, taking a large dose of a sleeping pill. When a patient takes a sleeping pill before bed and then does not remember awakening during the night, the usual interpretation is that the sleeping pill produced good sleep. Another possibility is that the sleeping pill abolished the memory of wakefulness and changed sleep very little. A person who does not remember being awake is less likely to complain of poor sleep.

Triazolam is in a family of drugs referred to as **benzodiazepines.** Physicians prescribe them primarily as sleeping and antianxiety medications. Although they are relatively safe, they have a number of potential side effects, including the memory problem. In some cases, anterograde amnesia actually may benefit patients, physicians, and hospitals. For example, a physician performing a colonoscopy, a procedure that entails inserting a tube through the rectum into the large intestine, may use the drug midazolam (Versed) to relax the patient. An unspoken benefit is that the patient is less likely to recall the unpleasantness of the procedure and be less hesitant to have a repeat procedure if needed later. Hospital administrators are pleased because the patient is less likely to talk about any unpleasant hospital experience. Some people use benzodiazepines for sinister and illegal purposes. The "date rape drug" flunitrazepam (Rohypnol) is so called, at least in part, because victims may have no recollection of what occurred. Mixing a large dose of flunitrazepam surreptitiously in a drink produces grogginess, sedation, and perhaps sleep. Like alcohol, it may also produce disinhibition. Victims may offer little resistance and have little or no recollection of what occurred.

My first experience with anterograde amnesia was in the late 1970s at Baylor College of Medicine. We were testing a new benzodiazepine drug for its effects on sleep. Its premarketing name was CG3033, one of the more than 3000 benzodiazepine-type drugs developed.

As more specific EEG mapping and functional brain-imaging techniques become widely employed in basic research, science will be able to look much more closely at the potential workings of memory, and possibly other cognitive functions, during sleep. A question that must be answered is, What functional mechanism is REM sleep serving in the devel-opment of the organism? Newborns spend half their sleeping time in this stage. REM plummets and can be nonexistent in old age. Is this also related to memory functioning? Sleep researcher Johnathon Winson thinks the changes in REM relate to a developmental trend in the need to build a basic foundation of memory in the first few years of life. It may even stimu-

The first marketed was chlordiazepoxide (Librium) in the 1960s. Our subjects, medical students, took the drug before going to bed in the Sleep Disorders Center. We attached sensors to monitor brain waves, eye movements, muscle tension, and heart rate. The students slept well except for less deep sleep than normal and slightly less REM sleep. All got up the next morning with no more difficulty than most young adults and left the center for their day of classes. Not until the following day did I begin to hear from them and realize that we had a problem. Reactions varied from being upset and frightened, to puzzled over the lack of any recollection of what they had done during the day after they left the center. I became concerned over the possibility that we had damaged the memory of several bright young medical students. Reports from their friends indicated that some acted normally, some dozed in class (perhaps the norm for medical students), and one slept most of the day in the student lounge. The drug CG3033 never reached the market. At the time we assumed it had unique effects on memory. Now I suspect that CG3033 probably differed little from other benzodiazepines and that our mistake was giving too large a dose. The drug remained active in the body during the next day and consequently affected memory of the day's events.

Benzodiazepine medications and some new nonbenzodiazepine sleeping pills, such as zolpidem (Ambien), facilitate activity of the major inhibitory neurotransmitter, gamma-aminobutyric acid (GABA). All benzodiazepines appear capable of suppressing recall of what occurred while the drug was in the body. Why? One possibility is that the amnesia stems from a state dependency. If that is correct, recreating the same physiological/pharmacological state by readministering the drug might have helped the students recall their missing day of medical school. That would suggest that the memory problem was one of retrieval rather than storage. A second possibility is that sedated subjects may pay less attention to detail and therefore have less information to recall. The authors of one recent study using aversive learning in rats, found that injecting a drug that blocks GABA (a GABAergic antagonist) into the amygdala blocked the memory-impairing effects of the benzodiazepine midazolam (Dickinson-Anson & McGaugh, 1997). In light of other studies, they interpreted their data as indicating that benzodiazepines disrupted memory consolidation.

Despite problems, benzodiazepine medications are remarkably safe compared to prebenzodiazepine drugs. Unlike earlier sleeping pills, an overdose of a benzodiazepine alone is not lethal. Primarily because of safety issues, physicians prescribe benzodiazepine medications, or those with effects mediated through the benzodiazepine pathways, more commonly than other types of sleeping pills. However, all benzodiazepines may produce dose- and concentration-dependent sedation, drowsiness, performance impairment, amnesia, and disinhibition. Because the person taking the drug may not recognize these effects, patients and their families need to know about these potential problems.

Although rare, benzodiazepines may have dramatic and lethal side effects. Several years ago in a neighboring town of Virginia Beach, one that ranks among the most crime-free U.S. cities, a physician gave an older woman a benzodiazepine sleeping pill. She took the prescribed dose and went to bed early. Her husband of many years fell asleep on the couch watching TV. Later she got out of bed and went into the kitchen. Then, with a butcher knife, she stabbed her husband to death on the couch. There was no motive and no other evidence of marital discord. She denied killing her husband and acted appropriately shocked and distraught. The evidence, however, was clear. In court, her lawyer claimed that the drug dose was too large, resulting in disinhibition and anterograde amnesia. Nevertheless, the jury found her guilty. In this case, the real problem was ignorance of sleep and sleeping medications. Her physician administered a dose too high for an elderly woman, and more importantly, did not appear to know how to deal with her insomnia through behavioral treatments.

---

late nerve growth. A question for future exploration is whether REM specifically enhances memory or whether it acts as a more general cognitive enhancer.

The Dreaming Mind

The aspects of consciousness discussed thus far involve the mind looking out. Dreams reflect the mind looking in. There is almost no physical input or output. Brains and minds are temporarily suspended from bodies. This is an amazing state, seemingly disjointed and illogical. Except for those who are "lucid" dreamers, dreaming minds wander from scene to scene with no conscious guidance. Dreamers are detached from their own self-consciousness and more critical selves.

Dreams may be intensely emotional to strangely devoid of emotion. After a history of much debate on the function that dreams may serve, scientists are returning to the premise that dreams have a psychological core.

Aspects of the mind state of dreams may correlate with the physical aspects of a brain temporarily divorced from a body. Noted sleep researcher J. Alan Hobson (1995) has suggested that dreamers may feel they move effortlessly during dream states because they are being moved or guided by internally generated states and active central motor neurons. Perhaps in some measure, dream experiences of floating or flying also result from the brain being allowed to "float free" from the body, or perhaps in combination with, as Hobson suggests, spontaneous stimulation of orientation and position control centers in the brain. Hobson notices that when dreamers try to "will" dream movement while trying to escape from a pursuer, their feet and bodies may become leaden because of the conflicting motor messages of "voluntarily commanded movement (saying go) and the involuntarily clamped muscles (saying stop)." He further suggests that this standoff may suddenly break off the dream, thrusting the person into wakefulness and vivid dream recall. Awakening from a particular terrifying dream is called a "sleep anxiety attack." In fact, a large percentage of reported dreams are "hostile," and the most frequent themes are those of being chased and falling.

There are probably many other correspondences between brain–body states and mind states in dreaming. This is an interesting area of study in its own right, and work in it will help to explain "how" people dream. Another question fundamental to understanding consciousness is "why" people dream. The brain activity occurring during REM sleep, such as memory consolidation, does not require conscious awareness. Biological functions of the brain could all occur without being brought to waking attention. Many dreams are not recalled. But why do some dreams bubble to the surface? This has been a matter of theoretical interest since Freud's revolutionary *The Interpretation of Dreams,* written in 1899. Since Freud's time, the history of dream theory has gone through a cycle from Freud's ideas that dreams represented unconscious sexual and aggressive urges, to the behaviorist movement's totally turning away from the study of subjective states. Francis Crick's utilitarian housekeeping notion that dreams may just be the images that float by as the brain rids itself of the day's mental garbage suggests that dreaming is nothing more than a random firing of neurons. But many dream researchers have come back to a version of psychological interpretations.

Freud laid some of the basic groundwork in thinking about the psychological function of dreams from which other theories could spring. Today, most dream theorists do not attribute the same negative sexual and aggressive motivations to dream images that Freud did, but some of his methods and ideas may still be useful in uncovering the psychological meaning of dreams for the dreamer. With expansion from recent conceptualizations, researchers may be closer to a neuropsychological understanding of dreaming. Freud divided mental processing into conscious and unconscious processes. He saw unconscious processes as primitive, ancient, and disguised. Dreams, he felt, arose from these "unconscious" areas of the brain. This conceptualization is not unlike recent ideas of explicit versus implicit information processing. That which is explicit is available to verbal conscious awareness. However, as in memory processing and in some disorders such as neglect, a level of processing and recognition may exist outside conscious awareness. Is this not unlike the unconscious or the subconscious? Freud did not have the ability to look deep into the brain, but his ideas that unconscious thoughts emerge from more primitive areas of the brain are not inconsistent with theories of implicit processing taking place in the more primitive subcortical and limbic centers of the brain.

Perhaps where modern dream interpretive approaches have advanced most is in moving away from Freud's idea that even remembered dream content is unavailable psychologically to the dreamer unless interpreted by someone, such as an analyst, who can slice through the manifest content, defense mechanisms, and symbols, to uncover the latent meaning. This is not to say that the perspectives of others regarding the meaning of one's dreams are useless. In fact, such perspectives may be quite revealing and helpful. However, some of the greatest understanding available of the meaning in a dream involves self-interpretation in light of personal current life circumstances. After all, the dream was generated by the person dreaming it. Self-interpretation may involve not only the content, but the associated emotion that the dream invokes.

Troubling life circumstances provide the fodder for sleep researcher Rosalind Cartwright (Cartwright, Lloyd, Knight, & Trenholme, 1984; Cartwright, Kavits, Eastman, & Wood, 1991). Her volunteers, all going through separation or divorce, agreed to go through psychological testing that examined coping styles, and consented to be awakened during REM sleep to report their dreams. Cartwright found that dream content and topics differed among subjects, but the themes were congruent with the waking response to the problem. Indeed, the content and themes of dreams may be useful in helping solve many personal problems. But sometimes dreams accompany remarkable changes in waking life. We once treated a patient for depression, who was also a smoker trying to kick the habit. One therapy session he reported a dramatic dream he had had. In his dream his whole body was turned grotesquely inside out, showing his lung, which was full of tumors and pus, to the outside world. After this dream the patient quit smoking.

An interesting exercise in exploring your own "dream consciousness" is to keep a dream journal for collecting and analyzing the content and themes of your dreams. What sensory processes are operating? Do you see, hear, feel, taste, or smell things in your dreams? As we mentioned earlier, sleep researcher J. Alan Hobson reminds us that the absurdity of dreams and the temporary "impairment" of judgment and cognition occurring during dreaming are very common phenomena. Temporary disinhibition of the cortex may very well represent a physiological disconnection of aspects of the frontal lobes from other cortical and limbic centers. This may help to explain our often bizarre logic and lack of self-reflection during dreams. But what of those brain-impaired individuals who have structural damage resulting in waking disinhibition. Will we find that their dreams are even more disinhibited? This is a question for future research.

SLEEP DISORDERS

For most people, sleep is a pleasurable event. For some people, however, sleeping can become a medical emergency, as during sleep apnea, or intrude into wakefulness, as in narcolepsy.

Sleep Apnea

Sleep apnea has become the most common disorder the sleep literature describes and the most common presenting problem sleep disorder centers evaluate (Guilleminault, 1982). **Sleep apnea syndrome (SAS)** is a serious disorder resulting from frequent episodes of apnea (cessation of airflow) during sleep. **Apnea** literally means "lack of breath." It is normal for muscles to relax during REM sleep. In some people, however, excessive muscle relaxation may disrupt breathing. The sleep apnea patient may actually stop breathing while asleep. This of course presents an immediate crisis for the body, because of the danger of hypoxia and of increased rapid heart rate and blood pressure. The apnea finally stops when, in an effort to breathe, the patient arouses, gasping for air. Each gasp for air is associated with a miniawakening as recorded on the EEG. If repeated apnea and awakening occur more than five times an hour, the patient is diagnosed with sleep apnea (see Figure 13.6 on p. 422).

SAS patients may actually experience hundreds of apnea episodes per night, lasting up to a minute or longer. Serious cases may show over 500 apneas per night each one lasting over 10 to 120 seconds and terminating with at least partial arousal. Besides markedly disrupted sleep characterized by a significant absence of the normal progression of sleep stages, dangerously low levels of oxygen to the brain may result. Apnea periods usually produce drops in sleep-related blood oxyhemoglobin saturation and increases in carbon dioxide. This condition, known as **hypoxia,** is associated with below-average levels of oxygenated blood, often below 60% (normal is 95%). These changes have a profound impact on numerous body systems. It is impossible to hold one's breath indefinitely, even when a person is sleeping. Essentially, a reflex controls breathing. But in young children this reflex has not yet developed, and cessation of breathing during

Neuropsychology in Action 13.3

Lucid Dreaming: A Paradox of Consciousness

by Mary V. Spiers

Often when one is asleep, there is something in consciousness which declares that what then presents itself is but a dream.

— *Aristotle*

Can one be simultaneously conscious and dreaming? Although an ancient phenomenon, documented in stories throughout history, lucid dreaming has only recently caught the attention of scientists who are exploring the frontiers of human consciousness. Throughout history, most of the major religions have used lucid dreaming as a spiritual practice. Examples within Christianity, Islam, Hinduism, and Tibetan Buddhism show how to use lucid dreaming as a path to enlightenment. The assertions are that the meditative masters can maintain conscious awareness throughout sleep. This ability may emanate from incredible mental control in waking life and from long years of practice in the meditative arts. However, many ordinary people also report lucid dreams. Children have lucid

dreams more naturally, without special training, but prevalence declines with age. Among 10-year-olds, 63% in one study reported lucid dreaming on a monthly basis, 58% of 11-year-olds and 36% of 12-year-olds (Armstrong-Hickey, 1991).

Most dreams occur in a state of unawareness of their illusory nature. In fact, sleep itself is generally characterized as unconscious. **Lucid dreaming** is the ability, while dreaming, to become conscious of the fact that one is in a dream state. The following is a description of the first lucid dream of one man:

> I was standing in a field in an open area when my wife pointed in the direction of the sunset. I looked at it and thought, "How odd; I've never seen colors like that before." Then it dawned on me: "I must be dreaming!" Never had I experienced such clarity and perception—the colors were so beautiful and the sense of freedom so exhilarating that I started racing through this beautiful golden wheat field waving

my hands in the air and yelling at the top of my voice, "I'm dreaming! I'm dreaming!" Suddenly, I started to lose the dream; it must have been the excitement. I instantly woke up. As it dawned on me what had just happened, I woke my wife and said, "I did it, I did it!" I was conscious within the dream state and I'll never be the same. Funny isn't it? How a taste of it can affect one like that. It's the freedom, I guess; we see that we truly are in control of our own universe. (LaBerge, 1990, pp. 1–2)

At once it is evident that lucid dreams differ from ordinary dreams. Lucid dreamers typically report vivid sensation and heightened imagery and clarity, not only visual sensation, but auditory and kinesthetic as well. Hearing music, seeing bright light, and flying are common. Joy and exhilaration often distinguish these dreams. What often triggers lucidity is awareness of inconsistency or oddity. The dreamer abruptly shifts into conscious awareness, sometimes ac-

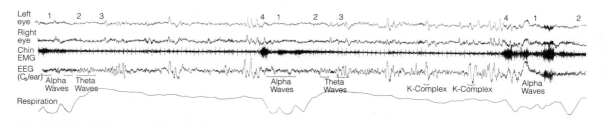

Figure 13.6 An EEG recorded episode of sleep apnea. The patient is fully awake at point 1 (EEG alpha waves). At point 2 he is starting to fall asleep (EEG theta waves). At point 3 the patient is fully asleep (notice the relaxation of the chin EMG (electromyogram) and absence of breathing). At point 4 the patient awakens and breathing resumes. The cycle then repeats. (From P. Hauri, *Current Concepts: The Sleep Disorders*, Peapack, NJ: Pharmacia & Upjohn, Inc. 1977, foldout. Reprinted by permission of the author and publisher)

companied by a feeling of mind expansion and greater self-knowledge. What is interesting in comparison to ordinary dreams is that lucid dreams are not disjointed, lacking in judgment, or irrational. The dreamer has control and free will in the sense of deciding where to go and what to do, but cannot totally control the plot or outcome. For example, the dreamer may decide to travel to a certain place or meet various people, but may be surprised by what occurs. The person may also decide to use the dream to face problems of living, which has ramifications for the study of lucid dreams in a healing or therapeutic manner. A person with a fear of water reported this dream:

> In reality I have a great fear of water, and swimming was one of the possible choices for me to try in a lucid dream. In the dream I'm in my backyard and am immediately aware that I'm dreaming. I decide that it would be great fun to swim. Instantly there is water all around me. I swim several hundred feet and make many adjustments to my swimming form. I start to stand up in what is chest deep water and start to feel fearful. I remind myself that in a dream there is no reason to fear. I immediately feel comfortable and start to walk back around the house,

when I observe that the water has disappeared. (LaBerge, 1990, p. 260)

The study of lucid dreams has revealed that dreams take place in real time, not in an instant or a blink of the eye. As dreamers, people may take shortcuts and transport themselves from place to place, but the story line of dream action occurs at ordinary speed. This is known because sleep researchers, such as the group at Stanford Sleep Research Center, have been able to correlate eye movement during lucid dreams with dream reports. First, a prearranged signal is set—for example, a light embedded in eye shades worn by the sleeper will flash three times when EEG recordings detect REM sleep. If the dreamer detects the light and becomes aware of the fact that this is the signal, he or she returns a signal by moving the eyes in a pattern that was practiced before sleep onset. This methodology is quite ingenious, because during the benign paralysis of REM sleep, the only way for the dreamer to signal to the external world is through the eyes. One lucid dreamer reported that in his dream he was walking along a beach when suddenly he saw the sun rise and set, rise and set, rise and set. He kept walking and then suddenly thought how odd that was. In an "aha" experience, he recognized that this was the prearranged signal and was able to signal back to the researchers with his eyes. His report of the dream, and the time period between the signal and the dreamer's response corresponded to the eye movement tracings.

Are lucid dreams a melding of the conscious and unconscious mind states? During lucid dreams, the dreamer has knowledge of normally available waking thoughts and memories as well as an awareness of the dream illusion. What is normally unconscious has become conscious. Lucid dreams have been described, and may reasonably be thought of, as a cocreation between the two mind states, sometimes marked by intense pleasure, but with a different twist from the Freudian idea of a naughty "id" in that the dreamer often experiences these as mind expanding growth opportunities filled with personal insight and a sense of personal accomplishment. The scientific study of lucid dreaming may very well represent the next wave of research in understanding the brain processes related to levels of consciousness.

---

sleep may result in death. This is one of the possible causes of **sudden infant death syndrome (SIDS)** and most often occurs between the ages of 2 and 4 months.

Two primary mechanisms are involved in sleep apnea. The first one is the more common **obstructive sleep apnea.** Apneas occur most often during REM sleep when either the upper airway collapses, not allowing air to pass, or the body weight of the patient on the chest compromises respiratory effort. In each case, the consequence is disordered breathing. In the second mechanism of sleep apnea, **central sleep apnea,** disordered breathing is related to the brain failing to send the necessary signals to breathe. This may reflect brain stem abnormalities that manifest only during sleep. In either case the disorder is serious and often associated with severe O_2 desaturation. The terms *central* and *obstructive* do not represent a strict dichotomy, because obstructive sleep apnea may impair CNS control of muscles, and episodes of obstructive sleep apnea often precede central apnea. Such episodes are called *mixed apnea.* Complications of apnea result in poor physical health and associated neuropsychological deficits of poor concentration and memory (Barth et al., 1993).

The etiology of sleep apnea is not well understood, although age, obesity, and being male are all risks. Generally, researchers consider sleep apnea episodes to be caused by a complex interaction of physiologic and anatomic factors. Clinical features that are characteristic of the syndrome include excessive daytime sleepiness, heart failure, hypertension, morning headaches, disturbing snoring, irritability, headaches, sleep disruption, and personality changes. The hypoxia of sleep apnea markedly affects central neurotransmitter function and cellular metabolism, disrupting the biochemical and hemodynamic (pertaining to blood circulation) state of the CNS. Hypoxia may also lead to disturbed fluid and electrolyte distribution within the sodium-potassium pump, and alters brain adenosine levels in animals. In addition, cerebral blood flow studies demonstrate abnormally decreased blood flow in the case of sleep apnea patients, which may further compromise neuropsychological functioning because of decreased neuronal activity (Guilleminault & Dement, 1978). Sleep apnea can have serious psychosocial effects as well, including significant changes in adaptive functioning (Zillmer, Ware, Rose, & Bond, 1989).

Most treatment efforts focus on relief of apneas through surgical and mechanical means. The most effective is CPAP (continuous positive airway pressure), which is a mask that "forces" air through the nose or mouth while sleeping. CPAP is not considered a "cure," but it abolishes sleep apnea by maintaining upper airway flow during sleep. One of the most successful and least invasive treatments for SAS, CPAP acts as a pneumatic splint to prevent upper airway collapse during the night. CPAP must be used every night by the patient, but has few side effects as long as one can actually sleep (one patient described CPAP as analogous to holding your head out of the car window while driving at 50 mph). Losing weight can also help, because obesity is a major risk factor in sleep apnea. More controversial treatments include surgery to increase the dimensions of the pharynx via **uvulopalatopharyngoplasty (UPPP)** and tracheotomy, to completely bypass the upper airway obstruction during sleep (Williams & Karacan, 1978). UPPP involves removing the uvula, the small, fleshy tissue hanging from the center of the soft palate, which may relax and sag, obstructing the upper airway. However, this treatment is not as successful as CPAP and may also alter the subject's voice. Patients who have undergone treatment for SAS often report an improvement in their cognitive functioning.

Narcolepsy

The most notable disorder resulting from impaired CNS control of the sleep–wake cycle is **narcolepsy** (Greek, "a taking hold of numbness"). Narcoleptics are afflicted with irresistible daytime "sleep attacks." They can fall asleep while at work, while driving a car, or during a conversation. Such sleep attacks can last from a few seconds to more than 30 minutes. Excessive daytime sleepiness is the primary symptom of narcolepsy, although patients are also subject to narcoleptic sleep attacks, cataplexy, sleep paralysis, and hypnagogic hallucinations. Narcolepsy is a central nervous system disorder of the region in the brain stem that controls and regulates sleep and wakefulness. Once the disorder is established, it typically persists for one's entire life. Narcolepsy occurs in 1 out of every 1000 people. Symptoms typically begin to appear between the onset of puberty and age 25.

Excessive Daytime Sleepiness Pathologic daytime sleepiness is often the first sign to emerge in narcolepsy, typically associated with normal amounts of sleep at night. Many narcoleptics are asleep or sleepy during much of the day. They often complain of poor concentration and memory. Especially during the afternoon, after a meal, or when watching TV, narcoleptics are at risk for falling asleep. It is as if no amount of sleep could satisfy the patient's frequent and irresistible need for sleep. Excessive daytime sleepiness is the most prominent and troublesome component of narcolepsy. The patient is typically miserable and fatigued, often demonstrating inappropriate sleep.

Cataplexy **Cataplexy** is the most debilitating of the narcoleptic symptoms. Cataplexy is a brief (seconds to minutes) episode of muscle weakness and/or actual paralysis. In a benign form of cataplexy, only the face and the head may droop. In a severe attack all the muscles may become limp, resulting in the victim falling to the floor. When the attack is over, the patient quickly regains alertness and muscle tone. Cataplectic attacks occur during periods of sudden excitement and emotional change, including laughter, anger, and athletic activity. The sleep paralysis of cataplexy is always associated with pathologic REM sleep. If a cataplectic attack lasts long enough, it often becomes full-blown REM sleep. Thus, you can think of cataplexy as an inappropriate attack of REM sleep. The pathological intrusion of REM sleep and associated motor inhibition relates to a variety of nervous system dysfunctions, including massive nonreciprocal excitation of spinal inhibitory interneurons and active inhibition of motor neurons.

Hypnagogic Hallucination **Hypnagogic hallucinations** are also a symptom of narcolepsy and occur in the transition between wakefulness and sleep onset. Most people do not experience imagery during the transition from waking to sleep, because they are moving into NREM sleep, a period of little imagery. Narcoleptics, in contrast, can experience hypnagogic hallucinations during their shorter transition from waking to REM sleep. Thus, narcoleptics may experience vivid, dreamlike intrusions into wakefulness. The hallucinations can be mundane or nightmarish, and can cause great anxiety.

Sleep Paralysis **Sleep paralysis** is the momentary paralysis on awakening or at sleep onset. Although the person may be able to see what is happening in the room, the body is totally unable to move for seconds to minutes. People without narcolepsy have also described this sleep paralysis on awakening from a REM period in the early morning hours. To "break out" of this paralysis, they may start by moving their eyes, then willfully moving a finger. As soon as the voluntary muscles engage, the person breaks out of the REM-controlled sleep paralysis.

Narcolepsy can be best conceptualized as an imbalance among the wake, REM, and NREM systems. In such patients, wakefulness is weak, and REM sleep, or parts thereof, can intrude into it. This imbalance among the three stages can range from mild to severe. Narcolepsy is not a psychological disorder, although the socioeconomic and psychological toll on the patients can be great. The casual observer often thinks narcoleptic attacks are related to epilepsy, but they are not. The cause is generally unknown, although a minority of patients manifest parts of the syndrome following encephalitis, severe head injury, or brain tumor. Clinicians often make the differential diagnosis in a sleep disorder center using a procedure known as the *multiple sleep latency test (MSLT)*. Interestingly, narcoleptics are asked to arrive at the sleep disorder center, not in the evening, but during the morning. Around 10 A.M. they are put to "rest." The reason for this, is that the early morning would be the least likely time for most well-rested people to fall asleep and proceed into REM sleep. To diagnose narcolepsy, the subject must fall asleep in less than 5 minutes (normal sleep latency is 15 minutes at nighttime), and show at least two sleep onset REM periods (see Figure 13.7 on p. 426). Treatment of narcolepsy includes counseling for patient and family, developing good sleep habits including frequent naps, and the administration of medication, typically stimulants (such as amphetamines) for sleepiness and tricyclics (such as imipramine) for cataplexy. Although narcolepsy cannot be cured, its symptoms can be controlled with proper behavioral and medical therapy.

The Runaway Brain: Seizure Disorders

Seizures, like sleep, are reversible alterations of consciousness. But seizures occur suddenly during periods of expected wakefulness. For reasons not fully explainable, groups of neurons fire spontaneously in synchronous oscillation. If the abnormal rhythm is confined to a particular brain area, the result will be a **partial seizure.** If it involves the entire brain, the event is a **generalized seizure** (or grand mal). Episodes can also begin as a partial seizure and secondarily generalize to involve the whole brain.

Epilepsy ("falling sickness") is not a disease itself, but a syndrome in which brain seizure activity is a primary symptom. Perhaps the majority who have had a seizure in fact do not show the full epileptic syndrome (Hauser, 1992). Adults may suffer "nonepileptic episodes" from such events as hyperventilation,

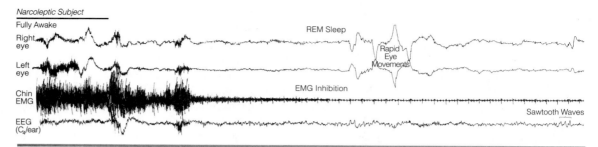

Figure 13.7   The narcoleptic goes quickly into REM sleep. (From P. Hauri, *Current Concepts: The Sleep Disorders*, Peapack, NJ: Pharmacia & Upjohn, Inc. 1977, foldout. Reprinted by permission of the author and publisher)

breath holding, migraines, ischemic attacks, drug toxicity, narcolepsy, and extreme emotion such as anger.

CLASSIFICATION OF SEIZURE TYPES

Seizures classifications depend on what is known of the origin or focus of the seizure within the brain. In contrast, the original French classification scheme was based on behavioral observations of what happened during a seizure. For example, people named **grand mal,** or "big bad" seizures for the most violent motoric abnormalities of stiffening (**tonic**) and jerking (**clonic**) episodes and the accompanying loss of consciousness. The **petit mal** or "little bad" seizures, in contrast, don't result in violent physical loss of control but do cause an altered state of consciousness. Today's seizure taxonomies are divided into two primary classifications: generalized and partial seizures. One main difference is that generalized seizures involve both cortical hemispheres, whereas partial seizures are confined to a specific area. As you may imagine, there are many different variations of partial seizures, depending on the site of origin. The epilepsy classification scheme presented in Table 13.3 shows some of the more common seizure types of both classifications.

Irrespective of the primary seizure type, up to 70% of people report having an **aura** before a seizure. This is the **prodromal phase,** in which one may experience odd transient symptoms such as nausea, dizziness, or numbness. Sensory alterations or hallucinations in any sensory domain may appear. For example, chemical sense disruptions may manifest as unpleasant metallic tastes or foul odors. Some people recognize their aura as an emotional change such as fear or anxiety. Others experience a temporary aphasia or a sense of forced thinking. Yet others describe auras as an otherworldly or surreal dream state, or a sense of déjà vu. These symptoms are highly idiosyncratic, but are likely to be consistent within a person. Most seizure sufferers become adept at recognizing their own auras; however, some auras occur without awareness, although they may be recognized by others. Auras may point to the genesis, or the eliptogenic focus, of the seizure within the brain (Cascino, 1992). Interestingly, some people are also able to arrest the progression of a seizure during this prodromal phase by learning to counteract the sensation with its opposite. For example, if a foul smell is part of an aura, a strong pleasant smell may halt the seizure (Efron, 1957). We explore this aspect of seizure control further in our discussion of epilepsy treatment.

Following a seizure episode is a **postictal phase** in which the person gradually emerges into full consciousness. Often symptoms of confusion, disorientation, depression, headache, or fatigue follow. Less commonly, the person may bite his or her tongue or lose bladder control. This phase may be momentary or may last for hours, somewhat depending on seizure type.

In the following sections we discuss seizure types according to the epilepsy classification scheme of Table 13.3. Clinical descriptions correlate with what

Table 13.3	*Seizure Classification*

Generalized Seizures

1. Absence	4. Tonic
2. Myoclonic	5. Tonic-clonic
3. Clonic	6. Atonic

Partial Seizures

1. Simple: focal motor, somatosensory or special-sensory, psychic, and autonomic
2. Complex partial: psychomotor, temporal lobe
3. Secondarily generalized: Jacksonian, grand mal

is known of their neurologic counterparts. A more generalized discussion of the brain mechanisms responsible for seizure activity follows.

Generalized Seizures

Generalized seizures, formally known as *grand mal seizures,* are bilaterally symmetric episodes characterized by a temporary lack of awareness, or what appears on observation to be complete loss of consciousness. The brain origin of these seizures has traditionally been considered unknown or generalized. Behaviorally, they typically have a motor component that onlookers consider frightening. The motor discharge is likely to consist of any combination of a *tonic* or *clonic* form. A number of seizures involve both aspects. The behavior that alerts others to a seizure onset is the tonic stage. Patients describe passing out, and onlookers are likely to witness a stiffening of the person's whole body, jaw clenching, and a blue appearance to the face. The blueness may look like a respiratory arrest, but during a seizure this actually occurs because peripheral blood vessel constriction allows more blood to flow to the brain. In any case, breathing stops only temporarily. After seconds to minutes, the second clonic stage appears. The body begins a rhythmic jerking of limbs and may involve the whole torso. This is followed by abrupt limpness (or **atonia**) and a gradual regaining of conscious awareness. Generalized seizures may take several forms, but

usually include components of irregular motor discharge in the form of tonic and/or clonic movement.

Absence seizures appear in some classification schemes as a partial seizure and in others as a generalized seizure. This may represent differences related to the brain areas responsible and the extent of cortical involvement. As you can see in the following case example described by a neurologist, the typical gross motor involvement of generalized seizures is absent and is replaced by ictal **automatisms.**

[A] mother brought her delightful red-headed eight-year-old daughter to see me. Because the girl seemed so attentive, intelligent, and well-behaved, it was hard for me to believe that she was having a difficult time at school. Her teacher reported that she made frequent mistakes on the blackboard and was often unable to answer simple questions. In my office, I asked her to take some rapid shallow breaths. After thirty seconds, she stared vacantly into space with her eyelids fluttering. Ten seconds later, she was back to her usual self. I had witnessed a classic absence seizure. Her EEG showed a pattern of 3 cps spike and dome activity during overbreathing, typical of absence epilepsy." (Richard & Reiter, 1990, p. 30)

Here the doctor precipitated a seizure by having the girl hyperventilate. This girl's fluttering eyelids are an important behavioral clue to seizure activity. Additional automatisms may include stereotyped hand movements or facial tics. Less typical for this type of seizure are a sudden myoclonic jerk or atonic loss of muscle tone. At the approach of an attack, some may just stop talking midstream, stare blankly into space for the duration of the attack, and then resume without noticing any lapse in consciousness. Absence attacks characteristically affect children from age 4 to 14. Interestingly, many children with absence attacks "outgrow" them, suggesting that a delay or anomaly in brain development plays an important role in their occurrence. It is rare for adults with no seizure or trauma history to develop absence attacks.

Partial Seizures

Partial or focal seizures may take several forms, but always begin as a local neuronal discharge that may generalize across the corpus callosum, eventually involving the entire brain in a secondarily generalized seizure. This seizure category represents the most common type, affecting about 800,000 people in the United States (Cascino, 1992). These seizures can be more frequently localized than generalized seizures, but still only a third of those afflicted have identifiable etiologies. Head trauma, stroke, viral brain diseases such as meningitis, and encephalitis are a few of the conditions that may lead to partial seizures.

Partial seizures consist of three main types. First, **simple seizures** are focal events that may involve sensory-motor expression or psychic expression (mood, emotion, or altered consciousness). The behavior experienced reflects the area from which the seizure emanates. For example, discharges from the motor strip can cause sudden or stereotypic movement, such as jerking or twitching. People have reported that their eyes may move to a certain position or that they turn their heads involuntarily. Occipital lobe foci can result in seeing vivid images or flashing lights. Memory and personality alterations can be a result of temporal lobe foci, and intensive mood experiences can occur with limbic system foci. The behavioral results vary widely from person to person but are closely tied to the site of seizure focus. Because there is no further involvement, the person can also experience these events as an aura.

The second type of partial seizure, a **secondarily generalized seizure,** is actually a variation of the first type. If a simple seizure spreads, this spreading can generalize throughout the whole brain as in the case of **Jacksonian seizures,** named for Jackson (see Chapter 1). Jacksonian seizures involve motor areas and have been called "marching seizures," because they begin with jerking or tingling of a single body area and spread to other areas. The symptoms reflect their corresponding brain regions, so diagnosticians consult maps of the motor homunculus. The third type are **complex partial seizures,** the most common forms being **psychomotor** or **temporal lobe epilepsy.** These are more "complex" than simple partial seizures in that they have an element of altered psyche or awareness in addition to sensory or motor components. About half of those with complex partial seizures experience an aura (Cascino, 1992). Complex partial seizures typically emanate from the temporal lobes, but can also occur as the result of a frontal lesion. The alter-

ation of consciousness can take several forms. It may include a sense of déjà vu ("already seen") in new environments or jamais vu ("never seen") in a familiar place. The person may experience a sense of forced thinking, illusions, panic, terror, or even ecstasy. The motor changes during the ictal phase often take the form of odd, catatonic-like posturing and automatisms such as lip smacking or undoing buttons. The shift into the ictal phase is abrupt, usually commencing with a motionless stare. The postictal period of confusion and drowsiness can be quite long with complex partial seizures. The case of the "sweeping lady" is a good example of what may happen with complex-partial seizures (see Neuropsychology in Action 13.4).

NEUROANATOMY AND NEUROPHYSIOLOGY OF SEIZURES

Partial and secondarily generalized seizures are the most likely to be localized because both the aura and the behavior during a seizure can point to a seizure's **eliptogenic focus** (the anatomic site of onset). Generalized seizures are difficult to localize, because they quickly disrupt the entire range of behavior involving all cortical neurons and may arise from a central mechanism capable of having a global effect on the brain. If there is an identifiable seizure focus, EEG recording is very useful in locating it if a seizure occurs spontaneously or can be induced during EEG monitoring.

Seizures are a symptom, similar to the concept of fever, that something is going on in the brain. A seizure may be localized to a particular anatomic area of the brain, and technicians may be able to image a corresponding structural pathology such as a lesion, a tumor, a vascular disease, or other anomaly. Because seizures also arise from metabolic disturbances and infections that affect the delicate physiological balance of the brain, neurologists cannot always find a structural location of injury or neuronal destruction in the brain. Although many normal people may experience a seizure, the occurrence may indicate significant brain pathology and medical consultation should always be sought.

Normally the brain maintains a balance of neuronal firing between excitatory discharges and inhibitory control of excessive firing. Single neurons and neuronal circuits fire according to their own direction and processing in what appear to be random patterns. Because so many different patterns are occurring simultaneously, and because the EEG represents a summation of neuronal firing, the resultant EEG tracing is fast and asynchronous. Seizures occur due to excessive excitatory synchronous neuronal firing. If you have ever been caught up in a "wave" in a packed football stadium, the analogy to the brain is similar. All the people represent individual neurons and are initially involved in their own behaviors. At first, although small groups of people may be involved in a rhythmic "give and take," the summation of "stadium behavior" appears random, with occasional synchronous bursts of cheering from one side or the other. But if a small group of people successfully initiate a wave, before long the entire stadium of 50,000 people synchronizes in a rhythm that sweeps through the crowd.

Absence seizures provide a good example of a generalized seizure that arises from a central mechanism. EEGs of classical absence seizures show characteristic synchronous bilateral spike-and-wave discharge (SWD) with a 3 cps frequency. This EEG frequency is within the same range as delta waves, characteristic of deep sleep. A reasonable description of absence seizures is that they force a temporary disconnection within the arousal system of the reticular activating system, thus pushing the whole cortex into a temporary sleeplike state.

Both animal and human studies point to the thalamocortical circuitry as the source for the primary aberrant mechanism involved in absence attacks. As we have discussed, during an alert state neurons in the thalamocortical loop are involved in continuous tonic firing. This allows signals from the external environment to pass through the thalamus to the cortex. External transmission to the cortex dampens when neurons begin firing according to an internally generated oscillating rhythm. Neurologists think that a group of neurons within the thalamus, the **nucleus reticularis thalami (NRT),** regulates oscillatory be-

havior of the thalamocortical loop. Direct recordings indicate that this is the source of rhythmic burst firing when the EEG becomes synchronized and also is a source of asynchronous firing during wakefulness. The NRT also projects to the contralateral dorsal thalamus, and thus have the ability to influence both hemispheres. The NRT mainly consists of GABAergic neurons that project to each other within the NRT and other areas of the thalamus. One of their main functions is in controlling cerebral excitability. Researchers report that during early development, one form of GABA receptors—the GABA-b type—increases and later is pruned to adult levels. Researchers also know that GABA agonist drugs make absence seizures worse. Some investigators believe that absence seizures in children may result from an error in development, resulting in a temporary overabundance of GABA receptors and therefore a temporary imbalance in the excitatory/inhibitory forces of the brain (Snead, 1995). They think what happens within this system of neurons that affects a shift between asynchronous and synchronous rhythms, is a change in the calcium potential of the cellular membrane. This may explain why some antiepileptic drugs such as ethosuximide and trimethadione, which act on the calcium current of the membrane, are effective.

In addition to the GABAergic neurons within the thalamus, numerous neurotransmitter systems may be involved in generalized absence seizures, because the ascending neuronal pathways to the cortex involve cholinergic, noradrenergic, dopaminergic, and serotonergic neurons. Acetylcholine and cholinergic projections emanating from the nucleus basalis to the cortex have an effect on arousal apart from the thalamocortical loop. Thus the regulation and control of arousal, and therefore seizures, represent a complex interaction of anatomic and physiologic systems.

NEUROPSYCHOLOGICAL PRESENTATION

Although neurologists may diagnose many seizures via EEG and other imaging measures, this is not always possible because seizures do not occur "at will." The interictal intervals can range from minutes to

Neuropsychology in Action 13.4

Epilepsy and the Case of the Sweeping Lady

by **Thomas L. Bennett** Ph.D., Professor of Psychology, Colorado State University, Clinical Director, Brain Injury Recovery Program, Fort Collins, Colorado.

Epilepsy is a common neurologic disorder, currently affecting over two million people in the United States (for a detailed discussion of epilepsy, see Bennett, 1992). Approximately 2.2% of the population has a single seizure at some time during life. Neurologists diagnose epilepsy only in cases where seizures recur. Diagnosis of epilepsy depends on clinical interview and EEG assessment showing abnormality in the interictal (between seizures) scalp electrode EEG tracings. The interictal spike is a marker for this disorder (McIntosh, 1992).

When psychic alterations occur, the seizures are called complex partial seizures. For neuropsychologists, these are the most interesting epileptic disorders (Bennett, 1987). They may be associated with motor automatisms consisting of stereotyped, repetitive movements such as chewing, blinking, lip smacking, pointing, or picking at one's clothes. Complex partial seizures, because of their frequent temporal lobe and limbic

system focus, may have an emotional component to the psychic alterations. The most common emotion is fear, but the person may also report pleasure, sadness, or vague familiarity. Individuals with complex partial seizures also commonly report sensory hallucinations or misperceptions. These sensations may range throughout the spectrum of visual, gustatory, olfactory, auditory, or somatic perceptions. Olfactory sensations are the most common type of sensory aura reported. These are typically quite displeasing (such as the smell of burning or rotting flesh), but may on occasion be pleasant (such as the smell of roses).

In the course of a complex partial seizure, the person may utter meaningless speech, laugh, or cry. Complex motor responses may also occur, including compulsive, purposeless writing, and even running. During a complex partial seizure, a person may be unaware of or unresponsive to her or his environment, failing to respond to questions by others.

The person may be vaguely aware of what is going on but unable to control it. While in a state of altered consciousness during a seizure, he or she may go into another room, wander through a public place, or leave a store and wander down the street. Imagine how upset you would be to find yourself in a different place from where you "just" were and to have lost several minutes or even hours of time, not knowing what you did during the interim. This is illustrated by the case of the sweeping lady.

This individual—let's call her Alice— has been a client of mine for almost 15 years. We meet on occasion as she continues to deal with the impact of her epilepsy on her life. Alice's epilepsy has never been completely controlled by antiepileptic drugs, a far too common experience for those with complex partial seizures. She has had to alter her lifestyle and goals in life significantly, but overall, she has adapted well to her disability. Before the onset of her seizure disorder

months to years. Neuropsychological evaluation can help determine the probability, by level and extent, that functional deficits are caused by seizure activity, and can therefore aid in diagnosis. Testing can also help determine the extent to which emotional components and stress may stem from seizures. Specialized testing with the Wada test (or technique) is also particularly useful before surgeries for partial complex seizures involving the temporal lobe (temporal lobe epilepsy/partial complex seizures), to determine

the likely effect of removing brain tissue on the functions of language and memory.

Neuropsychological presentation is highly individualistic, depending on seizure locus, type of seizure, and chronicity of disorder. No typical pattern of cognitive dysfunction is associated with epilepsy, and some patients may show few to no discernible problems. However, on testing many seizure sufferers exhibit attention and memory problems. This is particularly evident in tests requiring sustained or divided

in her early 20s, she was very active in sports and the community, and planned to return to college to complete a bachelor's degree. Alice has two daughters. She has worked in a couple of settings, but overstimulation and fatigue can increase seizure frequency, and she is currently not working. Diagnostic EEGs have produced some normal and some abnormal results. (Normal EEGs are also observed in others with complex partial seizures, showing that a normal EEG does not rule out epilepsy.) Her seizure pattern is interesting, because it typically contains many of the phenomena I have discussed.

Early in the development of her epilepsy, and when the seizures were less frequent with a fairly long interictal interval, Alice typically experienced epigastric sensations ("butterflies in the stomach") and nausea during the day before her seizures. This phenomenon, which was a seizure event, actually led her to seek evaluation from a gastrointestinal specialist before complex partial seizures were diagnosed. During this interval, her time perception was distorted so that everything seemed to slow down around her. She felt detached from her surroundings.

As the abnormal electrical activity spread and overt signs of the seizure

pattern began to develop, Alice experienced olfactory/gustatory sensations, including putrid, burning flesh, olfactory sensations, and the taste of soap. A blank stare preceded her motor automatisms, and she lost clear awareness of her surroundings at this point. She then began purposeless pacing and hand rubbing for two to three minutes. She reported that she was vaguely aware of these things happening, but she could not control them. She would typically emit a series of grunting and gasping sounds, which sounded to others as if she were having trouble getting enough air. Grimacing contorted her face. She laughed uncontrollably for several minutes, and then cried and rocked back and forth for several minutes more. The sequence ended when the spread of epileptic activity caused a generalized tonic contraction and she lost consciousness. This case illustrates the wealth of events that can occur during a complex partial seizure episode.

Several times Alice lost all awareness of what she had done for several hours. This happened when she went into a grocery store or large department store during the day when things were busy, noisy, and visually overstimulating. She later discovered that she must have just aimlessly wandered through the store,

perhaps repeatedly examining objects, because she had lost up to two to three hours of time for which she had no recollection. One of the most unusual experiences she had during a complex partial seizure occurred several years ago. I have thought of this as the "great fugue" or the "case of the sweeping lady."

It was the middle of the day in late spring or early summer, and Alice was home alone. She remembers that she was in her kitchen and had decided to sweep the floor. She vaguely remembers starting to sweep the floor, but nothing of the next 45 to 60 minutes. Apparently, she swept across the kitchen, down the hall, through the entry way, and out the front door! Her next memory was that she was lying on a stranger's porch. At first, she did not know who she was or where she was. Over the next few minutes, she became reoriented and realized she was on someone's porch. She stood up, walked down the sidewalk into the street, and recognized a friend's house several houses away. That enabled her to reorient to where she was. It turned out that she had walked several blocks from her home crossed several intersections, without awareness, while in an extended complex partial seizure fugue!

---

attention. In general, cognitive functioning tends to be more impaired with longer duration (younger age of onset) and increased frequency of seizures (Haynes & Bennett, 1990). Lowered cognitive functioning also links with greater EEG abnormality. In general, the type of seizure activity parallels the functional deficits expected. For example, generalized tonic-clonic seizures are more likely to result in widespread functional impairment of both hemispheres. Partial seizures (which have not generalized) are most likely

to be associated with lateralized impairment related to the side of abnormal discharge. As mentioned earlier, behavior during auras and the type of motor or sensory behavior evident during a seizure can also provide clues to seizure locus and are likely to correspond to neuropsychological assessment.

Patients with complex partial seizures involving the temporal lobe show the most consistent neuropsychological and behavioral pattern. This group most commonly reports problems with learning, memory, and language, and is less affected by attentional difficulties. Verbal fluency and verbal retrieval deficits are common manifestations of the interaction between memory and language. However, all aspects of memory encoding, organization, and retrieval may be affected. Emotional and behavioral disturbances, although prevalent among seizure sufferers in general, are most common with those who have complex partial seizures involving the temporal lobe. The pervasiveness of these problems during interictal (between seizures) time periods has led neuropsychologists to characterize them as temporal lobe epilepsy personality dysfunction. Although there is no one type of disturbance, this dysfunction may involve increased irritability, obsessions, and an interpersonal "stickiness" or difficulty in leaving conversations or places.

Neuropsychologists are typically involved in the administration of a specialized presurgery evaluation commonly called the **Wada test** (it is also referred to as the *intracarotid amobarbital procedure,* or *IAP*). Named after its developer, Juhn Wada (Wada & Rasmussen, 1960), this procedure involves the injection by a radiologist of a barbiturate, sodium amytal, through the patient's carotid artery to anesthetize one hemisphere at a time. The aim is to test the function of each hemisphere individually in regard to its relative dominance for language and its ability to support memory functioning before temporal lobectomy. If, for example, the Wada test shows that speech is atypically represented in the right hemisphere, then right temporal lobectomy is contraindicated. During the six to eight minutes while one hemisphere remains "paralyzed," the neuropsychologist tests the functioning of the "awake" hemisphere.

Many variations of the procedures are used during the Wada test, but the core involves brief testing of both expressive and receptive language and short and long-term memory in both the verbal and visual-spatial domains. The premise behind this assessment procedure is that the neuropsychological testing reveals the distribution of brain function and can help predict the sparing of memory and language functioning after temporal lobe resection. This aspect is usually quite helpful, however, there is some controversy over whether sodium amythal injections indeed anesthetize memory functions. For one reason, the injection into the anterior carotid artery only perfuses into the anterior portion of the hippocampus leaving posterior aspects free to function. To handle this problem, some medical centers also selectively inject the middle or posterior cerebral artery, although this is more risky. The change in a patient undergoing a Wada procedure is usually quite dramatic, in that the brain anesthetizes very quickly and speech abruptly halts if the dampened hemisphere is dominant for speech. Because many patients being considered for epilepsy surgery have a long-standing history of epilepsy, often dating back to early developmental years, cerebral representation of speech can show a variety of patterns presumably because the brain, responding to seizures, may have developed atypically. For example, there could be reversed dominance for speech with both expressive and receptive aspects controlled by the right hemisphere, equal disruption in each hemisphere, or a dissociation of expressive speech in one hemisphere and receptive speech in the other (for review, see Jones-Gotman, 1996).

TREATMENT OF EPILEPSY

The treatment of epilepsy is a collaborative effort between the patient and various health care professionals. As in many chronic diseases, patients are often the best experts on the symptoms of their conditions and the situations most likely to provoke a seizure. The various treatments available for epilepsy range from behavioral management, to nutritional therapy, to pharmacologic treatments, to neurosurgery.

The decision to take regular medication for seizures requires a neurologist's full evaluation as to its necessity, and a commitment from the patient. Seizures may occur in isolation but epilepsy denotes a pattern of seizure activity. People with a low seizure threshold may suffer an attack in combination with factors such as high stress, sleep deprivation, and overindulgence or withdrawal from alcohol. In these cases it is difficult to predict the risk of further seizures, and medication may not be necessary. Educational counseling regarding the possible precipitating factors for seizures and behavioral change to avoid the same situation in the future may be the best course of action, especially considering the potential for liver toxicity and blood problems with prolonged seizure medication. If a neurologist can establish a diagnosis of epilepsy, then a physician often prescribes specific drugs according to seizure type. For example, generalized tonic-clonic seizures often respond to anticonvulsants that prolong GABA's inhibitory action in the brain. These drugs include phenytoin (Dilantin), carbamazepine (Tegretol), or sodium valproate (Depakote) barbiturates and benzodiazepines. As described earlier, absence seizures appear to involve a mechanism that is pharmacologically different from GABA. Absence seizures are worsened by GABAergic drugs such as Dilantin, Tegretol, or barbiturates (Snead, 1995) and are treated by GABA-b antagonists ethosuximide (Zarontin), but may also be treated with sodium valproate (Depakote). Physicians may treat partial seizures with the preceding drugs or, for seizures involving motor disturbances, often use clonazepam (Klonopin) or acetazolamide (Diamox). In instances when drugs have not effectively controlled seizures, surgery as a treatment method has also been used. The pathologic brain area, if it can be localized, is simply cut out. Here is where the neuropsychological evaluation, and specifically the Wada test, can be particularly useful in advising the surgeon as to areas of function, such as speech and memory, that might be affected by the procedure.

Some people with seizures have also learned to control their attacks by noticing their auras and arresting the seizure before the ictal episode fully materializes. One pioneer in seizure research, Wilder Penfield, noticed that "When an attack is just beginning, strong stimulation of the part threatened may avert the further development of a seizure" (Penfield, 1975, p. 39). Sensory auras including smell, touch, and taste seem particularly amenable to natural arrest. For example, if the aura involves the sensation of a putrid smell, countering this with a pleasant smell may interrupt the progression of a seizure. In an early case study Robert Efron (1957) reported that one of his patients, a concert singer, had seizures preceded by the aura of a bad smell. He gave her a vial of essential oil of jasmine to sniff at the onset of her aura. The jasmine served as a natural counteractant to the hallucinated bad smell and apparently stopped the seizure. Through behavioral conditioning, Efron also taught her to arrest her seizures by imagining the odor of jasmine. In a similar vein, some patients find that they can halt gustatory auras such as metallic tastes by eating something pleasant tasting. Tactile auras have been stopped by such methods as tickling and squeezing. It is reasonable to assume that because the type of aura experienced by any one person is highly individual, patients would need to experiment to find what works for them. Efron's patient was able to control her seizures well enough that her medications could be reduced. In another interesting example (Pritchard, Holmstrom, & Giacinto, 1985), a patient with complex partial seizures developed his own technique of blinking or shutting his eyes and visualized himself fishing. What was most striking was that EEG monitoring corroborated the fact that he could arrest his seizure through this specific visualization but not through other mental tasks suggested to him such as mental arithmetic or reading. Interestingly, although a number of patients report that they have been able to stop a seizure, almost no formal research has been done to help people to control their own seizures. This is a promising area for neuropsychological study and intervention into the effect of mind control and natural arrestors in consciousness disorders.

Conclusion

Normal circadian peaks and valleys occur on about a 24-hour cycle in accordance with the sleep–wake cycle. In general, EEG indicates level of alertness, as seen in normal sleep and wakefulness patterns. However EEG, which is the outward measure of brain rhythm, is not necessarily an accurate indicator of mind state. Two people may show similar EEG patterns but have very different levels of conscious alertness. For example, although sleep is often called "unconscious," some people show "lucidity" during REM sleep. Slow delta waves accompany deep sleep and coma, but accomplished meditators can also produce this "deep" brain state while maintaining a more alert "mind" state. The mind state of dreaming during the brain state of REM has fascinated philosophers and scientists alike as they endeavor to understand potential connections to problem solving, memory, and psychological adjustment.

The hypothalamus, the thalamus, and the reticular activating system are particularly important in the sleep–wake cycle. When this clocklike rhythm is disrupted, sleep disorders such as life-threatening insomnia or narcolepsy can occur. Excessive daytime sleepiness occurs with most sleep disorders, often associated with complaints of poor memory and concentration.

Seizures suddenly alter consciousness during wakefulness and often result in abnormal movement and mentation. Seizures are the outward behavioral manifestation of excessive excitatory synchronous neuronal firing. The behavioral symptoms of seizures relate to the scope and the location of the brain focus, and the classifications of generalized and partial seizures are well documented. Neuropsychologists assess seizure patients for treatment planning and surgical evaluations. Although treatment of seizures primarily relies on medications, behavioral interventions may also be possible in the future as scientists and individuals learn more about controlling aspects of their own consciousness.

Critical Thinking Questions

- ◼ What is the biological or psychological function of "rhythms" of consciousness?
- ◼ How fluid are the boundaries between conscious and subconscious awareness?
- ◼ How do REM sleep and dreaming change in people who have various neurologic disorders?
- ◼ In what ways might neuropsychology be able to contribute to treatments for people with sleep disorders or epilepsy?

Key Terms

Consciousness
Epileptic syndrome
Circadian rhythm
Ultradian rhythm
REM sleep
NREM sleep
Nocturnal myoclonus
Suprachiasmic nucleus (SCN)
Reticular activating system (RAS)
Benzodiazepines
Sleep apnea syndrome (SAS)

Apnea
Hypoxia
Sudden infant death syndrome (SIDS)
Obstructive sleep apnea
Central sleep apnea
Lucid dreaming
Uvulopalatopharyngoplasty (UPPP)
Narcolepsy
Cataplexy
Hypnagogic hallucinations
Sleep paralysis

Seizures
Partial seizure
Generalized seizure
Epilepsy
Grand mal seizure
Tonic
Clonic
Petit mal seizure
Aura
Prodromal phase
Postictal phase
Atonia
Absence seizures

Automatisms
Simple seizure
Secondarily generalized seizure
Jacksonian seizure
Complex partial seizure
Psychomotor (temporal lobe epilepsy)
Eliptogenic focus
Nucleus reticularis thalami (NRT)
Wada test

Web Connections

http://www.stanford.edu/~dement/sleepinfo.html
Stanford University Sleep Center
A complete guide to various sleep disorders including all the disorders discussed in the text. In addition, discussions of the relationship of sleep disorders to specific psychiatric and medical diagnosis may provide an interesting link between previously discussed disorders and sleep disturbances.

http://www.sleepnet.com/index.shtml
SleepNet
Provides an overview of sleep, including sleep disorders, research, sleep labs, and more.

http://neuro.med.cornell.edu/NYH-CMC/ne-general.html
Cornell University Epilepsy Center
This overview of epilepsy covers the basics, such as the definition of a seizure, to more advanced discussions of treatment options and surgical procedures available for epilepsy patients.

http://neurosurgery.mgh.harvard.edu/epilepsy.htm
Harvard Epilepsy Site
Not only is this site an excellent source for discussions of surgical options in epilepsy, it also provides general resources and other links on this topic as well as the more general topic of epilepsy as a whole.

Part Five

NEUROPSYCHOLOGY IN PRACTICE

Chapter 14

NEUROPSYCHOLOGICAL ASSESSMENT

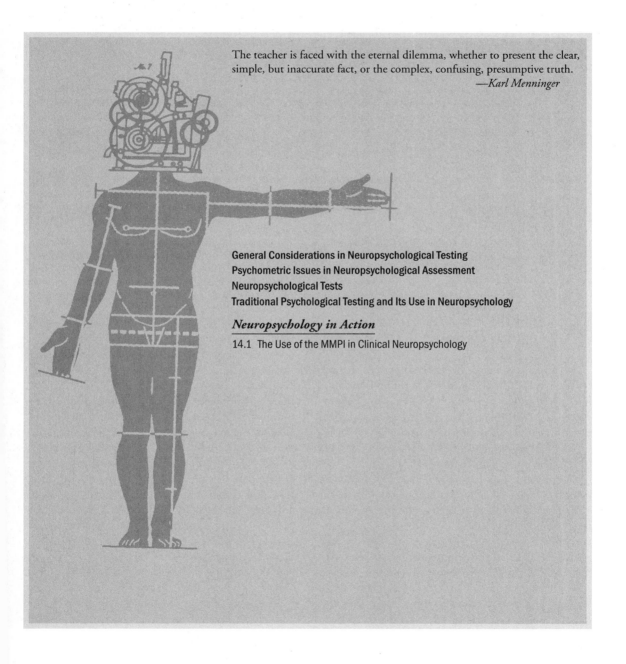

The teacher is faced with the eternal dilemma, whether to present the clear, simple, but inaccurate fact, or the complex, confusing, presumptive truth.
—*Karl Menninger*

General Considerations in Neuropsychological Testing

Psychometric Issues in Neuropsychological Assessment

Neuropsychological Tests

Traditional Psychological Testing and Its Use in Neuropsychology

Neuropsychology in Action

14.1 The Use of the MMPI in Clinical Neuropsychology

Keep in Mind

- What do clinical neuropsychologists do?

- How is clinical neuropsychology distinguishable from clinical psychology or from neurology?

- What makes a neuropsychological test reliable and valid?

- Will advances in neuroimaging techniques eventually replace the need for clinical neuropsychologists?

Overview

Does Dr. Grayson, a clinical neuropsychologist in the hospital, conduct only diagnostic "neuropsychological assessments"? Must the patient be referred to Dr. Smith, a clinical psychologist, for personality testing or psychotherapy? In other words, does clinical neuropsychology only play a narrow role in the diagnosis of brain dysfunction? How can behavioral tests aid understanding of brain dysfunction?

People often ask practicing neuropsychologists these questions. Not only do students and people new to the field ask, but also other psychologists, physicians, and hospital administrators. In this chapter on assessment, and in the next two chapters on interpretation and diagnosis, and on rehabilitation and intervention, we address these questions by providing an overview of the methods clinical neuropsychology uses. Specifically, we offer an overview on neuropsychological assessment, test selection, and interpretation and approaches to intervention and rehabilitation.

General Considerations in Neuropsychological Testing

This chapter describes the most frequently used assessment techniques in neuropsychology and outlines the scientific and theoretical principles of neuropsychological measurement. We stress that clinical neuropsychologists use a number of different methods to evaluate and treat individuals with brain dysfunction. Simply put, neuropsychologists are foremost clinical psychologists who have specialized in neuropsychological conceptualizations and methods. For neuropsychologists to understand the individual, they must view psychology as the expression of neuropsychology. From this perspective, neuropsychology is a broad field, and the neuropsychologist's roles span the range from evaluation to rehabilitation to research. This provides flexibility for employment in diverse settings. Figure 14.1 outlines representative employment settings of clinical neuropsychologists. Almost

half of all clinical neuropsychologists work in private practice, 24% in medical schools, 11% in rehabilitation hospitals, 5% in university settings, and 5% in Veterans Affairs (V.A.) medical centers. Other employment settings for clinical neuropsychologists include community mental health centers/clinics, school systems, military settings, and prisons/correctional facilities. Across all settings the "average" clinical neuropsychologist devotes 63% of his or her professional time to neuropsychology, has approximately 12 years of experience in practicing neuropsychology, is 45 years of age, and is predominantly male (73%; Gordon & Zillmer, 1997).

In private practice the role of the neuropsychologist is perhaps the most varied and flexible, but also the most ambiguous, because the amount of time devoted to neuropsychology depends on the type of patient population. Thus, neuropsychologists in private practice may provide neuropsychological evaluation and diagnosis as well as psychotherapy, family therapy, biofeedback, and other forms of traditional psychological services. Most often clinical neuropsychologists in private practice are generalists; that is, they have a grounding in clinical psychology with expertise in clinical neuropsychology. Some private practitioners have teaching or clinical appointments in universities or medical schools and participate to some degree in teaching and research.

In medical schools and hospitals, and in V.A. medical centers, clinical neuropsychologists most frequently work in psychiatry and rehabilitation departments and to a lesser extent in neurology or neurosurgery departments. The role of the neuropsychologist in the medical arena is typically neuropsychological diagnosis, evaluation, and intervention. The major difference, compared to the private practice setting, is the degree to which neuropsychologists participate in research. Particularly in medical schools, research plays an important role and neuropsychologists are often important participants in multidisciplinary research. In rehabilitation hospitals, neuropsychologists are essential in interventions for and remediation of disabilities related to brain impairment. In the academic setting, neuropsychologists predominantly teach undergraduate students in psychology and graduate students in clinical psychology. Academic neuropsychologists typically run active research programs. Clinical service delivery may play a minor role. Neuropsychologists in university settings may see patients in an integrated university neuropsychology clinic, or they may participate in a small private practice. Common to all employment settings is the emphasis on clinical diagnosis and evaluation, research, and rehabilitation and intervention.

The types of patient problems seen in any of the preceding settings reflect the changes in the population, eradication of some disease conditions, and new diseases that affect the brain, such as AIDS. Figure 14.2 outlines the typical patient populations that clinical neuropsychologists serve. A combined total of over 70% of the patients that neuropsychologists see are rehabilitation, psychiatry, or neurology patients. To a lesser degree they see patients referred with learning disabilities, forensic issues, dementia, general medical conditions, and patients suffering from seizure disorders.

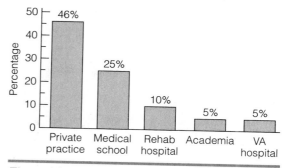

Figure 14.1 Distribution of neuropsychology practice, based on a survey of over 2000 members of the National Academy of Neuropsychology. (Gordon & Zillmer, 1997)

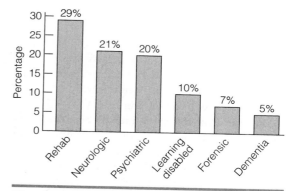

Figure 14.2 Types of patients seen by neuropsychologists. (Gordon & Zillmer, 1997)

WHY TESTING?

In the past, the interest in clinical neuropsychology and specifically in assessment reflected a perceived need to expand the clinical understanding of behavior to include effects on human functioning caused by brain dysfunction. As a result, evaluation of brain functioning through the development of neuropsychological testing has been a major contribution to psychology. Clinical neuropsychologists, however, have often been—not undeservedly—pigeonholed as "brain damage testers" or reductionistic "lesion detectors." But this notion is outdated. Clinical neuropsychology is a quickly evolving field in which the neuropsychologist can play several roles. One of those roles has traditionally been conducting psychological evaluations of brain-behavior relationships. Understand

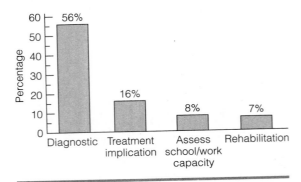

Figure 14.3   Overview of the neuropsychologist's role in assessment. (Gordon & Zillmer, 1997)

that neuropsychologists gain expertise in neuropsychological assessment and diagnosis over years of study and clinical practice, which they usually pursue at predoctoral and postdoctoral levels.

The purposes of administering psychological assessment instruments are to identify a patient's cognitive and behavioral strengths and weaknesses, to assist in the differential diagnosis of mental disorders, and to aid in treatment and discharge planning. You can review the neuropsychologist's role in assessment and diagnosis in Figure 14.3, which summarizes the general purposes of neuropsychological assessments.

A majority—over 50%—of all neuropsychological evaluations are diagnostic in purpose. In essence, the question is to understand if there are indications of a decline in cognitive abilities and whether they suggest a specific diagnosis or neuropathological condition. In many cases involving obvious pathology (such as brain tumor and stroke), neuropsychological evaluations are a precursor or are complementary to more in-depth neurologic or neuroimaging procedures that can establish the exact medical or neurologic diagnosis. In other cases (such as learning disabilities, attention deficit disorder, dementia, or minor head injury), the medical diagnosis is much more obscure and cannot be precisely verified by medical imaging techniques. Neuropsychological evaluations play a major role in assessing such conditions, because the diagnosis often rests largely on behavioral symptoms.

In some medical conditions (such as epilepsy, multiple sclerosis, and AIDS), neuropsychological assessments have only minor diagnostic value, but are used for documenting the extent of cognitive strengths and weaknesses, to outline effective treatment strategies and appropriate placements for school or vocational settings. Thus, many neuropsychological evaluations are conducted with more descriptive purposes in mind. As a result, neuropsychologists' roles have evolved from that of a strict diagnostician to providing descriptions of cognitive functioning, current adaptation, and future prognosis.

RATIONALE OF THE NEUROPSYCHOLOGICAL EXAMINATION

You cannot determine whether a certain function of the brain is impaired unless you test that function. The **neuropsychological evaluation** is an objective, comprehensive assessment of a wide range of cognitive and behavioral areas of functioning, which the neuropsychologist typically integrates with intellectual and personality assessments and evaluates within the context of CT and MRI scans. When based on a thorough description of abilities and deficits, neuropsychological testing leads to recommendations for rehabilitation and treatment. In using such tests, clinical neuropsychologists are interested principally in identifying, quantifying, and describing changes in behavior that relate to the cognitive integrity of the brain. Serial assessments can demonstrate gradual improvement or deterioration in mental status over time, allow better differentiation of cognitive deficits, and assist in treatment and disposition planning (Zillmer, Fowler, Gutnick, & Becker, 1990). Thus, the neuropsychologist may address issues of cerebral lesion lateralization, localization, and progress. Neuropsychological evaluations can provide useful information about the impact of a patient's limitation on his or her educational, social, or vocational adjustment. Because many patients with neurologic disorders, such as degenerative disease, cerebrovascular accidents, or multiple sclerosis, vary widely in the rate at which the illness progresses or improves, the most meaningful way to equate patients for severity of illness is to assess their behavior objectively, using neuropsychological procedures.

The neuropsychological evaluation has a number of advantages that many standard neurodiagnostic techniques do not share; for example, it is noninvasive and provides descriptive information about the patient. Specific tests employed in neuropsychological assessment batteries may vary, although most assessments include objective measures of intelligence, academic achievement, language functioning, memory, new problem solving, abstract reasoning, constructional ability, motor speed, strength, and coordination, and personality functioning (Zillmer & Ball, 1987).

You can conceptualize neuropsychological assessment as a method of examining the brain by studying its behavioral product. Because the subject matter of neuropsychological assessment is behavior, it relies on many of the same techniques and assumptions as does traditional psychological assessment. As with other psychological assessments, neuropsychological evaluations involve the intensive study of behavior by means of standardized tests that provide relatively sensitive indices of brain-behavior relationships. Neuropsychological tests have been used on an empirical basis in various medical and psychiatric settings, are sensitive to the organic integrity of the cerebral hemispheres, and can often pinpoint specific neurologic or psychological deficits. Neuropsychological assessment has also become a very useful tool for clinical service delivery and for research regarding the behavioral and cognitive aspects of medical disorders.

APPROPRIATE REFERRALS FOR NEUROPSYCHOLOGICAL EVALUATION

Because a neuropsychological workup may take anywhere from 30 minutes to 8 hours of professional time, health practitioners should request consultations with some discrimination for cost effectiveness and utility. The interpretation and diagnosis of the patient's profile ultimately depends on the referral question, the neuropsychologist's test selection, and the process by which the neuropsychologist interprets the data. Referrals should specify exactly what questions or problems prompted the referral, what the referral source hopes to obtain from the consultation, and the purpose for which the referrer will use the information. The advanced student in neuropsychology often feels frustrated by the failure of medical professionals to give a clear referral question. Note, however, that generating appropriate referral questions, as well as questions from the patient about the goals of the evaluation, is the responsibility of the neuropsychologist. Thus, it is often necessary to educate the professional community about the purpose and goals of a neuropsychological evaluation. Having the patients themselves ask specific questions about the goals of the evaluation (for example, whether they can go back to work) often makes the evaluation process more meaningful to patients, and typically motivates them to participate and attempt their best.

In a medical setting the neuropsychologist is most helpful to the treatment team as a neurobehavioral describer of functional strengths and weaknesses as well as a provider of neurodiagnosis (Zillmer & Passuth, 1989). As already mentioned, such disorders as mild head injuries, early stages of Alzheimer's dementia, or learning disabilities may show no symptoms beyond the cognitive dysfunction that formal neuropsychological testing assesses so well. The following are instances in which a neuropsychological consultation is generally useful:

- Differential neurologic diagnosis
    Acute versus static
    Focal versus diffuse
    Location of damage
- Establishment of a baseline for neuropsychological performance from which future evaluations can assess improvement or deterioration
- Descriptions of the effects of brain dysfunction on behavior
- Determinations of disability levels for compensation in personal injury litigation
- Evaluation of vocational potential
- Assessment of environmental needs after discharge from hospital (disposition planning)

- Development of remedial methods for rehabilitation of the individual brain-damaged patient
- Measurement of residual abilities during rehabilitation
- Patient management

Psychometric Issues in Neuropsychological Assessment

The science of standardized clinical psychological testing has evolved over the past 80 years to the point that there are now hundreds of psychological assessment instruments in use today. It is important for the neuropsychology student to understand the scientific principles of psychological measurement before examining neuropsychological assessment instruments in more detail.

Psychometrics, the science of measuring human traits or abilities, is concerned with the standardization of psychological as well as neuropsychological tests. A **standardized test** is a task or set of tasks administered under standard conditions and designed to assess some aspect of a person's knowledge or skill. Standardized psychological tests typically yield one or more objectively obtained quantitative scores, which permit systematic comparisons to be made among different groups of individuals regarding some psychological or cognitive concept. Most neuropsychologists agree that tests are rarely used alone and are not interpreted in a vacuum. Almost always, neuropsychological tests are only one of multiple components of information used to make important decisions about an individual. Neuropsychological assessment, then, depends on the complex interplay among the neuropsychologist, the patient, the context of the assessment, and the data from neuropsychological testing.

RELIABILITY

For any psychological test to be useful, it must be both reliable and valid. **Reliability** is the stability or dependability of a test score as reflected in its consistency on repeated measurement of the same individual. A reliable test should produce similar findings on each administration. If test scores show a great deal of variation when administered to the same individual on several occasions, the test scores are unreliable and there is concern about error. Interpretation of the scores becomes difficult. There are several different forms of reliability, including test–retest reliability, split-half reliability (the correlation between two halves of the test), or internal consistency (the degree to which items of a scale measure the same thing, also known as Cronbach's alpha). Thus, the concept of reliability is not as simple as it first appears, and test developers must present substantial detail when making claims of test reliability.

VALIDITY

The **validity** of a test is the meaningfulness of specific inferences made from the test scores; that is, does the test really measure what it was intended to measure? If a test is unreliable, it cannot be valid. For example, if you take the same language test on three different days and obtain three different scores, it is easy to conclude that there is no consistency and therefore the test can't possibly be used to predict anything about your language abilities. A reliable test is not necessarily a valid one. Let's say a test was purported to measure how well you make organized extemporaneous speeches. The test requires you to generate as many words as you can in one minute. On three different days you took the test, and on three days you got a similar score. The test has high reliability. But is it telling us about your ability to make impromptu speeches? Not necessarily; an analysis of the test's validity may show that it is primarily measuring your ability to search and retrieve words from memory. It may have very little to do with your ability to put your thoughts together and come up with a good speech.

Although the concept of a test accomplishing its purpose is easy to grasp, applying this concept often results in confusion. Many tests that neuropsychologists use were originally designed for other purposes or diagnostic groups for which they are used now. Rather than discuss validity in overgeneralized terms, scrutinize an evaluation of a test's validity in relation to the specific purpose and the specific population it is used in. In other words, never consider a test *generically* "valid" or "invalid." The question to ask is "Is this test valid for this particular purpose?"

You can use several different strategies for determining validity. **Construct validity** focuses primarily on the test score as a measure of the abstract, psychological characteristic or construct of interest (such as memory, intelligence, impulsiveness, and so forth). Construct validity would be most important if you wanted a demonstration of the cognitive or functional abilities a test measures (for example, visual-spatial problem solving or perceptual-motor functioning).

Content validity pertains to the degree to which a sample of items or tasks make conceptual sense or represent some defined psychological domain. Various items of the test should correspond to the behavior the test is designed to measure or predict, such as measuring how fast someone can tap a finger, to assess upper-extremity motor speed. Finally, **criterion validity** demonstrates that scores relate systematically to one or more outcome criteria, either now (concurrent validity) or in the future (predictive validity). Criterion-related validity has traditionally been an area of prime concern in neuropsychology related to the correct classification of diagnostic groups including brain-impaired, psychiatric, and normal individuals. It is also the issue if the test is being used as a measure to describe current everyday functioning. Criterion-related predictive validity is important if a test is designed to predict decline or recovery of function or future behavior of any type (such as medication management or ability to drive a car).

FALSE POSITIVES AND BASE RATES

A **false positive** (also known as a Type I error or false alarm) is a case in which a neuropsychological test erroneously indicates a pathologic condition—such as "brain damage"—in an individual who is actually "normal." In setting a cutoff score on neuropsychological tests, statisticians attend to the percentage of false rejects (or false positives) as well as to the percentages of successes and failures within the selected group. In most medical (life threatening) situations,

statisticians set the cutoff point low enough to exclude all but a few false rejections (such as on tests that detect the presence of cancer). When the selection ratio is not externally imposed, the cutting score on a test can be set at a point yielding the maximum differentiation between criterion groups. You do so, roughly, by comparing the distribution of test scores in the two criterion groups, including the relative seriousness of false rejections and false acceptances.

The validity resulting from the use of a test depends not only on the selection ratio but also on the base rate of the test. **Base rate** is the frequency with which a pathologic condition is diagnosed in the population tested. For example, if 10% of a psychiatric population of a hospital has organic brain damage, then 10% is the base rate of brain damage in this population. Although introducing any valid test improves predictive or diagnostic accuracy, the improvement is greater when the base rates are closest to 50% (closest to chance). With extreme base rates found in very rare pathological conditions (for example, <1%) an improvement with a neuropsychological test may be negligible. Under those conditions, the diagnostic use of a neuropsychological test is unjustifiable when you take into account the cost of its administration and scoring. When the seriousness of a condition makes its diagnosis urgent, as in Alzheimer's disease, neuropsychologists may often use tests of moderate validity in early stages of sequential decisions. Table 14.1 demonstrates a simple decision strategy for neuropsychological procedures. A single test is administered, and the decision to reject or accept a diagnosis is made with four possible outcomes.

Table 14.1 Decision Making in Neuropsychological Assessment		
Decision	**Positive** (presence of pathology)	**Negative** (absence of pathology)
CORRECT	Valid acceptance (hit)	Valid rejection (correct rejection)
INCORRECT	False positive (false alarm, Type I error)	False negative (miss, Type II error)

Neuropsychological Tests

Table 14.2 reviews the most frequently used types of neuropsychological measures in practice today. Different types of tests have different goals and applications. **Achievement tests** measure how well a subject has profited by learning and experience, compared to others. Typically, achievement is most influenced by past educational attainment. Achievement tests are not designed to measure the individual's future potential, which is typically measured by aptitude tests. **Behavioral-adaptive scales** examine what an individual usually and habitually does, not what he or she can do. Neuropsychologists most frequently use such scales in evaluating the daily skills of individuals who are quite impaired (such as the mentally retarded or the severely brain injured). **Intelligence tests** are complex composite measures of verbal and performance abilities that are in part related to achievement (factual knowledge) and in part to aptitude (for example, problem solving). **Neuropsychological tests** have been traditionally defined as those measures that are sensitive indicators of brain damage. Today, scientists consider a measure to be a neuropsychological test if a change in brain function is systematically related to a change in test behavior. Most available neuropsychological tests, therefore, have a broader function, and we describe them in more detail later in this chapter. Another area of psychological testing concerns the nonintellectual aspects of behavior. Tests designed for this purpose are commonly known as **personality tests**—most often, measures of such characteristics as emotional states, interpersonal relations, and motivation. Finally, **vocational inventories** assess opinions and attitudes that indicate the individual's interest in different fields of work or occupational setting.

Neuropsychologists generally recognize that there is considerable overlap among all types of psychological tests. For example, it is difficult to measure aptitude without measuring achievement, to measure vocational interest without measuring personality, or to measure intelligence without measuring neuropsychology. One way to deal with this overlap is to reduce the complexity to two basic neuropsychological constructs, "crystallized" and "fluid" functions. Psychologists consider **crystallized functions** to be most dependent on cultural factors and learning. They believe **fluid functions,** in contrast, to be culture free and independent of learning. Problem solving and abstract reasoning are abilities considered fluid, whereas spelling and factual knowledge are considered crystallized. Nevertheless, even this simple differentiation of psychological test properties is controversial. For example, much discussion concerns whether intelligence tests tap mostly crystallized or fluid forms of behavior. Actually, it is nearly impossible to measure all aspects of a complex skill or group of skills with a single test. As a result, neuropsychologists prefer to administer a number of different tests, known as a *test battery,* that address different areas of brain–behavior functioning. After all, testing behavior, whether vocational or adaptive, is mediated by brain function. Thus neuropsychologists use the preceding tests to some degree to evaluate specific questions about an individual.

The best way to understand the purpose of the neuropsychological assessment is to examine the evaluation process. Because neuropsychological assessment batteries typically evaluate a wide range of behaviors, they are considered multidimensional in their

Table 14.2   *Types of Tests Most Commonly Used by Psychologists*

Type of Test	Intended to Measure . . .
Achievement	Profit from past experience
Aptitude	Profit from future training and educational experiences
Behavioral/adaptive	Basic adaptive behaviors (for example, self-care, communication, socialization)
Intelligence	Ability to adapt to novel situations quickly
Neuropsychological	Brain–behavior relationships
Personality	Psychopathology and ability to adapt and cope with stress
Vocational	Success in a specific occupation or profession

Table 14.3 *Common Areas of Neuropsychological Assessment Grouped Hierarchically by Function*

Orientation
- Arousal
- Degree of confusion
- Disorientation
- Place
- Person
- Time
- Awareness of change/time

Sensation/Perception
- Recognition
- Familiarity of stimuli
- Relationship among features
- Visual acuity
- Auditory
- Taste/smell
- Tactile/proprioceptive
- Internal/environmental
- Awareness

Attention
- Span
- Selective attention
- Shifting
- Sustained attention
- Vigilance
- Neglect
- Fatigue

Motor
- Cerebral dominance
- Initiation and perseveration
- Manual dexterity
- Graphomotor skills

Motor (continued)
- Balance
- Ambulation
- Motor speed
- Speech regulation
- Motor strength

Visual Spatial
- Construction
- Route finding
- Spatial orientation
- Facial recognition

Language Skills
- Receptive speech (following directions, reading comprehension)
- Expressive speech (verbal fluency, naming, writing, math)
- Articulation (stuttering, stammering, articulation voice, fluency)
- Speech production (articulation fluency, voice)
- Syntax and grammar
- Aphasias: Broca's, Wernicke's, conduction, fluent, transcortical, subcortical

Memory
- Verbal
- Visual
- Immediate
- Short term
- Long term
- Recognition
- Encoding

Memory (continued)
- Storage
- Retrieval
- Chunking
- Declarative
- Procedural

Abstract Reasoning/Conceptualization
- Comprehension
- Judgment
- Calculations
- Problem solving
- Organizational abilities
- Higher-level reasoning
- Sequencing

Emotional/Psychological Distress
- Depression
- Attitude toward rehabilitation
- Motivation
- Locus of control
- Family relationships
- Group interaction
- One-to-one interaction
- Behavioral impulsivity
- Aggressive/confrontational

Activities of Daily Living
- Toileting
- Dressing
- Bathing
- Transferring
- Continence
- Feeding

approach to measuring higher cortical functions. Thus, the neuropsychological exam involves accurately evaluating multiple cognitive abilities (see Table 14.3). The usual categories of the neuropsychological examination include the following functional areas, which are listed hierarchically; that is, higher cognitive functions depend to a large degree on intact lower functions, which are listed first:

- Orientation (arousal)
- Sensation and perception
- Attention/concentration
- Motor skills
- Verbal functions/language
- Visual-spatial organization
- Memory
- Judgment/problem solving

Let's examine each of these areas in greater depth. For each neuropsychological domain, we present the neuropsychology student with an example to elucidate the construct measured and the method used to do so. The neuropsychological items we present here come from the Assessment of Impairment Measure (AIM; Zillmer, Chelder, & Efthimiou, 1995; Zillmer et al., 1993). In addition, we present examples of frequently used neuropsychological tests for each neuropsychological domain.

ORIENTATION (AROUSAL)

Brain impairment affects not only a person's intellect or muscle movement, but all other aspects of performance as well, including his or her level of consciousness. Patients who are lethargic or tired all the time tend to perform poorly compared to patients who have good energy. Lethargy is sometimes a symptom of brain damage and sometimes a symptom of depression. It is the psychologist's job to determine which factors are at work in a given case.

Alertness is the most basic aspect of cognition. Patients who cannot demonstrate adequate arousal may have difficulty participating in a neuropsychological evaluation and are perhaps unlikely to benefit from rehabilitation or psychological intervention. **Orientation** describes a patient's basic awareness of himor herself to the world around them. Specifically, in neuropsychology *orientation* refers to an individual's knowledge of who he or she is (orientation to person), what the date is (orientation to time), and where he or she is (orientation to place). If a patient is fully oriented, the neuropsychologist will say that he or she is "oriented times three," meaning that those three areas of awareness are intact.

Neuropsychological Items (Orientation)

The neuropsychological assessment typically involves the common evaluation of orientation in the three spheres; for example, "What is your full name?" (both first and last names are required) "Where do you live?" (specific town or city is required), or "How old are you?" In addition, neuropsychologists may also ask additional questions that relate to an individual's ability to recall his or her specific whereabouts, the purpose of the hospitalization, and any part of his or her address: "What is the name of the place you are in now?" (a response indicating that the patient knows he or she is in a hospital is considered correct), "What town or city are you in now?" (any response indicating adequate orientation to the hospital's location is scored). The following two items are examples of the patient's orientation to well-known current facts, in-

volving famous individuals: "Who is president of the United States right now?" and "Who was president before him?"

Neuropsychological Tests (Orientation)

To measure orientation, neuropsychologists frequently use the Galveston Orientation and Amnesia Test (GOAT; Levin, O'Donnell, & Grossman, 1979). This short mental status examination assesses the extent and duration of confusion and amnesia after traumatic brain injury. Like the Glasgow Coma Scale (GCS, see Chapter 10), it was designed for repeated measurements and can be used several times a day and repeated over days or week as necessary. The GOAT yields a score from 0 to 100, with a suggested cutoff score of 75 or better indicating relatively intact orientation and the capacity of the patient to undergo formal neuropsychological testing. Both the GCS and the GOAT are simple to administer, and therefore the treatment team often uses them. Because these scales quantify level of patient's arousal, researchers have frequently used them in examining outcome of brain injuries that involve an alteration in consciousness.

SENSATION AND PERCEPTION

Sensation is the elementary process of a stimulus exciting a receptor and resulting in a detectable experience in any sensory modality. For example, "I hear something." **Perception** depends on intact sensation and is the process of "knowing." For example, "I hear music, it is Pearl Jam." The perceptual process begins with arousal and orientation, sensation is the second stage, and perception the third. In assessing sensation and perception, the neuropsychologist is interested in quickly and grossly evaluating the patient's visual, auditory, and tactile functional levels. Screening for impaired sensation and perception yields important information by ruling out the contributions of dysfunctional visual or auditory sensation to test performance. In addition, discovering unilateral sensory deficits aids in diagnosis of lateralized brain injury. Understand that neuropsychologists are interested in a more-or-less general assessment of a patient's sensory functioning. Specialists, including audiologists (hearing) or neuro-optomologists (visual), perform diagnostic evaluations.

Neuropsychological Items (Sensation and Perception)

Sample items of testing the sensory and perception domain may include assessing the intactness of the patient's left and right visual fields (see Chapter 4 for a description of visual field deficits). This is achieved by administering a visual field exam, common in a neurologic examination. For this procedure, the examiner must sit facing the patient, at a distance of approximately 3 to 4 feet, asking, "I would like you to look straight at my nose. I am going to put my arms out like this, and I want you to tell me which finger I am moving. You can point to it if you like." The examiner extends the index finger of each hand in a vertical fashion with arms spread out at shoulder height and presents the stimuli by moving each finger slightly, waiting for the patient's response between trials. Discrimination of similar auditory, verbal stimuli may be tested by the examiner saying, "I am going to say two words, and I want you to tell me whether I am saying the same word twice or two different words," to assess auditory functioning:

house – house	(same)
people – peanut	(different)
bar – bar	(same)
first – thirst	(different)

To assess the patient's ability to sense or feel objects, the examiner may say, "I am going to place an object in one of your hands. I would like you to close your eyes, feel the object, and tell me what it is." This procedure measures stereognosis, recognition of objects by touch.

Neuropsychological Tests (Sensation and Perception)

Some neuropsychologists have standardized their procedures for examining sensory and perceptual functioning and developed scoring systems as well. For example, part of the well-known and often used Halstead-Reitan Neuropsychological Battery includes a sensory-perceptual examination that tests for finger agnosia, skin writing recognition, and sensory extinction in the tactile, auditory, and visual modalities (Reitan & Wolfson, 1993).

ATTENTION/CONCENTRATION

Attention is a critical requirement for learning. To remember, you first have to pay attention. Some patients are incapable of attending to their environment. Others may be able to attend to a learning task, but only for a limited amount of time. Still others may be able to attend to a task only if there are no distractions in the environment. Psychologists divide the concept of attention into separate categories such as sustained attention, paying attention to something over a prolonged period of time or sustained attention, and selective attention, paying attention to more than one thing at a time.

Neuropsychological Items (Attention/Concentration)

Tasks requiring mental control involve simple, over-learned information, but require the individual to maintain an adequate level of attention throughout the item. Errors in this area may indicate extreme fatigue or an impairment in concentration skills. For example,

"Count from 1 to 20 as quickly as you can."
"Recite the days of the week backward beginning with Sunday."
"Say the alphabet—A, B, C, . . .—all the way through."
"Count by threes, beginning with 1 and adding 3 to each number. For example, 1, 4, 7, and so on. (Stop when you reach 22.)"

Another form of attention in this cognitive skill area is attention span. Here the examiner asks the patient to attend to various verbal stimuli and repeat them. The stimuli become progressively more complex. In this manner, it is possible to evaluate a patient's span of attention for unfamiliar combinations of stimuli.
"I am going to say some numbers, and after I finish I would like you to repeat them:"

TRIAL 1	5	8	9		
TRIAL 2	9	2	7	5	
TRIAL 3	7	1	6	3	2

"Now I am going to say some more numbers, but this time when I finish, I want you to say them backward. For example, if I say 3 – 6, you say 6 – 3."

TRIAL 1	5	8	
TRIAL 2	2	6	1

Sustained attention is the ability to concentrate over a period of time. For example, you can assess verbal attention with the following task: "Tap on the table when you hear me say the number 4:"

2	3	5	4	7	4	6	4	4	2
1	8	1	7	8	4	5	4	2	3

Neuropsychological Tests (Attention/Concentration)

Standardized tests of attention include the Symbol Digit Modalities Test (SDMT; Smith, 1982), which requires the respondent to fill in blank spaces with the number that is paired to the symbol above the blank space, as quickly as possible for 90 seconds. The SDMT primarily assess complex scanning, visual tracking, and sustained attention. An interesting test of selective attention is the d2 Test of Attention (Brickenkamp & Zillmer, 1998). The d2 Test is a timed test of selective attention and is a standardized refinement of a visual cancelation test. It has been translated into four languages and is the most frequently used test of attention in Europe. In response to the discrimination of similar visual stimuli, the test measures processing speed, rule compliance, and quality of performance, allowing estimation of individual attention and concentration performance (see Figure 14.4). Originally developed in 1962 in Ger-

many and Switzerland as an assessment tool for driving efficiency, the test has recently been made available, by Hogrefe & Huber, psychological test publishers, to American neuropsychologists. Subjects who fail the d2 task tend to have difficulty concentrating, including difficulty in warding off distractions (Zillmer & Kennedy, 1999a, 1999b).

MOTOR SKILLS

Neuropsychologists are interested in assessing an individual's ability to demonstrate motor control in the upper and lower extremities. Simple motor skills require little coordination, whereas more complex items tap into higher motor processes. As items progress in difficulty, the patient must show more integration of cognitive skills to perform the task successfully. The following items measure varied aspects of a patient's motor functioning. The hierarchic nature of the item presentation can yield clues to the patient's limits in terms of motor functioning.

Neuropsychological Items (Motor)

Items involving gross motor movement assess one of the most basic cortically mediated motor responses such as a response to a single command: "Raise your right hand" or "Move your left leg." You can evaluate motor speed from the patient's ability to "Touch your thumb to your forefinger as quickly as you can" and fine motor ability from "Touch your thumb to each

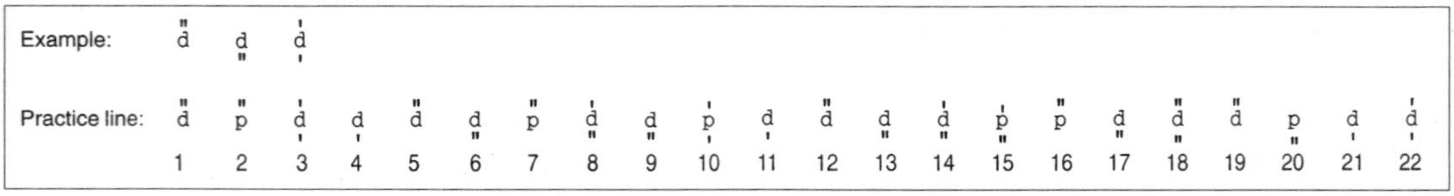

Figure 14.4   Practice line of d2 Test. The test items consist of the letters *d* and *p* with one to four dashes, arranged either individually or in pairs above and below the letter. The subject must scan across each line to identify and cross out each *d* with two dashes. In the manual these items (correct hits) are called "relevant items." All other combinations of letters and lines are considered "irrelevant," because they should not be crossed out. The one-page d2 Test form provides sections for recording identifying data and test scores, and provides a practice sample. On the reverse side is the standardized test, consisting of 14 lines, each with 47 characters, for a total of 658 items. The subject is allowed 20 seconds per line. (From R. Brickenkamp and E. A. Zillmer, *d2 Test of Attention*, Göttingen, Germany: Hogrefe & Huber, © 1998, p. 7; reprinted by permission)

finger, one after the other." These previous items assess the ability to perform a particular response; the following items tap the patient's ability to perform and inhibit motor behavior. Neuropsychologists consider this a higher-level cognitive process, because it requires the patient to shift between initiating and inhibiting behavior. "If I clap once, you clap twice." (Clap hands one time.) "Now, I clap twice, you clap once." (Clap hands two times.)

Neuropsychologists often examine graphomotor skills. The following items* assess the ability to copy shapes with increasing degrees of difficulty. They involve the integration of visual perception (input) and a complex motor response (output). "Copy these designs. Take your time and do your best." The patient's drawings are scored related to the correct shape, size, symmetry, and integration.

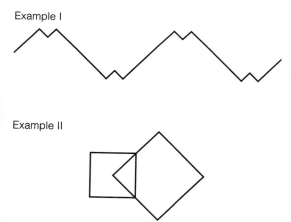

Example I

Example II

Motor apraxia items assess the intactness of common motor sequences. In general, the term *apraxia* refers to an inability to carry out purposeful sequences of motor behaviors. Although basic motor skills may be intact, the patient may be unable to perform even overlearned motor sequences. The form of apraxia assessed here is **motor apraxia** or **ideomotor apraxia.** Impairments in this area may stem from an inability to access a stored motor sequence or an inability to relay that information to the motor association areas.

*Both examples from E. A. Zillmer, M. J. Chelder, and J. Efthimiou, *Assessment of Impairment (AIM) Measure,* Philadelphia: Drexel University, 1995.

An example to test this is "Show me how you would make a telephone call from beginning to end."

Neuropsychological Tests (Motor)

Examples of standardized motor tests include a measure of grip strength and finger-tapping speed, both from the Halstead-Reitan Neuropsychological Battery. Grip strength simply measures the patient's ability to squeeze the dynamometer (see Figure 14.5) as hard as he or she can. The Finger Oscillation or Finger Tapping Test requires the patient to tap as rapidly as possible with the index finger on a small lever attached to a mechanical counter (see Figure 14.5).

VERBAL FUNCTIONS/LANGUAGE

Neuropsychologists screen for intactness of language. Initial items test the patient's ability to understand simple spoken language. More complicated areas of expressive language are then evaluated by assessing word repetition, naming, and word production.

Neuropsychological Items (Language)

Receptive speech evaluates the patient's ability to comprehend simple spoken commands such as "Wave hello" or a more difficult, three-step command: "Turn over the paper, hand me the pen, point to your mouth." Expressive speech focuses on vocabulary

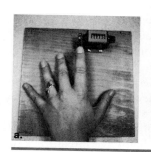
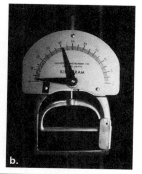

Figure 14.5 The Finger Tapping Test and Strength of Grip Test. (Jeffrey T. Barth, University of Virginia)

knowledge and recognition of concepts and objects, "Please tell me what the word *happiness* means." Additional tests involve word and phrase repetition ("Repeat: 'No ifs, ands, or buts'") and sentence generation ("Make up a sentence using the word *vacation*.") Deficits in verbal fluency and naming are also tested; for example, "Name all the animals that you can think of as quickly as you can." Visual naming can be evaluated by pointing to a picture and saying, "Tell me what this object is."

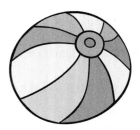

You can evaluate writing by assessing the quality of writing at the word and sentence level. You can also assess deficits in the motor component of writing (dysgraphia), simple reading (dyslexia), and spelling skills (spelling dyspraxia): "Please write down the name of this picture."

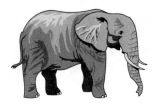

Neuropsychological Tests (Language)

Many standardized neuropsychological tests assess verbal and language functioning. A very simple but effective test of auditory comprehension (receptive language) is the Token Test (see, for example, Boller & Vignolo, 1966). Almost every nonaphasic person who has completed fourth grade should pass this test in its entirety. The test consists of a number of commands (such as "Touch the small yellow circle" or "Touch the green square and the blue circle") that relate to plastic tokens, which come in different shapes, sizes, and colors. This test is sensitive to disrupted linguistic processes that are central to aphasic disability.

The Controlled Oral Word Association test (COWA; Benton & Hamsher, 1989) assesses the subject's ability to use expressive speech. It measures verbal fluency by asking the subject to name as many words as possible that start with a specific letter. For example, within 60 seconds an undergraduate or graduate student should be able to name 15 words that start with the letter *R*. In the COWA, examiners administer three word-naming trials using the letters *C*, *F*, and *L*. These letters were selected on the basis of English word frequency. That is, words beginning with *C* have a relatively high frequency; the second letter, *F*, a somewhat lower frequency; and the third letter, *L*, a still lower frequency. Word fluency is a sensitive indicator of general brain dysfunction and expressive language dysfunction.

VISUAL-SPATIAL ORGANIZATION

In the visual-spatial domain, neuropsychologists assess various aspects of processing. They ask the patient to perform tasks of map skills, route finding, spatial integration and decoding, and facial recognition. The results of these neuropsychological tests can provide information about specific disorders of visual-spatial organization.

Neuropsychological Items (Visual-Spatial)

For example, neuropsychologists can evaluate spatial orientation with simple directional skills and mazes, and then proceed through clock drawing and motor-free constructional tasks: "If this were a compass on a map and you were facing north, which direction would be behind you?" Or "Draw the face of a clock, showing all the numbers, and set the hands to read ten minutes after 11." Testers may evaluate visual-spatial processing by asking, "Which of these sets of lines makes up this figure at the top, A, B, or C?"*

*From E. A. Zillmer, M. J. Chelder, and J. Efthimiou, *Assessment of Impairment (AIM) Measure*, Philadelphia: Drexel University, 1995)

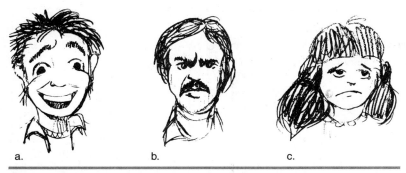

Figure 14.6 Test of facial recognition. (From E. A. Zillmer, M. J. Chelder, and J. Efthimiou, *Assessment of Impairment (AIM) Measure,* Philadelphia: Drexel University, 1995)

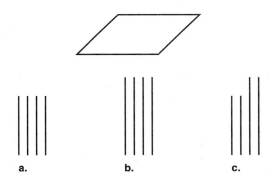

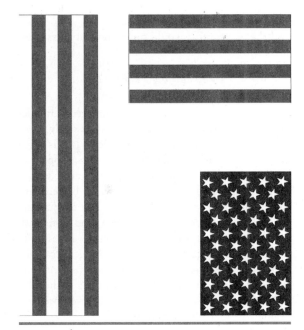

Figure 14.7 Spatial organization task.

Facial recognition is the patient's ability to recognize a familiar face, as well as to compare similar faces and identify facial affect. For example, the examiner may ask, "Show me 'the happy face, the sad face, the angry face'" (see Figure 14.6).

Spatial manipulation assesses the individual's ability to perceive and organize more complex and ambiguous visual stimuli. More than just a recognition task, these items require a more active cognitive process for success. For example, "This is a picture of an object that has been cut up and turned around. (An easy example of this is included here.) Tell me what the object is" (see Figure 14.7).

Visual sequencing also involves more integration and higher-order processing. The person must comprehend the overall meaning of the activity, and then be able to correctly assemble the pictures to form the sequence of steps. "This card has three pictures on it. If the pictures are put in the right order, they tell a story. Look carefully at the pictures, tell me the story, and point to the one you think comes first in the story. Now point to the one that would come second,

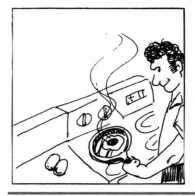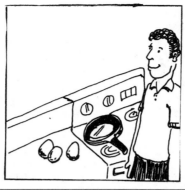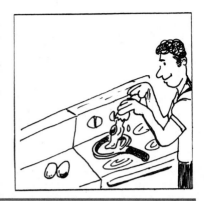

Figure 14.8   Example of picture arrangement. (From E. A. Zillmer, M. J. Chelder, and J. Efthimiou, *Assessment of Impairment (AIM) Measure,* Philadelphia: Drexel University, 1995)

and the picture that would finish the story" (see Figure 14.8).

Neuropsychological Tests (Visual-Spatial)

The Bender Gestalt test consists of nine geometric designs, which the patient must reproduce exactly (Bender, 1938; Hutt, 1985). The "Bender," as it is often called, is a popular measure of visual-spatial construction. It measures a patient's ability to organize visual-spatial material and has been shown to be sensitive to changes in neuropsychological status, particularly visual-graphic disabilities. Rey (1941) and Osterrieth (1944) devised another drawing test to investigate perceptual organization. The Rey-Osterrieth Complex Figure Test presents the subject with an intricate figure to reproduce. For both the Bender and the Rey-Osterrieth, scoring systems have been developed that evaluate specific copying errors.

MEMORY

You can look at memory in many ways. For example, as we noted earlier, to remember things people must pay attention first. After paying attention, people must encode the information (do something meaningful with the information such as rehearsing it), in order to put the information into more permanent storage.

Once information is in storage, people must be able to retrieve the information as needed.

Neuropsychological Items (Memory)

Neuropsychologists assess general memory and new learning skills in a variety of modalities. There are immediate and delayed memory tasks in both verbal and visual formats. Performance on free recall and recognition tasks can help identify different aspects of memory function and dysfunction. Multiple trials of a list learning task can assess immediate verbal memory. For example, the examiner presents the patient with five words, repeated over four trials regardless of the patient's success on the item's initial trials. "I'm going to say a list of five words. Please try to remember them, and repeat them when I finish: *train, radio, apple, fork, chair.*"

You can assess delayed verbal memory by asking the patient, at a later point during the examination (such as 30 minutes), to say whether or not each word had been included in the list "I am going to read a list of words. Tell me which of these words were in the earlier list I asked you to recall several times: *clock, **apple**, book, **train**, table, **fork**, sandwich, truck, **radio**, **chair**.*"

Delayed visual memory assesses the patient's ability to remember visual information the examiner pre-

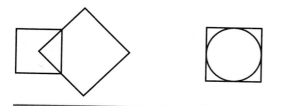

Figure 14.9 Example of design copy test.

sented earlier in the testing (an intermediate delay), as well as the ability to remember simple visual figures following a very short delay. The examiner presents these items in a recognition format rather than a free recall format, so the patient chooses between similar stimuli, one of which is the correct figure. "Earlier I asked you to copy four designs. Which of these designs was it?" (see Figure 14.9).

You can assess contextual or logical memory, immediate and delayed, by testing the patient's free recall ability. The examiner presents a short story to the patient, testing memory for information presented in a specific contextual structure. After an interference item, the examiner again asks the patient to tell the story. Slashes separate each unit of information in the following example.

I am going to read to you a short story. When I finish, I want you to tell me as much of the story as you can remember. Try to remember it in the same words as I have used: "Joseph / Green / left his house / and headed for the subway. /He was on his way / to the supermarket. / He purchased / wine, / steak, / and ice cream. / Later that day / he had dinner /with his boss /from the office./" Now tell me as much of the story as you can remember.

A completely verbatim response is not necessary, because neuropsychologists are mostly interested in whether the individual has formed a memory. For example, an acceptable substitution for /steak/ is *meat* or *beef*.

Neuropsychological Tests (Memory)

To provide thorough coverage of the varieties of memory disabilities, researchers have developed bat-

teries of memory tests. One of the most frequently used memory assessment instruments used by neuropsychologists is the Wechsler Memory Scale (WMS; first introduced by Wechsler in 1945), which is now in its third revision (WMS-III). The WMS consist of seven subtests, which include personal and current information, orientation, mental control, logical memory (which tests immediate recall of two verbal stories), digit span, visual reproduction (an immediate visual memory drawing task), and associate learning (which requires verbal retention). The WMS is sensitive to memory disorders and memory defects associated with aging.

JUDGMENT/PROBLEM SOLVING

A patient's ability to use abstract reasoning relates, in part, to his or her capacity to understand concepts. In determining a patient's ability to use abstract reasoning, the neuropsychologist examines the patient's ability to generalize from one situation to another. This skill is known as "transfer of learning." For example, if a rehabilitation patient can learn to transfer from the mat to the wheelchair with minimal assistance during physical therapy, one would normally expect the same patient to be able to generalize that skill from the physical therapy wing of the hospital to the nursing wing. Otherwise the patient's learning is circumstantial.

Often neuropsychologists are interested in evaluating insight specific to the patient's capacity to realize the implications of his or her disorder. At times a patient presents to a neuropsychologist, and says, "I'll be fine as soon as I get home" or "There is nothing wrong with me, I can drive a car." Initially, the neuropsychologist will measure his or her own evaluation against those by other team members. For example, if the patient has had a mild stroke, and is only hindered by his or her own dislike of the hospital setting, it may be true that the patient will be "fine" on discharge. If the patient has experienced a moderate or more severe brain injury, the patient's communication may be evaluated as demonstrating lack of insight. One of the jobs of the neuropsychologist is to evaluate the insight that a patient has in regard to the nature and the implications of his or her own disability.

Neuropsychological Items (Problem Solving)

You can evaluate higher-order cognitive functioning and abstract thinking skills by asking the patient to interpret proverbs, solve everyday problems, or perform mental arithmetic. For example, you can assess abstract reasoning by asking a patient to interpret a common proverb, scoring responses based on degree of abstraction. Proverb interpretations are a traditional feature of the neuropsychological exam, assessing the ability to reason beyond the concrete level. For example, "What does this saying mean: 'You can't judge a book by its cover?'" An abstract answer may be "Don't judge a person by their looks," and a concrete answer may be "You don't know what is inside the book, just by looking at its cover."

A common way to assess concept formation is to use a similarities–differences paradigm or analogies. The following items involve the abstract categorization of objects and concepts. They assess whether the patient can determine the appropriate abstract links between these objects and discriminate form and function. "How are an eagle and a robin alike?" Or "Please complete this sentence: 'Banana is a fruit, cat is an animal. Father is a man, mother is a . . . .'"

Problem-solving tasks tap the patient's ability to formulate solutions to a common, everyday situation. Responses can often reveal impulsivity and poor social judgment, as well as decreased functional independence or a need for supervision. "What should you do if you can't keep an appointment?" Sometimes tests present absurdities in order to evaluate reasoning skills, attention to abstract details, and the ability to formulate an abstract verbal response: "What is strange about this sentence: 'When the cook discovered that he had burned the meat, he put it in the refrigerator to fix it'?" Or "What is funny or strange about this picture?" (see Figure 14.10).

Neuropsychological Tests (Problem Solving)

Neuropsychologists have been very creative in developing assessment procedures that evaluate executive abilities, and literally dozens of tests measure this neuropsychological domain. Only a few are mentioned

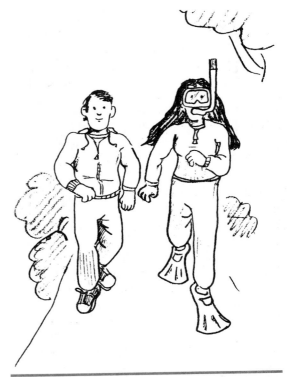

Figure 14.10   Example of a visual absurdity. (From E. A. Zillmer, M. J. Chelder, and J. Efthimiou, *Assessment of Impairment (AIM) Measure*, Philadelphia: Drexel University, 1995)

here. The Trail Making Test B, part of the Halstead-Reitan Neuropsychological Battery, requires the participant to draw lines to connect consecutively numbered and lettered circles by alternating the two sequences (1 to *A*, *A* to 2, 2 to *B*, and so on). This timed task necessitates complex visual scanning, motor speed, mental flexibility, and attention.

The Wisconsin Card Sorting Test (WCST; Berg, 1948) is widely used to study "abstract behavior" and "shifting sets." The examiner gives the subject a pack of 64 cards on which are printed one to four symbols, triangle, star, cross, or circle, in red, green, yellow, or blue. No two cards are identical. The patient's task is to place them one by one under four stimulus cards according to a principle that the patient must deduce from the pattern of the examiner's responses to the patient's placement of the cards. For example, if the principle is color, the correct placement of a red card is under one red triangle, regardless of the number of symbols. Thus, the subject simply starts placing cards and the examiner tells him or her whether the placement is correct. After 10 cards have been correctly placed in a row, the examiner shifts the principle, indicating the shift only to the patient by the changed patterns of "right" and "wrong" statements. A poor performance on this test often suggests that the patient has trouble organizing his or her own behavior or has difficulty applying one set of rules to different situations. The WCST is a sensitive neuropsychological measure, particularly for injuries to the frontal lobes.

Culbertson and Zillmer (1998a, 1998b, 1998c) designed the Tower of London–Drexel University (TOL^{dx}) as a neuropsychological measure of executive planning and problem solving based on the original Tower of London (Shallice, 1982). The TOL^{dx} measures executive planning that involves the ability to conceptualize change, respond objectively, generate and select alternatives, and sustain attention (Lezak, 1995). The frontal lobes, in systematic interaction with other cortical and subcortical structures, support executive planning. The TOL^{dx} test materials include two identical tower structure (see Figure 14.11), one for the subject and one for the examiner to use. Each structure consists of three pegs of descending lengths and three colored beads that the patient can place on the pegs in different configurations or patterns. The examiner asks the subject to move the beads of his or her tower structure to match bead configurations that the examiner presents. In solving the bead patterns, the subject must adhere to two strictly enforced problem-solving rules: Only move one bead at a time, and don't place more beads than fit on each peg. The examiner records number of moves, rule violations, and time the subject uses in solving the bead patterns. Interpreting the subject's performance involves an analysis of both quantitative and qualitative variables. Empirical studies (Culbertson & Zillmer, 1998a, 1998b; Culbertson, Zillmer, & Di Pinto, 1999; Zillmer, Culbertson, & Holda, 1997) show that the TOL–Drexel University is sensitive to a complex set of cognitive processes, including planning computations, working memory, mental flexibility, attention allocation, and response inhibition.

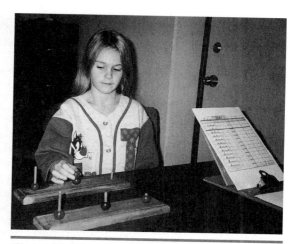

Figure 14.11 Administration of the Tower of London–Drexel University that evaluates frontal lobe functioning. (Eric Zillmer)

Table 14.4 reviews the most frequently administered neuropsychological tests, in a survey of over 2000 members of the National Academy of Neuropsychology (Gordon & Zillmer, 1997).

Traditional Psychological Testing and Its Use in Neuropsychology

Generic psychological evaluations are, for the most part, specifically concerned with identifying the nature and severity of maladaptive, abnormal, and bizarre behavior patterns and phenomena, as well as understanding the conditions that have caused and/or are maintaining such behavior. Researchers have designed numerous tests to measure such facets of intelligence and personality, and it is convenient to group these tests into the following two categories: tests of intelligence, and objective and projective personality techniques. Intelligence tests use items that measure abilities and are most closely related to neuropsychological tests. **Objective personality tests** typically use the questionnaire technique of measurement (for example, true/false or multiple choice), whereas **projective personality tests** rely on relatively

Table 14.4   *Frequently Used Neuropsychological Assessment Procedures, Grouped by Function*

Functional Domain	Name of Test	Frequency of Use
Orientation	Glasgow Coma Scale (GCS)	<5%
	Galveston Orientation and Amnesia Test	<5%
Sensation/Perception	Sensory/Perceptual Exam (from HRNB)	27%
Motor	Finger Tapping Test (from HRNB)	27%
	Hand Dynamometer (from HRNB)	27%
	Grooved Pegboard	6%
Attention/Concentration	Digit Span (from WAIS-R)	90%
	Stroop Color Word Test	27%
	Paced Auditory Serial Addition Task (PAST)	18%
	Symbol Digit Modalities Test (SDMT)	19%
	Continuous Performance Tests	<5%
	d2 Test of Attention	<5%
Verbal Functions	Vocabulary (from WAIS-R)	90%
	Controlled Oral Word Association Test (COWA)	61%
	Token Test	17%
	Boston Naming Test (BNT)	12%
Visual-Spatial Organization	Block Design (from WAIS-R)	90%
	Tactile Performance Test (from HRNB)	27%
	Bender Gestalt Visual Motor Test	27%
	Rey-Osterrieth Complex Figure Test	17%
	Ravens Progressive Matrices	8%
	Hooper Visual Organization Test	6%
	Judgment of Line Orientation	5%
	Beery Visual Motor Integration	<5%
	Clock Drawing	<5%
Memory	Wechsler Memory Scale-Revised (WMS-R)	71%
	California Verbal Learning Test (CVLT)	38%
	Rey Auditory Verbal Learning Tests (RAVLT)	30%
	Selective Reminding Test	11%
	Memory Assessment Scales (MAS)	<5%
Judgment/Problem Solving	Wisconsin Card Sorting Test (WCST)	51%
	Category Test (from HRNB)	27%
	Trail Making Test B (from HRNB)	27%
	Ravens Progressive Matrices	8%
	Tower of London–Drexel University (TOL^{DX})	<5%

Note: HRNB = Halstead-Reitan Neurological Battery; WAIS-R = Wechsler Adult Intelligence Scale, 3rd edition.

ambiguous, vague, and unstructured stimuli, such as inkblots.

INTELLIGENCE TESTING

The testing of intelligence has had a history of constant misuse, misunderstanding, and dispute. Although certainly valid criticisms can be raised against testing intelligence, it also offers a number of benefits. For example, one of the main assets of intelligence tests is their accuracy in predicting future behavior (such as academic achievement) and in identifying the present level of cognitive functioning, as well as cognitive strengths and weaknesses. However, considerable controversy has raged over the use of intelligence tests in clinical neuropsychology, specifically about their sensitivity to brain dysfunction.

Despite the common use of the word **intelligence** in psychology as well as in the English language, there are many definitions of intelligence. In fact, many investigators suggest, somewhat cynically, that intelligence is synonymous with the score on an intelligence test. The precise definition of intelligence, however, has remained elusive and is still debated. Wechsler (1944) has suggested that intelligence be defined as the "aggregate or global capacity involving an individual's ability to act purposefully, to think rationally, and to deal effectively with their environment" (p. 3). Although there are well over 100 different tests of intelligence, the scales David Wechsler developed have become widely used throughout the world and typically include a variety of scales measuring verbal comprehension skills and tests tapping perceptual organization abilities.

The Wechsler Intelligence Scales (Wechsler, 1981) are actuarial measures, like many other standardized psychological tests, and are interpreted in terms of averages and probabilities. In the case of IQ tests (IQ = intelligence quotient), examiners give the measure to a large number of people and then sort and tally the scores in a distribution that shows how many individuals earned each possible score. In the normal distribution, which is a particular mathematical form that often closely approximates actual score distributions (such as height, weight, as well as intelligence), about two-thirds of the scores deviate less than one standard deviation from the mean and about 95% of the scores are within two standard deviations. Thus, IQ scores are expressed as deviation units away from the norm. Each of the three Wechsler IQs (Verbal, Performance, and Full Scale IQ) has a mean of 100 and a standard deviation of 15. Table 14.5 presents a set of often-used classifications of Wechsler IQ scores together with corresponding numeric limits in terms of IQs and percentages. For example, only 2.2 percent of the population scored above an IQ of 128, suggesting a very superior range of intellectual functioning.

We present the following studies on IQ tests for comparison of estimated IQ among different normal and clinical groups. The mean WAIS-R Full-Scale IQ of a heterogeneous psychiatric inpatient population

Table 14.5 *Intelligence Classification According to IQ Scales, Including Percentages for the U.S. Standardization Sample for Each IQ Category*

Classification	IQ Limits	% Included
Very Superior	>128	2.2
Superior	120–127	6.7
Above Average	111–119	16.1
Average	91–110	50.0
Below Average	80–90	16.1
Borderline	66–79	6.7
Mentally Deficient	<65	2.2

Source: Wechsler (1981), p. 28.

is approximately 85 or Low Average (Zillmer, Fowler, Newman, & Archer, 1988; Zillmer, Ball, Fowler, Newman, & Stutts, 1991). The mean IQ of stroke patients who are hospitalized in a rehabilitation setting is about 87 or Low Average (Zillmer, Fowler, Waechtler, Harris, & Khan, 1992). College graduates score on average about 118 or in the High Average range, and doctoral students have a mean IQ score of 125, falling within the Superior range (Kole & Matarazzo, 1965).

The highest score obtainable on the Wechsler IQ test is approximately 150, that is, if the subject answers all items correctly. Although the concept of genius typically involves a capacity for creative and original thought, some have also defined it as having an extraordinarily high intelligence rating on a psychological test (IQs above 140). In a landmark study (Terman, 1925, 1959) of "geniuses," the Stanford psychologist Lewis M. Terman identified schoolchildren in California with an IQ higher than 140. Of the 250,000 eleven-year-old children screened, Terman found 1524 who fell into the "genius" bracket. Terman and his researchers followed the sample of geniuses over many decades and found that they were more likely to graduate from college and earn above-average incomes. Interestingly, the "genius" sample also included criminals, alcoholics, and prostitutes.

Similarly, serial killers Ted Bundy and Jeffrey Dahmer have tested with an IQ of 122 and 121, respectively (in the superior range of cognitive abilities). Clearly, intelligence and morality are not necessarily related.

The Wechsler scales are among the most commonly used tests in clinical neuropsychology today (Zillmer & Ball, 1987). For example, among members of the National Academy of Neuropsychology, 97% report using the WAIS-R as part of their neuropsychological evaluations (Gordon & Zillmer, 1997). It is clear that the Wechsler scales continue to be the cornerstone of the neuropsychological battery, but exactly how they are used with various neuropsychological populations is not well understood. Most criticism of the use of intelligence scales in neuropsychology comes from studies that show the IQ's limited sensitivity to even gross lesions such as stroke (for example, see Zillmer et al., 1992). Estimating intelligence may have little in common with determining brain impairment. This is related to the fact that intelligence scales measure mostly crystallized or learned aspects of intelligence, whereas neuropsychological procedures measure more fluid or biological measures of neurocognitive abilities (Zillmer et al., 1988). Clinical neuropsychologists are typically most interested in those aspects of higher cortical function reflecting fluid intelligence. Nevertheless, the Wechsler Scales remain popular assessment tools and, when appropriately used, provide the clinical neuropsychologist with an index of general intelligence, an estimate of premorbid functioning, age-corrected norms, and some insight into the patient's pattern of performance.

PERSONALITY ASSESSMENT

Neuropsychology has been defined as the study of the relationships between brain functions and behavior. In contrast, few scholars have agreed on a definition of personality, but characterize it variously as the structure of the mind; an individual's effort to adjust to his or her environment; the most striking or dominant characteristic of a human being; or a person's unique pattern of traits. Together, the fields of neuropsychology and personality assessment embrace variables that exist widely in the population and encompass almost all aspects of life and experience. The common denominator of both fields is that they measure behavior. More importantly, in both cases the behavior reveals critical information regarding brain processes. Thus, there is a great need to understand the manner in which these two diverse fields come together. The areas of neuropsychological and personality assessment have long and rich traditions, which in the past have been used to correlate brain functioning and personality/emotional adjustment. Only recently, however, have researchers realized that these two fields are inextricably linked. Both neuropsychology and personality are products of brain functioning (Perry & Zillmer, 1996).

Objective Personality Tests

The major clinical objective test in use today is the Minnesota Multiphasic Personality Inventory (MMPI), developed by Hathaway, a psychologist, and McKinley, a psychiatrist, in 1943 at the University of Minnesota (Greene, 1991). The MMPI consists of over 500 true/false items and has become the most widely employed objective measure of psychopathology in adolescents and adults (Zillmer & Ball, 1987). The subject endorses items that apply to him or her. Topics range from physical conditions to moral and social attitudes. The neuropsychologist then compares the patient's responses with the responses patients make in different diagnostic groups (such as schizophrenia, affective disorder, or hypochondriasis). Similarities in the pattern of responses can be very helpful in diagnosing mental disorders and in planning appropriate treatment strategies. The MMPI was revised and restandardized in 1989—to eliminate sexist wording, increase grammatical clarification, and modernize the test—and republished to form the 567-item MMPI-2. The MMPI-2 has built-in measures for detecting defensiveness or an exaggeration of problems on the part of the person taking the test as well as number of new content scales. Table 14.6 illustrates the major scale names for the 10 clinical and the 3 validity scales (Greene, 1991).

The MMPI has a controversial history in neuropsychology related to researchers' repeated efforts to diagnose brain damage using a personality test. Despite all this research activity, personality assessment instruments have not held up to empirical scrutiny,

Table 14.6 *Item Numbers of the Basic Validity and Clinical Scales of the MMPI-2*

Number of Items

VALIDITY SCALES	Lie (L)	15
	Infrequency (F)	60
	Defensiveness (K)	30
CLINICAL SCALES	1. Hypochondriasis (Hs)	32
	2. Depression (D)	57
	3. Hysteria (Hy)	32
	4. Psychopathic Deviate (Pd)	50
	5. Masculinity-Femininity (Mf)	56
	6. Paranoia (Pa)	40
	7. Psychasthenia (Pt)	48
	8. Schizophrenia (Sc)	78
	9. Hypomania (Ma)	46
	0. Social Introversion (Si)	69

Note: Many of the items overlap and are scored on more than one scale.
Source: Greene (1991), p. 2.

demonstrating little, if any, validity in terms of measuring or being related to neuropsychological processes (Zillmer & Perry, 1996, see Neuropsychology in Action 14.1).

Projective Personality Techniques

Projective tests rely on various ambiguous, vague, and unstructured stimuli, such as inkblots (see Figure 14.13), rather than on specific test questions and answers. By presenting ambiguous material in an unstructured testing situation, the examinee may project a good deal about his or her own conflicts, motives, coping techniques, and other aspects of his or her personality (Zillmer & Vuz, 1995). Thus, projective tests place greater emphasis on how an individual organizes and perceives the stimuli presented to him or her. For example, any stimulus situation that is not structured to elicit a specific class of responses (as do true/false inventories and the like) may invoke the projective process.

The Rorschach Inkblot Test is one of the first personality tests developed and one of the most researched and frequently used psychological techniques today, although only 11% of clinical neuropsychologist use it routinely in a neuropsychological evaluation (Gordon & Zillmer, 1997). Swiss psychiatrist Herman Rorschach (1884-1922) developed the test as an extension of earlier research using inkblots to study imagination. Since first described by Rorschach, the inkblot technique has enjoyed a rich, but often controversial history regarding the precise nature of the test's administration, scoring, and interpretation. This controversy relates, in part, to the developer of the test having died at the early age of 38, just a year after the test was published, and to the subsequent loss of leadership regarding the use of the test. Over the last 20 years, John Exner, Jr., has summarized and systematized the Rorschach Inkblot Test in an intensive effort to make the Rorschach technique more objective and empirical (1993). The resulting Rorschach Comprehensive System represents a significant step forward in standardizing and validating the administration, scoring, and interpretation of Rorschach responses (Piotrowski, Sherry, & Keller, 1985; Zillmer, 1991).

The early history of projective psychological testing also reflects a strong interest in attempting to diagnose brain impairment from psychological tests.

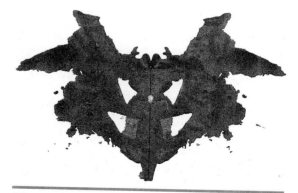

Figure 14.13 Card One of the Rorschach Inkblot Test. (Hermann Rorschach, Rorschach® Test. © Verlag Hans Huber AG, Bern, Switzerland, 1921, 1948, 1994.)

Neuropsychology in Action 14.1

The Use of the MMPI in Clinical Neuropsychology

by Eric A. Zillmer

As a result of the interaction between personality and ability factors in determining rehabilitation progress and ultimately psychosocial adjustment, neuropsychologists have increasingly added measures of personality to their assessment. This has prompted Rourke (1991) to predict that "There will be an intense interest in the investigation of the socio-emotional and personality correlates of brain disease" (p. 5). Although the MMPI is not used in the diagnosis of brain damage per se, it is frequently administered as part of a neuropsychological evaluation; that is, approximately 60% of neuropsychologists use the MMPI as part of a neuropsychological evaluation (Gordon & Zillmer, 1997). Neuropsychologists are interested in understanding a patient's personal adjustment after a head trauma, estimating the presence and severity of depression in dementia, and documenting the presence of psychopathology in individuals with neurological disorders. As such, personality testing tells the neuropsychologist how an individual deals with stress in an adaptive or maladaptive manner.

In general, there is no single personality profile of individuals who have brain dysfunction. For example, it is entirely possible that patients who have experienced head injury of the same severity may react very differently to it. One individual may become very depressed and lethargic in response to the trauma, whereas another person may become impulsive and labile. Still others may seem completely normal on personality testing. Figure 14.12 shows the five MMPI profiles of subjects who experienced emotional distress after they were exposed to chlordane pesticide and required medical treatment after their homes were treated for termites. Chlordane is a potent neurotoxin and animal carcinogen and results in cognitive deficits in humans ranging from mild to moderate on tasks requiring speeded processing, problem solving, and delayed memory. MMPI profile analysis indicated a mild to high level of overall psychological disturbance (scores of T = 50 to 70 are "average," scores above T = 70 are considered "pathological"). Elevated high-point scale combinations were apparent for the neurotic triad (scale 1, hypochondriasis, and scale 3, hysteria), indicating a preoccupation with bodily concern, excessive somatization, fatigue, dizziness, depression, and hysterical features. Similar MMPI profile configurations are, however, not at all uncommon in general medical patients (see, for example, Zillmer et al., 1988).

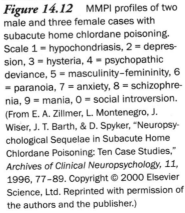

Figure 14.12   MMPI profiles of two male and three female cases with subacute home chlordane poisoning. Scale 1 = hypochondriasis, 2 = depression, 3 = hysteria, 4 = psychopathic deviance, 5 = masculinity–femininity, 6 = paranoia, 7 = anxiety, 8 = schizophrenia, 9 = mania, 0 = social introversion. (From E. A. Zillmer, L. Montenegro, J. Wiser, J. T. Barth, & D. Spyker, "Neuropsychological Sequelae in Subacute Home Chlordane Poisoning: Ten Case Studies," *Archives of Clinical Neuropsychology, 11,* 1996, 77–89. Copyright © 2000 Elsevier Science, Ltd. Reprinted with permission of the authors and the publisher.)

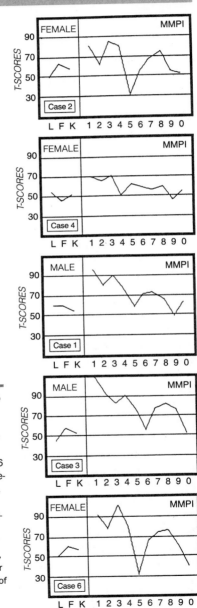

Clearly, an assessment of emotional functioning is important in the consideration of neurotoxic conditions. This is particularly the case in attempting to fully understand the impact of an individual's emotional and cognitive functioning on personal adjustment and quality of life following exposure to toxins. Interestingly, in some instances clinical neuropsychologists have noticed that the consequences of a maladaptive personality adjustment as a result of brain injury may be equally as, or more important than the cognitive sequelae of brain dysfunction. Diamond, Barth, and Zillmer (1988) did one of the first studies to examine the relationship between personality and neuropsychology. They administered the MMPI and a comprehensive neuropsychological battery to 50 mild head trauma patients and 50 patients, matched for age and education, with known, often serious neurologic disease including stroke, brain tumor, and dementia. Results revealed that at three months post injury, the mild head injury group demonstrated significant emotional distress similar to those individuals with long-standing neurologic damage, although the mild head trauma group was less neurologically and neuropsychologically impaired than the comparison group. The most important findings related to difficulties in returning to school or work. Results indicated that ratings of neuropsychological impairment used in conjunction with the MMPI, as an objective measure of emotional adjustment, was more highly indicative of difficulties in returning to the tasks of preinjury activity than was either measure used individually. These findings support a growing literature on the effects of brain disease or trauma on emotional adjustment in mild head injury, hypoxia, chemical poisoning, alcoholism, stroke, migraine headaches, and Lyme disease (for example, see Bundick et al., 1995; Zillmer et al., 1986).

For example, Rorschach himself (1942) suggested that it could be used for differential diagnosis of brain impairment: "It should be possible . . . in almost every case to come to a definite conclusion as to whether the subject is normal, neurotic, schizophrenic, or has organic brain disease" (p. 120). One early Rorschach pioneer was Molly Harrower, who as a research fellow of neurologist Wilder Penfield at the Montreal Neurological Institute in the 1930s, was asked on a regular basis to evaluate all "organic" patients suspected of brain tumor. Of course, the neuropsychology student should realize that sophisticated imaging techniques were not available and that a skilled clinician would probably have an equal or better chance to observe behavioral abnormalities compared to other health professionals. The interest in the differential diagnosis of brain damage was also a focus of Zygmunt Piotrowski (1940), who outlined 10 specific "organic personality signs" using the Rorschach inkblots.

The MMPI and Rorschach tests have not held up to empirical scrutiny, demonstrating little, if any, validity for measuring brain impairment. Thus, after years of research, there has been little convincing evidence that either the Rorschach or the MMPI could definitely identify specific neuropathological processes (Zillmer & Perry, 1996). As a result, very few investigators would use the Rorschach or the MMPI to diagnose neurologic conditions, but do administer them to understand how a subject may adapt to a brain injury. For a review of the most frequently used personality tests in neuropsychology, see Table 14.9.

PSYCHOLOGICAL VERSUS NEUROPSYCHOLOGICAL DIAGNOSIS AND EVALUATION

How do traditional psychological and neuropsychological assessments differ? How are they alike? Is it practical to categorize all clinical psychological tests into three groups: personality, intellectual, and

Table 14.9 *Frequently Used Personality Tests by Clinical Neuropsychologists*

Name of Test	Frequent Usage
MMPI/MMPI-2	60%
MCMI (Million Clinical Multiaxial Inventory)	13%
Rorschach Inkblot Test	11%
SCL-90 (Symptom Check List)	10%
TAT (Thematic Apperception Test)	6%

Source: Gordon and Zillmer (1997).

neuropsychological? Neuropsychologists have used all of those tests at one time or another to diagnose brain damage, although with varying success.

There is no strict definition for what test is a neuropsychological test and what test is not. One rule of thumb is to consider whether the measure's test score changes systematically with a change in brain integrity. If it does, the test is sensitive to brain changes, whether they are structural, metabolic, electrophysiological, or otherwise, and the procedure can be considered a neuropsychological test. If the test shows no predictable and systematic change, then it should not be considered a neuropsychological test. Sometimes the relationship between test data and changes in brain integrity is not clear, and then neuropsychologists argue about a test's sensitivity to brain functioning. This is the case for some measures of personality and often for tests of intelligence.

In general, traditional psychological and neuropsychological tests are alike in that they both employ the methods and standards of psychometric testing. Their general goal involves deficit measurement; that is, they assess deviation from the mean. Psychological and neuropsychological tests are dissimilar in that they require different forms of training. Particularly neuropsychological assessment involves a high degree of expertise in clinical neurosciences, neuroanatomy, and theories of brain functions. In contrast, generic psychological testing is grounded in more traditional theories of psychopathology, including those of psychodynamic and cognitive-behavioral theory. It should be obvious to the neuropsychology student that both traditional psychological and neuropsychological assessments relate to brain processes, and many neuropsychologists seek to conceptualize patient symptoms and problems by integrating data from both approaches.

Let's examine what two experts have to say on this topic. In one of the classic books on psychological assessment, Anne Anastasi (1988) suggested the first problem that stimulated the development of psychological tests was identifying the mentally retarded. To this day, detecting intellectual deficiency remains an important application of certain types of psychological tests. For most clinical neuropsychologists, the standard sourcebook on evaluation is Muriel Lezak's

Neuropsychological Assessment (Lezak, 1995). On this topic Lezak suggests that one distinguishing characteristic of neuropsychological assessment is its emphasis on identifying and measuring psychological deficits. Lezak indicates that it is primarily in deficiencies and dysfunctional alteration of cognition, emotionality, and self-direction and management (executive functions) that brain damage manifests behaviorally. Neuropsychological assessment, she adds, is also concerned with documenting and describing preserved functions, that is, the patient's behavioral competencies and strengths (Lezak, 1995).

It is interesting that both authors describe the motivation for testing as a search for problems or dysfunctions, which neuropsychologists often term "deficit measurement." A deficit implies comparison to some standard, either as an expectation of appropriate performance in relation to others or by an intraindividual comparison of strengths versus weaknesses or present versus past performance. Calculating the statistical probability of the expected versus observed performances for any tests in question then determines deficits. If the performance is reliably below expectations, then a deficit is likely to exist. Actually, all clinical psychology targets "abnormal" behavior or "pathology," so this is not specific to neuropsychology. Also interesting is that generic psychological and neuropsychological tests may be concerned with a wide range of behavioral functioning. The mainstay of psychological testing since World War II has been intellectual functioning, personality, and emotional assessment. Certainly this covers a wide domain. According to Lezak (1995), neuropsychological assessment concerns areas of emotion and behavioral functioning as well as cognition.

Yet brain damage always implies behavioral impairment. Even when psychological "changes after head injury or concomitant with brain disease are viewed as improvement rather than impairment, as when there is a welcome increase in sociability or relief from neurotic anxiety, a careful assessment will probably reveal an underlying loss" (Lezak, 1995, p. 97).

Unfortunately, people still make an arbitrary distinction between "functional" and "organic" problems, which serves to categorize all that is environmental, emotional, and personality as "functional," and all that arises from biology as "organic." It is usually more useful to frame problems of human behavior as having multiple and reciprocal causality. For example, a child with a developmental language delay begins life with a brain that is organized differently from those of other children. But brain development continues rapidly through the first few years of life. Whereas most children's language and brain development is shaped by what they hear around them, the continued inability to profit from correctly interpreting speech in the child with a language delay compounds the developing brain's dysfunction. Exposure to an appropriate enriched environment may help the brain to adapt and develop toward more "normal" language. And someone with posttraumatic stress disorder (PTSD), which is usually considered a "psychological" anxiety disorder, may result in considerable "organic" dysfunction. In addition to sleep disturbances and intrusions of flashbacks into consciousness, PTSD patients often complain of difficulties in attention and concentration. These difficulties reflect the brain's adaptation to an environmental stressor. In turn, this altered brain functioning may result in further "psychological" problems. Many disorders show this combination of biological and environmental influences. Each influence has the potential to further impact the other: heredity, genetic, development, and acquired metabolic and brain problems impact the environment, and vice versa. Many clinical psychologists and clinical neuropsychologists recognize this interplay of environment and biology and seek to understand patients in a comprehensive manner.

Conclusion

The neuropsychological evaluation is a method of examining the brain by studying its behavioral product. As with other psychological assessments, neuropsychological evaluations involve the comprehensive study of behavior by means of standardized tests that are sensitive to brain–behavior relationships. In effect, the neuropsychological exam offers an understanding of the relationship between the structure and the function of the nervous system. Thus, the goal of the clinical neuropsychological exam is to be able to evaluate the full range of basic abilities represented in the brain. In practice, the neuropsychological assessment is multidimensional (concerned with evaluating many different aspect of neurofunctioning from basic to complex), reliable (stable across different situations and time), and valid (meaningful). The next chapter presents a discussion that is relevant to the clinical neuropsychologist in areas of test selection, test interpretation, diagnosis, and test development.

Critical Thinking Questions

▪ Why are the concepts of reliability and validity so important in psychological and neuropsychological assessment?

▪ What kind of questions and tests do neuropsychologists use in a neuropsychological evaluation?

▪ How are neuropsychology assessment procedures the same, how are they different?

▪ What sort of recommendations and treatments can neuropsychologists give to brain-impaired people that will be useful in their daily lives?

Key Terms

Neuropsychological evaluation	Reliability	Criterion validity	Behavioral-adaptive scales
Psychometrics	Validity	False positive	Intelligence tests
Standardized test	Construct validity	Base rate	Neuropsychological tests
	Content validity	Achievement tests	Personality tests

Vocational inventories	Orientation	Motor apraxia	Projective personality tests
Crystallized functions	Sensation	Ideomotor apraxia	Intelligence
Fluid functions	Perception	Objective personality tests	

Web Connections

http://ericae.net
ERIC Clearinghouse on Assessment and Evaluation
Extensive site on psychological and educational testing and assessment; includes test locator, frequently asked questions, search engine for ERIC, and many other links.

http://www.unl.edu/buros
Buros Institute of Mental Measurement
Home page of the *Buros Mental Measurements Yearbook,* tests in print, test reviews, and test locators.

http://www.mindtools.com/page12.html
Psychometric Testing
Interactive page that lets you discover your learning style; provides "IQ test," Myers-Briggs Personality Test, and other measures.

http://www.brain.com/home.htm
Psychological Testing
An interactive site that distributes various levels of psychological facts (and fictions, so be careful). An excellent tool for the administration and understanding of web-based psychological assessment tools. Different "IQ" tests let you to critically evaluate their construction and validity compared to other measures offered at this site.

http://www.pangea.ca/~mwady/tests1.html
Tools
Brief summaries of commonly used psychological tests, including Bender Visual Motor Test, Intelligence Tests, and others.

Chapter 15

INTERPRETATION AND DIAGNOSIS

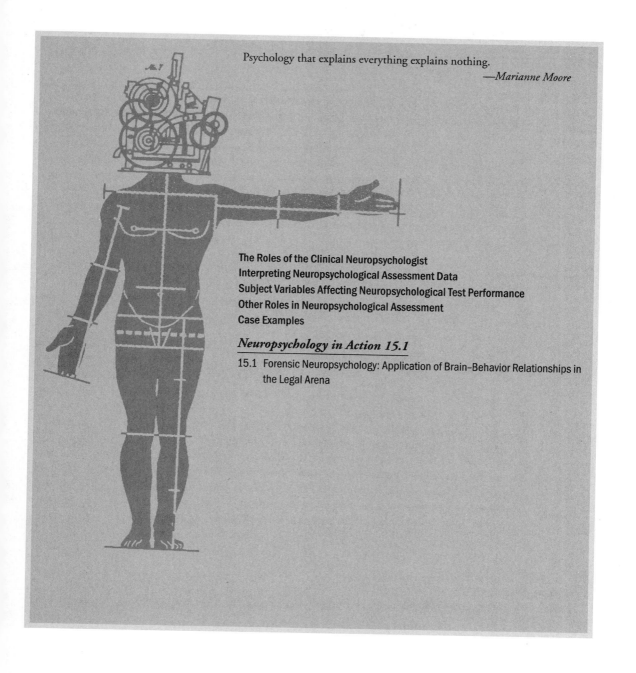

Psychology that explains everything explains nothing.

—*Marianne Moore*

The Roles of the Clinical Neuropsychologist
Interpreting Neuropsychological Assessment Data
Subject Variables Affecting Neuropsychological Test Performance
Other Roles in Neuropsychological Assessment
Case Examples

Neuropsychology in Action 15.1

Keep in Mind

- What different roles do neuropsychologists play?
- What major methods do neuropsychologists use in interpreting neuropsychological tests?
- What individual differences influence neuropsychological test interpretation?
- How can a neuropsychologist improve a patient's quality of life?

Overview

Jeanne was a passenger on a motorcycle with her husband when at an intersection a car ran a stop sign and hit them. Although her husband received only minor injuries, Jeanne was thrown about five feet. Luckily, she was wearing a helmet. However, Jeanne thinks she must have been knocked out, because she doesn't remember anything until the ambulance arrived. Emergency room personnel attended to her knee injury. She also had a terrible headache. MRI did not detect any contusions or lesions. The hospital released Jeanne that day and told her to see her general practitioner if she had any more problems.

Jeanne recovered for a week at home and then went back to her job as a medical records clerk. She also returned to school to enroll in coursework for a nursing degree. First, she noticed that she often forgot a client's seven-digit medical record number between the time she looked at it and went next door to get the chart. Her grades also started slipping. Before the accident, she was getting As and Bs. But on her first biology test a month after the accident, she got a D. She also continued to have headaches, which she had not had before. Four months after her injury, after several visits to her general practitioner and a neurologist, neither of whom could find anything medically wrong with her, her practitioner referred her for a neuropsychological evaluation. The request was to evaluate her to determine whether she had suffered a brain injury as a result of her accident or if her symptoms might be a psychosomatic reaction, that is, related to increased stress in dealing with the accident and the aftermath.

What can neuropsychology offer Jeanne? Many people who have head injuries or suffer whiplash injuries in car accidents, sports injuries, or falls may have a brief lapse of consciousness. They may feel temporarily confused or disoriented. They may or may not go to a doctor or the hospital, and if they do, they are usually released after a brief observation. CT or MRI results are quite likely to be negative for any small or microscopic contusions or lesions. Only after going home, and trying to resume the normal tasks of working or going to school, may someone such as Jeanne feel unable to concentrate or is forgetting things. The person may have other odd symptoms that he or she doesn't understand, such as becoming more easily frustrated or just not feeling "herself." If these problems do not resolve and if the person is persistent, or the physician perceptive, then the physician makes a referral for neuropsychological testing.

The Roles of the Clinical Neuropsychologist

The role of the clinical neuropsychologist in the past was almost exclusively that of a diagnostician. In the 1960s and 1970s, before the sophisticated neuroimaging techniques of today, physicians often asked neuropsychologists to assist in diagnosing "organicity"—whether a patient did or did not have brain damage. Because they could identify precise functional areas of the brain through specialized behavioral procedures, clinical neuropsychologists could often "localize" (locate) primary areas of brain damage. The classic test battery of the time, the Halstead-Reitan Neuropsychological Battery (Halstead, 1947; Reitan & Wolfson, 1993) was the main tool clinicians used to identify and localize brain damage. Since then, research in clinical neuropsychology has provided a greater theoretical understanding of brain–behavior relationships. The level of knowledge is now so immense that neuropsychologists could spend their whole careers becoming experts in one specific area of neuropsychology including language, memory, or executive functioning. Researchers are rapidly generating experimental and clinical measures to aid in describing brain–behavior function. No longer is there one primary testing approach or testing battery that most neuropsychologists use. At the same time, neuropsychology is expanding expertise to include new roles such as evaluating the quality of patients' lives and their ability to do well in their environment. The work of clinical rehabilitation specialists has focused more on intervention, remedial methods for rehabilitation, and discharge planning. Now medical teams often ask clinical neuropsychologists to describe current behavioral functioning and help determine such issues as whether a person can live independently. Neuropsychologists also help plan treatments and develop and manage entire rehabilitation programs (see Chapter 16). In this chapter we describe the roles of the neuropsychologist as they relate to interpreting neuropsychological assessment procedures and diagnosing neuropsychological dysfunction.

DIAGNOSIS

With the advent of modern medical diagnostic procedures (see Chapter 6), including single-photon emission computed tomography (SPECT), magnetic resonance imaging (MRI), computed transaxial tomography (CT), positron emission tomography (PET), angiography, and evoked potential, using behavior-based assessments to diagnose organic-functional etiologies has become less essential. It has become less important for neuropsychologists and psychologists to act in the capacity of "lesion detectors," and more important to document the precise effects of brain

dysfunction on behavior for purposes of remediation and treatment (Zillmer & Perry, 1996). Nevertheless, clinical neuropsychologists continue to figure prominently in uncovering the behavioral syndromes that correspond to impaired brain regions and neuronal circuits and may play an important role in diagnosing neuropathological conditions (for example, see Damasio, 1991; Fuster, 1991; Goldman-Rakic & Friedman, 1991; Stuss, 1992).

Medical teams still ask clinical neuropsychologists to aid in diagnosis, not merely confirming what might appear on PET or MRI images, but adding behavioral and descriptive information about a patient's cognitive strengths and weaknesses. If a neurologist wants to know if a patient has had a left hemisphere stroke, a CT scan or an MRI can reveal this. Neuropsychological testing would be redundant and not as precise as sophisticated imaging equipment in terms of exactly locating the lesion within the brain. Imaging technology, however, does not provide information about how brain damage may affect behavior. Clinical neuropsychologists provide invaluable and unique diagnostic information in areas where behavioral information provides an important piece of the diagnostic puzzle. Those areas include the diagnoses of mild head injury (MHI), attention-deficit/hyperactivity disorder (ADHD), learning disability (LD), or Alzheimer's disease (AD). Currently available imaging techniques are not sufficient to diagnose Alzheimer's. Brain biopsy after death is the only certain method. Thus, AD dementia is a diagnosis largely determined by behavioral methods. Through careful observation and history taking with the patient and family, the neuropsychologist documents the extent and probable progression of the behavioral deterioration. Then, through repeated evaluations spread out over time, the neuropsychologist charts the severity and course of the neuropsychological impairments. If the team can rule out all other medical causes of dementia, then the person can be diagnosed as having "possible" or "probable" Alzheimer's. In fact, the diagnosis of most dementia subtypes requires close collaboration between neurologists and neuropsychologists (see Chapter 11).

Mild to moderate head injuries also present diagnostic issues that neuropsychology can help clarify. With many head injuries, particularly of the mild variety (such as concussion), it is not immediately evident if the person has actually sustained a brain injury. In many cases the diagnostic aim of the neuropsychological evaluation is to determine the presence and severity of brain injury. The diagnosis is made, not to answer the outdated question "Is this patient 'organic'?" but to answer the question "Does this neuropsychological profile fit with what is known about the neuropsychological pattern of impairment following closed head injury?" CT and MRI may not reveal microscopic shearing, tearing, stretching, and bruising of axons. Even if they did, you could not predict clear behavioral symptoms from looking at radiological or imaging data. As in Alzheimer's disease, behavioral testing largely determines the diagnosis and severity of brain damage after closed head injury. Thus neuropsychologists play an important role in determining patterns of neuropsychological dysfunction characteristic with a variety of central nervous system disorders. In addition, and to address the entire diagnostic picture, many neuropsychologists conduct comprehensive examinations of emotion and personality, to understand how the patient is adapting. For example, they not uncommonly diagnose depression or significant deficits in stress tolerance in patients who have experienced a head injury. The neuropsychologist's diagnostic skills as a psychologist helps differentiate between the impact of emotional/personality problems and brain dysfunction.

Neuropsychological diagnosis remains an important component of the neuropsychologist's role. However, diagnosis is usually not the only question of interest when a patient comes in for neuropsychological testing. In the next section we discuss certain other issues that practicing neuropsychologists address.

DESCRIBING FUNCTION, ADAPTATION, AND PROGNOSIS

Describing behavioral functioning—that is, a patient's cognitive strengths and weaknesses—puts the "psychology" into neuropsychology. Psychology is the science of behavior; neuropsychology is the science of brain–behavior functioning. Although neuropsychology combines neurologic and psychological foci, the neurologic goal of detecting and classifying lesions

dominated clinical neuropsychology through the 1970s. Since then, emphasis has shifted to a more behavioral focus, assessment of the human person, ranging from assessing cognitive abilities to evaluating quality-of-life indicators. In this approach, the goal as a clinical neuropsychologist is to describe brain–behavior functioning in such a manner as to accurately depict the current and future adaptive capabilities of the individual. Such information is important in evaluating the rehabilitation needs of a patient to facilitate adaptive functioning and prognosis, or in assessing the degree and type of assistance needed in the home and work environment. This chapter addresses these important issues in neuropsychological description, its similarities to and differences from generic psychological description, how it seeks to describe current adaptation in the real world, and how neuropsychologists use it to predict the course of recovery or decline of an individual.

Interpreting Neuropsychological Assessment Data

By now it should be obvious that the neuropsychological examination is a complex undertaking. Not only are no two patients alike, but how neuropsychologists administer the tests and which tests they select often differ. In addition, many procedures we have reviewed measure more than one functional domain, making it difficult to interpret the neuropsychological construct and cause underlying an impaired performance. This section presents an overview of interpretative guidelines for the neuropsychologist. We provide quantitative and qualitative dimensions of neuropsychological performance as well as case studies, elucidate neuropsychological diagnosis and evaluation. Although this depends on the specific referral question, the clinical neuropsychologist is primarily interested in generating **interpretive hypotheses** about the patient as well as in answering specific questions about the test data, including the following:

■ Is there any cerebral impairment?
Evidence of behavioral deficits
Behavioral changes caused by lesion

■ How severe is the injury?
Medically significant
Does it impair the person's ability to function in his or her daily activities?

■ Is the lesion progressive or static?

■ Is the lesion diffuse or lateralized, or are there multiple lesions?

■ Is the impairment anterior or posterior? Can it be localized?

■ What is the most likely pathologic process, and what is the prognosis?

■ What are the individual's cognitive/behavioral strengths and weaknesses, and how do they relate to daily living skills, treatment, and rehabilitation?

■ Do the neuropsychological deficits influence the patient's quality of life?

■ What is the patient's reaction to the injury and/or impairment?

APPROACHES TO NEUROPSYCHOLOGICAL INTERPRETATION

Clinicians disagree somewhat in their approach to neuropsychological interpretation. These differences center on both practical and theoretical test issues and have become a source of debate. In making determinations regarding the evolution of a specific assessment and interpretation approach, practical and theoretical issues are often intertwined. A typical example is test selection and time needed for completing the neuropsychological exam. Neuropsychologists usually broaden information regarding a patient by administering a wider range of tests (such as memory, motor, learning, and language); they deepen information by administering a number of tests examining varying aspects of the same cognitive domain (such as selective attention or sustained attention). They must balance these theoretical considerations against the practical reality of exam length. Many patients cannot tolerate long testing sessions because of fatigue effects. Given the current climate in which managed health care reduces specialized services to pa-

tients, most clinicians are also concerned about cost effectiveness in time spent on evaluating the patient.

The approaches presented here include the major strategies of neuropsychological assessment and interpretation from which numerous variations have developed. We discuss the pros and cons of each approach in regard to both theoretical and practical issues.

Standard Battery Approach

Halstead (1947) and Reitan (1966) pioneered the use of a **standard battery approach** of tests for identifying brain damage. First Halstead and Reitan identified tests that were sensitive to the integrity of cortical functioning. Then they sought to incorporate the evaluation of all the major cognitive, sensory, motor, and perceptual skills that a neuropsychological exam should reflect. The purpose of the Halstead-Reitan Neuropsychological Battery was to allow the development of various principles for inferring psychological deficit as applied to results obtained on individual subjects (Reitan & Wolfson, 1993). In this approach, the clinician gives the same tests to all patients, regardless of his or her impression of an individual patient or the referral question. Typically a technician administers the neuropsychological procedures, rather than a doctoral-level psychologist, because the tests are administered according to standardized rules of procedure, without variations. Using technicians allows more testing for the same cost, because the more expensive time of a doctoral-level neuropsychologist is not needed.

This standard battery approach has several advantages. First, it can ensure that all subjects are evaluated for all basic neuropsychological abilities. This makes it unlikely that the diagnosis could overlook a condition of importance. Second, the neuropsychologist can use the data to identify objective patterns of scores that he or she can consider in diagnosing various neuropathological conditions. Patterns within the data can help in diagnosing the probability of certain causes of brain dysfunction. Knowledge of causes can be useful in providing the patient, physician, or treatment team with tentative diagnoses, as well as in predicting the course of a disorder. Finally, the standard battery approach lends itself to the teaching of neuropsychological assessment and interpretation, because the beginning neuropsychology student need not make decisions about test selection and the interpretation is objective and data driven. Finally, because the test instructions, test selection, and test interpretation are all standardized, this approach is particularly useful for empirical studies and facilitates comparison across different research projects.

There are also drawbacks to the test battery approach. The time involved in testing any patient can be considerable. Problems such as fatigue or loss of motivation may develop. The time involved forces the use of a testing technician to ensure a reasonable cost and reasonable use of the neuropsychologist's time. As a result, the neuropsychologist may have little contact with the patient outside of the interview and thus loses the opportunity to make a qualitative analysis of the patient's behavior. Obtaining qualitative impressions of the patient's appearance and behavior is often very important, however. For example, we once observed a neuropsychologist who used the standard battery approach make an interesting misdiagnosis. This particular neuropsychologist strictly favored the neuropsychological battery approach and therefore typically did not interview his patients. He claimed that the subjective presentation of the case would "contaminate" his ability to make an objective interpretation. During a neuropsychological exam of a patient, the neuropsychologist's psychometrician indicated on her data summary sheet that the patient's performance on the Finger Tapping test was zero. The neuropsychologist proceeded to interpret this score as "severe, right-sided, upper extremity motor slowing with possible corresponding left hemisphere cortical dysfunction." But visual inspection of the patient would have made obvious that the patient was not suffering from motor slowing and "brain damage"—instead, his right arm was amputated! The issue of using psychometricians to administer the neuropsychological tests remains very controversial in contemporary neuropsychology.

The original choice of tests to include in the battery heavily influences standard batteries. The theoretical beliefs of the person doing the choosing often biases the choice. A poorly chosen test battery, no matter how many times it is given, will continue to yield unsatisfactory results. In different situations, alternate areas of assessment may be more effective in providing information. However, because the user of a standard battery gives no additional tests, he or she would never discover this. For example, the Halstead-Reitan Neuropsychological Battery does not include a memory test.

You can see a common problem of interpreting the empirical approach in composite tests that require the examinee to have a number of cognitive skills. For example, the Hooper Visual Organization Test (Hooper, 1983) requires the subject to name or write more or less readily recognizable cut-up objects. The Hooper consists of 30 stimuli. The maximum score is 30, and a score below 20 typically indicates "organic brain pathology." Because examiners think the measure primarily measures perceptual integration, a function often associated with right hemisphere function, they often interpret low scores as perceptual fragmentation most likely related to dysfunction of the right hemisphere. However, left hemisphere stroke patients often make low scores on this test, not related to impaired perceptual functioning, but related to the patient's impairment in naming objects. Thus, critiques of the battery approach often suggest that understanding why a patient failed a task is as valuable as the fact that the person failed (Luria, 1966). Such information, they argue, can be often more useful than test scores in making intervention and diagnostic decisions. Furthermore, opponents of the empirical approach argue that complex behavior cannot and should not be reduced to a single number or test score. For example, the Hooper demands include comprehending the instruction, visually scanning the stimulus figure, mentally rotating the cut-up parts of the object to form a whole, and recognizing, naming, and articulating the object, either in writing or orally. Thus, this seemingly simple task actually requires the person to integrate a number of neuropsychological processes to generate a correct response.

The standard battery method also fails to recognize that altering a test procedure is sometimes valuable in determining a specific deficit. A standard battery may not be appropriate for all patients, especially when there are peripheral deficits, such as injury to the limbs, a serious visual loss, or spinal cord injury. Such patients's inability to complete a given test may reflect a peripheral motor or visual problem, rather than a dysfunction of the central nervous system. Consequently, data from such a patient on a standard battery may be useless for diagnosis, evaluation, and intervention. Finally, interpreting even a standard battery requires considerable skill, knowledge, and experience. Nevertheless, as standard rules and norms develop, standard batteries are somewhat easier to interpret and to teach.

Although the criticisms of the battery approach are valid, many psychologists remain faithful to administering a "core battery." As can be seen from Table 15.1, however, 55% of neuropsychologists favor a flexible, modified battery approach, suggesting that the type of patient seen and the nature of the referral question plays an important role in test selection.

Process Approach

The **process approach** to neuropsychological testing, often called the *hypothesis approach,* rests on the idea that the neuropsychologist should adapt each exam to the individual patient. Rather than employing a standard battery of tests, the neuropsychologist selects the tests and procedures for each exam, using hypotheses he or she has made from impressions of the patient and from information available about the patient. As a result, each examination may vary considerably from patient to patient in terms of length and test selection. The clinician may use standard tests, or may alter and adapt tests as he or she tries to form an opinion on the nature of the deficits (Christensen, 1979; Lezak, 1995). Altering tests to discover the patient's strategies is a popular method within the process approach to neuropsychological assessment (for example, see Milberg, Hebben, & Kaplan, 1986). Many conclusions reached in the exam follow the clinician's qualitative interpretations of the test results and the patient's behavior. The clinician also grounds the conclusions on his or her experience and knowledge of the clinical literature. The principal developers of the process approach are Alexander Luria and Edith Kaplan.

The process approach has several advantages. First, it acknowledges the individual nature of the patient's deficits and seeks to adapt the exam to this individuality. Under the proper condition, such a technique can yield more precise measurements of a subject's skill on a given ability than just the patient's score on a given test. Second, the exam can concentrate on those areas the neuropsychologist sees as most important for the patient. It can ignore areas not important for the patient's prognosis. Because the time for any exam is limited, this enables the clinician to more thoroughly investigate significant areas.

Perhaps most importantly, the flexible/process approach emphasizes in what manner a patient fails or succeeds in a specific cognitive task. For example, a patient is unable to answer the question "What is the capital of the United States?" Does this relate to the patient not understanding the question (speech comprehension), does it indicate an inability to answer verbally (expressive aphasia), or does the patient not know the answer (poor factual knowledge)? The standard battery approach does not allow a deviation from the standard instructions of the test, because deviating would invalidate the results. If the patient is unable to answer the question, the process approach allows for further investigation. For example, the examiner can show the patient a multiple-choice card with the

Table 15.1 *Frequently Used Neuropsychological Assessment Batteries/Composite Tests*	
Scale	Percentage of Total Usage
Wechsler Adult Intelligence Scale–Revised	89%
Partial/Modified Halstead-Reitan Neuropsychological Test Battery	55%
Wide Range Achievement Test (WRAT-III)	51%
Halstead-Reitan Neuropsychological Battery (HRNB)	27%
Dementia Rating Scale	16%
Woodcock-Johnson Psycho-Educational Battery	6%
Benton Tests	5%
Luria Nebraska Neuropsychological Battery	5%
Wide Range Assessment of Memory and Learning (WRAML)	5%

answer and several wrong alternatives. If the patient points to the correct answer, "Washington, D.C.," the neuropsychologist would interpret this response as meaning that the patient knows this factual knowledge, but cannot express this information either verbally or in writing. Thus, the process approach lets the clinician concentrate on tasks related to the most important deficits that the patient shows.

The process approach also has several disadvantages. Because the content of the exam emphasizes areas that the clinician feels are important, the exam may selectively confirm the clinician's opinion. Because the clinician may never test areas that he or she sees as irrelevant, no one may realize that a deficit has been missed. Because the test's focus just on the patient and his or her expected problems, the data may be biased toward confirming the original hypothesis. Thus many neuropsychologists feel this more subjective approach relies willy-nilly on clinical experience, hunches, colleagues' anecdotes, intuition, common sense, folklore, and introspection (Meehl, 1973).

Using tests not standardized for a clinical population, or tests that have been adapted, also presents potentially serious problems. The interpretation of a test that has not been adequately standardized is always questionable. The clinician's subjective impression of what a score should mean for a given patient may be quite wrong. A test that appears to measure one thing in a normal population may measure something entirely different in a brain-injured population. In each of these situations, the accuracy of the individual clinician's judgment becomes the accuracy of the test. Thus, in the process approach the opinion of the clinician is as good as his or her reputation. At present there are no measures of such accuracy, but probably this varies considerably among clinicians.

The use of different exams and procedures for each patient precludes the experimental validation of individual tests in applied clinical settings. It also precludes evaluation of the process as a whole, because conclusions do not come from test scores, but from the clinician's judgments. Clinicians may, in such a situation, continue using an ineffective test because it appears to work. The process approach, therefore, does not lend itself to large-scale research, but often relies on case studies.

Structuring an exam on an individual basis may mean that it assesses only some of the basic functions mediated by the brain. Rehabilitation and prognosis depend on the state of the brain as a whole; the lack of information on the entire brain can impede an intervention program or invalidate a prognosis. In practice, it is not unusual to see patients with secondary deficits that seem unrelated to their primary referral problem and to the impression that the patient gives. For example, it is not unusual for a patient with a major stroke to have had smaller, secondary disorders of cerebral circulation. The deficits may have existed before the patient's current problem arose. Whatever the source of the deficits, the clinician must identify and consider them in making any recommendations for a client. Finally, the flexible/process approach is more difficult to teach to students, because few "rules" and "procedures" exist. Test selection, adaptation, and interpretation depend largely on extensive clinical experience. This approach is also time consuming, because the neuropsychologist must perform the evaluation, rather than a technician. Table 15.2 reviews the pro and cons of the standard battery and process approaches.

Paul Meehl, a preeminent psychodiagnostician and former president of the American Psychological Association, addressed the complex decision-making process involved in psychological assessment. In 1957 he wrote a now classic essay entitled "When Shall We Use Our Heads Instead of the Formula?" (1973). With this question he examined the rationale for when to use more empirical (psychometric) compared to more clinical approaches (qualitative) to psychological assessment, interpretation, and diagnosis. By the term "formula," Meehl implied the scientific, empirical, and data-driven approach to psychology, consistent with those neuropsychologists who favor the fixed battery approach. By "using our heads," in contrast, Meehl was referring to the more clinical, common-sense, approaches typically used by the process approach in neuropsychology. Meehl suggested that the two answers to his question—"Always" and "Never"— were equally unacceptable. He also proposed that it would be silly to answer, "We use both methods, they go hand in hand." If the formula and your head invariably yield the same predictions about an individ-

Table 15.2 *Summary and Comparison of Approaches to Neuropsychological Interpretation*

Standard Battery Approach	Process Approach
Same tests or "core battery" given to all	Exam administered by a neuro-psychologist
Tests administered according to standardized rules	Tests not administered in a standard way
Interpretation based on standardized norms	Conclusions based on clinical experience
Advantages	
Comprehensive evaluation of abilities	Acknowledges the individuality of patient
Objective interpretation based on normative data	Exam focuses on most important deficits
Facilitates teaching because of standard rules/norms	Emphasizes how a task is failed or solved
Useful for empirical studies	Useful for clinical case studies
Disadvantages	
Time demanding and labor intensive	Test procedure may be biased by clinician
Tests only as good as standardization	Opinion of the clinician is subjective
Relatively inflexible approach to testing	Difficult to teach, because it requires experience
Scores may not reflect a single cognitive process	Does not lend itself to large-scale research

many different diagnostic problems. In the meantime, neuropsychologists continue to make descriptions, interpretations, and predictions about human behavior. How should neuropsychologists be making interpretive decisions? Should they use the process approach, or should they follow the empirical, psychometric approach? Mostly neuropsychologists will use their heads, because researchers have not developed adequate empirical batteries for every type of neuropsychological problem. In those cases in which there are good empirical approaches to neuropsychological problems (as in estimating intelligence), they should use an empirical approach. What if there is a case in which the formula disagrees with the clinical opinion of the process approach? Which approach should neuropsychologists use then? Meehl, a staunch scientist, suggested that in such a situation they should use their heads very, very seldom—except, of course, if the issue is as clear as a broken leg or amputated arm.

Considerable controversy has raged about the preceding approaches to performing and interpreting a neuropsychological evaluation. Although there are certainly schools of thought about this, almost 50% of neuropsychologists report using parts of both approaches (see Figure 15.1; Gordon & Zillmer, 1997). That is, a majority of neuropsychologists use a modified battery approach, in which they choose specific tests to answer a referral question. They may interpret some tests in an empirical fashion, and other test behavior in a more qualitative way. Approximately 25% report that they strictly adhere to a standard/fixed battery approach or a process/qualitative approach.

ual, you should use the less costly method, because the more costly one is not adding anything. If the methods *don't* always yield the same prediction—and most empirical studies show that they don't—then the psychologists can't use both, because they cannot predict in opposite ways for the same patient.

This discussion remains a central theme in any type of psychological assessment, although the empirical approach has been increasingly refined since Meehl wrote his famous paper. Empirical and theoretical considerations suggest that the field of neuropsychology would be well advised to continue to concentrate efforts on improving actuarial techniques rather than to focus on calibrating each clinician for each of

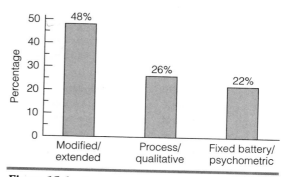

Figure 15.1 Approaches to neuropsychological test interpretation. (Gordon & Zillmer, 1997)

We caution the neuropsychology student that diagnostic and treatment decisions warrant integrating data drawn from a number of sources, including neuropsychological measures, pertinent neuromedical findings, and the patient's developmental and medical history. Neuropsychologists typically do not render diagnostic decisions based on a single neuropsychological measure. Obviously, site, nature, and severity of the injury/disease process, premorbid personality, and a host of other moderating variables affect neuropsychological test performance. Interpreting the neuropsychological data requires a thorough understanding of neuropsychological principles, developmental findings, and psychopathology.

Interpretation of the neuropsychological protocol can then proceed through several levels of analysis, including the following:

- Overall level of impairment
- Pattern of impairment
- Lateralizing and localizing signs
- Qualitative observations

Once interpretation proceeds through these levels, the neuropsychologist can then evaluate test data to determine consistency with a patient's known medical conditions and presenting diagnoses, as well as to predict functional abilities and limitations.

ASSESSING LEVEL OF PERFORMANCE

The Use of Norms in Neuropsychology

The use of norms in neuropsychology entails comparing an individual's test scores and available **normative data.** This approach provides the neuropsychologist with information regarding an individual's ability in comparison to others. This method compares the patient's score on a test to an expected score, or norm. The method determines the expected test score from the performance of a normative sample of patients and controls. Such norms may take into account such factors as age, sex, education, and intelligence. Many neuropsychological tests have a **cutoff score.** A patient scoring worse than the cutoff score is labeled as impaired; a patient scoring better is labeled as within normal limits (WNL).

The selection of any specific cutoff point relates to factors of test **specificity** and test **sensitivity.** When seeking to identify people whose cognitive abilities are abnormal (for example, brain damage), neuropsychologists prefer a sensitive test. In such cases, they set the cutoff score so that as few errors as possible arise in classifying a disease entity. However, sensitive tests that rely on measuring impaired cognitive functioning may also include false positive errors, for example, erroneously identifying psychiatric patients as brain damaged. Such a test is of little value to the neuropsychologist who wants to delineate the precise nature of a patient's deficits. Rather, the clinician needs tests that examine specific aspects of neuropsychological functions, that is, tests that have high specificity. Such tests may assess more general areas of cognitive functioning, including sustained attention or immediate memory. But they may miss patients who have impairments outside of those specific areas of cognitive functions, which results in false negative errors. Of course, tests that have high sensitivity as well as high specificity are most useful in neuropsychology. In reality, there is always a trade-off between aspects of how specific a procedure is versus its usefulness as a sensitive test. Thus, neuropsychologists often set cutoff scores at an intermediate point where the chances of misclassifying either impaired performance or normal performance are about equal.

Statistical Approaches

When administering a battery of tests, it is important to be able to compare performance on tests that measure widely different skills. As you gain enough experience with a set of tests, this skill often becomes automatic. However, the easiest way to accomplish this task is to use standardized scores rather than raw scores. A raw score is a score that is presented in terms of the original test units. It is simply the number of items passed or points earned. A standard score, in contrast, is a derived score that uses as its unit the standard deviation of the population on which the developers standardized the test. Thus a standard score is a deviation score. A standard deviation relates to the variability or scatter of test scores. This pattern is known as a *distribution* of test scores. The normal probability distribution (also known as the *bell-shaped curve*) represents the frequency with which many human characteristics are dispersed over the population. For example, intelligence and spatial reasoning ability are distributed in a manner that closely resembles the bell-shaped curve.

In the **normal distribution,** 68.2% of all cases fall between ±1 standard deviation (SD) from the mean; 95.4% of the cases fall between ±2SD from the mean, and 99.7% of the cases fall within ±3 SD from the mean. The normal distribution is the basis for the scoring system on many standardized tests. For example, on the Scholastic Aptitude Test (SAT) the developers set the mean at 500 and the standard deviation at 100. Hence, SAT scores reflect how many standard deviations above or below the mean a student scored. For example, a score of 700 means that you scored two standard deviations above the mean, exceeding approximately 97% of the population on which the test is normed. Thus, test scores that place examinees in the normal distribution can always be converted to percentile scores, which are often easier to interpret. A percentile score indicates the percentage of people who score below the score you obtained. For example, if you score at the 60th percentile, 60 percent of the people who take the test scored below you, and the remaining 40 percent scored above you. Tables are available that permit transformation from any standard deviation placement in a normal distribution to a percentile score.

Neuropsychologists use a variety of standard scores. They determine standard scores by a mathematical formula that can convert raw scores from tests to a standard scale. For example, Table 15.3 lists commonly used standardized scores in clinical neuropsychology. Once you know the test score frequency of a neuropsychological measure, you can easily compute a standard score. For example, determine the standard score (SS) by first subtracting the mean score from a normative group for a test from the person's actual score. Divide the result by the standard devia-

Table 15.3 *Examples of Different Standardized Scores*

Name of Standardized Score	Mean	Standard Deviation	Tests Used
Z-score	0	1	None
Sten score	5	1	16 personality factors
Scaled score	10	3	Wechsler subtests
T-score	50	10	MMPI, many norms
Standard score (SS)	100	15	Wechsler IQ scores

tion of the scores in the normative sample. Multiply this result by 15 (the standard deviation), and add 100 (the mean) to this answer. The formula for standard score is as follows:

$$SS = 100 + \frac{(\text{Score obtained minus average normative score})}{\text{Standard deviation (normative sample)}} \times 15.0$$

The standardized score approach to neuropsychological assessment has several advantages. First, all scores are roughly comparable. Second, you can make adjustments for such factors as age and education. You do this by determining normative means and standard deviations for different age or educational levels. You can then include the normative scores corresponding to a given person's age or education. Of course, not all neuropsychological measures result in normal test distributions. Some distributions skew in one direction or another. Some neuropsychological tests, particularly those which the process approach favors, are relatively "easy." That is, most "intact" individuals would have few problems passing the test. For example, "On a plain piece of paper, draw a clock with all the numbers and the hands of the clock positioned at 10 minutes after 11." Most individuals would pass this task, but patients with disturbances in visual-spatial perception or planning ability may "fail." Thus, the resulting test score distribution is dichotomous (pass–fail) and does not present a normal distribution. It is inappropriate to calculate standard scores from such a test distribution. A great pitfall of the statistical approach to neuropsychological interpretation is that developers have transformed to standard scores many tests that are not normally distributed, thus providing inexact estimations of performance.

DEFICIT MEASUREMENT

Deficit measurement, as an approach, is standardized and group oriented. It is useful for understanding general conditions and disease states. By comparing a person to "the norm," you can determine statistically probable deficits. By examining a battery of tests, you can examine an individual's pattern of strengths and weaknesses. You can compare these to known, general profiles. But clinicians are also concerned with the uniqueness and dynamic qualities of each individual. The adaptive approach to neuropsychology mirrors developments in other areas of psychology. To paraphrase Howard Gardner, the Harvard psychologist, neuropsychologists should not be asking, "How smart is this person?" but "How is this person smart?" In clinical neuropsychology, the focus is not only on the level of deficits and strengths to describe functioning, for example, "How adapted (normal) is this person?" but how does this person adapt to his or her condition? Neuropsychologists should question what is lost in terms of understanding the brain if they do not consider the range and extent of individual adaptations to injury, tumor, and disease.

Differential Score Approach

The deficit measurement approach compares a patient's score on two tests. One test is theoretically highly sensitive to brain damage (for example, a new problem-solving task); the second is theoretically insensitive to brain dysfunction (for example, a measure of factual language). The insensitive test is supposed to reflect the individual's ability before any brain injury occurred, whereas the sensitive test reflects the effects of brain damage. If the sensitive test score is significantly worse, the neuropsychologist assumes the difference is due to a brain injury. In general, you combine two test scores to get a single score measuring their difference. You may accomplish this by simply subtracting or dividing one score by the other.

Then analyze this single score by treating it as described in the section on level of performance.

Pattern Analysis

A modification of the differential score approach is **pattern analysis,** which examines the relationships among the scores in a test battery. It seeks to recognize patterns consistent with specific injuries and particular neurologic processes and has value in identifying mild disorders that cause relatively little disturbance in level of performance. For example, in early stages of Alzheimer's dementia neuropsychologists would expect a deficit in memory functioning compared to performance on verbal tests, which may be relatively normal. If you plot all the neuropsychological data on a standardized norm worksheet, a profile of cognitive skills may emerge. You can then observe the interrelationships among these differing cognitive skills areas. A basic method of pattern analysis involves observing strengths and weaknesses in the highest and lowest scores. You can evaluate cognitive strengths and weaknesses relative to the normative group by observing which scores fall above, below, or within the average range. You can also determine strengths and weaknesses relative to the individual's specific profile. Again, high and low scores are highlighted, but without regard for where they fall relative to the normative sample. Finally, you can integrate information about cognitive strengths and weaknesses with therapeutic suggestions to family and treatment team to improve the patient's recovery.

The differential score method and pattern analysis has the advantage of recognizing that each individual starts at a different level of performance. Thus, it avoids error of misclassifying all people with low ability as brain injured. But this approach has several potential sources of error. First, a sensitive test may fail to reflect the impairment present. At present, no test is sensitive to all forms of brain dysfunction. Second, the brain injury may lower a score on an insensitive test. Because all abilities depend on the brain, brain damage can affect all abilities. No test is fully insensitive to brain injury. Finally, relatively little is known about specific patterns of deficits that correlate with specific neurologic disorders or how to set any cutoff points to identify those conditions.

LATERALIZING SIGNS

The two cerebral hemispheres control the contralateral sides of the body for most sensory and motor behaviors. If one side of the body performs significantly worse than the other, the opposite hemisphere may have been injured. Lateralizing signs are specific test results or behaviors that suggest right or left cerebral hemisphere dysfunction. This approach resembles the differential score approach in that one side of the body serves as the control for the other. Generally, you subtract the scores from the two sides of the body to obtain a single difference score. You then treat this score as described in the level-of-performance approach. This approach may yield inaccurate conclusions, however, when an injury involves both hemispheres, or when an injury to the spinal cord is involved, because such injuries may also cause lateralized motor or sensory deficits or impair performance bilaterally.

PATHOGNOMONIC SIGNS (QUALITATIVE OBSERVATIONS)

Examining **pathognomonic signs** is a method clinical neurologists commonly use. In the medical model, the clinical exam often assumes that specific, distinctive characteristics of a disease or pathologic condition can be detected. These signs or symptoms are often labeled *pathognomonic* (Greek for "fit to give judgment"), because often a specific diagnosis can be made from them. The medical model is a causal model in which specific signs stem either from a specific medical condition, or from the disease itself. Thus a standard medical examination is often a series of medical tests for pathognomonic signs. Once a disease has been diagnosed, it can be treated. This model has served the field of medicine rather well. For example, the model attempts to fit (pigeonhole) the available information from the medical examination into often rigid and inflexible diagnostic criteria. Also if the signs from the medical exam do not precisely fit, or are contradictory, and if some symptoms are transient, the model does not work well, because no substantive diagnosis can be established and thus no treatment can be offered.

Pathognomonic signs occur rarely in normal individuals. In clinical neurology, this includes such signs as an eye that will not move from side to side. In neuropsychology, examples of pathognomonic signs include the rotation of a drawing or the failure to draw the left half of a figure. You can count the number of pathognomonic signs within a given test to get a summary number. You can treat this number as a level-of-performance score. In other cases, the simple presence of a particular pathognomonic sign is taken as indicating brain damage.

Subject Variables Affecting Neuropsychological Test Performance

Neuropsychologists cannot meaningfully interpret an individual's neurological integrity without thoroughly understanding subject variables that might influence that performance. Although some of the variables we present in this section are important to consider when conducting any type of psychological assessment, we present these variables in reference to their specific impact on neuropsychological functioning.

AGE

As individuals grow older, they often do less well on clinical tests measuring adaptive abilities. Many neuropsychological tests fall into this realm. As a result, older people tend to do less well on neuropsychological tests, specifically tests requiring flexible problem-solving skills and procedures that require perceptual and attentional skills. However, contrary to the intuitive notion that motor speed and strength show significant decrements with age, pure motor tests do not have a significant relationship with age. We outlined the specific nature of age-related changes on neuropsychological functioning in more detail in Chapter 11.

Using norms that are not age graded can easily result in older patients being misclassified as neuropsychologically impaired. Consequently, analyzing neuropsychology test scores from older patients by comparing them to younger normative groups is very questionable. In working with older patients, it is important to look more closely at the relationship of test scores to one another. If some test scores are considerably more depressed than others, this information is useful for diagnosis and evaluation. For example, the pattern of scores in brain-damaged patients can be the same for both younger and older patients. Over the last 10 years, test developers have normed many neuropsychological measures on older populations and have specifically designed and developed tests for older individuals. Nevertheless, very few normed tests are available for the oldest old, those over 85 years old.

PREMORBID FUNCTIONING

Premorbid functioning is the cognitive and neuropsychological status occurring before the development of disease or trauma. In establishing that a drop or decline in functioning from previously higher functioning has occurred, or to compare test performance in relation to expected performance, the neuropsychologist should consider variables such as education, occupation, and socioeconomic status, because they certainly influence interpretation of test performance. For example, someone without neurologic impairment who typically performs in the low average to borderline range on cognitive tests can be easily misclassified as having a brain impairment. Similarly, a research scientist with a doctorate may have a premorbid functioning in the high average to superior range of cognitive ability. If that subject after a head injury is now functioning in the average range, he or she may not appear impaired when compared to the "norm" without regard to premorbid status. You can easily appreciate this point in the following case study:

The importance in understanding premorbid functioning can be extremely important, as can be seen in the case of Jeff, who was a world-class violin player. Jeff was traveling in Texas and wanted to make a telephone call in a phone booth. Telephone booths in Texas are sometimes equipped with a ceiling fan that turn on automatically when someone steps into the booth. Unfortunately, when Jeff entered the booth the entire ceiling, including the fan, came tumbling down and fell on his head. Jeff was dazed, but otherwise able to continue his activities. Later, however, he noticed he was unable to concentrate as well as he was

used to. This became most apparent when he played and practiced violin for extended periods of time. On neuropsychological testing, Jeff's performance was extremely high, undoubtedly due to his high level of premorbid functioning. Thus, his tests scores were mostly above average, although he did show a drop in abilities, compared to his own level of functioning, on tasks that required sustained attention and concentration. From the neuropsychological testing, it was obvious that Jeff had sustained a mild head injury. Jeff sued the manufacturer of the telephone booth, but the jury did not award damages to Jeff. It must have seemed counterintuitive to them to give money to someone who was by all accounts in control of his faculties and functioning average to above average in all areas of abilities. It was difficult to explain to the jury that Jeff was one of only a few individuals who have attained a superior level of skill on the violin. Jeff never returned to his previous level of musical skill and resigned from the symphonic orchestra he played in. He now teaches music and violin.

In regard to occupation and socioeconomic status, the clinician must generally make individual judgments regarding the independent effects of these variables on cognitive performance. Although in most instances considering educational level will be important, in certain cases an individual's occupation may bear on interpretation of test results. A watch repairperson would be expected to possess a high level of visual-motor coordination, fine-hand motor skills, and problem-solving abilities. A literary editor should have high verbal comprehension skills. Test validation studies using different occupational groups are helpful in determining if skills necessary for certain occupations give some individuals clinically reliable advantages on certain tests. More recently, researchers have attempted to estimate premorbid level of functioning empirically, using mathematical regression models.

DOMINANCE

The term **dominance** may refer to hand (and to a lesser extent eye and foot) preferences and proficiencies in performing tasks or to the cerebral organization of the brain. Cerebral organization for speech is widely associated with dominant hand preference and proficiency in neuropsychological assessment. Milner

(1974) reported that 96% of the right-handed population is left hemisphere dominant for speech, as is 70% of the left-handed population. Clinical studies of aphasia in right-handed individuals indicate that the vast majority have left hemisphere lesions (Searleman, 1977). As researchers estimate the incidence of right-handedness to be between 90% and 95% of the general population, the majority of the population can be estimated to be left hemisphere dominant for speech.

Although you can generally consider strongly right-handed individuals to be left hemisphere dominant for speech, you can no longer assume that neuropsychological test interpretation for left-handers is a simple matter of reversing the pattern of localization seen for right-handers. Levy (1982) suggests that abilities such as speech and reading, which in right-handers the left hemisphere seems to control, may not necessarily completely lateralize to the right hemisphere in left-handers. Lezak (1995) suggests three different patterns of cerebral speech dominance among left-handed and ambidextrous individuals. The significant majority, as noted, show the same pattern of brain organization as seen in right-handers, but a full one-third of left-handers show a different organization. Of this group, about half show a lateralized reversal of that which is expected for right-handers, and the other half show evidence of bilateral speech representation.

Although specialized methods of identifying verbal cerebral dominance exist, such as sodium amytal injection to incapacitate a single hemisphere (Wada test), these methods are not feasible for standard neuropsychological assessment. Traditionally, neuropsychologists have inferred cerebral dominance for language according to patient's self-report and performance on motor tasks involving hand, eye, and foot. These tasks may involve writing, looking through a telescope, and standing on one foot. Because strength of preference and level of proficiency may relate to varying levels of cerebral dominance, particularly for left-handers, it is important to assess handedness by degree rather than in a dichotomous fashion. If an individual is not strongly right- or left-hand dominant, he or she may be "ambidextrous," showing right-hand superiority for some tasks and left-hand superiority for other tasks. If a person to be assessed is strongly right-handed, it usually suffices to assess handedness by self-report of preference in performing several different tasks such as writing, throwing a ball, and unscrewing a jar lid. If the person states a left-hand preference in some tasks or activities, that warrants a more thorough examination of dominance (for example, using the Edinburgh Handedness Inventory).

SEX

Until recently, the vast majority of neuropsychological investigations have focused on right-handed Caucasian men, with the assumption that these results may generalize to the rest of the population. There is now increasing evidence that cerebral organization in women may differ from that of men. Following the idea that the left hemisphere specializes for language and the right for visual-spatial perception, evidence suggests that women are less likely to be asymmetrically organized for language than are men, although information regarding lateralization of spatial functions is less clear.

Evidence of sex-associated strengths and weaknesses on neuropsychological test performance indicates that women generally perform better than men on tasks requiring verbal skills, verbal learning, and verbal fluency (Benton et al., 1983). Men often show a visual-spatial advantage (Dodrill, 1979). Tests of motor speed and strength, such as the finger-tapping test and the strength-of-grip test from the Halstead-Reitan Neuropsychological Battery, consistently reveal a male advantage (Yeudall, Reddon, Gill, & Stefanyk, 1987). But there are indications that women perform better on motor tests requiring both unimanual and bimanual speed and coordination. Lezak (1995) reports that women score higher on the Purdue Pegboard Test than do men.

The neurological student should take care in evaluating these results regarding sex differences on clinical tests. Most cognitive and neuropsychological tests do not separate norms by sex. In many cases, this indicates that even if statistically reliable differences appear in group studies, the differences may be too small to have much clinical meaning. However, in other cases they may indicate that sex was not addressed. In assessing the utility of available normative data and in developing new normative data, always consider sex. Do not overinterpret sex differences, particularly if the test developer used appropriate sex representation in norming the test.

MOTIVATIONAL VARIABLES

Interpreting neuropsychological test data assumes that the person has performed to the best of his or her ability. If this is not the case, test data cannot adequately represent ability and may be largely uninterpretable as an indicator of cognitive functioning.

Level of Cooperation

Malingering is the intentional exaggeration or presentation of neuropsychological symptoms. In cases of court settlements, insurance payments, or worker's compensation for injury and disability, a client may intend to present as impaired for monetary, social, or emotional gain. Unfortunately, little guidance is available for the neuropsychologist who is trying to detect malingering or faking. Unlike personality tests such as the Minnesota Multiphasic Personality Inventory–2 (MMPI-2), which have validity scales and detect deviant response sets, neuropsychological tests have no validated formal procedures to detect faking.

Nonoptimal test performance can be classified into two categories, simulation and dissimulation. In **simulation,** the patient is faking or exaggerating an illness or the severity of the symptoms, usually to gain some secondary gain (such as attention, hospitalization, or a financial settlement). This test bias on the part of the patient may range from outright malingering or consciously distorting the test performance to more subtle, nonoptimal, approaches to his or her performance. **Dissimulation** is the opposite condition. The patient is consciously denying that there is anything wrong, also for secondary gain (for example, to avoid hospitalization or to gain employment). In some instances these biased test-taking approaches actually stem from the patient's neurologic symptoms. For example, patients with right parietal-occipital stroke often have limited insight into their condition.

Thus, the neuropsychologist must also be expert in evaluating the test-taking approach and motivation of each individual.

Lezak (1995) suggests that neuropsychologists can detect malingering and functional disorders by finding performance patterns that are discrepant with known neuropsychological patterns. She suggests a procedure for assessing the validity of general or visual perceptual complaints involving the counting of increasingly longer patterns of dots. Although test givers expect that time to complete the task would increase in people who are showing good effort, others "not performing in good faith" may show a different pattern. Neuropsychologists currently use other such procedures in a qualitative manner, but researchers have not yet established the validity of these methods. Although many clinical neuropsychologists may assert that clinical experience and familiarity with symptom patterns is sufficient to determine if a patient is malingering, mounting evidence shows that this is not the case. Preadolescent children have been able to fake believable neuropsychological deficits with relatively little instruction so that 34 of 42 experienced clinical neuropsychologists classified the protocols as indicating abnormality suggestive of cortical dysfunction (Faust, Hart, & Guilmette, 1988).

Arousal

Behaviorally, you should assess a patient's level of arousal and changes in arousal level. Note how quickly fatigue occurs and if there is a relationship to the type of task the person is performing. Physical fatigue may compromise motor tasks requiring speed and dexterity. In cases of lowered cortical arousal, performance on tasks requiring speeded information processing and new learning may deteriorate most. You can also use fatigue as a diagnostic factor. Luria (1966) has observed that patients fatigue faster when working with material that reflects their deficits. If a patient shows more fatigue with particular tests, those tests may reflect his or her underlying disorder.

Medication

Always question patients regarding their current level of medication and drug use, the length of use, and their self-report of the drug effects on their functioning. In most cases medications that interfere with motivation and arousal should be discontinued in order to assess the individual's best level of performance. This decision should be made in consultation with the patient's physician. The length of time between discontinuation of medication and testing varies with the patient, dosage, and drug. Generally, one to three days eliminate acute effects, but residual effects may last longer. If a patient requires continual medication, as do most seizure patients, then the purpose of the assessment may be to address the individual's performance while on medication. Discontinuing the medication in such cases would result in an atypical situation and possibly lower performance. In this case interpretations of test data while the patient is off medication may not be valid indicators of the person's daily situation.

In conclusion, the neuropsychologist is responsible for identifying specific variables and patient characteristics that may influence test performance. The testing situations should take these factors into account. To offset some of those factors, breaks in testing may be scheduled according to the needs of the patient, to alleviate fatigue. Whereas many younger and physically healthy patients can tolerate an extensive testing session, older and more severely compromised individuals may not be able to tolerate more than a few hours of testing during one day. For these patients, testing may be scheduled over a period of several days.

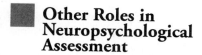

Other Roles in Neuropsychological Assessment

FORENSIC APPLICATION OF CLINICAL NEUROPSYCHOLOGY

The highly objective and quantitative nature of neuropsychological tests have become valuable assets in the courtroom to offer information to the jury or judge regarding the determination, effects, and prognosis of brain dysfunctioning. Because neuropsychol-

ogy assessment batteries typically evaluate a wide range of behaviors, this multidimensional approach to measuring higher cortical functioning has proven very helpful in quantifying disabilities resulting from head trauma or other neuropathological conditions. Neuropsychological evaluations are crucial for comprehensive understanding of the cognitive, behavioral, and emotional sequelae of a variety of neurologic conditions, particularly for legal documentation. Therefore, neuropsychologists are in a position to deal with varied aspects of brain dysfunction and are rapidly becoming an integral part of the doctor-lawyer team in testifying as expert witnesses on cases related to personal injury, disability determination, and worker's compensation (see Neuropsychology in Action 15.1).

NEUROPSYCHOLOGICAL ASSESSMENT AND RESEARCH

Neuropsychological assessment techniques also have become very useful as baseline and outcome measures in medical research. For example, studies that have benefited from such evaluations include the psychological and neuropsychological effects of sleep apnea, the cognitive concomitants of exposure to industrial toxins, the neuropsychological sequelae of mild head injury, and the cognitive benefits of ventricular shunting in normal-pressure hydrocephalus patients, to name just a few.

NEUROPSYCHOLOGICAL TEST DEVELOPMENT

Test validity is an important consideration at all stages of test development and test evaluation. It is essential for both the test developer and the testing consumer. This section presents factors and methods to consider specific to neuropsychological test development and validation.

As with any test, developers should conceive neuropsychological tests within a conceptual framework. Arguments abound as to whether tests should be developed via atheoretical empiricism focusing totally on criterion-related validity, or via theoretical

Neuropsychology in Action 15.1

Forensic Neuropsychology: Application of Brain–Behavior Relationships in the Legal Arena

by Jim Hom Ph.D., Editor, Journal of Forensic Neuropsychology, *and cofounder,* The Neuropsychology Center, Dallas, Texas.

Over the last several decades clinical neuropsychologists have been increasingly called on to provide important information regarding brain–behavior relationships in legal matters. Forensic neuropsychology is a rapidly emerging subspecialty of neuropsychology that directly applies the principles and practices of neuropsychology in cases where questions of brain injury are pertinent to civil or criminal issues. Frequently the court asks the clinical neuropsychologist to identify and delineate cognitive, behavioral, and emotional consequences of brain injury. The court uses this information to understand the impact of brain impairment on the function of the individual and to assist in settling the specific legal claims of the case. In civil cases, attorneys use neuropsychological test results and the neuropsychologist's professional opinions to provide credible evidence regarding the functional impact of brain injury on the daily activities of

the individual involved. Clinical neuropsychologists address such issues as how neurocognitive dysfunction will affect routine daily activities, work-related abilities and function, and social activities. Typically, the clinical neuropsychologist is asked to provide information concerning loss or changes in brain function as they relate to these issues. The neuropsychologist addresses clinical questions such as prognosis, treatment recommendations, rehabilitation potential, and future care of the individual as they relate to the claims of the case. An area of civil litigation in which clinical neuropsychologists have played an important role is that of personal injury claims involving head injury or exposure to toxic substances. In these cases, clear-cut neurologic and/or neuroradiologic evidence (such as physical neurologic examination, CT or MRI scans, EEG, and other traditional diagnostic procedures) are often either normal or equivo-

cal. However, the claimant is reporting neuropsychological impairments that are affecting his or her ability to function. Neuropsychological evidence assists in determining the legitimate basis for the claim and any financial compensation.

An example of a personal injury case in which the court may ask a clinical neuropsychologist for assistance is one where an individual sustained a closed head injury during a motor vehicle-pedestrian accident. With the injury, the pedestrian lost consciousness, had a skull fracture, and had multiple contusions of the body. She recovers completely from her physical injuries. However, after several months, she is fired from her job because of poor work performance. A lawsuit is pending against the driver of the motor vehicle that hit her. In such a case, the clinical neuropsychologist would be able to provide important information concerning the relationship of the head injury to the problems on the

constructs, thereby focusing on construct validity. Neuropsychology is moving away from a focus on test validity solely determined by its sensitivity in detecting brain damage. Neuropsychologists want tests that offer both criterion-related and construct validity. That is, tests must help neuropsychologists differentiate among groups of individuals or areas of functional abilities, and must help neuropsychologists describe behavior in relation to theories of knowledge in areas such as perception, learning, attention, memory, and problem solving, and theories of brain–behavior functioning. This approach often presents a dilemma to the test developer. Construct validity is

most adequately demonstrated if the concept is pure or homogeneous. However, many neuropsychological impairments, syndromes, and disease entities involve multiple and interactive abilities, which, if included in one test, may demonstrate good criterion-related validity but poor construct validity because of the seeming "hodgepodge" of concepts being measured. If developers are building single-construct tests, then multiple tests are necessary to diagnose multifunctional impairments. Another issue related to the "purity" of tests is that some impairments are not evident except when a complex task assesses a combination of abilities. As a result, it is clearly the

job. Clinical neuropsychological evaluation would help identify neurocognitive deficits as well as problems in psychological function. Further, such evaluation could address medical-legal issues such as the extent of her neuropsychological impairment, the contribution of pre-existing medical/psychological conditions, and her potential for rehabilitation. The court would use this neuropsychological information to determine whether the individual has a legitimate basis to sue the driver. Then, if the patient won the case, the court would use this information to help determine monetary compensation awards.

Clinical neuropsychologists also play an important role in criminal proceedings. In such cases, the issues the clinical neuropsychologist must address differ from those in civil cases. The clinical neuropsychologist helps determine whether brain injury has affected the defendant's competence to stand trial, his or her ability to understand his or her legal rights, to distinguish right from wrong, and to appreciate the consequences of his or her actions. Further, if the defendant is convicted, the court uses neuropsychological evidence in deciding on the final sentence. An example of a criminal case would be one in

which the accused sustained brain damage from a gunshot wound to the head five years before committing the present criminal act. The clinical neuropsychologist will aid in determining whether the defendant's brain damage has affected his ability to understand the legal proceedings against him and whether he can participate in his own defense. This includes determining whether the defendant understands the charges against him and his legal rights, and whether he appreciates right from wrong and the consequences of his actions. If the defendant is convicted, the court uses the neuropsychological information concerning the significance of brain damage in determining the type and/or term of the sentence. For example, if he were significantly impaired, he may not be sentenced to serve in a traditional facility, but rather in one more appropriate for his present condition.

Regardless of type of legal proceeding, the expert testimony that the clinical neuropsychologist gives in the courtroom is subject to judicial rules for admitting or excluding scientific evidence. Essentially, admissibility of scientific testimony by an expert is based on whether the technique or principle has sufficient scientific reliability and validity to assist the court

in understanding the evidence and in reaching accurate conclusions. As such, the neuropsychological evidence and professional opinions that the expert neuropsychologist offers in testimony should be scientifically tested, by peer reviewed, meet accepted professional standards, and be accepted as reliable and valid by the scientific community. Clearly, to satisfy these judicial requirements, the expert neuropsychologist must be prepared to demonstrate objectively that his or her findings are based on sound science and rely on methods that follow standard scientific procedures that the neuropsychological profession accepts. With the increasing participation of clinical neuropsychologists in the legal setting, stricter judicial scrutiny of neuropsychology will likely occur. The expert neuropsychologist will need to be knowledgeable about the field of neuropsychology and its relation to neurology, psychiatry, and medicine. The well-prepared neuropsychologist will also have to understand medical-legal issues to be an effective witness. Ultimately, adherence to scientific principles and methodology will best serve the clinical neuropsychologist who is involved in forensic work.

---

higher-level integration abilities that are impaired, rather than a pure skill.

Even within the domain of criterion-related validity, controversy exists over what criterion is most important for neuropsychological tests to measure. Some are of the opinion that neuropsychological tests should always be first judged on their ability to detect presence or absence of brain damage (for example, see Kane, Parsons, & Goldstein, 1985). Others argue that this criterion is no longer useful, because if brain functioning is considered as a continuum, then the pattern of results related to an individual's cognitive functioning is most important (Zillmer & Ball, 1987).

As with all tests, developers must always consider a neuropsychological test's validity in relation to its intended purpose. Is the purpose of the assessment measure to determine the specific location of brain damage? Is its purpose to discover the nature and complexity of the functional impairment? Or is the purpose to link structural damage to functional impairment? Regarding the first question, it is possible that developers may design some tests using an empirical strategy in which items selected are those most closely associated with specific areas of damage, even though the items may in fact be conceptually unrelated. This type of test may be most useful in determining lesion site. Its validity is determined by its ability to appropriately identify damaged structures.

In the second instance, developers typically design functionally or conceptually derived tests that usually measure a specific ability or set of abilities employing a theoretical strategy regarding the nature of the ability to be measured. They assess the validity of this type of test according to its ability to clearly describe function. As is readily apparent, the first type of test may result in high "localization" validity but low "construct" validity, whereas the second type of test may show just the opposite pattern. Neuropsychologists aim to develop tests that demonstrate both high structural localization validity and high functional conceptual validity, thus striving toward demonstrating a strong structure-function relationship. Although developers have built, and will continue to build, some tests that are good measures of a specific function related to a specific brain site, the human brain is not an organ containing tidy one-to-one relationships between structure and function. Thus, in many cases attempting to achieve one type of neuropsychological test validity may do so at the expense of another type of validity.

Case Examples

We present next two clinical case examples related to neuropsychological interpretation and diagnosis. Each case provides background information about the patient. We base the interpretation on the just mentioned strategies of performance level, using the standard score approach, the differential score approach (pattern impairment), lateralizing and localizing signs, and pathognomonic signs (qualitative observations). In each case, we use the functional domains outlined in Chapter 14 to illustrate the multidimensional nature of neuropsychological diagnosis and evaluation.

CASE 1: ACUTE POISONING BY CHLORDANE, A TERMITE PESTICIDE

Jim was a 31-year-old phone repairman with 12 years of education. Jim had just purchased a new home that

he and his pregnant wife moved into. He had asked a pesticide company to have the dwelling treated for termite control using subslab injection of chlordane, a potent pesticide. When Jim came home after work, obviously something was wrong, because the carpet was saturated with the pesticide and the air smelled of chemicals. Jim did not think much of it and used a towel to soak up the puddles of chlordane, not knowing that the poison is easily absorbed through unbroken skin. Within four days of being exposed, he developed headaches, fatigue, and numbness. He also complained of difficulties with memory, attention, eye–hand coordination, and changes in his personality. He went to see his family physician, who referred him to the toxicology research center of a large university medical center, where lab tests showed that Jim had elevated tissue levels of chlordane as estimated by blood and body fat analysis.

People have used chlordane (chlorinated hydrocarbon insecticides) extensively to combat household pests such as flies, cockroaches, fleas, termites, and mosquitoes as well as agricultural crop enemies. Chlordane is a heavy, dark-brown, oily liquid that is insoluble in water but soluble in common organic (carbon-based) solvents. Chlordane is chemically stable and persists in the environment. In fact, it maintains its effects for approximately 15 or more years after treatment and therefore offers an economically appealing long-term treatment against termites. Because of its chemical stability, investigators can detect chlordane in approximately 70% of U.S. homes today. Once absorbed, chlordane is an axon poison, disturbing the normal action of the sodium-potassium adenosinetriphosphatase (ATPase) pump, and interfering with transmission of nerve impulses. The internal medicine department requested neuropsychological testing to examine Jim's neuropsychological and emotional sequelae.

Table 15.4 shows the neuropsychological test scores representing general intellectual ability, academic skills, abstract reasoning, attention, and motor and sensory functioning. Performance was also rated in T-scores, which are in parentheses. This standardized scoring system provides age, sex, and educationally corrected T-scores for each measure, with T-scores of 39 and below indicating impairment.

Jim's WAIS-R Full Scale IQ score fell within the Average range (Full Scale IQ = 98, T-score = 51). In

Table 15.4	*Neuropsychological Profile of Patient with Chlordane Poisoning*
Age	31
Gender	Male
Education in years	12
Occupation	Phone repairman
Intellectual Functioning (WAIS-R)	
Verbal IQ	94 (45)
Performance IQ	105 (55)
Full-Scale IQ	98 (51)
Academic Skills	
PIAT Reading Comprehension (SS)[a]	95
Abstract Reasoning, Cognitive Efficiency, Mental Flexibility	
Category Test (errors)	65 (35)
Trail-Making Test A (seconds)	18 (60)
Trail-Making Test B (seconds)	72 (45)
Attention/Concentration	
PASAT % correct series 1/2[b]	49/37
PASAT % correct series 3/4	29/discontinued
Motor Speed and Coordination	
Finger-Oscillation DH	61 (64)
Finger-Oscillation NDH	41 (47)
Grooved-Pegboard (seconds) DH	57 (51)
Grooved-Pegboard (seconds) NDH	71 (42)

Note. [a]Mean = 100; SD = 15, PIAT = Peabody Individual Achievement Test (Dunn & Markwardt, 1970); SS = Standard Score; [b]PASAT=Paced Auditory Serial Addition Task—Norms Trial 1 >78%, Trial 2 >69%, Trial 3 >63%, Trial 4 >52% (Brittain, La March, Reeder, Roth, & Boll, 1991); DH = dominant hand; NDH = nondominant hand. T-scores in parentheses from Heaton, Grant, and Matthews (1991).

terms of the cognitive efficiency, this patient had a raw score of 65 errors (cutoff for impaired performance is ≥51) on the Category Test. The Category Test is part of the Halstead-Reitan Neuropsychological Battery and is a test of abstracting ability consisting of 208 visually presented items. Six sets of items,

each organized on the basis of different principles, precede a seventh set made up of previous shown items. The subject's task is to figure out the principle each set presents and to signal the answer. The score is the number of errors—in Jim's case, 65—which corresponded to a T-score of 35 and suggested mild impairment.

Thus, Jim, although exhibiting "normal" intelligence, was having difficulties with a task that required complex information processing, mental flexibility, and the ability to shift mental sets or rules. To test this deficit further, the Paced Auditory Serial Addition Task (PASAT) was administered. The PASAT (Gronwall, 1977) is a test that requires extensive sustained concentration and attention. Any problems Jim had with this type of cognitive skill would surely show up on this test. The PASAT requires the patient to add 60 pairs of randomized single digits so that each adds to the digit immediately preceding it. For example, if the examiner reads the numbers "2–8–6–1–9," the subject's correct responses, beginning as soon as the examiner says "8," are "10–14–7–10." The digits are presented at four different rates of speed, each differing by 0.4 sec and ranging from one every 2.4 sec to one every 1.2 sec (Lezak, 1995). On the first series of numbers presented at 2.4 sec, Jim could only respond with a 49% accuracy, compared to a normal value of >78%. During the fourth and fastest presentation (1.2 sec), the test had to be discontinued, because Jim could not keep track and became very frustrated.

The neuropsychology student is correct in assuming that this is a relatively "painful" way of eliciting attentional deficits. However, in Jim's case it appeared as if the tester needed to make the presence of subtle attentional deficits quantifiable, in the interest of the patient's health. In addition, neuropsychologists are trained to prepare the examinee about unpleasant procedures, by informing them that many tests are very difficult and they may not be able to pass them. Thus, they may feel that they are failing when they are not. The PASAT was consistent with the Category Test and the Intelligence test data, which indicated unsatisfactory ability for processing auditory information quickly and accurately.

On tests of motor speed, coordination, and strength, the overall level of performances were not significantly affected and were generally within normal limits. On the sensory perceptual examination, Jim had four errors on fingertip number writing, which may have been related to his difficulty in attending to the task at hand. The neuropsychologist administered a number of memory measures to Jim, and his test scores revealed generally adequate immediate recall for verbal passages and pictorial information. Asked to retrieve the information from both modalities 30 minutes later, however, Jim showed poor short-term memory in the verbal modality by demonstrating much less than normal 70% recall. Personality testing using the Minnesota Multiphasic Personality Inventory indicated a mild level of overall psychological disturbance. Jim was mildly preoccupied with bodily concern, excessive somatization, fatigue, dizziness, depression, and hysterical features. Of course, Jim was experiencing many of these symptoms, and similar personality configurations are not at all uncommon in other medical patients (for example, see Zillmer, Ware, Rose, & Maximin, 1988).

Taken together, the neuropsychologist considered that Jim's overall potential for abstract reasoning, hypothesis testing, and new learning was deficient, a cognitive deficit one would normally not expect in the absence of any CNS trauma. Although crystallized knowledge as assessed by general intelligence and academic skills measures is relatively unaffected by chlordane exposure, the findings clearly suggested neurotoxic effects in this exposure victim, with both cognitive and emotional functions being compromised. Areas of cognitive functioning affected included rapid information processing, mental flexibility, and memory.

This case demonstrates how a comprehensive neuropsychological evaluation can help identify areas of cognitive impairment and associated neurobehavioral changes by assessing subtle brain dysfunctions produced by chlordane intoxication. This in turn sheds light on the degree and pattern of neuropsychological deficits that may be associated with chlordane neurotoxicity and Jim's occupational plans, and serves as a baseline to which future neuropsychological assessments can be compared. Neuropsychological test batteries offer a promising tool for increasing knowledge about the effects of chlordane toxicity on the human CNS. Neuropsychological testing can also describe specific patterns of performance, and monitoring the course of treatment (Zillmer & Ball, 1987; for a more detailed description of the neuropsychological sequelae of chlordane poisoning, see Zillmer, Montenegro, Wiser, Barth, & Spyker, 1996). Jim had to evacuate his home, and his case ended up in compensation litigation against the involved pesticide company. The court awarded a large cash settlement to the plaintiff because of the obvious chlordane misapplication. Jim returned to work, but at a reduced level of responsibility, because he continued to experience difficulties in concentration and adapting to novel situations. His pregnant wife, who was also tested, did not show any evidence of poisoning or neuropsychological deficits.

CASE 2: THE NEUROPSYCHOLOGY OF LYME DISEASE

David was an active, 66-year-old, right hand–dominant, married, male who had completed 11th grade before joining the U.S. Armed Forces. Before retiring David was employed as a medical technician in a psychiatric hospital. His wife, a nurse, was his supervisor. In August 1992, David began experiencing periods of blurred vision, headaches, nausea and "feeling ill all over, as if I was coming down with the flu." The family doctor suspected a heart problem as David had a history of mild hypertension and angina beginning in 1987, but a 24-hour EKG monitor revealed no heart malfunction. Over the next month David experienced five similar episodes. Then, in September 1992, he awoke with numbness and weakness on the right side as well as slurred speech, and was subsequently hospitalized. Initial neurologic findings indicated that David was awake and alert with dysarthria and right hemiparesis. The examiner noted periods of paralysis, with the comment that the patient felt "locked in" when these occurred. Physicians at the hospital diagnosed him as having had a transient ischemic attack (TIA; see Chapter 9). After a 10-day course of treatment, the patient was sent home. Hospital records noted that he was "fully recovered" at this point.

MRI of the brain suggested prominence of the ventricular system and subarachnoid spaces consistent

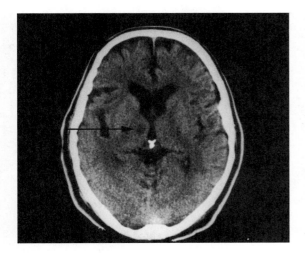

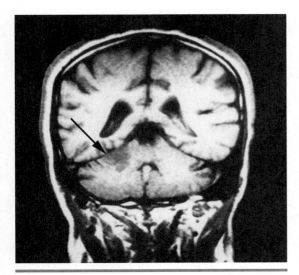

Figure 15.2 Horizontal CT (top) showing infarction in left thalamus. Coronal MRI (bottom) revealing subacute cerebellar infarct as well as moderate atrophy. (Eric Zillmer)

with moderate atrophy. The report also noted mild white matter changes on the periventricular region. MRI films of the coronal (see Figure 15.2) and sagittal (see Exhibit 9) planes revealed a subacute cerebellar infarct (stroke). CT scans of the head, without intravenous contrast infusion, confirmed the atrophy and previously visualized infarct in the left cerebel-

lum. Repeat CT scan of the head without contrast three weeks later revealed an additional new small infarction in the left thalamus (see Figure 15.2). Intracranial and neck angiogram sequences revealed no stenosis of the right or left carotid artery bifurcations. Taken together, radiological data suggested moderate atrophy, postacute left cerebellar infarct, a small left thalamic infarct, and minimal thickening of the common, internal, and external carotid arteries. The radiological studies did not indicate the presence of intracranial hemorrhage, or any significant stenosis or plaque in the right or left carotid system. Electroencephalogram revealed no definite focal or epileptogenic features.

David continued to have episodes of nausea and blurred vision, and in October 1992 he was again hospitalized with right hemiparesis, dizziness, and slurred speech. Initial diagnosis was that he had suffered another TIA. He was experiencing projectile vomiting and had episodes of high fever and brief periods during which he could only move one eye. He also had behavioral digressions where he would not recognize anyone and would pull out his IV tubes and exhibit other strange behaviors until he had to be restrained to the bed. The medical staff was mystified as to the causes of David's symptoms.

A few weeks into David's treatment, the Center for Disease Control (CDC) notified the hospital that David had tested positive for Lyme disease. Puzzled by the cause of David's symptoms, the family doctor had taken a blood serology before the second hospitalization and forwarded samples to the CDC. David was given a course of treatment appropriate for both stroke and Lyme disease. As a result, David's strange symptoms abated and have not returned, though the hemiparesis and dysarthria remain. The hospital physician did not agree that the Lyme disease was responsible for David's symptoms. David was discharged to a rehabilitation hospital for continued care, where he was referred for neuropsychological testing to evaluate his cognitive status and his ability to participate in speech therapy and physical therapy.

Table 15.5 reviews the results of the neuropsychological battery. Compared to Jim, David exhibited generalized deficits, with impaired performance across

Table 15.5   *Neuropsychological Profile of Patient with Lyme Disease*

Age	66
Gender	Male
Education in years	11
Occupation	Retired medical technician

Intellectual Functioning (WAIS-R)

Verbal IQ	91 (31)
Performance IQ	84 (28)
Full Scale IQ	87 (27)

Abstract Reasoning, Cognitive Efficiency, Mental Flexibility

Trail Making Test A (seconds)	109 (26)
Trail Making Test B (seconds)	255 (35)
Wisconsin Card Sort (in perseveration errors)	65 (34)

Memory: Wechsler Memory Scale–Revised

Logical Memory I	19 (36)
Logical Memory II	5 (11)

Motor Speed and Coordination

Finger Oscillation DH	Not attempted
Finger Oscillation NDH	31 (29)
Grooved Pegboard (seconds) DH	Not attempted
Grooved Pegboard (seconds) NDH	154 (34)

Note: DH = dominant hand; NDH = nondominant hand. T-scores in parentheses from Heaton, Grant, and Matthews (1991).

cognitive areas. His performance on the neuropsychological tests indicated impaired attentional capacity, motor slowness, and weakness in the nondominant upper extremity (the patient was unable to use his dominant hand), impaired fine motor ability, left auditory suppressions, impaired visual-constructional ability, deficient spatial memory, and poor executive functioning. David's memory performance revealed slightly impaired verbal recall, moderately impaired visual recall, and moderately to severely impaired delayed recall for both verbal and visual material. His intellectual performance, as measured by the WAIS-R, was in the Low Average range. David's WAIS-R scores indicated slightly higher verbal than performance ability, again partially because of his right hemiplegia, but also because of impaired perception of visual material, especially visual details. The visual impairment was further documented by his borderline performance on the Hooper Visual Organization Test. On the Wisconsin Card Sorting Task, David failed to complete any categories and used the maximum possible number of trials to complete the test. Results of clinical personality testing (MMPI) did not indicate significant psychopathology or psychological dysfunctioning. However, factors reflected in the protocol did suggest susceptibility to developing psychological problems including denial, somatic concern, and tension. Individuals with similar profiles are often mildly dysphoric, pessimistic about the future, and difficult to engage in psychological therapies because of their defensiveness and lack of insight.

The neuropsychological evaluation did not shed any light on whether Lyme disease was the "culprit" for David's medical problems (for a more detailed description of the clinical, radiological, and neuropsychological manifestations of Lyme disease, see Bundick, Zillmer, Ives, & Beadle-Lindsay, 1995). David's case analysis demonstrates that psychological and neuropsychological assessment may serve to aid in the more definite diagnosis and improved intervention/rehabilitation of patients exhibiting complex symptoms.

Conclusion

The neuropsychologist's role in evaluation has evolved from a diagnostic emphasis to one in which current neuropsychological functioning is described and the individual's adaptation to the unique demands of his or her environment is evaluated. The focus is on performance in the testing setting as well as on a task analysis of the cognitive requirements of home and work. Neuropsychological testing profiles can aid in identifying general categories of neurologic disease and conditions. The purpose of the neuropsychological evaluation examines the individual's strengths and weaknesses, ability to deal with stress, adaptation, and overall social and occupational functioning. It is in this latter more descriptive role that neuropsychologists have made their most recent advances. In the next chapter we focus on how results from neuropsychological testing are used to remediate and rehabilitate functions that relate to brain impairments.

Critical Thinking Questions

■ How do the major two approaches (process and battery) to interpreting neuropsychological data differ?
■ What role can neuropsychologists play in court?
■ What is a pathognomonic sign, and why is it so important?
■ How do neuropsychologists go about trying to make sense out of a neuropsychological evaluation?

Key Terms

Interpretive hypotheses	Cutoff score	Deficit measurement	Dominance
Standard battery approach	Specificity	Pattern analysis	Malingering
Process approach	Sensitivity	Pathognomonic signs	Simulation
Normative data	Normal distribution	Premorbid functioning	Dissimulation

Web Connections

http://www.neuropsychologycentral.com/interface/content/links/links_interface_frameset.html
Forensic Neuropsychological Testimony
Forensic links and literature, including article entitled "Admissibility of Neuropsychological Testimony" by Bruce H. Stern, with relevant court decisions linked to the social sciences.

http://dpa.state.ky.us/~rwheeler/wagner/wagner.htm
Forensic Neuropsychology
Includes article entitled "Neuropsychological Evidence in Criminal Defense: Rationale and Guidelines for Enlisting an Expert" by Dr. Marilyn M. Wagner, complete with references and associated links.

http://www.sportsci.org/resource/stats/index.html
A New View of Statistics
This site features a web-based book about the ins and outs of statistical procedures using simple sports analogies and common everyday problems. Within this site you can find concrete examples of the simple statistical terms and validity as well as reliability procedures discussed in this chapter on interpretation.

http://www.sas.com & http://www.spss.com
SPSS and SAS
Home pages for two of the most commonly used statistical packages in the social sciences.

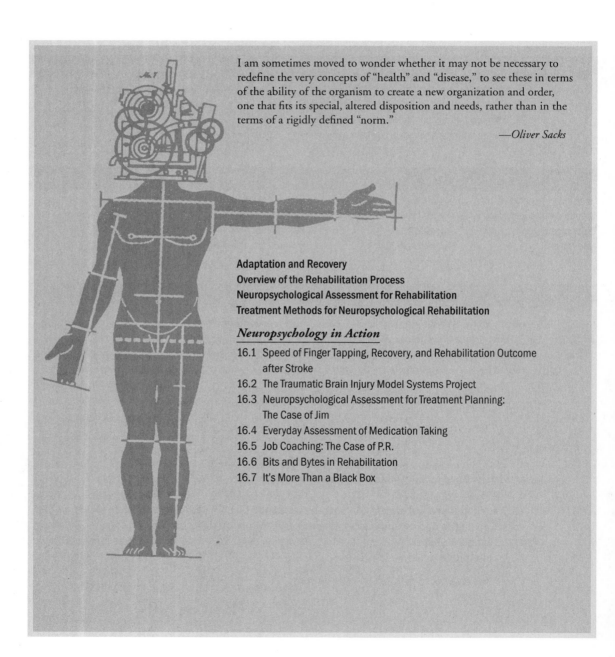

Chapter 16

RECOVERY, REHABILITATION, AND INTERVENTION

I am sometimes moved to wonder whether it may not be necessary to redefine the very concepts of "health" and "disease," to see these in terms of the ability of the organism to create a new organization and order, one that fits its special, altered disposition and needs, rather than in the terms of a rigidly defined "norm."

—*Oliver Sacks*

Adaptation and Recovery
Overview of the Rehabilitation Process
Neuropsychological Assessment for Rehabilitation
Treatment Methods for Neuropsychological Rehabilitation

Neuropsychology in Action

Keep in Mind

- How does the rehabilitation process work?
- Describe a rehabilitation program for attention.
- How do rehabilitation programs further the process of recovery and adaptation?
- What is the specific role of the neuropsychologist in the rehab team?

Overview

Oliver Sacks's story of Jonathan on the following pages speaks to the amazing resiliency of humans, the human brain, and the human will to adapt and make sense and meaning out of tragedy. Jonathan no doubt has "deficits" caused by brain damage. But his ability to compensate for his deficits and develop a new approach to painting attests to his resiliency to adapt and recover. Of course, Jonathan had a very circumscribed brain injury. Unfortunately, most patients presented in this chapter have suffered more widespread and devastating brain injuries. But the case of the color-blind painter raises interesting questions. What is the potential for the human brain to recover after brain injury? Are there areas or functions that may be able to repair themselves? Are other areas of the brain able to take over or compensate for destroyed brain functions? These are the first issues we consider in discussing brain damage and recovery.

With many types of brain damage some spontaneous recovery is expected, perhaps for a full year or longer. What, then, is the function of rehabilitation programs? How do they encourage the process of adaptation? We discuss these questions in the next section, covering the rehabilitation process. You will see how the team members work individually and together to foster the attainment of treatment goals. Specifically, we examine how neuropsychologists contribute to the team in rehabilitation settings: What is their role, and what services do they provide? Next we examine the theories and methods of neuropsychological rehabilitation, including selected strategies that rehabilitation neuropsychologists use to assess and achieve cognitive remediation of damaged functions or compensation for lost functions. Supported employment or "job coaching" and innovative uses of computers are some of the exciting new methods that hold great promise. We also stress the importance of psychotherapy and the rehabilitation of the "whole person."

THE CASE OF JONATHAN

I am a rather successful artist just past 65 years of age. On January 2nd of this year, I was driving my car and was hit by a small truck on the passenger side of my vehicle. When visiting the emergency room of a local hospital, I was told I had a concussion. While taking an eye examination, it was discovered that I was unable to distinguish letters or colors. The letters appeared "Greek" to me. My vision was such that everything looked to me as viewing a black and white television screen. Within days, I could distinguish letters and my vision became that of an eagle—I could see a worm wriggling a block away. The sharpness of my ability to focus was incredible. BUT— I AM ABSOLUTELY COLOR BLIND. I have visited ophthalmologists who know nothing about this color-blind business. I have visited neurologists, to no avail. Under hypnosis, I still can't distinguish colors. I have been involved in all kinds of tests. You name it. My brown dog is dark grey. Tomato juice is black. Color TV is a hodgepodge. (From Sacks, O., *An Anthropologist on Mars*, p. 3. © 1995 Alfred A. Knopf)

And so begins Oliver Sacks's (1995) clinical tale of "The case of the colorblind painter," the compelling tale of the artist Jonathan with **cerebral achromatopsia,** or total colorblindness. Although the neuroimaging techniques of CT or MRI were negative, extensive neuropsychological testing by Sacks, a neurologist with an interest in neuropsychology, estimated the damage was to a small part of the secondary visual cortex of the occipital lobe. This specific injury, to an area no bigger than the size of a "bean," devastated this artist's life.

The "wrongness" of everything was disturbing, even disgusting, and applied to every circumstance of daily life. He found foods disgusting due to their greyish, dead appearance and had to close his eyes to eat. But this did not help very much, for the mental image of a tomato was as black as its appearance. Thus, unable to rectify even the inner image, the idea of various foods, he turned increasingly to black and white foods—to black olives and white rice, black coffee and yogurt. These at least appeared relatively normal, whereas most foods, normally colored, now appeared horribly abnormal. His own brown dog looked so strange to him now that he even considered getting a Dalmatian. (Sacks, 1995, p. 3)

Sacks describes an overwhelming sense of loss in Jonathan, as a person who had lost the sense of beauty of the world—particularly devastating to an artist whose whole world had been awash in a sea of color. Immediately after the injury he was at times nearly suicidally depressed, he was fearful that he might lose more sight and was desperate in his hope that color would return. But within a month Jonathan began to show adaptation to his new condition. Two months after the accident, some of his agitation was calming down; he had started to accept, not merely intellectually, but at a deeper emotional level, too, that he was indeed totally color blind and might possibly remain so. His initial sense of helplessness began to give way to a sense of resolution—he would paint in black and white; indeed, he would live in black and white.

His first black-and-white paintings, done in February and March, gave a feeling of violent forces—rage, fear, despair, excitement—but these were held in control, attesting to the powers of artistry that could disclose, and yet contain, such intensity of feeling. In these two months he produced dozens of paintings, marked by a singular style, a character he had never shown before. In many of these paintings, there was an extraordinary shattered, kaleidoscopic surface, with abstract raging—and dismembered body parts, faceted and held in frames and boxes. They had, compared

with his previous work, a labyrinthine complexity, and an obsessed, haunted quality—they seemed to exhibit, in symbolic form, the predicament he was in. (Sacks, 1995, p. 14)

As time went on Jonathan's paintings became less macabre and more vital. He began sculpting and painting portraits, which he had not done before. Because he could only see in black and white, he became much more comfortable in the colorless world of the night.

"Jonathan," when he was not traveling, would get up earlier and earlier, to work in the night, to relish the night. He felt that in the night world (as he called it) he was the equal, or the superior, of "normal" people: "I feel better because I know then that I'm not a freak . . . and I have developed acute night vision, it's amazing what I see—I can read license plates at night from four blocks away. You couldn't see it from a block away."

Most interesting of all, the sense of profound loss, and the sense of unpleasantness and abnormality, so severe in the first months following his head injury, seemed to disappear, or even reverse. Although Jonathan does not deny his loss, and at times still mourns it, he has come to feel that his vision has become "highly refined," "privileged," that he sees a world of pure form, uncluttered by color. Subtle textures and patterns, normally obscured for the rest of us because of their embedding in color, now stand out for him. He feels he has been given "a whole new world," which the rest of us, distracted by color, are insensitive to. He no longer thinks of color, pines for it, grieves its loss. He has almost come to see his achromatopsia as a strange gift, one that has ushered him into a new state of sensibility and being. (Sacks, 1995, pp. 37, 39)

Jonathan changed in response to his damaged color system—so much so that he felt he had been able to develop extreme sensitivity to the colorless world. Interestingly, when someone suggested to him some time later that there might be a "cure," he was not interested. He was now comfortable with his new altered world and had trouble imagining anything else.

Adaptation and Recovery

Knowledge of brain damage and recovery comes from two sources, the study of animals in the laboratory and the study of human "cases." The study of animals offers insight into the immediate effects of injury on the brain and provides a way to study how the brain attempts to reorganize and repair itself at the neuronal level. Studying animals also allows direct examination of the brain at various stages of recovery.

For over a century, neuroscientists have been actively searching for means to transplant healthy central nervous system tissue into damaged animal brains. Human transplantation research began in the early 1980s. Surgeons have attempted to transplant fetal tissue in cases of Parkinson's disease, Huntington's disease, spinal cord injury, and brain injury. The theory of fetal transplantation proposes that immature cortical tissue shows the greatest potential for neuronal growth and differentiation. The mechanism by which grafted tissue operates, however, is not fully known. Maybe the yield of deficient neurotransmitter increases. Or neuronal tissue may act as a structural bridge between damaged areas. Finally, young tissue may function indirectly, stimulating surrounding tissue by secreting neuroprotective or neurogrowth factors. In addition to the difficult ethical questions fetal transplantation research raises, the work has achieved limited success. In brain injury, it may be necessary to match the fetal cortical area to the damaged cortical area. For example, fetal hippocampal tissue may be necessary to improve hippocampal functioning (Soares, Sinson, & McIntosh, 1995). In any transplantation procedure, the subject's immune system must be suppressed, thereby increasing vulnerability to infection. Also, because tissue from miscarried fetuses is ineffective for transplantation research (Hainline et al., 1995), neurosurgeons have used fetal cells from other animals, such as pigs. This usage carries the danger of cross-species infection.

Several promising directions for brain injury repair may emerge from research done on other disorders. For example, researchers seeking to increase dopamine levels in monkeys in which the researchers have induced Parkinson's disease, have found that dopamine-producing cells from the monkey's own carotid glands in the neck are useful alternatives to fetal tissue. Carotid cells transferred into the monkey putamen continued to produce dopamine throughout the duration of the three- to five-month experiment. These cells also appeared to secrete a growth factor that stimulated the poorly functioning cells into remanufacturing dopamine. Medical researchers

are also working on CNS tissue in the spinal cord. Most patients who have spinal cord injury lose muscle control beneath the break, because the severed nerve cells do not regrow across the damaged area. The damaged nerve cells actually produce proteins that prevent themselves from regrowing. By blocking these inhibitory proteins, researchers can induce cell regrowth and restore some movement. Eventually, this procedure could lead to better treatment for people paralyzed by spinal cord injury.

Brain damage in humans is our main interest, with the potential for recovery and rehabilitation as the end goal. Familiarity with the effects of damage and the process of neural and behavioral recovery is an invaluable aid in predicting the long-term course of intervention and recovery in the rehabilitation process. The case of Jonathan is a good example of how a very small site of injury can have a major effect on one's life. Brain damage causes not only cognitive effects, but emotional reactions to those effects as people struggle to make meaning out of their altered sense of self. Brain damage may occur suddenly or gradually, but the recovery process is inevitably gradual ranging from weeks to years. For example, although it is common to think that **coma** and wakefulness are two distinct states walled off from each other by a curtain of consciousness, people coming out of a coma do not just wake up, recognize their loved ones, and walk out of the hospital. The recovery from coma is a process of "emergence" in which the person gains greater and greater awareness of environmental stimuli.

Behind most theories of neuropsychological rehabilitation lies the premise that if functions are not completely ablated, there is a chance that they can be restored through the brain's ability to heal and adapt. To what degree functions may spontaneously recover versus needing aid via neuropsychological rehabilitation techniques is still unresolved. There is no doubt that some spontaneous recovery can occur, but how much does targeted training also help to restore function? We return to this question later in this chapter. What if a function is completely lost? In this case most neurobehavioral rehabilitation focuses on substitution, or the use of other behavioral strategies or devices to "work around" the problem or serve as an external prosthetic device to help take the place of the lost function. Automated reminder systems and the use of computers to produce speech are two good examples of prosthetic aids.

The major neurobiological theories of recovery and rehabilitation parallel the possible functional outcomes just outlined (Diller, 1987; Poppel & von Steinbuchel, 1992). These include (1) restitution of damaged neurons, (2) and substitution for lost neurons. These mechanisms do not operate in a mutually exclusive manner, but may explain the various ways the brain may adapt and attempt to recover function (restitution), and the mechanisms used to find alternate neuronal routes (substitution). It is important to note that neurologists typically use the terms *restitution* and *substitution* in a functional sense; for example, the function of expressive language may be restorable, or the function of expressive language may be lost and the patient must use an appropriate substitute for communication, such as writing. However, it is still speculative whether the underlying neurons and neuronal connections have somehow repaired themselves and restored the original connections, or if they have managed to reorganize to form new connections in the brain (neuronal substitution).

Both the consequences and the recovery process of brain injury are quite individual and depend on a number of factors. Biological factors such as maturity of the nervous system and its adaptability (plasticity), individual variation in brain anatomy, the location and extent of the damage, and physical health especially contribute to the brain's ability to restore itself. Psychosocial contributions to recovery and rehabilitation include motivation and the presence of external supports from family, professionals, and other prosthetic aids. These factors may affect recovery directly or may mediate actual brain changes.

The neuropsychologist should consider the following when considering influences on recovery:

1. Location and extent of damage
2. Duration of time since injury
3. Age (brain plasticity)
4. Premorbid intellectual level
5. Premorbid personality characteristics
6. Premorbid functional level
7. Medical health
8. Emotional health
9. Support system
10. Type of treatment

Restitution and substitution of brain function may be possible under several different scenarios. The neurobiological mechanisms of *diaschisis, redundancy of function,* and *brain reorganization* all appear to play important roles in recovery. These recovery mechanisms are not mutually exclusive, but may each contribute in various ways among different individuals. Various neural mechanisms seem to operate to restore lost functioning. Because restitution of function generally implies a partial deficiency (for example, if the function of expressive speech is not completely lost), inherent in this theory is the idea that an individual is left with some remaining functioning neurons, or partially working neurons for that function or that the brain is able to reorganize, restore, or replace that function. The process of recovery may in some cases appear spontaneous, and in others may benefit from training targeted for that function. Unfortunately, science has not yet been able to directly correlate recovery of behavioral function with concomitant recovery of neuronal functioning in humans. As discussed in Chapter 2, learning modifies neurons and neuronal connections. Therefore, scientists generally assume that any new learning corresponds to some change in neuronal structure.

DIASCHISIS

Diaschisis (first described by von Monakow, 1911) refers to an unmasking of function after temporary neuronal disruption. Monakow's theory of diaschisis (from Greek *schizein,* "to split") described the loss of function caused by cerebral lesions in areas that are remote from the lesion but that are neuronally connected to it. A depression in neuronal functioning can occur due to neuronal shock, intercranial pressure, edema, metabolic changes, or any condition that reduces blood flow. This transience of function inhibition implies that the neuronal systems have not been permanently damaged. Therefore diaschisis differs from restitution in that it is a passive process of uncovering working systems rather than an active process of repairing damaged systems. As the condition causing the dysfunction is removed, the behavioral function reemerges.

Researchers have proposed that diaschisis represents an imbalance between excitatory and inhibitory mechanisms (Poppel & Von Steinbuchel, 1992). An interesting demonstration in animals (Poppel & Richards, 1974) provides an example. If the right occipital lobe is damaged, blindness in the left visual field results; however, if the left superior colliculus is destroyed, sight is restored. How is this so? Apparently, the colliculi of each hemisphere serve to inhibit each other while each occipital lobe excites its ipsilateral colliculus. So in the normal brain, all is balanced. However, when the right occipital lobe is damaged, the right superior colliculus, which no longer is receiving input from its occipital lobe, cannot moderate the left superior colliculus. In fact, the right becomes overinhibited by the relative overactivity of the left. If the inhibitory input of the left is removed, the right becomes functional again and some sight is restored. This complicated interplay between excitatory and inhibitory functions repeats itself over and over again with different functional systems of the brain. According to the theory of diaschisis, this imbalance between excitation and inhibition resolves spontaneously. Other clues to diaschisis and recovery are discussed in Neuropsychology in Action 16.1.

BRAIN REORGANIZATION

Reorganization of brain function after injury has much to do with the brain's plasticity. **Plasticity,** the behavioral or neural ability to reorganize after brain injury, appears to be one of the more important factors contributing to the speed and level of final recovery. Most research on plasticity has tested animals, leaving the relation between neuronal reorganization and behavioral organization unclear in humans. Immature nervous systems are much more plastic than those of adults; children show less behavioral effect and recover faster from brain injury. Some have suggested that recovery from aphasia in prepubescent children may be caused by the adaptability of the short-axon Golgi type II cells (Hirsch & Jacobson, 1974; Kertesz, 1985). Whereas the long axon neurons of the brain seem preprogrammed genetically for cer-

tain functions, the more flexible Golgi type II cells appear to maintain flexibility until the onset of hormonal changes associated with puberty.

Axonal and Collateral Sprouting

One way in which the brain reorganizes is through the regrowth of neurons that have been only partially damaged. As mentioned earlier in Chapter 2, unlike axons in the peripheral nervous system, those in the CNS are not known to regenerate after total severing. However, axons that have been sheared may resprout, and collateral sprouting can occur from nearby intact neurons. Younger organisms seem to have the highest potential for axonal regrowth. Theoretically, sprouting could replace the lost function. Although researchers have documented that axonal and collateral sprouting does occur, they do not yet know if the "reconnections" rebuild the previous function. Excessive sprouting may even hinder behavioral functioning.

Denervation Supersensitivity

If an area of the brain is lesioned, any remaining neurons in that area may become hypersensitive to the neurotransmitters that act on them. The mechanism appears to act via a proliferation of postsynaptic receptor sites. This may result in a greater excitatory or inhibitory potential, depending on the type of neuron.

REDUNDANCY OF FUNCTION

Theoretically, the brain operates with a surplus of synapses within many neuronal systems such as attention, speech, or visual-spatial processing (for example, see Poppel & von Steinbuchel, 1992). During brain development, more synapses are produced than needed. The process of learning pares these synapses down; however, the potential for redundancy within neuronal systems remains active throughout life. After an injury, damaging one aspect of the system may activate previously nonfunctional system components. Generally, the "nonactivated" neurons are in close geographic proximity to the damaged neurons of the system. They then take over to substitute for the damaged neurons. However, if damage is too widespread, functional redundancy may not be

Neuropsychology in Action 16.1

Speed of Finger Tapping, Recovery, and Rehabilitation Outcome After Stroke

by George P. Prigatano Ph.D., Chair, Section of Neuropsychology, Barrow Neurological Institute, Phoenix, Arizona.

Sometimes the simplest observations provide the best clues for understanding complicated phenomena. Why, for example, do higher cerebral functions recover only partially after a severe and abrupt injury to the brain (such as a cerebrovascular accident, or CVA, or traumatic brain injury)? Von Monakow (1911) proposed a theory of diaschisis to help explain this observation. In its simplest form, the concept asserts that regions far removed from the lesion site may become temporarily dysfunctional. This "temporary inhibition" slowly resolves with time. Consequently, some behaviors (and cognitions) become "functional" again, creating the impression of recovery.

Positron emission tomography (PET) permits researchers to study the brain's use of oxygen and glucose during various stages of recovery. This technique can be used to test Von Monakow's theory.

Perani and coworkers (Perani, Vallar, Paulesu, Alberoni, & Fazio, 1993) noted that two patients who had suffered a right hemisphere stroke showed signs of hemineglect. One recovered; one did not. What was the difference? Both patients initially showed bilateral hypo-metabolic activity (decreased glucose use) after what appeared to be a unilateral lesion in the right cerebral hemisphere. The patient who showed recovery eventually demonstrated almost normal metabolism in the left hemisphere. The patient who did not recover from unilateral neglect continued to show bilateral hypometabolism (for no apparent reason). This observation suggests that if "temporary inhibition" resolves, certain higher cerebral functions may, in fact, recover.

Behavioral and neuropsychological studies also provide simple and useful information regarding recovery and

rehabilitation after stroke. Testing neuropsychological functions early after CVAs can be useful (Therapeutics and Technology Assessment Subcommittee of the American Academy of Neurology, 1996), despite beliefs to the contrary. For example, we studied speed of finger tapping and grip strength after unilateral CVA (Prigatano & Wong, 1997). Immediately after the stroke, CVA patients demonstrated the expected decrease in speed of finger tapping and grip strength in the hand contralateral to the cerebral hemisphere with the lesion. Interestingly, the hand ipsilateral to the lesion was also affected negatively but not to the same degree. After a mean of 30 days of inpatient rehabilitation, grip strength and speed of finger tapping tended to improve in both hands. Surprisingly, patients whose speed of finger tapping improved substantially in the so-called unaffected hand (the hand ipsilateral

possible. Whether new synaptic connections may be activated "spontaneously," or are aided by training and learning techniques focused at the particular system, is as yet unknown.

In addition to unilateral systems, it is also theoretically possible that a function, such as speech, has bilateral cortical representation, or the potential for such. After injury to one area, the homologous (corresponding) area in the opposite hemisphere may step in to take over. Because of the greater plasticity of children's brains, traumatic lesions to the speech areas suffered before age 5 may shift the affected speech function to the other hemisphere (Woods, 1980; Woods & Teuber, 1973). For example, if the left an-

terior speech area responsible for expressive speech (frontal operculum) were damaged, then expressive speech representation would shift to the frontal operculum of the right hemisphere. Even in adults who have suffered strokes to the left hemisphere speech areas, the right hemisphere is sometimes capable of taking over speech functions. In some patients who have recovered from left hemisphere strokes, later suppression of the right hemisphere (through Wada test sodium amytal injection) again produced aphasia (Kinsbourne, 1971). Although this shows an ability for speech to develop in two corresponding areas of different hemispheres, it may also be that some people have previously developed bilateral represen-

to the lesion) achieved rehabilitation goals at a higher frequency than those who did not. Typically, by the end of the rehabilitation these patients were within 1.5 standard deviations of the normal range of speed of finger tapping. Grip strength did not relate to rehabilitation outcome (goal attainment). As Figure 16.1 illustrates, more than 70% of patients whose speed of finger tapping with the "unaffected hand" (shown in light gray) was within this range achieved their rehabilitation goals. Speed of finger tapping in the affected hand (depicted in dark gray) was unrelated to goal attainment.

Why? PET studies suggest that the ability to move and coordinate finger movements rapidly actually involves many regions of the human brain, including the contralateral sensorimotor cortex, the ipsilateral sensorimotor cortex, the supplementary motor cortex, and the ipsilateral cerebellar hemisphere (Roland, 1993). Thus, the ability to tap one's fingers rapidly after a stroke is most likely adversely affected because both cerebral hemispheres are rendered dysfunctional, even after an acute unilateral lesion. With time, the so-called unaf-

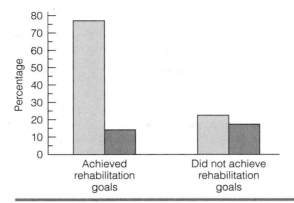

Figure 16.1 Improvement in finger-tapping speed after CVA. Patients whose speed of finger tapping with the "unaffected hand" (shown in light gray) was within a normal range achieved their rehabilitation goals. Speed of finger tapping in the affected hand (shown in dark gray) was unrelated to goal attainment.

fected hemisphere begins to regain functional capacity, and this recovery may be reflected by an increase in the speed of finger tapping in the hand ipsilateral to the lesion. Therefore, it may prove useful for neuropsychologists to find ways of improving motor functioning in the hand ipsilateral to a lesion as a method of facilitating rehabilitation outcomes in patients after acute CVA.

Clinical neuropsychologists can thus use neuropsychological tests not only to predict outcomes of rehabilitation but perhaps also to unlock some of the mysteries surrounding the recovery of function after a brain injury.

tation of speech and so are less affected by unilateral strokes.

What is the potential for the human brain to recover or adapt after brain injury? First, insult to the brain can result in different effects depending on the site and mechanism of damage. What is remarkable, however, is the brain's amazing ability to try to adapt to damage. If damage does not totally destroy neurons, the brain attempts to restore functioning. If the injury was caused by shock or some other temporary mechanism, diaschisis may serve to "unmask" functioning neuronal systems. When neurons are damaged through processes such as tearing and shearing, they may reorganize through axonal resprouting, col-

lateral sprouting, or developing supersensitivities to neurotransmitters. When neuronal damage is complete, depending to a large degree on plasticity, the brain may sometimes be able to substitute other functioning neurons or neuronal systems or rely on some redundancy to take over.

Overview of the Rehabilitation Process

Rehabilitation seeks to retrain and reeducate people with disabling injuries, to improve level of daily functioning. The philosophy of a rehabilitation center is very different from that of an acute care hospital. In the early stages after an injury or trauma, the hospital's goal is to medically stabilize the patient. The hospital provides care for the patient, and does not require the patient to be active in treatment. Rehab centers expect the patient and family to take a more active role in retraining, and to become partners in treatment planning. Rehab settings also use rehab teams of specialists who work together in setting goals and implementing treatment. In this section, we consider the various specialties in more depth. Traditionally, rehab treatment was set up over a period of weeks to months on an inpatient unit, then followed periodically on an outpatient unit. With the advent of managed care, inpatient rehabilitation has shortened, outpatient rehab has lengthened, and the role of the neuropsychologist has evolved to meet new demands for services. The final goal of rehabilitation is to reintegrate people back into the community at the highest level of functioning possible.

Rehabilitation psychology, like neuropsychology, is a distinct specialty area within psychology. Practicing rehabilitation psychologists may treat people who have suffered nonneurologic problems such as burns, chronic pain, amputation, or blindness as well as neurologic brain and spinal cord injuries and trauma. The focus is on applying psychological principles to recovery and adjustment to disability. More specifically for the psychologist working with brain disorders, neuropsychological rehabilitation—or brain injury rehabilitation, as it is more commonly known—represents the intersection of neuropsychology and rehabilitation. As such, the focus is on the process of recovery, adjustment, and rehabilitation of brain disorders. The conditions most often seen on brain injury units of rehab hospitals include traumatic brain injury (TBI) caused by head injuries from accidents and falls, and cerebral vascular accidents (CVAs). Less often rehab units see patients recovering from brain tumor or brain disease. With the increasing survival rate of heart attack victims, rehab centers are experiencing a greater influx of anoxic/hypoxic injuries resulting from loss of oxygen to the brain before resuscitation.

Rehabilitation hospitals are specialty hospitals, which admit patients who fit a restricted group of di-

agnoses, such as traumatic brain injury (TBI). Length of inpatient stay varies but has shortened dramatically since the advent of managed care. For example, during the late 1990s the typical length of stay for a TBI survivor declined from an average of 60 days to an average of 25 days (Hart, 1999). As inpatient stays shortened, the focus of treatment evolved to include a greater emphasis on outpatient treatment within a person's home, social, and occupational settings.

There are about 1600 TBI treatment programs in the United States (National Directory of Head Injury Services, 1992). A large proportion of neuropsychologists work in rehab settings where they apply knowledge of brain–behavior relationships and neuropsychological evaluation to the process of recovery and community reintegration. A challenge for neuropsychogists working in these settings is to translate level of functioning to appropriate treatments for problems of daily life. In comparison to the focus of the previous two chapters, which emphasize assessment, rehab neuropsychologists spend the majority of their time treating the patient and family. Those involved in research constantly wrestle with the issue of ecological validity—that is, with developing means of evaluation and treatment specific to common issues of rehabilitation such as driving, cooking, and return to work. Neuropsychologists may also collaborate in research projects aimed at studying the outcomes of rehabilitation programs and developing new standards of care (see Neuropsychology in Action 16.2).

ADMISSION TO REHABILITATION PROGRAMS

Although most neuropsychologists in rehabilitation work in specialty rehabilitation hospitals or treatment programs focus primarily on treatment, others work in large acute care hospitals that have rehabilitation units and focus on early evaluation before transfer to a specialized facility. Brain injury specialists working in acute care hospitals get the earliest view of a person's functioning, perhaps while emerging from coma or recovering from brain surgery. They conduct the first evaluations of alertness, attention, sensorimotor, and cognitive skills over the course of the first few days and weeks of recovery before being transferred to a longer-term rehabilitation hospital. The Glasgow Coma Scale, discussed in Chapter 10, is a good example of a measure used early in the process of recovery from head injury. Also, acute care rehabilitation neuropsychologists conduct pre- and post-surgery assessments to document the level of change in cognitive functioning. These first neuropsychological evaluations can serve as a valuable baseline and predictor of future level of recovery. Therefore, neuropsychological evaluation becomes a valuable part of the prescreening process. Neuropsychologists design the prescreening process for entry into a rehabilitation program to select patients whom they consider to have potential for treatment success and enough social support for postrehab care. In fact, admission to a rehabilitation program in itself suggests the absence of a medical life-threatening crisis and the potential for further recovery.

The rehabilitation hospital is the primary setting for learning the skills to return to a home setting. If rehab facilities did not exist, a large proportion of brain-damaged patients would go directly from the acute care hospital to a skilled nursing facility. This is because most patients admitted to rehabilitation hospitals cannot care for themselves and may still be in a state of significant cognitive confusion, and their families do not yet understand the condition and the care-taking responsibilities. The rehab hospital is an opportunity to take advantage of the skills of others and to practice practical skills with professional supervision. Therefore, it is quite normal for patients to spend some time getting used to the functioning and philosophy of a rehabilitation unit. The "team" approach is also a new concept for most people accustomed to acute care hospitals.

As patients move from the acute care hospital to a rehab program, they must make the transition from the hospital environment to the rehab environment. Rehabilitation patients need time to orient to the philosophy of empowerment that rehab programs advocate. The team teaches the means to maximize independence both for survivor and family caretaker. The goal for a patient is not to live in the rehabilitation hospital, but to get back to community life. Thus, patients in a rehabilitation hospital are not relegated

to the traditional "sick" role, or to a self-perception that earlier experiences on other acute care medical units may have been shaped.

There is much for a newly admitted patient to adapt to in the rehab environment, such as structured rehabilitation programs and new expectations. In addition, the sheer variety of patients of different ages recovering from myriad disorders can be overwhelming. Depending on the size of the facility and the extent of services, there are often separate units for orthopedic and brain injury patients, although sometimes the patients are mixed together. Where brain injury is involved, there are usually a preponderance of young men in their teens and 20s recovering from head injuries, gunshot wounds, or spinal cord injury. Elderly heart attack and stroke victims are also present, as well as tumor surgery patients. The brain injury patients can be expected to have significant cognitive compromise, often still involving, confusion, and posttraumatic amnesia as they arrive at a rehab facility.

THE REHABILITATION TEAM: GOAL SETTING, TREATMENT, AND EVALUATION

Once a patient is accepted for admission, the typical protocol assigns him or her to a rehabilitation team. Teams usually consist of specialists in rehabilitation nursing, social services, psychology/neuropsychology, **physiatry, speech therapy, occupational therapy, physical therapy,** and **therapeutic recreation.** Treatment teams are often directed by the physiatrist, but may also be directed by psychologists or speech therapists. A "physiatrist" is a physician who specializes in physical medicine and rehabilitation. Other related specialists may also become involved, including specialists in audiology, nutrition, orthotics, optometrics, and dentistry. A variety of medical specialists are also available to patients, such as internists, urologists, cardiologists, ophthalmologists, and pediatricians. These teams generally follow a multidisciplinary or transdisciplinary approach in which each discipline works together in a coordinated fashion to achieve specific treatment goals. More and more patients and their families are becoming integral members of their

Neuropsychology in Action 16.2

The Traumatic Brain Injury Model Systems Project

by **Tessa Hart** Ph.D., Clinical Neuropsychologist, Drucker Brain Injury Center, MossRehab; Institute Scientist, Moss Rehabilitation Research Institute.

The Traumatic Brain Injury (TBI) Model Systems of Care is a longitudinal multi-center study funded by the National Institute on Disability and Rehabilitation Research (NIDRR). Currently, 17 rehabilitation centers nationwide are contributing to a standard database and collaborating on a variety of research and demonstration projects intended to reinforce standards of care and develop more effective treatments for the unique needs of this disability group.

MossRehab in Philadelphia received a five-year TBI Model Systems award in 1997. Rehabilitating people with TBI has been a special focus at MossRehab since 1976, when a dedicated unit was founded. The establishment of the Moss Rehabilitation Research Institute (MRRI) in 1992 allowed formal integration of practice and science, in support of the TBI Model Systems and many other research projects designed for clinical impact.

One of the major activities of Moss-Rehab and the other TBI Model Systems is the contribution of longitudinal data to a comprehensive national database, initiated in 1987. Each Model System collects the same set of several hundred variables—encompassing medical, social,

and neuropsychological data—on every participant. Data collection begins in the emergency room, where personnel record information on the cause and severity of the injury, blood alcohol levels, and associated variables. The acute care hospital focuses on variables such as duration of loss of consciousness (coma), findings on the CT scan, and medical complications. In the rehabilitation hospital, where patients begin to relearn productive activities with the help of a team of therapists, the emphasis shifts to the patient's cognitive and functional status. Therapists give a battery of neuropsychological tests when the patient is able, and interview the family for social information. The rehabilitation team provides data on the patient's evolving level of independence and residual disabilities. In annual followup visits with participants and their caregivers or family members, therapists repeat the test battery and administer new measures to assess community reintegration, need for supervision at home, and incidence of neurobehavioral problems. As of mid-1999 the national database contained information from more than 1100 subjects, some of whom had been followed

for nine years after injury. More information and journal references based on this data set can be found at the TBI Model Systems web site (http://www.tbims.org).

In addition to collecting the standard data set, each Model System engages in its own program of research. Some of the studies funded under the Moss-Rehab TBI Model System award include the following.

Computer Technology in Rehabilitation

Survivors of severe TBI can be left with chronic psychosocial problems such as social isolation and inability to return to productive employment. Two studies are evaluating whether computer technology can help to alleviate these problems. In one project, people with TBI who have "practice" jobs are trained to use electronic personal organizers or palmtop computers to better plan and remember their new job responsibilities. In the other project, people with TBI are learning to explore Internet resources such as chat rooms, educational sites, and recreation listings. Program developers hope that the ability to access these resources, and to teach others how to do so, will help

own treatment teams. This approach includes them in all areas of treatment planning and evaluation of progress.

Initial treatment planning routinely puts patients on a schedule of daily "therapies"; for example, one hour each of physical therapy, occupational therapy, and speech therapy. As noted earlier, patients who cannot endure this daily training are generally not considered ready for comprehensive rehabilitation and may be sent to a continuing care center until they are more able. Beyond the minimum rehabilitation requirement, many rehab hospitals provide additional rehabilitation hours, which consist of whatever the patient most needs. Next we explore the individual

reduce social isolation and enhance quality of life.

Racial/Ethnic Bias in Outcome Measures

Previous Model System research has suggested that the outcome of TBI tends to be less favorable for members of minority groups than for Caucasians with equally severe injuries. The Moss Model System is exploring the possibility that minority outcomes appear to be worse partly because of bias in measuring "outcomes." For example, one measure of community reintegration asks how often people engage in activities such as going out to eat and attending sports events. If different racial or ethnic groups have unequal opportunities to engage in these activities, or place unequal value on doing them at all, this measure could provide a biased view of differential outcomes. This study will evaluate whether such measurement bias exists in Model Systems measures.

The Effects of Violence-Related Injury

Studies of people with other disabilities (such as spinal cord injuries) suggest that those who blame themselves for the injury, versus other people or random chance, actually cope better with the aftermath. Many people with TBI are injured by other people—for example, by a gunshot wound to the head or assault with a blunt object. The Moss Model System is studying the relationship be-

tween blame and coping in patients whose TBI was caused by another person, compared to those injured by random chance or by reckless behavior such as drunk driving.

Costs of Rehabilitation and Effects of Service Restrictions

Three projects of the Moss Model System relate to a special NIDRR priority, the study of the cost effectiveness of rehabilitation. One project evaluates the cost effectiveness of a long-term followup process for people with TBI who have received supported employment services (job coaching), and who may need "booster" sessions to prevent costly job loss. The second project analyzes hospital bills to determine the relative costs of medical treatments versus therapeutic interventions. The goal is to try to uncover patterns that will help hospitals keep their costs at a manageable level. The third project uses in-depth interviews of people with TBI and members of their families to determine the impact of rehabilitation service "denials" by insurance companies.

Collaborative Research

With 17 centers now involved nationwide, the Model System of Care provides an ideal setup for collaborative research. Three multicenter projects involving Moss are underway. First, Moss is collaborating with the Model System of Mississippi on the largest and most comprehensive study to date of impaired self-awareness

after TBI. Five centers, including Moss, are participating in a study comparing the effectiveness of two neurotransmitter-enhancing medications for treating posttraumatic agitation. Finally, Moss is leading a multicenter effort to validate a clinical rating scale for measuring impairments of attention after TBI.

Consumer Involvement

The Moss TBI Model System actively seeks the involvement of people with TBI and their families. For example, such people serve on three advisory boards working on program improvements at all levels of care. Consumers were also involved in both the planning and implementation phases of a special Model System project, a day-long conference called "Living with Brain Injury: Resources and Solutions." This event featured information booths, discussion groups, and workshops on such topics as coping with relationships and role changes, managing managed care, getting back to work and school, and staying fit and healthy.

In summary, the Model System project seeks not only to study the process of recovery after severe TBI, but also to find new ways of enhancing it. By establishing a national database, creating innovative treatments, giving special attention to cost–benefit analyses, and encouraging the involvement of rehabilitation consumers, NIDRR and the participating centers have made a promising start toward these ambitious goals.

---

contributions of neuropsychology, physical therapy, occupational therapy, speech therapy, and recreational therapy in greater detail. Although we discuss these as separate disciplines, as a treatment team works together over a period of time a degree of "cross-training" often occurs. In some rehab hospitals the lines between disciplines become totally blurred as each person is

referred to as a "brain injury therapist," although their individual contributions may be somewhat different.

Neuropsychology

Neuropsychologists are active in the rehabilitation process from admission to discharge. As mentioned previously, neuropsychologists on rehab units of acute care or comprehensive hospitals may provide baseline evaluations that help determine an individual's capability to participate in a rehab program. On a patient's admission to a rehab unit, a neuropsychologist may conduct a formal evaluation. He or she may also evaluate functional neuropsychological skills such as meal planning and preparation, ability to plan and self-administer medication, driving, or work-related tasks. The recommendations generated specifically aim at helping the treatment team form workable goals and objectives given an individual's pattern of cognitive and emotional strengths and weaknesses. These evaluations necessarily focus on the functional level of the individual and serve as a baseline to document impairment. Notice that the focus of this evaluation is not only on the pattern of deficits exhibited but on the strengths that may aid the person in compensating for losses in other areas. During treatment planning, it is the neuropsychologist's role to discuss specific recommendations with the team regarding potential remediation strategies. For example, would memory log training be likely to be successful? How will the person's level of frustration tolerance impact his or her ability to participate in various therapies? How feasible is this training, given the cognitive demands of the patient's home environment?

During the treatment process, the neuropsychologist continues to assess progress toward goals of daily living in conjunction with other team members. Neuropsychologists take part in individual patient counseling surrounding issues of loss and cognitive readjustment. Family education and counseling regarding the effects of brain damage on behavior, and strategies to cope with cognitive and behavioral deficits is also quite important to support the patient in return to the community. Finally, the neuropsychologist often coordinates compensatory strategies across settings from rehab, home, community, work, and school (see Figure 16.2). We discuss the neuropsychologist's assessment and rehabilitation methods in greater depth later in this chapter.

Physical Therapy

Physical therapists (PTs) focus on motor control with the aim of improving physical functioning to the highest degree possible. PTs evaluate each patient on ad-

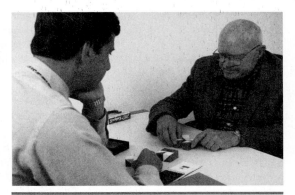

Figure 16.2   The neuropsychologist in the rehab setting. Neuropsychological assessment in the rehab setting uses in-depth analysis of qualitative performance. (Dan McCoy/ PictureQuest)

mission to assess performance of functional activities related to strength, balance, coordination, physical endurance, and range of motion. The evaluation also considers the neurologic status of the motor systems. For example, PTs evaluate activities such as rolling, standing, sitting, transferring, using a wheelchair, and walking. PTs develop and individualize treatment programs for each patient according to specific strengths and weaknesses. For example, treatment programs for those with motor disability, weakness, or paralysis may consist of the following: mat activities, developmental sequences, balance training, hydro/pool therapy, strengthening exercises, transfer and wheelchair training, walking, and use of adaptive equipment. PTs accomplish goals by teaching such activities as wheelchair management and wheelchair propulsion. They instruct patients how to transfer from their wheelchairs, bed, toilet, and car. To walk again may be a major goal. Physical therapists determine when a patient has sufficient strength, muscle control, and balance to attempt walking and to assess the need for assistive devices such as walkers, canes, crutches, braces, or splints.

Occupational Therapy

The term *occupational therapy* (OT) is confusing to some people who think that the training is specific to individuals who have an "occupation" and want to go back to work. This is not the only goal of OT. OT is concerned with self-care activities such as grooming, bathing, dressing, and feeding, commonly called "activities of daily living," or ADLs. Occupational therapists also focus on work activities ranging from home management, meal preparation, money management, household chores, and activities involved with "occupations" as well as "avocations"—hobbies.

The OT evaluates and treats the performance components that are necessary for functioning in ADLs, work, and leisure (see Figure 16.3). The performance components include many aspects of human functioning. Of great importance to the OT is an assessment of sensory and perceptual-motor functioning. The use of muscles to bend, move, and perform purposive action (praxis) lies within the domain of occupational therapy. Finally, issues of thinking, remembering, and problem solving for daily life hold special importance for the OT.

There are several ways to distinguish the difference in specialization between PT and OT. Both are concerned with muscle strength and coordination. However, in many hospitals PTs work primarily on the lower extremities (all muscles below the waist), and OTs work primarily on the upper extremities (everything above the waist). In those hospitals that do not distinguish between upper- and lower-extremity strength, the difference between PT and OT is usually broadly defined in terms of strength (PT) and function (OT). In regard to the latter definition, for example, a stroke survivor may be able to walk with strength and endurance. That same patient, however, may not be able to judge distances, determine left from right, or near from far. As a consequence, walking per se adds little to the patient's independence, because walking is not safe. The OT takes on the job of applying strength gained from PT to using that strength within everyday types of activities. For example, an OT therapy session may focus on teaching the patient to discriminate between things that are close and things that are far away (as in depth perception training) or things seen to the right versus things seen to the left (as in left neglect training). This therapy is referred to as *perceptual retraining,* or *perceptual remediation.*

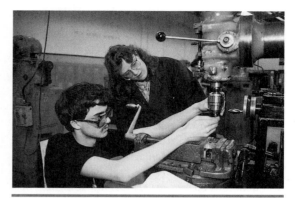

Figure 16.3 Occupational therapy. The occupational therapist assists patients with skills necessary to return to work. (Dennis McDonald/PhotoEdit)

Another area of OT concern among brain injury survivors is apraxia. Stroke victims often show this lack of purposive action. In practical terms, the OT will refer to, for instance, "dressing apraxia," indicating that the patient cannot dress on command, or "on purpose." This form differs somewhat from stroke patients who fail to dress one side of their bodies because of neglect. If you say to a stroke victim, "Let's go outside," she may automatically put on the sweater that is nearby. However, if you say, "Put on your sweater so we can go outside," she may either simply go outside without regard for the sweater or may sit there and fumble with the sweater because she can no longer put it on. OTs try to use activities to meet goals, so in this case the actions chosen will have the purpose or function of overcoming dressing apraxia.

Speech Therapy

Speech therapists provide therapy for patients experiencing a range of communication difficulties. These may include mechanical speech difficulties involving speech production, expressive language, hearing and understanding speech, reading, writing, and the social use of language. Speech therapists specifically trace communication problems from the basic level of auditory acuity and speech production to higher-level skills of communication and linguistic integration.

The ultimate goal is to design interventions to aid in speech production and understanding and to facilitate communication. This may be accomplished through practice and retraining or with prosthetics aimed at assisting communication through artificial means.

The speech problems most commonly treated deal with articulatory difficulties, or **dysarthrias,** caused by improper muscle control of tongue, lips, or cheeks for pronouncing words. If either the left hemisphere or right hemisphere is damaged, people with damage to the section of the motor strip controlling speech production will have contralateral impairment. Thus, one-half of the lips, cheeks, and tongue muscles used to articulate words may be weakened. Although it is not caused by a similar mechanism, if you have ever experienced slurred speech after a visit to a dentist who used Novocain, you will readily sympathize with the problems stroke survivors face in articulating speech. In the extreme case, such speech may sound garbled or unintelligible.

Neuropsychologists often design higher-order language and communicative evaluations to assess the presence and degree of aphasia, alexia, or agraphia. Speech therapists may specialize in evaluations to categorize aphasias (such as expressive, receptive, transcortical, and global), and to understand the nature of reading and writing difficulties such as alexia and agraphia (see Figure 16.4). At this level the interest is in cognitive-linguistic integration.

Therapeutic Recreation

Therapeutic recreation emphasizes the importance of recreational and leisure time activities. These activities serve a purpose beyond being just fun. For instance, patients are encouraged to use skills learned in PT or OT in completing craft projects. This helps in the "transfer" of learning. Therapeutic recreation also allows patients to begin socializing with each other in a structured, but less formal atmosphere than that afforded in other therapy settings.

At some facilities, the therapeutic recreational specialist takes patients on community outings. Community outings allow patients to practice their skills in real-life settings, among nonhospital people. This can help patients on the first important step in their transition from the hospital setting back to their home,

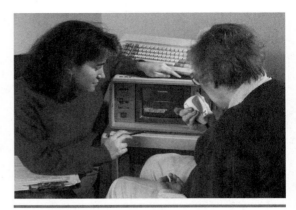

Figure 16.4   Speech therapy. A speech therapist assists a stroke patients in treatment for aphasia. (Frank Siteman/ PictureQuest)

friends, and family. The skills addressed in community outings may include

1. *Mobility:* Ramps, elevators, curbs, doorways, obstacles, transfers, and so on
2. *Daily living skills:* Money management, safety awareness, personal energy pacing, nutritional awareness, and problem solving

EVALUATION OF GOALS AND DISCHARGE PLANNING

The rehabilitation team begins planning discharge from the hospital and outpatient rehab from day 1. This idea sometimes confuses patients and families, who believe they cannot make discharge plans until they absolutely know the final functioning level of the brain injury survivor. It is often difficult to realize that no one can guarantee the exact level of functioning a person will attain by the end of a rehab program. However, rehab teams are in the business of estimating reasonable goals and can give a solid ballpark estimate of function level. Once this expected level of functioning is determined, then everyone can make appropriate plans for what will happen after the hospital stay.

Many brain injury survivors living at home before the injury choose to consider returning home after rehabilitation. As they contemplate this option, everyone must consider the feasibility of living at home safely and happily. The treatment team, patient, and family must consider the functional requirements of a person's current living situation and his or her resources to cope with that environment.

Increasingly, rehabilitation programs are incorporating shorter inpatient stays and longer outpatient treatment into their programs. Some impetus for this, of course, is due to the financial pressures of managed care. However, there is also a move to integrate people into the community as soon as possible. We return to a discussion of community integration programs, with the example of job coaching, later in this chapter. Next we turn to an in-depth look at the methods that neuropsychologists employ in rehabilitation settings.

In sum, the philosophy of treatment in a rehabilitation hospital requires that patients and families be active in rehabilitation. They are "trained" by multidisciplinary teams, which typically consist of specialists in areas of neuropsychology as well as physical therapy, occupational therapy, speech therapy, and therapeutic recreation. Each area contributes a unique expertise related to brain–behavior functioning. PTs focus on the motor system, OTs are concerned with applying motor functioning to daily life tasks and with other functional tasks of daily living, speech therapists evaluate and facilitate improvement in all aspects of communication, and therapeutic recreation specialists focus on leisure activities and on practicing skills in the community. Neuropsychologists provide initial and ongoing evaluation as well as treatment for cognition, mood, and behavior disorders. The training done by each team member necessarily focuses on parallel tracks: The first is to work directly with the patient to try to restore function or compensate for lost function, the second is to work with caregivers and family to ensure that treatment will continue after rehab ends. During outpatient treatment, where community reentry is the focus, the focus of the team turns to providing bridges to employment or other vocational endeavors. The next sections take an in-depth look at the role of neuropsychologists in rehabilitation settings: first the role in assessment, then the role in treatment.

Neuropsychological Assessment for Rehabilitation

In Chapter 14 we stressed that assessments are most useful when targeted to a specific purpose. In rehabilitation and intervention settings, the purpose is treatment. Neuropsychologists design evaluations to aid the team in treatment planning, goal setting, and treatment progress. The focus is more on strengths and the possibilities for adaptation than on a diagnosis. Assessments can also help predict success or failure in treatment. So the purpose is somewhat different, and so are the methods. In addition to traditional psychometric testing methods, neuropsychologists in rehabilitation settings often employ more functional methods that seek to link assessment to the daily needs of the patient. For example, a person's cognitive strengths and weaknesses can be directly assessed while he or she is attempting to prepare a meal, balance a checkbook, or assemble a piece of furniture from a diagram. Finally, in the rehab setting neuropsychologists also use behavioral methods to obtain baselines and chart progress as treatment progresses.

TREATMENT PLANNING

Successful treatment rests on appropriate evaluation. Assessments need to answer questions related to the possibilities of success in treatment and in returning to the "real world." What is the pattern of strengths and weaknesses according to the functional areas of verbal processing, visual-spatial processing, and so forth? Will the person be able to absorb the purpose of therapy and remember instructions? Does the patient appreciate the need for therapy? When deficits appear, what exactly is the nature of the problem? For example, in language are there more expressive difficulties, or receptive difficulties? How severe is the problem? Are there residual abilities that indicate the deficit can be strengthened through practice? Are there other areas of strength that can be trained to compensate or substitute for the problem? What is the likelihood that this person will be able to return home, return to work, return to independent functioning? These questions, in addition to describing patterns

Neuropsychology in Action 16.3

Neuropsychological Assessment for Treatment Planning: The Case of Jim

Jim, a 26-year-old man who had sustained a severe head injury in a motorcycle accident some 5 months earlier and who had been in a coma for 3 weeks, had been admitted to the rehabilitation center 4 weeks before he was referred for psychological treatment. He was referred by the occupational therapy department because of (a) poor concentration and (b) behavior problems. The notes from the referring hospital, where Jim had spent the 4 months since the accident, did not mention behavior problems. The physiotherapy department at the rehabilitation center reported that Jim was unsteady on his feet and had ataxia but was able to cooperate well in his physical therapy sessions, giving no cause for concern. The speech therapist reported that Jim had severe reading difficulties but that his other language skills were unimpaired.

The occupational therapist treating Jim presented a different picture, however. She reported that he was unable to concentrate and behaved disruptively. She explained that Jim could not work at the tasks set in occupational therapy but kept getting out of his seat and wandering around; he swore, shouted, and occasionally threw things to the floor. I arranged to see Jim for a neuropsychological assessment and also arranged to observe Jim in occupational and physical therapy before planning treatment.

Neuropsychological Assessment

The initial neuropsychological assessment took a total of 4½ hr over three occasions. Jim cooperated fairly well during these sessions, although he needed several short breaks. On the Wechsler Adult Intelligence Scale, Jim obtained a verbal IQ of 79, a performance IQ of 48, and a full scale IQ of 64. This large verbal performance discrepancy suggested greater damage to his right hemisphere than his left. He was also severely impaired on other tests of visuospatial functioning and on tests of visuoconstruction. For example, on a test in which he was asked to identify objects photographed from an unusual angle (Harrington, 1982), he scored only 6 out of 20, even though he identified 80% of the objects when they had been photographed from a conventional angle. This suggested the deficit was not due to poor eyesight or a naming disorder and that it was indicative of right parietal lobe damage.

Jim was also unable to copy or draw from memory any visual designs, although he could verbally describe the designs accurately, both when the designs were present and from memory. He was unable to write and could read only a few simple words. He could identify letters of the alphabet in upper and lower case when they were presented individually. A normal reader before

---

of neuropsychological functioning definitely require predictions. This forces the neuropsychologist to consider not only current level of functioning, but also the accumulated research and clinical knowledge regarding the probability and time course of recovery for the particular problem. Recovery depends on numerous factors: pattern of impairment, treatment program, degree of spontaneous recovery, physical and emotional state of the person, family support, and a number of other factors. Prediction becomes a quite challenging task.

The case of Jim presented in Neuropsychology in Action 16. 3 illustrates how neuropsychologists use both psychometric and behavioral assessment for treatment planning. This case was originally published by Barbara Wilson (1991), a rehabilitation neuropsychologist from England. The referral came to her because the occupational therapist noticed a problem. Although we present only the initial part of the original case presentation, Wilson also stresses ongoing evaluation to monitor progress toward goals and objectives.

ASSESSMENT OF EVERYDAY ACTIVITIES

Real-world tasks such as driving, cooking, balancing a checkbook, taking medication, or navigating an unfamiliar route require numerous cognitive compo-

the accident, Jim now appeared to have what Shallice and Warrington (1977) described as attentional dyslexia. In this condition, a patient can name individual letters when they are presented one at a time but typically makes errors when the letters are presented in strings.

Jim was oriented in time and place, his forward digit span was in the low to average range for his age, his immediate and delayed recall for the prose passages from the Wechsler Memory Scale (Wechsler, 1945) were within normal limits, and he was 100% correct on the easy pairs of the associate learning task form the Wechsler Memory Scale (though he managed to learn only one hard pair).

How did this information help us to understand Jim's problems as witnessed in occupational therapy, and how did we use the information to plan his future treatment? Jim's general intellectual functioning was impaired, and he had particular problems with visuospatial and visuoconstruction tasks. His reading and writing skills were compromised, yet his verbal memory skills were relatively unimpaired. One hypothesis was that the task set in occupational therapy had been too difficult for him and that this contributed to his behavior problems.

I decided to see Jim again to further investigate his attentional skills, but his relatively normal digit span and recall of prose passages suggested adequate attention for verbal material in the absence of competing demands.

When planning a treatment program for Jim, we needed to be aware of his limited intellect, his poor perceptual, visuospatial, and visuoconstruction skills, and his reading difficulties. (Because the reading difficulties might have been due to a perceptual difficulty, a more detailed investigation of them was planned.) Jim could learn new material when it was presented verbally, and he could remember verbal information.

Designing and Monitoring a Treatment Program

The behavioral assessment showed that on tasks on which Jim was expected to work alone, he typically spent no longer than 3 min working and often refused to start the task at all. Jim swore between 0 and 6 times a session and left his seat between 3 and 7 times a session, but he threw material to the floor only twice during the whole week. Interrater reliability ranged between 88% and 99% for behavior problems; ratings differed

by only a few seconds for time spent on tasks.

I met with the occupational therapist to draw up a treatment plan. This meeting was also attended by Jim's physical therapist, his social worker, one of the nurses from his ward, and one medical doctor. Although the occupational therapist had recognized the fact that Jim was intellectually impaired as a result of his head injury, she had not realized the full extent of his problems. Many of the tasks required of Jim in occupational therapy were beyond his abilities. His reading was almost nonexistent; he could not write, draw, or copy; and he could not fit paper into a typewriter or easily find the right key.

Treatment goals for Jim's concentration difficulties in occupational therapy were agreed on. Our long-term goal was to get Jim to work for 16 min before leaving his seat; our short-term objective was to ensure that Jim worked longer in each session than he had in the previous session. Our objectives for his disturbing behavior were to eliminate all swearing, throwing of materials and leaving of his seat during an activity.

Source: Barbara Wilson (1991), pp. 281–291. © by the APA. Reprinted by permission.

---

nents. Neuropsychological assessment often attempts to isolate the effects of functional areas such as divided attention, receptive language, or memory encoding. Although this is helpful in understanding the pattern of neuropsychological strengths and weaknesses, the "whole" of a process such as preparing a meal may be more than the sum of its generic cognitive "parts." Cooking certainly requires sustained attention, the ability to read and follow recipes, the ability to organize preparation of different dishes so they are finished at the same time, the necessity to monitor time so the cake won't burn, and of course basic visual-spatial abilities. A problem in any one of these areas may lead to a dining disaster. But does the

presence of basic skills ensure competence in cooking? A neuropsychological assessment that measures attention, reading, organization, and time monitoring may reveal deficits that pose problems for independent meal preparation. But if no problems are revealed, does this mean the person can prepare meals independently? Not necessarily. First of all, tests of general functional areas such as attention and memory may be too nonspecific to shed light on the exact neuropsychological requirements that make up successful meal preparation. Does a general test of organizational ability adequately predict organization of meals? This is a question of ecological validity. Second, even if we can identify the basic cognitive components involved, do the demands of combining and integrating these components into fluid action somehow change the nature of the task?

To deal with these issues, neuropsychologists who develop "ecologically valid" measures can take one of two approaches, and may take both. First, they may attempt a task analysis. This involves identifying all the relevant specific neuropsychological requirements of the task. Then they must devise tasks that measure components. The idea is that if any deficits appear there is a strong likelihood that the person cannot perform the task. The advantage of this method is that it may use paper-and-pencil measures and small, portable tasks to simulate the cognitive components. These tests can also be standardized using large populations. If the patient performs specific aspects of the test poorly, that pinpoints the deficits, which can be targeted for rehabilitation. The disadvantage is that this analytical approach may not totally capture the requirements of the whole task. The second method is to actually do the task or closely simulate it. Many rehabilitation hospitals use driving simulators to test driving skills. They may also build kitchens or apartments to directly test the functional skills of meal preparation or laundry, for example. If tasks can be recreated in a controlled environment, then the huge advantage is that they come closest to mimicking real life. Then performance on the task as an integrated whole can be assessed. Of course, the primary disadvantage is the initial expense of installing an entire working kitchen or a driving simulator. In addition, unless the key cognitive components of the task can be teased apart, doing poorly on a meal preparation task, for example, may not yield much information on how to intervene in training. Finally, because each kitchen is different, and the components of meal preparation may differ on any given day, success does not automatically translate into success at home.

Medication taking is an example of an everyday task that has implications for postrehab care. This task is usually more relevant for older patients, for whom it is not unusual to take four or more prescription medications per day. However, medication management is also relevant for younger neurologic patients, who may be on medications for seizure, cancer, or other medical conditions. An older stroke patient often must manage antihypertensive medications, some heart medications, and diuretics. A Parkinson's disease patient usually has three or more medications, which may have to be taken as frequently as every four hours around the clock. Independence in medication taking is often essential in the decision to allow a person to return to independent living. Therefore, appropriate assessment of medication self-management is crucial in determining if and where the patient has a problem in self-management.

In designing a test using the first method of assessment, the neuropsychologist must first lay out the specific cognitive components of medication taking. What skills does the patient need to remember to take a medication at the right time? To take the correct dosage, and follow any special instructions? What other skills does the patient need to coordinate multiple medications, some of which should be taken with food, some without? Most of us who have had to take any sort or medication over regular intervals, even just a short course of antibiotics, realize that one of the more difficult tasks is to remember to take the dosage at the correct time. This is a problem of **prospective memory,** or remembering to do something in the future. To be most effective, people generally have to set up reminder cues in advance, so that when they appear they are associated with remembering to take the medication. Most older medication takers use the strategy of trying to link pill taking to regular daily events such as meals and bedtime (Spiers & Kutzik, 1995). A test that attempts to measure the components of medication taking in daily life, the Cognitive Screening for Medication Self-Management (Spiers, 1995), is shown in Neuropsychology in Action 16.4.

The aims of psychometric testing and structured behavioral observations of daily activities are different but complementary. Whereas developers designed standardized psychometric testing to assess capacity, testing of everyday functional activities is at the level of the norm or what people would expect to be "usual" behavior. Of course, rehab teams can use these two methods in a complementary fashion. Treatment planning is likely to use standardized psychometric measurements as in the case of Jim (Neuropsychology

Neuropsychology in Action 16.4

Everyday Assessment of Medication Taking

by Mary Spiers

The Cognitive Screening for Medication Self-Management (CSMS) (Spiers, 1995) was specifically designed to test the cognitive components of successful medication taking in the elderly. We identified everyday tasks such as comprehension and memory for hypothetical prescription information, organization and planning of dosage and frequency, ability to remember a medication on cue (prospective memory), dosage calculations and basic sensory and motor tasks related to pill taking. This assessment takes approximately 30–45 minutes to administer (see Figure 16.5).

I designed this screening measure to pinpoint areas of difficulty in medication taking so that appropriate interventions can be used to target the problem areas. Together with a comprehensive medication review that evaluates the individual's knowledge of his or her medication regimen (correct dosage, timing, and purpose), the neuropsychologist can tailor interventions specifically to the individual.

The following are some representative tasks from the CSMS:

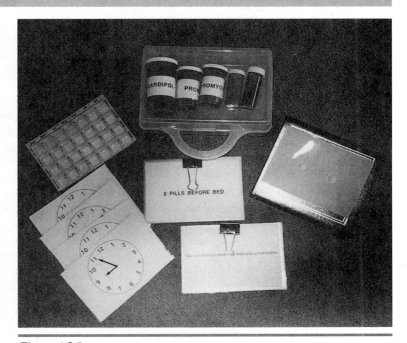

Figure 16.5 The Cognitive Screening for Medication Self-Management (CSMS). Tasks used to assess the components of medication taking. (Courtesy of Cate Price)

■ *Sensory*
  • Reading small-print prescription labels: "Take 2 tablets in the morning and 2 before bedtime"
  • Differentiating among differently colored pills (the aging cornea makes it more difficult to differentiate between yellow and white pills)

■ *Motor*
  • Opening pill bottles (child protected versus screw top or fliptop)

■ *General Cognitive*
  • Telling Time
  • Calculating dosages; for example, "If your doctor tells you to take 2 pills twice a day and 1 pill before bed, how many pills do you need for the day?"

■ *Memory*
  • Remembering prescription instructions
  • Prospective memory: Remembering to take out a pill on cue

■ *Strategy/Organization*
  • Organizing medications in a "pill organizer" for the week

in Action 16.3) to obtain a picture of a person's general cognitive strengths and weaknesses. In this example, behavioral assessment provided a complementary piece to aid in dealing with Jim's disruptive behavior during therapy sessions. Because of the need to translate knowledge of brain functioning to real problems of adjusting to home and work, testing of real-life functions is an emerging area of expertise for rehabilitation neuropsychologists. These types of tasks may attempt to tease apart the cognitive components of tasks such as meal planning or medication taking in an attempt to pinpoint the problem and develop targeted interventions. Real-life tasks may also rely on structured behavioral observations, or may actually assess progress in the context of home or work. In rehabilitation, assessment becomes much more of an ongoing process than it is with diagnosis. It monitors the progress of treatment and helps the team make decisions regarding the effectiveness of interventions and the prognosis for long-term outcome.

Treatment Methods for Neuropsychological Rehabilitation

Neuropsychologists use two primary approaches to brain injury rehabilitation that hearken back to our earlier discussion of **restitution** versus **substitution** of functioning: (1) approaches that stress retraining of an impaired skill, such as attention or memory, and (2) those which focus on searching for adaptations to the person's environment in the context in which the person will use them (Diller, 1994).

The first approach is cognitive remediation, or cognitive retraining. In this case, for example, computers may be used to provide practice exercises to attempt to strengthen memory or attention. In many instances, the underlying hope is that the brain may be able to rebuild axonal connections through retraining; that is, restitution. Approaches to cognitive remediation, however, do not necessitate proving structural changes to achieve functional success. For those functions that seem lost, cognitive remediation may focus on finding adaptive means, or "work-arounds," for lost memory or lost expressive speech, for exam-

ple. In other words, the idea is to find compensatory strategies for the lost process. Cognitive remediation approaches are usually practiced in a laboratory setting. They vary a great deal in the degree to which they seek to simulate real-life situations and in which situations they might generalize.

Cognitive retraining rests on theories of learning and pedagogy. Learning or relearning a skill or behavior is a building process that depends on an adequate base for establishing higher-order skills. If the aim is restitution, some neuronal functioning must be left. Whyte (1986) provides a useful hierarchical conceptualization for training. Basic mental activities such as focused attention or auditory processing represent the first level of cognitive operations. Cognitive processes, the next step, are combinations of cognitive operations. Flexible problem-solving and word fluency are two examples. A skill such as performing mental arithmetic or writing requires coordination of cognitive processes. Even more complex are metaskills that require the ability to sequence skills together, or to apply old skills to new situations. Finally, global functions such as working, driving, or managing a household are the most complex and integrative activities that depend on the integrity of the lower functions. The idea is to train in sequence from lower-order to higher-order operations.

Context-driven approaches (Diller, 1994) emphasize treatments that either involve actually training the person in his or her home or work environment or that are specifically tailored to the person's future needs outside the hospital, even though he or she may practice them in the rehab hospital. This is a relatively newer area of rehabilitation than is cognitive retraining. After it became evident that many people with brain injury fail to generalize or translate what they have learned in the laboratory environment to their own home or work environment, neuropsychologists recognized the need to train specific skills relevant to an individual's environment. Some of the approaches that train "in place" include the use of job coaches and supported employment, driver training, family training to aid in the home, or computers to assist scheduling or memory. Patients can also practice additional relevant skills for daily life in group therapy situations, in which groups of similarly impaired individuals may concentrate on social, orientation, or organizational skills (to name a few). Although in some cases the planners of training in the context where the skills will be used, may hope to restore function, usually the aim is compensatory.

Review of various treatment approaches makes apparent that practical, "ecologically valid," or contextual approaches to rehabilitation are increasingly the focus of many treatment programs. However, at this point there is still little outcome research to demonstrate their effectiveness. The largest number of studies have focused on such cognitive mediation efforts as documenting improvements in deficits such as attention or memory (Diller, 1994). Also, most approaches to rehabilitation combine deficit retraining and contextual methods in a more eclectic model. However, unless the neuropsychologist takes a conceptual approach toward the rehabilitation program, a combination of methods may be criticized for its resemblance to a shotgun approach to treatment (throw everything at the problem and see if something hits).

SPECIFIC FUNCTIONAL SYSTEM TRAINING

Much effort in cognitive rehabilitation has concentrated on attempting to retrain and restore specific functional or brain systems such as orientation, attention, memory, visual processing, and language. This type of cognitive retraining approach has been widely criticized in recent years, because although the patient can often demonstrate improvement on the task her or she is being trained to do, general neuropsychological evaluation of the same functional system will likely not show improvement. Even more importantly, generalization to global functions such as work and driving is questionable. We examine these issues next, using the example of attentional retraining.

Attentional Retraining

The Attention Process Training (APT) system is a computer program designed by Sohlberg and Mateer (1987, 1989) and intended to improve deficits in four areas of attention. It can present information visually or auditorily. Enough alternate forms of the task are developed so that it can be used over a period of weeks.

The basic idea behind repetition in the targeted area is to provide repeated stimulation to the brain's attentional system. Theoretically, this may facilitate strengthening and repair of the neuronal system via processes of restitution of function, as discussed earlier.

1. *Sustained attention.* To train sustained attention, the system presents a hierarchy of tasks that require constant attention. An easier task might require a response every time the number *3* is presented in a sequence (for example, *2, 7, 8, 3*, 2, 9, 3* . . .*). A harder task requires a response "every time you hear a number that is two less than the number before it" (for example, 1, 4, 8, 6*, 7, 2, 5, 3*, 1* . . .).

2. *Selective attention training.* Selective attention training incorporates distraction into tasks such as those used for sustained attention. In the auditory mode, training tapes with number sequences have taped background noise such as conversation, a newscast, or other types of sound. Visually presented numbers include other distracting designs or shapes in training. By comparing data from sustained attention and selective attention tasks, it is easy to determine if distraction significantly depresses performance.

3. *Alternating attention training.* Alternating attention requires flexible switching between two different types of attention demanding tasks. For example, Sohlberg and Mateer (1987, 1989) may use an "odd–even" letter cancelation task. In this instance the task is to cross out all "odd" numbers on successive lines of a sheet of paper, until told to switch. At this command the task is to continue by crossing out all "even" numbers. The examiner tells the person to switch at various intervals, and records his or her ability to do so. Sohlberg and Mateer (1987) also include a number of other tasks, which might require switching arithmetic operations from adding to subtracting a list of numbers, or reading the content words versus the size of type.

4. *Divided attention training.* Training divided attention entails simultaneous attention to two or more tasks. In daily life this may be akin to walking while chewing gum or driving while carrying on a conversation. This may be accomplished by first

training performance on two single sustained-attention tasks. When the person masters them, they are combined in a dual-task paradigm. For example, a person may have to attend and respond to both auditory and visual stimuli at the same time. Another approach to divided attention training is to ask the patient to keep track of two different stimulus properties at the same time. An everyday example in card games is to keep track of both suit and value of a card. Either property may be important, depending on the play.

There are three ways to evaluate retraining of a function or functional system. First, does the training improve performance on the trained tasks? Secondly, does training improve performance on similar types of tasks within the same domain? Finally, does training generalize to real-world functioning?

Task Improvement Effects   The effectiveness of attentional training on practiced tasks is generally good. Sohlberg and Mateer (1989) as well as others (for review, see von Zomeren and Brouwer, 1994) have been able to demonstrate improvement on their training measures for mild to severely impaired head-injured patients with attentional disorders. Practice over time may eventually yield performance in the normal range on the targeted tasks.

These results are encouraging, because they indicate that people with impairments can be trained to improve on specific task measures. The effects of training other domains such as memory or visual-spatial processing also yield similar positive results. Very importantly, most of the studies have trained patients who are more than one year post injury. This is past the time when the majority of spontaneous recovery should have occurred. These are important findings. However, before becoming overly optimistic, there are other questions to answer: Does the effect of training also show improvement on neuropsychological testing? Does training generalize?

Generalization to Neuropsychological Testing   Neuropsychological tests have demonstrated the effectiveness of attentional training, but researchers do not always report positive results. The training program just presented (Sohlberg & Mateer, 1987, 1989) did yield significant gains in other neuropsychological tests of attention (such as the PASAT test). These gains appeared to be long-lasting over a period of 8 months after training ceased. The improvements were also specific to attention. That is, there were no similar gains in other areas of neuropsychological functioning. Other studies too—in fact the majority—have reported that attention training results in improvement on other attention-related tasks (see, for example, von Zomeren & Brouwer, 1994, for review). However, it is difficult to make strong conclusions about the generalization of attentional training to other attentional tasks. Many of the studies have been based on small sample sizes and single cases. Also, many of these studies can be criticized for using neuropsychological tests that are similar to the trained tasks. For example, the PASAT test employed by Sohlberg and Mateer (1987, 1989) to show attentional generalization is very similar to the more difficult sustained-attention tasks they used for training. Is this merely "training to task" and not generalization? The preliminary work appears promising, and more studies are forthcoming to determine the scope of the generalization.

A difficulty in this type of research is to determine the degree of generalization that is appropriate. For example, is it feasible that training sustained attention should result in improvements on other tasks of memory or reading? Might training in alternating attention lead to improvements on other tests of flexible thinking (for example, WCST)? How far should we expect specific attentional training to generalize to real life? What sort of daily life tasks rely on the various types of attention? How would one measure these tasks?

Generalization to Daily Life Functioning   As yet, few studies have sought to test the generalization of attentional training to improvements in targeted aspects of daily functioning. When von Zomeren and Brouwer (1994) reviewed three studies that had measured aspects of daily functioning, such as rating behavior in rehab wards, on clerical tasks, and on driving, the patients did show improvements, but the improvements were difficult to attribute to the training. Other factors such as spontaneous improvement or improvement in other functions such as visual perception may have contributed to improvement on the global task.

To demonstrate a model of retraining based on the restitution approach to rehabilitation, we earlier gave an example of cognitive retraining in the functional domain of attention. The best approaches (such as Sohlberg & Mateer, 1987, 1989) base their training on a theoretical approach to neuropsychological functioning. In the area of attention, as in most areas of functional cognitive retraining, task-specific improvements can usually be demonstrated. In many cases, similar neuropsychological tests also show concomitant improvements. It appears that the jury is still out when it comes to how well specific functional training generalizes to daily life. Perhaps the difficulty lies in the fact that specific functions such as attention or speech are but individual building blocks that combine to determine higher-order skills and more global functions such as driving. These higher-order global functions of daily life are also more than the sum of their cognitive components. Some have suggested that training strategies is a better approach. This has also met with some success.

SUPPORTED EMPLOYMENT

Despite gains in some areas, brain injury survivors are often no longer able to compete in the job market at the level of which they are previously accustomed. This may be caused by various residual brain impairments resulting in poor time management, organizational difficulties or social inappropriateness with coworkers. Those who become employed post injury may be less than 30% (Brooks, McKinlay, Symington, Beatie, & Campsie, 1987). Moreover, even if they can work, most do not return to their previous level of employment. Many end up in sheltered workshops doing menial and repetitive tasks that are unchallenging and unfullfilling to many survivors, considering their preinjury aspirations and jobs.

Supported employment is a concept in brain injury rehabilitation modeled after programs designed for adults with mental retardation and developmental disabilities. Wehman has described this approach well (Wehman, 1991; Wehman & Kreutzer, 1990). This method bypasses traditional vocational rehabilitation approaches that focus on vocational aptitude testing, and work samples. Instead, individuals are introduced directly into a work environment with a "job coach" who works with the employer and the patient. The job coach provides training at the job site and tailors

the cognitive interventions to the specific job requirements. To do this, the job coach first conducts a task analysis of the job requirements. Table 16.1 provides a sample outline for conducting a task analysis for entry-level positions such as a food service worker or groundskeeper.

In this task analysis or "job inventory," it is important to understand the cognitive demands in each of the functional areas, from sensory-motor to higher cognitive skills demanded by the job. To do this, the job coach must have a good understanding of brain structure–function relationships and understand the effects of the specific injury on the person's functioning. In addition, it is important to evaluate the social milieu. For example, how must the person interact with supervisors, coworkers, and customers? How often is there contact with others, and will other staff

---

Table 16.1	*Outline for Conducting a Job Task Analysis (designed for entry-level jobs such as dishwasher, groundskeeper, and so on)*

I. General Information
  A. Reasons why persons with traumatic brain injury or other severe handicaps are considered for this job
  B. General description of the job
  C. General description of the work setting
  D. General description of the social environment
    1. Information related to fellow workers
    2. Information related to supervision
    3. Information related to special contingencies of the employer
II. Specific skill requirements of the job
  A. Listing of the basic physical/sensory motor skills required
  B. Listing of the basic interpersonal skills required
  C. Listing of the basic language skills (verbal and nonverbal) required
  D. Listing of the basic functional academic skills required
  E. Listing of the basic machine and tool skills required
  F. Listing of the basic hygienic skills required
III. Supportive skills and other useful information
  A. Transportation skills required
  B. Skills related to work preparation
  C. Basic money management skills useful
  D. Time-telling and time-judgment skills useful
  E. Health code requirements
  F. Informed consent and legal requirements

Source: Kreutzer, J. S., and Wehman, P. H. (eds.) (1991) *Cognitive Rehabilitation for Persons with Traumatic Brain Injury: A Functional Approach*, p. 271. Reprinted by permission of Paul H. Brookes Publishing Co.

Neuropsychology in Action 16.5

Job Coaching: The Case of P.R.

P.R. is a 33-year-old male who sustained a severe head injury in an alcohol-related automobile accident in 1975, which resulted in his becoming traumatically brain injured. Reportedly, P.R. had been a heavy drug and alcohol user. He had had many difficulties with the authorities and had a juvenile police record. As far as educational goals and expectations of himself, P. R. had none. He had dropped out of high school in the 9th grade, and stated that he could not see the value of continuing his education. He had found numerous jobs such as bricklayer's and carpenter's assistant, but had been unable to maintain these jobs for more than a few weeks at a time.

At the time of his injury, P.R. was 18. He remained in a coma for four months and continued to be hospitalized for three more months. Both physical and cognitive deficits were noted post injury. His physical deficits included functional blindness in his left eye and left-field cut in his right eye; left hemiparesis in his arm and leg, which was greater in his arm than in his leg; significant trunk deformity with spinal curvature; no sense of smell; and an unbalanced gait, which was

compounded by his obesity. His cognitive deficits included inattention, lack of concentration, poor organizational skills, short-term memory loss, lack of reasoning abilities, and inappropriate interpersonal skills.

At age 20, the state center for rehabilitation administered a vocational evaluation to P.R. The evaluation indicated that P.R. needed a sheltered employment-type placement. P.R. participated in a sheltered workshop for two months.

A neuropsychological evaluation was not done until 12 years later—on March 20, 1989, by the Department of Rehabilitation Medicine at the Medical College of Virginia. The purpose of the evaluation was to determine P.R.'s emotional status and the effects of his cognitive deficits on his vocational potential. The results of his emotional status evaluation showed that P.R. displays no evidence of significant depression or anxiety. However, he is still at risk for depression if his awareness of his deficits increases. Vocationally, P.R.'s problems with sustained attention and concentration, learning, memory, and motor/speed dexterity are felt to influence his work performance. Because of

these deficits, the evaluations suggested that he will take more time to complete tasks, have problems learning and retaining information, and have difficulty focusing on tasks requiring sustained attention. No psychiatric or psychological problems appeared evident. However, P.R. does display inappropriate behaviors at times. The behaviors include inappropriate verbalizations, invading personal space, and inappropriate touching.

Job Training

Initial job training began July 12, 1989, as a dining room attendant in a fast-food restaurant. His initial duties included wiping tables, emptying trash, cleaning lunch trays, stocking condiments, maintaining the upkeep of the bathrooms, and general maintenance of the dining area. The employment specialist was completing 60% of P.R.'s job, and he was completing 40%. After 6 weeks he had increased his percentage to 75%. By August 20, 1989, P.R. could perform tasks independently with one prompt. The employment specialist was finding that she could fade during some tasks

help support the brain-injured person when needed? Finally, what is the physical layout of the workplace? Are there any barriers that would make it difficult to maneuver? Is it a noisy or distracting place?

Effective supported employment includes several components according to Wehman (1991). We explain the components first and then present a case example to illustrate the process. Based on the task analysis and an assessment of the brain-injured person's strengths and weaknesses, the first step is to break the job skill into small steps that can be easily grasped.

Perhaps the person first masters one or two steps, and then they can be chained together in longer sequences until the skill is learned. Second, because many brain-injured people have difficulty organizing themselves because of executive functioning deficits, the job coach must structure the work environment. The coach may need to provide a "game plan," and it is important that guidance be consistent each time. Third, objective measurement of performance is key. If the coach can break tasks down into steps that are observable, or have measurable outcomes, then eval-

and return when he was finished. P.R. did not know what to do next until she gave him the next prompt. The employment specialist made a schedule for him to follow and posted it where it was accessible to him. P.R. liked the idea of the schedule and used it daily. Problems arose with the schedule because as P.R. performed tasks regularly, he increased his speed; therefore, when he looked at his schedule, he was ahead of time. He went to the next duty but was more confused as time went on. A new strategy needed to be implemented. The employment specialist then made a pocket schedule that had one task on each page. It had no times on it—just a number on the bottom corner so he would know what direction to turn the page after he completed a task. He was trained not to turn the page until he was finished with the task at hand. This pocket schedule was the answer to P.R.'s inability to organize himself. He no longer needed prompts to go to the next task. With the pocket schedule, he could now do it independently.

Another problem area for P.R. was that when leaving the dining room area, he would skip tables because he would jump from one row to another. What P.R. needed was to establish a set pattern. A specific route for him to follow was devised. He found that if he followed this route, he improved his accuracy and speed because he did not have to go back and wipe the missed tables. Another adaptation that was added to his route was the use of a caddy. In this caddy, he could put his cleaning supplies on one side and the small trash he picked up on the other. This made him more efficient because he did not have to stop his cleaning to throw a piece of trash away. He could just put it in the caddy and go on to the next table.

Another job duty–stocking the condiment stand–presented two obstacles for P.R. The first problem was that P.R. did not know when it needed to be stocked. This was easily resolved by putting red tape with the name of the item imprinted on it and attaching it to the inside of the bin. When the item needed restocking, P. R. would see the red tape. If he did not see the tape, the item was adequately stocked.

The other obstacle regarding the condiment stand was stocking it quickly. The supplies were stored in the stockroom, which meant that P.R. had to walk to the stockroom, get the needed item, and replace it on the stand. This was not a problem, except when he needed seven or eight items. Because of his left upper extremity paralysis, he could not carry everything. A small cart was purchased, and he was taught to stock it with everything he needed for the day, and to push it out to the stand, filling all bins and placing left-over supplies under the counter for later use in the day. This adaptation increased his efficiency and speed. Due to the increase in job duties, P.R.'s inappropriate behaviors, and a changeover in management, the employment specialist could not begin a set fading schedule until October 9, 1989. She began fading for the first hour and has since faded for the first hour and a half. She checks in on him to see if he is on schedule. If he is on schedule, she leaves for another hour and then returns. At that time, he should be cleaning the dining room and the lunch rush should be over. The employment specialist watches to make sure he stays on task and gets his work completed. During this time, P.R. has displayed inappropriate behaviors such as talking too much to customers, joking too much with coworkers, and neglecting his job duties. A behavioral contract was drawn up; when P.R. displayed any of these behaviors, he was reminded of the contract and its consequences. The managers at the restaurant have gotten very good at redirecting P.R. and getting him back on task.

He was given more responsibilities along with more hours on October 23, 1989, and now his duties also include stocking and maintaining the cold and hot food bars. He is now working a total of 5½ hours per day.

Source: Adapted with permission from Kreutzer, J. S., and Wehman, P. H. (eds.) (1991). *Cognitive Rehabilitation for Persons with Traumatic Brain Injury: A Functional Approach*, pp. 274–276. Paul H. Brookes Publishing Co.

---

uating and correcting trouble spots becomes easier. The coach can graph behaviors to show improvement over time and provide positive feedback to the worker. Finally, building in a way to wean the worker from the job coach is necessary. Supporting employment through job coaching is a time-intensive and expensive process in the beginning but is cost effective in the long run. Job coaches can use behavioral techniques moving from a continuous to intermittent schedule of reinforcement. To encourage generalization, after the brain-impaired worker masters initial tasks, coaches may have the person attempt slightly different tasks, to evaluate whether transfer of learning can take place. The eventual goal is for the job coach to fade out of the picture and to have supervisors and other staff continue to provide support and structure as needed. So during this final step the job coach needs to include other work site staff in the training. Job coaches return for "checkups," but if all goes well the brain-injured person can now function in a job that would have been difficult, or nearly impossible, to master alone (see Neuropsychology in Action 16.5).

COMPUTERS AS COMPENSATORY AIDS

Many of the approaches to rehabilitation we have discussed use computers with specially designed software in some manner (for example, see Sohlberg and Mateer's APT model). However, if a group of rehabilitation psychologists gather, use of computers in rehabilitation is apt to provoke a spirited debate. With the advent of the computer revolution in the 1980s, optimism abounded for the promise of computers as a rehabilitation aid. Perhaps the technology of the computer "wowed" people initially into thinking anything on a computer must be impressive. Computer programs proliferated for cognitive retraining and orthotics. Although some of the programs were well grounded in theory and practice, many programs were better off in the garbage heap. This resulted in a backlash against computers and a tendency to "throw the baby out with the bath water." Levin (1991) provides an apt analogy for how best to view computers in rehabilitation.

We do not ask whether a scalpel is or is not effective in surgery. Whether it is useful or not depends upon how it is used, under which conditions. A hammer and nails can help build a house, or can ruin it. Similarly, computer software may or may not augment the rehabilitation endeavor, depending on how it is applied. While it is certainly appropriate, and necessary, to question the cost-effectiveness of current cognitive rehabilitation methods, it is a diversion to focus on the worth of the tools of the method. (p. 163)

Computers and computer software are often used in the context of assessment and cognitive retraining. This is the area in which the majority of computer applications exist. Many focus on restitution of functioning by providing a way to generate many alternate forms of a task for repeated drill and practice. Although they may be more interactive and flexible than paper-and-pencil measures, many are little more than tests presented on a computer screen. Each of these programs are better evaluated in the context of the particular goals they are intended to achieve. How well do they improve task performance? How well do they reduce apparent functional deficits on neuropsychological testing? How well do they help a patient become self-sufficient in daily activities?

An exciting area in assessment and retraining is the development of computer simulations of real-life tasks such as driving (see Neuropsychology in Action 16.6). The obvious advantage, as any high school student in driver's education can attest, is that the person can practice driving in a protected environment. Complex tasks can be practiced, and the rehabilitation specialist can systematically add or remove component variables to control the complexity of the task. These real-life tasks are also inherently more interesting and motivating than other types of "drill and practice" tasks on the computer. With technologies such as virtual reality, the range of tasks that can be practiced in the safety of a simulated environment is greatly expanded. Computer simulations can be developed for operations from navigating through a house or neighborhood, to practicing job and social skills. As more simulations are developed, they will provide rich opportunities for observing the learning skills of brain-damaged individuals.

For the remainder of this section we deal specifically with the use and effectiveness of computers as compensatory or prosthetic aids to functioning. Prosthetics for cognitive functioning are external aids, much like an artificial leg for an amputee. They fall under the category of compensatory strategies. In other words, if a function such as speech or memory is lost or minimally retained, then computer-driven devices may provide artificial speech, or reminders. The idea is to "offload" to the environment as much of the cognitive demand for a task as possible. A low-tech example is the common use of daily planners to organize and provide reminders for appointments. Computers can provide "high-tech" assistance. As computer-assisted devices such as palm-tops and electronic organizers become easier to use, people can also use them as compensatory devices for memory and organization.

A computer, as a prosthetic device, should not be thought of only as a system on a desk, a laptop, or a palm-top organizer, any of which may require significant learning to master. Also, many older people are intimidated just by the idea of a computer. Luckily, today's computers can be fairly invisible components of aids, or require minimal learning. Computer chips run the electronics in cars, microwaves, stereos, and possibly the climate control and security systems in many homes. Much of the operation is fairly invisible. Once set up, the computer runs in the background. Also, many "off-the-shelf" systems that can aid a person in his or her daily activities. An exiting new area is the development of systems especially designed for cognitively impaired people.

For example, systems are needed that help keep brain-impaired people safe when they are in their homes. People with attentional or memory problems may forget to turn off the stove or the water, potentially risking a fire or flood. Installing automatic systems that turn off the stove or the water following a preset time period can effectively remove these hazards. Safety from the outside world is another concern for families of brain-impaired people. Anyone may forget to lock a door or window, risking danger from intruders. Safety locks and special locking systems can be used in this instance. But in other instances many families of brain-injured and Alzheimer's patients are just as concerned with someone wandering out. The solution is a "wandering cuff" to alert others when an AD patient has left an area of safety.

Another safety concern, especially for older brain-impaired adults on medication, is adequate medication management. Cognitively, these problems occur either through misunderstanding, forgetting to take a dose (errors of omission), or not remembering that a dose has been taken and taking extra doses (errors of commission). Most older adults attempt to remember to take their medications by associating medication with other daily activities such as meals and bedtime. Some use low-tech pill-organizing devices, but less than 1% of community-dwelling older adults on medication use high-tech devices that include timer reminders (Spiers & Kutzik, 1995). Much of the problem with currently available pill timers is that they are difficult to program and reset, and were not designed to accommodate more than one to two doses. For cognitively impaired older adults who may have to take four to five doses per day, managing off-the-shelf reminder systems can be nearly impossible. What is needed is to offload this memory task to an external device in the environment that not only can provide reminders for multiple medications but also can check to see if the medication has been taken, and provide appropriate reminders or warnings to others if it has not. Such systems are currently being developed and will provide a tremendous aid to cognitively impaired older people when they are commercially available.

PSYCHOTHERAPY IN REHABILITATION

Neuropsychological rehabilitation is concerned not only with rehabilitating cognition, but also with personality, emotion, and awareness. Of course, the brain is also the mediator of these functions. Altered self-awareness and personality after brain injury may, in fact, represent some of the most complicated and higher-order brain processes that a neuropsychologist and rehabilitation team attempts to treat. (For a case discussion, see Neuropsychology in Action 16.7.) Psychotherapy can aid by discussing frustrations in progress and providing motivational strategies. But more importantly, and more profoundly, brain-damaged individuals who have suffered more than mild impairment often report they no longer feel "normal" and have to go through a readjustment process to adapt to their new level of functioning. Those who have suffered brain injuries complain that their social life has declined (Elsass & Kinsella, 1987) and rank loneliness as their most frequent complaint (Thomsen, 1974). Relatives and significant others often describe a "personality change" (Jennett & Teasdale, 1981). Poor social interaction is evident in ratings of close others and direct behavioral observations (Newton & Johnson, 1985). These losses are perhaps the most tragic and far-reaching aspects of brain injury.

Frontal lobe damage, as we discussed earlier in this book, is a common result of moderate to severe head injury due to bony skull projections and shearing. Frontal lobe damage is typically suspect when certain qualities of psychosocial functioning are observed after injury. Among the difficulties co-occurring with frontal lobe injury are impulsivity, disinhibition, lack of initiation, rigidity, loss of abstract attitude, poor social judgment, and loss of personal and social awareness (Lezak, 1995). Prigatano (1992) argues that

Neuropsychology in Action 16.6

Bits and Bytes in Rehabilitation

by **Douglas L. Chute** Professor of Neuropsychology, Drexel University.

The application of computers to neuro-rehabilitation has had both successes and failures that have shaped the development of neuropsychology as a leading health care discipline. Successes have included the use of computational technologies in both assessments and treatments. I have selected here a couple of examples to illustrate such emerging technologies in neuropsychology.

Although the application of new technologies to neuropsychological problems offers hope and promise for the future, it would be an error not to recognize some inherent limitations and past difficulties. In general, these have arisen from overestimating the capabilities of technology, the lack of a satisfactory theory and science of rehabilitation, and the perception among practitioners that "high tech" is somehow counterproductive in comparison to "high touch" treatment methods. In that sense, the problems in the use of technology in rehabilitation closely resemble the problems in the use of technology in education (Chute, 1993a, 1993b).

The ability of the personal computer to approximate various types of "virtual reality" has led to entirely new neuropsychological tests. For example, if someone is unfortunate enough to have had a head injury, most jurisdictions require them to pass a new driving test. How should such a person be evaluated? Traditional neuropsychological tests such as Trail Making only correlate weakly with driving skill following a head injury. Even driving on a closed course around pylons or on a local street doesn't seem to represent very well the ecological environment of cognitively complex driving situations. To address these shortcomings, Maria Garay used the experiment-authoring tool Power-Laboratory to create more ecologically valid driving scenarios (Garay, 1996). Figure 16.6 shows a sample screen where the subject "drives" the computer through a variety of challenging driving situations.

Although technology has opened new views of assessment, it has also provided new pathways to rehabilitation. The personal computer offers a customizable cognitive adjunct (an **orthotic**) or cognitive replacement (a **prosthetic**). For example, Marilyn Bergman and Gail Kemmerer at the Lankenau Hospital in Philadelphia report long-term positive case outcomes for people who have brain injuries and who use computer as an orthotic providing assistance with such everyday living tasks as money management, memory organization, communication, and scheduling (Bergman & Kemmerer, 1996). In a project developed for Hanspeter Albisser, a sufferer of **amyotrophic lateral sclerosis** (ALS, or Lou Gehrig's disease), we expanded some earlier software to serve as a speech prosthesis, word processor, and home environment controller (Chute, Conn, Dipasquale, & Hoag, 1988). ALS is a disease of the motor systems where patients lose control of the muscles for speech as well as the muscles in their limbs. "SpeechWare," or its Swiss version "MacSprache," offered Albisser single-click control enabling slow and arduous communications, word processing, and home control. Unfortunately, Albisser died before the project

---

self-awareness requires the highest integration of "thought" and "feeling" areas of the brain, combining inputs from sensory-motor areas, limbic and paralimbic areas. The common perception that people with closed head injuries have an "egocentric" or "unempathic" attitude (Newton & Johnson, 1985; Elsass & Kinsella, 1987; Grattan & Eslinger, 1989) is usually attributed to various manifestations of these and frontal lobe difficulties. The specific inability to see a

situation from another's viewpoint may be one of the cognitive dysfunctions underlying apparent egocentric or unempathic behavior. This skill, labeled *cognitive perspective taking,* varies among moderately to severely injured people (Spiers, Pouk, & Santoro, 1994; Santoro & Spiers, 1994). The general ability to recognize and appreciate one's own functional and cognitive changes also varies over individuals and time since injury. However, those who have greater

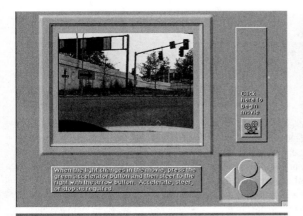

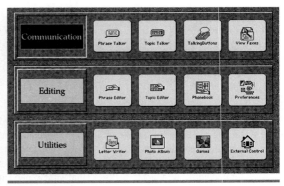

Figure 16.6 A Neurocognitive Driving Assessment screen. Simple "virtual" techniques create ecologically valid driving evaluations for the cognitively impaired. (Doug Chute, Ph.D., and Maria Schultheis, Ph.D., Drexel University, by permission)

Figure 16.7 A SpeechWare screen. For single-click operation with a mouse button or eyeblink, the program strobes through its various functions until a specific module is selected. Within a module, single-click operation permits word processing, speech, or home control that would otherwise be unavailable without computer technology. (Doug Chute, Ph.D., and Maria Schultheis, Ph.D., Drexel University, by permission)

was completed, but his foundation made copies available for others. Figure 16.7 shows the main control screen where communications or home control modules were selected.

The broader application of the concept of the personal computer as orthotic or prosthetic holds promise for helping such people as the elderly live effectively in their own homes or for otherwise assisting anyone with the various activities of daily living. The computer is flexible and readily customized to each person's needs. However, at this time few rehabilitation professionals are trained in this emerging field.

The neuropsychology of rehabilitation is essentially an individualized empirical clinical trial where little theory—and sometimes little evidence—shapes assessments and interventions. For example, it is widely held that early sensory and motor stimulation, even of a comatose patient, promotes recovery from neurological damage. Yet only recently have researchers published data bearing on the practice, and such data show that timing is critical and that stimulation can be too early (Nudo, Wise, SiFuentes, Milliken, 1996; Freund, 1996). Similarly with computer applications, it will be incumbent on neuropsychology to provide suitable research protocols to demonstrate the effectiveness and appropriateness of technology in neurorehabilitation. Psychologists are used to working quite independently, however, with technologies becoming so complex, it appears we will need to discover new ways and means to promote collaboration to develop this field (Chute & Westall, 1996).

awareness of their dysfunction typically show higher levels of emotional distress (Nockelby & Deaton, 1987).

Psychotherapy in the rehab setting often targets these neuropsychology-based issues of self-awareness, egocentricity, and empathy. Psychotherapy can be useful not only to aid coping and adjustment, but also for very practical reasons. Difficulty in psychosocial functioning and poor self-awareness is one of the prime reasons for poor vocational outcomes. If therapy targeting affective issues is provided, another 20 to 30% of patients may become productive workers (Prigatano, 1992). Beh-Yishay and Prigatano (1990) found that three factors largely predicted vocational outcome: involvement with others, ability to regulate affect, and acceptance of cognitive limitations. All three of these factors are mainly influenced by psychotherapy.

Neuropsychology in Action 16.7

It's More Than a Black Box

Cecil R. Reynolds Ph.D., *Department of Educational Psychology, Texas A&M University.*

A very popular means of treating disorders of learning and behavior in children is behavior therapy and derivative approaches that capitalize on changing behavior by implementing specific reinforcement programs. Clinically, this approach derived from work by the Russian physiologist Ivan Pavlov on classical conditioning (known sometimes as Pavlovian conditioning) and the American psychologist B. F. Skinner, who developed theories of operant conditioning (Skinnerian conditioning). Pavlov is best known for teaching, quite by accident, a dog to salivate on hearing the sound of a bell. Skinner taught rats to press levers for food and pigeons to peck keys to be fed. Early clinicians such as Joseph Wolpe were able to take these phenomena and translate them into methods to cause humans to alter their behavior by altering the so-called reinforcement systems they believe control a specific person's behavior.

As behavioral approaches to treating disorders of learning and behavior grew in schools and clinics around the world,

peaking in the late 1970s, understanding brain functioning faded into the background. Skinner and other radical proponents of behavior therapies argued that what went on in the brain was irrelevant. Only input and output were important, and people need not understand the brain's function further; it was treated as a black box, a euphemism for a space in which some transformation may occur through processes not understood but also that are irrelevant to the understanding of behavior and learning. As late as 1977, I had a professor in graduate school, teaching a course in learning, make the pronouncement in class that "the brain has nothing to do with learning; learning is all accomplished through change or continuance of reinforcement paradigms." Such views were not uncommon.

Behavioral approaches to the management and alteration of behavior in children with developmental disorders are often, but far from always, effective. And as it turns out, brain systems are crucial in mediating reinforcement

schedules and learning. Let me provide an example. At age 11, Deanna attended a program for gifted and talented children at her local public school, with a measured IQ in excess of 130. She played piano and had won a trophy as star player of her soccer team a year earlier. In spring of that year, Deanna was riding in the passenger seat of her dad's car when a drunk driver ran a stop sign, striking the car at Deanna's door. She suffered many injuries, including a broken pelvic bone and numerous cuts and bruises. Most devastating, however, was her head injury. Deanna had suffered a massive right frontal lobe injury, producing a large subdural hematoma that was evacuated in neurosurgery. Her cerebral bleeding extended through the right superior parietal areas, and much microscopic shearing and tearing of neurons occurred throughout her brain. She spent 11 days in a deep coma, and her parents were warned that she might not even recognize them if she came out of the coma at all. Deanna did revive and had a miraculous recovery.

Conclusion

Rehabilitation is clearly becoming one of the major areas of practice for neuropsychology. The rehabilitation process is complex and depends on many mechanisms, including biological, personal, and environmental factors. Throughout this book we have seen the brain's amazing ability to attempt to adapt to damage. It is the neuropsychologist's job to assess the degree to which spontaneous recovery will occur, functioning can be restored, or other means of adaptation must take place. Rehabilitation is best thought of as following a continuum from inpatient care to outpatient treatment to community reentry and followup. As the length of acute care and rehab stays shrink, the focus in rehabilitation has shifted from hospital level inpatient treatment to outpatient-, home-, family-, and job-centered assessment and treatment strategies. Rehabilitation of the brain-

After six months in a rehabilitation hospital, Deanna returned to school. Over the next two years, additional cognitive recovery was evident. Her IQ, measured in the 60s (mentally deficient) 6 months post injury, gradually increased to nearly 100 (average) and her academic skills in reading, writing, and arithmetic came to grade level. A far cry from their prior, or premorbid, status, but all in all, a very positive outcome. However, this once popular, socially adept young girl was now ostracized by her peers due to her now obnoxious behavior patterns.

She had few social skills and just did not seem to know how to interact positively with others. She was extremely impulsive, as she acted most often without thought, was constantly reaching out to touch whomever she talked to, and had no clear sense of personal space. Her social judgment was severely impaired, and she often blurted inappropriate and embarrassing comments to others. Deanna came to my attention after a consult request from the University Clinic, where a doctoral student had been working with the family for over a year to develop a behavioral treatment plan to change these many socially inappropriate behaviors. Such problems are common among patients of all ages with frontal lobe damage, especially prefrontal and orbitomedial damage, all

of which were present in this case. The early images of her brain injury, taken via MRI in the first few weeks and months following her injury, documented these lesions well. However, Deanna seemed resistant to behavioral intervention.

After a careful review of her case, another MRI was requested and obtained, now more than 30 months post injury. The new pictures revealed an injury that had not appeared before. Deanna had a lesion and scar tissue on the posterior portion of her hippocampus just above the fourth ventricle of the brain. The importance of such a lesion may not be immediately obvious; however, the hippocampus is a component of the limbic system and is crucial to memory functions. These brain systems, the frontolimbic system and particularly the hippocampus, are very involved in learning reinforcement systems. Individuals with posterior hippocampal damage are especially resistant to reinforcement schedules that are anything less than a one-to-one ratio reinforcement schedule.

The mediation systems that allow reinforcement to be recalled and to mediate learning had been irreparably damaged in Deanna. Despite the protestations of the devotees of Skinnerian conditioning, the brain does matter! Behavior therapies can be very effective in treating TBI and developmentally

disordered children with behavior problems, even with frontal lobe systems that are impaired. However, once limbic system and specifically hippocampal funtions are also damaged, such interventions fail.

With this knowledge and evidence, Deanna's insurance carrier was persuaded to fund a different, more intensive intervention. An in vivo therapeutic approach was devised in which a therapist went with Deanna to local shopping malls for several hours several times a week. Deanna's behavior was constantly monitored and redirected in this setting by a therapist, who also devised a set of verbal cues and self-talk strategies. In doing so we took advantage of her stronger verbal skills, given that most of her injuries were in the right hemisphere, as Deanna learned social skills in real-life setting, in vivo, or "on the job," so to speak. Being a teenager is a tough job; being a teenager with frontal lobe injury who does not respond to changes in the reward-and-punishment systems of life is nearly impossible. Deanna did graduate from high school, a year late, and is now employed in a clerical assistant position at a university library. She still hopes to attend college.

---

injured patient is one of the best examples of a neuropsychologist working with a multidisciplinary team to gain a comprehensive picture of an individual within his or her environment. The neuropsychologist may play many important roles in the rehabilitation process, including developing a thorough understanding of the status of the impaired individual; developing strategies for remediation and rehabilitation given the person's family and economic situation; providing education and therapy for the patient, family, and treatment team.

The assessment and evaulative methods used necessarily focus on functional, or "real life" tasks of daily living. Treatment requires that patients and families be active in rehabilitation and work as "trainees" of the team. In rehabilitation, assessment is an ongoing process, monitoring the progress of treatment, and aiding decision making regarding the effectiveness of interventions and the prognosis for long-term outcome.

The methods of treatment currently being developed by neuropsychologists provide exciting and creative ways to help ameliorate dysfunction of brain-impaired individuals. With specialized knowledge of the brain and behavior, as well as technical advances, neuropsychologists are uniquely positioned to guide individuals and their famililies to their highest potential for recovery and functioning.

Critical Thinking Questions

- What is the potential for the human brain to adapt and recover after brain injury?
- What are the challenges for rehabilitation in the 21st century?
- Will technology eventually be able to compensate for lost neural function?
- Is the quest for the search of the organ of the soul completed?

Key Terms

Cerebral achromatopsia	Physiatry	Therapeutic recreation	Substitution
Coma	Speech therapy	Dysarthria	Orthotic
Diaschisis	Occupational therapy	Prospective memory	Prosthetic
Plasticity	Physical therapy	Restitution	Amyotrophic lateral sclerosis

Web Connections

http://www.neuropsychologycentral.com
Neuropsychology Central
A great site that keeps you up to date on the latest in neuropsychological links and resources. Internal search engine allows you to determine what topic you would like to focus on and provides you with detailed summaries of each link that has been found. Provides links to neuropsychological assessment, forensic, treatment, and other related areas.

http://www.tbims.org
Traumatic Brain Injury (TBI) Model Systems
Learn about TBI's National Database, the diagnosis of TBI, the Center for Outcome Measures, and more.

http://www.healthpsych.com
Health Psychology and Rehabilitation Web Site
Comprehensive site that provides information on health and rehabilitation psychology.

http://www.neuro.pmr.vcu.edu
National Resource Center for Traumatic Brain Injury (TBI)
Guide for TBI survivors, tips on rehabilitation, and on living and working productively with traumatic brain injury.

REFERENCES

Abel, E. L. (1995). A update on incidence of FAS: FAS is not an equal opportunity birth defect. *Neurotoxicology and Teratology, 17,* 437–443.

Adams, R. D., & Victor, M. (1993). *Principles of neurology* (4th ed.). New York: McGraw-Hill.

Albert, M. L., Feldman, R. G., & Willis, A. L. (1974). The "subcortical dementia" of progressive supranuclear palsy. *Journal of Neurology, Neurosurgery, and Psychiatry, 37,* 121–130.

Allison, M. (1992). The effects of neurologic injury on the maturing brain. *Headlines, 3,* 2–10.

Alzheimer, A. (1907). Über eine eigenartige Erkrankung der Hirnrinde. *Allgemeine Zeitschrift für Psychiatrie, 64,* 146–148.

Alzheimer, A. (1987). About a peculiar disease of the cerebral cortex. L. Jarvik & H. Greenson, trans. *Alzheimer's disease and associated disorders, 1,* 7–8. (Originally published 1907.)

American Psychiatric Association. (1980). *Diagnostic and statistical manual of mental disorders* (3rd ed.). Washington, DC: Author.

American Psychiatric Association. (1987). *Diagnostic and statistical manual of mental disorders* (3rd ed., rev.). Washington, DC: Author.

American Psychiatric Association. (1994). *Diagnostic and statistical manual of mental disorders* (4th ed.). Washington, DC: Author.

Anastasi, A. (1988). *Psychological testing* (6th ed.). New York: MacMillan.

Andreasen, N. C., (1988). Brain imaging: Applications in psychiatry. *Science, 239,* 215–226.

Armstrong, C., Corn, B., Ruffer, J., Pruitt, A., Mollman, J., & Phillips, P. (2000). Radiotherapeutic effects on brain function: Double dissociation of memory systems. *Neuropsychiatry, Neuropsychology, Behavioral Neurology, 13*(2), 101–111.

Armstrong-Hickey, D. (1991). A validation of lucid dreaming in school age children. *Lucidity, 10,* 250–254.

Ashford, J. W., & Zec, R. F. (1993). Pharmacological treatment in Alzheimer's disease. In R. W. Parks, R. F. Zec, & R. S. Wilson, eds., *Neuropsychology of Alzheimer's disease and other dementias.* New York: Oxford University Press.

Ashford, J. B., Lecroy, C. W., & Lortie, K. L. (1997). *Human behavior in the social environment: A multidimensional approach.* Pacific Grove, CA: Brooks/Cole.

Asperger, H. (1991). "Autistic psychopathy" in childhood. U. Frith, trans. In U. Frith, ed., *Autism and Asperger's syndrome* (pp. 37–92). (Original work published 1944, Die 'Autistischen

Psychopathen' im Kindesalter. *Archiv für Psychiatrie und Nervenkrankheiten, 117,* 76–136.)

Aylward, E. H., Reiss, A. L., Reader, M. J., Singer, H. S., Brown, J. E., & Denckla, M. B. (1996). Basal ganglia volumes in children with attention-deficit hyperactivity disorder. *Journal of Child Neurology, 11,* 112–115.

Babinski, J. & Joltran, E. (1924). Un nouveau cas d'anosognosie. *Revue Neurologique, 31,* 638–640.

Baddeley, A. (1986). *Working memory.* New York: Oxford University Press.

Baddeley, A. (1990). *Human memory: Theory and practice.* Allyn and Bacon.

Bailey, A., Phillips, W., & Rutter, W. (1996). Autism: Towards an integration of clinical, genetic, neuropsychological, and neurobiological perspectives. *Journal of Child Psychology and Psychiatry, 37,* 89–126.

Balasubramanian, V., & Ranamurthi, B. (1970). Stereotaxic amygdalotomy in behavior disorders. *Confinia Neurology, 32,* 367.

Ball, G. F., & Hulse, S. H. (1998). Birdsong. *American Psychologist, 53,* 37–58.

Banich, M. T. (1997). *Neuropsychology: The neural basis of mental function.* New York: Houghton Mifflin.

Bannister, R. (1992). Disorders of the cerebral circulation. In R. Bannister, ed., *Brain and Bannister's clinical neurology* (7th ed.). New York: Oxford University Press.

Barakat, L. P., Kazak, A. E., Meadows, A. T., Casey, R., Meeske, K., & Stuber, M. L. (1997). Families surviving childhood cancer: A comparison of posttraumatic stress symptoms with families of healthy children. *Journal of Pediatric Psychology, 22*(6), 843–859.

Barkley, R. A. (1990). *Attention deficit hyperactivity disorder.* New York: Guilford Press.

Barkley, R. A. (1997a). *ADHD and the nature of self-control.* New York: Guilford Press.

Barkley, R. A. (1997b). Behavioral inhibition, sustained attention, and executive functions: Constructing a unifying theory of ADHD. *Psychological Bulletin, 121,* 65–94.

Barkley, R. A. (1997c). Update on a theory of ADHD and its clinical implications. *The ADHD Report, 5,* 10–16.

Barkley, R. A. (1998). *Attention deficit hyperactivity disorder* (2nd ed.). New York: Guilford Press.

Barnett, H. J. M., Mohr, J. P., Stein, B. M., & Yatsu, F. M. (1986). *Stroke: Pathophysiology, diagnosis, and management,* Vols. 1 & 2. New York: Churchill Livingstone.

Barth, J. T., Findley, L. J., Zillmer, E. A., Gideon, D. A., & Surrat, P. M. (1993). Obstructive sleep apnea, hypoxemia, and personality functioning: Implications for medical psychotherapy assessment. *Advances in Medical Psychotherapy, 6,* 29–36.

Barth, J. T., Macciocchi, S. N., Boll, T. J., Giordani, B., Jane, J. A., & Rimel, R. W. (1983). Neuropsychological sequelae of minor head injury. *Neurosurgery, 13,* 529–533.

Basso, A., Spinnler, H., Vallar, G., & Zanobio, M. E. (1982). Left hemisphere damage and selective impairment of auditory verbal short-term memory. A case study. *Neuropsychologia, 20,* 263–274.

Bear, M. F., Connors, B. W., & Paradiso, M. A. (1996). *Neuroscience: Exploring the brain.* Baltimore: Williams & Wilkins.

Beatty, J. (1995). *Principles of behavioral neuroscience.* Chicago: Brown & Benchmark.

Becker, R. O., & Seldon, G. (1985). *The body electric: Electromagnetism and the foundation of life.* New York: William Morrow.

Beh-Yishay, Y., & Prigatano, G. P. (1990). Cognitive remediation. In E. Griffith & M. Rosenthal, eds., *Rehabilitation of the adult and child with traumatic brain injury* (2nd ed.). Philadelphia: F. A. Davis.

Bell, M. A., & Fox, N. A. (1994). Brain development over the first year of life: Relations between electroencephalographic frequency and coherence and cognitive and affective behaviors. In G. Dawson & K. W. Fischer, eds., *Human brain and the developing brain* (pp. 314–345). New York: Guilford Press.

Bender, B. G., Linden, M. G., & Robinson, A. (1994). Neurocognitive and psychosocial phenotypes associated with Turner syndrome. In S. H. Broman & J. Grafman, eds., *Atypical cognitive deficits in developmental disorders* (pp. 197–216). New York: Oxford University Press.

Bender, L. (1938). *A visual motor gestalt test and its clinical use.* Research Monograph No. 3. New York: American Orthopsychiatric Association.

Benes, F. M. (1997). Corticolimbic circuitry and the development of psychopathology during childhood and adolescence. In N. A. Krasnegor, G. R. Lyon, & P. S. Goldman-Rakic, eds., *Development of the prefrontal cortex: Evolution, neurobiology, and behavior* (pp. 211–240). Baltimore: Paul H. Brookes.

Bennett, T. L. (1987). Neuropsychological aspects of complex partial seizures: Diagnostic and treatment issues. *International Journal of Clinical Neuropsychology, 9,* 37–45.

Bennett, T. L. (1992). *The neuropsychology of epilepsy.* New York: Plenum Press.

Bensen, D. F. (1991). The role of frontal dysfunction in attention-deficit hyperactivity disorder. *Journal of Child Neurology, 6,* S9–S12.

Benton, A. L. (1965). *Sentence Memory Test.* Iowa City, IA: Author.

Benton, A. L. (1972). The "minor" hemisphere. *Journal of History of Medicine and Allied Sciences, 27,* 5–14.

Benton, A. L.(1994). Four neuropsychologists. *Neuropsychology Review, 4,* 31–44.

Benton, A. L., & Hamsher, K. deS. (1989). *Multilingual Aphasia Examination.* Iowa City, IA: AJA Associates.

Benton, A. L., Hamsher, K. deS., Varney, N. R., & Spreen, O. (1983). *Contributions to neuropsychological assessment.* New York: Oxford University Press.

Berg, E. A. (1948). A simple objective treatment for measuring flexibility in thinking. *Journal of General Psychology, 39,* 15–22.

Bergman, M. M., & Kemmerer, A. G. (1996). Adaptive software design for people with cognitive deficits: A case illustration. *Society for Cognitive Rehabilitation, Inc.* (Special Edition: Focus on uses of computers in cognitive rehabilitation), *3,* 4–7.

Bernstein, J. H., & Waber, D. P. (1997). Pediatric neuropsychological assessment. In T. E. Feinberg & M. J. Farah, eds., *Behavioral Neurology and Neuropsychology* (pp. 721–728). New York: McGraw-Hill.

Biederman, J., Faraone, S., Mick, E., Wozniak, J., Chen, L., Ouellette, C., Marrs, A., Moore, P., Garcia, J., Mennin, D., & Lelon, E. (1996). Attention-deficit hyperactivity disorder and juvenile mania: An overlooked comorbidity? *Journal of the American Academy of Child and Adolescent Psychiatry, 35,* 997–1008.

Bigler, E. D. (1987). The clinical significance of cerebral atrophy in dementia. *Archives of Clinical Neuropsychology, 2,* 177–190.

Bigler, E. D. (1996). *Neuroimaging,* Vols. 1, 2. New York: Plenum.

Bigler, E. D., Yeo, R. A., & Turkenheimer, E. (1989). *Neuropsychological function and brain imaging.* New York: Plenum Press.

Birkmayer, W., & Hornykiewicz, O. (1961). Der L-dioxyphenalalanin L-DOPA Effekt bei der Parkinson Akinese. *Wiener Klinische Wochenzeitschrift, 73,* 787–793.

Blakemore, C. (1977). *Mechanics of the mind.* Cambridge, England: Cambridge University Press.

Boller, F., & Vignolo, L. A. (1966). Latent sensory aphasia in hemisphere-damaged patients: An experimental study with the Token Test. *Brain, 89,* 815–831.

Bond, M. R. (1976). Assessment of psychosocial outcome of severe head-injury. *Acta Neurochirurgica, 34,* 57–70.

Bond, M. R. (1986). Neurobehavioral sequelae of closed head injury. In I. Grant & K. M. Adams, eds., *Neuropsychological assessment of neuropsychiatric disorders.* New York: Oxford University Press.

Bornstein, R. A., King, G., & Carroll, A. (1983). Neuropsychological abnormalities in Gilles de la Tourette's syndrome. *Journal of Nervous and Mental Disease, 171,* 497–502.

Borod, J. C. (1993). Cerebral mechanisms underlying facial, prosodic and lexical emotional expression: A review of neuropsychological studies and methodological issues. *Neuropsychology, 7,* 445–463.

Borod, J. C., Haywood, C. S., & Koff, E. (1997). Neuropsychological aspects of facial asymmetry during emotional expression: A review of the normal adult literature. *Neuropsychology Review, 7,* 41–60.

Bowen, D. M., Benton, J. S. Spillane, J. A. Smith, C. C. T., & Allen, S. J. (1982). Choline acetyltransferase activity and histopathology of frontal neocortex from biopsies of demented patients. *Journal of Neurological Science, 57,* 191–202.

Bradshaw, J. L., & Mattingly, J. B. (1995). *Clinical neuropsychology: behavioral and brain science.* San Diego, CA: Academic Press.

Brandt, J. A., & Bylsma, F. W. (1993). The dementia of Huntington's disease. In R. W. Parks, R. F. Zec, & R. S. Wilson, eds., *Neuropsychology of Alzheimer's disease and other dementias* (pp. 265–282). New York: Oxford University Press.

Brazier, M. A. B. (1959). The historical development of neurophysiology. In J. Field, H. W. Magoun, & V. E. Hall, eds., *Handbook of physiology,* Vol. 1. Washington, DC: American Physiological Society.

Bressler, S. L., Coppola, R., & Nakamura, R. (1993). Episodic multiregional cortical coherence at multiple frequencies during visual task performance. *Nature, 366,* 153–156.

Brickenkamp, R., & Zillmer, E. A. (1998). *d2 Test of Attention.* Göttingen, Germany: Hogrefe & Huber.

Brittain, J. L., La March, J. A., Reeder, K. P., Roth, D. L., & Boll, T. J. (1991). Effects of age and IQ on Paced Auditory Serial Addition Task (PASAT) performance. *The Clinical Neuropsychologist, 5,* 163–175.

Broca, P. (1861). Perte de la parole. *Bull Soc Anthropol, 2,* 1.

Brodal, A. (1981). *Neuroanatomy in relation to clinical medicine* (3rd ed.). New York: Oxford University Press.

Brodmann, K. (1909). *Vergleichende Lokalisationslehre der Grosshirnrinde in ihren Prinzipien dargestellt auf Grund des Zellenbaues.* Leipzig: Barth.

Brooks, D. N., McKinlay, W., Symington, C., Beatie, A., & Campsie, L. (1987). Return to work within the first seven years of severe head injury. *Brain Injury, 1,* 5–19.

Brookshire, B. L., Fletcher, J. M., Bohan, T. P., Landry, S. H., Davidson, K. C., & Francis, D. J. (1995). Verbal and nonverbal skill discrepancies in children with hydrocephalus: A five-year longitudinal follow-up. *Journal of Pediatric Psychology, 20,* 785–800.

Brown, G. L., & Linnoila, M. I. (1990). CSF serotonin metabolite (5-HIAA) studies in depression, impulsivity, and violence. *Journal of Clinical Psychiatry, 54,* 31–41.

Brown, G., Baird, A. D., & Shatz, M. W. (1986). The effects of cerebrovascular disease and its treatment on higher cortical functioning. In I. Grant & K. M. Adams, eds., *Neuropsychological assessment of neuropsychiatric disorders.* New York: Oxford University Press.

Bruce, D. (1985). On the origin of the term "neuropsychology." *Neuropsychologia, 23,* 813–814.

Buchanan, L., Pavlovic, J., & Rovet, J. (1998). A reexamination of the visuospatial deficit in Turner syndrome: Contributions of working memory. *Developmental Neuropsychology, 14,* 341–368.

Bundick, W. T., Zillmer, E. A., Ives, D., & Beadle-Lindsay, M. (1995). Neurobehavioral sequelae and neurological complications of acute Lyme disease: Case studies of two adults. *Advances in Medical Psychotherapy and Psychodiagnosis, 8,* 145–160.

Burns, A., Jacoby, R., & Levy, R. Computed tomography in Alzheimer's disease: A longitudinal study. *Biological Psychiatry, 29,* 383–390.

Burt, A. M. (1993). *Textbook of neuroanatomy.* Philadelphia: Saunders.

Butters, N., Salmon, D. P., Munro Culum, C., Cairns, P., Troster, A. I., Jacobs, D., Moss, M., & Cermak, L. S. (1988). Differentiation of amnestic and demented patients with the Wechsler Memory Scale–Revised. *The Clinical Neuropsychologist, 2,* 133–148.

Cajal, R. (1937). *Recollections of my life.* Memoirs of the American Philosophical Society, Vol. 8. (Original work published 1901–1917.)

Cannon, W. B. (1927). The James-Lange theory of emotion: A critical examination and an alternative theory. *American Journal of Psychology, 39,* 106–124.

Cantu, R. C. (1996). Head injuries in sport. *British Journal of Sports Medicine, 30,* 289–296.

Cantwell, D. P. (1996). Attention deficit disorder: A review of the past 10 years. *Journal of Child and Adolescent Psychiatry, 35,* 978–987.

Cardon, L. R., DeFries, J. C., Fulker, D. W., Kimberling, W. J., Pennington, B. F., & Smith, S. D. (1994). Quantitative trait locus for reading disability on chromosome 6. *Science, 265,* 276–279.

Carlson, N., & Buskist, W. (1994). *The science of behavior* (5th ed.). Boston: Allyn and Bacon.

Carlson-Green, B., Morris, R. D., & Krawiecki, N. (1995). Family and illness predictors of outcome in pediatric brain tumors. *Journal of Pediatric Psychology, 20*(6), 769–784.

Carmichael Olson, H., Streissguth, A. P., Sampson, P. D., Barr, H. M., Bookstein, F. L., & Thiede, K. (1997). Association of prenatal alcohol exposure with behavioral and learning problems in early adolescence. *Journal of the American Academy of Child and Adolescent Psychiatry, 36,* 1187–1194.

Cartwright, R. D., Kravits, D. O., Eastman, C. I., & Wood, E. (1991). REM latency and the recovery from depression: Getting over divorce. *American Journal of Psychiatry, 148,* 1530–1535.

Cartwright, R. D., Lloyd, S., Knight, S., & Trenholme, I. (1984). Broken dreams: A study of the effects of divorce and depression on dream content. *Psychiatry, 47,* 251–259.

Cascino, G. D. (1992). Complex partial seizures: Clinical features and differential diagnosis. *Psychiatric Clinics of North America, 15*(2), 373–382.

Casey, B. J., Castellanos, F. X., Giedd, J. N., Marsh, W. L., Hamburger, S. D., Schubert, A. B., Vauss, Y. C., Vaituzis, A. C., Dickstein, D. P., Sarfatti, S. E., & Rapoport, J. L. (1997). Implication of right frontostriatal circuitry in response inhibition and attention-deficit hyperactivity disorder. *Journal of Child Psychology and Psychiatry, 36,* 374–383.

Castellanos, F. X. (1997). Toward a pathophysiology of attention-deficit hyperactivity disorder. *Clinical Pediatrics, 36,* 381–393.

Castellanos, F. X., Giedds, J. N., Eckburg, P., Marsh, W. L., Vaituzis, C. V., Kaysen, D., Hamburger, S. D., & Rapoport, J. L. (1994). Quantitative morphology of the caudate nucleus in attention deficit hyperactivity disorder. *American Journal of Psychiatry, 151,* 279–281.

Castellanos, F. X., Giedds, J. N., Marsh, W. L., Hamburger, S. D., Vaituzis, A. C., Dickstein, D. P., Sarfatti, S. E., Vauss, Y. C.,

Snell, J. W., Rajapakse, J. C., & Rapoport, J. L. (1996). Quantitative brain magnetic resonance imaging in attention-deficit hyperactivity disorder. *Archives of General Psychiatry, 53*, 607–616.

Cenci, M. A., Kalen, P., Mandel, R. J., & Bjoerklund, A. (1992). Regional differences in the regulation of dopamine and noradrenaline release in the medial frontal cortex, nucleus accumbens and caudate-putamen: A microdialysis study in the rat. *Brain Research, 581*, 217–228.

Chamberlain, R. S., & Herman, B. H., (1990). A novel model linking dysfunctions in brain melatonin, proopiomelanocortin peptides, and serotonin in autism. *Biological Psychiatry, 28*, 773–793.

Changeux, J.-P., & Chavaillon, J. (1995). *Origins of the human brain.* Oxford, England: Clarendon Press.

Chapman, L. F., & Wolff, H. (1959). The cerebral hemispheres and the highest integrative functions of man. *Archives of Neurology, 1*, 357.

Charman, T. (1997). The relationship between joint attention and pretend play in autism. *Development and Psychopathology, 9*, 1–16.

Christensen, A-L. (1979). *Luria's neuropsychological investigation* (2nd ed.). Copenhagen: Munksgaard.

Churchland, P. S. (1993). *Neurophilosophy: Toward a unified science of the mind/brain.* Cambridge, MA: MIT Press.

Chusid, J. G. (1982). *Correlative neuroanatomy and functional neurology.* Los Altos, CA: Lange Medical.

Chute, D. L. (1993a). The Classroom 2000 Project: A personal view of what the past tells us about the future. *Social Science Computer Review II, 4*, 477–486.

Chute, D. L. (1993b). MacLaboratory for psychology: Success, failures, economics, and outcomes over its decade of development. *Behavior Research Methods, Instruments, and Computers, 25*, 180–188.

Chute, D. L. (1996). Things I wish they had told me about technology. *Psychology Software News* (Center for Technology and Instruction, York, England), *5*(1), 2–12.

Chute, D. L., Conn, G., Dipasquale, M. C., & Hoag, M. (1988). ProsthesisWare: A new class of software supporting the activities of daily living. *Neuropsychology, 2*, 41–57.

Chute, D. L., & Westall, R. F. (1996). Fifth generation research tools: Collaborative development with PowerLaboratory. *Behavior Research Methods Instruments and Computers, 25*, 180–188.

Ciesielski, K. T., & Harris, R. J. (1997). Factors related to performance failure on executive tasks in autism. *Child Neuropsychology, 3*, 1–12.

Cohen, J. D., Noll, D. C., & Schneider, W. (1993). Functional magnetic resonance imaging: Overview and methods for psychological research. *Behavior Research Methods, Instruments, & Computers, 25*, 101–113.

Cohen, N. J. (1984). Preserved learning capacity in amnesia: Evidence for multiple memory systems. In L. R. Squire & N. Butters, eds., *Neuropsychology of memory.* New York: Guilford Press.

Cohen, R. A. (1993). *The neuropsychology of attention.* New York: Plenum Press.

Cook, E. H., Jr., Stein, M. A., Krasowski, M. D., Cox, N. J., Olkon, D. M., Kieffer, J. E., & Leventhal, B. L. (1995). Association of attention-deficit disorder and the dopamine transporter gene. *American Journal of Human Genetics, 56*, 933–998.

Corder, E. H., Saunders, A. M., Strittmatter, W. J., Schmechel, D. E., Gaskell, P. C., Small, G. W., Roses, A. D., Haines, J. L., & Pericak-Vance, M. A. (1993). Gene dose of apolipoprotein E type 4 allele and the risk of Alzheimer's disease in late onset families. *Science, 261*, 921–923.

Corkin, S. (1965). Tactually guided maze learning in man. Effects of unilateral cortical excisions and bilateral hippocampal lesions. *Neuropsychologia, 3*, 339.

Corn, B. W., Yousem, D. M., Scott, C. B., Rotman, M., Asbell, S. O., Nelson, D. F., Martin, L., & Curran, W. J. (1994). White matter changes are correlated significantly with radiation dose. *Cancer, 74*, 2828–2835.

Cote, L., & Crutcher, M. D. (1991). The basal ganglia. In E. R. Kandel, J. H. Schwartz, & T. M. Jessell, eds., *Principles of neural science* (3rd ed.), (pp. 647–659). New York: Elsevier Science.

Cowan, W. C. (1979). The developing brain. In W. C. Cowan, ed., *The brain* (pp. 56–69). San Francisco: W. H. Freeman.

Cowan, W. M. (1990). The development of the brain. In R. R. Llinas, ed., *The workings of the brain: Development, memory, and perception.* New York: W. H. Freeman.

Cowart, B. J., Young, I. M., Feldman, R. S., & Lowry, L. D. (1997). Clinical disorders of smell and taste. In G. K. Beauchamp & L. Bartoshuk, eds., *Tasting and Smelling.* San Diego, CA: Academic Press.

Coyle, J. T. (1985). The cholinergic systems in psychiatry. In R. E. Hales & A. J. Frances, eds., *Psychiatry Update: American Psychiatric Association Annual Review,* Vol. 4. Washington, DC: American Psychiatric Press.

Crick, F., & Koch, C. (1990). Towards a neurobiological theory of consciousness. *Seminars in the Neurosciences, 2*, 263–275.

Crosson, B. (1992). *Subcortical functions in language and memory.* New York: Guilford Press.

Culbertson, J. L., & Edmonds, J. E. (1996). Learning disabilities. In R. L. Adams, O. A. Parsons, J. L. Culbertson, & S. J. Nixon, eds., *Neuropsychology for clinical practice: Etiology, assessment, and treatment of common neurological disorders* (pp. 331–408). Washington, DC: American Psychological Association.

Culbertson, W. C., & Zillmer, E. A. (1998a). The construct validity of the Tower of London–Drexel University as a measure of the executive functioning of ADHD children. *Assessment, 5*, 215–226.

Culbertson, W. C., & Zillmer, E. A. (1998b). *TOL-DX Tower of London–Drexel University.* Chicago: Multi-Health Systems.

Culbertson, W. C., & Zillmer, E. A. (1998c). Tower of London[DX]: A standardized approach to assessing executive functioning in children. *Archives of Clinical Neuropsychology, 13*, 285–301.

Culbertson, W. C., & Zillmer, E. A. (2000). Tower of London^{DX}: Research version (TOL^{DX}:RV). North Tonawanda, NY: Multi-Health Systems.

Culbertson, W. C., Zillmer, E. A., & Di Pinto, M. (1999). The relationship of a neuropsychological model of inhibitory control to the TOL–Drexel performance of ADHD children. *Archives of Clinical Neuropsychology, 8,* 691–692.

Cullum, C. M., Harris, J. G., Waldo, M., Smernoff, E., Madison, A., Nagamoto, H., Adler, L., & Freedman, R. (1993). Neurophysiological and neuropsychological evidence for attentional dysfunction in schizophrenia. *Schizophrenia Research, 10,* 131–141.

Cummings, J. L. (1986). Subcortical dementia: Neuropsychology, neuropsychiatry, and pathophysiology. *British Journal of Psychiatry, 149,* 682–697.

Cummings, J. L. (1993). Frontal-subcortical circuits and human behavior. *Archives of Neurology, 50,* 873–880.

Cummings, J. L. (1994). Depression in neurologic diseases. *Psychiatric Annals, 24,* 525–531.

Cummings, J. L., & Benson, D. F. (1984). Subcortical dementia: Review of an emerging concept. *Archives of Neurology, 41,* 874–879.

Cummings, J. L., Benson, D. F., Hill, M., & Read, S. (1985). Aphasia in dementia of the Alzheimer type. *Neurology, 35,* 394–397.

Cytowic, R. E. (1993). *The man who tasted shapes: A bizarre medical mystery offers revolutionary insights into reasoning, emotion, and consciousness.* New York: Putnam's.

Damasio, A. R. (1994). *Descartes' error.* New York: Putnam's.

Damasio, H. C. (1991). Neuroanatomy of frontal lobe in vivo: A comment on methodology. In H. S. Levin, H. M. Eisenberg, & A. L. Benton, eds., *Frontal lobe functioning and dysfunction.* New York: Oxford University Press.

Damasio, H., Grabowski, T., Frank, R., Galaburda, A. M., & Damasio, A. M. (1994). The return of Phineas Gage: Clues about the brain from the skull of a famous patient. *Science, 264,* 1102–1105.

Danta, G., & Hilton, R. (1975). Judgement of the visual vertical and horizontal in patients with Parkinsons. *Neurology, 25,* 43–47.

Darwin, C. (1968). *On the origin of species.* New York: Penguin Books. (Originally published 1859).

Davidson, R. J. (1994). Temperament, affective style, and frontal lobe asymmetry. In G. Dawson & K. W. Fischer, eds., *Human brain and the developing brain* (pp. 518–537). New York: Guilford Press.

Davis, K. L., Kahn, R. S., Ko, G., & Davidson, M. (1991). Dopamine and schizophrenia: A review and reconceptualization. *American Journal of Psychiatry, 148,* 1474–1486.

Dawson, M. E., & Nuechterlein, K. H. (1984). Psychophysiological dysfunctions in the developmental course of schizophrenic disorders. *Schizophrenia Bulletin, 10*(2), 204–232.

DeAngelis, L., Delattre, J. Y., & Posner, J. (1989). Radiation-induced dementia in patients cured of brain metastases. *Neurology, 39,* 789–796.

deGroot, J. (1991). *Correlative neuroanatomy* (21st ed.). Norwalk, CT: Appleton & Lange.

Del Bigio, M. R. (1993). Neurpathological changes caused by hydrocephalus. *Acta Neuropathologica, 85,* 573–585.

Denckla, M. B. (1996). A theory and model of executive function: A neuropsychological perspective. In G. R. Lyon & N. A. Krasnegor, eds., *Attention, memory, and executive function* (pp. 263–278). Baltimore: Paul H. Brookes.

Denckla, M. B., & Reiss, A. L. (1997). Prefrontal-subcortical circuits in developmental disorders. In N. A. Krasnegor, G. R. Lyon, & P. S. Goldman-Rakic, eds., *Development of the prefrontal cortex: Evolution, neurobiology, and behavior* (pp. 283–294). Baltimore, MD: Paul H. Brookes.

Dennis, M., & Barnes, M. (1994). Developmental aspects of neuropsychology: Childhood. In D. W. Zaidel, ed., *Neuropsychology* (2nd ed.), (pp. 219–246). New York: Academic Press.

Descartes, R. (1664). *Traité de l'Homme* [Treatise on man]. Paris: Angot.

Devinsky, O. (1983). Neuroanatomy of Gilles de la Tourette's syndrome. *Archives of Neurology, 5,* 447–453.

Diamond, A. (1981). Retrieval of an object from an open box: The development of visual-tactile control of reaching in the first year of life. *Society for Research in Child Development Abstracts, 3,* 78.

Diamond, A. (1991). Neuropsychological insights into the meaning of object concept development. In S. Carey & R. Gelman, eds., *The epigenesis of mind: Essays on biology and cognition* (pp. 67–110). Hillsdale, NJ: Erlbaum.

Diamond, A., & Gilbert, J. (1989). Development as progressive inhibitory control of action: Retrieval of a contiguous object. *Cognitive Development, 12,* 223–249.

Diamond, R., Barth, J. T., & Zillmer, E. A. (1988). An investigation of the psychological component of mild head injury: The role of the MMPI. *International Journal of Clinical Neuropsychology, 10,* 35–40.

Diller, L. (1987). Neuropsychological rehabilitation. In M. J. Meier, A. L. Benton, & L. Diller, eds., *Neuropsychological rehabilitation.* Edinburgh: Churchill Livingstone.

Diller, L. (1994). Finding the right treatment combinations: Changes in rehabilitation over the past five years. In A. Christensen & B. P. Uzzell, eds., *Brain injury and neuropsychological rehabilitation: International perspectives.* Hillsdale, NJ: Erlbaum.

Dodrill, C. B. (1979). Sex differences on the Halstead-Reitan Neuropsychological Battery and on other neuropsychological measures. *Journal of Clinical Psychology, 35,* 236–241.

Dool, C. B., Stelmack, R. M., & Rourke, B. P. (1993). Event-related potentials in children with learning disabilities. *Journal of Clinical Child Psychology, 22,* 387–398.

Doty, R. L. (1990). Olfaction. In F. Boller & J. Grafman, eds., *Handbook of neuropsychology,* Vol. 4. Amsterdam: Elsevier.

Doty, R. L., Shaman, P., & Dann, M. (1984). Development of the University of Pennsylvania Smell Identification Test. A standard microencapsulated test of olfactory function. *Physiology of Behavior, 32,* 489–502.

Douglas, R. J., & Pribram, K. H. (1966). Learning aids and limbic lesions. *Neuropsychologia, 4,* 197.

Dr. Robert Ley's brain. (1946). *Medical Record, 159,* 188.

Drachmann, D. A. (1977). Memory function in man: Does the cholinergic system have a specific role? *Neurology, 27,* 783–790.

Dubois, B., Boller, F., Pillon, B., & Agid, Y. (1991). Cognitive deficits in Parkinson's disease. In S. Corkin, J. Grafman, & F. Boller, eds., *Handbook of neuropsychology,* Vol. 5 (pp. 195–240). Amsterdam: Elsevier.

Duffy, F. H. (1989). Clinical value of topographic mapping and quantified neurophysiology. *Archives of Neurology, 46,* 1133–1135.

Dunn, L. M. (1965). *Expanded manual for the Peabody Picture Vocabulary Test.* Minneapolis, MN: American Guidance Service.

Dunn, L. M., & Markwardt, F. C. (1970). *Peabody Individual Achievement Test.* Circle Pines, MN: American Guidance Service.

Dunnet, S. B. (1991). Neural transplants as a treatment for Alzheimer's disease? *Psychological Medicine, 21,* 825–830.

Earle, K. M. (1955). Metastatic brain tumors. *Disorders of Nervous System, 16,* 86.

Ebers, G. C., & Sadovnick, A. D. (1993). The geographic distribution of multiple sclerosis. *Neuroepidemiology, 12,* 1–5.

Ecobichon, D., & Joy, R. (1982). *Pesticides and neurological diseases.* Florida: CRC Press.

Eden, G. F., Stein, J. F., Wood, M. H., & Wood, F. B. (1995). Verbal and visual problems in reading disability. *Journal of Learning Disabilities, 28,* 272–290.

Efron, R. (1957). The conditioned inhibition of uncinate fits. *Brain,* 251–261.

Ehlers, S., Nyden, A., Gillberg, C., Sandberg, A. D., Dahlgren, S. O., Hjlemquist, E., & Oden, A. (1997). Asperger's syndrome, autism and attention disorders: A comparative study of the cognitive profiles of 120 children. *Journal of the American Academy of Child and Adolescent Psychiatry, 38,* 207–217.

Eiraldi, R. B., Power, T. J., & Nezu, C. M. (1997). Patterns of comorbidity associated with subtypes of attention-deficit/hyperactivity disorder among 6- to 12-year-old children. *Journal of the American Academy of Child and Adolescent Psychiatry, 36,* 503–514.

Eisenmajer, R., Prior, M., Leekam, S., Wing, L., Gould, J., Gelham, M., & Ong, B. (1996). Comparison of clinical symptoms in autism and Asperger's disorder. *Journal of the American Academy of Child and Adolescent Psychiatry, 35,* 1523–1531.

Elliott, F. A. (1992). Violence—the neurologic contribution: An overview. *Archives of Neurology, 49,* 595–603.

Elliott, T. K., Watkins, J. M., Messa, C., Lippe, B., & Chugani, H. (1996). Positron emission tomography and neuropsychological correlations in children with Turner's syndrome. *Developmental Neuropsychology, 12,* 365–386.

Elsass, L., & Kinsella, G. (1987). Social interaction following severe closed head injury. *Psychological Medicine, 17,* 67–78.

England, M. A., & Wakely, J. (1991). *Brain and spinal cord: An introduction to normal neuro-anatomy.* Aylesbury, England: Mosby-Wolfe.

Ernst, M., Liebenauer, L. L., Jons, P. H., & Zametkin, A. J. (1994). Cerebral glucose metabolism in adolescent girls with attention-deficit/hyperctivity disorder. *Journal of the American Academy of Child and Adolescent Psychiatry, 36,* 1399–1406.

Ernst, M., Liebenauer, L. L., King, A. C., Fitzgerald, G. A., Cohen, R. M., & Zametkin, A. J. (1994). Reduced brain metabolism in hyperactive girls. *Journal of the American Academy of Child and Adolescent Psychiatry, 33,* 858–868.

Eslinger, P. J., Biddle, K. R., & Grattan L. M. (1997). Cognitive and social development in children with prefrontal cortex lesions. In N. A. Krasnegor, G. R. Lyon, & P. S. Goldman-Rakic, eds., *Development of the prefrontal cortex: Evolution, neurobiology, and behavior* (pp. 295–336). Baltimore: Paul H. Brookes.

Exner, J. E. (1993). *The Rorschach: A comprehensive system, Vol. 1: Basic foundations* (3rd ed.). New York: Wiley.

Farah, M. J. (1990). *Visual agnosia: Disorders of object vision and what they tell us about normal vision.* Cambridge, MA: MIT Press/Bradford.

Farrer, L. A. (1986). Suicide and attempted suicide in Huntington's disease: Implications of preclinical testing for persons at risk. *American Journal of Medical Genetics, 24,* 305–311.

Faust, D., Hart, K., & Guilmette, T. J. (1988). Pediatric malingering: The capacity of children to fake believable deficits on neuropsychological testing. *Journal of Consulting and Clinical Psychology, 56,* 578–582.

Fein, D., Joy, S., Green, L. A., & Waterhouse, L. (1996). Autism and pervasive developmental disorders. In B. S. Fogel, R. R. Schiffer, & S. M. Rao, eds., *Neuropsychiatry* (pp. 571–614). Philadelphia: Williams & Wilkins.

Feldman, R. S., Meyer, J. S., & Quenzer, L. F. (1997). *Principles of neuropsychopharmacology.* Sunderland, MA: Sinauer Associates.

Fibiger, H. C. (1991). The dopamine hypothesis of schizophrenia and mood disorders: Contradictions and speculations. In P. Willner & J. Scheel-Krüger, eds., *The mesolimbic dopamine system: From motivation to action.* Chichester, England: Wiley.

Filipek, P. A. (1996). Structural variations in measures of developmental disorders. In R. W. Thatcher, G. R. Lyon, J. Rumsey, & N. Krasnegor, eds., *Developmental neuroimaging: Mapping the development of brain and behavior* (pp. 169–186). San Diego, CA: Academic Press.

Filipek, P. A., Semrud-Clikeman, M., Steingard, R. J., Renshaw, P. F., Kennedy, D. N., & Biederman, J. (1997). Volumetric MRI analysis comparing subjects having attention-deficit hyperactivity disorder with normal controls. *Neurology, 48,* 589–601.

Fisher, N. J., DeLuca, J. W., & Rourke, B. P. (1997). Wisconsin Card Sorting Test and Halstead Category Test performances of children and adolescents who exhibit the syndrome of nonverbal learning disabilities. *Child Neuropsychology, 3,* 61–70.

Fletcher, J. M., Brookshire, B. L., Landry, S. H., Bohan, T. P., Davidson, K. C., Francis, D. J., Levin, H. S., Brandt, M. E., Kramer, L. A., & Morris, R. D. (1996). Attention skills and executive functions in children with early hydrocephalus. *Developmental Neuropsychology, 12,* 53–76.

Fletcher, J. M., Francis, D. J., Thompson, N. M., Brookshire, B. L., Bohan, T. P., Landry, S. H., Davidson, K. C., & Miner, M. E. (1992). Verbal and nonverbal discrepancies in hydrocephalic children. *Journal of Clinical and Experimental Neuropsychology, 14,* 593–609.

Flowers, D. L., Wood, F. B., & Naylor, C. E. (1991). Regional cerebral blood flow correlates of language processes in reading disability. *Archives of Neurology, 48,* 637–643.

Foley, B., Barakat, L. P., Herman-Liu, A., Radcliffe, J., & Molloy, P. (In press). The impact of childhood hypothalamic/chiasmatic brain tumors on child adjustment and family functioning. *Children's Health Care.*

Ford, C. E., Jones, K. W., Polani, P. E., de Almeida, J. C., & Briggs, J. H. (1959). A sex-chromosome anomaly in a case of gonadal dysgenesis (Turner syndrome). *Lancet, 2,* 711–713.

Forstl, H., & Hentschel, F. (1994). Contribution to the differential diagnosis of dementias: Neuroimaging. *Reviews in Clinical Gerontology, 4,* 317–341.

Frackowiak, R. S. J. (1996). Plasticity and the human brain: Insights from functional imaging. In E. L. Bjork & R. A. Bjork, eds., *Memory.* NY: Academic Press.

Freedman, A. M., Kaplan, H. I., & Sadock, B. J. (1978). *Modern synopsis of comprehensive textbook of Psychiatry II.* Baltimore: Williams & Wilkins.

Freeman, W., & Watts, J. W. (1950). *Psychosurgery in the treatment of mental disorders and intractable pain.* Springfield, IL: Charles C Thomas.

Freud, S. (1891). *Zur Auffassung der Aphasien* [An understanding of aphasia]. Vienna: Deuticke.

Freud, S. (1959). On narcissism: An introduction. In S. Freud, *Collected papers* (pp. 30–59). New York: Basic Books. Originally published 1914.

Freund, H.-J. (1996). Remapping the brain. *Science, 272,* 1754.

Frith, U. (1989). *Autism: Explaining the enigma.* Cambridge, MA: Blackwell.

Frith, U. (1991). Asperger and his syndrome. In U. Frith, ed., *Autism and Asperger syndrome* (pp. 1–36). New York: Cambridge University Press.

Frombonne, E., Bolton, P., Prior, J., Jordon, H., & Rutter, M. (1997). A family study of autism: Cognitive patterns and levels in parents and siblings. *Journal of Clinical Psychology and Psychiatry, 38,* 667–683.

Fuster, J. M. (1991). Role of prefrontal cortex in delay tasks: Evidence from reversible lesion and unit recording in the monkey. In H. S. Levin, H. M. Eisenberg, & A. L. Benton, eds., *Frontal lobe functioning and dysfunction.* New York: Oxford University Press.

Gaddes, W. H. & Edgell, D. (1993). *Learning disabilities and brain function* (3rd ed.). New York: Springer.

Gajdusek, D. C. (1988). Transmissible and non-transmissible amyloidoses: Autocatalytic post-translational conversion of host precursor proteins to fl-pleated configurations. *Journal of Neuroimmunology, 20,* 95–110.

Galaburda, A., & Livingstone, M. (1993). Evidence for a magnocellular defect in developmental dyslexia. *Annals of the New York Academy of Sciences, 682,* 70–82.

Garay, M. (1996). Neurocognitive Driving Assessment System. In D. L. Chute & R. F. Westall, eds., *B/C PowerLaboratory.* Pacific Grove, CA: Brooks/Cole.

Gazzaniga, M. S. (1966). Interhemispheric communication of visual learning. *Neuropsychologia, 4,* 183.

Gennarelli, T. A. (1983). Head injury in man and experimental animals: Clinical aspects. *Acta Neurochirugica, Suppl., 32,* 1–13.

Gennarelli, T. A. (1984, October 9). From the experimental head injury laboratory. *Almanac,* 6–7.

Geschwind, N. (1965). Disconnexion syndromes in animals and man. *Brain, 88,* 237–294.

Geschwind, N., & Levitsky, W. (1968). Human brain: Left-right asymmetries in temporal speech region. *Science, 161,* 186–187.

Giedd, J. N., Castellanos, F. X., Casey, B. J., Kozuch, P., King, A. C., Hamburger, S. D., & Rapoport, J. L. (1994). Quantitative morphology of the corpus callosum in attention deficit hyperactivity disorder. *American Journal of Psychiatry, 151,* 665–669.

Gilman, S., & Newman, S. W. (1996). *Essentials of clinical neuroanatomy and neurophysiology* (9th ed.), Philadelphia: F. A. Davis.

Gilman, S., & Newman, W. S. (1996). The cerebrospinal fluid. In *Manter & Katz's Clinical neuroanatomy and neuropsychology* (9th ed.). Philadelphia: F. A. Davis.

Glaser, G. H., & Pincus, J. H. (1969). Limbic encephalitis. *Journal of Nervous Mental Disorder, 149,* 59.

Glidden, R. A., Zillmer, E. A., & Barth, J. T. (1990). The long-term neurobehavioral effects of prefrontal lobotomy. *The Clinical Neuropsychologist, 4,* 301.

Goldberg, E. (1992). Introduction: The frontal lobes in neurological and psychiatric conditions. *Neuropsychiatry, Neuropsychology, and Behavioral Neurology, 5,* 231–232.

Goldberg, E., & Costa, L. (1981). Hemispheric differences in the acquisition and use of descriptive systems. *Brain and Language, 14,* 14–22.

Goldberg, E., Bilder, R. M., Hughes, J. E. O., Antin, S. P., & Mattis, S. (1989). A reticulo-frontal disconnection syndrome. *Cortex, 25,* 687–695.

Goldberg, E., Podell, K., Harner, R., Lovell, M., & Riggio, S. (1994). Cognitive bias, functional cortical geometry, and the frontal lobes: Laterality, sex, and handedness. *Journal of Cognitive Neuroscience, 6,* 276–296.

Golden, C. J. (1978). *The Stroop Color and Word Test.* Chicago: Stoelting.

Golden, C. J., Zillmer, E. A., & Spiers, M. V. (1992). *Neuropsychological assessment and intervention.* Springfield, IL: Charles C. Thomas.

Goldenberg, G., Wimmer, A., Auff, E., & Schnaberth, G. (1986). Impairment of motor planning in patients with Parkinson's disease; evidence for ideomotor apraxia. *Journal of Neurology, Neurosurgery, and Psychiatry, 49,* 1266–1272.

Goldman, S., & Nottebohm, F. (1983). Neuronal production, migration, and differentiation in a vocal control nucleus of the adult female canary brain. *Proceedings of the National Academy of Sciences, USA, 80,* 2390–2394.

Goldman-Rakic, P. S. (1987a). Circuitry of primate prefrontal cortex and representation of behavior by representational memory. In F. Plum, ed., *Handbook of physiology: The nervous system Vol. V.* Bethesda, MD: American Physiological Society.

Goldman-Rakic, P. S. (1987b). Development of cortical circuitry and cognitive function. *Child Development, 58,* 601–622.

Goldman-Rakic, P. S. (1988). Topography of cognition: Parallel distributed networks in primary association cortex. *Annual Review of Neuroscience, 11,* 137–156.

Goldman-Rakic, P. S. (1993). Working memory and the mind. In *Mind and brain: Readings from* Scientific American. New York: W. H. Freeman.

Goldman-Rakic, P. S., & Friedman, H. R. (1991). The circuitry to working memory revealed by anatomy and metabolic imaging. In H. S. Levin, H. M. Eisenberg, & A. L. Benton, eds., *Frontal lobe functioning and dysfunction.* New York: Oxford University Press.

Goldstein, E. B. (1994). *Psychology.* Pacific Grove, CA: Brooks/Cole.

Gordon, A., & Zillmer, E. A. (1997). Integrating the MMPI and neuropsychology: A survey of NAN membership. *Archives of Clinical Neuropsychology, 4,* 325–326.

Gould, S. J. (1981). *The mismeasure of man.* New York: Norton.

Graf, P., & Schacter, D. L. (1985). Implicit and explicit memory for new associations in normal and amnesic subjects. *Journal of Experimental Psychology: Learning Memory & Cognition, 2,* 501–518.

Grant, D. A., & Berg, E. A. (1948). A behavioral analysis of degree of reinforcement and ease of shifting two new responses in a Weigl-type card sorting problem. *Journal of Experimental Psychology, 38,* 404–411.

Grattan, L. M., & Eslinger, P. J. (1989). Higher cognition and social behavior: Changes in cognitive flexibility and empathy after cerebral lesions. *Neuropsychology, 3,* 175–185.

Greene, R. (1991). *The MMPI-2/MMPI: An interpretative manual.* Boston: Allyn and Bacon.

Grigorenko, E. L., Wood, F. B., Meyer, M. S., Hart, L. A., Speed, W. C., Shuster, A., & Pauls, D. L. (1997). Susceptibility loci for distinct components of developmental dyslexia on chromosome 6 and 15. *American Journal of Human Genetics, 60,* 27–39.

Gronwall, D. M. A. (1977). Paced Auditory Serial-Addition Task: A measure of recovery from concussion. *Perceptual and Motor Skills, 44,* 367–373.

Gronwall, D., & Wrightson, P. (1975). Cumulative effect of concussion. *Lancet, 2,* 995–997.

Guilleminault, C. (1982). *Sleeping and waking disorders: Indications and techniques.* Menlo Park, CA: Addison-Wesley.

Guilleminault, C., & Dement, W. C. (1978). Sleep apnea syndromes and related sleep disorders. In R. L. Williams & I. Karacan, eds., *Sleep disorders: Diagnosis and treatment.* New York: Wiley.

Gur, R. C., Gur, R. E., Obrist, W. D., Hungerbuhler, J. P., Younkin, D., Rosen, A. D., Skolnick, B. E., & Reivich, M. (1982). Sex and handedness differences in cerebral blood flow during rest and cognitive activity. *Science, 217,* 659–660.

Gur, R. E., Levy, J., & Gur, R. C. (1977). Clinical studies of brain organization and behavior. In A. Frazer & A. Winokur, eds., *Biological bases of psychiatric disorders.* New York: Spectrum.

Haeger, K. (1988). *The illustrated history of surgery.* New York: Bell.

Haines, D. E. (1997). *Fundamental neuroscience.* New York: Churchill Livingstone.

Hainline, B. E., Padilla, L.M., Chong, S. K., Heifetz, S. A., Palmer, C., & Zhou, F. C. (1995). Fetal tissue derived from spontaneous pregnancy losses is insufficient for human transplantation. *Obstetrics and Gynecology, 85*(4), 619–624.

Hallgren, B. (1950). Specific dyslexia (congenital word blindness): A clinical and genetic study. *Acta Psychiatrica et Neurologica, Suppl., 65,* 1–28.

Halstead, W. C. (1947). *Brain and intelligence: A quantitative study of the frontal lobes.* Chicago: University of Chicago Press.

Hari, R. (1994). Human cortical functions revealed by magnetoencephalography. *Progress in Brain Research, 100,* 163–168.

Harlow, H. F. (1952). Functional organization of the brain in relation to mentation and behavior. In Milbank Memorial Fund, ed., *The Biology of Mental Health and Disease.* New York: Hoeber.

Harlow, J. M. (1868). Recovery from the passage of an iron bar through the head. *Publications of the Massachusetts Medical Society, 2,* 327–347.

Harnadek, M. C. S., & Rourke, B. P. (1994). Principal identifying features of the syndrome of nonverbal learning disabilities in children. *Journal of Learning Disabilities, 27,* 144–154.

Harris, J. C. (1995). *Developmental neuropsychiatry.* New York: Oxford University Press.

Harrower, M. (1991). Inkblots and poems. In C. D. Walker, ed., *Clinical psychology in autobiography* (pp. 125–170). Pacific Grove, CA: Brooks/Cole.

Hartman, D. E. (1988). *Neuropsychological toxicology: Identification and assessment of human neurotoxic syndromes.* New York: Pergamon Press.

Hasselbalch, S. G., Oberg, G., Sorensen, S., Andersen, A. R., Waldemar, G., Schmidt, J. F., Fenger, K., & Paulson, O. B. (1992). Reduced regional cerebral blood flow in Huntington's disease studied by SPECT. *Journal of Neurology, Neurosurgery, and Psychiatry, 55,* 1018–1023.

Hauri, P. (1997). *The sleep disorders.* Kalamazoo, MI: Upjohn Company.

Hauser, P., Zametkin, A. J., Martinez, P., Vitiello, B., Matochik, J. A., Mixon, A. J., & Weintraub, B. D. (1993). Attention deficit-hyperactivity disorder in people with generalized resistance to thryroid hormone. *New England Journal of Medicine, 328,* 997–1001.

Hauser, W. A. (1992). Seizure disorders: The changes with age. *Epilepsia, 33*(Suppl. 4), S6–S14.

Haynes, S. D., & Bennett, T. L. (1990). Cognitive impairments in adults with complex partial seizures. *International Journal of Clinical Neuropsychology, 12,* 74–81.

Heaton, R. K., Chelune, G. J., Talley, J. L., Kay, G. G., & Curtis, G. (1993). *Wisconsin Card Sorting Test manual: Revised and expanded.* Odessa, FL: Psychological Assessment Resources.

Heaton, R. K., Grant, I., & Matthews, C. G. (1991). *Comprehensive norms for an extended Halstead-Reitan battery: Demographic corrections, research findings, and clinical applications.* Odessa, FL: Psychological Assessment Resources.

Hebb, D. O. (1949). *The organization of behavior: A neuropsychological theory.* New York: Wiley.

Hebb, D. O. (1959). Intelligence, brain function and the theory of mind. *Brain, 82,* 260.

Hebb, D. O. (1983). Neuropsychology: Retrospect and prospect. *Canadian Journal of Psychology, 37,* 4–7.

Hécaen, H., & Albert, M. L. (1978). *Human neuropsychology.* New York: Wiley.

Heilman, K. M., Watson, R. T., & Valenstein, E. (1993). Neglect and related disorders. In K. M. Heilman & E. Valenstein, eds., *Clinical Neuropsychology* (3rd ed.). New York: Oxford University Press.

Heindel, W. C., Salmon, D. P. , Shults, C. W., Wallcke, P. A., & Butters, N. (1989). Neuropsychological evidence for multiple implicit memory systems: A comparison of Alzheimer's and Parkinson's disease patients. *Journal of Neuroscience, 9,* 582–587.

Heller, K. W. (1996). *Understanding physical, sensory, and health impairments.* Pacific Grove, CA: Brooks/Cole.

Hinshaw, S. P. (1992). Academic underachievement, attention deficits, and aggression: Comorbidity and implications for intervention. *Journal of Consulting and Clinical Psychology, 60,* 893–903.

Hirsch, H. V. B., & Jacobson, M. (1974). The perfect brain. In M. S. Gazzaniga & C. B. Blakemore, eds., *Fundamentals of psychobiology.* New York: Academic Press.

Hobson, J. A. (1995). *Sleep.* New York: Scientific American Library.

Hodges, J. R., Salmon, D. P., & Butters, N. (1991). The nature of the naming deficit in Alzheimer's and Huntington's disease. *Brain, 114,* 1547–1558.

Hoehn, M. M., & Yahr, M. D. (1967). Parkinsonism: Onset, progression, and mortality. *Neurology, 17,* 427–442.

Hooper, H. E. (1983). *Hooper Visual Organization Test (VOT).* Los Angeles: Western Psychological Services.

Hooper, S. R., Willis, W. G., & Stone, B. H. (1996). Issues and approaches in the neuropsychological treatment of children with learning disabilities. In E. S. Batchelor & R. S. Dean, eds., *Pediatric neuropsychology: Interfacing assessment and treatment in rehabilitation* (pp. 211–248). Boston: Allyn and Bacon.

Hornak, J. (1992). Ocular exploration in the dark by patients with visual neglect. *Neuropsychologia, 30,* 353–384.

Hubel, D. H. (1988). *Eye, brain, vision.* New York: Scientific American Library.

Hudspeth, W. J., & Pribram, K. H. (1990). Stages of brain and cognitive maturation. *Journal of Educational Psychology, 82,* 881–884.

Hudspeth, W. J., & Pribram, K. H. (1992). Psychophysiological indices of cerebral maturation. *International Journal of Psychophysiology, 12,* 19–29.

Hughes, C., Russell, J., & Robbins, T. W. (1994). Evidence for executive dysfunction in autism. *Neuropsychologia, 32,* 477–492.

Hutt, M. L. (1985). *The Hutt adaptation of the Bender-Gestalt Test: Rapid screening and intensive diagnosis* (4th ed.). Orlando, FL: Grune & Stratton.

Huttenlocher, P. R. (1990). Morphometric study of human cerebral cortex development. *Neuropsychologia, 28,* 517–527.

Huttenlocher, P. R., & Dabholkar, A. S. (1997). Developmental anatomy of prefrontal cortex. In N. A. Krasnegor, G. R. Lyon, & P. S. Goldman-Rakic, eds., *Development of the prefrontal cortex: Evolution, neurobiology, and behavior* (pp. 69–84). Baltimore: Paul H. Brookes.

Hynd, G. W., & Hiemenz, J. R. (1997). Dyslexia and gyral morphology variations. In C. Hulme & M. Snowling, eds., *Dyslexia: Biology, cognition and intervention* (pp. 38–58). London: Whurr.

Hynd, G. W., & Willis, W. G. (1988). *Pediatric neuropsychology.* Boston: Allyn and Bacon.

Hynd, G. W., Hall, J., Novey, E. S., Eliopulos, D., Black, K., Gonzales, J. J., Edmonds, J. E., Riccio, C., & Cohen, M. (1995). Dyslexia and corpus callosum morphology. *Archives of Neurology, 52,* 32–38.

Hynd, G. W., Hern, K. L., Novey, E. S., Eliopulos, D., Marshall, R., Gonzalez, J. J., & Voeller, K. K. (1993). Attention deficit-hyperactivity disorder and asymmetry of the caudate nucleus. *Journal of Child Neurology, 8,* 339–347.

Hynd, G. W., Morgan, A. E., & Vaughn M. (1997). Neurodevelopmental anomalies and malformations. In C. R. Reynolds & E. Fletcher-Janzen, eds., *Handbook of clinical child neuropsychology* (2nd ed.), (pp. 42–61). New York: Plenum Press.

Hynd, G. W., Semrud-Clikeman, M., Lorys, A. R., Novey, E. S., & Eliopulos, D. (1990). Brain morphology in developmental dyslexia and attention deficit disorder/hyperactivity. *Archives of Neurology, 47,* 919–926.

Hynd, G. W., Semrud-Clikeman, M., Lorys, A. R., Novey, E. S., Eliopulos, D., & Lyytinen, H. (1991). Corpus callosum morphology in attention deficit-hyperactivity disorder: Morphometric analysis of MRI. *Journal of Learning Disabilities, 24,* 141–146.

Jacobson, S. W., Jacobson, J. L., Sokol, R. J., Martier, S. S., & Ager, J. W. (1993). Prenatal alcohol exposure and infant information processing ability. *Child Development, 64,* 1706–1721.

James, E. M., & Selz, M. (1997). Neuropsychological bases of common learning and behavior problems in children. In C. R. Reynolds & E. Fletcher-Janzen, eds., *Handbook of clinical child neuropsychology* (2nd ed.), (pp. 157–189). New York: Plenum Press.

Jastak, J. F., & Jastak, S. R. (1965). *The Wide Range Achievement Test.* Wilmington, DE: Guidance Associates.

Jenkins, M. R., & Culbertson, J. L. (1996). Prenatal exposure to alcohol. In R. L. Adams, O. A. Parsons, J. L. Culbertson, & S. J. Nixon, eds., *Neuropsychology for clinical practice: Etiology, assessment, and treatment of common neurological disorders* (pp. 407–452). Washington, DC: American Psychological Association.

Jennett, B., & Teasdale, G. (1981). *Management of head injuries.* Philadelphia: F. A. Davies.

Jensen, P. S., Martin, D., & Cantwell, D. P. (1997). Comorbidity in ADHD: Implications for Research, Practice, and DSM-V. *Journal of the American Academy of Child and Adolescent Psychiatry, 36,* 1065–1079.

Johansson, B. (1991). Neuropsychological assessment in the oldest-old. *International Psychogeriatrics, 3*(Suppl.), 51–60.

Johansson, B., Zarit, S. H., & Berg, S. (1992). Changes in cognitive functioning of the oldest old. *Journal of Gerontology: Psychological Sciences, 47,* 75–80.

Johnson, S. C., Bigler, E. D., Burr, R. B., & Blatter, D. D. (1994). White matter atrophy, ventricular dilation, and intellectual functioning following traumatic brain injury. *Neuropsychology, 8,* 307–315.

Jones, A. W. R., & Richardson, J. S. (1990). Alzheimer's disease: Clinical and pathological characteristics. *International Journal of Neuroscience, 50,* 147–168.

Jones, E. (1981). *The life and work of Sigmund Freud: The formative years and the great discoveries,* Vol. 1. New York: Basic Books.

Jones, K. L., Smith, D. W., Ulleland, C. N., & Streissguth, A. P. (1993) Pattern of malformation in offspring of chronic alcoholic mothers. *Lancet, 1,* 1267–1271.

Jones-Gotman, M. (1996). Psychological evaluation for epilepsy surgery. In S. Shorvon, F. Dreifuss, D. Fish, & D. Thomas, eds., *The treatment of epilepsy.* Oxford, England: Blackwell Science.

Jonides, J., Smith, E. E., Koeppe, R. A., Awh, E., Minoshima, S., & Mintun, M. A. (1993). Spatial working memory in humans as revealed by PET. *Nature, 363,* 623–625.

Jordan, B. D. (1987). Neurologic aspects of boxing. *Archives of Neurology, 44,* 453–459.

Jurko, M. F., & Andy, O. J. (1973). Psychological changes correlated with thalamotomy site. *Journal of Neurology, Neurosurgery, and Psychiatry, 36,* 846.

Kagan, J. (1964). *The Matching Familiar Figures Test.* Unpublished. Harvard University, Cambridge, MA.

Kalat, J. W. (1995). *Biological psychology* (5th ed.). Pacific Grove, CA: Brooks/Cole.

Kalat, J. W. (1998). *Biological psychology* (6th ed.). Pacific Grove, CA: Brooks/Cole.

Kandel, E. R., Schwartz, J. H., & Jessell, T. H., eds. (1991). *Principles of neural science* (5th ed.). New York: Elsevier Science.

Kane, R. L., Parsons, O. A., & Goldstein, G. (1985). Statistical relationships and discriminative accuracy of the Halstead-Reitan, Luria-Nebraska, and Wechsler IQ scores in the identification of brain damage. *Journal of Clinical and Experimental Neuropsychology, 7,* 211–223.

Kanner, L. (1943). Autistic disturbances of affective contact. *Nervous Child, 2,* 9–33.

Karni, A., Tanne, D., Rubenstein, B. S., Askenasy, J. J. M., & Sagi, D. (1994). Dependence on REM sleep of overnight improvement of a perceptual skill. *Science, 265,* 679–682.

Kass, C. E. (1964). Auditory closure test. In J. J. Olson & J. L. Olson, eds., *Validity studies on the Illinois Test of Psycholinguistic Abilities.* Madison, WI: Photo.

Katzman, R., Lasker, B., & Bernstein, N. (1988). Advances in the diagnosis of dementia: Accuracy of diagnosis and consequences of misdiagnosis of disorders causing dementia. In R. D. Terry, ed., *Aging and the brain,* Vol. 32 (pp. 17–61). New York: Raven Press.

Kaushall, P. I., Zetin, M., & Squire, L. R. (1981). Single case study: A psychosocial study of chronic, circumscribed amnesia. *Journal of Nervous and Mental Disease, 169,* 383–389.

Kay, D. W. K. (1995). The epidemiology of age-related neurological disease and dementia. *Reviews in Clinical Gerontology, 5,* 39–56.

Kennedy, C. H. (1999). Assessing competency to consent to sexual activity in the cognitively impaired population. *Journal of Forensic Neuropsychology, 1,* 17–33.

Kennedy, C. H., & Zillmer, E. A. (1999). Predicting sexual consent: A neuropsychological model. *Archives of Clinical Neuropsychology, 8,* 750.

Kenyon, T. (1994). *Brain states.* Naples, FL: United States Publishing.

Kerns, K. A., Don, A., Mateer, C. A., & Streissguth, A. P. (1997). Cognitive deficits in nonretarded adults with fetal alcohol syndrome. *Journal of Learning Disabilities, 30,* 685–693.

Kertesz, A. (1985). Recovery and treatment. In K. M. Heilman & E. Valenstein, eds., *Clinical Neuropsychology.* New York: Oxford University Press.

Kety, S. S. (1979). Disorders of the human brain. *Scientific American, 241,* 202–214.

Kinsbourne, M. (1971). The minor cerebral hemisphere as a source of aphasic speech. *Archives of Neurology, 15,* 530–535.

Kinsbourne, M. (1993). Orientational bias model of unilateral neglect: Evidence from attentional gradients within hemispace. In I. H. Robertson & J. C. Marshall, eds., *Unilateral neglect: Clinical and experimental studies* (pp. 63–86). Hove, England: Erlbaum.

Kleist, K. (1933). *Gehirnpathologie.* Leipzig: Barth.

Klove, H. (1963). Clinical neuropsychology. In F. M. Forster, ed., *The medical clinics of North America* (pp. 1647–1658). New York: Sanders.

Kolb, B. (1995). *Brain plasticity and behavior.* Mahwah, NJ: Erlbaum.

Kolb, B., & Fantie, B. (1997). Development of the child's brain and behavior. In C. R. Reynolds & E. Fletcher-Janzen, eds.,

Handbook of clinical child neuropsychology (2nd ed.), (pp. 17–41). New York: Plenum Press.

Kolb, B., & Whishaw, I. Z. (1990). *Fundamentals of human neuropsychology* (3rd ed.). New York: W. H. Freeman.

Kole, D. M., & Matarazzo, J. D. (1965). Intellectual and personality characteristics of two classes of medical students. *Journal of Medical Education, 40,* 1130–1143.

Koller, W., et al. (1987). Relationship of aging to Parkinson's disease. In M. D. Yahr & K. J. Bergmann, eds., *Advances in neurology,* Vol. 45 (pp. 317–321). New York: Raven Press.

Korkman, M., Kirk, U., & Kemp, S. (1998). *NEPSY: A developmental neuropsychology assessment manual.* San Antonio, TX: Psychological Corporation.

Krakauer, J. (1997). *Into thin air.* New York: Villard.

Kramer, D. A. (1983). Post-formal operations? A need for further conceptualization. *Human Development, 26,* 91–105.

Krech, D. (1962). Cortical localization of function. In L. Postman, ed., *Psychology in the making.* New York: Knopf.

LaBerge, S. (1990). *Exploring the world of lucid dreaming.* New York: Ballantine Books.

Lainhart, J. E., Piven, J., Wzorek, M., Landa, R., Santangelo, S., Coon, H., & Folstein, S. E. (1997). Macrocephaly in children and adults with autism. *Journal of the American Academy of Childhood and Adolescent Psychiatry, 36,* 282–290.

Lange, C. G. (1922). *The emotions.* Baltimore: Williams & Wilkins.

Larsen, J. P., Hoien, T., & Odegaard, H. (1992). Magnetic resonance imaging of the corpus callosum in developmental dyslexia. *Cognitive Neuropsychology, 9,* 123–134.

Larson, J., & Lynch, G. (1986). Induction of synaptic potentiation in hippocampus by patterned stimulation involves two events. *Science, 232,* 985–988.

LaRue, A. (1992). *Aging and neuropsychological assessment.* New York: Plenum Press.

Lashley, K. S. (1929). *Brain mechanisms and intelligence.* Chicago: University of Chicago Press.

LeDoux, J. E. (1992). Brain mechanisms of emotion and emotional learning. *Current Opinion in Neurobiology, 2,* 191–197.

Lees, A. J., & Smith, E. (1983). Cognitive deficits in the early stages of Parkinson's disease. *Brain, 106,* 257–270.

Lemire, R. J., Loeser, J. D., Leech, R. W., & Alvord, E. C. (1975). *Normal and abnormal development of the human nervous system.* New York: Harper & Row.

Lemoine, P., Harrowsseau, H., Borteryu, J. P., & Menuet, J. C. (1968). Les enfants de parents alcooliques: Anomalies observees a propos de 127 cas. [The children of alcoholic parents: Anomalies observed in 127 cases.] *Quest Medicale, 21,* 476–482.

Lemonick, M. (1997). Heroes of medicine. *Time* Magazine.

Levin, B. E., Tomer, R., & Rey, G. J. (1992). Cognitive impairment in Parkinson's disease. *Neurologic Clinics, 2,* 471–485.

Levin, H. S., & Eisenberg, H. M. (1979). Neuropsychological outcome of closed head injury in children and adolescents. *Child's Brain, 5,* 281–292.

Levin, H. S., Benton, A. L., & Grossman, R. G. (1982). *Neurobehavioral consequences of closed head injury.* New York: Oxford University Press.

Levin, H. S., Culhane, K. A., Hartmann, J., Evankovitch, K., Mattson, A. J., Harward, H., Ringholz, G., Ewing-Cobbs, L., & Fletcher, J. M. (1991). Developmental changes in performance on tests of purported frontal lobe function. *Developmental Neuropsychology, 7,* 377–395.

Levin, H. S., Eisenberg, H. M., & Benton, A. L. (1989). *Mild head injury.* New York: Oxford University Press.

Levin, H. S., O'Donnell, V. M., & Grossman, R. G. (1979). The Galveston Orientation and Amnesia Test. A practical scale to assess cognition after head injury. *Journal of Nervous and Mental Disease, 167,* 675–684.

Levin, M. (1953). Reflex action in the highest cerebral centers: A tribute to Hughlings Jackson. *Journal of Nervous Mental Disorder, 118,* 481.

Levin, W. (1991). Computer applications in cognitive rehabilitation. In J. S. Kreutzer & P. H. Wehman, eds., *Cognitive rehabilitation for persons with traumatic brain injury.* Baltimore: Paul H. Brookes.

Levy, J., & Heller, W. (1992). Gender differences in human neuropsychological function. In A. A. Gerall, H. Moltz, & I. L. Ward, eds., *Handbook of behavioral neurobiology: Sexual differentiation.* New York: Plenum.

Lezak, M. D. (1995). *Neuropsychological assessment* (3rd ed.). New York: Oxford University Press.

Lifton, R. J. (1986). *The Nazi doctors: Medical killing and the psychology of genocide.* New York: Basic Books.

Lisowksi, F. P. (1967). Prehistoric and early historic trepanation. In D. Brothwell & A. T. Sandison, eds., *Diseases in antiquity* (pp. 651–672). Springfield, IL: Charles C. Thomas.

Little, S. S. (1993). Nonverbal learning disabilities and socioemotional functioning: A review of recent literature. *Journal of Learning Disabilities, 26,* 653–665.

Lowther, J. L., & Wasserman, J. D. (1994, November). *Use of Mirsky's neurocognitive model of attention in identifying DSM-IV disorders of attention.* Poster session presented at the annual meeting of National Academy of Neuropsychology, Orlando, FL.

Luria, A. R. (1964). Neuropsychology in the local diagnosis of brain injury. *Cortex, 1,* 3.

Luria, A. R. (1966). *Higher cortical functions in man.* New York: Basic Books.

Luria, A. R. (1968). *The Mind of a mnemonist.* New York: Basic Books.

Luria, A. R. (1971). Memory disturbances in local brain lesions. *Neuropsychologia, 9,* 367.

Luria, A. R. (1990). *The neuropsychological analysis of problem-solving.* Orlando, FL: Paul M. Deutsch Press.

Macmillan, M. (1996). Phineas Gage: A case for all reasons. In C. Code, C. Wallesch, Y. Joanette, & A. R. Lecours, eds., *Classic cases in neuropsychology* (pp. 243–262). Sussex, England: Psychology Press.

Maertens, P. (1998). Inborn errors of metabolism. I: Neurologic degenerative diseases. In R. B. David, ed., *Child and adolescent neurology* (pp. 295–358). New York: Mosby.

Mai, J. K., Assheuer, J., & Paxinos, G. (1997). *Atlas of the human brain.* San Diego, CA: Academic Press.

Majovski, L. V. (1997). Mechanisms and development of cerebral lateralization in children. In C. R. Reynolds & E. Fletcher-Janzen, eds., *Handbook of clinical child neuropsychology* (2nd ed.), (pp. 102–119). New York: Plenum Press.

Marie, P. (1906). The third left frontal convolution plays no special role in the function of language. *Sem. Medical, 26,* 241.

Marshall, J. C., & Halligan, P. W. (1988). Line bisection in a case of visual neglect. *Nature, 336,* 766–777.

Marshall, L. F., & Ruff, R. M. (1989). Neurosurgeon as a victim. In H. S. Levin, H. M. Eisenberg, & A. L. Benton, eds., *Mild head injury.* New York: Oxford University Press.

Martin, J. H., & Jessell, T. M. (1991). Development as a guide to the regional anatomy of the brain. In E. R. Kandel, J. H. Schwartz, & T. M. Jessell, eds., *Principles of neural science* (3rd ed.), (pp. 296–308). New York: Elsevier Science.

Matarazzo, J. (1990). Psychological assessment versus psychological testing. *American Psychologist, 45,* 999–1017.

Matousek, M., & Petersen, I. (1973). Frequency analysis of the EEG background activity by means of age dependent quotients. In P. Kellaway & I. Petersen, eds., *Automation of clinical electroencephalography* (pp. 75–102). New York: Raven Press.

Mattingly, J. B. (1996). Paterson & Zangwill's (1944) case of unilateral neglect: Insights from 50 years of experimental inquiry. In C. Code, C. Wallesch, Y. Joanette, & A. R. Lecours, eds., *Classic cases in neuropsychology* (pp. 243–262). Brighton, Sussex, England: Psychology Press.

Mattson, S. N., Riley, E. P., Delis, D. C., Stern, C., & Jones, K. L. (1996). Verbal learning and memory in children with fetal alcohol syndrome. *Alcoholism: Clinical and Experimental Research, 20,* 810–816.

Mattson, S. N., Riley, E. P., Gramling, L., Delis, D. C., & Jones, K. L. (1998). Neuropsychological comparison of alcohol-exposed children with or without physical features of fetal alcohol syndrome. *Neuropsychology, 12,* 146–153.

Mattson, S. N., Riley, E. P., Sowell, E. R., Jenigan, T. L., Sobel, D. F., & Jones, K. L. (1996). A decrease in the size of the basal ganglia in children with fetal alcohol syndrome. *Alcoholism: Clinical and Experimental Research, 20,* 1088–1093.

Maurer, K., Volk, S., & Gerbaldo, H. (1997). Auguste D. and Alzheimer's disease. *Lancet, 349,* 1546-1549.

Mayeux, R., et al. (1992). A population-based investigation of Parkinson's disease with and without dementia. *Archives of Neurology, 49,* 492–497.

McCarthy, R. A., & Warrington, E. K. (1990). *Cognitive neuropsychology.* San Diego, CA: Academic Press.

McDonough, L., Stahmer, A., Schreibman, L., & Thompson, S. J. (1997). Deficits, delays, and distractions: An evaluation of symbolic play and memory in children with autism. *Development and Psychopathology, 9,* 17–41.

McIntosh, G. C. (1992). Neurological conceptualizations of epilepsy. In T. L. Bennett, ed., *The neuropsychology of epilepsy.* New York: Plenum Press.

McKhann, G., et al. (1984). Clinical diagnosis of Alzheimer's disease. Report of the NINCDS-ADRDA Work Group. *Neurology, 34,* 939–944.

McLardy, T. (1970). Memory function in hippocampal gyri but not in hippocampi. *International Journal of Neuroscience, 1,* 113.

Meehl, P. (1973). *Psychodiagnosis: Selected papers.* New York: Norton Press.

Merz, P. A., Somerville, R. A., Wisneiwski, H. M., & Iqbal, K. (1981). Abnormal fibrils from scrapie-infected brain. *Acta Neuropathologica, 54,* 63–74.

Mesulam, M. M. (1981). A cortical network for directed attention and unilateral neglect. *Annals of Neurology, 10,* 309–325.

Mesulam, M. M. (1985). *Principles of behavioral neurology.* Philadephia: F. A. Davis.

Mesulam, M. M. (1990). Large-scale neurocognitive networks and distributed processing for attention, language and memory. *Annals of Neurology, 28,* 597–613.

Milberg, W. P., Hebben, N., & Kaplan, E. (1986). The Boston process approach to neuropsychological assessment. In I. Grant & K. M. Adams, eds., *Neuropsychological assessment of neuropsychiatric disorders.* New York: Oxford University Press.

Milner, B. (1968). Visual recognition and recall after right temporal lobe excision in man. *Neuropsychologia, 6,* 191.

Milner, B. (1974). Hemispheric specialization: Scope and limits. In F. O. Schmitt & F. G. Worden, eds., *The neuroscience third study program.* Cambridge, MA: MIT Press.

Milner, B. (1982). Some cognitive effects of frontal lesion in man. In D. E. Broadbent & L. Weiskrantz, eds., *The neuropsychology of cognitive function.* London: The Royal Society.

Milner, B., Corkin, S., & Teuber, S. C. (1968). Further analysis of the hippocampal amnesic syndrome: 14 year follow-up study of H.M. *Neuropsychologia, 6,* 215–234.

Minshew, N. J. (1997). Pervasive developmental disorders: Autism and similar disorders. In T. E. Feinberg & M. J. Farah, eds., *Behavioral neurology and neuropsychology* (pp. 817–826). New York: McGraw-Hill.

Minshew, N. J., Goldstein, G., & Siegel, D. J. (1995). Speech and language in high-functioning autistic individuals. *Neuropsychology, 9,* 255–261.

Mirsky, A. F. (1995). Perils and pitfalls on the path to normal potential: The role of impaired attention. Homage to Herbert G. Birch. *Journal of Clinical and Experimental Neuropsychology, 17,* 481–498.

Mirsky, A. F. (1996). Disorders of attention: A neuropsychological perspective. In G. R. Lyon & N. A. Krasnegor, eds., *Attention, memory, and executive function* (pp. 71–96). Baltimore: Paul H. Brookes.

Mishkin, M., Malamut, B., & Bachevalier, J. (1984). Memories and habits: Two neural systems. In G. Lynch, J. L. McGaugh, & N. M. Weinberger, eds., *Neurobiology of learning and memory.* New York: Guilford Press.

Mishkin, M., Ungerleider, L., & Macko, K. A. (1983). Object vision and spatial vision: Two cortical pathways. *Trends in Neurosciences, 6,* 414–417.

Moore, K. L., & Persaud, T. V. N. (1993). *Before we are born: Essentials of embryology and birth defects* (4th ed.). Philadelphia: Saunders.

Nairne, J. S. (1997). *Psychology: The adaptive mind.* Pacific Grove, CA: Brooks/Cole.

National Directory of Head Injury Services. (1992). Southbridge, MA: National Head Injury Foundation.

Naugle, R. I., Cullum, C. M., & Bigler, E. D. (1998). *Introduction to clinical neuropsychology: A casebook.* Austin, TX: Pro-Ed.

Nauta, W. J. H., & Feirtag, M. (1986). *Fundamental neuroanatomy.* New York: W. H. Freeman.

Neff, W. D., & Goldberg, J. M. (1960). Higher functions of the central nervous system. *Annual Review Psychology, 22,* 499.

Newman, A. C., Barth, J. T., & Zillmer, E. A. (1986). Serial neuropsychological assessment in an adult with Tourette's syndrome. *International Journal of Clinical Neuropsychology, 9,* 135–139.

Newton, A., & Johnson, D. A. (1985). Social adjustment and interaction after severe head injury. *British Journal of Clinical Psychology, 24,* 225–234.

Noback, C. R., & Demarest, R. J. (1975). *The human nervous system.* New York: McGraw-Hill.

Nockleby, D. M., & Deaton, A. V. (1987). Denial versus distress: Coping patterns in post head trauma patients. *International Journal of Clinical Neuropsychology, 9,* 145–148.

Nottebohm, F. (1981). A brain for all seasons: Cyclical anatomical changes in song-control nuclei for the canary brain. *Science, 214,* 1368–1370.

Nudo, R. J., Wise, B. M., SiFuentes, F., & Milliken, G. W. (1996). Neural substrates for the effects of rehabilitative training on motor recovery after ischemic infarct. *Science, 272,* 1791–1794.

Nuland, S. B. (1993). *How we die.* New York: Vintage.

Ogden, J. A. (1985). Anterior-posterior interhemispheric differences in the loci of lesions producing visual hemineglect. *Brain and Cognition, 4,* 59–75.

Ojemann, G. A. (1980). Brain mechanisms for language: Observation during neurosurgery. In J. S. Lockard & A. A. Ward, Jr., eds., *Epilepsy: A window to brain mechanisms.* New York: Raven Press.

Olson, L. (1990). Grafts and growth factors in CNS. Basic science with clinical promise. *Stereotactic Functional Neurosurgery, 54,* 250–267.

Ommaya, A. K., & Gennarelli, T. A. (1974). Cerebral concussion and traumatic unconsciousness. *Brain, 97,* 633–654.

Ornitz, E. M. (1992). Autism. In B. Smith & G. Adelman, eds., *Neuroscience year—supplement 2 to the encyclopedia of neuroscience* (pp. 15–17). Boston: Birkhauser.

Osterrieth, P. A. (1944). Le test de copie d'une figure complexe. *Archives de Psychologie, 30,* 206–356. J. Corwin & F. W. Bylsma, trans. (1993). *The Clinical Neuropsychologist, 7,* 9–15.

Ozonoff, S., Pennington, B. F., & Rogers, S. J. (1991). Executive function deficits in higher-functioning autistic individuals: Relationship to theory of mind. *Journal of Child Psychology and Psychiatry, 32,* 1081–1105.

Papalia, D. E., & Olds, S. W. (1995). *Human development* (6th ed.). New York: McGraw-Hill.

Papez, J. W. (1937). A proposed mechanism of emotion. *Archives of Neurology & Psychiatry, 38,* 725–743.

Papez, J. W. (1958). Visceral brain, its component parts and their connections. *Journal of Nervous Mental Disorder, 126,* 40.

Paterson, A., & Zangwill, O. L. (1944). Disorders of visual space perception associated with lesions of the right cerebral hemisphere. *Brain, 67,* 331–358.

Pavlides, C., & Winson, J. (1989). Influences of hippocampal place cell firing in the awake state on the activity of these cells during subsequent sleep episodes. *Journal of Neuroscience, 9,* 2907–2918.

Pearson, D. A., Yaffee, L. S., Loveland, K. A., & Norton, A. M. (1995). Covert visual attention in children with attention deficit hyperactivity disorder: Evidence for developmental immaturity? *Development and Psychopathology, 7,* 351–367.

Penfield, W. (1975). *The mystery of the mind.* Princeton, NJ: Princeton University Press.

Penfield, W., & Jasper, H. H. (1954). *Epilepsy and the functional anatomy of the human brain.* Boston: Little, Brown.

Penfield, W., & Milner, B. (1958). Memory deficit produced by bilateral lesions in the hippocampal zone. *Archives of Neurology Psychiatry, 79,* 475.

Pennebaker, R. B. (1982, December 5). Lobotomies: Surgery of the soul. *The Daily Progress,* Charlottesville, VA, pp. E1, E4.

Pennington, B. F. (1991). *Diagnosing learning disorders: A neurological framework.* New York: Guilford Press.

Pennington, B. F. (1997a). Attention deficit hyperactivity disorder. In T. E. Feinberg & M. J. Farah, eds., *Behavioral neurology and neuropsychology* (pp. 803–807). New York: McGraw-Hill.

Pennington, B. F. (1997b). Dimensions of executive functions in normal and abnormal development. In N. A. Krasnegor, G. R. Lyon, & P. S. Goldman-Rakic, eds., *Development of the prefrontal cortex: Evolution, neurobiology, and behavior* (pp. 265–282). Baltimore: Paul H. Brookes.

Pennington, B. F., & Ozonoff, S. (1996). Executive functions and developmental psychopathology. *Journal of Child Psychology and Psychiatry, 37,* 51–87.

Pennington, B. F., & Smith, S. (1983). Genetic influences on learning disabilities and speech and language disorders. *Child Development, 54,* 369–387.

Pennington, B. F., Heaton, R. K., Karzmark, P., Pendleton, M. G., Lehman, R., & Shucard, D. W. (1985). The neuropsychological phenotype in Turner syndrome. *Cortex, 21,* 391–404.

Penny, J. B., & Young, A. B. (1993). Huntington's disease. In J. Jankovic & E. Tolosa, eds., *Parkinson's disease and movement disorders* (2nd ed.), (pp. 205–216). Baltimore: Williams & Wilkins.

Perani, D., Vallar G., Paulesu, E., Alberoni, M., & Fazio, F. (1993). Left and right hemisphere contribution to recovery from neglect after right hemisphere damage: A PET study of two cases. *Neuropsychologia, 31,* 116–25.

Perry, W., & Zillmer, E. A. (1996). Overview: Neuropsychology and personality assessment. *Assessment, 3,* 207–209.

Petersen, S. E., Robinson, D. L., & Morris, J. D. (1987). Contributions of the pulvinar to visual spatial attention. *Neuropsychology, 25,* 97–105.

Pfefferbaum, A., Mathalon, D. H., Sullivan, E. V., Rawles, J. M., Zipursky, R. B., & Lim, K. O. (1994). A quantitative magnetic resonance imaging study of changes in brain morphology from infancy to late adulthood. *Archives of Neurology, 51,* 874–887.

Piaget, J. (1971). *Biology of knowledge.* Chicago: University of Chicago Press.

Pincus, J. H., & Tucker, G. J. (1985). *Behavioral neurology.* New York: Oxford University Press.

Pinel, P. J., & Edwards, M. (1998). *A colorful introduction to the anatomy of the human brain.* Boston: Allyn and Bacon.

Piotrowski, C., Sherry, D., & Keller, J. W. (1985). Psychodiagnostic test usage: A survey of the Society of Personality Assessment. *Journal of Personality Assessment, 49,* 115–119.

Piotrowski, Z. (1940). Positive and negative Rorschach organic reactions. *Rorschach Research Exchange, 4,* 147–151.

Piven, J., Arndt, S., Bailey, J., & Andreasen, N. (1996). Regional brain enlargement in autism: A magnetic resonance imaging study. *Journal of the American Academy of Child and Adolescent Psychiatry, 35,* 530–536.

Piven, J., Berthier, M. L., Starkstein, S. E., Nehme, E., Pearlson, G., & Folstein, S. (1990). Magnetic resonance imaging evidence for a defect of cerebral cortical development in autism. *American Journal of Psychiatry, 147,* 734–739.

Polster, M. R. (1993). Drug-induced amnesia: Implication for cognitive neuropsychological investigations of memory. *Psychological Bulletin, 114,* 477–493.

Poppel, E., & Richards, W. A. (1974). Light sensitivity in cortical scotomata contralateral to small islands of blindness. *Experimental Brain Research, 21,* 125–130.

Poppel, E., & vonSteinbuchel, N. (1992). Neuropsychological rehabilitation from a theoretical point of view. In N. vonSteinbuchel, D. Y. von Cramon, & E. Poppel, eds., *Neuropsychological rehabilitation* (pp. 3–19). Berlin: Springer.

Popplestone, J. A., & McPherson, M. W. (1994). *An illustrated history of American psychology.* Madison, WI: Brown & Benchmark.

Portin, R., & Rinne, U. (1986). Predictive factors for cognitive deterioration and dementia in Parkinson's disease. *Advances in Neurology, 45,* 413–416.

Posner, M. I. (1988). Structures and function of selective attention. In T. Boll & B. K. Bryant, eds., *Clinical neuropsychology and brain function: Research, measurement and practice* (pp. 169–202). Washington, DC: American Psychological Association.

Posner, M. I. (1992). Attention as a cognitive and neural system. *Current Directions in Psychological Science, 1,* 11–14.

Posner, M. I., & Petersen, S. E. (1990). The attention system of the human brain. *Annual Review of Neuroscience, 13,* 25–42.

Potegal, M. (1971). A note on spatial motor deficits in patients with Huntington's disease: A test of a hypothesis. *Neuropsychologia, 9,* 233–235.

Powers, W. J. (1990). Stroke. In A. L. Pearlman & R. C. Collins, eds., *Neurobiology of disease.* New York: Oxford University Press.

Price, B. H., Gurvit, H., Weintrub, S., Geula, C., Leimkuhler, E., & Mesulam, M. (1993). Neuropsychological patterns and language deficits in 20 consecutive cases of autopsy-confirmed Alzheimer's disease. *Archives of Neurology, 50,* 931–937.

Prigatano, G. P. (1992). Neuropsychological rehabilitation and the problem of altered self-awareness. In N. vonSteinbuchel, D. Y. von Cramon, & E. Poppel, eds., *Neuropsychological rehabilitation.* Berlin: Springer.

Prigatano, G. P., & Wong, J. L. (1997). Speed of finger tapping and goal attainment after unilateral cerebral vascular accident. *Archives of Physical Medicine and Rehabilitation, 78,* 847–852.

Pritchard, P. B., Holmstrom, V. L., & Giacinto, J. (1985). Self-abatement of complex partial seizures. *Annals of Neurology, 18,* 265–267.

Pruisiner, S. B. (1982). Novel proteinaceous infectious particles cause scrapie. *Science, 216,* 136–144.

Ragland, J. D., Gur, R. C., Raz, J., Schroeder, L., Smith, R. J., Alavi, A., & Gur, R. E. (2000). Hemispheric activation of anterior and inferior prefrontal cortex during verbal encoding and recognition: A PET study of healthy volunteers. *NeuroImage, 11,* 624–633.

Raichle, M. E. (1983). Positron emission tomography. *Annual Review of Neuroscience, 6,* 249–267.

Raichle, M. E., Fiez, J. A., Videen, T. O., MacLeod, A. K., Pardo, J. V., Fox, P. T., & Petersen, S. E. (1994). Practice-related changes in human brain functional anatomy during nonmotor learning. *Cerebral Cortex, 4,* 8–26.

Rakic, P., & Lombroso, P. J. (1998). Development of the cerebral cortex: I. forming the cortical structure. *Journal of the American Academy of Child and Adolescent Psychiatry, 37,* 116–117.

Ramachandran, V. S., Rogers-Ramachandran, D., & Steward, M. (1992). Perceptual correlates of massive cortical reorganization. *Science, 258,* 1159–1160.

Randall, C. (1996). Modern FAS research in perspective. In J. Weinberg (Chair), Symposium: New directions in fetal alcohol syndrome research. *Alcoholism: Clinical and Experimental Research, 20,* 72A–77A.

Raskin, S. A., Borod, J. C., & Tweedy, J. (1990). Neuropsychological aspects of Parkinson's disease. *Neuropsychology Review, 1,* 185–221.

Rebok, G. W., & Folstein, M. F. (1993). Dementia. *Journal of Neuropsychiatry and Clinical Neurosciences, 5,* 265–276.

Rees, J. R. (1948). *The case of Rudolf Hess; a problem in diagnosis and forensic psychiatry.* New York: Norton.

Reiss, A. L., & Denckla, M. B. (1996). The contribution of neuroimaging to behavioral neurogenetics research: Fragile X syndrome, Turner's syndrome, and neurofibromatosis. In G. R. Reid & J. M. Rumsey, eds., *Neuroimaging: A window to the neurological foundations of learning and behavior in children* (pp. 147–168). Baltimore: Paul H. Brookes.

Reiss, A. L., Freund, L., Plotnick, L., Baumgardner, T., Green, K., Sozer, A. C., Reader, M., Boehm, C., & Denckla, M. B. (1993). The effects of X monosomy on brain development: Monozygotic twins discordant for Turner's syndrome. *Annals of Neurology, 34,* 95–107.

Reiss, A. L., Mazzocco, M. M. M., Greenlaw, R., Freund, L. S., & Ross, J. L. (1995). Neurodevelopmental effect on X monosomy: A volumetric imaging study. *American Neurological Association, 38,* 731–738.

Reitan, R. M. (1966). A research program on the psychological effects of brain lesions in human beings. In N. R. Ellis, ed., *International review of research in mental retardation* (pp. 153–218). New York: Academic Press.

Reitan, R. M. (1984). *Aphasia and sensory-perceptual deficit in children.* Tucson, AZ: Neuropsychological Press.

Reitan, R. M., & Davison, L. A. (1974). *Clinical neuropsychology: Current status and applications.* Washington, DC: V. H. Winston.

Reitan, R. M., & Wolfson, D. (1993). *The Halstead-Reitan Neuropsychological Test Battery: Theory and clinical interpretation* (2nd ed.). Tucson, AZ: Neuropsychology Press.

Rey, A. (1941). Psychological examination of traumatic encephalopathy. *Archives de Psychologie, 28,* 286–340. Section translated by J. Corwin & F. W. Bylsma. (1993). *The Clinical Neuropsychologist, 7,* 3–22.

Rhodes, R. (1997). *Deadly feasts.* New York: Simon and Schuster.

Richard, A., & Reiter, J. (1990). *Epilepsy: A new approach.* New York: Prentice Hall.

Richters, J. E., Arnold, L. E., Jensen, P. S., Abikoff, H., Conners, C. K., Greenhill, L. L., Hechtman, L., Hinshaw, S. P., Pelham, W. E., & Swanson, J. M. (1995). NIMH collaborative multisite multimodal treatment study of children with ADHD: Background and rationale. *Journal of the American Academy of Child and Adolescent Psychiatry, 34,* 987–1008.

Rilke, R. M. (1996). *Rilke's book of hours: Love poems to God.* A. Burrows & J. Macy, trans. New York: Riverhead Books. Originally published in R. M. Rilke, *The book of monastic life.*

Rimel, R. W., Giordani, B., Barth, J. T., Boll, T. J., & Jane, J. A. (1981). Disability caused by minor head injury. *Neurosurgery, 9,* 221–228.

Rimel, R., Eisenberg, M., & Benton, A. L. (1989). Disability caused by minor head injury. *Neurosurgery, 9,* 221–228.

Roeser, R. J., & Daly, D. D. (1974). Auditory cortex deconnection associated with thalamic tumor. *Neurology, 24,* 555.

Roland, P. E. (1993). *Brain activation.* New York: Wiley-Liss.

Roland, P. E., Larsen, B., Lassen, N. A., & Skinholf, E. (1980). Supplementary motor area and other cortical areas in organization of voluntary movements in man. *Journal of Neurophysiology, 43,* 118–136.

Rolls, E. T. (1986). Neuronal activity related to the control of feeding. In R. Ritter & S. Ritter, eds., *Neural and humoral controls of food intake.* New York: Academic Press.

Romans, S. M., Roeltgen, D. P., Kushner, H., & Ross, J. L. (1997). Executive function in girls with Turner's syndrome. *Developmental Neuropsychology, 13,* 23–40.

Rorschach, H. (1942). *Psychodiagnostics: A diagnostic test based on perception.* Bern, Switzerland: Huber.

Rosenblum, J. A. (1974). Human sexuality and cerebral cortex. *Disorder of the Nervous System, 35,* 268.

Ross, E. (1985). Modulation of affect and nonverbal communication by the right hemisphere. In M. M. Mesulam, ed., *Principles of behavioral neurology* (pp. 239–257). Philadelphia: F. A. Davis.

Rosvold, H. E., Mirsky, A. F., Sarason, I., Bransome, E. D., & Beck, L. H. (1956). A continuous performance test of brain damage. *Journal of Consulting Psychology, 20,* 343–350.

Rourke, B. B., & Del Dotto, J. E. (1994). *Learning disabilities: A neuropsychological perspective.* Thousand Oaks, CA: Sage.

Rourke, B. P. (1989). *Non-verbal learning disabilities: The syndrome and the model.* New York: Guilford Press.

Rourke, B. P. (1991). Human neuropsychology in the 1990s. *Archives of Clinical Neuropsychology, 6,* 1–15.

Rourke, B. P. (1993). Arithmetic disabilities, specific and otherwise: A neuropsychological perspective. *Journal of Learning Disabilities, 26,* 214–226.

Rourke, B. P. (1995), The NLD syndrome and the white matter model. In B. P. Rourke, ed., *Syndrome of nonverbal learning disabilities: Neurodevelopmental manifestations* (pp. 1–26). New York: Guilford Press.

Rourke, B. P., & Conway, J. A. (1997). Disabilities of arithmetic and mathematical reasoning: Perspectives from neurology and neuropsychology. *Journal of Learning Disabilities, 30,* 34–46.

Rourke, B. P., & Fuerst, D. E. (1996). Psychosocial dimensions of learning disability subtypes. *Assessment, 3,* 277–290.

Rourke, B. P., Bakker, D. J., Fisk, L. J., & Strang, J. D. (1983). *Child neuropsychology: An introduction to theory, research, and clinical practice.* New York: Guilford Press.

Rourke, B. P., Fisk, J. L., & Strang, J. D. (1986). *Neuropsychological assessment of children: A treatment-oriented approach.* New York: Guilford Press.

Rovee-Collier, C. (1993). The capacity for long-term memory in infancy. *Current Directions in Psychological Science, 2,* 130–135.

Rovet, J. F. (1993). The psychoeducational characteristics of children with Turner syndrome. *Journal of Learning Disabilities, 26,* 333–341.

Rowland, L. P., Fink, M., & Rubin, L. (1991). Cerebrospinal fluid: Blood–brain barrier, brain edema, and hydrocephalus. In E. R. Kandel, J. H. Schwartz, & T. M. Jessell, eds., *Principles of neural science* (3rd ed.), (pp. 1050–1060). New York: Elsevier Science.

Roy, A., De Jong, J., & Linnoila, M. (1989). Cerebrospinal fluid monoamine metabolites and suicidal behavior in depressed patients. *Archives of General Psychiatry, 46,* 609–612.

Rubens, A. B., & Benson, D. F. (1971). Associative visual agnosia. *Archives of Neurology, 24,* 304–316.

Rudel, R. G. (1981). Residual effects of childhood reading disabilities. *Bulletin of the Orton Society, 31,* 89–102.

Rumsey, J. M. (1996a). Neuroimaging in developmental dyslexia. In G. R. Lyon & J. M. Rumsey, ed., *Neuroimaging: A window to the neurological foundations of learning and behavior in children* (pp. 57–78). Baltimore: Paul H. Brookes.

Rumsey, J. M. (1996b). Neuroimaging studies of autism. In G. R. Lyon & J. M. Rumsey, eds., *Neuroimaging studies of autism* (pp. 119–146). Baltimore: Paul H. Brookes.

Rumsey, J. M., Andreason, P., Zametkin, A. J., Aquino, T., King, A. C., Hamberger, S. D., Pikus, A., Rapoport, J. L., & Cohen, R. M.. (1992). Failure to activate the left temporoparietal cortex in dyslexia. *Archives of Neurology, 49,* 527–534.

Russell, W. R., & Espir, M. L. E. (1961). *Traumatic aphasia.* London: Oxford University Press.

Ryan, T. V., Crews, W. D., Cowen, L., Goering, A., & Barth, J. T. (1998). A case of Triple X syndrome manifesting with the syndrome of nonverbal learning disabilities. *Child Neuropsychology, 4,* 225–232.

Sacks, O. (1987). *The man who mistook his wife for a hat.* New York: Harper & Row.

Sacks, O. (1995). *An anthropologist on Mars.* New York: Knopf.

Sagar, H., Sullivan, E., Gabrieli, J., Corkin, S., & Growdon, J. (1988). Temporal ordering and short-term memory deficits in Parkinson's disease. *Brain, 111,* 525–539.

Samango-Sprouse, C. (1999). Frontal lobe development in childhood. In B. L. Miller & J. L. Cummings, eds., *The human frontal lobes: Functions and disorders* (pp. 584–604). New York: Guilford Press.

Santoro, J. M., & Spiers, M. V. (1994). Social cognitive factors in brain injury associated personality change. *Brain Injury, 8,* 265–276.

Schacter, D. L. (1987). Implicit memory: History and current status. *Journal of Experimental Psychology: Learning, Memory and Cognition, 13,* 501–518.

Scheibel, A. B. (1990). Dendritic correlates of higher cognitive function. In A. B. Scheibel & A. F. Wechsler, eds., *Neurobiology of higher cognitive function* (pp. 239–270). New York: Guilford Press.

Schiller, F. (1982). *Paul Broca: Explorer of the brain.* New York: Oxford University Press.

Scott, A. M., Fletcher, J. M., Brookshire, B. L., Davidson, K. C., Landry, S. H., Bohan, T. C., Kramer, L. A., Brandt, M. C., & Francis, D. J. (1998). Memory functions in children with early hydrocephalus. *Neuropsychology, 12,* 578–589.

Scoville, W. B. (1968). Amnesia after bilateral mesial temporal-lobe excision: Introduction to case H.M. *Neuropsychologia, 6,* 211–213.

Scoville, W. B., & Milner, B. (1957). Loss of recent memory after bilateral hippocampal lesions. *Journal of Neurology, Neurosurgery, and Psychiatry, 20,* 11.

Searleman, A. (1977). A review of right hemisphere linguistic capabilities. *Psychological Bulletin, 84,* 503–528.

Segalowitz, S. J., & Hiscock, M. (1992). The emergence of a neuropsychology of normal development: Rapprochement between neuroscience and developmental neuropsychology. In I. Rapin & S. J. Segalowitz, eds., *Handbook of neuropsychology: Child neuropsychology.* Amsterdam: Elsevier.

Semrud-Clikeman, M., Filipek, P. A., Biederman, J., Steingard, R., Kennedy, D., Renshaw, P., & Bekken, K. (1994). Attention-deficit hyperactivity disorder: Magnetic resonance imaging morphometric analysis of the corpus callosum. *Journal of the American Academy of Child and Adolescent Psychiatry, 33,* 875–881.

Semrud-Clikeman, M., Hooper, S. R., Hynd, G. W., Hern, K., Presley, R., & Watson, T. (1996). Prediction of group membership in developmental dyslexia, attention deficit hyperactivity disorder, and normal controls using brain morphometric analysis of magnetic resonance imaging. *Archives of Clinical Neuropsychology, 11,* 521–528.

Shaffer, D. R. (1999). *Developmental psychology: Childhood and adolescence* (5th ed.). Pacific Grove, CA: Brooks/Cole.

Shallice, T. (1982). Specific impairments of planning. *Philosophical Transactions of the Royal Society of London, B, 298,* 199–209.

Shallice, T., & Warrington, E. K. (1970). Independent functioning of verbal memory stores: A neuropsychological study. *Quarterly Journal of Experimental Psychology, 22,* 261–273.

Shallice, T., & Warrington, E. K. (1977). The possible role of selective attention in acquired dyslexia. *Neuropsychologia, 15,* 31–41.

Shaywitz, B. A., Shaywitz, S. E., Pugh, K. R., Skudlarski, P., Fulbright, R. K., Constable, R. T., Bronen, R. A., Fletcher, J. M., Liberman, A. M., Shankweiler, D. P., Katz, L., Lacadie, C., Marchione, K. E., & Gore, J. C. (1996). Functional magnetic resonance imaging as a tool to understand reading and reading disability. In R. W. Thatcher, G. R. Lyon, J. Rumsey, & N. Krasnegor, eds., *Developmental neuroimaging: Mapping the development of brain and behavior* (pp. 157–167). San Diego, CA: Academic Press.

Sherin, J. E., Shiromani, P., McCarley, R. W., & Saper, C. B. (1996). Ventrolateral preoptic neurons that innervate the tuberomammillary nucleus are activated during sleep. *Science, 271,* 216–219.

Sigelman, C. K., & Shaffer, D. R. (1995). *Life-span human development* (2nd ed.). Pacific Grove, CA: Brooks/Cole.

Sigman, M. (1994). What are the core deficits in autism? In S. H. Broman & J. Grafman, eds., *Atypical cognitive deficits in developmental disorders* (pp. 139–158). New York: Oxford University Press.

Silver, J. M., Yudofsky, M. D., & Hales, R. E. (1994). *Neuropsychiatry of traumatic brain injury.* Washington, DC: American Psychiatric Press.

Sitaram, N., Moore, A. M., & Gillin, J. C. (1978). Experimental acceleration and slowing of REM ultradian rhythm by cholinergic agonist and antagonist. *Nature, 274,* 490–492.

Skottun, B. C., & Parke, L. A. (1999). The possible relationship between visual deficits and dyslexia: Examination of a critical assumption. *Journal of Disabilities, 32,* 2–5.

Smith, A. (1966). Intellectual functions in patients with lateralized frontal tumors. *Journal of Neurology, Neurosurgery, and Psychiatry, 29,* 52.

Smith, A. (1982). *Symbol Digit Modalities Test (SDMT). Manual* (revised). Los Angeles: Western Psychological Services.

Smith, D. V., & Vogt, M. B. (1997). The neural code and integrative processes of taste. In G. K. Beauchamp & L. Bartoshuk, eds., *Tasting and smelling.* San Diego, CA: Academic Press.

Snead, O. C. (1995). Basic mechanisms of generalized absence seizures. *Annals of Neurology, 37,* 146–157.

Snowdon, D. A., Greiner, L. H., Kemper, S. J., Nanayakkara, N., & Mortimer, J. A. (1999). Linguistic ability in early life and longevity: Findings from the Nun Study. In J. M. Robine, B. Forette, C. Franceschi, & M. Allard, eds., *The paradoxes of longevity.* Berlin: Springer.

Snyder, A. Z., Petersen, S., Fox, P., & Raichle, M. E. (1989). PET studies of visual word recognition. *Journal of Cerebral Blood Flow and Metabolism, 9*(Suppl. 1–S576).

Soares, H. D., Sinson, G. P., & McIntosh, T. K. (1995). Fetal hippocampal transplants attenuate CA3 pyramidal cell death resulting from fluid percussion brain injury in the rat. *Journal of Neurotrauma, 12*(6), 1059–1067.

Sohlberg, M. M., & Mateer, C. A. (1987). Effectiveness of an attention training program. *Journal of Clinical and Experimental Neuropsychology, 9,* 117–130.

Sohlberg, M. M., & Mateer, C. A. (1989). *Introduction to cognitive rehabilitation: Theory and practice.* New York: Guilford Press.

Soliveri, P., Brown, R. G., Jahanshahi, M., & Marsden, C. D. (1992). Procedural memory and neurological disease. *European Journal of Cognitive Psychology, 4,* 161–193.

Spiers, M. (1995). The cognitive screening for medication self-management. Unpublished test, Drexel University, Philadelphia.

Spiers, M. V., & Kutzik, D. M. (1995). Self-reported memory of medication use by the elderly. *American Journal of Health-System Pharmacy, 52,* 985–990.

Spiers, M. V., Pouk, J. A., & Santoro, J. M. (1994). Examining perspective-taking in the severely head-injured. *Brain Injury, 8,* 463–473.

Spreen, O., Risser, A. T., & Edgell, D. (1995). *Developmental neuropsychiatry.* New York: Oxford University Press.

Springer, S. P., & Deutsch, G. (1993). *Left brain, right brain* (4th ed.). New York: W. H. Freeman.

Squire, L. R. (1987). *Memory and brain.* New York: Oxford University Press.

Squire, L. R. (1994). Declarative and nondeclarative memory: Multiple brain systems supporting learning and memory. In D. L. Schacter & E. Tulving, eds., *Memory systems* (pp. 203–232) Cambridge, MA: MIT Press.

Squire, L. R., & Butters, N., eds. (1984). *Neuropsychology of memory* (2nd ed.). New York: Guilford Press.

Squire, L. R., & Cohen, N. J. (1984). Human memory and Amnesia. In G. Lynch, J. L. McGaugh, & N. M. Weinberger, eds., *Neurobiology of learning and memory.* New York: Guilford Press.

Steinhausen, H. C., Willms, J., & Spohr, H. L. (1993). Long-term psychopathological and cognitive outcome of children with fetal alcohol syndrome. *Journal of the American Academy of Child and Adolescent Psychiatry, 32,* 990–994.

Steuer, F. B. (1994). *The psychological development of children.* Pacific Grove, CA: Brooks/Cole.

Stevens, J. (1992). Evidence for a genetic etiology in hyperactivity in children. *Behavioral Genetics, 22,* 337–344.

Streissguth, A. (1997). *Fetal alcohol syndrome.* Baltimore: Paul H. Brookes.

Streissguth, A. P., Barr, H. M., Bookstein, F. L., Sampson, P. D., & Carmichael Olson, H. (1999). The long-term neurocognitive consequences of prenatal alcohol exposure: A 14-year study. *Psychological Science, 10,* 186–190.

Stroop, J. R. (1935). Studies of interference in serial verbal reactions. *Journal of Experimental Psychology, 18,* 643–662.

Stuss, D. T. (1992). Biological and psychological development of executive functions. *Brain and Cognition, 20,* 8–23.

Stuss, D. T., & Benson, D. F. (1986). *The frontal lobes.* New York: Raven Press.

Swanson, H. L., Mink, J., & Bocian, K. M. (1999). Cognitive processing deficits in poor readers with symptoms of reading disabilities and ADHD: More alike than different? *Journal of Educational Psychology, 91,* 321–333.

Swanson, H. L., Posner, M., Potkin, S., Bonforte, S., Youpa, D., Fiore, C., Cantwell, D., & Crinella, F. (1991). Activating tasks for the study of visual-spatial attention in ADHD children: A cognitive anatomic approach. *Journal of Child Neurology, 6,* S119–S127.

Swillen, A., Fryns, J. P., Kleczkowska, A., Massa, G., Vanderschueren-Lodeweyck, M., & Van den Berghe, H. (1993). Intelligence, behaviour and psychosocial development in Turner syndrome. A cross-sectional study of 50 preadolescent and adolescent girls (4–20 years). *Genetic Counseling, 4,* 7–18.

Symonds, C. (1966). Disorders of memory. *Brain, 89,* 625.

Szatmari, P., Archer, L., Fisman, S., Streiner, D. L., & Wilson, F. (1995). Asperger's syndrome and autism: Differences in behavior, cognition, and adaptive functioning. *Journal of the American Academy of Child and Adolescent Psychiatry, 34,* 1662–1671.

Talland, G. A. (1965). *Deranged memory.* New York: Academic Press.

Teasdale, G., & Jennett, B. (1974). Assessment of coma and impaired consciousness. *Lancet, 2,* 81–84.

Teicher, M. H., Polcari, A., Anderson, C. M., Andersen, S. L., Glod, C. A., & Renshaw, P. (1996). Dose-dependent effects of methylphenidate on activity, attention, and magnetic imaging measures in children with ADHD. (Abstract). *Society for Neuroscience Abstracts, 22,* 1191.

Temple, C. M., & Carney, R. A. (1993). Intellectual functioning of children with Turner syndrome: A comparison of behavioral phenotypes. *Developmental Medicine and Child Neurology, 35,* 691–698.

Temple, C. M., Carney, R. A., & Mullarkey, S. (1996). Frontal lobe function and executive skills in children with Turner's syndrome. *Developmental Neuropsychology, 12,* 343–363.

Terman, L. M. (1925). *Genetic studies of genius,* Vol. 1. Stanford, CA: Stanford University Press.

Terman, L. M. (1959). *The gifted group at midlife.* Stanford, CA: Stanford University Press.

Terry, R. D., & Davies, P. (1980). Dementia of the Alzheimer type. *Annual Review of Neuroscience, 3,* 77–95.

Terry, R. D., Peck, A., DeTeresa, R., Schechter, R., & Horoupian, D. S. (1981). Some morphometric aspects of the brain in senile dementia of the Alzheimer type. *Annals of Neurology, 10,* 184–192.

Terry, R., & Katzman, R. (1992). Alzheimer disease and cognitive loss. In R. Katzman & J. W. Rowe, eds., *Principles of geriatric neurology* (pp. 207–265). Philadelphia: F. A. Davis.

Teuber, H.-L., Battersby, W. S., & Bender, M. B. (1960). *Visual field defects after penetrating missile wounds.* Cambridge, MA: Harvard University Press.

Teuber, H.-L. (1950). Neuropsychology. In M. R. Harrower, ed., *Recent advances in psychological testing* (pp. 30–52). Springfield, IL: Charles C Thomas.

Teuber, H.-L. (1959). Some alterations in behavior after cerebral lesions in man. In A. D. Bass, ed., *Evolution of nervous control.* Washington, DC: American Association for the Advancement of Science.

Thatcher, R. W. (1991). Maturation of the human frontal lobes. *Developmental Neuropsychology, 7,* 397–419.

Thatcher, R. W. (1994). Cyclic cortical reorganization: Origins of human cognitive development. In G. Dawson & K. W. Fischer, eds., *Human brain and the developing brain* (pp. 232–268). New York: Guilford Press.

Thatcher, R. W. (1997). Human frontal lobe development: A theory of cyclical cortical reorganization. In N. A. Krasnegor, G. R. Lyon, & P. S. Goldman-Rakic, eds., *Development of the prefrontal cortex: Evolution, neurobiology, and behavior* (pp. 85–116). Baltimore: Paul H. Brookes.

Therapeutics and Technology Assessment Subcommittee of the American Academy of Neurology. (1996). Assessment: Neuropsychological testing of adults: Considerations for neurologist. *Neurology, 47,* 592–599.

Thomsen, I. V. (1974). The patient with severe head-injury and his family—A follow-up study of 50 patients. *Scandinavian Journal of Rehabilitation Medicine, 6,* 180–183.

Toole, J. F. (1990). *Cerebrovascular diseases* (4th ed.). New York: Raven.

Torg, J. S. (1982). *Athletic injuries to the head, neck, and face.* Philadelphia: Lea & Febiger.

Träskmann, L., Asberg, M., Bertilsson, L., & Sjöstrand, L. (1981). Monoamine metabolites in CSF and suicidal behavior. *Archives of General Psychiatry, 38,* 631–636.

Tschirgi, R. D. (1960). Chapter 78. In J. Field & H. W. Magoun, eds., *Handbook of physiology, Section 1: Neurophysiology, Vol. 3* (pp. 1865–1890). Washington, DC: American Physiological Society.

Tulving, E. (1972). Episodic and semantic memory. In E. Tulving & W. Donaldson, eds., *Organization of memory.* New York: Academic Press

Turing, A. M. (1981). Computing machinery and intelligence. In D. R. Hofstadter & D. C. Dennett, eds., *The mind's I: Fantasies and reflections on self and soul.* New York: Basic Books.

Turner, H. H. (1938). A syndrome of infantilism, congenital webbed neck, and cubitus valgus. *Endocrinology, 23,* 566–574.

Tysvaer, A. T., Storli, O. V., Bachen, N. I. (1989). Soccer injuries to the brain. A neurologic and electroencephalographic study of former players. *Acta Neurologica Scandinavica, 80,* 151–156.

Valenstein, E. S. (1973). *Brain control.* New York: Wiley.

Vallar, G., Sandroni, P., Rusconi, M. L., & Barbieri, S. (1991). Hemianopia, hemianesthesia, and spatial neglect: A study with evoked potentials. *Neurology, 41,* 1918–1922.

Van Hoesn, G., & Damasio, A. R. (1987). Neural correlates of cognitive impairment in Alzheimer's disease. In V. B. Brooks, ed., *Handbook of physiology. The nervous system, Vol. V.* Bethesda, MD: American Physiological Society.

Van Raalte, J. L., & Brewer, B. W. (1996). *Exploring sport and exercise psychology.* Washington, DC: American Psychological Association.

van Zomeren, A. H., & Brouwer, W. H. (1994). *Clinical neuropsychology of attention.* New York: Oxford University Press.

Verona, J. W., & Williams, J. M. (1992). *Head injury and surgical intervention in pre-Columbian Peru.* Unpublished manuscript. Hahnemann University Medical School, Philadelphia.

Vilkki, J., & Laitinen, V. (1974). Differential effects of left and right ventrolateral thalamotomy on receptive and expressive verbal performances and face matching. *Neuropsychologia, 12,* 11.

Villardita, C., Smirni, P., LaPira, F., Zappala, G., & Nicoletti, F. (1982). Mental deterioration, visuoperceptive disabilities and constructional apraxia in Parkinson's disease. *Acta Neurologica Scandinavica, 66,* 112–120.

Voeller, K. K. S. (1996). Brief report: Developmental neurobiological aspects of autism. *Journal of Autism and Developmental Disorders, 26,* 189–193.

Volkmar, F. R., Klin, A., Schultz, R., Bronen, R., Marans, W. D., Sparrow, S., & Cohen, D. J. (1996). Asperger's syndrome. *Journal of the American Academy of Child and Adolescent Psychiatry, 35,* 118–123.

von Monakow, C. (1911). Lokalisation der Hirnfunktionen. *Journal of Psychiatry and Neurology, 17,* 185–200.

von Stockert, F. G. (1932). Subcortical dementia. *Archives of Psychiatry, 97,* 77–100.

Vonsattel, J. P. (1992). Neuropathology of Huntington's disease. In A. B. Joseph & R. R. Young, eds., *Movement disorders in neuropathology and neuropsychiatry* (pp. 186–194). Oxford, England: Blackwell Scientific.

Vygotsky, L. S. (1965). Psychology and localization of functions. *Neuropsychologia, 3,* 381.

Waber, D. P., & Tarbell, N. J. (1997). Toxicity of CNS prophylaxis for childhood leukemia. *Oncology, 11,* 259–264.

Wada, J., & Rasmussen, T. (1960). Intracarotid injection of sodium amytal for the lateralization of cerebral speech dominance: Experimental and clinical observations. *Journal of Neurosurgery, 17,* 266–282.

Walton, J. N. (1994). *Brain's diseases of the nervous system* (10th ed.). Oxford, England: Oxford University Press.

Wapner, W., Judd, T., & Gardner, H. (1978). Visual agnosia in an artist. *Cortex, 14,* 343–364.

Warren, R. P., Odell, J. D., & Warren, W. L. (1995). Reading disability, attention deficit hyperactivity disorder, and the immune system. *Letters of Science, 268,* 786–787.

Waterhouse, L., Fein, D., & Modahl, C. (1996). Autism. *Psychology Review, 103,* 457–489.

Wechsler, D. (1944). *The measurement of adult intelligence* (3rd ed.). Baltimore: Williams & Wilkins.

Wechsler, D. (1945). A standardized memory scale for clinical use. *Journal of Psychology, 19,* 87–95.

Wechsler, D. (1974). *Wechsler Intelligence Scale for Children–Revised.* New York: Psychological Corporation.

Wechsler, D. (1981). *Wechsler Adult Intelligence Scale–Revised.* New York: Psychological Corporation.

Wechsler, D. (1991). *Manual for the Wechsler Intelligence Scale for Children–Third Edition (WISC-III).* San Antonio, TX: Psychological Corporation.

Wehman, P. H. (1991). Cognitive rehabilitation in the workplace. In J. S. Kreutzer & P. H. Wehman, eds., *Cognitive rehabilitation for persons with traumatic brain injury.* Baltimore, Paul H. Brookes.

Wehman, P., & Kreutzer, J. (1990). *Vocational rehabilitation for persons with traumatic brain injury.* Rockville, MD: Aspen.

Weiss, G., & Hechtman, L. T. (1993). *Hyperactive children grown up* (2nd ed.). New York: Guilford Press.

Weiten, W. (1994). *Psychology: Themes and variations* (2nd ed.). Pacific Grove, CA: Brooks/Cole.

Weiten, W. (1998). *Psychology: Themes and variations* (4th ed.). Pacific Grove, CA: Brooks/Cole.

Wells, S. (1869). *How to read character: New illustrated hand-book of phrenology and physiognomy.* New York: Fowler & Wells.

Welsh, M. C. (1991). Rule-guided behavior and self-monitoring on the Tower of Hanoi disk-transfer task. *Cognitive Development, 6,* 59–76.

Welsh, M. C., Pennington, B. F., & Groisser, D. B. (1991). A normative–developmental study of executive function: A window on prefrontal function in children. *Developmental Neuropsychology, 7,* 131–149.

Wexler, A. (1995). *Mapping Fate: A memoir of family, risk, and genetic research.* New York: Random House.

White, B. J. (1994). The Turner syndrome: Origin, cytogenetic variants, and factors influencing the phenotype. In S. H. Broman & J. Grafman, eds., *Atypical cognitive deficits in developmental disorders* (pp. 183–196). New York: Oxford University Press.

Whyte, J. (1986). Outcome evaluation in the remediation of attention and memory deficits. *Journal of Head Trauma Rehabilitation, 1,* 43–53.

Wilkins, R. H., & Brody, I. A. (1970). Wernicke's sensory aphasia. *Archives of Neurology, 22,* 279.

Willerman, L., Schultz, R., Rutledge, N., & Bigler, E. (1992). Hemisphere size asymmetry predicts relative verbal and nonverbal intelligence differently in the sexes: An MRI study of structure-function relations. *Intelligence, 16,* 315–328.

Williams, P. L., & Warwick, R. (1975). *Functional neuroanatomy of man.* Philadelphia: Saunders.

Williams, R. L., & Karacan, I. (1978). *Sleep disorders: Diagnosis and treatment.* New York: Wiley.

Williams, R. W., & Herrup, K. (1988). The control of neuron number. *Annual Review of Neuroscience, 11,* 423–453.

Willis, K. E. (1993). Neuropsychological functioning in children with spina bifida and/or hydrocephalus. *Journal of Clinical Child Psychology, 22,* 247–265.

Wilson, B. (1991). Theory, assessment, and treatment in neuropsychological rehabilitation. *Neuropsychology, 5,* 281–291.

Wilson, S. A. K. (1912). Progressive lenticular degeneration: A familial nervous disease associated with cirrhosis of the liver. *Brain, 34,* 296–508.

Winson, J. (1972). Interspecies differences in the occurrence of theta. *Behavioral Biology, 7,* 479–487.

Witelson, S. F., Kigar, D. L., & Harvey, T. (1999). The exceptional brain of Albert Einstein. *Lancet, 353,* 2149–2153.

Witol, A., & Webbe, F. (1993). Neuropsychological deficits associated with soccer play. *Archives of Clinical Neuropsychology, 9,* 204–205.

Woods, B. T. (1980). The restricted effects of right-hemisphere lesions after age one; Wechsler test data. *Neuropsychologica, 18,* 65–70.

Woods, B. T., & Teuber, H.-L. (1973). Early onset of complementary specialization of cerebral hemispheres in man. *Transactions of the American Neurological Association, 98,* 113–117.

World Health Organization. (1992). *The ICD-10 classification of mental and behavioral disorders: Clinical descriptions and diagnostic guidelines.* Geneva: World Health Organization.

Wright, R. (1994). *The moral animal.* New York: Vintage.

Yeterian, E. H., & Van Hoesen, G. W. (1978). Cortico-striate projections in the rhesus monkey: The organization of certain cortico-caudate connections. *Brain Research, 139,* 43–63.

Yeudall, L. T., Reddon, J. R., Gill, D. M., & Stefanyk, W. O. (1987). Normative data for the Halstead-Reitan neuropsychological tests stratified by age and sex. *Journal of Clinical Psychology, 43,* 346–367.

Zaidel, D., & Sperry, R. W. (1973). Performance on Raven's Colored Progressive Matrices Test by subjects with cerebral commissurotomy. *Cortex, 9,* 34.

Zametkin, A. J., Liebenauer, L. L., Fitzgerald, G. A., King, A. C., Minkunas, D. V., Herscovitch, P., Yamada, E. M., & Cohen, R. M. (1993). Brain metabolism in teenagers with attention-deficit hyperactivity disorder. *Archives of General Psychiatry, 50,* 333–340.

Zametkin, A. J., Nordahl, T. E., Gross, M., King, A. C., Semple, W. E., Rumsey, J., Hamburger, S., & Cohen, R. M. (1990).

Cerebral glucose metabolism in adults with hyperactivity of childhood onset. *New England Journal of Medicine, 323,* 1362–1365.

Zangwill, O. L. (1960). *Cerebral dominance and its relation to psychological function.* Edinburgh: Oliver & Boyd.

Zec, R. F. (1993). Neuropsychological functioning in Alzheimer's disease. In R. W. Parks, R. F. Zec, & R. S. Wilson, eds., *Neuropsychology of Alzheimer's disease and other dementias.* New York: Oxford University Press.

Zeki, S. (1992). The visual image in mind and brain. *Readings from* Scientific American. New York: W. H. Freeman.

Zihl, J. (1995). Eye movement patterns in hemianopic dyslexia. *Brain, 118,* 891–912.

Zillmer, E. A. (1991). Rorschach Interpretation Assistance Program–Version 2 (Review). *Journal of Personality Assessment, 57*(2), 381–383.

Zillmer, E. A. (1995). The case of Aaron B. In D. L. Chute & M. E. Bliss, eds., *Exploring psychological disorders* (pp. 115–124). Pacific Grove, CA: Brooks/Cole.

Zillmer, E. A. (1996, November 14). *Mind over matter: Brain Research in the next millennium.* Invited paper to Congressional staff on Capitol Hill, Washington, D.C.

Zillmer, E. A., & Ball, J. D. (1987). Psychological and neuropsychological assessment in the medical setting. *Staff & Resident Physician, 33,* 602–609.

Zillmer, E. A., & Ball, J. D. (1989). Behavioral gerontology: Cognitive changes associated with normal and abnormal aging. *Staff & Resident Physician, 35,* 79–86.

Zillmer, E. A., & Kennedy, C. H. (1999a). Construct validity for the d2 Test of Attention. *Archives of Clinical Neuropsychology, 8,* 728.

Zillmer, E. A., & Kennedy, C. H. (1999b). Preliminary United States norms for the d2 Test of Attention. *Archives of Clinical Neuropsychology, 8,* 727–728.

Zillmer, E. A., & Passuth, P. M. (1989). Predicting functional ability from mental status among nursing home residents. *The Gerontologist, 29,* 142A.

Zillmer, E. A., & Perry, W. (1996). Cognitive-neuropsychological abilities and related psychological disturbance: A factor model of neuropsychological, Rorschach, and MMPI indices. *Assessment, 3,* 209–224.

Zillmer, E. A., & Resnick, D. A. (1994). Mind over matter: The study of neuropsychology. *Graduate Studies, 4*(1), 45–46.

Zillmer, E. A., & Vuz, J. (1995). Factor analysis with Rorschach data. In J. E. Exner, Jr., ed., *Methods and issues in Rorschach research* (pp. 251–306). Hillsdale, NJ: Erlbaum.

Zillmer, E. A., & Wickramaserkera, I. (1987). Biofeedback and hypnotizability: Initial treatment considerations. *Clinical Biofeedback and Health, 10,* 51–57.

Zillmer, E. A., Archer, R. P., & Castino, B. (1989). The Rorschach records of Nazi war criminals: A reanalysis using current scoring and interpretation practices. *Journal of Personality Assessment, 53,* 85–99.

Zillmer, E. A., Ball, J. D., Fowler, P. C., Newman, A. C., & Stutts, M. L. (1991). Wechsler Verbal-Performance IQ discrepancies among psychiatric inpatients: Implications for subtle neuropsychological dysfunctioning. *Archives of Clinical Neuropsychology, 6,* 61–71.

Zillmer, E. A., Chelder, M. J., & Efthimiou, J. (1995). *Assessment of Impairment (AIM) Measure.* Philadelphia: Drexel University.

Zillmer, E. A., Culbertson, W. C., & Holda, B. (1997). The relationship of temporal variables to the Tower of London–Drexel performance. *Archives of Clinical Neuropsychology, 4,* 434.

Zillmer, E. A., Efthimiou, J., McClain, M., Harris, B., Resh, R., & Chelder, M. J. (1994). Neuropsychological screening in stroke patients with unilateral and bilateral strokes. *Archives of Clinical Neuropsychology, 9,* 209–210.

Zillmer, E. A., Fowler, P. C., Gutnick, H. N., & Becker, E. (1990). Comparison of two cognitive bedside screening instruments in nursing home residents: A factor analytic study. *Journal of Gerontology: Psychological Sciences, 45,* 69–74.

Zillmer, E. A., Fowler, P. C., Newman, A. C., & Archer, R. P. (1988). Relationships between the WAIS and neuropsychological measures for neuropsychiatric inpatients. *Archives of Clinical Neuropsychology, 3,* 33–45.

Zillmer, E. A., Fowler, P. C., Waechtler, C., Harris, B., & Khan, F. (1992). The effects of unilateral and multifocal lesions on the WAIS-R: A factor analytic study of stroke patients. *Archives of Clinical Neuropsychology, 7,* 29–41.

Zillmer, E. A., Harrower, M., Ritzler, B., & Archer, R. P. (1995). *The quest for the Nazi personality: A psychological investigation of Nazi war criminals.* Hillsdale, NJ: Erlbaum.

Zillmer, E. A., Lucci, K., Barth, J. T., Peake, T., & Spyker, D. (1986). Neurobehavioral sequelae of subcutaneous injection with metallic mercury. *Journal of Toxicology: Clinical Toxicology, 24,* 100–110.

Zillmer, E. A., Montenegro, L., Wiser, J., Barth, J. T., & Spyker, D. (1996). Neuropsychological sequelae in subacute home chlordane poisoning: Ten case studies. *Archives of Clinical Neuropsychology, 11,* 77–89.

Zillmer, E. A., O'Connor, B., McClain, M., Stein, L., Harris, B., Resh, R., Chelder, M. J., & Efthimiou, J. (1993). A factor analytic study of the Assessment of Impairment Measure (AIM). *Archives of Clinical Neuropsychology, 8,* 278.

Zillmer, E. A., Ware, J. C., Rose, V., & Bond, T. (1989). An examination of the Symptom Checklist 90–Revised (SCL-90-R) in the assessment of personality function in sleep disorders. *Sleep Research, 18,* 189.

Zillmer, E. A., Ware, J. C., Rose, V., & Maximin, A. (1988). MMPI characteristics of patients with different severity of sleep apnea. *Sleep Research, 17,* 136.

Zola-Morgan, S., & Squire, L. R. (1993). Neuroanatomy of memory. *Annual Review of Neuroscience, 16,* 547–563.

Zubenko, G. S., Moossy, J., Martinez, A. J., Rao, G. R., Kopp, U., & Hanin, I. (1989). A brain regional analysis of morphologic and cholinergic abnormalities in Alzheimer's disease. *Archives of Neurology, 46,* 634–639.

GLOSSARY

Ablation experiment Developed by Pierre Flourens, and involved removing parts of the brain of pigeons and hens. Flourens reported that excising any part of the brain in birds led to generalized, not localized, disorders of behavior.

Absence seizures Occur when the normally asynchronous waking state is abruptly interrupted by low-wave synchronous activity; characterized by synchronous bilateral spike-and-wave discharge.

Acceleration The brain experiencing a significant physical force that propels it quickly, from stationary to moving.

Acetylcholine (Ach) Also called *choline;* the first neurotransmitter to be identified; plays a prominent role in the PNS, influencing motor control, and in autonomic nervous system functioning.

Achievement tests Most influenced by past educational attainment; measures how well a subject has profited by learning and experience as compared to others.

Achromatopsia The complete loss of ability to detect color.

Acidophilic adenoma A functioning type of pituitary tumor that usually appears in the anterior lobe of the pituitary gland. The acidophilic adenoma gives rise to excessive secretion of growth hormones often resulting in giantism (excessive growth of hands and feet).

Acoustic neuroma Progressively enlarging, benign tumor within the auditory canal arising from Schwann cells of the VIIIth cranial nerve.

Action potential An electrical potential across the neuron membrane. The action potential spreads down the axon as the voltage-controlled sodium channels open up sequentially, like falling dominoes.

Affective significance of stimuli The binding or attachment of emotion to novel and social stimuli.

Afferent nerves (sensory nerves) Convey incoming messages from the sensory receptors to the CNS.

Agenesis Complete or partial failure of an organ to develop.

Agnosia An absence of knowing. The distinction between the ability to recognize an object and the inability to name it. Term first coined by Sigmund Freud.

Aguesia Inability to recognize tastes.

Agyria, or **lissencephaly** A congenital disorder in which the normal gyri and sulci of the brain fail to develop. Believed to occur between the third and fourth month of gestation.

Air encephalogram or **pneumoencephalography** The radiographic visualization of the fluid-containing structures of the brain, the ventricles, and spinal column. It is similar to the x ray, but it involves the withdrawal of cerebrospinal fluid (CSF) by lumbar puncture, which is then replaced with a gas including, air, oxygen, or helium.

Akinetopsia The specific inability to identify objects in motion.

Alcohol-related neurodevelopmental disabilities (ARND) See **Fetal alcohol effect**.

Alternating attention The ability to switch back and forth between tasks.

Alzheimer's disease (AD) An irreversible cortical dementia, not due to an identifiable cause, that is characterized by neuropathologic markers including neurofibrillary tangles and senile plaques.

Amino acids A group of neurotransmitters that plays a major role in the more basic type of neuronal transmission that depend on rapid communication among neurons.

Amygdala Literally "almond," because of its shape; has a specific role in fear conditioning and impacts the strength of stored memory.

Amyotrophic lateral sclerosis (ALS) Disease of the motor system in which people experience a gradual to total loss of muscle control and muscle function.

Anastomosis Communication between blood vessels by collateral channels. See **Collateral blood vessel**.

Anencephaly A congenital condition characterized by a failure in development of the two hemispheres, mesencephalon, and diencephalon of the brain. The brain is represented by a vascular mass. The condition produces severe neurologic deficits and is incompatible with life.

Aneurysms   Weak areas in the walls of an artery that cause the vessel to balloon.

Angiography   X-raying blood vessels in the brain after introducing contrast material into the arterial or venous bloodstream. Angiography is the most useful technique for examining the blood supply to and from the brain.

Anomia   Problems in word finding. Only a word or two, here and there, is lost, and the communication can proceed pretty much as normal. In more severe cases, most or all words can be lost.

Anopsias   Term for visual difficulties.

Anosmia   Total loss of smell.

Anosognosia   A term first coined by Babinski to indicate the inability or refusal to recognize that one has a particular disease or disorder.

Anoxia   The complete cessation of oxygen supply to the brain. Anoxia often occurs with stroke or other severe traumas of the brain, such as are often seen in gunshot wounds to the head.

Anterior attention system   An attentional system of the brain mediating the voluntary control of attention that is supported by the frontal and medial cortexes of the brain.

Anterior cerebral artery   Resulting from one-half of the division of an internal carotid artery, it supplies the anterior medial portion of its corresponding cerebral hemisphere.

Anterior commissure   Minor intercerebral fibers.

Anterior communicating artery   Connects the left and right anterior cerebral arteries.

Anterior   Toward the front or front end.

Anterograde amnesia   The loss of memory for events after trauma or disease onset.

Anterograde degeneration   The degeneration of the axon after the cell body has been damaged.

Anticholinergics   Treatment for Parkinson's disease; act by blocking the action of acetylcholine.

Anton's syndrome   Actual denial of cerebral blindness; a behavioral mirror of apperceptive agnosia.

Aortic arch   Arises from the left ventricle of the heart.

Aphasia   A disturbance of language usage or comprehension. It may involve the impairment of the power to speak, write, read, gesture, or to comprehend spoken, written, or gestured language.

Apnea   The cessation of airflow; literally means "a lack of breath."

Apperceptive visual agnosia   A visual problem with object perception as the primary difficulty.

Apraxia   An absence of action, but the term is most often used to describe a variety of missing or inappropriate actions that cannot be clearly attributed to primary motor deficits, the lack of comprehension or motivation. Thus *apraxia* refers to an inability to perform voluntary actions despite an adequate amount of motor strength and control.

Arachnoid granulations   Small "pockets" of cauliflower-like veins within the subarachnoid space, which serve as pathways for the subarachnoid cerebrospinal fluid to be absorbed and reenter the venous circulation.

Arachnoid membrane   a "spiderlike" avascular membrane of the meninges.

Aristotle   Greek, 384–322 B.C.; a disciple of Plato, erroneously believed that the heart is the source of all mental processes. Aristotle argued that because the brain is bloodless, it fills the function of a "radiator," cooling hot blood ascending from the heart.

Arteriovenous malformations (AVM)   Abnormal, often redundant vessels that result in abnormal blood flow. Because AVMs have inherently weak vessel walls, they may lead to slow bleeding or to inadequate distribution of blood in the regions surrounding the vessels.

Articulation   The ability to form phonetic sounds of vowels and consonants, which then are placed in different combinations to form words and sentences.

Articulatory phonological loop   A working memory "slave system" that stores speech-based information and is important in the acquisition of vocabulary.

Ascending spinal-thalamic tract   Carries sensory information related to pain and temperature and runs in parallel to the spinal cord. It synapses over a wide region of the thalamus, primarily on the intralaminar and ventral posterior nuclei of the thalamus and then to the somatosensory cortex.

Asociality   Denotes a lack of social interest and relatedness. This anomaly is hypothesized to be one of the mechanisms responsible for autistic behaviors.

Asperger's syndrome   A pervasive developmental disorder characterized by symptoms of autism, including impairments in social relatedness and atypical patterns of behavior, interest, or activity. However, in contrast to autism, impairment in language, adaptive skills (with the exception of social skills), and curiosity about the environment are not pronounced. The disorder tends to have a later age of onset than autism.

Associative visual agnosia   A visual problem having to do with difficulty in assigning meaning to an object.

Astereognosia   Inability to recognize an object by touch.

Astereognosis   See **Tactile agnosia**.

Astrocytes   Nonneural, star-shaped glia cells that are highly branched and occupy much space between neurons in the gray matter. Their multiple functions include supporting neurons by interweaving among nerve fibers, contributing to the metabolism of synaptic transmitters, and regulating the balance of ions. Astrocytes join together to provide a barrier between parts of the CNS and non-CNS tissue.

Astrocytomas   A form of malignant tumors composed primarily of astrocytes, a type of glia cell.

Atharva-Veda   700 B.C. Indian text that proposed that the soul was nonmaterial and never died.

Atherosclerosis   A neuropathological process characterized by irregular distributed, yellow, fatty plaques in large and medium-sized arteries.

Atonia   Lack or reduction of muscle tone.

Atrophy   Brain shrinkage.

Attention-deficit/hyperactivity disorder (ADHD)   A neuropsychological developmental disorder characterized by age-inappropriate inattention, impulsivity, and overactivity.

Aura   A neurologic event that occurs before the onset of a migraine or a seizure. The aura presents usually as a visual symptom including flashing lights, zigzag lines, or blurred or partial loss of vision.

Autism   Previously referred to as *infantile autism* or *Kanner's autism*. A pervasive developmental disorder, evident before age 3, involving impaired communication, socialization, and behavioral adaptation. Atypical behaviors, preoccupations, or interests are frequently evident. The etiology of the disorder is unknown, and the prognosis is poor.

Autistic aloneness   A term proposed by Leo Kanner in his description of autistic children, referring to one of the central symptoms of the disorder, namely, the profound separation and disconnection of autistic individuals from other people.

Automatisms   Stereotyped hand movements or facial tics often seen during a absence seizure.

Autonomic nervous system (ANS)   Provides the "automatic" neural control of internal organs (such as heart, intestines). Most autonomic organs receive both sympathetic and parasympathetic input.

Axon   Extends from cell body. Its main function is to transmit information in the form of an action potential.

Babinski, Joseph   1857–1932; founder of British neurology.

Ballint's syndrome   Related to damage of the parietal-occipital area of both hemispheres; includes visual agnosia along with other visual-spatial difficulties such as misreaching and left-sided neglect.

Basal forebrain   Structure of the telencephalon, surrounding the inferior tip of the frontal horn; strongly inter-

connects with limbic structures; includes various structures such as the amygdala and the septum.

Basal ganglia   Also called the *basal nuclei;* deep nuclei of the telencephalon. Structures include the caudate nucleus, putamen, globus pallidus, substantia nigra, and subthalamic nuclei. Important relay stations in motor behavior (for example, the striato-pallido-thalamic loop). Coordinate stereotyped postural and reflexive motor activity.

Basal nuclei   See **Basal ganglia.**

Base rate   The frequency with which a pathologic condition is diagnosed in the population.

Basilar artery   Formed from a joining of the two vertebral arteries at the level of the brain stem.

Basolateral circuit   Anatomic circuit centered around the amygdala; its most likely role is in emotional processing.

Basophilic adenomas   A functioning type of tumor of the pituitary gland in the anterior lobe of the pituitary gland, which gives rise to excessive secretion of ACTH, which can cause Cushing syndrome.

Behavioral-adaptive scales   Tests that examine what an individual usually and habitually does, not what he or she can do. Such scales are most frequently used in evaluating the daily self-care skills of people who are quite impaired.

Benign   Describes cell growth that is usually surrounded by a fibrous capsule, is typically noninfiltrative (that is, noninvasive), and will not spread to other parts of the body.

Benton, Arthur   American neuropsychologist who pioneered the role of the right cerebral hemisphere in behavior.

Benzodiazepines   A family of sedating drugs used to treat anxiety and sleep disorders.

Beta-amyloid   Amino acid peptide protein core found in the center of senile plaques. Also written as β-*amyloid.*

Bipolar neurons   Neurons with two axons.

Blood–brain barrier   Affords protection from potentially harmful substances circulating in the body through the bloodstream. It bars certain drugs totally from the brain, and other substances require an active transport system across the blood–brain barrier.

Bradykinesia   A poverty of movement that is not only slowed but reduced in magnitude; negative motor symptom of Parkinson's disease.

Bradyphrenia   Extremely slow information processing speed characteristic of patients with subcortical dementias.

Brain abscesses   A "walled-off," localized pocket of pus within the brain often related to an infection.

Brain herniation   A pathologic process associated with increasing intracranial pressure that occurs in the cranium, which may result in a displacement and deformation of the brain.

Brain hypothesis   Suggests that the brain is the source of all behavior.

Brain stem   Evolutionary old brain structure involved in regulating brain activation. It emerges from the uppermost portion of the spinal cord and includes all the subdivisions below the telencephalon (that is, the diencephalon, the mesencephalon, the metencephalon, and the myelencephalon), except for the cerebellum.

Broca, Paul   1824–1880; French anthropologist and scientist, who advanced surgery, neuroanatomy, neurophysiology, and neuropathology.

Brodmann's areas   Cytoarchitectural scheme dividing the cortex into 52 sections.

Canalesthesia   The fragmentation of the processing of incoming information from the sensory modalities. The anomaly is believed to be one of the etiological factors of autistic behaviors.

Cannon-Bard theory   Opposite of James-Lange theory. Walter Cannon, and later Philip Bard, argued the conscious emotional experience can be divorced from bodily sensation or expression. Although today most scientists agree that there is a correspondence between cognitive experience of emotion and sensory experience, types of emotion, emotional intensity, and individual variation appear to vary considerably.

Cardiac hypothesis   Proposed that the heart was the seat of such emotions as love and anger.

Cataplexy   The most debilitating of the narcolepsy symptoms; a brief episode of muscle weakness and/or actual paralysis.

Caudal   Toward the rear, away from the head.

Caudate nucleus   Structure of the basal ganglia.

Cell doctrine   A hypothesis that assumed the ventricles were the location of the mind. Today, the cell doctrine is known to be entirely inaccurate.

Central executive   Concept from the theory of working memory in which the central executive is an attention-controlling system; supervises and coordinates slave systems and is the proposed deficit in Alzheimer's disease.

Central nervous system (CNS)   The CNS includes the brain and the spinal cord. It is located within and protected by the bony cavities of the skull and the spine.

Central sleep apnea   Apnea that occurs most often during REM sleep in which disordered breathing is related to the brain failing to send the necessary signals to breathe. This may reflect brain stem abnormalities that manifest only during sleep.

Central sulcus   Separates the frontal and parietal lobes.

Cerebellar peduncles   Large neural tracts connecting the cerebellum to the midbrain.

Cerebellum   Means "little brain"; sits posterior to the brain stem, and inferior to the telencephalon, functions in coordinating motor and sensory information.

Cerebral (or Sylvian) aqueduct   A narrow channel passing through the midbrain connecting the third to the fourth ventricle.

Cerebral achromatopsia   Total color-blindness.

Cerebral hemispheres (cerebrum)   Includes structures of the frontal, parietal, occipital, and temporal lobes; plays a role in higher cognitive functioning.

Cerebrospinal fluid (CSF)   A protective fluid that surrounds and supports the brain and spinal cord.

Cerebrovascular accident (CVA)   A technical term for stroke; describes a heterogeneous groups of vascular disorders associated with damage to the brain's blood vessels and decreased blood flow within and to the brain.

Chemoreceptors   Structures that respond to various chemicals on the surface of the skin and mucous membranes. They range from detecting levels of stomach acidity to skin irritations. Smell and taste are special examples of chemoreception and are discussed separately. Thermoreceptors detect heat and cold.

Chorea   Twisting, writhing, undulating, grimacing movements of the face and body. Commonly associated with Huntington's disease.

Choroid plexus   A highly vascularized network of small blood vessels that protrude into the ventricles from the pia mater and secretes CSF.

Chromophobic adenoma   A functioning type of tumor of the pituitary gland localized in the anterior aspects of the pituitary gland and is often associated with hyper- or hypopituitarism.

Cingulate gyrus   A structure of the limbic system, the medial cortex surrounding the corpus callosum.

Cingulum   A major intracerebral fiber.

Circadian rhythm   Daily biorhythm oscillation of heightened and lowered brain arousal observed throughout the wake and sleep cycle.

Circle of Willis   A spiderlike arterial structure formed by the anterior cerebral branches of the internal carotid artery and its connections, the anterior communicating artery, the posterior communicating artery, and the posterior cerebral branches of the basilar artery. It allows for a certain degree of redundancy among blood vessels and blood supply to the various areas of the brain.

Cisterns Cavities that are expansions of the subarachnoid space in the CNS.

Clonic Motoric jerking.

Closed head injuries A type of head injury that is associated with a blow to the head, but that does not penetrate the skull.

Cocktail party syndrome Hyperverbal; a form of speech featuring excessive verbiage that is lacking in clarity, organization, depth, and relevance.

Collateral blood vessel Allows redundant blood supply to take more than one route to a given region. The term *collateral* describes redundant blood flow present in the vascular network after occlusion of an artery. If one vessel is blocked, a given region might be spared an infarct because the blood has an alternative route.

Coma Loss of consciousness.

Communicating hydrocephalus A form of hydrocephalus that includes the presence of blood or blood products that are mixed with cerebrospinal fluid. This is most often caused by a hemorrhage or infection. Also see **Nonobstructive hydrocephalus.**

Complex partial seizure A type of seizure that has an element of altered psyche or awareness in addition to sensory or motor components.

Computed transaxial tomography (CT scan) An imaging process that renders an anatomic image of brain density based on multiple x-ray images of the brain. CT, which is readily available and can be used with almost anyone, provides a three-dimensional perspective of the brain with acceptable differentiation of brain structures.

Consciousness Awareness, level of mental alertness and level of attention; the mind's subjective experience of brain states and processes that are available to perception.

Construct validity Focuses primarily on a test score as a measure of the psychological construct of interest. If a neuropsychological test measures a specific construct (memory, attention, for example), then it has construct validity.

Content validity Pertains to the degree to which a sample of items or tasks make conceptual sense or represent some defined psychological domain.

Contralateral On the opposite side.

Coronal plane A plane (y axis) that shows the brain as seen from the front (frontal section). Typically this plane is viewed from behind in order to provide consistency for right and left directions of the brain and the picture.

Corpus callosum A large set of myelinated axons connecting the right and left cerebral hemisphere, functions in information exchange between the two hemispheres.

Cortical dementias Dementias affecting the cerebral cortex.

Corticogenesis The development of the cortex of the brain.

Countercoup injury A type of closed head injury sustained at the pole opposite from where the primary injury occurs because the brain "tears" away from the skull.

Cranial nerves Carry specific sensory and motor information directly to the brain, bypassing the spinal cord. These nerves are also very old from an evolutionary point of view.

Creutzfeldt-Jakob disease (CJD) A subcortical dementia characterized by a quick progression; connected to "mad cow disease"; transmitted between humans via transplants of affected neural tissue, through cornea transplants or contamination via medical procedures, and its variants can cross species through consumption of tainted meat containing neural tissue.

Criterion validity Demonstrates that scores are related systematically to one or more outcome criteria, either now (concurrent validity) or in the future (predictive validity).

Crystallized functions Thought to be most dependent on cultural factors and learning. Spelling and factual knowledge are examples of crystallized functions.

Crystallized intelligence An accumulation of acquired skills and general information, most related to formal education or diverse social experiences.

Cubitus valgus A deformity of the arm in which the forearm deviates laterally, resulting in an increased carrying angle at the elbow.

Cushing's syndrome Named after Boston surgeon Harvey Cushing (1869–1939); a severe systemic illness most often seen in females, which includes neurologic symptoms and changes in bone structure, hypertension, and diabetes. The ACTH-secreting tumor is the most serious condition encountered by any of the pituitary tumors and can result in a necessary complete removal of the tumor, including the pituitary gland.

Cutoff score Often used in neuropsychology to determine a range of impaired functioning. A patient scoring worse than the cutoff score is labeled as impaired;

a patient scoring better is labeled as *within normal limits (WNL)*.

Cytoarchitectonic dysplasia   A focal pathologic change of the cellular organization of brain cells.

da Vinci, Leonardo   1452–1519; Italian painter, sculptor, architect, and scientist.

Deceleration   Describes an event in which the brain is in motion traveling at a certain speed and then stops abruptly.

Declarative memory   A form of memory that is explicit, verbalizable, and accessible to conscious awareness.

Decussating   Switching the transmission of information from one side of the body to the contralateral side of the brain.

Deficit measurement   An approach to neuropsychological assessment for understanding general conditions and disease states about a patient by examining scores that are impaired and comparing them to other factors known about the patient.

Delirium   A transient cognitive problem associated with a confused state caused by specific organic problems.

Dementia   A pattern of impairment with varying causes characterized by a deteriorating progression in memory as well as other areas of cognitive functioning.

Dendrites   Feathery extensions that branch from the neuron into the immediate neighborhood of the cell body.

Dendritic spines   Short outgrowths on the dendrites that contain synapses for gathering information to be sent to the neurons.

Descartes, René   (French, 1596–1650); proposed a strict split or schism between mental processes and physical abilities. He hypothesized that the mind and body are separate, but interact with each other.

Diaschisis   A passive process of uncovering working neural systems after temporary neuronal disruption in areas far removed from the lesion site.

Diencephalon   Composed primarily of the thalamus and hypothalamus and a structure of the brain stem, also known as the *interbrain* or "between brain."

Digital subtraction angiography   A procedure in which the x-ray image of the brain is stored and subtracted after the images of the contrast material has been acquired. The process is particularly effective in enhancing the visualization of blood vessels, including the morphological and physiological states of the arterial, capillary, and venous phases of the cerebral circulation.

Disengage attention   The withdrawal or decoupling of attentional focus from a stimulus.

Disinhibition   Impulsivity and inappropriate behavior; may result from losing inhibitory neurons to trauma or disease.

Dissimulation   A form of malingering in which the patient is consciously denying that there is anything wrong with him or her, in order to achieve some secondary gain (for example, to avoid hospitalization, to gain employment).

Dissociation   A separation between functional contributions of two different brain areas.

Distal   Away from the center, toward the periphery, away from the origin of attachment.

Divided attention   Partialing out one's attentional resources at the same time rather than switching back and forth, however quickly.

Dominance   Hand (and to a lesser extent eye and foot) preferences and proficiencies in performing tasks or to the cerebral organization of the brain.

Dopamine   A neurotransmitter that plays an important role in the organization of motor behavior.

Dorsal column medial lemniscal pathway   Carries information pertaining to touch and vibration. It is so named because it is routed up the dorsal aspects of the spinal cord to a white matter tract termed the *medial lemniscus* that courses through the contralateral side of the brain stem through the medulla, pons, and midbrain to be routed up through the thalamus (ventral posterior nucleus, VP) and on to the primary somatosensory cortex.

Dorsal simultagnosia   A visual disorder related to damage of the parietal-occipital area of both hemispheres. Even though parts of a picture may be recognized, the whole is not perceived.

Dorsal   Toward the back. The top of the brain is dorsal in humans.

Dorsolateral prefrontal cortex   This area is located, functionally, in the prefrontal cortex, which is responsible for orchestrating and organizing many functions of the brain. The dorsolateral prefrontal cortex is not a "movement center" in and of itself, but is instrumental in deploying movement. Sensory information from the integrative association area of the parietal lobes is relayed to this motor planning area.

Double dissociation   A logical progression of scientific assumptions in localizing functional areas in the brain. For example, if symptom A appears with lesions in brain structure X, but not with those in Y, and symptom B appears with lesions of Y but not of X, then those specific areas of the brain each have a specific function.

Dura mater   "Tough mother"; a dense, inelastic, double-layered, vascularized membrane of the meninges that adheres to the inner surface of the skull.

Dysarthria   A specific motor apraxia involving the vocal musculature. People with dysarthria differ from pure aphasiacs, although the two conditions may occur together in that such patients know what they want to say, but are unable to formulate words because of a problem with motor control.

Dyscalculia   A disorder of mathematics involving impaired ability to comprehend number concepts, spatially orient numbers, reason mathematically, or perform mathematical operations.

Dysgenesis   Abnormal or defective development of an organ.

Dysgraphia   An impairment of the ability to write or express oneself in writing. Deficits are evident in one or more of the following areas: (1) letter formation, speed of writing, and spatial organization of writing; (2) written expression; (3) mechanical knowledge of spelling, grammar, punctuation, and capitalization; and (4) organization and thematic construction of written expression.

Dysguesia   Distorted taste sensation.

Dyskinesia   Uncontrolled involuntary movement.

Dyslexia   A developmental or acquired disorder of reading involving the disruption of one or more of the component skills of reading. Central reading skills include letter identification, phonological awareness and processing, and decoding of the written word.

Dysosmia   Distorted smell sensation.

Dysphonia   Loss of vocal emotional expression resulting in a monotonous voice tone.

Echolalia   An atypical communication behavior characterized by the repetition or "echoing" of the words or phrases just spoken by another person. Often displayed by children with pervasive developmental disorders.

Ectopias   Also referred to as "brain warts." Small areas of abnormally placed brain neurons.

Edema   The swelling of the brain

Efferent nerves   Motor nerves carry outgoing signals for action from the CNS to the muscles.

Electroconvulsive therapy (ECT)   Shock therapy; administering a large amount of electricity to the skull causing the collective firing of neurons: an induced seizure. ECT sometimes improves severe forms of depression within a few days. Although the mechanism is not clearly understood, therapists use ECT when it is important to intervene quickly to prevent the patient from acting on suicidal thoughts.

Electrocorticogram (ECoG)   A form of EEG in which electrodes are placed directly on the exposed cortex during surgery to isolate a precise location of brain pathology.

Electroencephalography (EEG)   One of the most widely used techniques in neurology. In EEG the electrical activity of nerve cells of the brain are recorded through electrodes attached to various locations on the scalp.

Eliptogenic focus   The anatomic site of onset.

Embolism   From *embolos,* Greek for "plug" or "wedge"; a type of occlusion of an artery in which the clot forms in one area of the body and travels through the arterial system to another area, in this case the brain, where it becomes lodged and obstructs cranial blood flow. Approximately 14% of all CVAs are caused by an embolism.

Emotional perception   The ability to identify and comprehend the emotions of others from both verbal and nonverbal behavioral cues.

Encode attention   An element of attention that is involved in short-term or working memory.

Endorphins   The most prominent neuropeptide with opioid properties. Endorphins have received much scientific attention for their analgesic effects and their possible role in a pain-inhibiting neuronal system.

Endothelium   The layer of epithelial cells that line the blood vessels. When the endothelium is breached, the blood-clotting properties of the platelets are activated. They change shape and adhere to the vessel wall, each other, and red blood cells. If this occurs pathologically (that is, in a normal vessel), it leads to a thrombosis, ultimately occluding the vessel.

Engaging attention   The attentional operation of focusing, or centering of attention on a stimulus.

Enhanced CT   A CT scan that involves the injection of a contrast agent to provide better visualization of brain structures, particularly bleeds.

Enuresis   The continuation of frequent bed-wetting beyond the age of 5 that is not a consequence of a physiological dysfunction.

Ependymal glioma   A bulky, solid, firm vascular tumor of the fourth ventricle.

Epidural hematoma   Represents a bleed between the meninges and the skull and occurs in 1 to 3% of major closed head injuries. The cause of an epidural is most often related to the rupture of an artery.

Epidural space   The space between the two dural layers of the meninges.

Epilepsy   "Falling sickness"; a syndrome in which brain seizure activity is a primary symptom.

Epileptic syndrome   Most people with repeat seizures are considered to have an epileptic syndrome, which is more serious than a single seizure.

Episodic memory   Individual episodes, usually autobiographical, that have specific spatial and temporal tags in memory.

Equipotentiality   Term first coined by Flourens to describe the notion that mental abilities depend on the brain functioning as a whole. Thus, the effects of brain injury are determined by the size of the injury rather than its location.

Evoked potential (EP)   Also called *event-related potentials (ERPs);* a electrophysiological diagnostic test that involves the stimulation of specific sensory fibers, which in turn generate electrical activity along the central and peripheral pathways as well as the specific primary receptive areas in the brain.

Excessive daytime sleepiness   Pathological daytime sleepiness; the most frequent first sign in narcolepsy.

Excitatory postsynaptic potential (EPSP)   Depolarization that increases the probability of the postsynaptic cell to reach its threshold and fire.

Executive functions   Higher-order regulatory and supervisory functions that researchers believe are subserved, in part, by the frontal lobes. Cognitive operations such as planning, mental flexibility, attentional allocation, working memory, and inhibitory control are considered executive functions.

Executive planning   Higher-order problem solving necessary for the generation and organization of behavior to achieve a goal. Executive planning requires the ability to anticipate change, respond objectively, generate and select alternatives, and sustain attention.

Expressive aphasia   A disorder of speech output.

Extended paraphasia   See **Word salad.**

Extended selective attention   Overly extended attentional focus and an inappropriate delay in shifting attention. The anomaly is considered one of the etiological factors in the symptoms of autism.

Extradural hematoma   Less frequent than the subdural hematoma, a bleed that occurs between the skull and the dura. Extradural hematomas are most likely caused by a tearing of the large middle meningeal arteries.

Extrapyramidal motor system   Responsible for stereotyped postural and reflexive motor activity. The system also acts to keep individual muscles ready to respond.

False positive   Also known as a *Type I error* or *false alarm.* Refers to a case in which a neuropsychological test erroneously indicates the presence of a pathologic condition.

Femorocerebral angiography   Angiography that introduces a catheter into the arterial system via the femoral artery.

Festinating gait   The rapid, shuffling gait characteristic of Parkinson's disease.

Fetal alcohol effects (FAE)   A developmental disorder that involves the cognitive and behavioral deficits associated with FAS, but without the physical stigmata of FAS. Also see **Fetal alcohol syndrome.**

Fetal alcohol syndrome (FAS)   A developmental disorder caused by the pregnant mother ingesting alcohol. The disorder is characterized by recognizable physical stigmata, neurologic abnormalities, and cognitive and behavioral impairments. Unlike many of the congenital disorders, FAS is preventable.

Fibers   See **Tracts.**

Finger agnosia   Inability to recognize or orient to one's own fingers.

Fissure   A very deep sulcus in the cortex.

Flicker fusion rate   Denotes the speed at which two separate visual images appear to fuse visually into a single image.

Flourens, Pierre   French, 1794–1867; the foremost early advocate of an alternative to localizationist theories.

Fluent aphasia   A disorder of speech in which the patient remains able to talk, but his or her speech makes no sense, often sounding like some unknown foreign language.

Fluid functions   Believed to be culture-free and independent of learning. Problem solving and abstract reasoning are considered fluid functions.

Fluid intelligence   Novel reasoning and the efficiency of solving new problems or responding to abstract ideas.

Focused attention   A form of selective attention involving the restriction of attention to a specific feature, or set of features, to the exclusion of other features.

Focus-execute attention   The ability to respond and pick out the important elements or "figure" of attention from the "ground" or background of external and internal stimulation. Also implies a measure of concentration or effortful processing.

Fontanelles   Literally "small springs or fountains," membranous gaps between the bony skull plates that are evident in newborns.

Foramen magnum   The largest of the foramina; provides a large median opening in the occipital bone for the spinal cord to pass through to the brain stem.

Foramen of Magendie   The middle opening, of three, of the membranous roof of the fourth ventricle, allowing the CSF to flow outside the brain and recirculate.

Foramen of Monro A small opening connecting the lateral ventricles.

Foramina More-or-less symmetrical orifices in the base of the skull that provide passage for nerves and blood vessels.

Foramina of Luschka The two lateral openings, of three, of the membranous roof of the fourth ventricle, allowing the CSF to flow outside the brain and recirculate.

Forebrain, or prosencephalon The topmost division of the developing brain.

Fornix A structure of the limbic system that contains nearly 1 million fibers, it rises out of the hippocampal complex and arches anteriorly under the corpus callosum. The fornix relays information to the mammillary bodies.

Fossae Conspicuous ridges in the base of the skull that hold the brain in place.

Fragile X A genetic disorder frequently associated with mental retardation and other cognitive deficits and distinctive physical features. The disorder is related to a compression or break of the X chromosome.

Freud, Sigmund Austrian, 1856–1938; best known as the founder of psychoanalysis and the father of clinical psychology. Freud's initial love was neurology and investigating the secrets of the central nervous system.

Frontal lobe One of the four cortical lobes; contains the primary motor cortex and the prefrontal lobe. Its functions are motor processing and executive, including planning, inhibition, and formulation of behavior.

Frontal operculum Broca's area.

Functional systems A concept first formulated by Luria, in which behavior results from interaction among many areas of the brain.

Functioning adenomas Pituitary tumors that play an "uninvited" role in the operation of the pituitary gland, often affecting the release of the gland's hormones.

Galen A.D. 130–201; Roman anatomist and physician who identified many of the major brain structures and described behavioral changes as a function of brain trauma.

Gall, Franz 1758–1828; Austrian anatomist who postulated that mental faculties were innate and related to the topical structures of the brain.

Gamma-amino butyric acid (GABA) One of over 20 amino acids, GABA is a neurotransmitter known to have strong inhibitory properties.

Ganglia (singular, *ganglion*) A strategic collection of nerve cells in the PNS.

Generalized seizure A seizure caused by an abnormal rhythm of the entire brain; formally known as "grand mal"; bilaterally symmetrical episodes characterized by a temporary lack of awareness, or what appears on observation to be a complete loss of consciousness.

Gerstmann-Straussler-Scheinker syndrome (GSS) An extremely rare familial Creutzfeldt-Jakob disease variant that results in a "fatal insomnia."

Geschwind, Norman 1926–1984; American neurologist who proposed that behavioral disturbances were based on the destruction of specific brain pathways that he called *disconnections.*

Gigantocellular tegmental field (GTF) Located in the higher pons; appears to generate brain waves. Left unchecked, the neurons fire spontaneously, producing a high level of activity. One particular set of discharges are termed *PGO spikes* because they travel from the pons (P) to the lateral geniculate (G) nucleus of the thalamus and to the occipital (O) cortex.

Gilles de la Tourette syndrome See **Tourette syndrome.**

Glasgow Coma Scale (GCS) A three-item scale often used in the medical setting to assess the severity of coma. The GCS ranges from 3 to 15 points, with lower scores indicating severe coma and higher scores suggesting a confusional state.

Glia Greek for "glue"; glia cells outnumber neurons and provide supportive structure and metabolic function to the neuron.

Glioblastoma multiforme (GBM) A particularly destructive and fatal glioma.

Gliomas A type of brain tumor, gliomas are a relatively fast growing brain tumor that arises from supporting glia cells. Gliomas are the most common infiltrative brain tumor, which make up approximately 40 to 50% of all brain tumors. The term *glioma* is often used to describe all primary, intrinsic neoplasms of the brain and the spinal cord.

Globus pallidus A structure of the basal ganglia.

Glutamate One of over 20 amino acids, glutamate is the major excitatory neurotransmitter of the brain.

Golgi, Camillo 1843–1926; Italian physician who made the discovery in the early 1870s that silver chromate stained dead neurons black. This allowed people for the first time to visualize individual neurons.

Gonadotropins Hormonal substances that stimulate the functions of the testes and ovaries.

Grading of tumors A method of evaluating the malignant features of brain tumors. Grading is from 1 to 4, with a grade 1 tumor representing a slow-growing tumor accompanied by few neuropsychological deficits. Grades 2 and 3 represent intermediate rates of growth and neuropsychological dysfunction. Grade 4 tumors are fast growing and typically have a poor prognosis for recovery.

Grand mal seizure   Literally "big bad" seizure; consist of violent motoric abnormalities of stiffening and jerking episodes and the accompanying loss of consciousness.

Gray matter   Areas of the brain that are dense in cell bodies such as the cortex and that appear gray in color.

Gyri (singular, gyrus)   Ridges of the cortex between sulci.

Halstead-Reitan Neuropsychological Battery (HRNB)   The first neuropsychology laboratory in the United States was founded in 1935 by Ward Halstead at the University of Chicago. Halstead worked closely with neurosurgery patients and developed assessment devices that differentiated between patients with brain damage and those without. Halstead later developed, with Ralph Reitan, the HRNB, which represented an empirical approach to the assessment of brain damage.

Hécaen, Henry   French neuropsychologist (born 1912) who made important contributions to brain–behavior relationships in health and disease, especially the role of the right hemisphere.

Hematoma   The massive accumulation of blood within the cranium.

Hemianopsia   Also called *homonymous hemianopsia;* half-blindness. Partial blindness on the same side, or visual field, of each eye. The partial blindness is not related to a malfunction of the eye, but to the brain connection to the occipital lobes. This problem is also attributed to unilateral damage to the right or left occipital lobes.

Hemispheric asymmetry   The differentiation in morphology and physiology of the brain between the right and left hemispheres.

Hemorrhage   Type of stroke related to a significant bleed in the brain. Hemorrhages are the most severe form of stroke and often result in permanent brain damage or death.

Heraclitus   6th century B.C.; Greek philosopher who referred to the mind as an enormous space whose boundaries could never be reached.

Herpes encephalitis   An infection that aggressively attacks the medial temporal and orbital frontal areas, resulting in the destruction of much of the limbic system, especially the hippocampus.

Heschl's gyrus   A gyrus of the superior temporal lobes known as the *primary auditory cortex;* often larger in area in the right hemisphere because two gyri are often present. Plays a role in nonspeech and musical processing.

Hindbrain   Also called *rhombencephalon;* the lower division of the developing brain.

Hippocampal commissure   Minor intercerebral fibers.

Hippocampal formation   A set of structures of the limbic system centered around the hippocampus; includes the hippocampus, dentate gyrus, and subiculum.

Hippocampus   Anatomic brain structure of the limbic system thought to be involved in consolidating memory.

Hippocrates   460–377 B.C.; Greek physician who has been honored as the father of medicine, also shared the belief that the brain controlled all senses and movements. He was the first to recognize that paralysis occurred on the side of the body opposite the side of a head injury.

Homonymous   Same-sided.

Homonymous hemianopsia   Same-sided half-blindness. Partial blindness on the same side, or visual field, of each eye. The partial blindness is not related to a malfunction of the eye, but to the brain connection to the occipital lobes. This problem is also attributed to unilateral damage to the right or left occipital lobes.

Horizontal plane   A plane (x-axis) that shows the brain as seen from above or parallel to the ground.

Horseradish peroxidase (HRP)   An enzyme, found in the roots of horseradish, that allows mapping of neuronal pathways using an axonal transport mechanism.

Human immunodeficiency virus (HIV)   The HIV/AIDS virus has a wide effect on the brain as it progressively destroys the immune system. The virus itself may have direct consequences for the brain. It also opens the brain to opportunistic infections and other diseases that can attack the brain.

Humors   Medieval physicians believed that humors, body liquids, were influential in health and disease.

Huntington's disease (HD)   Also called *Huntington's chorea.* A genetic, autosomal dominant progressive subcortical dementia that inflicts devastating motor impairment in the form of chorea as well as cognitive decline on adults in the prime of their life.

Hydrocephalus (HC)   A condition in which the ventricles become abnormally enlarged, most often related to a problem with cerebrospinal fluid flow, production, or absorption.

Hyperdensity   Increased density of brain tissue that typically signals an abnormal density such as seen in tumor or bleeding.

Hyperlexia   Early reading acquisition (decoding) without adequate comprehension. An anomaly exhibited by some children with developmental disorders, such as autism.

Hypnagogic hallucinations   Vivid, dreamlike intrusions into wakefulness; occur in the transition between wakefulness and sleep onset.

Hypodensity   Low density of brain mass.

Hypoguesia   Diminished taste sensitivity.

Hypokinesia   Reduced motor initiation; negative motor symptom of Parkinson's disease.

Hyposmia   Diminished smell sensation.

Hypothalamus   A structure of the diencephalon, part of the limbic system; considered instrumental in controlling the autonomic system. Activates, controls, and integrates the peripheral autonomic mechanisms, endocrine activity, and somatic functions, including body temperature, food intake, and development of secondary sexual characteristics.

Hypoxia   The reduced oxygenation of brain. Hypoxia is typically not associated with cell death, but some possible interference in the functioning of the neuron. Hypoxia is usually related to inadequate breathing, such as experienced during sleep apnea, can occur at high altitude, or be related to carbon monoxide poisoning.

Ideomotor apraxia   See **Motor Apraxia.**

Impact injury   A type of closed head injury in which the physical forces act on the brain tissue at the point of impact.

Implicit memory   Demonstrated by means whereby conscious awareness is not always necessary, such as implicit priming, skill learning, and conditioning.

Implicit priming   The phenomenon in which, if "primed" with three-letter word stems, people are more likely to complete the stem with a word they have already seen.

Infarction   A severe loss of blood caused by a blockage of an artery, often resulting in more lasting neuropsychological deficits.

Inferior colliculi   Two elevations within the roof of the tectum, which serve as an important relay center for the auditory pathway.

Inferior   Toward the bottom, or below.

Infiltrative tumors   Tumors that take over or infiltrate neighboring areas of the brain and destroy its tissue.

Inhibitory control   Inhibition of behavior through involuntary and voluntary neuropsychological processes. At a voluntary level, this capacity is considered an executive function, and connotes the volitional capacity to withhold behavior, particularly when invoking environmental contingencies are evident.

Inhibitory postsynaptic potential (IPSP)   The presence of an ionic current flow that hyperpolarizes the postsynaptic neuron. As a result, a greater depolarization than normal is required for excitation and there is only a small probability that there will be an action potential.

Intelligence tests   Complex composite measures of verbal and performance abilities that are in part related to achievement (for example, factual knowledge) and in part to aptitude (for example, problem solving). Although there are well over 100 different tests of intelligence, the scales that David Wechsler developed have become widely used throughout the world and typically include a variety of scales measuring verbal-comprehension skills and tests tapping perceptual-organization abilities.

Intelligence   The aggregate or global capacity involving an individual's ability to act purposefully, to think rationally, and to deal effectively with the environment.

Intercerebral fibers   Connect structures between two hemispheres.

Interference control   The ability to screen or block out internal or external distractions that could intrude into and disrupt attentional focus.

Interictal   Between seizures.

Internal carotid arteries   Two of the four major arteries to the brain, supplying the anterior portions of the brain.

Interneurons   Neurons with short axons or no axons.

Interpretive hypotheses   Inferences about the patient's cognitive status that the neuropsychologist makes in the process of interpreting neuropsychological assessment data.

Intracerebral fibers   Fibers that connect regions within one hemisphere.

Intracerebral   "Within the cerebrum" or brain.

Intracranial pressure (ICP)   Related to the presence of a bleed (or hemorrhage) within the cranium (skull) usually associated with the development of a space-occupying mass or pocket of blood, which may press on nearby brain structures, affecting their integrity.

Intraventricular hemorrhage (IVH)   Bleeding within the ventricles of the brain. A common cause of hydrocephalus in premature infants. Vessels in the area surrounding the ventricles rupture, and the blood and cellular debris obstruct the structures that allow for the reabsorption of the cerebrospinal fluid into the bloodstream.

Ions   Atoms or molecules that have acquired an electrical charge by gaining or losing one or more electrons. Four ions that are important in neuronal communication are sodium (NA^+), potassium (K^+), calcium (Ca^{++}), and chloride (Cl^-).

Ipsilateral   On the same side.

Ischemia   "Temporary" strokes caused by an insufficiency of blood supply to an area of the brain. These events are often only short-lasting, with transient deficits.

Isochromosome   An abnormal karotype characterized by identical arms on the X (female) chromosome. The chromosomal anomaly is associated with Turner's syndrome.

Jackson, Hughlings   British neurologist (1835–1911) who wrote on the integration of the localization and equipotentiality models of brain function. He suggested that behavior resulted from interactions among all areas of the brain, but that each area in the nervous system had a specific function that contributed to the overall system.

Jacksonian seizure   Involves motor areas; such events have been called marching seizures because they begin with jerking or tingling of a single body area and spread to other areas.

James-Lange theory of emotion   Promoted by American psychologist William James and Danish psychologist Carl Lange, postulating that emotion is consciously experienced as a reaction to physical sensory experience. In other words, we feel fear *because* our hearts are racing; we are sad *because* we are crying. Although critics saw this as an overstatement, the James-Lange theory did correctly insist that sensory and cognitive experiences were intimately entwined and couldn't be separated from each other.

Joint attention   The reciprocal attention evident in the interaction of individuals. Disruption of this interactional capacity of mother and child has been associated with autism.

Karyotype   A visual representation of an individual's chromosomes that displays the structural components and integrity of the chromosomes.

Kennard principle   A principle of neural recovery that bears the name of its originator, Margaret Kennard. The principle holds that earlier brain injury is associated with less impairment and better recovery of functions than injury occurring later in development. Subsequent clinical and experimental studies have not fully supported this principle.

Kinesthetic sense   A sense of one's physical body is supplied by a combination of vision, the vestibular organs, and the proprioceptive sense.

Kuru   A spongiform encephalophy suffered by the Fore people of New Guinea.

Lancisi, Giovanni   1654–1720; an Italian clinician who contributed greatly to the knowledge of aneurysm: abnormal blood-filled ballooning of an artery in the brain.

Lashley, Karl   1890–1958; American neuropsychologist who was one of the first to combine behavioral sophistication in experiments with neurological sophistication, thereby creating the field of experimental neuropsychology.

Lateral   Toward the side, away from the midline.

Lateral fissure   Separates the frontal and parietal lobes.

Lateralization   With *dominance,* refers to the differences in functional specialization between the two brain hemispheres.

Lesions   From Latin *laesio,* "to hurt"; any pathological or traumatic discontinuity of brain tissue. Depending on their size and location, lesions result in minor or major behavioral effects.

Lewy bodies   Small, tightly packed granular structures with ringlike filaments, found within dying cells.

Lexicon store   A "storehouse" of words that an individual knows or understands.

Lezak, Muriel   American neuropsychologist who pioneered the assessment approach in clinical neuropsychology.

Limbic system   Includes the fornix; some brain stem areas, particularly the mammillary bodies of the hypothalamus; and specific basal forebrain structures, including the amygdala ("almond" because of its shape) and the septum.

Lissencephaly   See **Agyria.**

Localization theory   Assigns specific functions to particular places in the cerebral cortex.

Locus ceruleus   Located below the wall of the fourth ventricle, it has been implicated as an important norepinephrine pathway.

Longitudinal fissure   The space between the two hemispheres.

Long-term memory (LTM)   Theoretically of unlimited capacity and relatively permanent except for models suggesting that loss of information through forgetting is possible.

Lucid dreaming   The ability while dreaming to become conscious of the fact that one is in a dream state.

Lumbar puncture   Also known as a *spinal tap;* a medical technique for collecting a specimen of cerebrospinal fluid surrounding the spinal cord for diagnostic study.

Luria, Alexander   1902–1977; Russian neuropsychologist who was responsible for the most profound changes in the scientific understanding of the brain and mind.

Magnetic resonance imaging (MRI)   A visualization procedure that provides the most detailed images of brain structures. The advantage of functional MRI over other functional procedures, such as PET, is that it provides good spatial resolution and images in very short time periods or "real time."

Magnetoencephalogram (MEG)   The magnetic equivalent of the EEG in which a three-dimensional magnetic field of the brain can then be calculated. Superconducting quantum interference device (SQUID) detect the small magnetic fields in the brain that are a marker of neural activity. A disadvantage of MEG is related to the fact that it is expensive and not readily available for clinical applications.

Magnocellular visual system   One of the two visual systems that extends from the eyes to the visual cortex. It consists of large cells that are inferiorly located in the lateral geniculate bodies that are highly sensitive to movement, low contrast, and spatial location.

Magnus, Albertus   German, about 1200; de-emphasized the role of the ventricles in brain functioning.

Malignant tumors   Tumors whose cells invade other tissue and are likely to regrow or spread.

Malingering   The intentional exaggeration or presentation of neuropsychological symptoms.

Mammillary bodies   Two small nuclei on the floor of the posterior hypothalamus.

Masked facies   Used to describe the masklike expression of Parkinson's patients.

Mass action   The extent to which behavioral impairments are directly proportional to the mass of the removed brain tissue.

Materialism   A theory that brain–behavior functions are produced by matter in motion, favoring a mechanistic view of the brain as a machine.

Mechanical receptors   Structures that transduce energy from touch, vibration, and the stretching and bending of skin, muscle, internal organs, and blood vessels.

Medial lemniscus   A white matter tract that courses through the contralateral side of the brain stem through the medulla, pons, and midbrain to be routed up through the thalamus (ventral posterior nucleus, VP) and on to the primary somatosensory cortex.

Medial   Toward the middle/midline, away from the side.

Medulla oblongata   Mylencephalon; a structure of the brain stem.

Medulloblastoma   A brain tumor seen most frequently in children; rapidly growing and very malignant; located in the inferior vermis close to the exit of cerebrospinal fluid from the fourth ventricle. This type of tumor accounts for about two-thirds of all tumors in children and produces increased intracranial pressure caused by obstructive hydrocephalus.

Membrane potential   See **Resting potential.**

Meninges   Protective covering of the brain and spinal cord consisting of the pia mater, the arachanoid membrane, and the dura mater.

Meningiomas   Highly encapsulated, benign tumors that arise from the arachnoid layer of the meninges. Meningiomas represent approximately 15% of all brain tumors.

Meningitis   Inflammation of the meninges caused by bacterial infection or viral infection. It can progress quickly, within 24 hours, from a respiratory illness, with fever, headache, and a stiff neck, to changes in consciousness including stupor, coma, and death.

Mesencephalon   One of the five principal divisions of the brain, part of the brain stem.

Metacognition   A higher-order cognitive ability that enables an individual to examine and analyze the manner in which he or she thinks, solves problems, encodes and retrieves information, and performs cognitive operations.

Metacognitive awareness   An ability to monitor one's own behavior and performance.

Metastasis   A form of tumor spreading in which tissue from a malignant tumor "travels" to other organs in the body through the blood stream. The capacity for metastasis is a characteristic of all malignant tumors. Metastatic brain tumors typically originate from sites other than the brain, most frequently the lung or the breast.

Metastatic tumors   Growths that arise secondarily to cancerous tumors that have their primary site in other parts of the body, such as the lungs, breasts, or the lymphatic system. The secondary growths arise because cancer cells from the primary neoplasm detach and travel to other sites through the blood system.

Metencephalon   One of the five principal divisions of the brain, part of the brain stem.

Microcephaly   A congenital disorder characterized by an abnormally small head in relation to the rest of the body. The head is more than two standard deviations below the average circumference for a child of a similar age and gender. The size of the brain is also subnormal, and the condition is associated with mental retardation.

Micrographia   Small handwriting; a common motor symptom of Parkinson's disease.

Midbrain (mesencephalon)   The middle division of the developing brain.

Middle cerebral artery   Resulting from one-half of the division of an internal carotid artery, it supplies the lateral hemisphere and most of the basal ganglia of its corresponding cerebral hemisphere.

Migraine stroke   A rare type of stroke in which a transient ischemic attack, typically associated with classic migraine, is severe enough to cause a stroke.

Mind-blindness   A neuropsychological deficit in which an animal's behavior suggests that it can "see" objects—that is, the test subjects do not bump into the object—but fail to recognize its significance (for example, as an object of fear).

Monopolar neurons Unipolar neurons; neurons with a single axon.

Mosaic karyotypes The presence of both structurally normal and abnormal female chromosomes that produces one form of Turner's syndrome.

Motor apraxia Ideomotor apraxia; an inability to access a stored motor sequence or an inability to relay that information to the motor association areas. An example is the inability to show me how you would make a telephone call from beginning to end.

Motor neurons Neurons responsible for contracting muscles or changing the activity of a gland.

Move attention A cognitive-attentional operation involving the shifting, or movement of attentional focus from one stimuli to the next.

Multi-infarct dementia A dementia caused by multiple small strokes or ischemic attacks.

Multipolar neurons Neurons with more than two axons.

Munk, Hermann German, 1839–1912; found that experimental lesions in the visual association cortex produced temporary mind-blindness in dogs.

Muscarinic choline One of two main subtypes of acetylcholine (ACh), a neurotransmitter known to stimulate receptors.

Myelencephalon One of the five principal divisions of the brain; part of the brain stem.

Myelin A lipid sheath that surrounds and insulates the axons of the central and peripheral nervous systems. It serves to increase the speed of nerve conduction.

Myelin sheath Fatty-type covering of axons that increases the speed of axonal transmission.

Myelin staining Selectively dyes the sheaths of myelinated axons. As a result, white matter, which consists of myelinated axons, stains black, unlike other areas of the brain that consist mostly of cell bodies and nuclei.

Narcolepsy A disorder that consists of irresistible daytime "sleep attacks"; a central nervous system disorder of the region of the brain stem that controls and regulates sleep and wakefulness. The primary symptom of this disorder is excessive daytime sleepiness.

Necrosis (or neuronal cell death) A direct result of a critical interference with the cellular metabolism of the neuron. In general, a period of four to six minutes of anoxia may cause necrosis

Neologism Atypical language characterized by the generation or production of words that are meaningless.

Neoplasm Literally, new tissue. The neurologic term for tumor.

Neostriatum This structure, also known as the *striatal complex,* includes the caudate and putamen, and receives projected information from cortical sensory areas. From the neostriatum, information is then funneled through the globus pallidus, then on to the thalamus, where it projects to the premotor and prefrontal areas.

Nerves A large collection of axons located in the PNS, primarily composed of white matter.

Neural tube The embryonic tube that develops into the central nervous system, specifically the brain and spinal cord. The neural tube develops during the third week of gestation. Abnormalities in neural tube development can lead to congenital developmental disorders.

Neurofibrillary tangles Excessive collections of tau proteins resembling entwined and twisted pairs of rope within the cytoplasm of swollen cell bodies in the brain. These are pathological markers of Alzheimer's disease.

Neurogenesis The congenital process by which the neurons of the brain develop.

Neurologic exam A routine introductory evaluation performed by a neurologist—a physician who has specialized in evaluating and treating neurologic disorders. Although there are many variations, in principle the neurologic exam involves a detailed history of the patient's medical history, and a careful assessment of the patient's reflexes, cranial nerve functioning, gross movements, muscle tone, and ability to perceive sensory stimuli.

Neuromas Tumors or new growths that are largely made up of nerve cells and nerve fibers.

Neurons Specialized nerve cells that allow complex information exchange.

Neuropsychological evaluation Involves a detailed examination, often using standardized tests, to describe an individual's cognitive strengths and weaknesses. Often used in conjunction with other pertinent information, for diagnosis, patient management, intervention, rehabilitation, and discharge planning.

Neuropsychological tests Traditionally defined as those measures that are sensitive indicators of brain functioning.

Neuropsychology The study of the relationships between brain functions and behavior; specifically, changes in thoughts and behaviors that relate to the structural or cognitive integrity of the brain.

Neurotransmitters Chemicals that influence neuronal behavior.

Neurotrophins Neuron-feeding nutrients.

Neurulation The congenital process involving the formation and closure of the neural tube that subsequently develops into the brain and spinal cord.

Nicotinic choline One of two main subtypes of acetylcholine (ACh), a neurotransmitter named after nicotine (from tobacco, *Nicotiana tabacum*), a bitter-tasting alkaloid that stimulates receptors.

Nissl, Franz 1860–1919; German histologist who discovered in the 1880s that a simple dye can stain the cell bodies in neurons. The Nissl method is particularly useful for detecting the distribution of cell bodies in specific regions of the brain.

Nocioceptors From the Latin *nocere,* "to hurt." Receptors that serve as monitors to alert the brain to damage or threat of damage. They can be mechanical or chemical but are specifically activated by potentially damaging stimulation such as heat or cold, painful pressure or pricking, or chemical damage such as exposure to noxious chemicals.

Nocturnal myoclonus Restless leg syndrome; twitching of muscles that occurs during NREM sleep. In severe cases, this will wake up the subject.

Nodes of ranvier Regular gaps along the axon where the myelin is interrupted.

Noncommunicating hydrocephalus See **Obstructive hydrocephalus.**

Nonfluent aphasia A difficulty in the flow of articulation, so that speech becomes broken or halting.

Nonfunctioning adenomas Benign neoplasms of the pituitary gland.

Noninfiltrative tumors Invasive tumors; encapsulated and differentiated (easily distinguished from brain tissue); cause dysfunction by compressing surrounding brain tissue.

Nonobstructive hydrocephalus Also referred to as *communicating hydrocephalus.* A form of hydrocephalus produced by blockage that disrupts reabsorption of cerebrospinal fluid into the bloodstream.

Norepinephrine (NE) A neurotransmitter that is important to the regulation of mood, memory, hormones (via the hypothalamus), cerebral blood flow, and motor behavior.

Normal distribution A frequency distribution in which the values or scores group around a mean. In neuropsychological testing, many test scores display such distributions.

Normative data These data compare the patient's score on a test to an expected score, or norm. The expected test score is determined from the performance of a normative sample of patients and controls.

NREM sleep (nonrapid eye movement sleep) Includes sleep stages 1 through 4.

Nuclei (singular, nucleus) A strategic collection of nerve cells in the CNS.

Nuclei of the raphe A collection of neurons located throughout the midline of the brain stem; implicated in serotonin pathways.

Nucleus basalis of Meynert Named after its discoverer; a collection of neurons implicated in Alzheimer's disease.

Nucleus reticularis thalami (NRT) A group of neurons within the thalamus that regulate oscillatory behavior of the thalamocortical loop.

Object permanence A cognitive capacity described by the developmental psychologist Jean Piaget, which is initially absent in the infant, but subsequently develops. The infant is unable to store in memory a representation of an object that is removed from view: In essence, what is out of sight is "out of mind."

Objective personality tests Typically use the questionnaire technique of measurement (for example, true/false or multiple choice).

Obstructive hydrocephalus Also referred to as *noncommunicating hydrocephalus.* A form of hydrocephalus produced by obstruction within the ventricular system of the brain. The obstruction can be a consequence of congenital malformation, tumors, or scarring.

Obstructive sleep apnea Apnea that occurs most often during REM sleep when either the upper airway collapses, not allowing air to pass, or the body weight of the patient on the chest compromises respiratory effort.

Occipital lobe One of the four cortical lobes, primarily dedicated to visual processing.

Occipital notch Sulci within the medial occipital lobe.

Occupational therapy Rehabilitation specialty that focuses on improving self-care activities such as grooming, bathing, dressing, and feeding, as well as activities concerned with a person's occupation and avocation.

Oligodendrocytes A type of nonneural cells; the projections of the surface membrane of each such cell fan out and coil around the axon of neurons in the CNS to form the myelin sheath.

Oligodendroglioma A rare, slowly growing tumor that mostly affects young adults and is derived from and composed of oligodendrogliocytes.

Optic gliomas A slowly growing glioma of the optic nerve or optic chiasm; associated with visual loss and loss of ocular movement.

Orientation A patient's basic awareness of him- or herself in relation to the world around.

Orthotic   Customizable cognitive adjunct, such as a computer, used in rehabilitating people with brain injury.

Overcorrection   An aversive behavior modification technique that involves having a child practice a positive response that is incompatible with an inappropriate behavior. Overcorrection is particularly effective in reducing self-stimulating and other inappropriate behaviors.

Palilalia   Compulsive word or phrase repetition.

Pallidotomy   A surgical treatment for Parkinson's disease; in this technique the ventral, or internal portion, of the globus pallidus is lesioned via heat coagulation of the neurons.

Papez circuit   Anatomic circuit centered around the hippocampus; plays a role in declarative memory processing.

Papillae   Bumps on which lie from one to several 100 taste buds consisting of between 50 to 150 taste receptor cells.

Paragrammatism   See **Word salad.**

Parahippocampal gyrus   Structure of the limbic system.

Parasympathetic nervous system   Division of the autonomic nervous system; functions to store energy by facilitating functions such as digestion through gastric and intestinal motility.

Paresthesia   Spontaneous crawling, burning, or "pins and needles sensation."

Parietal lobe   One of the four cortical lobes, concerned with the integration of information from sensory areas.

Parkinson's disease (PD)   A progressive disease process characterized by a dopamine deficiency of the substantia nigra; results in resting tremors and allied motor symptoms; may cause a subcortical dementia.

Parkinsonism   A behavioral syndrome marked by motor symptoms including tremor, rigidity, and slowness of movement.

Partial seizure   A seizure caused by an abnormal rhythm confined to a particular brain area; also known as *focal seizures;* always begins as a local neuronal discharge; the most common type of seizure.

Parvocellular visual system   One of the two visual systems extending from the eyes to the visual cortex. It consists of small cells dorsally located in the lateral geniculate bodies that are sensitive to viewing stationary objects, high contrasts, and fine spatial details.

Pathognomonic signs   Neurologic symptoms from which a specific diagnosis can be made.

Pathways   See **Tracts.**

Pattern analysis   Examines the relationships among the scores in a test battery.

Penetrating head injury   A type of head injury associated with a penetrating mechanism such as a bullet from a gun, a knife, or scissors.

Peptides   A group of neurotransmitters, peptides are short chains of amino acid. More than 60 neuroactive peptides have been identified.

Perception   The process of "knowing"; depends on intact sensation.

Peripheral nervous system (PNS)   The PNS includes all the portions of the nervous system outside the central nervous system (CNS). The PNS consists of the somatic nervous system and the autonomic nervous system (ANS).

Peripheral neuropathy   Peripheral nervous system dysfunction causing sensory loss (as in diabetes).

Personality tests   Measures of such characteristics as emotional states, interpersonal relations, and motivation.

Petit mal seizure   Literally "little bad" seizure; causes an altered state of consciousness, but lacks the violent physical loss of control seen during the grand mal seizure.

Phantoguesia   Experience of a phantom or hallucinatory taste.

Phantom limb pain   A feeling of pain in a nonexistent limb.

Phantosmia   Experience of a phantom or hallucinatory smell.

Phenylketonuria (PKU)   A genetic disorder affecting the metabolism of phenylalanine. If untreated, mental retardation and other cognitive deficits can result. Dietary control, particularly if started early, can reduce or eliminate the negative effects of the disorder.

Phonemic paraphasias   Errors of word usage of similar-sounding words (for example, using the word *bark* for *tarp*).

Phonological processing   The application of codes for translating letters and letter sequences into the appropriate speech–sound equivalents. Deficits in this processing have been linked to dyslexia.

Phrenology   An obsolete theory proposing that if a given brain area was larger in an individual, then the corresponding skull at that point should be enlarged, indicating a well-developed area of the brain. Conversely, a depression signaled an underdeveloped area of the cortex. Phrenology involved, in its most popular form, the reading of cranial bumps to ascertain which of the cerebral areas were largest.

Physiatry   The medical specialty of combining physical medicine and rehabilitation.

Physical therapy   A rehabilitation specialty that focuses on improving motor control and physical functioning.

Pia mater   Literally, "pious mother"; a vascularized part of the meninges that directly adheres to the surface of the central nervous system.

Pinealoma   A type of tumor of the pineal body.

Pituitary adenoma   Tumors of the pituitary gland that are often classified into functioning (changing the secretion of the pituitary gland) and nonfunctioning (benign).

Pituitary tumors   Tumors that arise from the pituitary gland. It is traditional to divide pituitary tumors into functioning and nonfunctioning adenomas.

Planum temporale   Region of the posterior surface of the temporal lobes between the Heschl's gyrus and the Sylvian fissure. The planum temporale of the left hemisphere is involved in mediating phonological processing and language comprehension.

Plasticity   Behavioral or neural ability to reorganize after brain injury.

Platelets   Disk-shaped cells found in the blood of all mammals. They are important for their role in blood coagulation and are produced in large numbers in the bone marrow. From there they are released into the bloodstream, where they circulate for approximately 10 days.

Plato   Greek (420–347 B.C.); suggested that the soul can be divided into three parts: appetite, reason, and temper. Plato also discussed the concept of health as being related to the harmony between the body and the mind. Thus he has been credited as being the first to propose the concept of mental health.

Pluripotentiality   The multiple, functional role of the brain. That is, any given area of the brain can be involved in relatively few or relatively many behaviors.

Polymicrogyria   A congenital disorder that can be traced to a disruption of the structure of the developing brain during the fifth to sixth month of gestation. As a consequence of this disruption, the gyri fail to develop appropriately. On inspection, the gyri are found to be small and crowded together. Learning disorders, mental retardation, epilepsy, and other neuropsychological anomalies are linked to the disorder.

Pons   Metencephalon; a "bridge" resembling two bulbs, a structure of the brain stem.

Positron emission tomography (PET)   A visualization technique that tracks blood flow, which is associated with brain activity. It is mostly used to assess brain physiology, including glucose and oxygen metabolism, and the presence of specific neurotransmitters.

Posterior attention system   One of the attentional systems of the brain that mediates visual-spatial orienting and is supported by the parietal, midbrain, and thalamic regions.

Posterior cerebral arteries   Formed by a division of the basilar artery.

Posterior communicating arteries   Arise from the internal carotid arteries and connect the middle and posterior cerebral arteries.

Posterior   Toward the back or tail.

Postictal phase   Phase in which the person gradually emerges into full consciousness; follows the seizure episode.

Posttraumatic amnesia (PTA)   A patient's memory of events surrounding an accident.

Pragmatics of language   Aspects of language that extend beyond the literal.

Precursor or progenitor cells   Early cells lining the neural tube that proliferate to create the neurons and glia cells of the brain.

Prefrontal motor cortex   Section of the frontal lobe. This area is considered to be the "conductor" or "executor" of the brain. Also called *prefrontal cortex.*

Premorbid functioning   The cognitive and neuropsychological status occurring before the development of disease or trauma.

Premotor cortex   Also known as *premotor area*. Located in Brodmann's area 6 of the frontal lobes; receives neuronal input from posterior parietal areas, secondary somatosensory areas, and cerebellum; plays a role in motor planning and sequencing, and may aid in the procedural aspects of carrying out motor plans.

Prepotent response   A response that has been "primed" to occur through reinforcement, repeated use, habit, or reflex.

Prestriate cortex   See **Secondary association.**

Primary motor cortex   Part of the frontal lobe, concerned with the initiation, activation, and performance of motor activity.

Procedural memory   Memory that is usually implicit and is demonstrated via performance. Procedural memory's domain is that of rules and procedures rather than information that can be verbalized, although procedural memory has not been clearly operationally defined and includes a hodgepodge of tasks such as motor skill learning, mirror reading, and verbal priming.

Process approach   Also known as the "hypothesis approach"; based on the idea that each examination should be adapted to the individual patient. Rather than employing a standard battery of tests, the neuropsychologist selects the tests and procedures for each exam, based on hypotheses made from impressions of the patient and from information available about the patient. As a result, each examination may vary considerably from patient to patient in terms of length and test selection.

Prodromal phase   A phase prior to the seizure, in which an aura occurs; odd, transient symptoms such as nausea, dizziness, or numbness may occur, as well as sensory alterations or hallucinations in any sensory domain.

Progenitor cells   See **Precursor cells.**

Projective personality tests   Tests that rely on relatively ambiguous, vague, and unstructured stimuli, such as inkblots.

Proprioception   The position of the body in extrapersonal space. Sensory dysfunctions that result in proprioceptive disorders include altered sense of bodily sensation and bodily position.

Proprioceptive disorder   Loss of body position sense.

Proprioceptors   From the Latin *proprius,* "one's own"; structures on skeletal muscles that detect movement via degree of stretch, angle, and relative position of limbs. Proprioceptors on the hands help identify the shapes of objects via touch.

Prosencephalon. See Forebrain.

Prosody   An aspect of speech that conveys meaning through intonation, tempo, pitch, word stress, fluency, and rhythm. It augments the meaning of spoken language and is important in communicating the emotional content of language.

Prosopagnosia   The special case of inability to recognize people by their faces.

Prospective memory   The intention to remember to perform an action in the future.

Prosthetic   Cognitive replacement, such as a computer, used in the rehabilitation of people with brain injury.

Proximal   Near the trunk or center, close to the origin of attachment.

Pruning   The process of eliminating excessive neurons and synapses in the developing brain. The elimination appears to reflect a purposeful "sculpting" of the brain to promote neural efficiency.

Psychology   The study of describing, explaining, predicting, and modifying behavior.

Psychometrics   The science of measuring human traits or abilities. Concerned with the standardization of psychological as well as neuropsychological tests.

Psychomotor epilepsy.   See Temporal lobe epilepsy.

Purkinje cells   A specific type of neuron that is found in the cerebellum. The dendrites characteristically spread out in one plane.

Putamen   Structure of the basal ganglia.

Pyramidal cells   A specific type of neuron that is found in all areas of the cerebral cortex. These cells have bodies that are pyramidal or conical in shape.

Pyramidal motor system   This system originates in the cerebral cortex and controls voluntary movement.

Pythagoras   About 580–500 B.C.; a Greek scholar who suggested that the brain is at the center of human reasoning and plays a central role in the "soul's life."

Receptive aphasia   A difficulty in auditory comprehension. Also see **Wernicke's aphasia.**

Receptor cells   Receptor cells detect numerous stimuli, including sight, sound, pressure, pain, chemical irritation, smell, and taste. Not technically neurons, although they create energy that is transduced into an electrical stimulus that is carried to neurons and then processed in the brain.

Receptor sites   Sites on the postsynaptic neuron to which neurotransmitters are delivered.

Reductionism   Investigating complex phenomena by dividing them into more easily understood components. Related to brain research, reductionists argue that behavior is no more than the results of chemical and structural relationship among neurons.

Refractory period   A recovery period after a neuron has fired. During this time period, which lasts one or more milliseconds (msec), the neuron resists re-excitation and is incapable of firing.

Reliability   The stability or dependability of a test score as reflected in its consistency on repeated measurement of the same individual. A reliable test should produce similar findings on each administration.

REM sleep   Rapid eye movement sleep; state of sleep where dreams occur.

Remote memory   Memory for long-past events.

Response cost   A behavioral modification technique that involves removing or taking away an already present positive reinforcer contingent on the display of a specific undesirable behavior. The technique is employed to inhibit or suppress a specific behavior.

Response inhibition   Three interrelated control processes: (1) stopping an ongoing response, (2) blocking or screening out distractions, and (3) restraining a response primed for release.

Resting potential   Membrane potential; a slight electrical imbalance between the inner and outer surfaces of the membrane caused by the separation of electrically charged ions.

Resting tremor   Rhythmic shaking that often occurs in one hand first; positive motor symptom of Parkinson's disease; characterized as "pill rolling."

Restitution One of two primary approaches to brain injury rehabilitation; stresses the retraining of an impaired skill in the hope that the brain can rebuild axonal connections through retraining.

Reticular activating system (RAS) Also called *reticular formation;* a neural network located within the lower brain stem transversing between the medulla and the midbrain. Functions in nonspecific arousal and activation, sleep and wakefulness.

Retrograde amnesia In this disorder, the patient has no recollection of the interval preceding the injury; the loss of old memories prior to an event or illness.

Retrograde degeneration The degeneration of the axon back to the cell body, once the axon has been damaged. This process may lead to cell death.

Rhinencephalon Evolutionarily old "smell brain."

Rhombencephalon See **Hindbrain.**

Rigidity Tightening of muscles and joints; positive motor symptom of Parkinson's disease.

Ring X karyotypes A relatively rare karyotype that is associated with one variant of Turner's syndrome. Mental retardation frequently occurs in this form of Turner's syndrome.

Röntgen, Wilhelm Conrad 1845–1923; a physicist who made a remarkable discovery that an invisible ray that, unlike heat or light waves, could pass through wood, metal, and other materials. This ray, also called x-ray, gave rise to radiology.

Rostral Toward the head.

Saccadic eye movements Quick eye movements made when the eye moves from one point of fixation to the next.

Sagittal plane From *sagitta,* Latin for "arrow." A plane (z-axis) that shows the brain as seen from the side or perpendicular to the ground, bisecting the brain into right and left halves.

Savant skills Extraordinary skills possessed by an individual who otherwise displays limited capacity. For example, the ability of a retarded child to mentally calculate complex square roots is a savant skill.

Schwann cells Type of nonneural cells. The projections of the surface membrane of each of those cells fan out and coil around the axons of neurons in the PNS to form myelin sheaths.

Secondarily generalized seizure A simple seizure that crosses the corpus callosum and eventually involves the entire brain.

Secondary association Prestriate cortex; processes primary features of visual information such as light wavelength, line orientation, and features of shape.

Secondary motor cortex Functions in strategic planning of the specific aspects of movement. The intention to move is also a function of this area.

Seizures Massive waves of synchronized nerve cell activation that can involve the entire brain. Seizures may have dramatic behavioral manifestations, including uncontrolled muscles contractions, changes in perception, and alterations in mood and consciousness.

Semantic memory Memory for information and facts that have no specific time-tag reference.

Senile plaques Also called *neuritic plaques.* Round aggregates of beta-amyloid that on disintegrating leave holes and misshapen neurons where there once were active connections.

Sensation The elementary process when a stimulus has excited a receptor and results in a detectable experience in any sensory modality.

Sensitivity How sensitive a test is in measuring a particular neuropsychological construct.

Sensory association area An area of the cortex that functions to integrate information from different sensory areas.

Sensory neurons Neurons that respond directly to changes in light, touch, temperature, or odor.

Septum In general refers to a thin plate of brain tissue separating two cavities or tissue areas. The septal area stretches between the fornix and the corpus callosum, forming one of the walls of the lateral ventricle's frontal horn. The septal area interconnects with the hippocampus and the hypothalamus.

Serotonin A neurotransmitter that is involved in sleep, depression, memory, and other neurologic processes.

Shift attention An element of attention involving the movement of attentional focus from one stimuli or task to another.

Short-term memory (STM) Memory of limited capacity (7 ± 2 bits of information); degrades quickly over a matter of seconds if information is not held via a means such as rehearsal or transfer to long-term memory.

Shunt A medical procedure to drain excessive cerebrospinal fluid from the ventricular system to the stomach. The procedure is employed with people who have developed hydrocephalus.

Simple seizures Focal events that may involve sensory-motor expression or psychic expression (mood, emotion, altered consciousness).

Simulation A form of malingering in which the patient is faking or exaggerating an illness or the severity of the symptoms, usually in order to gain some secondary gain (such as attention, hospitalization, or a financial settlement).

Single-photon emission computed tomography (SPECT) A visualization technique that measures blood flow, a correlate of brain activity. Because it takes the radioactive tracer almost two days to be eliminated from the body, SPECT cannot be used to monitor the brain's mental activity "moment to moment."

Sleep apnea From *a pnoia,* Greek for "negative breathing"; refers to breathing that is disturbed while sleeping and often completely stops for periods as long as a minute.

Sleep apnea syndrome A serious sleeping disorder resulting from frequent episodes of apnea.

Sleep paralysis Momentary paralysis on awakening or at sleep onset; the body is totally unable to move for seconds to minutes.

Social emotional learning disability Disturbed socioemotional behavior that is directly related to neuropsychological processing deficits, and does not reflect a secondary reaction to a learning disability such as dyslexia.

Sodium–potassium pump An active transport system across the membrane of the axon that exchanges three sodium ions for every two potassium ions.

Somatic nervous system (SNS) That part of the PNS that provides "voluntary" neural control with the external environment. Communicates with the CNS through spinal nerves and cranial nerves.

Somatopic organization Organization that follows the distorted figure of the sensory homunculus mapped onto the primary somatosensory cortex, which represents the relative importance and distribution of touch in various areas of the body rather than the actual size of the body part.

Somatosensory cortex Structure found in the anterior portion of the parietal lobe, concerned with primary tactile sensory processing.

Somatosensory system Body system that involves two types of sensory stimulation, external and internal. The somatosensory system can monitor sensations such as cold and heat, whether the sensation comes from the handling of an ice cube or from a fever. So the system processes external stimulation of touch (pressure, shape, texture, heat) in recognizing objects by feel and is also concerned with the position of the body in extrapersonal space (proprioception).

Specificity A factor in setting a cutoff score on a test. Neuropsychological tests with high specificity examine specific aspects of neuropsychological functions; that is, they are not correlated with other tests or factors.

Speech apraxia See **Dysarthria.**

Speech therapy A rehabilitation specialty that focuses on communication difficulties such as deficits in speech production, understanding speech, reading, and writing.

Spina bifida A congenital developmental disorder characterized by an opening in the spinal cord, commonly found in the lower region of the cord. The disorder is a consequence of a failure of the posterior end of the neural tube to close during gestation.

Spinal cord Part of the CNS that acts as the conduit for the majority of sensory and motor information to and from the body.

Spurzheim, Johann Austrian, 1776–1832; student of Gall; lectured extensively on phrenology in the United States.

Stable attention An element of attention referring to the consistency of atttentional performance over time.

Standard battery approach In this approach, the same tests are given to all patients, regardless of the clinician's impression of the patient or the referral question. Typically, a technician gives the tests and administers them according to standardized rules of procedures.

Standardized test A task or set of tasks administered under standard conditions. Designed to assess some aspect of a person's knowledge or skill. Standardized psychological tests typically yield one or more objectively obtained quantitative scores, which permit systematic comparisons to be made among different groups of individuals regarding some psychological or cognitive concept.

Stenosis Narrowing of an artery.

Striatal complex This group of structures includes the caudate and putamen and receive projected information from cortical sensory areas. From the striatum, information then funnels through the globus pallidus, then on to the thalamus, where it projects to the premotor and prefrontal areas. Also see **Neostriatum.**

Striate cortex A collection of brain structures involved in the motor system named after their striped or striated appearance. It is located in the most posterior aspect of the occipital lobes, but a major portion of it extends onto the medial portion of each hemisphere. Also see **Striatal complex.**

Striatum A collection of brain structures (including the caudate nucleus and the putamen) involved in the motor system; named after their striped or striated appearance. It is located in the most posterior aspect of the occipital lobes, but a major portion of it extends onto the medial portion of each hemisphere.

Stroke A neurologic event, also known as *cerebrovascular accident (CVA),* that always occurs in the brain and is the most common type of cerebrovascular disease.

Stuck-in-set perseveration Maintenance of a problem-solving approach when changing demands signal the need for an altered or modified approach or response.

Subarachnoid hemorrhage Occurs when a blood vessel on the surface of the brain bursts and blood flows into the small cavity that surrounds the brain, the subarachnoid space.

Subarachnoid space Space containing cerebrospinal fluid; below the arachnoid membrane.

Subcortical Below the cortex.

Subcortical dementia Dementia that primarily affects subcortical areas of the brain; characterized by slowness of cognitive processing, executive dysfunction, difficulty retrieving learned information, and abnormalities of mood and motivation; examples include Parkinson's disease, Huntington's disease, and Creutzfeldt-Jakob disease.

Subdural hematoma Bleeding into the subdural space; often encountered after a head injury.

Subdural space The space between the dura and the arachnoid parts of the meninges.

Substantia nigra Structure of the basal ganglia. A collection of neurons and nuclei known to be important dopamine pathways.

Substitution One of two primary approaches to brain injury; focuses on searching for adaptations to the person's environment in the context in which they will be used.

Subthalamic nucleus Structure of the basal ganglia.

Sudden infant death syndrome (SIDS) Death caused by the cessation of breathing during sleep.

Sulci (singular, sulcus) Valleys formed by infolding of the cortex.

Superior colliculi Two elevations within the roof of the tectum functioning as important reflex centers for visual information.

Superior sagittal sinus Large sinus of the brain.

Superior Toward the top or above.

Supplementary motor area Located on the dorsal and medial portion of each frontal lobe, functions as a motor sequencer and planner. It receives input from the somatosensory strip and the basal ganglia.

Suprachiasmic nucleus (SCN) A nucleus of the hypothalamus, hypothesized to be a biological clock that calibrates the sleep–wake cycle.

Sustained attention The ability to maintain an effortful response over time. A form of attention involving the maintenance of attentional focus over time. Sometimes referred to as "time-on-task performance," or "behavioral persistence."

Sylvian aqueduct See **Cerebral aqueduct.**

Sylvian fissure The large fissure separating the frontal from the temporal and parietal lobes.

Sympathetic nervous system Division of the ANS that mobilizes the energy necessary for psychological arousal in response to, or anticipation of, a stressful event based on the "fight or flight" response. Sympathetic activation includes an increase in blood flow, blood pressure, heart rate, and sweating; and a decrease in digestion and sexual arousal.

Synapse The tiny gap between the terminal button and the receptors of the two neuron. Neurons communicate through synapses. The anatomic location of this communication is known as the *synapse.*

Synaptic knobs Ends of neurons that have characteristic swelling to increase the area of contact with the postsynaptic neuron.

Synaptic vesicles Oval structures within the terminal that typically cluster close to the presynaptic membrane and where neurotransmitters are synthesized.

Synaptogenesis The developmental process by which the synapses and dendrites of the brain form.

Tachiphemia Segmented accelerated bursts of speech.

Tactile agnosia Also called *astereognosis;* a disorder in which there is an inability to recognize objects by touch.

Tactile extinction/suppression/inattention Suppression of touch sensation on one side of body.

Tardive dyskinesia A disorder with Parkinson-like symptoms, including writhing movements of the mouth, face, and tongue often develops in schizophrenics after long-term medication use.

Tectum "Roof"; structure of the midbrain.

Tegmentum "Covering"; a structure of the midbrain that surrounds the cerebral aqueduct.

Telencephalon Also called the *endbrain;* one of the five principal divisions of the brain; consists of the two cerebral hemispheres, which are connected by a massive bundle of fibers, the corpus callosum.

Temporal lobe One of the four cortical lobes, concerned with the reception and interpretation of auditory information; also plays a role in memory.

Temporal lobe (psychomotor) epilepsy A form of seizure originating from the temporal lobe; emotional symptoms often present (such as changes in mood).

Tensile strength The amount of physical, longitudinal stress that an axon can withstand before it ruptures.

Teratogen Any agent that disrupts the normal development of the embryo and fetus.

Terminal buttons Also called *axon terminals.* The site of interneuronal contact, where neurochemical information is transmitted from one neuron to another.

Teuber, Hans-Leukas American, 1916–1977; credited for first using the term *neuropsychology* in a national forum during a presentation to the American Psychological Association in 1948.

Thalamus A structure of the diencephalon, an important sensory relay station.

Thalotomy A surgical treatment for Parkinson's disease and other disorders causing tremor; used to attack tremor by lesioning the thalamus.

Theory of mind The cognitive capacity to understand, attribute, and predict the mental state of others, and the relationship of these mental states to behavior. Deficits in this capacity have been observed in autistic children and other developmental disorders.

Therapeutic recreation An approach to treatment that emphasizes the importance of recreational and leisure time activities in brain injury rehab, to help in the "transfer" of learning. Therapeutic recreation also allows patients to begin socializing with each other in a structured, but less formal atmosphere than that afforded in other therapy settings.

Thermoreceptors Receptors that serve as monitors to detect heat and cold throughout the body.

Thrombosis A type of occlusion in which a clot or thrombus (Greek for "clot") forms in an artery and obstructs blood flow at the site of its formation. This is the most common form of stroke and accounts for approximately 65% of all cerebrovascular accidents.

Tonic Motorically stiffened.

Tonotopic map Projected onto the auditory cortex in a manner similar to the retinopic mapping of the visual system. Because the cortical bands can respond to multiple frequencies, there is no strict one-to-one correspondence, but bands are more attuned to certain frequencies than others.

Tourette's syndrome A tic disorder defined by multiple involuntary motor and vocal tics. The disorder appears familial in origin. The etiology is unclear, but dysfunction of the basal ganglia has been implicated. Also called *Gilles de la Tourette syndrome.*

Tracts Also known as *pathways* or *fibers.* Large collection of axons located in the CNS. Primarily composed of white matter.

Transduction From the Latin *transducere,* meaning "to lead across." An environmental stimulus activates a specific receptor cell, and this energy is transduced into an electrical stimulus, which is then carried to neurons to be processed by the brain.

Transient ischemic attack (TIA) A temporary (transient) lack of oxygen (ischemia) to the brain, which may cause a time-limited set of neuropsychological deficits. TIAs are technically not considered a stroke, because neuronal death typically does not occur.

Transtentorial herniation Associated with high intracranial pressure and generalized swelling of the brain. As a result the brain is displaced downward.

Tremor Involuntary shaking, usually of a limb, tremors may be resting or occur with intentional movement.

Trephination An ancient procedure in which small holes were scraped or cut into the skull deliberately for either surgical or mystical reasons.

Tumor The morbid enlargement or new growth of tissue in which the multiplication of cells is uncontrolled and progressive. The tumor growth is often arranged in nonorganized ways, does not serve any functional purpose, and often grows at the expense of surrounding intact tissue.

Turner's syndrome (TS) A syndrome characterized by a failure to develop secondary sexual characteristics, short stature, webbed neck, and cubitus valgus. It is caused by an anomaly in the X chromosome (female).

Ultradian rhythm Ninety-minute cycles of heightened and lowered brain arousal observed throughout the wake and sleep cycle.

Ultrasonography A procedure for imaging the internal structures of the body by introducing and recording the reflection of high-frequency sound waves.

Uvulopalatopharyngoplasty (UPPP) The removal of the uvula, the small, fleshy tissue hanging from the center of the soft palate, which may relax and sag, obstructing the upper airway. A surgical approach to the treatment of sleep apnea.

Validity The validity of a test is the meaningfulness of the test scores. Validity gauges whether a specific test really measures what it was intended to measure. There are different types of validity: construct, content, and criterion validity.

Vascular system The blood supply system of arteries and veins.

Ventral Toward the belly. The bottom of the brain is ventral in humans.

Ventricles Four interconnected, fluid-filled cavities in the brain.

Ventricular localization hypothesis Theory that postulated that mental as well as spiritual processes were located in the ventricular chambers of the brain.

Ventricular system Four interconnected, fluid-filled cavities in the brain.

Vermis A structure of the cerebellum; two large, oval hemispheres connected by a single median portion.

Vertebral arteries Two of the four major arteries to the brain, supplying the posterior portions of the brain.

Vesalius, Andreas Italian anatomist (1514–1564) who advanced neuroanatomy through continual dissections and careful scientific observations.

Vestigial ovarian streaks A failure of gonadal development characteristic of Turner's syndrome. Reproductive cells are evident in the gonads of Turner's syndrome embryos, but begin to deteriorate late in fetal development. By early childhood the gonads consist only of fibrous streaks.

Vigilance attention system One of the attentional systems of the brain that mediates sustained attention.

Visual agnosia Inability to recognize a person or object by sight.

Visual object agnosia Failing to recognize objects at all, or in milder cases, confusing objects if they are observed from different angles or in different lighting conditions.

Visual-spatial sketch pad A working memory "slave system" that manipulates visual and spatial images.

Vitalism A theory that suggests that behavior is only partly controlled by mechanical or logical forces.

Vocational inventories Tests that measure opinions and attitudes indicating an individual's interest in different fields of work or occupational settings.

Wada technique Also known as the *Wada test,* after its developer. Similar to the angiogram in that it places a catheter, typically in the left or right internal carotid artery. Then sodium amytal, a barbiturate, is injected, which temporarily anesthetizes one hemisphere. In this way neuropsychologists can study the precise functions of one hemisphere while the other one "sleeps." Also called the *intracarotid sodium amytal procedure (IAP).*

Wernicke, Carl German, 1848–1904; announced that the understanding of speech was located in the superior, posterior aspects of the temporal lobe. Wernicke noted that a loss of speech comprehension due to damage in this area was not accompanied by any motor deficit; only the ability to understand speech was disrupted.

Wernicke's aphasia Damage to the left hemisphere auditory processing areas results in the partial or total inability to decipher spoken words. This condition is also known as *receptive aphasia.*

Wernicke's area A structure that includes the secondary auditory cortex and is located on the posterior aspect of the superior temporal gyrus. It is responsible for auditory processing of speech.

Wernicke-Korsakoff's syndrome A disorder associated with memory function of the limbic system, typically observed in severe alcoholics who show multiple nutritional deficiencies. Such patients may develop a confusional state over time as well as severe new-learning and motor difficulties.

White matter Myelinated axons. Areas of the brain that are mostly made up of myelinated axons, such as neuronal tracts and pathways, which are characteristically white in appearance.

Willis, Thomas 1621–1675; English anatomist best known for his work on the blood circulation of the brain.

Word salad Unconnected words and word sounds. This feature of Wernicke's aphasia is a deficit in placing words together in proper grammatical and syntactical form. This condition is more formally known as *paragrammatism* or *extended paraphasia,* and is characterized by running speech that is logically incoherent, often sounding like an exotic foreign language.

Working memory A concept introduced by Alan Baddeley, also referred to as *short-term memory,* or "working on memory." Working memory directs the temporary storage of information being processed in any range of tasks from reading, to math to problem solving. It includes the concepts of the central executive, the articulatory phonological loop, and the visual-spatial sketch pad.

X rays A type of light ray that is very useful for clinical work of various parts of the body, because they reveal the presence and position of bones, fractures, and foreign bodies. A clinical disadvantage of x rays, and specifically x-ray films of the brain, is that there is little differentiation between the brain structures and the cerebrospinal fluid, making the clinical use of this procedure ineffective.

Zangwill, Oliver A British neuropsychologist (born 1913) who contributed significantly to an understanding of the nature of neuropsychological deficits associated with unilateral brain disease or injury.

ANSWERS TO
CRITICAL THINKING QUESTIONS

CHAPTER 1

How does localization brain theory differ from equipotentiality brain theory? What is each one's lasting contributions?

Localization brain theory assumes that detailed brain processes in specific anatomic locations give rise to specific mental processes. Phrenology is a good example of localization theory. Equipotentiality brain theory assumes that the brain functions more or less as a unit. One proponent of equipotentiality brain theory is Flourens, who suggested that the entire brain is greater than the sum of its parts. The lasting contribution of localization theory is that, indeed, some brain functions seem to be localized to a specific brain region. For example, Broca's area specifically controls verbal motor output. However, many functions, such as thinking and problem solving, do not seem to have a strict or precise anatomic representation in the brain. The lasting contribution of equipotentiality theory is the idea that redundancy may be built into the brain and that if one area of the brain is damaged, another area may be able to compensate for the function.

Is the quest for the search of the organ of the soul completed?

Yes and no. Yes, the search for the organ has been completed. There is no question that the healthy brain gives rise to the mind and the soul. The question that is not yet answered is, How exactly does the brain accomplish this? We have learned much from recent research involving neuropsychology and modern imaging technology, but the precise mechanism—that is, how the soul arises from brain matter—has remained elusive.

Why is Luria's functional model of the brain such an important step in understanding brain functions?

Luria combined both the localization and equipotentiality approaches to neuropsychology into one model. As with equipotential theory, Luria regards behavior as the result of an interaction of many different areas of the brain. As with localization theory, Luria also assigns a specific role to each area of the brain. In Luria's functional model, each function depends on the interaction of specific brain systems. Luria suggests that behavior is the result of the brain operating as a whole. At the same time, each area within the brain has a specific role in the formation of behavior. The importance of any one area depends on the behavior to be performed. This model has been very useful in rehabilitating patients with neuropsychological disorders, such as stroke and brain trauma, where one function may be damaged, but another function may compensate for the loss.

In the year 2025, what will the most important future concepts about the brain be, and how will they relate to society?

The U.S. population will become educated consumers, understanding the critical importance of having a healthy brain in order to enjoy a healthy life. As a result, more educational resources will be available on the functioning brain as well as on how to protect the integrity of the brain.

CHAPTER 2

What are the limitations of the neuron hypothesis?

The neuron hypothesis suggests that behavior has an underlying neural correlate. Some have argued that the mind's range of functions and experiences is produced by the healthy and mature brain, and that this process is correlated to a precise biological phenomenon. The problem with the neuron hypothesis is that studying the individual neuron tells us little about behavior. Intelligent behavioral properties can only be understood by studying networks of interacting neurons, rather than individual neurons in isolation. Although the study of neuronal networks has shown some promise, there are inherent limitations in examining the nervous system by analyzing its parts.

Actor Christopher Reeves has pledged that one day in the future he will walk again, even though he has a severe spinal cord injury that has left him paraplegic. What are the odds that he will fulfill his pledge? Why?

A commercial during a recent NFL Super Bowl showed a computer simulation of Christopher Reeves walking again, presumably healed after his spinal cord injury. This commercial and Reeves's pledge that he will walk again are controversial. At the present the recovery from neuronal damage of the spinal cord presumes that little healing occurs once a neuron in the brain or the spinal cord has been damaged. A process called *collateral sprouting,* which occurs in nearby intact neurons, may facilitate a functional reorganization. But the complexities involved in the regrowth of neurons and its millions of projections to other neurons are daunting and at present not well understood. Consider that it takes the brain five years to develop millions of intricate connections that allows its owner to understand written language. All these connections can be lost within a split second due to brain trauma. The likelihood that these connections regrow spontaneously is, at the present, very small. Thus, it is unlikely that Reeves will ever walk again, although his pledge has created much media interest in spinal cord injuries and an influx of research funds. Of course, we would love to be proven wrong on this argument.

What are the anatomic and electrophysiological constraints of a neuron? How can they affect behavior?

We know that individual neurons send electrical impulses that trigger the release of chemicals or neurotransmitters, which in turn induce an electrical impulse in adjacent neurons. This interaction of electrical and chemical processes is the basis of brain communication. The anatomical constraints are related to the fact that once damaged, neurons in the CNS do not heal. Because neurons depend on a specific electrophysiological and chemical environment, changes to that environment may influence neuronal processes and in turn influence behavior. For example, the collective firing of neurons can cause a seizure, and drugs that act at the level of the synapse can change a person's perception or mood and in some cases cause death.

What is the connection between drugs and neurotransmitters?

Our brains are affected not only by internally produced chemical messengers, but also by externally originating chemicals that find their way to the synapse. Such chemicals are known as *psychoactive drugs* and include caffeine, cocaine, nicotine, and alcohol, among many others. Certain drugs, however, are totally barred from the brain, and other substances require an active transport system to cross the blood–brain barrier. Most psychoactive drugs act at the level of the synapse. One discovery of interest to neuropsychologists is that the nervous system has specific receptor sites that bind drugs such as nicotine and opiate compounds. In general, drugs at the synapse either increase or decrease the likelihood of neuronal transmission.

CHAPTER 3

To what extent can behavioral functions be localized to specific brain structures?

The structures presented in this chapter represent important topographical features on which the various processing systems of the brain depend. Aspects of behavior can be attributed directly to many of these structures. In general, the structures described in depth here, such as the brain stem structures, are responsible for very rudimentary aspects of behavior. Many of the structures are necessary for sustaining life, for controlling wakefulness and sleep, and for controlling other drive states. As a general rule, more basic and fundamental aspects of behavior are more easily traced to specific structures. In the next chapters it will become evident that as behavior becomes more complex students must move from specific structure–function correspondence to an emphasis on larger functional systems that subserve the complexities of human behavior.

What level of brain mapping is most useful to the neuropsychologist?

When it comes to understanding the relationship of the human brain to behavior, mapping at the level of the cell or the neuron is usually considered too minuscule to provide an accurate picture of the complexity of human behavior. Also, some functions are basic and automatic, and of less interest related to their psychological functions, such as the role of CSF as a waste product remover. Finally, understanding the complex organization of the brain, as a whole, would not provide useful information for neuropsychologists, who are often asked to respond to questions such as "What effect does an injury to the basal ganglia have on behavior?" or "If a person has poor motor coordination, which areas of the brain are most likely to be affected?" In general, researchers tend to think of behavior related to its function, so it is most useful to consider the brain structures and systems that relate to that function. In this chapter, basic structures were presented with ties to function. However, in the next chapters more complex functions such as visual perception or memory, as well as more complex and interconnected systems within the brain, emerge as the most useful level in describing most human behavior.

If a human is born without cerebral hemispheres, would the resulting behavior be like that of a comparable animal on the phylogenetic scale?

Certainly some animals function quite well with little to no cortical material. Reptiles, for example, have little more tissue than a brain stem, yet they show complex motor, sensory, instinctual, and learned behaviors. It is relatively rare for a human to be born alive with only a brain stem, and if this happens it is rare for the person to live long. However, there are remarkable stories of people who may have only one hemisphere. If one hemisphere is lost at a young age, the other hemisphere is sometimes able to take over the functions of both hemispheres.

Are there adaptive reasons why the cerebral hemispheres would gravitate toward either a bilateral or asymmetrical organization? Explain.

Although science does not provide a definitive answer to this issue, in order to approach this question it is important to think about what factors lead to differences in hemispheric organization. One of these factors is handedness. About 90% of the population is right-handed, with a tendency toward left hemisphere dominance for speech. Another factor is gender. Sex hormones affect brain organization starting during fetal development. Women tend to be more bilaterally organized than men. Considering these two factors, it is interesting to speculate if, for example, men needed to have more lateralized brains for stereotypically "male" activities such as visual-spatial abilities, and women needed to have more bilaterally organized brains for stereotypically "female" activities such as superior language function. And what advantages might right-handers have, if any?

CHAPTER 4

What does the neuropsychology of sensory-perceptual processing have to contribute toward the idea that there is an objective reality related to object perception?

This question is the fodder for philosophical debate. However, from a neuropsychological point of view, consider that we started the chapter by saying, "The range of what humans can detect is unique to our species." The sensory detectors of other species may result in detection of different stimuli or experiences in a wider or narrower range than humans. For example, many animals do not detect color, but can detect faint smells or have visual acuity that is far superior to humans. Whose actuality is real? Even if this question is limited to human experiences, consider that being "objective" implies being unbiased by personal experience. Sensory information comes in fragments. Meaning, such as an object's name, the intensity of pain, or the pleasantness of a smell, must be attached at secondary and higher processing centers. At each level of processing, more aspects of interpretation are required. So, are there aspects of sensory perception where general agreement can constitute

objective reality? Where would you draw a line between the seeming "realness" of sensation and the "personal experience" of perception?

In what ways does the study of sensory-perceptual and motor disorders inform us about intact brain functioning? In what instances might the study of damaged brains lead us astray?

The study of individuals with damaged brains has provided important clues to the workings of brain systems. For example, by examining patients with lesions in Broca's or Wernicke's areas, or damage to area V4 (occipital cortex), functions of language and vision, respectively, have been mapped. However, this strategy can lead to erroneous information because a lesioned area does not always "contain" the function, but may act as a "cable" in the network that serves to join two or more functions.

Do conditions such as phantoms, neglect, and synesthesia represent distortions of conscious awareness?

Phantoms, such as phantom limbs, appear as sensory-perceptual "hallucinations." A neglect patient can show a total unawareness of the left side of the body and even deny the ownership of a limb. A synesthete can feel jaggedness when eating chocolate. These examples appear to be distortions from the "norm" of conscious awareness. They are deviations of "reality testing," yet we don't label these people as psychotic. Why not? Perhaps the most interesting fact here is the variations one can experience in conscious awareness. And for some, such as synesthetes, the melding of sensory perceptions may have constituted a natural reality since birth.

Does intact motor output require intact sensory-perceptual input? Explain.

Consider the example of speech presented in this chapter. To what extent does speaking require the ability to understand speech? This chapter discusses the extent to which expressive speech is damaged in those with Wernicke's aphasia. Would this be more or less of a problem in a child who is born with a difficulty in understanding speech? Do you think this is the case in all sensory modalities? Can you think of any exceptions?

CHAPTER 5

Do the higher cognitive functions discussed in this chapter represent more intelligent thought processes than those functions discussed in previous chapters? Explain.

The implication is that "higher" cognitive processes indicate the pinnacle of intellectual functioning, given that we often equate abstract and complex thought with the highest levels of human achievement. This may well be the case from the human point of view. Can you think of examples to dispute this statement from what you have read in previous chapters?

Are animal minds other than humans also conscious? Explain.

At this point, what is your definition of consciousness? Does it include the ability to verbalize? To show awareness? Are there things that animals may be "conscious of" that humans may not be? David Chalmer raised the issue of the "why" of consciousness. Is consciousness important to animal functioning?

Do disorders of higher cognitive functioning represent a greater disability for humans than sensory-perceptual and motor disorders? Why or why not?

Although some may answer unequivocally yes, it may also be argued that with sensory-perceptual and motor disorders, the building blocks of functioning may be so compromised that intact higher functions may not be able to be expressed adequately. What arguments can you make for each case?

Do emotions represent a higher cognitive function or a lower basic function? Explain.

In many ways, emotions represent the most basic of functions evolutionarily. Fear, anger, and other primary emotions are shared with the most primitive of creatures. We included emotions in the chapter on higher cognitive functioning because in humans, the interpretation and higher perception of emotions, particularly social emotions, by the cortex requires a high degree of cortical processing.

CHAPTER 6

What are the differences among electrical, magnetic, and metabolic technologies in imaging?

Electrical measures record the electrical activity of nerve cells of the brain through electrodes attached to various locations on the scalp. This procedure, known as *electroencephalography,* or *EEG,* is most sensitive to the actual firing rate of large collections of neurons. Magnetic imaging measures the concentration of the hydrogen nucleus, which is present in high concentration in biologic systems and generates a small magnetic field. This procedure is known as *magnetic resonance imaging,* or *MRI.* With MRI researchers can accurately calculate brain tissue densities and can generate a computer-constructed anatomic representation. The imaging of brain metabolism provides a completely different approach to the examination of the brain. For example, measuring glucose metabolism is a direct cor-

relate of neuronal activity and can lead to a clearer understanding of the functioning brain. Medical technologies that use this approach are single-photon emission computed tomography (SPECT) and positron emission tomography (PET).

Why is the coregistration—that is, the use of multiple assessment using different technologies—an important advancement in neuropsychology?

A major advancement in imaging technology has been to merge different assessment technologies, such as MRI's anatomic detail with PET's ability to localize function using the imaging of brain metabolism. Such coregistration of different approaches has resulted in multimodal approaches to neuroimaging, often providing new insights as well as corroborating established findings.

Which medical technology would you volunteer for to examine your brain? Why?

We personally do not mind having our brains imaged using different technologies. There is always a risk associated with this, however, namely that some previously unknown pathology may be detected, but those chances are relatively small. The only other risk, then, is the inconvenience of an invasive procedure. On a continuum from least to most invasive those procedures are (in our opinion); x-ray, EEG, EP, MRI, MEG, SPECT, PET, EMG, lumbar puncture, and angiography. Because MRI is relatively noninvasive but allows for precise anatomic pictures of the brain, it would be the procedure we would volunteer for first.

Will neuropsychology be outdated because of the increase in sophisticated brain imaging technology? Why or why not?

No, modern imaging technologies and the study of neuropsychology are compatible. Certainly, the advances in modern imaging technology have been spectacular in showing us the brain's anatomy. Furthermore, the domains previously held by neurologists and that by neuropsychologists are getting much closer, and both disciplines have much to learn from each other. But neuropsychologists are bringing special knowledge to the area of brain research and are participating in the research using this technology because of their expertise in the functional aspects of neuroanatomical structures, their knowledge of neuropsychological tests, and their background in scientific methodology and design. Thus, neuropsychologists play an important role in providing functional assessments of brain-injured patients. Neuropsychologists also diagnose conditions (such as concussions) that are not easily detected using modern imaging technologies, and evaluate a patient's potential for adapting to a specific neurologic disorder, their capacity to work, and their quality of life.

CHAPTER 7

In light of the devastating effects of many genetic and chromosomal disorders, do you think that potential parents should seek genetic counseling prior to having children? Explain.

Genetic and chromosomal disorders can have devastating effects on the developing brain and other body systems of the child. Many of these disorders are not currently detectable prior to the child's conception, so genetic counseling would not necessarily prevent their occurrence. Fortunately, only a small percentage of children are afflicted. However, it is advisable that individuals with family histories of genetic/chromosomal disorders, or of ethnic or regional origins often associated with specific disorders such as Tay-Sachs disease, seek genetic counseling.

Why are executive functions important in adaptation?

We are beginning to realize the centrality of executive functions to adaptation insofar as they are implicated in the (1) development of new and flexible behavior in response to changing, complex, and challenging demands; (2) guidance of behavior by mental representations; (3) synthesis of past, present, and future information in the development and implementation of goal-directed behavior; (4) monitoring and evaluation of behavior; and (5) integration, modification, and regulation of the cognitive-emotional-social elements of behavior.

In recent years, an increasing number of teratogens have been identified in the environment. Are our children at greater risk for brain anomalies than children of earlier generations? Why or why not?

An increasing number of teratogens have been identified, suggesting, at first glance, greater risk to our children. Although many of these teratogens have been present for years, the injurious effects to the unborn child have only recently been recognized. The identification of previously existing and new agents helps reduce birth defects by prompting appropriate control, avoidance, or elimination of these agents. Ideally, greater attention should be given to identifying and regulating potential teratogens before they are released into the environment. Unfortunately, identifying and regulating teratogens does not necessarily prevent their impact on our children. For example, the intrauterine teratogenic effects of alcohol have been documented for years; yet children affected with FAS/FAE continue to be born.

What steps could be taken to prevent FAS?

The use of alcohol is an established fact in our society, and moderate use does not necessarily lead to deleterious effects. Unfortunately, some women fail to make the necessary modifications in drinking patterns when pregnant because they lack awareness or understanding of the potential effects of alcohol consumption on the developing child. In other cases, women continue drinking because alcohol consumption is a lifestyle preference or because they are struggling with alcoholism. Improving prevention would involve increasing public awareness of FAS, starting with early and appropriate education provided by medical agencies, schools, social agencies, and public health alerts. Women with chronic drinking problems require special attention because of difficulty in altering established drinking patterns. These individuals should be advised to forestall pregnancy until they can abstain from alcohol, and treatment options should be provided. If pregnancy has occurred, the risk of continued drinking should be explained and treatment options quickly identified and provided.

CHAPTER 8

Why are the symptoms of the NVLD syndrome and ADHD so often displayed by children exhibiting a wide range of developmental disorders?

As we have discussed, Rourke and associates hypothesize that white matter tissue damage causes the NVLD syndrome. Insofar as white matter damage is suggested across a number of developmental disorders, NVLD symptoms would be expected to occur, varying in number and intensity, depending on the extent and location of the impairment. Likewise, the functional neural systems that support attention and behavioral regulation are distributed throughout the brain and, accordingly, the injurious effects to different regions or circuits of the brain could result in behaviors of inattention, impulsivity, and overactivity. Thus, the symptoms of ADHD could potentially be evident across a variety of developmental disorders.

Can an autistic or Asperger's syndrome child develop normal social awareness and attachment? If so, how would this be accomplished?

A primary impairment of both autism and Asperger's syndrome is significant deficits in social awareness and attachment. Unfortunately, these social deficits rarely, if ever, are fully resolved. Although therapists have used social skill training and other interventions, they have met little success. The amelioration of social impairments of autism and Asperger's syndrome is hampered by lack of understanding, knowledge of the neuropsychological basis, and etiology of social functioning. Specifically, neuropsychologists need to identify the developing relationships of neural systems to special classes of social behavior (such as attachment), the effects of environmental influences on neural-social development, the etiologies specific to different types and forms of social impairments, and the malleability of and means of modifying neural-social behaviors necessary for altering social deficits. Once they gain this knowledge, people should be able to develop interventions necessary for the development of normal social relatedness and interaction.

How would you respond to the comment "ADHD does not exist, it is merely a diagnosis to excuse lazy and undisciplined children?"

Some challenge the very existence of ADHD as an excuse for lazy and undisciplined children. To counter this challenge, cite the voluminous research that supports the existence of the disorder, the converging clinical and empirical studies that delineate the key symptoms and potential etiologies of the disorder, and the outcome studies showing significant improvement in regulatory control for children with ADHD who receive appropriate medical and psychological treatment. Finally, present specific differences between the child who is exhibiting ADHD and one who is showing lazy/undisciplined behaviors.

As understanding of the neural correlates of learning and neuropsychiatric disorders expands, what impact will this have on traditional psychological and educational treatment?

As people increasingly identify neural correlates of learning and neuropsychiatric disorders, significant changes will become evident in psychological and educational interventions. Although the potential changes are both numerous and unknown, several of the following are predicted: (1) The discovery of genetic and chromosomal links to specific developmental disorders and accompanying neurogenetic interventions will enable children to be born relatively free of neuropsychological deficits. The need for traditional medical and psychological services specific to these disorders will be rendered virtually obsolete. (2) Neurogenetic, molecular, and chemical advances will guide the development of medical interventions to repair and regenerate damaged brain tissue. In such cases, neuropsychological treatment will primarily focus on developing plans and interventions to enable parents and other caretakers to provide the experiences necessary to stimulate development and recovery of functions. (3) Advances in the understanding of brain–behavior relationships will encourage the development of increasingly complex neuropsychological models to predict appropriate treatment options for specific brain disorders as affected by socioenvironmental factors, age, gender, health status, cognitive abilities, and other variables. (4) As understanding of brain–cognitive functioning expands, people will be able to develop specific educational strategies and interventions that will expand and maximize the learning of children, both disabled and nondisabled.

CHAPTER 9

What are the neurological, behavioral, and emotional symptoms of a stroke?

The initial neurological symptoms of stroke include a sudden headache, nausea, and loss of behavioral function, which may be relatively specific in nature. Because a stroke can affect many different areas of the brain, the neurological symptoms can vary, but there can be an associated loss of consciousness. Behavioral symptoms relate to the precise area of the brain that has been affected. For those affected with left hemisphere stroke, a common behavioral symptom is difficulty in understanding and expressing speech. Visual symptoms indicate posterior or basilar involvement, but a precise understanding of the behavioral symptoms is often not possible until a comprehensive neuropsychological evaluation is completed. Emotional symptoms can include depression for left hemisphere stroke, or irritability for right hemisphere stroke. Again, a comprehensive neuropsychological evaluation may include a measure of emotional and personality functioning.

What are the major forms of treatment for stroke?

The acute treatment of the stroke patient involves medical stabilization and control of bleeding, through medication or surgery. Common medications include anticoagulants to dissolve blood clots or prevent clotting, vasodilators to dilate or expand the vessels, and blood pressure medication and steroids to control cerebral edema. Surgery can include clipping a bleeding aneurysm or evacuating blood to control the intracranial pressure often associated with a hemorrhage. Treatment for TIA symptoms is more difficult because of the ambiguous nature of the symptoms and is often restricted to pharmacologic intervention with anticoagulants. Long-term treatment of stroke patients may include intensive rehabilitation, including speech therapy, occupational training, and vocational training. Often basic activities of daily living must be "relearned." Periodic reevaluation by a neuropsychologist may determine treatment and rehabilitation progress and outcome.

Why is it possible that some stroke victims downplay their illness, whereas others go into a deep depression?

The symptoms of a right hemisphere stroke are very different from those of a left hemisphere CVA because of the lateralization of many functions in the brain. A right hemisphere stroke may result in a "lack of awareness" associated with very poor insight and disinhibition. Right brain–damaged individuals tend to be unaware of their dysfunction associated with the consequences of the stroke. In fact, such patients often deny that there is anything wrong with them. Many patients with right brain damage display a range of emotions from indifference to euphoria. This contrasts to the depression that patients with left brain damage often show. Therefore it is easy to assume that deficits from right brain damage are not as serious as those from left brain damage. As a result, right hemisphere stroke patients may be blamed for being "rude," "disruptive," or "inappropriate" when they are actually exhibiting symptoms of right brain injury, including impulsivity, verbosity, inattention, and poor judgment. Obviously these problems can be highly disruptive to patient and family alike, often even exceeding the problems associated with left hemisphere CVAs. Because right hemisphere stroke patients and their families underestimate the severity of the condition, those patients are not diagnosed as rapidly as are left hemisphere stroke patients.

Describe the most common neuropsychological deficits associated with stroke.

Almost always, neuropsychological disruption appears in stroke survivors and thus neuropsychologists often evaluate stroke patients. Both the right and left hemispheres are associated with changes in motor and sensory functioning after a stroke. Those changes can be as benign as mild motor slowing to effects as debilitating as complete paralysis, particularly if there are lesions in the thalamic area or the motor and premotor area of the frontal lobes. Right hemisphere stroke motor deficiencies, however, are generally less severe, because the nondominant left hand is not as important for skilled tasks. Deficits affecting the right cerebral artery involve areas responsible for spatial, rhythmic, and nonverbal processing. Right hemisphere symptoms, although serious in the patient's overall functioning, can be less striking in the acute phase, particularly if they do not involve motor dysfunction. Research has shown consistently that patients with right hemisphere stroke are hospitalized longer in rehabilitation facilities, than are patients with left hemisphere strokes. This fact is related to the pervasive deficits that right hemisphere patients present with in the area of visual-spatial abilities and the extended rehabilitation process that is required in rehabilitating these patients in areas of dressing, ambulating, and other self-care behaviors. The capacity to drive after a stroke continues to be one of the most sensitive issues facing health care workers, and the stroke victims and their families.

CHAPTER 10

Would you want to know what type of cell a tumor arises from, if a family member of yours had brain cancer? Why? Should physicians routinely inform their patients of such medical details?

Yes, I (EAZ) would like to know. The reason for knowing is that the more information the patient and family has the easier it is to make personal decisions, such as estate management, issues of quality of life, and life expectancy. The specific type of brain tumor, and the type of cell it has arisen from, often signals a clear course of the disease. For example, the glioblastoma multiforme (GBM) is a particularly destructive and fatal glioma. Conversely, the presence of a meningioma often has little consequences to one's long-term well-being. Many physicians share detailed medical information with their patients and treat them as educated consumers. But many do not. My Aunt Edna died of a brain tumor, but the doctors never told her and her family what kind of tumor she had, even though clearly (to me) it was a GBM. As a result the family had great hopes for her recovery, which unfortunately was not realistic; she passed away within eight months. Would you like to know?

How do children who suffer from brain tumors react differently to their disease from the way adults do? How do their families react?

In general, children are quite resistant to the psychological consequences of life-threatening diseases. When they are adolescents, the burden on them physically and psychologically may manifest itself by experiencing depressed mood and irritability. But young children seem to cope surprisingly well when confronted with cancer. The parents of those children seem to absorb much of the psychological distress, however, often feeling guilty and being overprotective. Families often view the cancer and its consequences as severe and insurmountable. As a result, it has become essential to work with the entire family when a child is diagnosed with a brain tumor, in order to understand the subjective appraisals or perspectives of the child and the family and to provide a realistic but optimistic framework. This crisis is not only the child's but also the entire family's. Thus, diagnosis and treatment of cancer in children affects family functioning in subtle ways, and family functioning affects cancer and its treatment in children. Psychologists play an important role in managing the emotional consequences of the families and children with brain tumor.

Can a head injury change a person's life?

Yes, often dramatically. The consequences of moderate and severe traumatic head injury can be profound, with obvious emotional and cognitive changes in the head injury survivors. It is not unusual in such cases that a spouse complains that a head injury victim is not the person that he or she married. Their quality of life, marital status, and employment status often change significantly. The consequences of mild head injury (MHI) and concussions are more subtle, even to the patients themselves. Nevertheless, they can change a person's life, because the mild cognitive deficits that are often associated with MHI affect the victim's quality of life. Often depression and somatic complaints appear in mild head injury survivors, as do cognitive deficits in memory and attention. However, many individuals who have sustained an MHI completely recover. Often neuropsychologists can determine the level of recovery by making a neuropsychological assessment.

What is the neuropsychologist's role in diagnosing and treating the victims and their families who suffer from brain tumors?

Since the advent of modern imaging technologies neuropsychologists play a minor role in the diagnosis of brain tumors. CT and MRI technology can often pinpoint the precise location and size of a brain tumor. If the tumor is thought to be fatal, neuropsychologists often provide counseling and education to brain tumor patients and their families. If the brain tumor is operable and recovery is likely, neuropsychologists can provide a baseline assessment to which future evaluations (postoperation) can be compared. Treatment choices are complex and should have input from a team of oncological professionals including neurosurgeon, oncologist-hematologist, radiation therapist, neuroradiologist, neurologist, and neuropsychologist. In general, neuropsychologists can play an important role in assessing brain tumor survivors, and in providing rehabilitation care and intervention. As with other neurological disorders, neuropsychologists can play an important role in helping people to understand the cognitive changes associated with brain tumor diagnosis and treatment.

CHAPTER 11

Will exercising one's mind help ward off dementia? Must one "use it or lose it?"

There is increasing consensus among researchers that maintaining flexibility of thought and keeping mentally active contributes to one's cognitive reserve. Although some people who don't "use it" may not be prone to dementia, an active, healthy lifestyle, both mentally and physically, appears to help ward off many disorders of aging.

How is Alzheimer's disease best identified in life?

Because AD is a diagnosis of exclusion, only confirmed later by biopsy at autopsy, behavioral and cognitive profiles are crucial to the differential diagnosis of AD and of various dementia subtypes. In addition to differentiating between AD and normal aging, the next chapter makes clear that different dementia subtypes show distinct neuropsychological profiles. Knowing the behavioral and cognitive profile is one of the best means of differentiating between some types of cortical (AD) and vascular dementias, and normal aging. This is because once all other medical causes have been ruled out, imaging and physiological testing often cannot detect minute vascular changes or patterns of brain necrosis. This is also because, as we have said, degree of cortical shrinkage is not reliably associated with declines in cognitive functioning. Changes in behavioral functioning, however, are the hallmark of dementia and they must be carefully documented.

How can a neuropsychological profile aid dementia sufferers and their families?

As is evident from the previous question, in addition to aiding in diagnosis, one of the best things a cognitive profile can provide is a picture of the person's pattern of strengths and weaknesses, and an estimation of degree of decline from former abilities. This picture is a "snapshot in time," but it serves to educate patients and caretakers about the degree to which the person is currently able to manage independently and in what areas he or she is likely to need assistance. The neuropsychological profile can also serve as a planning aid for future caretaking and treatment needs. Although there is no "cure" for AD, ameliorative treatments can help the AD patient. Knowing, for example that an AD patient has preserved nondeclarative motor skill learning means that the person may be taught relaxation techniques requiring progressive muscle relaxation even though they retain no declarative knowledge of learning. Such behavioral treatments, used by psychologists, show promise in calming restlessness and agitation that can occur in later stages of the disease. In sum, the neuropsychological profile helps reveal the problematic brain functioning, educate regarding strengths and weaknesses, plan for individualized caretaking needs, and suggest possible behavioral treatments.

How does the Alzheimer's disease patient's concept of self change with the progression of the disease?

This question allows speculation, given what has been presented of the neuropsychological profile of the AD sufferer. If you look at each area where decline is evident, how do you think this would affect a person's self-concept? New learning deficits and declarative memory loss are hallmarks of the disease. Considering the possibility that aspects of our selves are built on memories of our own experiences, do you think a person's self-concept would change as they lose aspects of their memory, as they have increasing trouble learning, or as they are having trouble doing certain things they once did well? Are there certain people whose sense of self may be more affected than others by AD?

CHAPTER 12

It may soon be possible to test for many neurologic diseases. Would you want to be tested for the possibility of future dementia?

A positive genetic test for Huntington's disease indicates almost certain manifestation of the disease. But what about other neurologic diseases, where a positive test could indicate much lower odds of disease certainty? There are cases of AD patients with normal identical twins. Factors other than inheritance play into whether one develops dementia. Would you want to know about your tendency toward a certain disease? Would you want others to know? Why do you think most people at risk for HD have declined to be tested?

How is the behavioral quality of subcortical motor disorders presented in this chapter similar or different from the cortical motor disorders such as apraxia presented in Chapter 4?

Is the behavioral quality of the motor dysfunction of Parkinson's, Huntington's, or Creutzfeldt-Jakob disease different from that of, say, apraxia (see Chapter 4)? Most clinicians would say yes. With subcortical motor problems, the movement is usually not orchestrated or regulated well, but apraxia is a problem of not "knowing." For example, if asked to pantomime "pouring and serving tea," an apraxic patient may have no idea of how to demonstrate this or may mime a wrong action. In contrast, a PD patient is more likely to demonstrate the correct movement, but may have trouble initiating the movement or show slowness in performing the movement (tremor may be evident in later stages of the disease during intentional movements). In what other ways might the behavioral quality of subcortical motor disorders differ from that of cortical motor disorders?

How do the subcortical and cortical motor systems work together?

In Chapter 4 we described two theories of how the motor system may work. One, the hierarchy theory states that the primary motor cortex sits at the top and is the funnel for all bodily information. A competing theory suggests that the motor system works in a parallel processing mode with several motor processing circuits working in coordination with the primary motor cortex. Although these theories remain debatable, we also know that much of the initiation for motor behavior and executive programming for movement originates in the higher association area of the prefrontal cortex, which is responsible for orchestrating and organizing motor behavior. The dorsolateral prefrontal cortex (contained within) is not a "movement center" in and of itself, but is instrumental in deploying movement. Much of the input to this area comes from the subcortical motor centers. So the subcortical motor functions and the cortical motor functions must coordinate and may do so through the dorsolateral prefrontal cortex. Although there appears to be some hierarchy of functioning, it may also be that parallel circuits relate to different aspects of motor behavior within this hierarchy.

What are the ethical and scientific issues in the treatment of dementias?

This chapter and the preceding one discussed a number of different treatments for dementias. These included drug, behavioral, and even surgical interventions. The most ethically controversial treatments include genetic treatments and surgical interventions with "young" brain tissue. Also, to what extent should society go to develop drugs to ameliorate symptoms of dementia? What are the costs versus the benefits?

CHAPTER 13

What is the biological or psychological function of "rhythms" of consciousness?

We began this chapter by discussing the idea that there are preset circadian rhythms of human consciousness. We discussed how these operate in normal waking, sleeping, and dreaming. It is also apparent that narcolepsy disrupts the flow of this rhythm so that sleep attacks may occur during wakefulness. Also, the rare circadian rhythm disorder can be life threatening (see "The Case of the Last Coronation"). Given what you know of this, can you speculate on the biological reasons for daily and 90-minute periods of relatively more active and more quiet brain activity? Does this somehow "tone" the brain, as some suggest? Psychologically, is it adaptive for humans to alternate between periods of activity and quiet?

How fluid are the boundaries between conscious awareness and the subconscious?

This question concerns not only this chapter, but also ideas of conscious awareness, which we have presented throughout the book, as well as general ideas of consciousness debated in psychology. To approach this issue, it appears first necessary to conceptualize and operationalize a definition of "conscious awareness" with particular attention to how conscious awareness is demonstrated. Must this always be in a verbal manner? Can one demonstrate awareness just through performance of an action? When one is in a state of consciousness, which is other than being "fully awake," what sense of awareness can there be? How does your knowledge of the functional and dysfunctional brain help to inform your ideas of consciousness?

How do you think REM sleep and dreaming change in people who have various neurological disorders?

This issue presents an exciting and relatively underexplored area in neuropsychology. There are a number of case reports of people with abnormalities in dreaming from global cessation of dreaming to decreased or odd qualities of dreaming, to problems in remembering dreams. How do you think dreams of people with frontal lesions differ from those with parietal lesions? Do you think that people with motor problems will also have motor problems in their dreams?

In what ways might neuropsychology be able to contribute to treatments for people with sleep disorders or epilepsy?

If you consider the range of behavioral treatments of clinical psychology and the neuropsychological problems represented by the disorders we have presented in this chapter, you can see that a number of treatment strategies are possible. For example, memory and concentration problems are common in sleep apnea, and to a certain extent, in narcolepsy. Do you think strategies that aid memory will be useful for sleep apnea patients? Narcolepsy patients may have sleep attacks in response to emotional stimuli. Might relaxation techniques help them? With seizure patients, if auras are related to the foci of the seizure, might visualization techniques help to ward off visual auras, and therefore the seizure? What else can you think of? These areas are ripe for future investigation.

CHAPTER 14

Why are the concepts of reliability and validity so important in psychological and neuropsychological assessment?

If a test is not repeatable, it is not reliable and thus can provide no consistent score on a specific dimension. Think of weighing yourself on a scale that gives you a different weight every time you step on it. Such a scale could not be trusted, could it? Validity is important because it relates to the meaningfulness of a psychological test score. What if a psychological measure of depression does not really measure depression, but something else, such as stress? Such a scale would not be an appropriate measure of depression. Let's go back to the example of the scale. This time it is reliable (remember if a test is not reliable, it cannot be valid). A scale would not be a valid measure for anything else besides estimating weight. For example, you would not use a scale to determine what the temperature is. This is the assumption of validity, that is, whether a psychological or neuropsychological test is really designed to measure what it is supposed to measure in a meaningful way.

What kind of questions and tests do neuropsychologists use in a neuropsychological evaluation?

Neuropsychologists use mostly standardized tests and questions in a neuropsychological exam. That is, they may use specific tests and scales that have questions that every subject receives more or less in the same way. As a result, the neuropsychologist knows what it means if a person may not know the answer to a particular set of questions. Neuropsychologists use many different tests, tasks, puzzles, and questions to get an overview of an individual's cognitive strength and weaknesses. Thus, it is not uncommon to have a battery of tests that include measures of memory, attention, intelligence, personality functioning, and so on. The neuropsychologist uses a specific set of procedures to answer the referral question. For example, he or she may treat a referral question about diagnosis differently from a referral question about employment capacity, in terms of selecting neuropsychological tests.

How are neuropsychology assessment procedures the same? How are they different?

All neuropsychological assessment procedures are similar in that the same rules of reliability and validity bind them. Also, almost all neuropsychological tests are given in a standardized format and environment, and are administered to the patient individually. They are different in that they measure different aspects of behavior. There are tests that measure memory, problem solving, and attention, to name just a few. Some tests measure personality functioning, adaptive skills, intelligence, vocational, and educational attainment. These types of tests are strictly not neuropsychological tests, even though they depend on brain functioning, because they are not sensitive indicators of cortical dysfunction. A test is considered a neuropsychological test if a change in brain function systematically relates to a change in test behavior.

What sort of recommendations and treatments can neuropsychologists give brain-impaired people that will be useful in their daily lives?

How to make recommendations to individuals about their everyday lives has become a very important issue in neuropsychological assessment. This is important because many neuropsychological tests seem to be somewhat abstract on the surface. For example, a test of driving capacity has not been developed yet, so neuropsychologists rely on traditional measures of attention, memory, and eye–hand coordination to make inferences about whether a brain-injured individual should be allowed to drive. Besides driving, there are many instances in which neuropsychologists can help their patients regarding activities that have a cognitive component, but are performed almost every day. Those can range from balancing a checkbook, going shopping, and finding one's way around, to more basic activities such as getting dressed, taking a bath, or brushing one's teeth. Neuropsychologists can determine what everyday tasks brain-injured individuals may have problems with. Neuropsychologists then recommend what task may be strengthened through rehabilitation or through compensation of other intact skills. For example, if a right hemisphere patient has trouble finding his or her way around a hospital and often gets lost, the patient may learn specific right/left directions and also compensate by learning to ask bystanders about directions. The patient may also rely on a notepad that always reminds him or her what the destination is. Thus neuropsychologists play an important role in treating and rehabilitating individuals with brain injury.

CHAPTER 15

How do the major two approaches (process and battery approach) to interpreting neuropsychological data differ?

The two approaches are different in a variety of ways (see Table 15.2), so that it is almost a philosophical difference in terms of neuropsychological assessment. The principal difference is that the battery approach is a standardized approach to assessment, whereas the process approach is a clinical analysis of a patient. The former is akin to having a patient undergo a series of tests and standardized questions to understand their abilities and deficits. The latter is based on the idea that each patient's presentation is so unique that it is of most importance to understand the unique problems that a patient is presenting with, and thus to tailor the exam to the individual. The standard battery approach has evolved through empirical analysis and the extensive testing history of psychological testing. The process approach has evolved in the clinical setting. Although proponents of the process approach would disagree with this conclusion, research supporting the process approach is not as robust as the empirical foundation of the standard battery approach. As with most issues that are so polarized, most neuropsychologists borrow certain aspects from each approach in their own approach to neuropsychological assessment.

What role can neuropsychologists play in court?

A neuropsychologist can work closely with the legal profession, and in fact, this is a very exciting aspect of the practice of neuropsychology. Neuropsychologists perform court-ordered psychological evaluations, evaluate the competency of individuals to stand trial, and are consulted as expert witnesses. The role of the expert witness is particular interesting for neuropsychologists who do not mind the adversarial climate in courts. Expert witnesses can provide opinions to the court, and neuropsychologists are often sought after to give such opinions on either the plaintiff's or the defendant's side on issues of head injury, toxic conditions, and insanity. Obviously, neuropsychologist who work in this capacity should have extensive training in neuropsychology and clinical psychology.

What is a pathognomonic sign, and why is it so important?

Pathognomonic symptoms occur rarely in normal individuals. Pathognomonic symptoms are especially important to detect, because the presence of such symptoms often yields clues of a specific pathologic condition or diagnosis, and thus often a specific diagnosis or course of treatment can be suggested. *Pathognomonic* is Greek for "fit to give judgment." What pathognomonic signs can you list, having read some of the clinical chapters in this book?

How do neuropsychologists go about trying to make sense out of a neuropsychological evaluation?

Neuropsychologists examine and evaluate, among other pertinent information, the patient's behavioral presentation, presenting problem, and history, as well as the results of a neuropsychological exam. One of the most exciting aspects of neuropsychology practice is integrating and synthesizing all this information. The goal is to adequately describe an individual's cognitive strengths and weaknesses, to answer the referral question, and in some cases to provide a diagnosis. This complex, delicate process requires not only a doctoral degree in psychology with extensive work in neuropsychology, but also state licensure as a practicing psychologist.

CHAPTER 16

What is the potential for the human brain to adapt and recover after brain injury?

In this chapter, as well as in previous chapters of this book, we have presented cases in which people had to adapt to the devastating effects of brain injury. Some patients have adapted very well even in the face of little to no recovery. Other patients, particularly younger children, have made dramatic recoveries of function. The practicing neuropsychologist must weigh multiple factors, including injury severity, age, previous level of functioning, available resources as well as the person's psychological state and level of motivation in predicting potential for recovery. This remains an inexact science, but neuropsychologists are often surprised by the ability of people to adapt to their injuries.

What are the challenges for rehabilitation in the 21st century?

After reading this chapter, where do you think neuropsychological rehabilitation should head in this century? Should it be in the area of technology? Inpatient treatment? Community reintegration and job skills? Family and patient counseling related to adapting to the injury or illness?

Will technology eventually be able to compensate for lost neural function?

This question allows for creative speculation. Right now scientists can program the nervous system of only the most simple invertebrates. However, changes in technology are occurring at lightning speed. Will actor Christopher Reed, paralyzed from the neck down, walk again through the aid of technology? We posed this question in Chapter 2. What do you think now?

Is the quest for the search of the organ of the soul completed?

We posed this question in Chapter 1. After completing this book, have your thoughts about the relationship of the mind and the brain changed? How should we now understand the mind? Is it synonymous with the brain? Is it a larger concept than the brain? Is it different from the brain? Do we now have more questions than we started with?

NAME INDEX

SUBJECT INDEX

Note: Page numbers in **boldface** type indicate pages on which terms are defined or introduced.

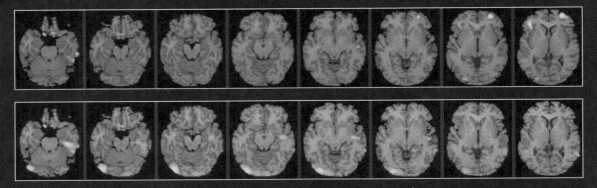

Exhibit 6 (Chapter 6)

Verbal encoding using PET cerebral blood flow. Brain images show differences in regional blood flow between word encoding and averaged baseline for 23 healthy volunteers (top) and 23 patients with schizophrenia (bottom). Note activation in left and right prefrontal cortex for healthy volunteers, and in right temporal and left occipital cortex for patients. Deactivation is visible in left precentral and occipital areas for healthy volunteers, and in left precentral area for patients. The inability to activate prefrontal regions during encoding may underlie learning difficulties in patients with schizophrenia (Ragland et al., 2000; Ragland, Gur, Raz, Schroeder, Smith, Alavi, & Gur, University of Pennsylvania, by permission)

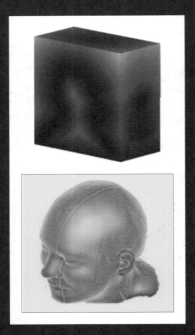

Exhibit 7 (Chapter 6)

Three-dimensional imaging of objects. (Top) Cuboid of scalp surface for which distance map was computed. Darkest color represents scalp surface (distance = 0); lightest color indicates farthest distance from scalp. (Bottom) 3-D geometric alignment of scalp surface. (Dorota Kozinska, Ph.D., University of Warsaw, Poland, by permission)

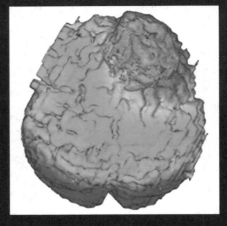

Exhibit 8 (Chapter 6)

Sensory-evoked response examination with MRI. With this technique, electrical activity and anatomic detail can be co-registered for clinical analysis. Image includes visualization of right frontal tumor. (Dorota Kozinska, Ph.D, University of Warsaw, Poland, by permission)

SO-BCU-466

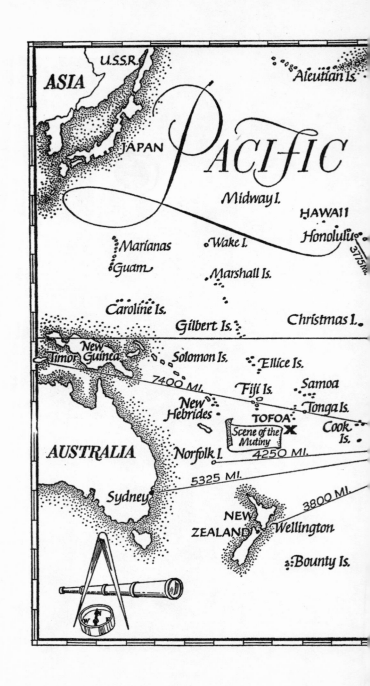

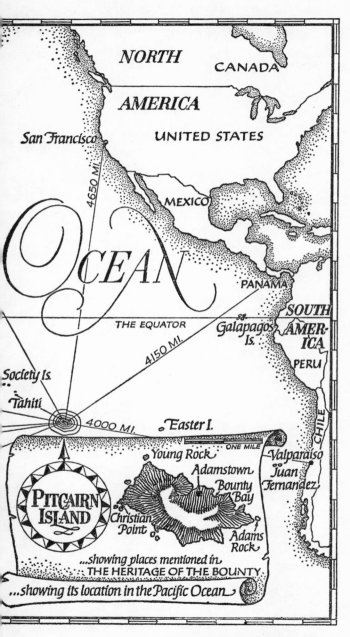

MAP DRAWN BY STEPHEN KRAFT

THE PITCAIRN ISLANDERS

HARRY L. SHAPIRO

[Formerly *The Heritage of the Bounty*]

REVISED WITH A NEW POSTSCRIPT

ILLUSTRATED WITH PHOTOGRAPHS

A CLARION BOOK
PUBLISHED BY SIMON AND SCHUSTER

A Clarion Book
Published by Simon and Schuster
Rockefeller Center, 630 Fifth Avenue
New York, New York 10020
All rights reserved
including the right of reproduction
in whole or in part in any form
Copyright © 1936, 1962 by Harry L. Shapiro

First Clarion printing 1968

Manufactured in the United States of America
Printed by Murray Printing Company, Forge Village, Mass.
Bound by Electronic Perfect Binders, Inc., Brooklyn, N.Y.

ACKNOWLEDGMENTS

Chiefly I am indebted to Mr. Templeton Crocker not only for my visit to Pitcairn but also for his invaluable aid in recording island documents.

To all the Pitcairn Islanders I owe my best thanks for their patience and coöperation. It would be impossible, where everyone was so uniformly kind, to distinguish one above another.

To Mr. Cooze I am obliged for many hours of tedious clerical assistance.

To my colleagues, Dr. James Chapin, Mr. Lee Jaques, and Dr. George Lyman, I am grateful for many kindnesses.

TABLE OF CONTENTS

CONTENTS

VI. POSTSCRIPT

EPISTLE DEDICATORY

[*To Professor E. A. Hooton*]

DEAR EARNEST:

This book on the Pitcairn Islanders has every right to claim you as its godfather. Because it all started, you may remember, one winter morning back in 1922 in the classroom on the second floor of the Peabody Museum. On that occasion you happened to relate the story of Pitcairn Island. I don't know how many times you had told that yarn before, or have told it since, but for me it was marvelously new and exciting.

I had been lolling on one of those hard, wooden benches gnawed with the graffiti of generations of anonymous Harvard undergraduates; my attention was about equally divided between the intricate pattern of bare winter branches against the warm, red brick of the Agassiz and the tedious business of recording in grotesque, lecture-note English your erudite remarks on race mixture. If I remember correctly, the Rehobother Bastards had been occupying our attention for the past several lectures. We had, following your lead, delved into the genetics of those Hottentot-Boer hybrids, drab offspring of dull unions. Then with all the magic of the movies the scene shifted, and we were in the warm, vibrant Pacific, on the Cytherean shores of Tahiti, amidst the turmoil of a mutiny on board the *Bounty* and stranded on a forgotten speck of land called Pitcairn, where human folly was succeeded by inhuman virtue.

That unique narrative of an eighteenth-century bread-fruit expedition resolving itself into mutiny, court-martial, hanging, crime, murder, and, finally, a new population of mixed bloods made a glorious text, and no one realized it better than you.

The traceries of the old trees were forgotten, and my notebook still shows a lacuna for that day. Who could dream of arboreal designs, and what memory needed jogging for such events? I distinctly recall that you paused, after the narrative, and commented that you would rather go to Pitcairn than anywhere else in the world. I was impressed. But you were, to use an inelegant analogy, like a hen who, on finding a particularly juicy morsel, was calling on her little chicks to come and get it. I was one of those chicks and, with the selfishness of the very young, grabbed at it while you complacently looked on, quietly pleased. After all, what could have made a more absorbing subject for research than the heredity of the hybrid Anglo-Polynesian children of the *Bounty?*

When the arrangements to go to Pitcairn were finally made possible in the following spring by a Bishop Museum Fellowship from Yale, I was scarcely more elated than you, and when I started out on my journey in July, 1923, your benediction made the task seem lighter. You know most of what happened on that trip: the negotiations for a means of reaching inaccessible Pitcairn, the voyage to Panama where the best I could do was to take passage on the ill-fated *Paparoa* (she was later burned at sea) on the chance that she might break the long, slow voyage to New Zealand by a brief call at Pitcairn. But I don't know whether I ever told you that the captain, a tough, old, red-faced Englishman, refused point-blank to drop me at the island. I didn't have the proper papers. His reason was that since Pitcairn was not an official point of call, he had no authority to discharge passengers there, and under the circumstances would have to present a full passenger list at his destination in

Auckland. Nor have I ever revealed that in desperation I had plotted to jump ship when we reached the island. One of the passengers was in my confidence and ready to aid my plans. The day before we were due to arrive at Pitcairn I secretly packed, and we hoped that I and my belongings might be surreptitiously lowered into one of the island boats and taken ashore without the captain's knowledge. I hadn't come all those thousands of miles to be cheated of my goal when it was almost within my grasp.

Then fate or "something" intervened. Just before we were scheduled to sight Pitcairn, a brief but severe tropical storm descended on us. The sun vanished behind clouds as thick and gloomy as any Ryder ever painted, the glass fell alarmingly, and the aged joints of the *Paparoa* began to groan. The captain, fearful of the dangers of approaching Pitcairn in a storm, altered his course, and I passed the island without even a glimpse of what I had come to see.

A couple of weeks later I found myself at Auckland, New Zealand, facing a choice. I could return to Panama and try again to reach Pitcairn (at that time only outward-bound ships, I was informed, ever stopped there). Or I could go on to Norfolk Island, where the larger part of the descendants of the mutineers of the *Bounty* now live. The lack of time and money, principally the latter, forced me to choose Norfolk. From Sydney, Australia, I made the six-day trip in a small Burns-Philp steamer to Norfolk where I remained about five months gathering material for a study of the descendants of the mutineers of the *Bounty* and their Tahitian wives.

The kindliness of the Norfolk Islanders, their hospitality, their affection indeed gratified me, beset as I was with the weighty responsibilities of my first independent piece of research. But they were not Pitcairn Islanders. And my desire to visit Pitcairn, though thwarted, did not die. It certainly received little encouragement. After each of my successive trips to Polynesia, I sighed regretfully that I was still unable to voyage to that isolated rock in the middle of the south Pacific. Pitcairn seemed like an unrealizable dream.

When, therefore, Templeton Crocker invited me in the spring of 1934 to join his expedition to the eastern Pacific for the American Museum of Natural History, I was naturally delighted to accept. And when he generously asked me where I wished in particular to go, I promptly answered Pitcairn.

We left San Francisco September 13, 1934, on board the *Zaca*, veteran of a world cruise and a number of scientific voyages. This time I was duly armed with official documents from the High Commissioner of the Western Pacific, in whose jurisdiction Pitcairn lies. I was informed that it was necessary to receive the unanimous consent of the islanders before anyone could land on Pitcairn. Since we encountered no opposition to our sojourn I assume that we had been thoroughly approved of before our arrival.

The *Zaca*, as you have seen from her photographs, is a handsome, two-masted gaff-rigged schooner built on the lines of a Newfoundland Bank fisherman. She is 118 feet long over all, is 96 feet at the water line, and has a 23-foot beam and a draft of 14 feet. The gross tonnage is 84. Power is furnished by two Diesel engines of about 120 H.P. each. She is beautifully equipped and very comfortable.

The first leg of our itinerary landed us, after twenty-one perfect days such as only the Pacific can provide, in the Marquesas. From these islands we proceeded to the brimming coral atolls called the Tuamotus, to Tahiti, to the Austral Islands, to Rapa famous for its Polynesian Amazons, to Mangareva, once the scene of an amazing hierarchy, and then to Pitcairn which we reached December 23, 1934. That day was the one hundred and forty-seventh anniversary of the sailing of the *Bounty* from Spithead, England. For ten days the *Zaca* lay off the rocky coast of Pitcairn while I lived ashore. The story of that visit and the account of my researches are contained in the following pages which are, as I started by saying in the beginning, dedicated to you. Rarely is a duty so felicitously contained in a pleasure or a debt so blessed to a debtor as mine are to you.

Affectionately,

H.L.S.

New York City
October, 1935

I. PERSONAL

1

MY FIRST DAY ON PITCAIRN

It was curious not feeling elated, not even feeling a trace of exaltation. Yet here, at last, was Pitcairn, the island where a part of the mutinous crew of H.M.S. *Bounty* sought refuge and found death. The fabulous island which had nurtured the children of these mutineers and their children's children. It was, at first, a mere smudge, scarcely more perceptible than a cloud on the horizon, too mirage-like to be the goal at the end of 9000 miles, the attainment of a passionate desire nursed for twelve years. As I contemplated this shadow of an island I wondered at my strange anesthesia where there should have been a wild, leaping excitement. I supposed, now that the moment I had anticipated so long was here, that the increasing tension of the past three months had created its own antidote, that my reactions, like those of an over-trained athlete, had gone stale. Besides, I was really terrified that I might be disappointed. The numerous books I had read, the many pictures I had created from this reading, had shaped in my mind a Pitcairn that I couldn't bear to have altered by the inexorable impact of reality. But there it was at last before me, ready for me, with unguessed impressions and experiences to be added to my store.

As I watched the dim gray shadow my solid resistance melted in proportion as Pitcairn slowly thickened into a deeper gray, then to purple and green, and a more natural excitement succeeded my lethargy.

That silhouette, remembered from ancient woodcuts, inky plates, and blurred photographs, was familiar. But, despite its familiarity, it had a character that no representation had ever conveyed. It was chunky, solid, and massive as I had anticipated. But from a distance its cliffs did not appear as impregnable as the Gibraltar I had imagined. Later I was to discover that I was mistaken. From the angle of our approach it looked like an inverted canoe, and strangely un-Polynesian. To me a Polynesian island is either a lofty volcanic pile, eroded into deep mysterious valleys and unscalable pinnacles, or else it is next to nothing—the merest coral reef rising just enough above the level of the sea to support its comb of cocoanut trees. But Pitcairn had neither the wild picturesque quality of a Mooréa nor the ineffable sadness of a coral atoll.

Pitcairn is situated in the south Pacific in latitude 25° 4′ S and longitude 130° 19′ W. It is roughly about 4000 miles west of Valparaiso, Chile, and about 2500 miles southeast of Tahiti. Only slightly more than two miles in length, it seemed lilliputian on the vast plain of the Pacific. No wonder the mutineers of the *Bounty* who landed here in 1790 had been lost to the world. It was a lump of an island, but its associations cast a glamour about it that made me forget its insignificance in a rapidly increasing anxiety to reach the shore, to make the famed and perilous landing, and to see the children of Christian, Adams, and Young—the progeny of the mutineers of the *Bounty*.

I had ample time from 7 a.m., when I first saw Pitcairn, until 10 a.m., when we dropped anchor off Bounty Bay, to review the story of this extraordinary island or, more exactly, of these extraordinary islanders, whom we saw coming out to us in two huge dories built on the lines of a whale boat. But their history and their significance to my scientific mission faded before the prospect of actually seeing them, which became more and more imminent as their boats rapidly devoured the half mile or so which separated the *Zaca* and the shore. The boats were full of men, two or three to a seat with the rest standing between. Twenty-eight oars, fourteen to each boat, rose and dipped with a steady rhythm, an obvious power, and the efficiency if not the grace of a racing crew. Then suddenly and swiftly they were alongside, shouting hearty greetings in a strange intonation, and, like a horde of invaders, some forty men swarmed onto the deck of the *Zaca*. Without waiting for a ladder they eagerly clambered aboard. They filled the decks. In their pleasure to see us they grasped every hand: sailors', cook's, captain's, and guests'. The social distinctions of a yacht vanished without a trace, and the *Zaca* succumbed to a wave of simple and hearty good-fellowship.

I found myself, with the others in the *Zaca's* party, besieged by a seemingly interminable succession of hands. One after another each of the islanders pressed forward, extended a hand, gave a hearty shake, uttered a pleasant greeting, and was pushed aside by another eager applicant. The confusion gradually subsided, and soon every member of our party was surrounded by a group of island men, each of us answering almost identical questions.

"Where do you come from?"

"Are you staying long?"

"When are you coming ashore?"

Then followed numerous queries about the *Zaca*, her size, engines, and speed.

With somewhat more leisure, after the confusion of the first greeting, I began consciously to inspect our visitors. My first impression was slightly disappointing. I had expected to see definite indications of the Tahitian contribution to their mixed Anglo-Polynesian origin. Instead, the men, *en masse*, were more like a group of Englishmen—dock workers—with ugly, knobby hands and feet, roughened and calloused by labor. They wore nondescript garments, the gifts of passing vessels or bartered from the crew of the New Zealand Shipping Company steamers. Battered officers' caps were clapped on mops of shaggy hair. Blue sea-jackets rubbed shoulders with ancient tweed coats. And hardly a pair of trousers matched its companion jacket. Shirts, open at the throat, revealed strong muscular necks and hairy chests. A glance at their bare feet explained why shoes were unnecessary. To rough, callous, padded feet like these, shoes could only be an encumbrance, at best an adornment, never a protection where nature had so amply fulfilled her function.

But I was not interested in their clothes. I was more concerned with their faces and their physical structure. I was examining them with a professional eye, picking out traits reminiscent of their English and Tahitian ancestors. What I saw seemed at once heterogeneous and curiously repetitious. On the whole, as I had remarked, they were rather English-looking, though varied in type. But in all of them a similar pattern was discernible—large prominent noses slightly beaked, heavy brows defined by bony bars above the eyes, giving the forehead a pronounced slope in profile. The complexion was ruddy and weather-beaten and the hair dark, although with a suggestion of fairer color here and there. The almost universal loss of teeth had produced a curious sucking-in of the cheeks and a collapse of the mouth. Several in my rapid survey reminded me of the bird man in Barnum and Bailey's circus—thin prominent nose, retreating brow, and atrophied, edentulous jaws.

In my examination of these faces I was suddenly arrested by one that was strangely familiar, then by another. For a moment I had difficulty in associating them with a persistent memory. Then I had it. They were the two Young brothers Sir Arthur Keith had photographed twenty years before on their visit to London as sailors on the *Mana*. I spoke to Edward Young.

"Aren't you the man that Sir Arthur Keith examined in London?"

"Why yes," he replied. "How did you know?"

"I recognized you from the photograph he published," I replied.

After about an hour spent in becoming acquainted with our visitors, I prepared to go ashore. I had elected to live with one of the islanders, Burley Warren. He had pressed his hospitality so warmly that despite the disappointment of others who had also put forth claims, I had arranged to stay at his house. With my bags and instruments in Burley's safe custody, I dropped into the island boat as it rose in the swell. It was a stout, heavy boat and very roomy. As soon as it was packed, we pushed off and started for shore.

Everything was at once so strange and fascinating that I found myself consciously watching every gesture and every item of behavior. I noticed that these men were so accustomed to their duties that, without a word of command or a show of authority, oars were promptly taken up and a man sprang to the guiding stern-sweep. As we rowed to shore they kept up a chatter of conversation, frequently lapsing into a dialect unintelligible to me.

Although the weather was exceptionally calm, I became apprehensive as we neared the shore. Former callers had described so vividly the hazards of landing at Bounty Bay that despite the universal praise of the islanders' skill in maneuvering their boats I could not but feel somewhat uneasy. Instruments immersed in the sea might rust or even be lost, and cameras bathed in brine suffered no improvement. Besides, I did not relish getting wet myself. Experience on other islands had led me to expect someone to assume command as we reached the danger point, but even though we were now close in shore, the men seemed almost phlegmatic, even disorganized, to my apprehensive frame of mind. Ahead of us were rocks and more rocks, then the narrow shingle at the base of a steep cliff. This so-called Bounty Bay was no bay to me. It was not even a cove. Nothing protected it from the swelling pulsations of the Pacific, as they rhythmically threw masses of surf and spray against the rocks. At last, as I had finally decided that these were not superskilled boatmen but foolhardy idiots, the rowing ceased without a spoken command. We paused. Wave after wave came up, lifted our boat high on its crest, passed on again as we dropped down into the trough. Once or twice a voice cried, "Now." But apparently the men recognized it as premature, or else they waited for the command of a more trusted voice, for suddenly someone yelled, "Now," and eagerly the word was taken up. "Now, now," "pull, pull," came from all parts of the boat. In response to the exhortations, oars were dug into the sea, and the boat gathered a momentum to match the oncoming swell. With a turn and a skilful pointing of the boat we had rounded the huge boulders into a narrow channel hardly visible to an inexperienced eye, and carried by the force of the awaited swell we were thrown straight and true down the short, narrow channel and hard onto the pebbly shingle.

The force of the impact of the boat on the shore threw me forward and onto my feet. Briskly the men began leaping into the shallow water. Scorning to use the arms lifted up to bear me dry-shod to the beach, I leaped for a point beyond the edge of the nibbling waves. To my chagrin I fell flat on my face. But no one laughed at the ridiculous figure I must have cut. Instead, several rushed up to assist me. Recovering my dignity and nursing a wrenched ankle, I took a position well up on the sharply sloping beach. From there I could examine the landing place and watch the activities of the men.

The beach itself is but a very narrow pebbly ramp. On one side stretches a rock-strewn shore impossible for launching or beaching any craft; on the other a shoulder of the cliff juts forward and drops its bulk directly into the sea. From below the level of the tide up to the boat-houses a fan-shaped runway of logs—like a corduroy road—has been laid down. On this the heavy dories are pulled up or lowered by main force. Its convenience is obvious to anyone who has tried to drag a heavy boat through sand and gravel. A cluster of about a dozen open-ended, thatched roofed sheds serve as boat-houses. I saw housed within their narrow confines only two kinds of craft—a heavy dory and a small dugout used for fishing.

Back of the boat-houses loomed the cliff. It rose sheer from the narrow beach on which I stood to a height of several hundred feet. Across its face of reddish-black volcanic rock a broad smear of an alien white stone stood out sharply. And high above I could see the green of a foliage securely rooted on the plateau. I scanned the precipice for a possible ascent, but although I knew from the published accounts of its difficulty that a trail existed, I could see none. I turned to watch the islanders. The scene, flanked by huge spray-wet rocks, was a very active one. Pitcairn urchins, boys and girls, in wet clothes which clung to their firm and supple little bodies were splashing in the water and clambering over boulders fallen from the cliff. The men, having deposited their cargo on the shore, were hauling the boat up the way. All muscles were enlisted and taxed to their utmost to budge the heavy bulk. At first it did not move, but by repeated efforts and by pulling in rhythm, they started it on its progress to the boat-house. Watching the effort necessary to beach their boats, I decided that only pressing need would persuade me to call on the islanders for transportation to the yacht.

As I stood entranced by the scene, Burley, the well-named, came up to where I stood and in a gentle, shy, and somewhat deprecatory voice that I came to recognize as characteristic of this stout, simple-hearted man, asked me if I were ready to go home. Assenting, I turned to follow my guide and host. Walking to the rear of the boat-houses we came upon the path which had been hidden from my view. About as wide as a narrow lane and rutted by the wear of innumerable bare feet and by rivulets of rain water, it now, during a dry spell, was hard and gravelly. We followed this path as it

sharply climbed the narrow talus to the point where it
reached the sheer face of the rocky precipice. Turning,
the path now hugged the wall-like side of the cliff. Like
a fire escape on a New York tenement house it mounted
sharply and flat against the precipice. Breathless but
less exhausted than I had anticipated, I gained the midway point which was rather more horizontal and permitted me to catch my second wind for the final and
steepest climb. I noted with satisfaction that some of the
natives also had found this a taxing ascent, for rough
stone steps were crudely let into the grade. Observing
the ease with which Burley and the others climbed, I
secretly exonerated my own red-faced, blown, and puffy
condition on the ground that months on a yacht had un-
fitted me for so sudden and strenuous an exertion.

In no condition to exchange graceful amenities after
this climb, I came face to face with the female and the
senile sections of the colony. There in front of us and
above us, seated on rocks and standing in groups, were
the women and the old folks. Several came forward, the
older ones with considerable poise, the younger ones
rather shyly, to shake my hand and offer a hearty or
mumbled greeting, depending on their age. The women,
barefooted like their husbands and brothers, were clad
in simple cotton dresses. Most of them were bareheaded,
although one or two, either more fortunate or vainer
than the others, wore hats—toques—of an outmoded
fashion. Like the men, they had lost many of their
teeth, and so at first sight they were by no means pre-
possessing.

Pausing here at the top of the ascent, we could enjoy
the cool breezes which swept in off the Pacific and contemplate the climb we had just accomplished. Several
hundred feet below, in open view, lay the waters on
which the *Zaca* had been rolling and plunging for days
and weeks. Even now with my feet firmly planted on the
earth the sight of the long, fascinating undulations of
the sea brought sharply back to some sympathetic nerve

the rhythm of its measured beat. The deep pure blue faded into the hazy horizon, and an overpowering feeling of constriction and isolation welled up from its sparkling, impersonal surface. Directly below, the rocky coast of the island caught the sea in a firm white line of broken surf. I could see the minute figures of men at the landing and watch some of them making the ascent.

I now turned to see the island itself. The clear, cloudless sky poured down a bath of brilliant sunlight that caused every blade and every leaf to reflect its radiance. At my feet the red-brown road open to the sky wound its sinuous course, making a narrow terrace along the side of a slope. Above, as well as below the lane, the slope was steep. On a ridge, cocoanut palms wove their fragile tracery against the sky. Closer at hand was a rich and varied growth of green, though unfortunately in my botanical ignorance I could recognize only a few species. Among them I did notice the close, umbrageous orange, the lemon, the stiff-armed breadfruit, and the *miro*. In effect, however, the thick growth that covered the slopes and softened the angles of the hills endowed the island with an appearance of rank fertility.

Burley, to whom these sights were as natural as breathing and as little thought-provoking, stood waiting for me to tear myself away. We now struck off down the main road which was more like a curving swath through the green foliage than a tunneled avenue, and soon espied the outlying houses of the village which is about a quarter of a mile distant from the cliff overlooking the landing at Bounty Bay. These structures were simple, unpainted dwellings, one story high, with walls of roughly cut, horizontal planks overlapping like clapboards. The roofs were covered by corrugated iron which though aesthetically inferior to thatch is more durable and collects rain water more effectively.

Finally the road made a turn and led downward to the village itself. About fifty houses were clustered in a compact group, only their roofs and walls showing through the masses of green trees and shrubbery. My notions of Adamstown, as the settlement is sometimes called, were definite. From early descriptions I had expected to see the houses neatly arranged about a village green. Beechey in 1825 had so described it. Nothing could have been more different. There was no trace of arrangement or order of any kind. Branching off from the main road were a succession of smaller paths, and from these stemmed others, no one of which kept to a straight line. Curving, twisting, crossing back and forth, these lanes, determined by convenience, formed a veritable maze in which I later often found myself wandering helplessly. Along these lanes, so close to the roadway that a passerby could peep through the window or door, the sprawling houses of the islanders were scattered, according to no regular pattern that I could detect. We followed one of these paths downward into a thicket of dwellings. A mere footpath, its narrow, hard surface pounded firm by the patter of countless feet, it was edged by miniature gullies cut into the unprotected earth by the run-off of rain storms. Where its course met the dry and shallow bed of some rain-born stream a neat bridge of a couple of logs spanned the break. Rounding the corners of houses and cutting across back yards we followed the trail to the third or fourth house—the last on that bypath. This was the home of Burley Warren.

Not knowing our destination, I had no time to scrutinize the house, before we arrived at the door. Standing on the threshold was Eleanor, Burley's wife, daughter of David Young and great-great-granddaughter of Edward Young of the *Bounty*. Above medium height, with a well-built upstanding body, she made a pleasant figure. Her masses of almost black hair, caught simply in a knot at the back of her head, her rather wide brow and face shaded and relieved by a natural sweep of hair, and her dark brown eyes, wide set and full, added a definite charm to her habitual expression of pleasant simplicity. Shyly, with a suspicion of embarrassed awkwardness,

Eleanor made me welcome and ushered me into her home. Crossing a threshold, two low steps above the ground, I entered the family living room. Wide, roughly-cut, but smooth boards covered the floor. The walls and ceiling were hung with wall paper which needed replacing. But so hard is wall paper to come by that no doubt Burley preferred retaining his tattered paper to having none at all, even though torn spots revealed the burlap beneath on which it was hung. A homemade, slat-bottomed, cushionless couch occupied one corner. A table was set between two windows on the side wall, and an old and elaborate bureau shared another wall with a harmonium of the same vintage. Besides crippled kitchen chairs, the only other furniture was a stout chest whose nicked and battered condition lent a nautical air to the room.

The hospitality of Burley and Eleanor was so warm-hearted, so generous, that I immediately felt at home, and I knew that I should like them. In their unpretentious way, with the native good manners of unpremeditated simplicity, they had the art of welcoming a stranger. Although the morning was practically gone and it was an hour when, under ordinary circumstances, I would be thinking of lunch, Eleanor asked me if I wanted "breakfast."

Preferring to put my things in order, I was shown to a narrow room which led directly from the living room. It was just wide enough for the length of a bed set against a single window. At the other end of the room were two more sea chests. A few hang-headed nails, which needed readjustment each time I ventured to trust my garments to them, sufficed for a closet. I took this to be the room of one or two of the three sons of the family, since it was the only other bedroom besides Burley's and Eleanor's. Theirs was a much larger one opening off mine and contained two beds. I must have dispossessed the boys who retired to their parents' room to make way for the guest. But since they never seemed to display any resentment, I concluded that the shift was accepted with the resignation children sometimes accord to their parents' arrangements.

The islanders were too excited and disorganized by the unaccustomed visit of a yacht for me to begin my investigations on the day of arrival, even had my own state of mind permitted. Consequently, I felt that I was not losing precious time when I decided to accept Burley's invitation to accompany him to the plantation where he wished to gather a basket of pineapples. The *Ruahine*, a New Zealand Shipping Company steamer on her way to Panama, was expected soon, and during her brief stay the men were accustomed to board her in order to sell curios to the passengers or to barter fruits and vegetables for clothing or foreign foodstuffs.

Burley and I set out once more, accompanied this time by his eight-year-old son, named (like an echo) Curley. Weaving our way around the neighboring houses, we were stopped frequently by islanders who shook my hand and passed a pleasant welcoming word. One elderly lady reminded me so forcefully of my own New England that it was with difficulty that I recollected her origin. Tall and flat-chested, with a high curved beak of a nose, she enhanced her similarity to a well-known type of New England spinsterhood almost to caricature by keeping up a steady and voluble chatter of unsolicited reminiscences and genealogical lore. Burley finally saved me from the burden of my politeness, and we continued to climb the footpath up the slope to the main village road. Just above the spot where this path abutted onto the road, I caught a glimpse of the only place that might be called a community center—a flat open area about one hundred feet square and about six to ten feet directly above the road. Here were a two-storied, many-windowed church, like a New England meeting house without a steeple, the courthouse, and the signal bell suspended on a crossbar. Not stopping to examine these buildings we proceeded on our way. The road led down into a slight hollow and then climbed again steadily until it reached the plateau which forms the top of the island. Part way up we met some men descending with an underslung wheelbarrow full of gnarled and knotted lumps of wood. We all stopped to rest and sinking down onto the grass alongside the narrow road, I lit my pipe.

Since the history of the Pitcairn Islanders was uppermost in my mind and since I had been, as I walked with Burley, silently checking my illusions acquired from reading against what I was actually seeing, I fell to questioning these roadside companions on the events of the first years on Pitcairn. It was natural to expect that John Adams, last survivor on Pitcairn of the *Bounty* mutineers, and the ten surviving Tahitian women of those who had accompanied them would have frequently retold their exploits to an eager audience of children, and those listeners would transmit the story in turn to a newer crop of ears—and so on unto the present. But expectation overran the facts. I was told almost to the very phrases the accounts I had read for myself, and I discovered that these modern islanders learned their yarn not from some rich local tradition handed down inviolate through generations, but from the very books I had myself consulted. In fact, my own information proved to be wider than theirs, since their sources were derived from only two or three accounts while mine included every item that twelve years of search had revealed.

When I reflected later on this strange absence of a contemporary tradition, the reason suddenly seemed clear to me. The situation here bore no analogy to our own conditions. Tradition is born of reminiscence, and reminiscence generally flourishes where there are at least two companions both of whom have taken a part in its making, for otherwise one would inevitably become a bore. The Civil War veterans around the village stove, each enjoying the yarn for his own contribution's sake, must have repeated their story so often that the younger generation could not escape its memory. On Pitcairn,

Adams had no companion with whom to warm over ancient grudges or lament the turn of events. Certainly, the women who spoke an aborted English and Adams who spoke a similar Tahitian could hardly have settled down to a comfortable chat about old times. And during the long years before the growing infants were old enough to constitute an audience, Adams must have learned the peace of silence. But whatever the cause of this poverty of historical detail, the comfort of my resting place was delightful and compensation enough for loitering. The tall grass on the bank was soft, and above my head lofty, full-leaved trees, leaning down from the slope above the road, spread a pleasant shade against the sun. In front of me I could see over the descending curve of the hill and spy the tin roofs of the village glistening in the sun. Not far away, a mountain spring trickled through a greener, richer foliage than that around us.

Fragrant both of nature and of romance as our station was, Burley had still his pineapples to gather, and regretfully I tore myself away to continue the laborious climb. With each advancing step more and more of the island presented itself, and the temptation to stop was strong. Finally we attained a bluff which offered an incomparable view. To our right and below us lay the tree-tufted carpet of the precipitous valley in which the village snuggled. From this distance only the roofs of the houses were visible, and each one made a spangle of light in the thick green.

To the left, a tower of rock lifted its solid mass against the heavens. Facing us and the sea, one side of the escarpment formed a wall-like precipice. As I stood gazing at it Burley said,

"See that cave."

Now that it was pointed out to me, I did see a darker patch on the wall of rock and studying it more closely I discerned its character.

"That," said Burley, "is Christian's cave."

My merely mild interest in caves in general was replaced instantly by a vivid interest in this particular one.

"Sixty or seventy people can live in that comfortably," Burley added, for my information. As he was not one of those who are historically or antiquarianly-minded, I did not tax his anxiety to please by asking for information concerning Christian's use of this retreat. I already knew the tradition that here Fletcher Christian, the leader of the mutiny on the *Bounty*, retired alone and, from that niche high above the sea, often sat and pondered over the same waters that had borne him here, far from his native Isle of Man. It took no great flight of the imagination to reconstruct that scene nor did I find it difficult to guess the gnawing thoughts, the resignation, the wild revolt the sea must have induced in turn in the mind of that unfortunate man. Here he sat, no doubt, rehearsing his grievances against Bligh, his captain, whipping himself anew to a fury against the insults endured on the *Bounty*, and justifying his actions as natural to any man in similar circumstances. But he must have had moments when a bitter regret seized him that he had ever led the mutiny which ended with an honorable career in the Royal Navy snuffed out like a candle, and himself yoked forever to a crew of tough sailors and a band of alien women and, worst of all, severed eternally from family and friends. The time had not yet come when a South Sea island was automatically regarded as a romantic retreat, for Rousseau's association of the Savage Man with the ideal life had not affected the philosophy of the sailor. To Christian his fate must have been awful to contemplate, and relief must have come to him in the form of a vain hope that some day a chance sail would release him from his prison.

And there before me were perhaps the only things that had remained unchanged for one hundred forty-five years, since the days when Fletcher Christian seated in his cave had dreamed over them and hated them—the sea and the sky.

But again pineapples, like a persistent theme song,

once more banished other melodies. Dogging after Burley, I continued to climb. Soon we came upon a group of little cabins. These, explained Burley, were the "camps," and I discovered that several weeks a year many of the families take a vacation by moving into these camps on the plateau. They were empty now, and I did not hesitate to peek into their interiors. They consisted mainly of one or two rooms, fitted with roughly constructed beds and similarly made tables and chairs. Cooking appeared to be carried on either at outdoor fireplaces or in sheds. Passing these dwellings we finally reached some of the plantations. We went through patches of Irish potatoes, pineapples, and *kumara,* a kind of sweet potato. Burley's destination was a fair-sized patch, about an acre in extent, entirely devoted to pineapples, and there he rapidly selected enough ripe fruits to fill his basket. He cut an extra one for us, and never did pineapple taste sweeter or pour more juice from its flesh than this one. Warm with the sun it gave off a delicious fragrance, but its juices drying on my hands left them uncomfortably sticky until I washed them on our return.

The descent was rapid and uninterrupted, the steep decline lending speed to our legs. Again I was entering the village, somewhat more familiar this time. We went straight to Burley's house. On our arrival Eleanor began preparing a meal. This time I did not refuse. We sat down to a long table, I on a chair at the head, the rest on benches. On my left were Burley and Eleanor and opposite were Lyndon, Curley, and Douglas, the three Warren lads, silent, shy, and watchful. The youngest, Douglas, had, in addition to his shyness, an ingratiatingly pert expression.

I remembered at least one custom of the Pitcairn Islanders. I therefore waited. When we were all seated, Burley in a low voice said a simple grace. That devout act was as effective as anything I had seen in symbolizing Pitcairn. Indeed, each visitor to Pitcairn in turn had recorded the solemn effect of this simple and invariably

observed act of piety. It was, in effect, a link with home
—and with the customs of an innocent youth. To one of
my generation, saying grace belongs to a remembered
past, and so this act, aside from its peculiarly Pitcairn
flavor, was poignantly nostalgic.

But the smell of wholesome, simple food stimulating
an already hungry digestive system did not permit me
to linger long over these musings. As the Pitcairn Islanders would say, I fell to and tucked away a fair share
of the grub. There were soup, boiled potatoes, Irish and
sweet, chicken, bread, jam, and a drink brewed from
bran husks. The service was of the simplest character:
thick unmatched plates stamped with the insignia of
the New Zealand Shipping Company, blackened metal
knives, forks, and spoons, for which one reached to an
old jam jar in which they were arranged business end up
like a murderous bouquet.

After lunch, I sought out Parkins Christian, the chief
magistrate, to ask him to call a general meeting that evening at which I intended to explain the purpose of my
visit as tactfully as possible. I found Parkins at home surrounded by his family. I had already met him on board
the *Zaca*, but that did not prevent my being impressed
again by his truly extraordinary personality. Tall, lean,
and muscular, his mere physical presence was enough to
dominate a crowd. But in addition, his rather handsome
face, distinctly Polynesian in its brown swarthiness, and
his deep brown eyes, set off by graying hair, had an alert
repose that inspired confidence and respect. Spoken
rather slowly and in a vibrant drawl, his words had humor and pertinence. It was remarkable to see this man,
raised on a remote island, far from contact with the
world, and lettered only to the extent provided by an inadequate island school, conduct himself with poise and
dignity. Parkins agreed to assemble the island population
at the courthouse where I could address them after
supper.

Retiring once more to Burley's house which I had

come by now to regard as home, I spent the afternoon greeting callers and arranging my paraphernalia. I found myself repeating so often the same admiring phrases about Pitcairn that I came to mistrust the sincerity of my emotions. But the visitors so obviously expected the praise that I could not bring myself to refuse it, nor did I wish to. As my acquaintance with the islanders widened I suddenly remembered Mary Ann McCoy. Norman Hall had met her and he had reported in his *Tale of a Shipwreck* her hope that I might visit Pitcairn and complete a study of the descendants of the mutineers of the *Bounty* that I had commenced twelve years before on Norfolk Island. In fact, Hall had entrusted to my care the delivery of a book and a letter to Miss McCoy. With the double purpose, therefore, of discharging my duty and of making the acquaintance of Mary Ann McCoy, I prepared to call on her. I found her living in a little three-room house whose interior was scrupulously neat and clean. She had been expecting my visit, and, as she rose to greet me, I realized that she was blind. Her blindness was provocative of an overwhelming tenderness. She moved with such care and gentle confidence, her aged and wrinkled face was brushed with so tender a smile, and her appearance of fragility was so poignant that I felt that she was as delicate and precious as an ancient porcelain. I wish I could convey the feeling she invoked. She was a small woman, shortened further by a stoop, with soft hands twisted by age. Her face was rather large, with prominent cheek bones and with a nose somewhat wide at the nostrils but saved from coarseness by a high curving bridge. Her forehead was heavy and had a pronounced slope, but the rugged character of the brow was softened by delicate white hair. I couldn't see her eyes which were concealed by a pair of blue spectacles, but her voice and her smile of chastened patience compensated for the veiling of those features.

I was particularly eager to meet "Aunt" Ann, as I called her, following the universal island custom, because

she was one of the very few survivors of the third generation born on Pitcairn. Born in 1851, her eighty-four
years represented more than half the history of the colony, and I hoped to receive information from her that
otherwise would die with her.

"I've heard of you," she said, "from Mr. Hall."

"And I have come to talk to you about the old folks,"
I answered.

"I am so glad," she continued. "For after I am gone,
no one will remember. It is such a pity that none of the
young people take an interest."

Aunt Ann was the only islander who had ever visited
the other branch of the colony at Norfolk, and her eagerness to hear from me some word about her relatives
there led us into conversation along that channel. When
the afternoon had almost gone, I left Aunt Ann with a
promise to return soon and set to work on genealogies.

On my return to Burley's I did what was to happen
frequently for the next day or two—I became lost in the
tangled skein of paths. One of the children, quickly observing my bewilderment, came and guided me to the
door. Supper was ready on my arrival, and again I sat
down to food substantially like that at luncheon.

We had just finished supper, and the twilight was rapidly deepening, when I heard the sharp stroke of a bell.
Associations were so strong that I turned to Burley and
stated more than asked, "Church?" "No," he responded.
"Your meetin'."

Taking an electric torch to light our homeward path,
we picked our way along shadowy lanes towards the
courthouse. We were among the first arrivals at the meeting place. Someone unrecognizable in the waning light
hailed me and invited me to a seat. Along the road side
of the square was a long narrow bench on the very edge
of a ten-foot bank which dropped vertically to the road
below it. Here sat the slowly assembling islanders, awaiting the opening of the meeting. Parkins soon appeared
and, after a wait of about fifteen minutes, he sang out in

his rich drawl, "All in, everybody," and led the way to the courthouse. This was a single large room, one end of which was partitioned off as a post office. The remainder of the room contained about fifteen long benches. Over one hundred men and women crowded into the room until every bench was full and every chair occupied. A single kerosene lamp on the speaker's table threw an uncertain light which left the further corners of the room in darkness. I could see directly in front of me a glowing mass of faces with intent eyes and—back of these—only eyes. Suddenly and unbidden the thought came to me that the success of my work depended on the coöperation of these people, and immediately fear seized me that they might not understand, might even be hostile and resent strangers, however scientific in aim, prying into their intimate lives. For a moment I longed for the godlike power of the entomologist or the zoölogist who had no need to placate his subjects or to consult their convenience. To my mind these eyes had taken on a hostile look. And I had to tell them that I had come from America to study their heredity, probe into their genealogies, and determine the results of race mixture between English and Polynesian.

I hardly heard Parkins' introduction. Something about "come from far away" and "hospitality." And then I was on my feet and speaking. Without plan, I began telling these unblinking eyes that I was quite nervous and deeply moved to be here at last, addressing Pitcairn Islanders. That confession seemed to break the fixity of those eyes, for I noticed some smiles and a general relaxation. I proceeded to tell of my visit to Norfolk Island among their cousins twelve years ago and to recall names familiar to them. I lingered on the hospitality I had received from the Norfolk Islanders. Introducing the purpose of my visit I was relieved to detect an alert interest in my plans to study among them the consequences of race mixture, and when I illustrated my points by the studies I had made in Norfolk I knew I had won their approval. Their assent was definitely clinched when I promised that medical assistance would be given to all those in need of it by the *Zaca's* physician, Dr. George Lyman.

Immediately after I concluded, a number of men and women rose to ask questions. In clear, unembarrassed voices and with the manners of people accustomed to speaking their minds in public meetings, they framed their queries with skill. Having answered these questions, I was then surrounded by a number of the men who displayed a keen interest in the genealogical charts collected on Norfolk. I very soon discovered, however, that their interest centered on whether or not their own lines were represented. Before closing the meeting, someone suggested a rising vote of thanks, for what I couldn't fathom, and I knew that the first encounter had been won. But taught by experience in these matters, I was not yet counting chickens. The laborious work of catching every islander on the wing and examining physically each in turn would be no easy task.

I was glad to start for home at last, and the thought of the bed awaiting me there occupied my mind. But I did not earn my rest so soon, for a number of men and women followed me right into Burley's house. Passersby, seeing the light and hearing the voices, joined the party, and thus we conversed until ten o'clock. When our guests saw that I could scarcely keep my eyes open, they laughingly rose and departed. Needless to say, I did not linger in preparing for sleep, and even the springless bed and grass-stuffed mattress offered no hindrance to the almost immediate oblivion that rounded off my first day on Pitcairn.

II. HISTORICAL

MUTINY ON THE *BOUNTY*

The story of the mutiny on the *Bounty* and of the subsequent settlement on Pitcairn is a perennial in an old-fashioned garden of favorite yarns. But even standard perennials undergo successive waves of popular approval and comparative neglect. Although the Pitcairn adventure has never been completely forgotten, it has suffered periods of obscurity only to be revived by its mere telling. Sir John Barrow's *Mutiny and Piratical Seizure of H.M.S. Bounty*, published in 1831, was one of the first narratives to create a wide interest in Pitcairn. About twenty years later, the Rev. Thomas Boyles Murray issued *Pitcairn* of which, by 1860, 30,000 copies had been sold. At this time Sunday schools throughout the United States were glutted with tracts in which the lesson of Pitcairn was neatly pointed. Murderers and cutthroats might found a modern Eden, ran the parable, evil might produce good, and the simple and primitive might harbor the true righteousness, if the voice of God were heeded as on Pitcairn.

Again another burst of general interest in Pitcairn was started in the seventies by Lady Belcher's account. And at the turn of the century the *Story of Pitcairn by a Native Daughter*, ran through a number of editions. But it remained for that admirable combination of Nordhoff and Hall to capture the virility and romance of this unique story. The appeal of their narratives has secured them a very large audience, and already they have taken their place as classics in the literature of romantic adventure.

The story of Pitcairn properly begins with the breadfruit tree. Fabulous, if not miraculous, to the eighteenth-century Englishman, that tree started the chain of events to be recounted here. The explorers of the Pacific had carried back to the civilized world many a tale of the wonders they witnessed: islands devoted to Venus, savage man in the lap of a bountiful nature, giant statues on Easter Island, and a godlike race descended from Homeric heroes. But it was the breadfruit which stimulated most the practical imagination; at least it caused a group of Englishmen, interested in the West Indian plantations, to petition their sovereign, George III, patron of geographical exploration, to dispatch an expedition to Tahiti in the South Seas and to bring back specimens of this extraordinary tree. The breadfruit is a tropical plant, large-leaved and stately, and bears abundantly round green fruit about the size of a large grapefruit. When baked in a native underground oven it tastes like hot bread, or perhaps more like a cross between hot bread and potatoes. In Polynesia where it is indigenous, it is a staple food, since it requires little attention, bears the year round, and has a large crop. For plantation slaves, thought British planters, the fruit of such a tree would be nutritious, and for British pockets decidedly advantageous. Therefore, the petition begged that these plants be transplanted to the West Indies. The proposal had the weighty support of Sir Joseph Banks, president of the Royal Society.

In due course, Lieutenant William Bligh of His Majesty's Navy was assigned in August, 1787, to this task. Bligh was selected because he had an excellent reputation as a seaman and because of his experience in the South Seas, acquired as one of Captain James Cook's officers on the ill-fated third voyage. Although only about thirty-three years old, Bligh had already had a long and hard experience in that brutal school—the British Navy in the eighteenth century. Contemporary portraits picture a small-featured gentleman of pleasant mien, not the fierce-browed, heavy-featured sea dog carelessly associated with the sailor of those times.

Already the fame of Otaheite, as the English then spelt Tahiti, or of la Nouvelle Cythère, as the more romantic French called it, was widespread. Wallis in 1767, and Bougainville in 1768, had reported its discovery. Cook had contributed to its glamour by returning with Omai, a native of the island, who created a sensation in London's drawing rooms, sang Tahitian love songs at the Burneys', and charmed sophisticated ladies. Even the great Johnson met Omai, and Boswell has recorded the master's apt comment, fitting for more than one Tahitian.

"Sir," said Johnson, "he had passed his time, while in England, only in the best company; so that all that he had acquired of our manners was genteel. As a proof of this, Sir, Lord Mulgrave and he dined one day at Streatham. They sat with their backs to the light fronting me, so that I could not see distinctly; and there was so little of the savage in Omai, that I was afraid to speak to either, lest I should mistake one for the other."

Gouty gentlemen at the Crown and Anchor roared, no doubt, at the frank stories of love in the islands, and over coffee cups and between puffs at their pipes must have envied Bligh, the lucky dog, his opportunities. But no record remains of what Bligh himself thought as he unknowingly faced the supreme adventure of his life.

The *Bounty* had been designated for the voyage. She was of 215 tons burden, 90 feet in length, and with a beam of 24 feet 3 inches. Refitted at Deptford, the great cabin was converted into a conservatory to house the plants that were to be gathered at Tahiti. A false floor was laid down, with holes designed to secure the pots from shifting. The ship's complement consisted of Captain Bligh, one master, three warrant officers, one surgeon, two master's mates, two midshipmen, thirty-four petty officers and seamen, one botanist, and one gardener, making in all forty-six. Of the officers Fletcher Christian, the master's mate, was an old shipmate of Bligh who had personally selected him for the post. Peter Heywood and George Stewart, midshipmen, were appointed through family influences. The sailors were all carefully chosen for the mission.

By December of the same year, the *Bounty* was finally ready for her journey. Her holds were filled with provisions for eighteen months, and, in addition, articles for trade with the Tahitians were taken aboard. Bligh knew the eagerness with which the natives sought, and when occasion offered stole, iron nails, mirrors, and axes.

The sailing directions recommended the passage around the Horn. Therefore after laying on wine and other provisions at the Canaries, Bligh, setting his course for South America, sailed from Spithead, December 23, 1787. The voyage proceeded with the usual encounters of weather. Periods of rain and storm were succeeded by calm and relaxation during which the ship's stores were aired, and the men repaired the damages suffered.

There are two accounts of the voyage. One is Bligh's own which he published in his defense immediately on his return to England. The other is by James Morrison, boatswain's mate. Mr. Rawson casts doubt on the validity of the latter as a contemporary report. He recalls that Morrison not only went through a mutiny, lived on Tahiti for months, was chained aboard the *Pandora*, was wrecked on the Great Barrier Reef, but endured other vicissitudes, a combination of events which makes it improbable that the author had either the writing materials or the means to preserve a journal. Besides these documentary evidences, there are the testimony of the men court-martialed in England, Adams' stories, and the bits of tradition which have survived.

In all this contradictory body of evidence it is difficult to ascertain the truth, and, undoubtedly, eye witnesses might honestly record varying reactions according to their points of view. There is no question, however, that on several occasions Bligh used blunt quarter-deck methods in handling his crew. Most of his difficulties with the crew were concerned with food, and the accusation has been made that his double function as master and purser encouraged him to shave the ship's victualing to his own advantage. In any event, except for some disciplinary measures that Bligh well knew how to administer, and with which the crew were familiar, nothing of obvious moment occurred during the voyage to Tahiti to disturb Bligh's peace of mind.

In April, 1789, after an unsuccessful attempt to round the Horn, Bligh was forced to change his plans. He had feared boisterous weather at the Horn and had been foresighted enough to secure discretional orders from the Admiralty. He now proceeded to the Cape of Good Hope on the other side of the Atlantic. In the bald way of the sailor, Bligh briefly touches on the remainder of the outward voyage. After departing from Africa, the *Bounty* touched at Van Diemen's Land (now Tasmania), black aborigines were observed and described, and once more the ship was on her way. Finally, ten months after leaving England, the *Bounty* found a resting place at Matavai Bay, Tahiti. It was then October 26, 1788.

Despite Bligh's traditional reputation, he was capable of actions of remarkable consideration. Before arriving at Tahiti he had had posted a list of instructions governing the behavior of the crew in their commerce with the natives. Among other provisions his experience at Tahiti had taught him to demand of each sailor a physical examination. At a time when most captains were criminally negligent of the havoc that their crews might cause among an unprotected people, Bligh thus attempted to forestall the spreading of venereal disease among the Tahitians.

The sailors were also enjoined from bartering independently lest it interfere with the procural of the ship's necessities—and no mention was to be made of Cook's death. Bligh knew the veneration with which the Tahitians regarded Cook, or "Toote" in the native tongue, and he wished to avail himself of whatever magic that name might invoke.

If the modern visitor to Tahiti is amazed to see the crowds of curious islanders throng the pier for the scheduled and long-established visits of a mail steamer, what must have been the reception the *Bounty* received? The dozen or so European vessels to reach these shores before the arrival of Bligh had not satiated the curiosity of a people always interested in nautical innovations, and fascinated, moreover, by white men who were regarded as of partly divine origin.

As for the *Bounty's* crew, their pleasure must have been unbounded. Ten months at sea! They were young and hungry for fresh food and the company of women. Barter was immediately commenced with the hordes of natives who surrounded the ship in their canoes. Some of them even swam out, too impatient to await a place in a canoe. It was not long before intimacies were established with the natives. It was customary to select some applicant as a special friend, or "tyo," from among the islanders who eagerly presented themselves for the honor. One's *tyo* brought fruits and presents of native manufacture and in return expected nails, mirrors, and bits of iron. Bligh recorded that scarcely one of his people was without his *tyo*. And so whole-heartedly were the demands of *tyo*ship and barter indulged that the *Bounty* was soon in danger of falling apart from the removal of her nails.

Scenes of festivity frequently occurred. The quick-witted Tahitians soon adjusted themselves to the social idiosyncrasies of their visitors and discovered that an infallible way to fill their beakers with wine was to rise and shout, "Te arii no Pretanie" (the King of England). Oberreah, a prominent chieftainess, came out to visit Bligh and unknown to him, native machinations were under way to utilize his prestige in island politics.

But Bligh had not forgotten his mission. Suspecting that the islanders might refuse an honest, frank request for breadfruit plants, he laid an indirect approach. Presenting gifts to Tinah, the chief of Matavai, from the King of England, Bligh asked him, "And will you send something to King George in return?" "Yes," replied Tinah, "I will send him anything I have." Whereupon Bligh immediately suggested breadfruit plants as an adequate gift to King George. Being thus under obligation according to his own code, Tinah had no alternative but to assent. It seems strange that it never occurred to Bligh that all this maneuvering might be unnecessary, and that breadfruit might be forthcoming for the mere asking.

At all events, the work of slipping, potting, and transferring the plants was soon under way. For the next six months gardening was the principal concern of Mr. Nelson, the botanist, and Mr. Brown, the gardener. It is needless to mention what occupied the attention of the ship's company.

During these months two episodes occurred which assume significance in the light of subsequent events, although they probably have no direct bearing on them. At four o'clock on the morning of January 5, 1789, a small cutter was found missing, together with three men. Bligh immediately dispatched a searching party, and the men were retaken at the island of Taha, one of the Society group. The deserters were punished by lashes and imprisonment. A month later, the ship's cable was found severed, except for one strand. Bligh, in retrospect, came to believe that this was an intentional act on the part of one of his own men who hoped thereby to put the ship ashore, thus prolonging a pleasant stay at Tahiti. But at the time he suspected the natives and made a strict search for the culprit among them. No one, however, was found guilty. It seems more likely that the cable was severed neither by natives nor crew, but was chafed by the coral heads which abounded in the lagoon.

By March 31, all the plants were aboard: 774 pots, 39 tubs, and 24 boxes, containing in all 1,015 breadfruit plants besides other specimens of Tahitian flora, filled the cabin prepared for their reception. Four days later, on April 4, the *Bounty* was ready to depart. The farewells were long and no doubt tearful. Six months are a long time. With banana stalks hanging from the yardarms, and with cocoanuts piled, and pigs squealing, on the decks, the *Bounty* spread her canvas and, passing through the opening in the reef, set sail on her homeward voyage. But before making for the West Indies and England, Bligh set his course for Endeavour Straits and Java where he had been directed to secure additional botanical specimens.

Twenty-three days later, on the night of April 27, the *Bounty* was standing between Tofoa and Kotoo in the Tonga group. The watch had been divided into three parts: the master, Mr. Fryer, having the first; the gunner, the middle; and Fletcher Christian, the master's mate, the morning watch. Captain Bligh had retired for the night with his "mind entirely free from suspicion." But he was not destined to awaken to the same state of mind. He was actually aroused by Fletcher Christian and Thomas Burkitt to find himself a prisoner. This day, April 28, saw a mutiny on the high seas, gave birth to a series of adventures of the most incredible character, and resulted in the establishment of a unique settlement that to this day remains its tangible result.

We shall never know the exact circumstances surrounding the birth of the mutiny. Many stories survive. Christian is represented as having carefully planned the *coup* and, on the other hand, as having acted on impulse. Uncle Cornish Quintal once related to me a story handed down in his family from his mutineer ancestor, Matthew Quintal. According to this account Fletcher Christian, during his watch, was gloomily leaning over the rail of the ship when Matthew Quintal approached him and asked him what was the matter. Christian declared vehemently that he was unable to bear Bligh's abuse any longer and was contemplating casting adrift in a cutter. Quintal then counseled that they take the ship, a suggestion that Christian was quick to adopt.

The following account in Bligh's own words may be accepted as substantially correct, although he probably erred in attaching blame to some of the men and may well have heightened the effect of his story by several judicious brush strokes.

"Just before sun-rising, Mr. Christian, with the Master-at-arms, gunner's mate, and Thomas Burkitt, seaman, came into my cabin while I was asleep, and seizing me, tied my hands with a cord behind my back, and threatened me with instant death, if I spoke or made the least noise. I, however, called so loud as to alarm everyone: but they had already secured the officers who were not of their party, by placing centinels at their doors. There were three men at my cabin door, besides the four within; Christian had only a cutlass in his hand, the others had muskets and bayonets. I was hauled out of bed, and forced on deck in my shirt, suffering great pains from the tightness with which they had tied my hands. I demanded the reason for such violence, but received no other answer than threats of instant death, if I did not hold my tongue. Mr. Elphinston, master's mate, was kept in his berth; Mr. Nelson, botanist, Mr. Peckover, gunner, Mr. Ledward, surgeon, and the master, were confined to their cabins; and also the clerk, Mr. Samuel, but he soon obtained leave to come on deck. The fore hatchway was guarded by centinels; the boatswain and the carpenter were, however, allowed to come on deck, where they saw me standing abaft the mizen-mast, with my hands tied behind my back, under a guard, with Christian at their head.

"The boatswain was now ordered to hoist the launch out, with a threat, if he did not do it instantly, to take care of himself.

"The boat being out, Mr. Hayward [not to be confused with Peter Heywood, who remained with Christian] and Mr. Hallet, midshipmen, and Mr. Samuel, were ordered into it; upon which I demanded the cause of such an order, and endeavoured to persuade someone to a sense of duty; but it was to no effect.

" 'Hold your tongue, Sir, or you are dead this instant,' was constantly repeated to me.

"The master, by this time, had sent to be allowed to come on deck, which was permitted; but he was soon ordered back again to his cabin.

"I continued my endeavours to turn the tide of affairs, when Christian changed the cutlass he had in his hand for a bayonet, that was brought to him, and, holding me with a strong grip by the cord that tied my hands, he, with many oaths, threatened to kill me immediately if I would not be quiet: the villains around me had their pieces cocked and bayonets fixed. Particular people were now called on to go into the boat, and were hurried over the side: whence I concluded that with these people I was to be set adrift.

"I, therefore, made another effort to bring about a change, but with no other effect than to be threatened with having my brains blown out.

"The boatswain and the seamen, who were to go in the boat, were allowed to collect twine, canvas, lines, sails, cordage, an eight and twenty gallon cask of water, and the carpenter to take his tool chest. Mr. Samuel got 150 pounds of bread, with a small quantity of rum and wine. He also got a quadrant and a compass into the boat; but he was forbidden, on pain of death, to touch either map, ephemeris, book of astronomical observations, sextant, time-keeper, or any other of my surveys or drawings.

"The mutineers now hurried those they meant to get rid of into the boat. When most of them were in, Christian directed a dram to be served to each of his own crew. I now unhappily saw that nothing could be done to effect the recovery of the ship: there was no one to assist me, and every endeavour on my part was answered with threats of death.

"The officers were called, and forced over the side into the boat, while I was kept apart from everyone, abaft the mizen-mast; Christian, armed with a bayonet, holding me by the bandage that secured my hands. The guard around me had their pieces cocked, but, on my daring the ungrateful wretches to fire, they uncocked them.

"Isaac Martin, one of the guards over me, I saw, had an inclination to assist me, and, as he fed me a shaddock (my lips being quite parched with my endeavours to bring about a change), we explained our wishes to each other by our looks; but this being observed, Martin was instantly removed from me; his inclination then was to leave the ship, for which purpose he got into the boat; but with many threats they obliged him to return.

"The armourer, Joseph Coleman, and the two carpenters, McIntosh and Norman, were also kept contrary to their inclination and they begged of me, after I was astern in the boat, to remember that they declared that they had no hand in the transaction. Michael Byrne, I am told, likewise wanted to leave the ship.

"It is of no moment for me to recount my endeavours to bring back the offenders to a sense of their duty: all I could do was by speaking to them in general; but my endeavours were to no avail, for I was kept securely bound, and no one but the guard was suffered to come near me.

"To Mr. Samuel I am indebted for securing my journals and commission, with some material ship papers. Without these I had nothing to certify what I had done, and my honour and character might have been suspected, without my possessing a proper document to have defended them. All this he did with great resolution, though guarded and strictly watched. He attempted to save the time-keeper, and a box with all my surveys, drawings, and remarks for fifteen years past, which were very numerous, when he was hurried away, with 'Damn your eyes, you're well off to get what you have.'

"It appeared to me, that Christian was some time in doubt whether he should keep the carpenter or his mates; at length he determined on the latter, and the carpenter was ordered into the boat. He was permitted, but not without some opposition, to take his tool chest.

"Much altercation took place between the mutinous crew during the whole business; some swore, 'I'll be damned if he does not find his way home, if he gets anything with him' (meaning me); others, when the carpenter's chest was carried away, 'Damn my eyes, he will have a vessel built in a month.' While others laughed at the helpless situation of the boat, being very deep, and so little room for those who were in her. As for Christian, he seemed meditating instant destruction on himself and everyone.

"I asked for arms, but they laughed at me, and said that I was well acquainted with the people where I was going, and therefore did not want them; four cutlasses, however, were thrown into the boat, after we were veered astern.

"When the officers and men, with whom I was suffered to have no communication, were put into the boat, they only waited for me, and the master-at-arms informed Christian of it; who then said, 'Come, Captain Bligh, your officers and men are now in the boat, and you must go with them; if you attempt to make the least resistance you will instantly be put to death'; and, without any further ceremony, holding me by the cord that tied my hands, with a tribe of armed ruffians about me, I was forced over the side, where they untied my hands. Being in the boat we were veered astern by a rope. A few pieces of pork were then thrown to us, and some clothes, also the cutlasses I have already mentioned; and it was now that the armourer and carpenters called out to me to remember that they had no hand in the transaction. After having undergone a great deal of ridicule, and been kept some time to make sport for these unfeeling wretches, we were at length cast adrift in the open ocean.

"Notwithstanding the roughness with which I was treated, the remembrance of past kindnesses produced some signs of remorse in Christian. When they were forcing me out of the ship, I asked him if this treatment was a proper return of the many instances he had received of my friendship. He appeared disturbed at my question, and answered, with much emotion, 'That, Captain Bligh, that is the thing; I am in hell—I am in hell.'"

Morrison, however, reports this differently. According to him, Bligh begged of Christian to desist in his course, saying: "I'll pawn my honour, I'll give my bond, Mr. Christian, never to think of this, if you'll desist," urging, at the same time, consideration at least for his wife and family.

Christian replied, "No, Captain Bligh, if you had any honour, things would not have come to this; and if you had any regard for your wife and family, you should have thought of them before, and not behaved so much like a villain."

When the boatswain, Mr. Cole, also attempted to plead with Christian, he was told, "It is too late, I have been in hell for this fortnight past, and I am determined to bear it no longer, and you know, Mr. Cole, that I have been used like a dog all the voyage."

The motivation of Christian's leadership in the mutiny has been variously interpreted. Morrison's account, which vaguely resembles the Quintal tradition reported by Uncle Cornish, relates that Christian, being hurt by the insensitive treatment he had endured at Bligh's hand, had quietly determined to leave the ship. To this end he had arranged to be supplied with part of a roast pig, nails, beads, and other articles of trade, all of which he had stowed in a bag hidden in the clue of Midshipman Tinkler's hammock. His accomplices were the boatswain, the carpenter, and two midshipmen (Stewart and Hayward). As a means of navigation, Christian had constructed a rude raft of some staves and stout planks. When the opportunity of escaping did not present itself during the first and middle watch of the fateful day, he laid down at half past three in the morning to sleep until the time was propitious. Morrison continues his narrative by reporting that at four o'clock when Mr. Stewart came to relieve Christian, he found the latter asleep and urged him to abandon his plans. But Christian, anticipating no interference from Hayward, the mate of his watch, asleep on the arms chest, or from Hallet, the other midshipman, who was absent, suddenly conceived the idea of forcibly taking the ship. Christian first spoke of his intentions to Matthew Quintal and Isaac Martin, who had suffered floggings from Bligh. These men readily fell in with Christian's plan, and to them were added a number of other seamen who had no love for Bligh. The arms chest was then secured, and Christian and his mutineers proceeded to place Bligh under guard and to restrain all others not in his party.

Bligh's prompt defense published on his return to England presents a different picture. Unable to conceive his own actions as inspiring mutinous and bitter resentment, he deduces that the mutiny was a carefully laid conspiracy to enable the men to return to the licentious idleness of Tahiti. Moreover, he marvels at the diabolic secrecy which prevailed, since none of the sailors who accompanied him were cognizant of Christian's plans.

The truth is probably somewhere between these divergent views. Bligh's record is a black one. He was the victim of another mutiny years later at Botany Bay in New South Wales. His treatment of his crew was harsh, even though it can be justified as common enough in the period. He did publicly and repeatedly insult Christian, an officer. On the other hand, Tahiti must have been a sailor's dream of heaven. And among these rough sailors, there must have been some ready enough, with-

out special provocation, to exchange their lots for softer
berths ashore at Tahiti. To this tinder in the crew was
applied the fire of Christian. Geoffrey Rawson describes
him as an "unusual type of man." Of superior birth and
breed to the rough seamen of the forecastle, he was at
the same time of an ardent and passionate nature. He
was "a great man for the women, and Lamb, with whom
he sailed in the *Britannia,* said of him that 'he was then
one of the most foolish young men I ever knew in regard
to the sex.'"

There is nothing to show that Christian had cold-
bloodedly arranged a mutiny, except Bligh's deductions.
There is the entire circumstantial setting to convince us
that an accumulated bitterness and resentment on the
part of Christian against Bligh spontaneously meshed
into a natural regret among the men at leaving Tahiti.
Thus geared, these motives were sufficient and complementary.

In the voluminous discussion of the direct and indirect
circumstances leading to the mutiny on the *Bounty,* the
ages of the mutineers have been curiously neglected.
Christian was only twenty-four. The youngest was seventeen and the oldest forty. The average age of all twenty-
five mutineers was about twenty-six and a half years.
These figures are based on Admiralty records which were
perhaps entered at the outset of the voyage. But even
an allowance of a year and a half from the date of the
record to the time of the mutiny, still leaves the mutineers a youthful crew. Had the crew consisted of older
and less responsive men, perhaps no mutiny would have
occurred.

It is tempting to divert this narrative from the main
current of the history of Pitcairn and to pause for Bligh's
adventure in the *Bounty's* cutter. But that is a story in
itself. There were nineteen men, including Bligh, scantily
supplied with 150 pounds of bread, 32 pounds of pork,
6 quarts of rum, 6 bottles of wine, and 28 gallons of
water. They were crowded into an open boat and set

down in an uncharted sea. Despair and the courage born of extremity must have filled every heart as the men watched the *Bounty* sail away. And had they known the agony they were to endure, they might not have had the hardihood to face it. The true temper of Bligh appeared now and persisted through the next forty-one days. Through trackless seas, under broiling suns, with gnawing hunger in their bellies and with swollen tongues in hot, choking throats, these men, under the firm, watchful command of Bligh, made one of the most extraordinary voyages on record. They met hostile natives, they navigated dangerous waters, they sailed 3,618 miles to a haven in Timor. Of the nineteen men only twelve reached England and home.

The others, the mutineers, were twenty-five in number. Not one of the seamen elected to go with Bligh. In addition, three of the midshipmen and some of the petty officers remained on the *Bounty*. This is the full list of mutineers:

FLETCHER CHRISTIAN, *master's mate*
PETER HEYWOOD, *midshipman*
EDWARD YOUNG, *midshipman*
GEORGE STEWART, *midshipman*
CHARLES CHURCHILL, *master-at-arms*
JOHN MILLS, *gunner's mate*
JAMES MORRISON, *boatswain's mate*
THOMAS BURKITT, *able seaman*
MATTHEW QUINTAL, *able seaman*
JOHN SUMNER, *able seaman*
JOHN MILLWARD, *able seaman*
WILLIAM McCOY, *able seaman*
HENRY HILLBRANT, *able seaman*
MICHAEL BYRNE, *able seaman*
WILLIAM MUSPRAT, *able seaman*
ALEXANDER SMITH, *able seaman*
JOHN WILLIAMS, *able seaman*
THOMAS ELLISON, *able seaman*

ISAAC MARTIN, *able seaman*
RICHARD SKINNER, *able seaman*
MATTHEW THOMPSON, *able seaman*
WILLIAM BROWN, *gardener*
JOSEPH COLEMAN, *armorer*
CHARLES NORMAN, *carpenter's mate*
THOMAS McINTOSH, *carpenter's crew*

With Fletcher Christian in command, the course of the *Bounty* was directed toward the island of Tubuai, about 300 miles south of Tahiti. This in itself might be taken to indicate that the lure of Tahiti was not the primary motivation of the mutiny. On May 25, 1789, they reached Tubuai. All the breadfruit plants laboriously collected and carefully nurtured for six months were now discarded, and the mutineers appropriated the property of the departed men.

The Tubuaians on close acquaintance proved less hospitable than the Tahitian experience had led the mutineers to expect. Unable to obtain from the suspicious natives the supplies necessary for a settlement, Christian was forced to make his way once more to Tahiti where he could anticipate a warmer reception.

An episode occurred at this stage which impressed on Christian the possibility that one mutiny might lead to another. A plot was hatched to relieve Christian of the command, but it was discovered in time. From then on the keys to the arms chest were carefully guarded. Morrison, to whom we owe a knowledge of this attempt, adds, however, that Christian never lost the respect of his men even though they might disagree with him.

When the *Bounty* arrived at Tahiti on June 6, Christian took a leaf from Bligh's book. He informed the natives that Bligh had met Cook and that the *Bounty* had been sent back to obtain additional supplies. The name of the heroic and already mythical Cook procured within a few days 312 hogs, 38 goats, and 8 dozen fowl in addition to the bull and cow deposited by Bligh. The livestock Bligh had taken such pains to bring was given up willingly enough. Besides this, quantities of breadfruit, plantain, bananas, and other fruit were brought aboard. Heavily stocked, the *Bounty* sailed again two weeks later for Tubuai. Morrison states that native stowaways were discovered: nine women, twelve men, and eight boys.

Assisted by their native companions, the mutineers had better luck this time in establishing a *rapport* with the Tubuaians. These islanders are closely related to the Tahitians and speak almost identical dialects. The chief of the island coöperated with his uninvited guests by giving them a plot of ground. Christian's first act was to build a fort 50 yards square, surrounded by walls and a ditch 20 feet broad. The guns of the *Bounty* were mounted as further protection. This elaborate fortification seemed more than ominous to the natives who naturally showed signs of resentment at the hostile gesture. Added to this, dissension broke out among the Englishmen. Those who had no active part in the mutiny looked askance at this digging which had all the signs of permanency. They wanted to go home. Finally, the matter was put to a vote, and the decision was reached to abandon the attempt to settle at Tubuai.

Three months after the last departure from Tahiti the *Bounty* was back again, landing at Matavai Bay, September 22. The crew of twenty-five was divided into two parties. One, consisting of sixteen men, elected to land at Tahiti. The other of nine men decided to seek another island where they might escape the increasingly long arm of British justice. Their names are as follows:

FLETCHER CHRISTIAN
EDWARD YOUNG
JOHN MILLS
MATTHEW QUINTAL
WILLIAM McCOY
ALEXANDER SMITH (later known as JOHN ADAMS)
JOHN WILLIAMS

Isaac Martin
William Brown

At dawn the next day, after spending his last few hours ashore with Stewart and Heywood at the home of a friendly chief, Christian bade his youthful companions a sad farewell. And as the *Bounty* slowly gained speed the two midshipmen on the beach watched her disappear forever.

Tahiti welcomed the sixteen men left behind by Christian. Contact with white men had not yet engendered a feeling of contempt or indifference. Wherever they went, the Englishmen were surrounded by an eager band. Chieftains welcomed the prestige of their friendship. And natives of a lower order accepted them with traditional Polynesian hospitality, not unmixed with a love of novelty. Morrison and Millward became the protégés of Poenoo, a landowner at Matavai Bay. Stewart and Heywood were received into the household of Tippaoo, with whose daughter Stewart fell in love. The others scattered to various districts and households.

Not long after the arrival of the mutineers, the Tahitians experienced an example of the brutal conduct of which the Englishmen were capable. Matthew Thompson, who had adopted an overbearing attitude toward the natives, commanded one of them, whom he encountered walking with his wife and child, to stop. Not comprehending the order, the native advanced on his way. Thompson, infuriated by the indifference to his command, raised his musket and deliberately shot to death the unoffending native. Forced to retire into the interior to escape the anger of the islanders, Thompson joined Charles Churchill who had assumed the title of chief on the death of his *tyo* or patron. In a short time, Thompson quarreled with Churchill and slew him also. For this crime he was murdered by the enraged subjects of Churchill.

Morrison, however, soon grew dissatisfied with the

prospects of a life of exile and, joined by eight others, undertook to build a boat by which they might work their way back to civilization. To avoid obstacles from the natives, they explained that the craft was intended for cruising around the island. The boat was finally launched on July 30, 1790. She was a stoutly made boat, 30 feet long, with a beam of 9 feet 6 inches, and was named *Resolution*. Her builders, however, were never to employ her for their escape. On March 23, 1791, H.M.S. *Pandora* anchored at Matavai Bay, prepared to capture and return the mutineers to England for trial.

Edwards, captain of the *Pandora,* soon had the mutineers aboard, even though he had to chase Morrison, Ellison, and Norman, who had tried a get-away in the *Resolution.* The instructions delivered to Edwards were "to keep the mutineers as closely confined as may preclude all possibility of their escaping, having, however, proper regard to the preservation of their lives, that they may be brought home to undergo the punishment due to their demerits." There is nothing, however, in these orders which justifies the actual measures taken by their instrument, Captain Edwards. He had constructed on the quarter deck of the *Pandora* a cage about 11 feet long, entered only from the top through an opening 18 inches square. Into this chamber, known as "Pandora's box," were pressed fourteen men, heavily shackled with irons that were not supposed "to fit like gloves," as Mr. Larkin, the lieutenant, put it when the men complained of the swellings on their legs caused by their fetters. The only provision for air and light, except for the small entrance, was two nine-inch scuttles in the bulkhead of the box. Under these inhuman conditions fourteen men were forced to live and to perform the necessities of nature. Only once a week was this infernal trap cleaned with a hose. No commentary is necessary on the character of a man capable of confining fellow creatures in such a cesspool.

What must have been the horror of the natives when

they saw their friends treated in such fashion by their own countrymen. Many of the Tahitians loyal to their *tyo*ship brought daily supplies for the comfort of the mutineers, but only a few were permitted to visit them. Hamilton, the surgeon of the *Pandora*, was deeply moved by the sight of the reunion of the men and their native wives. "The prisoners' wives visited the ship daily and brought their children, who were permitted to be carried to their unhappy fathers. To see the poor captives in irons, weeping over their tender offspring, was too moving a scene for any feeling heart. Their wives brought them ample supplies of every delicacy the country afforded while we lay there, and behaved with the greatest fidelity and affection to them."

The grief of Peggy, Stewart's wife, was so heart-rending that, unable to bear the daily ordeal, he begged the captain not to allow her to visit him. The missionaries who arrived eight years later reported that Peggy died of a broken heart a few months after Stewart's departure.

On May 8, the *Pandora* left Tahiti. After a fruitless search among the neighboring islands for the remaining nine mutineers, Edwards gave up the hunt and started on the homeward voyage. While traversing the passage between Australia and New Guinea, the *Pandora* was wrecked on the Great Barrier Reef. Trapped like rats in Pandora's box, the men might have all drowned had not their despairing cries attracted the attention of the boatswain's mate. He was only able to draw some of the bolts before the ship lurched to her doom. Skinner and Hillbrant were drowned, still fastened to their chains. Stewart and Sumner, freed at the last moment, were struck by the gangway and sank. The folly of Edwards was colossal, and to him must be attributed these four violent deaths.

The surviving men of the *Pandora* and the ten captives made their way with much suffering to Timor where Bligh had preceded them two years earlier. Finally, on September 12, 1792, almost five years after their departure, the ten mutineers were held at Newgate for court-martial.

The trial lasted five days. Each man in his turn told his story, was cross-examined, and was then retired to await the decision of the Court. Norman, Coleman, McIntosh, and Byrne were acquitted. The remaining six, Heywood, Morrison, Ellison, Burkitt, Millward, and Musprat, were condemned to death, but the first two, Heywood and Morrison were recommended to the King's mercy. They were pardoned by a King's warrant. Musprat was also liberated. No hope, however, sustained the other three. Aboard the *Brunswick*, on October 29, 1792, Ellison, Burkitt, and Millward were hanged, thus expiating the crime of the mutiny on the *Bounty*.

Like a fallen rider who remounts, Heywood reëntered the service and distinguished himself under Lord Hood. When he retired after an honorable career, he was near the head in the list of captains. Morrison likewise saw service again and lost his life as gunner on the *Blenheim*. The others vanish into anonymity.

REDEMPTION ON PITCAIRN

When Christian, accompanied by eight mutineers and a number of natives, sailed from Tahiti, he sailed out of the world. As he watched the island blur with the distance, it was the last glimpse of what must have subsequently seemed like civilization. And how poignant a glimpse that was! Tahiti, with its deep, rich purples and greens, wet with the dawn, pouring down its spires and pinnacles, and with scarves of mist rising in the fiordlike valleys as the morning sun emerged.

Tight-lipped concerning his plans, or silent possibly because he had none, Christian left no clue to follow. When the punitive Edwards arrived on the *Pandora*, no one in Tahiti could give him any information about the hiding place of the leader of the mutiny. And none of the islands Edwards visited in the vicinity revealed traces of the vanished crew. In England, all expectation of ever seeing the departed was abandoned by the government, and after the single attempt of the *Pandora*, no further effort was made to apprehend them. As far as the world was concerned they were forgotten.

Then, in a letter dated Nantucket, 1813, Captain Mayhew Folger of Boston reported to the British Admiralty the discovery of Christian's retreat. He related that in 1808, while on a sealing voyage in the *Topaze*, he ran close to an island that he took to be Pitcairn, an uninhabited morsel of land, first sighted in 1767 by En-sign Pitcairn sailing with Carteret. Putting over two boats, Folger started for shore to seek water and seals. His surprise was great when he observed a small boat being launched from what he supposed was a deserted shore. Even greater was his astonishment when he was hailed in excellent English as the boats drew together. There were three youths in the boat, and they asked for the captain of the ship to whom they presented a gift of cocoanuts. At the same time they invited Folger to visit a white man who lived on the island.

Folger, in logbook style, records that he went on shore and found there an Englishman by the name of Alexander Smith, the only survivor of the nine Englishmen who last sailed the *Bounty*. In this manner was the last of the mutineers accounted for about eighteen years after their disappearance.

The events of the years intervening between their departure from Tahiti and Folger's visit were related by Alexander Smith to his visitor. When the Englishmen left Tahiti they took with them native wives and six men as servants. Smith did not indicate whether Pitcairn was the definite objective of Christian or was met by chance. At any rate, Pitcairn appeared to be satisfactory, and the Englishmen and their native followers landed with all their goods and chattels. To prevent any desertion Christian had the *Bounty* run on the rock-strewn shore of Bounty Bay where the surf completed the dismemberment begun by the men. This event took place in 1790. A short time later the colony lost two of her Englishmen. One ran mad and hurled himself into the sea. The other died of fever. About four years later, the native men, brutally treated by the seven Englishmen, rose in rebellion and attacked their masters. They murdered six of the Englishmen, leaving only Alexander Smith desperately wounded by a pistol ball in his neck. Then Smith and the widows combined, according to this version, to destroy utterly the native men. There now remained only Smith, eight or nine native women, and an unspecified number of children. Smith in his story to Folger concluded simply by saying that he went to work tilling the ground so that it produced plenty for them all and that he lived comfortably as commander-in-chief of Pitcairn's Island.

This, the first story of the events surrounding the settlement of Pitcairn, does not jibe with either the later accounts narrated by Smith himself or with the island tradition reported by Shillibeer and Miss Young. Shillibeer, a young lieutenant on board the *Tagus*, visited Pitcairn in 1815, and he describes his visit with enthusiasm.

Natives came out to greet the new arrivals. When requested to come alongside, the Pitcairn youths replied, "We have no boat hook to hold on by."

"I will throw you a rope," answered the captain.

"If you do we have nothing to make fast to," came the reply.

In spite of these difficulties, the islanders came on board. After the first few minutes of greeting and curious inspection on both sides, young McCoy asked, "Do you know one, William Bligh, in England?" In turn he was asked if he knew one Christian.

"Oh, yes," responded McCoy, "very well. His son is in the boat there, coming up. His name is Friday Fletcher October Christian. His father is dead now—he was shot by a black fellow."

The story extracted from these sons of the mutineers by cross-examination is given by Shillibeer as follows:

QUESTION: Christian, you say, was shot?

ANSWER: Yes he was.

QUESTION: By whom?

ANSWER: A black fellow shot him.

QUESTION: What cause do you assign for the murder?

ANSWER: I know no reason, except a jealousy which I have heard existed between the people of Otaheite and the English. Christian was shot in the back while at work in his yam plantation.

QUESTION: What became of the man who killed him?

ANSWER: Oh! that black fellow was shot afterwards by an Englishman.

QUESTION: Was there any other disturbance between the Otaheitians and English, after the death of Christian?

ANSWER: Yes, the black fellows rose, shot two Englishmen, and wounded John Adams, who is now the only remaining man who came in the *Bounty*.

QUESTION: How did Adams escape being murdered?

ANSWER: He hid himself in the wood, and the same night, the women enraged at the murder of the English, to whom they were more partial than their countrymen, rose and put every Otaheitian to death in their sleep. This saved Adams, his wounds were soon healed, and although old, he now enjoys good health.

QUESTION: How many men and women did Christian bring with him in the *Bounty*?

ANSWER: Nine white men, six from Otaheite, and eleven women.

QUESTION: And how many are there now on the island?

ANSWER: In all we have forty-eight.

QUESTION: And what became of the *Bounty*?

ANSWER: After everything useful was taken out of her, she was run ashore, set fire to, and burnt.

QUESTION: Have you ever heard how many years it is since Christian was shot?

ANSWER: I understand it was about two years after his arrival at the island.

QUESTION: What became of Christian's wife?

ANSWER: She died soon after Christian's son was born, and I have heard that Christian took forcibly the wife of one of the black followers to supply her place, and which was the chief cause of his being shot.

Not only does this story of the first years of the colony at Pitcairn differ materially from the narrative told to Captain Folger, but they both depart from the version recorded by Captain Beechey on his visit in 1825. This last is by far the most convincing on account of its greater detail, some of which Beechey quotes from Edward Young's diary. This journal seems to have been examined only by Beechey, and it has since disappeared.* The story follows:

"The mutineers now bade adieu to all the world, save the few individuals associated with them in exile. But where that exile should be passed, was yet undecided; the Marquesas Islands were first mentioned, but Christian, on reading Captain Carteret's account of Pitcairn Island, thought it better adapted to the purpose, and accordingly shaped a course thither. They reached it not many days afterwards; and Christian, with one of the seamen, landed in a little nook, which we afterwards found very convenient for disembarkation. They soon traversed the island sufficiently to be satisfied that it was exactly suited to their wishes. It possessed water, wood, a good soil, and some fruits. The anchorage in the offing was very bad, and landing for boats extremely hazardous. The mountains were so difficult of access, and the passes so narrow, that they might be maintained by a few persons against an army; and there were several caves to which, in case of necessity, they could retreat, and where, as long as their provision lasted, they might bid defiance to their pursuers. With this intelligence they returned on board, and brought the ship to an anchor in a small bay on the northern side of the island, which I have in consequence named 'Bounty Bay,' where everything that could be of utility was landed, and where it was agreed to destroy the ship, either by running her on shore, or burning her. Christian, Adams, and the majority, were for the former expedient; but while they went to the forepart of the ship, to execute this business, Matthew Quintal set fire to the carpenter's store-room. The vessel burnt to the water's edge, and then drifted upon the rocks, where the remainder of the wreck was

* A recent letter in the London *Times* reports the existence of Edward Young's Journal in England, but inquiry has not succeeded in bringing it to light.

burnt for fear of discovery. This occurred on the 23rd
of January, 1790.

"Upon their first landing they perceived, by the remains of several habitations, *morais*, and three or four
rudely sculptured images, which stood upon the emi-
nence overlooking the bay where the ship was destroyed,
that the island had been previously inhabited. Some ap-
prehensions were, in consequence, entertained lest the
natives should secrete themselves, and in some un-
guarded moment make an attack upon them; but by degrees these fears subsided, and their avocations proceeded without interruption.

"A suitable spot of ground for a village was fixed
upon, with the exception of which the island was divided into equal portions, but to the exclusion of the poor
blacks, who being only friends of the seamen, were not
considered as entitled to the same privileges. Obliged to
lend their assistance to the others in order to procure a
subsistence, they thus, from being their friends, in the
course of time became their slaves. No discontent, however, was manifested, and they willingly assisted in the
cultivation of the soil.

"In clearing the space that was allotted to the village,
a row of trees was left between it and the sea, for the
purpose of concealing the houses from the observation
of any vessels that might be passing, and nothing was
allowed to be erected that might in any way attract attention. Until these houses were finished, the sails of the
Bounty were converted into tents, and when no longer
required for that purpose, became very acceptable as
clothing. Thus supplied with all the necessaries of life,
and some of its luxuries, they felt their condition comfortable even beyond their most sanguine expectation,
and everything went on peaceably and prosperously for
about two years, at the expiration of which Williams,
who had the misfortune to lose his wife about a month
after his arrival, by a fall from a precipice while collecting birds' eggs, became dissatisfied, and threatened to

leave the island in one of the boats of the *Bounty,* unless he had another wife; an unreasonable request, as it could not be complied with, except at the expense of the happiness of one of his companions: but Williams, actuated by selfish considerations alone, persisted in his threat, and the Europeans not willing to part with him, on account of his usefulness as an armourer, constrained one of the blacks to bestow his wife upon the applicant. The blacks, outrageous [sic] at this second act of flagrant injustice, made common cause with their companion, and matured a plan of revenge upon their aggressors, which, had it succeeded, would have proved fatal to all the Europeans.

"Fortunately, the secret was imparted to the women, who ingeniously communicated it to the white men in a song, of which the words were, 'Why does black man sharpen axe? to kill white man.' The instant Christian became aware of the plot, he seized his gun and went in search of the blacks, but with a view only of showing them that their scheme was discovered, and thus by timely interference endeavouring to prevent the execution of it. He met one of them (Ohoo) at a little distance from the village, taxed him with the conspiracy, and in order to intimidate him, discharged his gun, which he had humanely loaded with powder only. Ohoo, however, imagining otherwise, and that the bullet had missed its object, derided his unskilfulness, and fled into the woods, followed by his accomplice Talaloo, who had been deprived of his wife. The remaining blacks, finding their plot discovered, purchased pardon by promising to murder their accomplices, who had fled, which they afterwards performed by an act of the most odious treachery. Ohoo was betrayed and murdered by his own nephew; and Talaloo, after an ineffectual attempt made upon him by poison, fell by the hands of his friend and his wife, the very woman on whose account all the disturbance began, and whose injuries Talaloo felt he was revenging in common with his own.

"Tranquillity was by these means restored, and preserved for about two years; at the expiration of which, dissatisfaction was again manifested by the blacks, in consequence of oppression and ill treatment, principally by Quintal and M'Coy. Meeting with no compassion or redress from their masters, a second plan to destroy their oppressors was matured, and unfortunately, too successfully executed.

"It was agreed that two of the blacks, Timoa and Nehow, should desert from their masters, provide themselves with arms, and hide in the woods, but maintain a frequent communication with the other two, Tetaheite and Menalee; and that on a certain day they should attack and put to death all the Englishmen, when at work in their plantations. Tetaheite, to strengthen the party of the blacks on this day, borrowed a gun and ammunition of his master, under the pretence of shooting hogs, which had become wild and very numerous; but instead of using it in this way, he joined his accomplices, and with them fell upon Williams and shot him. Martin, who was at no great distance, heard the report of the musket, and exclaimed, 'Well done. We shall have a glorious feast today,' supposing that a hog had been shot. The party proceeded from Williams' towards Christian's plantation, where Menalee, the other black, was at work with Mills and M'Coy; and, in order that the suspicions of the whites might not be excited by the report they had heard, requested Mills to allow him (Menalee) to assist them in bringing home the hog they pretended to have killed. Mills agreed; and the four, being united, proceeded to Christian, who was working at his yam-plot, and shot him. Thus fell a man, who, from being the reputed ringleader of the mutiny, has obtained an unenviable celebrity, and whose crime, if anything can excuse mutiny, may perhaps be considered as in some degree palliated, by the tyranny which led to its commission.

"M'Coy, hearing his groans, observed to Mills, 'There was surely some person dying,' but Mills replied, 'It's only Mainmast (Christian's wife) calling her children to dinner.' The white men being yet too strong for the blacks to risk a conflict with them, it was necessary to concert a plan, in order to separate Mills and M'Coy. Two of them accordingly secreted themselves in M'Coy's house, and Tetaheite ran and told him that the two blacks who had deserted were stealing things out of his house. M'Coy instantly hastened to detect them, and on entering was fired at; but the ball passed him. M'Coy immediately communicated the alarm to Mills, and advised him to seek shelter in the woods; but Mills, being quite satisfied that one of the blacks whom he had made his friend would not suffer him to be killed, determined to remain. M'Coy, less confident, ran in search of Christian, but finding him dead, joined Quintal (who was already apprised of the work of destruction, and had sent his wife to give the alarm to the others), and fled with him to the woods.

"Mills had scarcely been left alone, when the two blacks fell upon him, and he became a victim to his misplaced confidence in the fidelity of his friend. Martin and Brown were next separately murdered by Menalee and Tenina; Menalee effecting with a maul what the musket had left unfinished. Tenina, it is said, wished to save the life of Brown, and fired at him with powder only, desiring him, at the same time, to fall as if killed; but, unfortunately rising too soon, the other black, Menalee, shot him.

"Adams was first apprised of his danger by Quintal's wife, who, in hurrying through his plantation, asked why he was working at such a time? Not understanding the question, but seeing her alarmed, he followed her, and was almost immediately met by the blacks, whose appearance exciting suspicion, he made his escape into the woods. After remaining there three or four hours, Adams, thinking all was quiet, stole to his yam-plot for a supply of provisions; his movements, however, did not escape the vigilance of the blacks, who attacked and shot him through the body, the ball entering at his right shoulder, and passing out through his throat. He fell upon his side, and was instantly assailed by one of them with the butt end of the gun; but he parried the blows at the expense of a broken finger. Tetaheite then placed his gun to his side, but it fortunately missed fire twice. Adams, recovering a little from the shock of his wound, sprang on his legs, and ran off with as much speed as he was able, and fortunately outstripped his pursuers, who seeing him likely to escape, offered him protection if he would stop. Adams, much exhausted by his wound, readily accepted their terms, and was conducted to Christian's house, where he was kindly treated. Here this day of bloodshed ended, leaving only four Englishmen alive out of nine. It was a day of emancipation to the blacks, who were now masters of the island, and of humiliation and retribution to the whites.

"Young, who was a great favourite with the women, and had, during this attack, been secreted by them, was now also taken to Christian's house. The other two, M'Coy and Quintal, who had always been the great oppressors of the blacks, escaped to the mountains, where they supported themselves upon the produce of the ground about them.

"The party in the village lived in tolerable tranquillity for about a week; at the expiration of which, the men of colour began to quarrel about the right of choosing the women whose husbands had been killed; which ended in Menalee's shooting Timoa as he sat by the side of Young's wife, accompanying her song with his flute. Timoa not dying immediately, Menalee reloaded, and deliberately despatched him by a second discharge. He afterwards attacked Tetaheite, who was condoling with Young's wife for the loss of her favourite black, and would have murdered him also, but for the interference of the women. Afraid to remain longer in the village, he escaped to the mountains and joined Quintal and M'Coy, who, though glad of his services, at first received him with suspicion. This great acquisition to their force enabled them to bid defiance to the opposite party; and to show their strength, and that they were provided with muskets, they appeared on a ridge of mountains, within sight of the village, and fired a volley which so alarmed the others that they sent Adams to say, if they would kill the black man, Menalee, and return to the village, they would all be friends again. The terms were so far complied with that Menalee was shot; but, apprehensive of the sincerity of the remaining blacks, they refused to return while they were alive.

"Adams says it was not long before the widows of the white men so deeply deplored their loss, that they determined to revenge their death, and concerted a plan to murder the only two remaining men of colour. Another account, communicated by the islanders, is that it was only part of a plot formed at the same time that Menalee was murdered, which could not be put in execution before. However, this may be, it was equally fatal to the poor blacks. The arrangement was, that Susan should murder one of them, Tetaheite, while he was sleeping by the side of his favourite; and that Young should at the same instant, upon a signal being given, shoot the other, Nehow. The unsuspecting Tetaheite retired as usual, and fell by the blow of an axe; the other was looking at Young loading his gun, which he supposed was for the purpose of shooting hogs, and requested him to put in a good charge, when he received the deadly contents.

"In this manner the existence of the last of the men of colour terminated, who, though treacherous and revengeful, had, it is feared, too much cause for complaint. The accomplishment of this fatal scheme was immediately communicated to the two absentees, and their return solicited. But so many instances of treachery had occurred, that they would not believe the report, though delivered by Adams himself, until the hands and heads of the deceased were produced, which being done, they returned to the village. This eventful day was the third October, 1893. There were now left upon the island, Adams, Young, M'Coy, and Quintal, ten women, and some children. Two months after this period, Young commenced a manuscript journal, which affords a good insight into the state of the island, and the occupations of the settlers. From it we learn, that they lived peaceably together, building their houses, fencing in and cultivating their grounds, fishing, and catching birds, and constructing pits for the purpose of entrapping hogs, which had become very numerous and wild, as well as injurious to the yam-crops. The only discontent appears to have been among the women, who lived promiscuously with the men, frequently changing their abode.

"Young says, March 12, 1794, 'Going over to borrow a rake, to rake the dust off my ground, I saw Jenny having a skull in her hand: I asked her whose it was? and was told it was Jack Williams's. I desired it might be buried: the women who were with Jenny gave me for answer, it should not. I said it should; and demanded it accordingly. I was asked the reason why I, in particular, should insist on such a thing, when the rest of the white men did not? I said, if they gave them leave to keep the skulls above ground, I did not. Accordingly when I saw M'Coy, Smith, and Mat. Quintal, I acquainted them with it, and said, I thought that if the girls did not agree to give up the heads of the five white men in a peaceable manner, they ought to be taken by force, and buried.' About this time the women appear to have been much dissatisfied; and Young's journal declares that, 'since the massacre, it has been the desire of the greater part of them to get some conveyance, to enable them to leave the island.' This feeling continued, and on the 14th of April, 1794, was so strongly urged, that the men began to build them a boat; but wanting planks and nails, Jenny, who now resides at Otaheite, in her zeal tore up the boards of her house, and endeavoured, though without success, to persuade some others to follow her example.

"On the 13th of August following, the vessel was finished, and on the 15th she was launched: but, as Young says, 'according to expectation she upset,' and it was most fortunate for them that she did so; for had they launched out upon the ocean, where could they have gone? or what could a few ignorant women have done by themselves, drifting upon the waves, but ultimately have fallen a sacrifice to their folly? However, the fate of the vessel was a great disappointment, and they continued much dissatisfied with their condition; probably not without some reason, as they were kept in great subordination and were frequently beaten by M'Coy and Quintal, who appear to have been of very quarrelsome dispositions; Quintal in particular, who proposed 'not to laugh, joke, or give anything to any of the girls.'

"On the 16th August they dug a grave, and buried the bones of the murdered people; and on October 3rd, 1794, they celebrated the murder of the black men at Quintal's house. On the 11th November, a conspiracy of the women to kill the white men in their sleep was discovered; upon which they were all seized, and a disclosure ensued; but no punishment appears to have been inflicted upon them, in consequence of their promising to conduct themselves properly, and never again to give any cause 'even to suspect their behavior.' However, though they were pardoned, Young observed, 'We did not forget their conduct; and it was agreed among us, that the first female who misbehaved should be put to death; and this punishment was to be repeated on each offence until we could discover the real intentions of the women.' Young appears to have suffered much from mental perturbation in consequence of these disturbances; and observes of himself on the two following days, that 'he was bothered and idle.'

"The suspicions of the men induced them, on the 15th, to conceal two muskets in the bush, for the use of any person who might be so fortunate as to escape, in the event of an attack being made. On the 30th November, the women again collected and attacked them; but no lives were lost, and they returned on being once more pardoned, but were again threatened with death the next time they misbehaved. Threats thus repeatedly made, and as often unexecuted, as might be expected, soon lost their effect, and the women formed a party whenever their displeasure was excited, and hid themselves in the unfrequented parts of the island, carefully providing themselves with fire-arms. In this manner the men were kept in continual suspense, dreading the result of each disturbance, as the numerical strength of the women was much greater than their own.

"On the 4th of May, 1795, two canoes were begun, and in two days completed. These were used for fishing, in which employment the people were frequently successful, supplying themselves with rockfish and large mackerel. On the 27th of December following, they were greatly alarmed by the appearance of a ship close in with the island. Fortunately for them there was a tremendous surf upon the rocks, the weather wore a very threatening aspect, and the ship stood to the S.E., and at noon was out of sight. Young appears to have thought this a providential escape, as the sea for a week after was 'smoother than they had ever recollected it since their arrival on the island.'

"So little occurred in the year 1796, that one page records the whole of the events; and throughout the following year there are but three incidents worthy of notice. The first, their endeavour to procure a quantity of meat for salting; the next, their attempt to make syrup from the tee-plant (*dracaena terminalis*) and sugar-cane; and the third, a serious accident that happened to M'Coy, who fell from a cocoa-nut tree and hurt his right thigh, sprained both his ankles and wounded his side. The occupations of the men continued similar to those already related, occasionally enlivened by visits to the opposite side of the island. They appear to have been more sociable; dining frequently at each other's houses, and contributing more to the comfort of the women, who, on their part, gave no ground for uneasiness. There was also a mutual accommodation amongst them in regard to provisions, of which a regular account was taken. If one person was successful in hunting, he lent the others as much meat as they required, to be repaid at leisure; and the same occurred with yams, taros, etc., so that they lived in a very domestic and tranquil state.

"It unfortunately happened that M'Coy had been employed in a distillery in Scotland; and being very much addicted to liquor, he tried an experiment with the teeroot, and on the 20th April, 1798, succeeded in producing a bottle of ardent spirit. This success induced his companion, Matthew Quintal, to 'alter his kettle into a still,' a contrivance which unfortunately succeeded too well, as frequent intoxication was the consequence, with M'Coy in particular, upon whom at length it produced fits of delirium, in one of which, he threw himself from a cliff and was killed. The melancholy fate of this man created so forcible an impression on the remaining few, that they resolved never again to touch spirits; and Adams, I have every reason to believe, to the day of his death kept his vow.

"The journal finishes nearly at the period of M'Coy's death, which is not related in it; but we learned from Adams, that about 1799 Quintal lost his wife by a fall from the cliff while in search of birds' eggs; that he grew discontented, and, though there were several disposable women on the island, and he had already experienced the fatal effects of a similar demand, nothing would satisfy him but the wife of one of his companions. Of course, neither of them felt inclined to accede to this unreasonable indulgence; and he sought an opportunity of putting them both to death. He was fortunately foiled in his first attempt, but swore he would repeat it. Adams and Young having no doubt he would follow up his resolution, and fearing he might be more successful in the next attempt, came to the conclusion, that their own lives were not safe while he was in existence, and that they were justified in putting him to death, which they did with an axe.

"Such was the melancholy fate of seven of the leading mutineers, who escaped from justice only to add murder to their former crimes; for though some of them may not have actually imbrued their hands in the blood of their fellow-creatures, yet all were accessory to the deed.

"As Christian and Young were descended from respectable parents, and had received educations suitable to their birth, it might be supposed that they felt their altered and degraded situation much more than the seamen who were comparatively well off; but if so, Adams says, they had the good sense to conceal it, as not a single murmur or regret escaped them; on the contrary, Christian was always cheerful, and his example was of the greatest service in exciting his companions to labour. He was naturally of a happy, ingenuous disposition, and won the good opinion and respect of all who served under him; which cannot be better exemplified than by his maintaining, under circumstances of great perplexity, the respect and regard of all who were associated with him up to the hour of his death; and even at the period of our visit, Adams, in speaking of him, never omitted to say, 'Mr. Christian.'

"Adams and Young were now the sole survivors out of the fifteen males that landed upon the island. They were both, and more particularly Young, of a serious turn of mind; and it would have been wonderful, after the many dreadful scenes at which they had assisted, if the solitude and tranquillity that ensued had not disposed them to repentance. During Christian's lifetime they had only once read the church service, but since his decease this had been regularly done on every Sunday. They now, however, resolved to have morning and evening family prayers, to add afternoon service to the duty of the Sabbath, and to train up their own children, and those of their late unfortunate companions, in piety and virtue.

"In the execution of this resolution Young's education enabled him to be of the greatest assistance; but he was not long suffered to survive his repentance. An asthmatic complaint, under which he had for some time laboured, terminated his existence about a year after the death of Quintal, and Adams was left the sole survivor of the misguided and unfortunate mutineers of the *Bounty*. The loss of his last companion was a great affliction to him, and was for some time most severely felt. It was a catastrophe, however, that more than ever disposed him to repentance, and determined him to execute the pious resolution he had made, in the hope of expiating his offences."

Thus at Folger's arrival in 1808 the colony consisted of one surviving mutineer, eight or nine Tahitian women, and twenty-five children. These last were the progeny of the Englishmen and their Tahitian wives, the native men having left no offspring. The eldest was Thursday (Friday in the island records) October Christian, then eighteen years old and already a tall, powerfully built man. While still infants, these twenty-five children lost their fathers, and they turned to Smith, or John Adams as he preferred to be called, for guidance and paternal support. On him devolved the responsibility of their training and education which he attempted to execute to his best ability. Fortunately, just before his death of asthma, sometime about 1800, Young sought to make use of his education by instructing the children. Morning and evening family prayers were made a regular practice and services were held on Sabbath. Another and no doubt apocryphal story relates that Adams had two vivid dreams in which were reënacted his past transgressions and the dire punishment awaiting him. In one, he saw a terrible being, a devil, threaten him with a spear, and in the other were painted the lurid details of hell. These so terrified Adams that he resolved to mend his ways and bring up the guiltless children in the true light. His success has been abundantly testified by the first visitors to Pitcairn. Beechey found them "a happy and well-regulated society."

Adams,* whose formal education had been extremely limited, was just able to write his own name, and he could, with some difficulty, spell out the words of the *Bounty's* Bible and prayer book. What little he knew he imparted to the children with the aid of the King James version, a text that could hardly have been better.

From 1790, the year of the landing on Pitcairn, until 1808, four ships were seen by the islanders—one every four and a half years. None of them stopped, and it was not until 1808, as has already been mentioned, that Folger discovered the settlement of some forty-five people on the island. The next visitor arrived in 1815. Captains Staines and Pipon, in the *Tagus,* were in the South Pacific under orders to track down Porter who had ravaged British shipping in the Pacific until the British Admiralty had been forced to take notice of his depredations. Staines and Pipon were only dimly aware of the colony on Pitcairn, Folger's report having been received skeptically in England, so that when the *Tagus* approached Pitcairn those aboard were surprised to see a small boat come out to welcome them. The officers were impressed by the stalwart, vigorous youths who visited their ship. Although the eager curiosity of the islanders betrayed an intelligent and lively interest which, however, never overstepped the bounds of good breeding, the new world that these ships from the ends of the earth represented could sometimes be terrifying. Young McCoy, seeing a small black terrier for the first time, became very alarmed and ran to one of the officers for protection. Somewhat ashamed at his display of timidity,

---

* John Adams (Alexander Smith in the Admiralty records) was, according to tradition, the son and brother of London lightermen. I have, however, received from Mrs. J. F. Mc-Gowan, of Pittsburgh, a letter in which she claims descent from Alexander Smith, who she says lived in County Armagh, Ireland, until he deserted his family. Mrs. McGowan doubts that he ever saw London.

he pointed to the animal, saying, "I know what that is, it is a dog. I never saw a dog before—will it bite?" And then, turning to another islander, he remarked, "It is a pretty thing too to look, is it not?" But the slight condescension of the officers turned to embarrassed shame when, before eating breakfast to which they had been invited, the islanders said their usual grace.

Here is the scene in Shillibeer's own words. "I must here confess I blushed when I saw nature in its most simple state, offer that tribute of respect to the Omnipotent Creator, which from an education I did not perform, nor from society had been taught its necessity. 'Ere they began to eat; on their knees, and with hands uplifted did they implore permission to partake in peace what was set before them, and when they had eaten heartily, resuming their former attitude, offered a fervent prayer of thanksgiving for the indulgence they had just experienced. Our omission of this ceremony did not escape their notice, for Christian asked me whether it was not customary with us also. Here nature was triumphant, for I should do myself an irreparable injustice, did I not with candour acknowledge, I was both embarrassed and wholly at loss for a sound reply, and evaded this poor fellow's question by drawing his attention to the cow, which was then looking down the hatchway, and as he had never seen any of the species before, it was a source of mirth and gratification to him."

Folger, the discoverer of the Pitcairn colony, being an American, created no misgivings among the islanders. Staines and Pipon, however, were the first Englishmen to confront Adams since the mutiny, and his sense of guilt at the sight of officers in His Majesty's Navy was keen. Hannah, the daughter of John Adams, met the visitors at the top of the cliff overlooking Bounty Bay. The visitors had an intuition that she had come to test out the situation so that ample warning might be given her father to escape if their attitude seemed hostile. Reassured of their kindly intentions she led the guests to her parent. The younger officers evinced as much if not more interest in Hannah than in her rather more notorious father. In the words of one of them, "She was arrayed in nature's simple garb, and wholly unadorned, but she was beauty's self, and needed not the aid of ornament. She betrayed some surprise—timidity was a prominent feature."

Although the English officers suspected that Hannah's fears reflected a similar state of mind in Adams, they discovered that he had a longing to see England before he died. He was offered a passage home with any of his family who chose to go. But this proposal was met with an emotional outbreak. Hannah, in tears, cried, "Oh, do not, sir, take from me my father!" To her sobs were added those of the aged Tahitian wife of Adams and other members of the community. The possibility of losing their patriarch filled them with dread and sorrow. Reassured that Adams would not be removed contrary to their wishes, calm was again restored, and our smitten officer noticed that Adams' "daughter too had gained her usual serenity, but she was lovely in her tears, for each seemed to add an additional charm."

The susceptible British described the young women as "having invariably beautiful teeth, fine eyes, and open expression of countenances, and looks of such simple innocence, and sweet sensibility, that renders their appearance at once interesting and engaging, and it is pleasing to add, their minds and manners were as pure and innocent, as this impression indicated. No lascivious looks, or any loose, forward manners, which so much distinguish the characters of the females of the other islands."

The little colony which aside from Adams and the surviving Tahitian women consisted of twenty-odd youngsters, none more than twenty-five years old, made a deep impression on the visitors. The patriarchal Adams was the father of this flock, adored by all, and their instructor in religion and learning. Everyone looked to him for guidance, and his word was the final appeal. Happily it was not necessary, since quarrels were rare. Those which in the natural course of human affairs did arise were trivial and were "nothing more than a word of mouth quarrel."

Ten years later, Captain Beechey in the *Blossom* found little change. Adams had grown older, fatter, and even more patriarchal, more of the children of the mutineers had married, and a thriving crop of grandchildren had appeared. Adams, his fears allayed that he might be punished for his part in the mutiny of thirty-five years ago, came out to the ship this time. His old fo'c'sle manners reasserted themselves automatically, and he respectfully reached to his bald head for a forelock long since vanished. The young men of the island aroused a friendly response from Beechey. He found them "tall, robust and healthy, with good-natured countenances." Their manners were simple and their patent anxiety to give no offense was effective in promoting good-will. "Please may I sit down?" "Please may I open the door?" and similarly polite and, no doubt, tedious requests disarmed the officers of the *Blossom*. As Staines and Pipon were bombarded by questions, so Beechey found himself exploited as an encyclopedia for the eager curiosity of the islanders.

In their desire to emulate the costume of their visitors and to show off their few prized articles of European clothing acquired from their previous visitors, the islanders were a "perfect caricature." Some wore long black coats on bare torsos, others a simple waistcoat without shirt or coat. And all lacked shoes and stockings.

The charm of those islanders aboard his ship, added to the romance surrounding their origin, intensified Beechey's desire to see more of the natives and the manner in which they lived. The hazardous landing was willingly relinquished to the hands of the Pitcairn islanders who landed their guests two by two. That fascinating young lady, Hannah Adams, who had already conquered at least one Englishman's heart, was waiting to greet the newcomers who thereby felt themselves rewarded for the dangers of the landing. Clad in the island cloth manufactured from the bark of the mulberry tree, she was a graceful and charming figure. Hannah's demonstrative and unpremeditated affection for her father pleased the officers. Under her guidance, they proceeded to climb the arduous cliff, clinging to tufts of grass as they laboriously advanced. Having arrived at the neat village of five houses, Beechey found himself engulfed in the warm and simple hospitality of the island. He spent that day and the next in exploring the island and enjoying the homely life of the natives. Among the services he was able to render his hosts in return for their generosity was one specially requested by old John Adams. Having lived thirty-five years in unsanctified union, it was Adams' desire that he now be formally married to his aged Tahitian consort. As captain of the *Blossom*, Beechey had the power to satisfy this request.

The islanders had been educated, according to the traditions of their fathers, to look to England as their mother country. The display of their loyalty to the Crown touched a sentimental chord in the hearts of the visiting Englishmen. This devotion to England and the eagerness of the islanders to identify themselves with the Empire, even though only with the ragged hem of her skirt, led them to view the visiting men-of-war as a tangible thread with "home." Already they had initiated the custom, later to become traditional, of appealing to the captain of a British man-of-war for final decision in disagreements they could not decide themselves.

One of the first cases brought to Captain Beechey was the affair of George Adams vs. Polly Young. Old John Adams had trained the youth to regard their word once given as sacred. This lofty standard had resulted in an unforeseen and difficult situation. George Adams, having become deeply smitten by Polly Young, a young lady slightly older than he, proposed marriage to her. Polly, for reasons known only to herself, had firmly and emphatically stated that she *never* would give her hand to George. But George, either from lack of choice (girls being scarce) or from a divine persistency common to lovers, plied Polly with all the blandishments in his armory. There was no problem until the efforts of George began to make an impression on Polly, and she found herself regretting her rash statement. But so well had Adams taught that Polly felt herself bound to her foolish vow, and for want of a solution the lovesick couple languished in the bonds of honor. Beechey remarks that "the weighty case was referred" to him for consideration, "and the fears of the parties were in some measure relieved by the result, which was, that it would be better to marry than continue unhappy, in consequence of a hasty determination made before the judgment was matured." But so strong were these early habits that the couple, though yearning for each other, could not be prevailed upon to accept the inevitable at once.

The reader, curious about the solution of this impasse, may rejoice to know that my records show that George married Polly on All Fools' Day, 1827. He had three sons: John, Jonathan, and Josiah; and after Polly's death in 1843, he found consolation in Sarah McCoy.

When Beechey went on shore, he discovered that the population had been increased by normal multiplication and by the arrival of two Englishmen. The colony now contained sixty-six persons of whom thirty-six were males. The two Englishmen were John Buffett, who hailed from Bristol, and John Evans, the son of a Longacre watchmaker. Both these men had been sailors aboard the *Cyprus* of London which touched at Pitcairn in 1823. The simplicity and harmony of the little colony had strongly appealed to Buffett who had secured permission to remain behind. When the *Cyprus* had departed, Evans was discovered ashore, having jumped ship.

Buffett, a man of some education, undertook to teach the children, to maintain a register of island affairs, and to conduct the religious exercises. Beechey found his sermon to be very good but tedious, since it was repeated three times in succession in order to fix it firmly in the minds of the islanders. This passion for exhaustive performance also led Adams to read not only the appropriate prayer but also all those intended only as substitutes.

Even at this early date, 1825, the nightmare of overpopulation had troubled Adams. He anticipated serious difficulties if the population continued to grow as rankly as it had commenced. Consulting with Beechey he requested the British government to come to their assistance. On Beechey's representations, the Admiralty and the Colonial Office prepared to take steps to remove the population to a more commodious place. But the reluctance of the islanders, when it came to actual removal, to leave their beloved though constricted Pitcairn caused the plan to remain in abeyance.

Three years after Beechey's memorable sojourn on Pitcairn, a momentous event in the colony's history occurred. In November, 1828, George Hunn Nobbs came to reside among the islanders. Nobbs is a somewhat mysterious person. Nothing very definite is known about his origin. It has been averred without evidence that he was the illegitimate son of a daughter of the Irish gentry and fathered by a marquis. The following brief account of his life and adventures is drawn from the pious pages of the Reverend Thomas B. Murray.

Nobbs was born in Ireland in 1799, and at an age now regarded as tender entered in the British Navy. In 1813 he sailed on the *Indefatigable* to New South Wales and Van Diemen's Land. On the succeeding voyage he journeyed to Valparaiso where he served in the Chilean navy under Lord Cochrane, later Earl of Dundonald, and was rewarded with a lieutenancy for his services. From Chile Nobbs, whose itinerary reads like a modern aviator's, proceeded to Naples. Wrecked *en route* from that city to Messina, he endured a voyage in an open boat to Messina. In 1823, he went back to England, but not for

long. The lust had gripped him again, and he was off for
Sierra Leone as chief mate of the *Gambia*. Again Providence saved him for Pitcairn, for of the nineteen men
who manned the ship, only the captain, Nobbs, and two
Negroes survived. On the next voyage of the *Gambia*
Nobbs was in command. This time fever nearly took him
off. In the course of his globe-trotting Nobbs had heard
of the already famous Pitcairn colony, and true to form
he conceived a passion for visiting the island. We next
find him aboard the *Circassian* in November, 1825,
bound for Pitcairn via Calcutta. At this point the Reverend Mr. Murray points out that Nobbs had already
been four times around the world and that he wished to
lead a life of peace and usefulness. Detained at Calcutta
until August, 1827, Nobbs finally obtained a passage on
an American ship, *Ocean*, for Valparaiso. Again shipwreck threatened in the Straits of Sunda, but no doubt
Nobbs was able by this time to regard it with non-
chalance. At Callao, Nobbs fell in with an American
named Noah Bunker, with whom he secured, for £150,
an 18-ton bark. These two after a six-week voyage
reached Pitcairn in November, 1828. The charmed
Nobbs survived the arrival, but his companion succumbed.

Nobbs' education and aggressiveness were superior to
those of anyone else's on the island, and he took it upon
himself to act as registrar, schoolmaster, and pastor. For
these services he expected to be supported by the natives.
This poaching on the preserves of John Buffett caused
some dissension, though the island soon settled back to
its wonted if not impervious calm.

But not for long. On March 5, 1829, John Adams, the
last survivor of the mutiny, died. A chapter ended, but
so well had he labored and so amenable to his precepts
were his "children" that something of his spirit carried
over to the next generation. Adams was sixty-five when
he died, but he seemed much older to his flock. Just before his death, he called in the islanders and urged them

to select a head who would maintain harmony and order. His wise counsel was not adopted, however, and Nobbs extended and consolidated his influence. Although the character of Nobbs was not wholly ingratiating, his addition to the colony was not entirely regrettable. He was the best schoolmaster available, and under his tutelage the children acquired a quite adequate education. At worst, he encouraged some of the natives to adopt an attitude of odious cant and self-conscious religiosity, though this phenomenon is perhaps not to be laid entirely at Nobbs' door. No doubt, the uniform reaction, the universal praise that their simple and unpremeditated devotion had excited in their visitors encouraged some to a more calculated effort to achieve this sweet adulation. Witness the Pitcairn woman who met Waldegrave on his visit in 1830.

"I have brought you a clergyman," announced the captain.

"God bless you, God bless you!" came the response. "To stay with us?"

"No," replied Captain Waldegrave.

"You bad man, why not?"

"I cannot spare him, he is the clergyman of my ship. I have brought you clothes, which King George sends you," explained Captain Waldegrave.

"We rather want food for our souls," came the reply.

Fortunately, this tendency was not universal, nor is it just to create the impression that the Pitcairn Islanders were given to sanctimony. There is decisive evidence that their piety was genuine. Waldegrave was able to confirm all previous impressions of the people. He wrote, "It was with great gratification that we observed the Christian simplicity of the natives. They appeared to have no guile. Their cottages were open to all, and all were welcome to their food."

In the five years since Beechey's visit, Waldegrave found that fifteen people had been added to the population. When he asked the islanders their total number, they replied eighty-one. But on the actual counting of names the answer persistently came to seventy-nine. Finally one of them quietly solved the difficulty by giving the Christian names of two others previously withheld. But the parents' names were not divulged. "It would be wrong to tell my neighbors' shame," was the explanation. This lapse from the celebrated chastity of the Pitcairn Islanders was a source of great shame to the natives who had already come to take pride in their virtue. In defense of the islanders, it should be placed on record that John Buffett was the father of at least one of these two illegitimates. This episode illustrates two things of interest; one, that the genealogical records were being kept with care and were therefore reliable for modern research, second, that the serpent had made its entrance into the South Sea Eden.

The specter of a water shortage and of famine never left the subconscious minds of the leaders of the colony, so that when in 1830 a severe drought and failure of crops occurred, the islanders decided that the time had come to migrate to a larger island. Pomare, King of Tahiti, offered to set aside a fertile tract of land for these stepchildren of Tahiti, and arrangements were made by the British admiralty to remove the population of Pitcairn to their new home. Captain Sandilands, H.M. sloop *Comet,* was dispatched together with a transport bark, the *Lucy Anne,* to Pitcairn, where they arrived on February 28, 1831. Assembling the heads of the families, Captain Sandilands explained his mission. One half of them gave their names immediately as ready to depart, but the others proved reluctant to quit their homes. The next morning, however, the opposition had disintegrated, and the entire colony prepared to abandon their world for another, rendered attractive by distance and legend. Eighty-seven persons, with their most cherished lares and penates, embarked on the *Lucy Anne* on the 7th of March. During the voyage of sixteen days,

Lucy Anne Quintal was born, making a total of eighty-eight returning to one of the homes of their ancestors.

The arrival at Papeete, Tahiti, found Pomare dead and his daughter on the verge of a civil war with rebellious chiefs. But the gentlemanly and chivalrous Tahitians temporarily laid aside their quarrels to greet the newcomers. Natives from all the districts came to seek among the little band the girls and the men who had left them forty-two years before. One old lady found a sister among the four surviving Tahitian women who had accompanied the mutineers so bravely long ago. Sandilands arranged subsistence for the islanders until their first crops might mature and then departed, leaving them established on a rich stretch of land.

But the Pitcairn Islanders were not to remain for long in their happy state. Tahiti requires more resistance to withstand her sweet and poisonous blandishments than these innocents could muster. The Pitcairn recorder notes "soon after arrival at Tahiti the Pitcairn people were taken sick." And the more responsible of the party viewed with distinct and mounting alarm the debauching of the youthful and even some of the older members of the group. On April 21, Thursday October Christian died. On the 24th, John Buffett and family, Robert Young, Joseph Christian, Edward Christian, Charles Christian 3rd, Matthew Quintal, and Fredine Young decided to leave Tahiti and sailed on a small schooner for Pitcairn. Adverse winds, however, forced them to land at Lord Hood Island where they remained until they were rescued by a French brig and carried to Pitcairn on June 27. Meanwhile the deaths continued at an alarming rate, finally driving the remainder of the colony to charter the American brig *Charles Dogget* of Salem, with the copper bolts of the *Bounty* as part payment. On September 2, the last of the surviving islanders had returned to their haven on Pitcairn. Aside from other losses, this adventure had exacted a toll of, perhaps, seventeen lives.

This misadventure need not have taken place had the

Pitcairn Islanders not feared to displease the British government by refusing to accept its offer of transportation. Or so the islanders declared to Captain Freemantle in 1833, when he found them "not improved by their visit to Otaheite (Tahiti), but on the contrary much altered for the worse, having, since their return, indulged in intemperance to a great degree, distilling a spirit from the tee root, which grows in great quantities on the island." The most intelligent of the men "agreed that they never had been happy or contented" since leaving Pitcairn, and they affirmed their intention never to leave it again. Despite their joy at returning home, "They had nothing to complain of respecting their treatment at Otaheite, but disliked the character of the people, and were alarmed at the sickness which prevailed among themselves."

"It is impossible," wrote Captain Freemantle in a long summary, "for any person to visit this island without being pleased with a people generally so amiable, though springing from so guilty a stock, and brought up in so extraordinary a manner. And although I have no hesitation in saying that they have lost much of that simplicity of character which has been observed in them by former visitors, they are still a well-disposed, well-behaved, kind, hospitable people, and, if well advised and instructed, would be led to anything; but I fear, if much left to themselves, and visited by many ships, which now is not an uncommon occurrence, that they will lose what simplicity they have left, and will partake of the character of their neighbors the Otaheitians. I found even now that it was a difficult matter to obtain the truth on any point which told at all to their prejudice; and it was only by cross-questioning them that I could arrive at it. The present generation of children is the finest I ever saw; and out of the whole number, seventy-nine, there are fifty-three under twenty years of age, who appear to have been well instructed, many of them capable of reading, and nearly on a par with children of the same age in England. It certainly is desirable that this system of instruction should be kept up, and that a clergyman should be sent to them, who would be most acceptable. The Englishmen who have been on the island have on the contrary done much harm, particularly Buffett, who, although a married man, has seduced one of the young girls, by whom he has two children."

This censure, mixed with praise, is somewhat unjust. For my part, I cannot find fault with a people who object to retailing to every comer the scandal concerning their companions.

4

DICTATORSHIP: CHAPTER AND VERSE

Despite its isolation a century ago, life on Pitcairn was far from dull. At the end of 1832, an elderly gentleman, named Joshua Hill, arrived from London with letters, subsequently discovered to be spurious, giving him authority to act as governor of the island. Recognizing in the Englishmen Nobbs, Buffett, and Evans possible adversaries to his ambitions, he commenced activities calculated to remove them from the island. On Captain Freemantle's arrival four or five months later, he informed him that Nobbs was habitually drunk. One of Hill's first moves was to form a temperance society to eradicate the growing practice of imbibing intoxicants. To punish Buffett who opposed him, he had the poor unfortunate publicly flogged and even threatened similar chastisement to some women who, he said, had gossiped about him. Finally Hill's despotism went to the extreme of banishing the three Englishmen from Pitcairn: Buffett and Evans to the Gambiers, Nobbs to Tahiti. The plight of these men is revealed by their own statements.

*The humble Petition of George Hunn Nobbs, late
Teacher at Pitcairn's Island**

"Sheweth,—That your petitioner went to Pitcairn Island in 1828, with the intention of assisting the late John
Adams in teaching and schoolkeeping; that, on your petitioner's arrival, he was kindly received by the natives,
and, at their request, and with the consent of John
Adams, your petitioner immediately commenced keeping school. On the death of John Adams your petitioner,
at the desire of the natives, undertook the charge of their
spiritual affairs, and your petitioner's conduct gave general satisfaction, as will appear by the accompanying
certificate. For the space of two years things went on in
an amicable manner, when H.M.S. *Comet* arrived, for
the purpose of removing the inhabitants to Tahiti. After
some deliberation, the natives determined to remove.
Your petitioner, thinking he could be of no further service to them (as they would be under the guidance of
the missionaries at Tahiti), wished to remain with his
wife and family on the island of Pitcairn. This the islanders objected to, and insisted on your petitioner accompanying them to Tahiti. Your petitioner complied
with their desires; and, previous to Capt. Sandilands (of
H.M.S. *Comet*) quitting Tahiti, he (Capt. S.) sent for
your petitioner, and told him he must not quit the Pitcairn people, but continue to be their teacher, under the
direction of the missionaries: adding, 'You have been of
service to them, and may be so still; you are married
amongst them, and in fact become as one of themselves;
therefore you ought not, and it is my request you will
not, leave them.' After the departure of H.M.S. *Comet*,
sickness appeared among the late inhabitants of the Pit-

* This, together with the following appeals by Buffett
and Evans, were apparently directed to the commanding
naval officer of the British station on the Western coast of
South America and were transmitted to the Admiralty.

cairn's, and ultimately twelve died. During their sickness the attention paid them by your petitioner obtained the approbation of the missionaries and other gentlemen residing in Tahiti. Your petitioner was also indefatigable in obtaining subscriptions to assist them in returning to their native land. Previous to their departure from Tahiti, they went, of their own accord, to the missionaries, and requested your petitioner should be appointed 'their sole minister and teacher,' which the missionaries agreed to, and signed a paper to that effect, a copy of which accompanies this petition.

"A short time after our return to Pitcairn's Island, some of the natives (Edward Quintal, William Young, and Fletcher Christian), determined to re-commence distilling rum—a practice they had been accustomed to in John Adams's time. Your petitioner remonstrated with them on the impropriety of their conduct, but to no purpose; the answer they gave to your petitioner's advice was, 'We are our own masters; we shall do as we like; no one shall control us.' Many times your petitioner talked with them, and begged them to desist from distilling spirits; but your petitioner always received abuse in return, and twice narrowly escaped a beating from Edward Quintal. Afterwards a Mr. Hill arrived, who assumed great authority, said he was sent out by the British Government to adjust the internal affairs of the island, and the British ships of war on the coast were under his direction.

"He furthermore told the natives that he had resided for a considerable time at Oahu, where he possessed great influence, by reason that your Honour had served under him on board one of the Honourable East India Company's ships, which he (Mr. Hill) commanded.

"Believing these things to be true, your petitioner gave Mr. Hill an apartment in your petitioner's house, and used every means to make him comfortable; but, before one month had expired, Mr. Hill had succeeded, by villainous misrepresentations, atrocious falsehoods, and magnificent promises of presents, to be obtained through his influence from the British Government and several British of Mr. Hill's acquaintance, in ejecting your petitioner from his house. Mr. Hill then told the natives he should act as their teacher, until a qualified teacher was sent out from England. Soon after, H.M.S. *Challenger* touched at Pitcairn's Island from Tahiti. Capt. Freemantle assembled the inhabitants, and informed them that Mr. Hill was not acting under the authority of the British Government; also, that he, Capt. Freemantle, came on shore with the intention of removing Mr. Hill from the island; but, on hearing that your petitioner had partaken of the spirits distilled by the natives, he, (Capt. F.) informed your petitioner that he could not re-instate him in the situation of which Mr. Hill had deprived him; at the same time Capt. F. told Mr. Hill he did not approve of his (Mr. H.'s) conduct, as he acted without authority. Capt. F. also told Mr. Hill he must not interfere with the laws, as the administration of them was vested in the natives.

"Capt. F. asked your petitioner what he intended to do. Your petitioner replied, it was his wish to leave the island. Capt. F. said he thought it was the best thing your petitioner could do, under existing circumstances, but that he certainly might remain if he chose. Before Capt. F. departed, he told the natives it was his belief that Mr. Hill wished to get the other Europeans off the island, that he, Mr. Hill, might make himself king over them. Capt. F. also sharply reprimanded Mr. Hill for calling the other British residents, 'lousy foreigners,' etc.; and bade him desist from doing so. Mr. Hill promised to obey, but never kept his promise. Shortly after Capt. F.'s departure, Mr. Hill began again to oppress your petitioner and the two other Englishmen. He ordered the natives to turn us out of their houses; and our nearest relatives dared not come and visit us.

"As soon as a ship appeared off the island, a canoe was dispatched on board, forbidding the officers and crew coming to our houses, and we were threatened with stripes if we offered to go on board. In May last, an act was passed (by force) to deprive our children of their mothers' inheritance, merely because their fathers were foreigners (Englishmen). In August Mr. Hill sent his colleagues to seize the muskets of those persons whom, he said, were opposed to the governor of the commonwealth. As soon as Mr. Hill obtained possession of the muskets, he loaded them with powder and ball, and deposited them in his bedroom, for the use of the magistracy of the island. Every Sunday a loaded musket is placed beneath his seat in church, to intimidate his hearers. Since that period your petitioner has been in continued alarm for the lives of himself and family. Your petitioner dared not go out of his house after dark, nor up to his plantation at any time, by himself, for fear of being maltreated by the colleagues of Mr. Hill. Several of the natives protested against such conduct; Mr. Hill threatened to give them a flogging, and, moreover, said, that if they did not obey him, he would cause a military governor to be sent out from England, with a party of soldiers, who would take their land from them and treat them as slaves. In the month of November last your petitioner was seized with the dysentery, and for three months was confined to his bed. Your petitioner could not obtain medicine, although there was a medicine-chest on the island, and of which your petitioner was a part proprietor. In fact, it was the declared intent of Joshua Hill and his colleagues to bring about the death of your petitioner, either by hanging, flogging, or starvation.

"Your petitioner at last, by sickness, deprivation of common necessaries, and anxiety of mind, occasioned by Joshua Hill's wicked counsel and conduct, was brought to the verge of the grave, when, providentially, a ship appeared in sight, which proved to be the *Tuscan* of London, Capt. Stavers; who, on seeing the miserable condition of your petitioner, kindly consented, at your petitioner's earnest request, to give him a passage to Tahiti. Owing to the professional and benevolent endeavours of Dr. Bennett, surgeon of the *Tuscan*, your petitioner is recovering, and hopes, ere long, to be re-instated in health. And now, Honoured Sir, will you permit your unfortunate petitioner to implore your Honour's protection? Driven from family and home by an unauthorized person, without friends or money, and almost without clothes, your petitioner is at a loss what course to pursue. Your petitioner cannot support the idea of being separated for ever from his wife and family; but, alas! he can scarcely hope to see them again unless your Honour condescends to espouse his cause. Convinced that his cause is just, and knowing that Capt. Stavers and Dr. Bennett can corroborate the most material statements in this petition, the fervent prayer of your petitioner, and the other two unfortunate Englishmen with him, to be restored to their families and possessions on Pitcairn's Island; and your petitioner, in duty bound, will ever pray, etc.

"Your petitioner has no desire to be replaced as teacher, but simply to employ himself in agricultural pursuits, for the support of his family."

To this should be added the following complaints of John Buffett and of John Evans.

"HONOURED SIR,—I hope you will excuse the liberty I take in writing to you, which I doubt not you will, when you are informed in what critical circumstances I am placed. In December, 1823, on our return to England, we touched at Pitcairn's Island, and by desire of the natives and consent of our captain, I went on shore to teach their children to read, etc., which I did to their satisfaction. Mr. Nobbs arriving soon after, became their teacher; since then I have lived as a private individual, on good terms with the natives. After going to Tahiti with them, and remaining there about three weeks, I procured a passage for myself, my wife, and family and arrived at Pitcairn's Island about three months before the rest of the natives. After they all arrived, we all lived together upon friendly terms, until the arrival of Mr. Joshua Hill from Tahiti, in October, 1832, who stated that he had been sent out by the British Government, and whatever he was in want of he would procure from England, New South Wales, or Valparaiso.

"By means of such promises, and by his making them believe that whatever heretofore has been sent out, was by his influence, he has gained the favour of a few natives, and appointed three elders and two privy councillors. He has framed laws and built a prison; and should any of the natives refuse to obey him, let his proposals be ever so unjust, he tells them he will send to England for a governor and a regiment of soldiers. By such means he has persuaded the natives to sign a petition to Government to deprive us Englishmen and our children of their lands; and I am ordered, with my wife and five children, to leave the island. His plea (J. H.'s) is, that there is not land sufficient. At the same time, he has proposed to send to England for English ladies, for wives for the youth of the island; and because I made known his plan of sending my wife and family off the island, I had a mock-trial, on which Mr. Hill was judge, jury, and executioner.

"After Mr. Hill's beating me over the head, breaking it in two places, likewise my finger, I was suspended by my hands in the church, and flogged until I was not able to walk home, and confined to my bed for two weeks, and it was several weeks before I was able to work or have the use of my hand; my wife, at the same time, was ill and not able to work, and Mr. J. Hill would not allow the natives to visit me or my wife, not even her own sister, but literally tried to starve us. Charles Christian, the oldest man on the island, was brutally treated, and turned out of his house, for trying to prevent my being flogged; and because the women assembled crying shame on his (Mr. J. H.'s) proceedings, he, Mr. J. Hill, on the Sunday following read the riot act, and told them, should they do so again, the authorities would be justified in shooting them. He then sent his colleagues, as he is pleased to call them, to take possession of our fire-arms, which they loaded with ball, and Mr. J. Hill has since kept them in his possession.

"Since this, Sir, not only the lives of us English residents, but some of the natives, have been in danger from the malicious temper of Mr. J. Hill. He has been the means of depriving one of my children of the land left her by her grandfather, and he proposes to deprive the others also, and as they grow up to send them to sea as cabin boys, etc. He wished Capt. Freemantle, of H.M.S. *Challenger,* who touched at Pitcairn's Island, in February, 1832, to remove me from the island; but he (Capt. F.) would not. Since that he has been trying all in his power to prejudice the natives against me. Capt. T. Stavers has been so kind as to give me a passage to Tahiti, when I shall endeavour to get a passage for my family, either to Lord Howe's Island or Rappa. In the meantime, I humbly hope, Sir, you will use your influence to get Mr. Hill removed from Pitcairn's Island; it is the desire of most of the inhabitants. The land that Mr. Hill wishes to deprive my children of, is their mother's portion, left by her father (Edward Young of the *Bounty*). If, Sir, you would condescend to write me a few lines, informing me how to act, to the care of Mr. Pritchard, Tahiti, you would greatly oblige your most humble servant,"

(*Signed*)   J. BUFFETT.

The humble Petition of John Evans, two (sic)
years resident on Pitcairn's Island

"*Sheweth,*—That your petitioner landed on Pitcairn's in the year 1823, and after a residence of twelve months was united in marriage with the second daughter of the late John Adams (by his consent). From that period your petitioner continued to live in peace and harmony with the natives, and maintained himself and family in a comfortable manner. Your petitioner accompanied the Pitcairn people to Tahiti, and while there, assisted them as much as lay in his power. At their return, the natives were perfectly agreeable that your petitioner should return with them, and resume possession of his wife's land, etc. Things went on in their usual train for twelve months after our return, when a Mr. Joshua Hill arrived at Pitcairn's, who informed your petitioner he was come by authority of the British Government to adjust the internal affairs of the island, and that he had sent orders to Valparaiso for H.M.S. *Dublin* to come and take him on board, and convey him to the Marquesas Islands in a diplomatic capacity.

"Your petitioner gave credit to Mr. Hill's assertions, and treated him with all possible respect, also cheerfully contributed to his support; but scarcely had Mr. Hill been on shore three weeks, when he attempted to persuade your petitioner's wife to leave him, saying he would take her under his protection, and supply her with everything she wanted; adding, 'I will cause the first captain of a man-of-war who arrives to remove these lousy foreigners from the island.' My wife refused to do as he wished, and from that time forth he became her declared enemy. Shortly after a ship of war arrived, the captain of which declared he knew nothing of Mr. Hill, neither had he (Mr. Hill) any authority from the British Government.

"Mr. Hill used every means in his power, by misrepresentation and gross falsehood, to induce Capt. Freemantle to remove me from the island. This Capt. F. refused, saying, he had a good opinion of me, and should not separate me from my family. Capt. Freemantle severely reprimanded Mr. Hill for his conduct towards the

English residents, and desired him to alter his conduct towards them; this Mr. Hill promised to do, but malice and falsehood are prominent traits in the character of Joshua Hill. No sooner was Capt. Freemantle gone, than Mr. Hill (vexed that he had not gained his point) became more outrageous than ever; he still asserted he was sent out by the British Government, that Capt. F. was no gentleman, and denounced vengeance on every native that did not join with him in oppressing the lousy foreigners. Whenever a ship appeared in sight, two confidential men were dispatched on board to forbid the captain and officers holding any communication with foreigners on shore; and we were prohibited, under pains and penalties, from going on board. In May last a prison was built, for the avowed purpose of confining the Englishmen and their friends, and a law passed (by force) depriving our children of their mothers' inheritance; and all the genuine natives, from seven years and upwards, were compelled to sign a paper, declaring they would never intermarry with the foreigners—a term applied to our children as well as ourselves. In July a law was enacted relative to high treason.

"Your petitioner requested a copy as a guide for his future conduct; Mr. Hill refused to give him one, flew into a violent rage, and shortly after, your petitioner was dragged to the church, underwent a mock-trial, no witnesses being allowed, and received one dozen lashes with a cat-o'-nine-tails, each tail being the size of a man's little finger. Your petitioner was so much hurt about the head, eyes, and ribs, as to be confined to his bed for ten days. From this time the state of things became desperate, and your petitioner was under continual alarm for the lives of himself and family. Mr. Hill and his colleagues were continually threatening the life of someone or other, and your petitioner firmly believes, had it not been for the opportune arrival of the ship *Tuscan,* Capt. R. T. Stavers, murder would have been shortly committed. Capt.

Stavers, seeing the untoward state of affairs, humanely consented to give your petitioner a passage to Tahiti. And now, Honoured Sir, will you permit your petitioner to hope you will commiserate my unhappy condition? Neither the natives nor Mr. Hill can bring any serious charge against me, as Capt. Stavers and Dr. Bennett can certify, and yet your petitioner is banished from family and home, merely to gratify the malevolence of Mr. Hill. Your petitioner humbly begs that your Honour will restore your petitioner again to his wife and family, that he may support them by his labour.

"And your petitioner as in duty bound, will ever pray."

But so completely had Hill deluded the simple-minded, unsophisticated islanders that either of their own volition or out of fear, some of them signed the following petition addressed to Hill. The style of this extraordinary document suggests, however, that its composition was the product of Hill himself.

Copy of a Letter, dated Pitcairn's Island, 3rd October 1833, from the Public Functionaries and others, to Captain Joshua Hill, Teacher, etc.

"RESPECTED SIR.—We, the undersigned, being all public authorities, as well as other natives, who are earnestly desirous for the prosperity and welfare of our dearly beloved island, beg not only that you will be pleased to accept our most sincere gratitude for all which you have done for us, in various respects, both before your arrival here in October last, and since, especially in thus saving and snatching us so providentially, as it were, from the brink of infidelity itself, and as well as other crying and besetting sins (now too painful for us to contemplate), which otherwise must have been our entire and total ruin. But, moreover, we entreat that you will not think of leaving us yet awhile, or until we become, with the blessed Lord's help, settled somewhat in safety. For, indeed, we have too good reason to know, that so long as one of these profligate foreigners is among us on Pitcairn's, we never shall be able to go on aright, or resist their corrupting or destructive practices. Hence we implore you, dear friend, to consider our unfortunate case; and remember that, on your arrival here (aforesaid), we had two cursed stills up—without a school, without a church!—and, alas! alas!—'tell it not in Gath'— we were living without God, in the world!

"We pray you, therefore, leave us not thus to the enemy, or we fear again that we shall be for ever lost!

"We hereto subscribe ourselves, respected Sir, your most sincere friends, and very obedient servants."

(*Signed etc., by all.*)

Hill's reply sounds curiously like the petition itself.

J. Hill's Answer to the foregoing, dated Pitcairn's Island, October 4th, 1833

"My very dear Friends,—The lively interest which, from the beginning, I have taken in your welfare is well known to our mutual friends in England. And thus, since my arrival here, on the 28th October, 1832, you know yourselves. I can only observe, at this moment, in answer to the request which you have deemed requisite thus to reiterate, that is repeat, in your joint letter to me of the 3rd instant, which you handed to me at our prayer-meeting yesterday, P.M., in reference to my continuing a while longer with you, etc., I would say that, notwithstanding the importance of time, I shall not, with the blessed Lord's will, think of leaving you until hearing from home; i.e. from the British Government, nor until my presence becomes no longer necessary in furtherance

of the established welfare of your commonwealth and beloved little island. Being always,
            "My friends, really and faithfull,
                "Your well-wisher,"
        (*Signed*)   JOSHUA HILL,
                                Teacher, etc.

Having assumed the reins of government, such as they
were, Hill appointed from among the principal men on
the island four elders, three subelders, and four cadets.
He continued to dominate the island, while correspondence to, from, and about him passed back and forth
across the Pacific. I am tempted to extract additional
documents relating to the extraordinary Mr. Hill, but
I shall conclude these engrossing quotations with a
lengthy self-testimonial by Joshua Hill himself.

"I am aware that pedantry and egotism become no
one, and myself perhaps less than any. (Pro. xxvii. 2.)
But for certain reasons, the following credentials, as a
memorandum, I hope will be pardoned on the present
occasion—they are truths.

"I observe, *in limine*, that I have visited the four quarters of the globe, and it has ever been my desire to maintain, as far as lay in my power, the standing of an English gentleman. I have lived a considerable while in a
palace, and had my dinner parties with a princess on my
right, and a General's lady upon my left. I have had a
French cook, a box at the opera. I have drove my dress
carriage (thought the neatest then in Paris, where I
spent five or six years; as well I have known Calcutta),
and the handsomest lady (said), Madame R——, to grace
my carriage. I have drove a curricle with my two out-
riders, and two saddle-horses, besides a travelling-car-
riage. A valet, coachman, footman, groom, and, upon
extraordinary occasions, my *maître d'hôtel*. I have (at
her request) visited Madame Bonaparte, at the Tuileries,
St. Cloud, and Malmaison. I might thus mention many
others of note abroad.

"I have frequently dined with that remarkable woman, Madame Carburas, afterwards the Princess de C——. I have had the honour of being in company; i.e. at the same parties, with both his late Majesty George IV. then Prince Regent, and his present Majesty William IV. then H.R.H. Duke of Clarence, as well with their royal brothers. I have ridden in a royal Duke's carriage, with four horses and three footmen, more than once, and have dined at his table, and drunk the old hock of his late father, George III. I have visited and dined with some of our first families, and have been visited by a Duke, and others of the first noblemen. I have known and dined with (abroad and in England), Madames Catalini, Grassini, Georges, etc. And I have given the arm to Lady Hamilton (of Naples renown), whom the hero of the Nile has given his (one) to more than once. I have dined with a Viceroy Governor (who was a General and a Count), and with Admirals, both on board their ships and on shore. I have entertained Governors, Generals, Captains (R.N.), on board my ship, more than once. And I have commanded several ships, and went to sea at the beginning of the French Revolution.

"I have been acquainted with many military and naval officers. I have since 1807, my admittance, from the late President, Sir Joseph Banks, to the sittings of the Royal Society. I have occasionally breakfasted with Sir Joseph, and visited, and even presented a friend (the actual President of the bank of the N.N.S. of America) to his evening parties. My admittance to the Royal Society has always admitted me to similar institutions abroad. I received the dress sword, and nautical instruments, etc. of a noble lord (at his death), a Vice-Admiral of the Red. I sailed from England (Portsmouth, May 1st, 1794) to the East Indies and China, in the largest fleet, possibly, that ever was; it was under Lord Howe, down the British Channel, just one month before his great victory. I have visited the Falls of Niagara and Montmorency, the natural bridge in Virginia, the great Reciprocating Fountain in East Tennessee, the great Temple of Elephants at Bombay.

"I have dined with a prince, as well as with a princess; and with a count, a baron, an ambassador, a minister (ordinary and extraordinary), and have dined with a Chargé d'Affaire, and lived with consuls, etc. I have visited and conversed with 'Red Jacket,' the great Indian warrior. I have visited and been visited by a bishop. I have frequently partook of the delicious Hungarian wine (tokey), Prince Easterházy's; as also of Prince Swartzerburgh's old hock, said to have been 73 years old; and I was intimate with the brother-in-law of this last German nobleman. I have dined with a principal Hong merchant at Canton. I have sat next to the beautiful Madame Recamier and Madame Carbanus, at the great dinner parties. I have written to the Prime Minister of England; and have received the (late Earl of Liverpool's) answer with his thanks, etc.

"I was at Paris when the allies were made there. I have visited and breakfasted with the late Warren Hastings, Esq., at his seat in Gloucestershire. I have had permission with a party of friends to hunt over his grounds. Entertained etc. two or three days at the sporting lodge of an Earl, now a Marquis. I have made a crimson silk net for a certain fashionable Marchioness, which she actually wore at her next great party of five or six hundred persons. I have danced with the Countess Bertand; i.e., Mademoiselle Fanny Dillon, before she married the Marshall. I was at Napoleon's coronation. I have been invited to the Lord Mayor's, and to the dinner of an Alderman of London; to those also of the first merchants and bankers, as the late Mr. Thelusson (afterwards Lord Rendlesham), the formerly rich Messrs. A. and B. Goldsmiths, etc. And at Paris I have had a credit of 400,000 francs, at one time, on the house of Perregan, Lafitte, etc., and other bankers at Paris for considerable sums. Delepent and Co. for 40,000 francs, and Recamier's, at one time, for upwards of 100,000 francs. Lafitte's house at another time for 50,000 francs; again for 12,000 francs. I have had at a time, nearly 5000 sterling at the Bank of England.

"I wrote and published in the London *Morning Post* (7th March, 1811), on naval power. I have seen the Vestrises, father, son, and grandson, at once (the only time), dance on the stage at the opera at Paris. I have given a passage to many on board my ship, but never in my life received a farthing as passage-money from any person. I am decidedly against the use of ardent spirit (malt liquor may do for those who like it), tobacco, etc. And as for wine, that only at dinner; it even then ought to be good, if not the very best, as the Gourmet would have it, when speaking of Clas-Vangeat, and Romance, etc. I have had a fine band of music on board my ship, and my four kinds of wine on my table. (I am not sleeping on a 'bed of roses' now, but in a humble hut or cabin.) After all, what does the foregoing amount to?— vanity of vanities. I will merely add, that I have had a year in the Church of Christ, and that I am a life member of the Bible Society. That I am looking with the blessed Lord's help to something of far more intrinsic worth and consideration—'the price of our high calling' —the life to come. I am now in my sixty-second year of age, and of course it is high time that I should look upon this world as nearly to close on me. I might perhaps say much more, but must stop. I am now an humble teacher upon Pitcairn's Isle for the time being.

"June, 1834."

(*Signed*)   J. HILL.

The entire tragi-comedy ended ignominiously for Joshua Hill when Captain Lord Edward Russell visited Pitcairn on H.M.S. *Actaeon* in 1837. Hill had let it be known that "he was a very near relative of the Duke of Bedford, and that the Duchess seldom rode out in her carriage without him." Nemesis at last appeared in the guise of Lord Edward, who was the son of the Duke of

Bedford. Unable to remove Hill without instructions from London, Lord Edward immediately reported to his superiors. In the following year, H.M.S. *Imogene* arrived and quietly removed Hill to Valparaiso.

Released from the domination of the magnetic and grandiloquent Hill, the principal men of the island now signed a petition to restore the exiled Englishmen in their adopted homes. And in due course Nobbs, Buffett, and Evans were returned to their families and to their former occupations.

5

HEGIRA

The year of Mr. Hill's downfall, 1838, also marked a definite regularization of the island's official position and the formal establishment of an internal organization. These events were engineered by Captain Elliott, H.M. sloop *Fly,* who landed at Pitcairn in November, 1838, but their need had long been recognized by the islanders. The episode of Joshua Hill had made apparent the wisdom of an ordered government. And the increasing contact with the outside world, represented by whaling ships, made some formal authority imperative.

It is necessary to pause here to describe the relationship of the Pitcairn colony to the whaling industry. The discoverer of the settlement, in 1808, was the first in a wave that was to mount to extraordinary proportions. The American whalers, having exhausted the Atlantic of its cetaceans in the eighteenth century, had already found a new and rich field in the Pacific by the beginning of the nineteenth. In increasing numbers, hundreds of little harbors up and down the New England coast were sending out whaling expeditions, financed by "stocking" capital. Of these centers Nantucket and New Bedford were the most flourishing. By 1849, the peak year, some 4000 whalers from New England ports were at sea, mainly in the Pacific. Out often four years at a stretch, the captains greatly needed convenient ports of call where they might secure water and fresh provisions and where they might shelter their wives during parturition. Pitcairn, lying near one of the South Pacific whaling grounds, proved to be so handy that the number of ships calling there annually increased enormously. The island's register gives a list from which the following figures are derived:

NUMBER OF SHIPS		NUMBER OF SHIPS		NUMBER OF SHIPS	
1823	1	1833	6	1843	29
1824	3	1834	4	1844	18
1825	4	1835	2	1845	22
1826	3	1836	7	1846	49
1827	3	1837	4	1847	19
1828	2	1838	10	1848	9
1829	7	1839	13	1849	18
1830	4	1840	10	1850	47
1831	6	1841	20	1851	24
1832	5	1842	30	1852	14

These figures represent all ships that called at the island, but the great majority were American and practically all of these were whalers. The honesty and friendliness of the islanders were so renowned that most of the captains welcomed the opportunity to visit Pitcairn. Lady Belcher quotes one sailor "that if any insult were to be offered to any of them (the Pitcairn Islanders), and especially to the female part of the community, a man would not be long alive after he came on board." Laudable as this sentiment was and typical as it might have been, unfortunately whaling crews did not always measure up to such standards. Melville's description of at least one job lot complement leads one to suspect that some rather tough customers sailed on those "stinking trypots." On one occasion on Pitcairn part of "the ruffian crew of a whale ship were on shore for a fortnight, during which time, they offered every insult to the inhabitants, and threatened to violate any woman whose protectors they could overcome by force." To eliminate recurrence of such raids, Captain Elliott formally declared the island to be under the protection of the British crown; and both to protect them from successors to Mr. Hill, and to preserve them from taunts that they had no government or country, he endowed the islanders with a simple form of self-government. To administer the affairs of the island, Edward Quintal was elected the first magistrate.

For the most part the annals of the island, preserved in the *Pitcairn Island Register*, record with monotonous regularity the births of the new Janes and Mary Anns, Edwards and Arthurs, varied by arrivals of ships and attacks of illness. But in 1845, the chronicler had three subjects worthy of his pen. The first concerned the *Bounty's* guns. "January 19th. During the past week we have been employed fishing up two of the *Bounty's* guns (long nines, I believe). For fifty-five years they had been deposited at the bottom of the sea on a bed of coral guiltless of blood—(during the time so many thousands of mankind in Europe became 'Food for Cannon'); but on Saturday last one of these guns resumed its original vocation; at least the innocuous portion of it, to wit, belching forth fire and smoke, and causing the island to reverberate with its bellowing: the other gun is condemned to silence having been spiked by someone of the *Bounty's* crew."

The second event called forth an essay on the "salubrity" of Pitcairn. The islanders for some years past had been suffering, as many island populations suffer after the visits of ships, from recurrent epidemics of influenza. In 1845, another hit the colony, and its course was faithfully recorded in the Register. "March 27th. The fever is on the decline, cheerful faces are again seen, and I hope grateful hearts are praising God whose mercies endureth for ever.

"I will now say a few words respecting the salubrity of the island: it is generally supposed to be a healthy spot;

indeed, appearances seem to justify such a conclusion; but the reverse is found by experience, to be the fact. Asthmas, Rheumatism, Consumption, Scrofula and last but not least Influenza under various modifications is prevalent. Five times within the last four years have the fever been rife among us, and though it has not been so severe latterly as it was on its first appearance, this, I think, may be accounted for by the teacher becoming more acquainted with the nature of the disease (thanks to Dr. Gunn [*hiatus*]) and also with the appropriate remedies—when the influenza first appeared among us it did not spread so rapidly as it has done on its subsequent reappearance, but the cough was more violent then, than it has been since. This I attribute to the teacher's not giving them emetics as soon as the disease attacked them; since then he has invariably given them vomits on the first appearance of the disease; which seems to prevent any considerable degree of cough. But there is one particular in which the recent fever differs from the previous ones; viz. in the total absence of a cold fit at the very commencement. I have seen some of the patients when first attacked tremble as violently, and apparently from the same causes, as ever I saw anyone under the influence of ague.

"Now, in this last sickness it was not thus; only one person complained of cold and he was but slightly affected. The first person attacked was a man of full habit of body, plethoric and subject to fits, he had attended Divine service in the morning, it being the Sabbath, after evening service I found him under the influence of a raging fever; his eyes seemed ready to start from their sockets and the heat of his skin caused a disagreeable sensation to those who touched him;—he complained of violent pains in his head, back and thighs and said he felt as if 'live things were creeping between his flesh and skin.' Fearing it might bring on one of the fits to which he was subject the teacher bled him, and gave him a sudorific which had a good effect; the next day a dose of

calomel and jalap was administered, and two days after
that he was well; though very weak.

"I do not think the fever was infectious; and though in
the space of six days not less than sixty out of one hundred and twenty-two were attacked yet I attribute it
solely to the peculiar state of the atmosphere: whenever
we have been visited by this epidemick the circumstances, as respects the weather have been invariably the
same. A long drought succeeded by two or three weeks
of wet; and the wind settling into the north west; in fact
a north west wind is always the precussor [sic] of rheumatism, catarrh, and slight febrile affection. Bleeding is
not to be recommended; vomits are the sovereign
remedy, for certainly no community of persons secrete
greater quantities of bile than the inhabitants of this island. March 31st. There is now but one person sick and
she is recovering,—a few have a slight cough but that is
wearing away.

"And now it behoves us to offer up our grateful thanksgiving to Almighty God, Father, Son and Holy Spirit,
to Whom be glory now and for ever. Amen."

The third occurrence to exercise Mr. Nobbs' pen was
a phenomenon startling to the islanders. During the
night of April 16, "a perfect typhon" raged over the island, "the whole concave of the heavens" being in a "continued blaze and roar of the thunder." "Very frequently
through the night loud crashes were heard, which we
supposed were the trees in the higher parts of the island
yielding to the fury of the storm;—the noise did proceed
from the falling, and smashing of trees, but from a cause,
of which we were, at that time happily ignorant.

"At daylight a man, much alarmed, came to my house
saying, 'A part of the island had given way and was
going into the sea;—' From the door of my house I obtained an imperfect view of the spot from which a portion of the earth had been detached and felt certain it
was an avalanche occasioned by the wind acting upon
the trees, and the torrents of rain which fell detaching

the earth from the parts above it. So great was the consternation and amazement of many of the natives that although they had seen the spot from which the earth had slidden almost every day of their lives, yet they could not so far collect their ideas as to remember the original appearance of the place, whose property it had been; nor the locality of the parts near it;—As to the cause of the disruption various opinions prevailed some said it was occasioned by a waterspout, others that a thunderbolt had fallen there and a third party were anxiously enquiring if it were not probable the sea had perforated a hole from the under side of the island and so washed it away.—That they had considerable occasion for alarm cannot be disputed, and what may easily be referred to natural causes (and those not very recondite either) would by persons so inexperienced as our community, appear mysterious and awful.

"I will endeavour, in a few words, to describe what presented itself to our view at daylight. On going out of doors we saw that a considerable portion of the earth had been detached from the side of the [?] but to what extent we could not then ascertain;—the place in question was situated at the head of a ravine which debouched into the sea; the rain mixing with the falling earth (which was of clayey nature) brought it to the consistancy of thick mud but sufficiently liguified to glide very slowly down the inclined plane of the valley;—nothing with which it came in contact could resist its force,—the large trees at the head of the ravine, and immense pieces of rock, were borne slowly but unresistingly along and about three hundred cocoa nut trees were torn up by the roots and swept into the sea.

"So tenacious was the heterogeneous stream that some of the cocoa nut trees from forty to fifty feet in height, after being displaced from their original situation remained in an upright position some minutes, and when they fell it was many yards from the spot in which they had come to maturity.—A considerable portion of this aquatic lava (for indeed its appearance had a distinct resemblance to the molten streams of an active volcano) had reached the sea before daylight: and when some of our people ventured to the edge of the precipice, they found to their dismay the boat houses, and boats left there, had disappeared. Two families whose houses were adjacent to the ravine removed their household goods, fearing the foundation of their dwellings might become undermined, and whelm them in the ruin;—but in a few hours the stream ceased to flow, and confidence was in a measure restored. We had now time to turn our attention to other parts of the island; at Bounty Bay a great quantity of earth had been washed away, a yam ground containing a thousand yams totally disappeared, several fishing boats destroyed, the *Bounty's* guns washed to the edge of the surf and large pieces of rock so encumbered the harbour that if a ship should come it is doubtful whether a passage could be found for her boat to pass through.

"In the interim all the plantain patches are levelled, about four thousand plantation trees are destroyed, one half in full bearing; the other half designed for the year 1846 so that this very valuable article of food we shall be without for a long time to come. The fact is, from this date until August we shall be pinched for food; but 'God tempers the wind to the shorn lamb.' I humbly trust the late monitions of providence viz. Drought sickness and storm which severally have been inflicted upon us this year may be sanctified to us, and be the means of bringing us, one and all, into a closer communion with our God; may we remember the rod and who hath appointed it; may we flee to the cross of Christ for safety and for succour in every time of need; always bearing in mind our heavenly Father doth not willingly afflict the children of men."

On January 23, 1850, the islanders celebrated the sixtieth anniversary of the founding of the Pitcairn community. Everyone enjoyed the event so fully that it was decided to repeat it annually.

"This day was observed as the anniversary of the settlement of the colony, sixty years since. One survivor of that strange event and its sanguinarry results; witnessed the celebration. At daylight one of the *Bounty's* guns was discharged and wakened the sleeping echoes and the more drowsy of the inhabitants. At ten o'clock divine service was performed. Text [*hiatus*]. After the sermon the various letters received from the British Government and principal Friends were read from the pulpit and commented upon. At twelve a number of musketteers assembled under the 'Flag Staff' and fired a volley in honor of the day. After dinner the community male and female assembled in front of the church, where the British flag was flying and gave three cheers for Queen Victoria, three for the Government at Home, three for the Majestrates here, three for absent friends, three for the Ladies and three for the community in general; amid the firing of the muskets and the ringing of the Bell.—At sunset the gun of the *Bounty* was fired again and the day closed in harmony and peace—Much, very much have we to be grateful for, both to God and man.—It is voted that an annual celebration be observed."

In July of the same year Susannah, a Tahitian woman, died—the last link with the *Bounty* and her crew.

Since 1819 the Society for Promoting Christian Knowledge had taken a deep interest in the welfare of the Pitcairn Islanders. Presents of religious books, clothing, and other articles were frequently sent from England to this remote spot from the Society and its friends. Through the officers of the Society and others in England interested in the island, the wishes of the islanders, and of Nobbs himself, to have a pastor duly accredited by the Church of England, were finally granted. Admiral Moresby arrived in 1852 and, substituting his own chaplain, Mr. Holman, gave Nobbs passage to Valparaiso *en route* to England where, after some months of instruction, he was first ordained a deacon by the Bishop of Sierra Leone, then a priest by the Bishop of London. Before quitting England, Nobbs was appointed a missionary with a small salary by the Society for Promoting Christian Knowledge. Nine months after his departure Nobbs once more landed on Pitcairn, May 16, 1853.

Through their benefactor, Admiral Moresby, whose name has been preserved in the memory of the community as a given name among their own members, the Pitcairn Islanders presented a gift to Queen Victoria. The letter of presentation bears its own stamp of authenticity. A part of it follows:

"We humbly trust we may be allowed to consider ourselves your Majesty's subjects; and Pitcairn's Island a British Colony as long as it is inhabited by us in the fullest sense of the word. Several years since the Capt. of your Majesty's ship *Fly* took formal possession of our little Island; and placed us under your Majesty's protection; and if your Majesty's government would grant us a document declaring us part of your Majesty's dominion; we should be freed from all fears (perhaps groundless) on that head; and such a gracious mark of Royal favour would be cherished by us to an exertion in the discharge of the various duties incumberent on British subjects. . . .

"At the suggestion of our worthy benefactor Rear Admiral Moresby we have ventured to present your gracious Majesty with a small chest of drawes of our own manifacture from the Island wood; the native name of the dark wood is *miro*; the bottoms of the drawers is made of the breadfruit tree; our means are very limited; and our mechanical skill also; and we will esteem it a great favour if your Majesty would condersend to except of it; as a token of our loyalty and respect to our gracious Queen."

The memory of Tahiti and the activities of Mr. Hill had been effective for a time in banishing all thought of leaving Pitcairn. As late as 1849 Captain Wood had of-

fered to move the islanders, an offer which was refused
after some deliberation. In the same year Captain Fanshawe wrote: "I could not trace in any of them the slight-
est desire to remove elsewhere. On the contrary, they expressed the greatest repugnance to do so, whilst a sweet
potato remained to them." But even while the islanders
were expressing themselves so strongly, a change in attitude was appearing. If the island was regarded as
cramped for the 1831 population of eighty persons, now
that it contained twice that number the need for a larger
island began to seem inevitable. Each year the leaders
of the community noted another crop of babies to be
supported. The hive was full, and the bees must swarm.

A year after the visit of Captains Fanshawe and
Wood, the community's views tended to removal. We
read in Mr. Brodie's account of a brief visit in 1850 that
Pitcairn was inadequate for its population, and that
practically nothing was left for barter after the limited
acreage supplied the needs of the islanders.

The decision to be made no longer was whether or not
to move, but where to go. A large tract of land in Hua-
hine, one of the Society Islands, had been inherited by
the Pitcairners through one of the wives of the mutineers, but this did not suggest a solution. The islanders
still retained a vivid memory of the disastrous experiment at Tahiti, another of the Society Islands. Once bit-
ten twice shy. The choice of the community favored an
uninhabited island where they could develop as a homogeneous community, unimpeded and unmolested. Juan
Fernandez appealed to them, but Selkirk's hermitage belonged to Chile and was not available.

A famine and scarcity of water now forced the colony
to act, and a petition was directed to the British Government to remove them as a body. Norfolk Island, abandoned in 1855 by Great Britain as a penal colony, was
the island suggested, because there they expected to find
a climate similar to their own and because there they
could continue to be isolated and untrammeled. The

British government, ever complaisant to the requests of
its subjects on Pitcairn, decided to grant the request and
informed the governor of Norfolk to hold the island for
the Pitcairners, not allowing squatters to settle on it.

Norfolk Island is situated roughly in latitude 29° S and
longitude 167° 50' E, about one thousand miles northeast of Sydney, Australia, and over four thousand miles
west of Pitcairn. It is a volcanic island about twenty miles
in circumference, five to six miles at its greatest breadth,
and contains upward of eight thousand acres. The highest point, Mt. Pitt, has an altitude of one thousand feet.
The soil is very rich, bearing a wide variety of tropical
and subtropical fruit and vegetables, and the surrounding waters abound in edible fish. The island also contained a large number of buildings: compounds for the
prisoners, a government house, two churches, and various small cottages, the quarters of the officers and the
barracks for the soldiers. Most of these structures were
solidly built of gray stone, their dour institutionalism emphasized by an austere type of Georgian architecture.
Livestock, consisting of cattle, sheep, and horses, were
also left for the benefit of the new tenants of the island.

The transfer from Pitcairn took place in 1856. Captain Mathers, the *Morayshire*, arrived at Pitcairn in
April and, after the natural reluctance of the islanders
was overcome, sailed with the entire population of 187
persons. The *Morayshire* reached Norfolk thirty-six days
later. The first view of Norfolk was a severe disappointment to some of the islanders. They missed the rugged
beauty of Pitcairn and their cozy little houses embow-
ered in a rich foliage; they wanted the snug security
that their own island gave them. The parklike tranquillity of Norfolk seemed immense. It lacked the dramatic beauty of their wild and romantic Pitcairn. One
could, to be sure, slip off a precipice into the sea at Pitcairn, but one couldn't get lost in pathless forests or
swampy gullies. On Norfolk, one could wander for days

without seeing another friendly human. It was uncomfortable.

The three-storied stark stone buildings, the oxen, and the horses filled the islanders with astonishment. But a mere two weeks later Nobbs* noted a change. He wrote, "Some are employed tending sheep, some driving cattle, and two or three at the wind-mill grinding maize; and it is really wonderful with what facility our people comprehend the details of these complicated employments." Sir William Denison, governor of New South Wales, urged the inhabitants to build habits of self-reliance in their new home. There was sufficient, he maintained, for their needs without the gifts of charity that had become increasingly necessary to support life on Pitcairn.

Doctor Selwyn, Bishop of Melanesia, had secured permission to establish his Melanesian mission at one corner of the island, and the colony found a new teacher in Mrs. Selwyn, his wife. Arrangements were made in England to send out Thomas Rossiter as teacher, James Darve as miller, wheelwright, and smith, and H. J. Blinman as mason and plasterer. Of these new settlers, only Rossiter remained. Thus the new life of the Pitcairn colony was established auspiciously on Norfolk. The land was divided into fifty-acre allotments, one for each family. A thriving trade was commenced with the whalers, dripstones were manufactured from a suitable rock discovered on the island, and offshore whaling became a possibility where beaches were accessible.

* Nobbs continued as the spiritual guide of the colony on Norfolk until his death. He raised twelve children who in turn have helped swell the population of Norfolk Island.

HOME SWEET HOME

Even though some were tending sheep, some driving cattle, and two or three working the windmill, still others
were finding it difficult to forget Pitcairn and "home."
There are always such. Nowadays we have a glib word
for these people. And we call their nostalgia a fixation.
Towards the end of 1858, after a two-year trial of Norfolk, two families decided that they preferred to return
to their former home—to the Pitcairn they loved. These
were Moses Young with his wife and five young children,
and Mayhew Young and his wife together with seven
children. Of these last, six were the offspring of Mrs.
Mayhew Young by a former marriage to Matthew Mc-
Coy. The sixteen pilgrims took passage on the *Mary Ann*
and reached Pitcairn in January, 1859.

Aunt Mary Ann, who was one of the children returning to Pitcairn, told me that the little band arrived at the
island just in time, for, according to her tale, soon after
their landing a French man-of-war appeared with the
intention of claiming the abandoned island for France.
Having saved Pitcairn for the Empire, they climbed the
cliff eagerly anxious to see their beloved homes. But a
ruin faced them. Most of the houses had been destroyed,
the gardens had run wild, and desolation chilled their
hearts. Later the returning islanders discovered that during their absence on Norfolk a crew of sailors had landed
from neighboring Oeno, where they had been ship-

wrecked. That desert island offered no asylum, and the shipwrecked crew had made their way to Pitcairn only to find it abandoned. After living on the island for a short time, and tiring of the pastime of carving their names on the school benches, the shipwrecked sailors decided to construct a craft by which they might sail to Tahiti. The planks and nails of the houses were handy to their purpose, and, without much compunction, they wrecked what was necessary.

With fortitude and increasing joy, the little band of islanders fell to the task of rebuilding their dwellings and planting their crops. The plantations, fallow for more than two years, now yielded crops more abundant than ever before in the memory of that generation. The elder girls, profiting by Mrs. Selwyn's instruction, undertook to preserve among the younger ones the few elements of learning they possessed.

Five years after the arrival of the first lot, a second arrived. News of the successful resettlement of Pitcairn had reached Norfolk and stirred up dormant longings in others to return to the island of their birth. This time four families deserted Norfolk. These were Thursday October Christian, 2nd, wife, nine children, and mother-in-law (the aged Mrs. Young, *née* Elizabeth Mills, the only child of John Mills of the *Bounty*); Robert Buffett and wife; Simon Young, his mother Hannah (the daughter of John Adams), his wife, and their eight children; and finally a newly married couple, Samuel Warren and his wife Agnes Christian. The last man, Samuel Warren, was a sailor who had recently joined the colony at Norfolk. Hailing from Providence, R. I., he had found life among the islanders more seductive than that aboard a whaler. Throwing in his lot with the Norfolk Islanders, he married a daughter of Thursday October Christian, and when the latter decided to return to Pitcairn, daughter and son-in-law determined to accompany him. Samuel Warren left a large brood of prolific children who have in turn added to the island population. It was a grandson of old Samuel, Burley Warren, who was my devoted host on Pitcairn, and it was Burley's quarter of American ancestry that gave him first claim to a fellow American.

No dissuasion had any effect on the second lot, although much pressure was brought to bear on these diehards to remain on Norfolk. Amid sad partings which the participants knew were for ever, the little band of thirty-one set sail on the *St. Kilda*. They left Norfolk on December 18, 1863, and on February 2, 1864, joined their predecessors at Pitcairn. Thus in all forty-seven, about one quarter of the total colony, found their way back to the place from which they had started.

Unknown to the islanders ashore, the *St. Kilda* arrived at night with her load of homesick passengers. In the joy of reaching their destination and in their eagerness to announce their coming, a terrific din of shouts and musket fire was let loose to attract the attention of the friends and relatives ashore. But it had the unforeseen effect of creating stark terror in the hearts of the children and devastating dread in the parents. The next morning brought a doubled rejoicing—the removal of fear and the discovery of friends.

Among the newcomers was Simon Young, a man of superior parts and with a high sense of social responsibility. With a keen realization of the needs of the rising generation, he established a school, revivified the religious services, and in general took a leading part in guiding the growth of the tree cut back to its stump. Not the least of his influence was felt by his young daughter, Rosalind Amelia. This girl was the most apt of her father's pupils and ultimately became the most literate of all the children of Pitcairn.

The succeeding years were full of peace and calm, broken only by the visits of passing ships. As the years passed and with them the prosperity of the whaling industry, fewer ships brought the world to Pitcairn's shore. The time had almost come when Pitcairn once more was nearly as isolated as it had been at the beginning of the century.

In 1868, the Norfolk Islanders for the last time attempted to entice the Pitcairn Islanders to rejoin them. Their letters offered every inducement even to paying for the charter of a transport; but although some of the experimental youth were ready to try another trek, the conservative judgment of their elders prevailed, and the offer was refused.

The year 1875 was marked by two shipwrecks. The first was that of the *Cornwallis*, which crashed on the rocks of Pitcairn Island itself. The second took place on the nearby coral island, Oeno, where the *Khandeish* ran aground. One of the crew settled for a time on Pitcairn and married one of the women. This shipwreck of the *Khandeish* proved profitable to the natives, for the stories of their kind reception that the crew told on their return to San Francisco inspired its citizens to send to Pitcairn quantities of gifts, among them an organ which created great enthusiasm on the island.

So rapidly had the colony been increasing that at the time of Admiral de Horsey's call at Pitcairn in 1878, the population, consisting of ninety persons, had almost doubled itself since 1864.

In 1880 the islanders underwent a psychological experience that left a deep impression and that was regarded at the time as a "visitation." We are indebted to Rosalind Amelia Young for the account. Only eleven or twelve of the younger members of the colony were affected. The victim first became subject to hallucinations of a terrifying but unspecified nature. In some cases they heard voices calling. Then apparently exhausted by these emotional crises, the subjects were unable to recall the memory of past events, the power of speech was temporarily lost, and their faces froze into an empty rigidity as though the mind had flown from its abode. Usually the victim was not violent. A peculiarity often accompanying this state was the seeming transformation of large objects into miniature ones or the reverse, so that children grew miraculously to gigantic size and full-grown men shrunk to dwarfs.

The "visitation" was not confined to the natives alone. A shipwrecked youth, who was confined to the island until he might find passage on a ship, was also a victim. He began by seeing his mother's coffin pass above his head and out the window. Soon after he became oblivious to the world about him and lost the power of speech. When speech and consciousness returned, he started to seek an unjustly persecuted friend who had been thrown into prison. Later he was found by a search party at the opposite side of the island sleeping under a rock and rolled in a scout's blanket. At that stage, he was Davy Crockett on the trail of Indians.

The last case was the longest. One of the girls fell under this strange spell in 1884 and was not restored to normality until 1886.

No explanation of this series of mental disturbances has ever been offered. Once at a meeting of physicians, I cited these cases, and a friend of mine, Dr. Ramsay Spillman, suggested that a noxious weed might conceivably have induced the phenomena described. He cited the effect of the Jimson weed on the settlers of Jamestown who, unfamiliar with its qualities, became temporarily deranged on eating it. It is not impossible, however, that most of the seizures on Pitcairn might have been the result of suggestion. Such an explanation is probable when we remember the youth of the victims.

Three more outsiders joined the colony at this time when the *Acadia* was wrecked on Ducie Island, a coral atoll about three hundred miles away. When the *Edward O'Brien* arrived a short time after the shipwreck and removed the sailors, three elected to remain on Pitcairn. Two of these married Pitcairn girls, one remaining on the island, the other after three years returning with his wife and two children to Wales. The third man left by the *Acadia* aroused a hornet's nest by winning the affections of a girl already betrothed to an island man. The family of the fickle young lady was infuriated by this state of affairs and succeeded in antagonizing the chief magistrate against the newcomer, who was subsequently dismissed from the island at the first opportunity. Captain Clark of H.M.S. *Sappho* was the *deus ex machina*, and as a sequel to this affair he officially forbade, at the request of the islanders, all marriages with strangers. The law was afterwards amended to permit marriage with anyone whose admission might be deemed beneficial to the community.

In 1886, a major event in the religious life of the Pitcairn Islanders took place. John I. Tay, a missionary of the Seventh Day Adventists, came among them. This visit had been well prepared, for ten years earlier, Elders James White and J. N. Loughborough had sent to Pitcairn a box of literature concerning the tenets of the Seventh Day Adventists. These writings were regarded first with horror, then tolerated, and at last embraced. The islanders, always interested in churchly affairs and devoted to the reading of religious tracts, could hardly resist the temptation to examine the documents of this new sect. Nothing, however, was done to change their academic interest into one of active faith until the arrival of Tay in October, 1886. During a brief stay of six weeks he was able to persuade a large part of the colony to adopt the new articles of belief. A minority, however, at first refused to abandon the church of their fathers, thereby threatening a schism in the community. So closely knit, however, was the community that the reluctant minority wisely decided to adopt the new faith in order to preserve a unanimity in religious observances.

The islanders, ever sensitive to the opinion of their friends in England and America and fearful of criticism, were concerned about the reception the news of their conversion would receive. They were not long in waiting, for after the visit of H.M.S. *Cormorant* in 1887, they discovered that many "viewed with regret" and the rest lamented their religious "debauch."

Partaking easily of the prevailing opinion in the mother country, the Pitcairn Islanders had assumed with the most loyal of Englishmen a reverential attitude toward Queen Victoria. Prayers for her welfare were never forgotten, and inquiries as to her health and happiness were punctiliously made of all visiting British ships. None of her subjects bestowed a greater devotion on Queen Victoria than did these, the least important of them. It was, therefore, a labor of love for the islanders to add their mite to the bounty showered on the Queen on the occasion of her jubilee in 1887. A box of island curios together with a letter of presentation was prepared and dispatched to Her Majesty by the Pitcairn Islanders.

Queen Victoria, who took a keen interest in the colony, replied to their gift by sending a present of commemoration coins, ranging from six-penny to four-shilling pieces. These were distributed among the women and girls who cherished the token of their Queen's remembrance.

In 1890 the inhabitants celebrated the centenary of the settlement on Pitcairn. Although the affairs of the island were of no importance to the world, and the life of the community was but slightly affected by the historical events of the century; yet within the microcosm of the colony much had happened, and far beyond most isolated communities, this one had enjoyed the attention of the world. They had undertaken in a body two remarkable migrations. To their shores had come a long list of ships, many of them containing men distinguished in their day, and within their island they had suffered oppression and had experienced release.

To celebrate the one hundredth birthday of their community the islanders characteristically chose a hymn as the most appropriate form of verse in which to sing their thanks to God. The following was composed by a native and sung by the participants in the celebration:

Our Father, God, we come to raise
Our songs to thee in grateful praise;
We come to sing. Thy guiding hand,
By which supported still we stand.

To this fair land our fathers sought
To flee their doom their sins had brought,
In vain—nor peace nor rest was found,
For strife possessed th' unhallowed ground.

Darkness around their path was spread;
Their crimes deserved a vengeance dread;
When, lo! a beam of hope was given
To guide their erring feet to heaven.

The holy word, a beacon light,
Had pierced the shade of sin's dark night.
And poured a flood of radiance where
Had reigned the gloom of dull despair.

We own the depths of sin and shame,
Of guilt and crime from which we came;
Thy hand upheld us from despair,
Else we had sunk in darkness there.

We, their descendants, here today
Meet in thy house to praise and pray,
And ask thy blessing to attend
And guide us to life's journey's end.

Oh, that our lives henceforth may be
More consecrated, Lord, to thee!
Thy boundless favours to us shown
With gratitude we humbly own.

Thou know'st the depths from whence we sprung;
Inspire each heart, unloose each tongue,
That all our powers may join to bless
The Lord, our Strength and Righteousness.

The Pitcairn Islanders, eager for fresh tides rolling in from the world, were thrown into considerable excitement their centennial year by the news that the Seventh Day Adventist missionary ship, *Pitcairn*, was bound for the island where it would make its first "parochial" call. The visit meant more to them than visits of other ships, welcome as these were. It was a flattering recognition by the mother church and an unusual opportunity for religious and social diversion. The *Pitcairn* arrived on November 25, 1890, bearing Elders Gates and Read, their wives, and Mr. and Mrs. John I. Tay. The entire community was baptized, and a rich fare of theology was easily digested by the communicants. After a short visit the *Pitcairn* departed, taking three island men aboard.

In July, 1892, the ship was back again, and this time Elder Gates remained on the island. This gentleman injected into the quiet waters of Pitcairn life a current of activity which was strong enough to bear the burden of a class, a literary society attended by over forty members, and the first newspaper. This periodical had a somewhat collegiate name, the *Monthly Pitcairnian*, and consisted of laboriously hand-written pages. Its reportorial staff was overburdened by six news gatherers whose lack of activity explained their abundance. Rosalind Amelia Young, who no doubt was energetic and prolific in her contributions, described the paper as having its first page devoted to an original poem, followed by an editorial page over which Elder Gates presided. Moral and Religious Topics, the Home Circle, News Items, Pleasantries, and All Sorts constituted the remaining departments. It would be interesting to see a copy of Pitcairn's solitary journalistic effort, but I have never come across one. Perhaps they suffered the usual fate of all old newspapers.

The zeal of Mrs. Gates spent itself in schemes of dubious utility. She started a kindergarten according to the latest pedagogical methods; and perhaps from exuberance attempted to teach stenography to some of the young people who, wiser than their instructress, lost interest in the impractical endeavor.

Having disposed of their religious welfare, the islanders turned now to their political housekeeping. For some time they had wanted a change in the form of local government, and when H.M.S. *Champion,* Captain Rookes, arrived on October 3, 1892, the principal men of the group took the opportunity to consult with this official representative of Great Britain. The result of the conference produced this resolution and a modification in the number of government officials.

RESOLUTION

"Whereas, we have witnessed in the past, that thro' lack of strength and firmness, on the part of the government officers, some evil has resulted, and, Whereas, we believe that a larger number of officers would tend to make a stronger government, and that plans for the public welfare would be executed with better success, therefore,

"Resolved, that we heartily endorse the plan of having a government consisting of a parliament of seven, with power to legislate, to plan for the public good, to execute all decisions of the court, and to see that all public demands are attended to without unnecessary delay."

Then follow a list of duties pertaining to various offices and a list of laws. These will be described in detail later. The resolution with its attendant features was approved on January 1, 1893, by the voters.

This code and the administrative offices were modified later in 1904 and, with the exception of minor changes since then, have endured to the present time.

In February, 1893, the missionary ship *Pitcairn* again touched at the island. Mr. Gates took passage on this trip, but his place was taken by a newcomer, Hattie André. This young lady, fresh from college, had come to teach school on the island. She started classes for adults as well as for the children and very soon won the affection of the islanders.

When the *Pitcairn* departed, she carried a manuscript history of the island written by Rosalind Amelia Young. A daughter of the gentle and devoted Simon Young, she had inherited from her father a love of learning and a sweetness of character that still make her name blessed among the Pitcairn Islanders. Miss Young had literary ambitions and, besides the account of Pitcairn published by the Seventh Day Adventist Press, was also the author of numerous verses. She is the best example of a type common in the colony: a deeply religious nature schooled to a gentle and deprecating tolerance for the weaknesses of the less rigorously faithful members of the community. For the best part of her life, Rosalind Young continued her father's task: the teaching and guiding of the children. But in 1907, Miss Young married David Nield, a minister of the Seventh Day Adventist Church. The couple had met three years before at Tahiti, where Miss Young had gone to attend a church conference. This meeting led to a correspondence in which, says the Reverend Mr. Nield, "All points of Doctrine, Health Reform, Food, Ages, Business, and Mission work were carefully considered." Rosalind Young, emerging without blemish from this inspection, arrangements were made for her to join her prospective husband in Auckland, N. Z., where they were joined in holy wedlock. She threw herself into her husband's work and, until her death in 1924 while visiting Pitcairn, maintained a deep interest in churchly affairs.

At the beginning of the present century, Pitcairn was again an almost forgotten island. The whaling days with their stream of free-lancing ships had passed, the World War inhibited the visits of British men-of-war, and the opening of the Panama Canal diminished the use of the route around the Horn. Fewer and fewer ships paid their friendly calls. Rapid voyages and refrigerating systems eliminated the lure of the fresh vegetables that Pitcairn had to offer. This increasing isolation made the fewer visits paid the island greater events.

When Mr. and Mrs. Routledge called at Pitcairn on their yacht, *Mana*, in 1915, they were welcomed with enthusiasm. Two island youths, Edward and Arthur Young, shipped aboard the yacht and accompanied the Routledges to London. This sort of temporary seafaring was no novelty among adventurous Pitcairn boys. Bred to the sea and fearless of her moods, they make excellent sailors. Many of the older Pitcairn men now alive have traveled widely among the islands of the Pacific. The Youngs' sortie was, therefore, no cause for wonder, but seeing the United States and England was a bit of good fortune that made the two lucky ones the envy of their fellows.

Within the last few years, Pitcairn once more has been brought into more regular communication with the world. The New Zealand Shipping Company steamers on their way to and from Panama stop for about a half hour as a diversion for their passengers. The natives come out to sell their curios, and the passengers have an opportunity to inspect the "strange creatures" and to ask impertinent and ill-advised questions.

III. CULTURAL

EARLY VICTORIAN EDEN

The attention that Pitcairn has received during the last century and more arises mostly from the romance and the drama of its history and a little from the appeal that all isolated and lonely communities exert, especially when they are situated on a lovely Pacific islet. For some the chords of the imagination vibrate more readily to the story of the mutiny; others respond more keenly to the tale of crime and the toll of murder that accompanied the first days on Pitcairn. An older and more godly generation succumbed to the spectacle of redemption rising like a sweet flower from a dung heap. But varied as the human interest of Pitcairn is and wide as the range of emotions in its history, it has still another claim that has been strangely neglected. The very sequence of events which produced a unique and absorbing story in its own right also created, as a by-product, a social and biological experiment of profound importance. My desire to study the mixture of races on Pitcairn led to my earlier attempt to reach the island in 1923 and to my successful try about twelve years later. Therefore, I shall now turn to Pitcairn in its scientific aspect. In the present chapter, however, I intend to consider only the "social experiment."

Perhaps I should begin by explaining exactly what I mean by the somewhat pretentious phrase *social experiment*. Pitcairn was not the scene of a Utopia or an

Erewhon. No social or political theories stimulated its founding. But it was an unconscious and spontaneous experiment none the less. The problems it illuminates are those of culture contact. This is a phenomenon as ancient and as widespread as the existence of culture itself, and some of its more dramatic phases are represented by the contacts of European civilization with those of the native peoples with whom it collided during the European expansion of the last four centuries. Classic Attica itself was the fruit of a grafting of a sophisticated Cretan civilization on a rude Greek culture. So, too, the civilization of France has grown from the fertilization of Gallic culture by the seed of Rome.

America, North and South, illustrates dramatically nearly all phases of culture contact. The Europeans arriving on these shores came to grips with a preëxisting, firmly established population living according to a cultural pattern inimical or antithetical to that the invaders brought. The Europeans automatically proceeded to establish various types of contact depending on the character of their culture, the nature of the country, and reaction of the Indians. They came as exploiters, colonizers, conquerors, traders, and missionaries. As a result of these varied forms of impingement, some Indian tribes folded up and vanished, if not like a mist into thin air, then into the less favored areas. A few tribes resisted and were able to preserve their integrity. A great many resisted but were conquered and absorbed. Still others, and by far the most important, were normally conquered but never really digested by their conquerors. These last, however, unlike those who had vanished, or had been absorbed, integrated their native culture with that of their conquerors and are now undergoing a renascence of the utmost significance. The Mexican is such a rebirth of Indian culture. In the dynamics of culture the importance of the phenomenon is self-evident.

Similarly in Polynesia culture contact with Europeans, beginning in the eighteenth century, has had a tremendous effect on native life. Here the contact was largely trading and missionary in origin, and—I need not add—amorous. Military conquest has played a very minor part. And yet, except for Samoa and Tonga, where native life has been protected, Polynesian culture has been almost completely destroyed. The expert can still find a few fragments surviving into modern times, but to a Captain Cook the present culture would bear about as much resemblance to what he saw in the eighteenth century as would life in his native Yorkshire to that in Chicago. He would find the once sacred *maraes* now tumbled piles of rocks overgrown with brush and trees; he would recognize in the modern outrigger canoe a sad degeneration from the skill that built the ancient war canoes; he would see no connection between the modern Tahitian woman in her European clothing and the *tapa*-clad houri of his day.

At the risk of overwhelming little Pitcairn with these mighty examples, I have expatiated somewhat on this theme to illustrate a fact of great importance in all cultures. On Pitcairn, we see an experiment in culture contact—the impact of European, or English, civilization and Polynesian. It occurs, to be sure, on a small scale, but it is a reduction in degree only. Here we have a number of advantages for the study of the phenomenon. The situation has been simplified to its basic elements. Most of the imponderables which affect other foci of culture contact and the complex reactions that obscure the design are absent on Pitcairn.

The Englishmen and Tahitian women who set up housekeeping on Pitcairn were completely shut off from the rest of the world for eighteen years and practically so for the thirty-five years from the date of landing in 1790 to Beechey's arrival in 1825. The initial ingredients, therefore, in the Pitcairn pudding were allowed to set without an added pinch of salt from England or an extra spoonful of sauce from Tahiti. Moreover, the stigmata and the disabilities, invariably attached to such "experiments" as these, did not exist. No social pressure, no external economic forces, no cultural reinforcements were brought to bear.

In addition to the importance of isolation in this social experiment, there is the added advantage of contact not only between two divergent cultures but between cultures relatively well known. Between Polynesian and English customs there is a gulf as wide as the geographical distance which separates them. Such contrast makes the resulting pattern easier to decipher.

We must not neglect to point out still another element in this unique set-up. That is the attitude of the culture-bearers themselves. Today we have become familiar through novels and cinemas with Polynesia; or if not familiar, at least cognizant. The romantic literature of escape has inflamed the heated imaginations of countless readers, many of whom would be ready to abandon everything for a cocoanut tree, a blue lagoon, and a brown maiden, voluptuous if not fair. The inherited culture of such romantics would have but little chance against the Polynesian. The English sailor, however, of the eighteenth century, much as he might enjoy the comfort of Polynesian life, was not conditioned by his reading, if he ever read, to regard the adoption of Polynesian life as the highest good. Therefore psychologically the mutineers on Pitcairn were ready to put up a good strong plea for England and the way they did things back home. I regard this state of mind as an element of incalculable importance. Few realize the revolution in the attitude of the white man towards native people. Familiarity has brought not contempt but a greater tolerance and even an insight that has led to a more profound appreciation of the achievements of people once held hardly better than slaves.

Pitcairn itself should not be omitted in this description of the birth of Pitcairn life. The very nature of the island, the fruit and vegetables it produced, its climate, all contributed to the character of the new colony. Had the

Bounty wandered farther south to a more inhospitable island or to one whose aspect was less like Tahiti, the inherited lore of the women would surely have been less useful and therefore less effective in shaping the manners of the colony.

Pitcairn was settled by a group of twenty-seven or twenty-eight persons, consisting of nine British mutinous seamen, six Polynesian men from Tahiti, and twelve, or by some counts thirteen, Tahitian women. Consider what that meant. Here was a group of Englishmen, hardly knowing the simplest elements of the Tahitian language and totally ignorant of the unguessed subtleties of that speech. Nor was this the extent of their ignorance of Polynesia, for they knew next to nothing of Polynesian life, its conventional manners and customs, and its rich traditional lore for supporting existence—a knowledge which was second nature to their native companions. Living in a more complex civilization where the activities of life were more specialized and divided into compartments, they lacked the knowledge to reproduce it entirely, even had they wished to do so. But if the mutineers had cherished such an ambition, they would have been immediately discouraged. The little group was confronted by a world without tools, equipment, or any of the necessities with which we manufacture other necessities. Even the fruits and vegetables of the land and the fish in the surrounding sea were not the varieties to which they were accustomed at home.

On the other hand, the Tahitians, both men and women, found Pitcairn similar enough to their own beloved Tahiti to feel at home. Living habitually closer to nature and employing simpler means of obtaining their livelihood, they were less at a loss as to how to take up the same pursuits here.

With such a set-up certain eventualities are predictable. It takes no profound insight to see that the mechanics of living would be Tahitian in origin. *Tapa*-making, underground cooking, and basketry were merely Polynesian transferals. But even though the first settlers derived much from Tahiti, the English stamped their character on the community life. And to this were added certain original developments, in response to local conditions.

Before describing the life of the Pitcairn Islanders of today, let us go back a century or more, before contact with Europe and America had begun to change the habits of the islanders, to a period when their existence and customs represented the products of their inherited culture plus the ingenuity of their wit. We are indebted to Captain Beechey for the most nearly complete account of the island in those days and to others, too numerous to mention, for additional details.

Since the first things to capture the attention of the stranger are usually the material manifestations, I shall begin by describing those aspects of the Pitcairn of one hundred years ago. The village was unlike the present one. The first settlers and their children built their houses around a rectangular plot of level ground, like a village green. The houses bore no resemblance to anything ever seen before in Polynesia, having been built by the Englishmen who naturally turned to familiar models. A Polynesian house is a light structure, consisting of a framework lashed together and covered with thatch or mats. Those on Pitcairn were solid, substantial cottages with sturdy plank walls. But there the resemblance to English cottages ceased. Lacking nails, glass, cut stone, mortar, cement, and similar building materials, the ingenious mutineers overcame these obstacles by evolving a house like a tree rooted to the ground. The few that have survived the hand of the wrecker are still sound.

The following account gives a brief description of the principal features of these houses. Since cellars and foundation walls were impossible, large rocks were set at each corner with a few more at intervals between to serve as supports. On these the builders laid heavy, roughly dressed logs, into which they mortised square uprights. Besides one upright at each corner, others were set at regular intervals along the sides. The tops of these uprights also were tenoned into cross pieces. The sides of the uprights were grooved so that a wall could be added without nails, and boards cut to the proper length were slid into these facing grooves. Shutters made in the same way, tongue and groove, were built into slots and could be pushed aside in good weather or closed in bad. The roofs were covered by thatch made in the Tahitian fashion. This consisted of folding a series of overlapping pandanus leaves around a palm stem or a similar stick. These leaves were then secured by a long wooden sliver which joined all the leaves like a simple running stitch. Lengths such as these were then laid on the roof in neat overlapping rows and made a very picturesque as well as practical covering.

The interior usually consisted of one long room divided by one or two partitions. Bunks like those on ships were built along the inner wall, while on the opposite wall was the long row of shuttered openings. A few houses had an upper story used for sleeping and reached by a ladder through a central trap door. The houses naturally were unpainted and soon weathered to a pleasing soft gray-brown, which blended into the rich, green foliage surrounding them.

The climate made fireplaces unnecessary, and the houses had no chimneys. For cooking, an outhouse, less substantially built, was attached to the main house, and the wide cracks in the walls permitted the smoke to escape. Besides the bakehouse, other outhouses included a poultry shed and a pigsty.

The furniture of these locally modified European houses was naturally of a very simple order. Cabinet work is a special craft. The best results require practiced hands and a series of tools that the islanders lacked. What furniture was made, therefore, was crude but sturdy. But note that the models were English. It is easy to understand why. Polynesians sit and sleep on the ground; they even squat on the ground when they eat.

Except for beautifully woven mats their house interiors are bare and simple. But the mutineers were accustomed to postures which require chairs, tables, and beds, and they proceeded to manufacture these articles of furniture as best they could. The beds or bunks, built against the inner wall of the main room, were usually raised about eighteen inches from the floor. Furnished with mattresses, consisting of palm leaves and about three layers of *tapa*-cloth, they were not uncomfortable. To these the children of the household retired, the parents shielding their own quarters by a partition.

The main room, always on the ground floor even in a two-storied house, had a large table and stools as its principal furnishings. Strangely enough, mats so indispensable in a Polynesian household were not used on Pitcairn. But sea chests were common articles of household furnishings. They were requisite for the storage of *tapa* and the scanty clothes of European origin.

In the evening, which comes soon after six o'clock on Pitcairn, these snug interiors were illuminated by the faltering light of the *doodoee* or candle nut. The use of these nuts for lighting once widespread in Polynesia today still lingers on remote islands such as Rapa. The oily kernels were strung on the midstem of the palm leaf, and as one nut burnt low the next would be ignited, thus producing a candlelike illumination satisfactory except for the cracking and spitting that Beechey found disconcerting.

Having housed themselves in ingenious dwellings the construction of which was variously derived from English, Tahitian, and native resource, the islanders revealed less eclecticism and ingenuity in the matter of their garb. In one respect choice played no part. Woven cloth was not available beyond the limited supply with which they arrived. Some source of apparel was absolutely essential, for even though the climate of Pitcairn is benign through the greater part of the year, there are periods of chill and damp. Moreover, the nights are cool and fresh, and bedclothes are a necessity. Fortunately there existed on Pit-cairn the breadfruit and the paper mulberry tree whose bark is suitable for making *tapa*, a kind of paper cloth. In the manufacture of this fabric, the women, trained as good Polynesian housewives, were expert.

The technique of *tapa*-making consists first of strip-ping the bark from the paper mulberry or, in some cases, from the breadfruit tree. The essential inner bark is removed and soaked in water until it becomes soggy and the fibers loosened. Then, kneeling before a stout log, the women beat the pulpy mass to the appropriate thickness with a *tapa*-beater. This implement, about a foot and a half long, is square in cross section except for the round, smooth handle. The four faces of the working end of the beater are grooved with longitudinal ribbings of different thicknesses on the various faces, the coarser ones being used for the early stages and the finer ones for the final beating. The work was laborious and slow, and much of the women's time was occupied in making rolls of *tapa* not only for clothing but for sheets as well. Some of the *tapa* was dyed a rich red brown with pig-ment obtained by steeping the *doodoee* nut in water. Al-though the *tapa*-cloth was stiff when fresh from the beater, it acquired softness after the repeated washings that its toughness and durability permitted.

Lack of needles and thread may explain why the men were forced to abandon the use of trousers. Or, possibly, paper pants seemed a ridiculous solution, for on their first discovery they were disclosed in heathen costumes. The men wore, Polynesian fashion, a *maro*, which was simply a length of *tapa* passed around the waist, with one end drawn between the legs and then tucked in at the waist. This garment, though abbreviated, was very comfortable, modest, and convenient. In fact, even when European clothing had been introduced and was acces-sible to all the men, they frequently preferred to wear the *maro* when there were no visitors on the island.

The costume of the women, although more voluminous than the male attire, had a classic simplicity. A skirt or "petticoat," reaching from waist to ankle, was made by wrapping a length of *tapa* around the hips. It was then snugly secured by rolling down the top like the stocking of the erstwhile flapper.

Both men and women wore a subsidiary garment like the Tahitian *ahu buu,* which was simply a mantle thrown around the shoulder. The women dressed their hair like their Tahitian mothers, either braided or flowing unbound save for a wreath of flowers. Says Beechey, "It must be remembered, that these people, as with other Islanders of the South Seas, the custom has generally been to go naked, the *maro* with the men excepted, and with the women, the petticoat, or kilt, with a loose covering over the bust, which, indeed, in Pitcairn's Island, they are always careful to conceal; consequently, an exposure to that extent carried with it no feeling whatever of indelicacy; or, I may safely add, that the Pitcairners would have been the last persons to incur the charge."

Both sexes wore hats, for protection against the sun, cocoanut leaves and pandanus furnishing the fiber as in Tahitian hats. Friday October Christian, Folger's first visitor, had his headgear decorated with a black cock's feathers. And Captain Pipon, captivated by Pitcairn graces, exclaimed that the bonnets of the women would please a fashionable London dressmaker by their simplicity and good taste.

The women naturally took charge of another department of the island economy and practised an art acquired from Tahiti. This was the preparation and cooking of food. The principal method of cooking employed the underground oven—a device not unlike the clambake known and valued in New England. A pit was filled with stones and heated red-hot by a wood fire. After the embers had been removed, the meat or fish, wrapped in *ti*-leaves and surrounded by vegetables, was placed on the stones, and then covered by a matted layer of leaves and sticks. To retain the heat more effectively a final blanket of earth was placed over the whole. After an hour or two the removal of the covering layers revealed a superbly baked meal with all its delicate flavors retained.

Meals were generally prepared only twice a day, once late in the morning and again in the early evening after the day's labor. Such is the custom in Polynesia, and thus did the Pitcairn housewives plan their culinary labors. The main source of food was vegetable: yams, taros, sweet potatoes (*kumara*), pumpkins, peas, *yappai*, and sugar cane. In addition, there were abundant fruits such as bananas, oranges, plantain, breadfruit, cocoanuts, and watermelons. Once or twice a week fish was served and even more rarely meat, the principal source being the pigs which were kept in a sty adjacent to the house. Eggs, from chickens and from the sea birds that frequented the island at certain seasons, were another adjunct to the Pitcairn table.

Only one recipe for a blended dish has come down to us. It may be that on Pitcairn food was preferred in its simplest and purest elements. But it is more likely that the canons of the primitive Polynesian cuisine, which eschews mixed concoctions, also governed the Pitcairn kitchens. At any rate, I have discovered only one mixed dish. This is known on Pitcairn as *pillihai*, and is still in high favor on the island. It is made from boiled yams which are grated and mixed with cocoanut meat. The resulting paste is baked in a cake. A variant of this employs mashed bananas and cocoanut. These *pillihai* cakes are often sweetened with a molasseslike syrup extracted from the *ti*-root.

"Raw fish," a delectable dish that is widely appreciated not only in Polynesia but throughout Oceania even to Japan, seemingly was neglected in Pitcairn. According to the Tahitian ritual, the firm flesh of special species of fish is cut into small pieces, soaked for an hour or two in sea water flavored with lime juice, and then eaten with the fingers after each piece is dipped in a sauce of cocoanut milk. The more impatient Polynesians have been known to attack their fish while still wriggling on the hook. As the Russian yearns for *borscht*, the Marseillaise for the rich *bouillabaisse*, the Strasbourger for his *pâté* oozing goose fat, so the Polynesian craves raw fish. I have seen a look of positive beatitude on the face of a Samoan who, after months of deprivation, was able at last to satisfy his longing for this delicacy. It is therefore a matter of wonder that this form of fish consumption is absent on Pitcairn where raw-fish eaters controlled the kitchen. Had it once become established in the island diet, nothing could have shaken its hold, and it would have survived to this day among the islanders as one of the major requisites to the enjoyment of life.

Poë, another universally Polynesian article of food, is made by various methods in different parts of this island world. There is the breadfruit *popoë* of the Marquesas, the most obnoxious of all to the uncultivated taste. It is the habit, among these islanders, to reduce the breadfruit to a paste leavened with the yeasty remains of a more aged batch. Then after acquiring the proper ripeness in a subterranean pit it is served in a huge wooden bowl blackened by age and the polish of "poëy" hands. Just as the taste for it is a matter of cultivation, the trick of eating it requires skill. The participants, seated in a circle about the bowl, dip two fingers into the sticky viscous paste, the color of an ancient dish cloth, and with a practiced twist extract a mouthful which is adroitly speeded to the mouth, eagerly opened to receive it. The novice, however, requires a bath and a strigil after the banquet.

On other islands taro instead of breadfruit forms the base of *poë*. And in Tahiti *poë* has undergone numerous refinements to tickle the European palate. On Pitcairn, however, the only trace of it lingers, fittingly enough, in the name of the food on which infants are weaned. This, called *popoë* on Pitcairn, was a paste made from ripe plantains and boiled taro.

The principal beverage of the Pitcairn Islanders was and, for that matter, still is, water. Stronger drink had proved disastrous among the mutineers. William McCoy, lacking a more orthodox material for the exercise of his Scotch instincts, found a worthy substitute in the *ti*-plant, and his retentive mind reproduced from a youthful experience an efficient distillery that left an indelible impression on Pitcairn tradition. *Ti*-whiskey, if it may be so termed, was abhorred, and, until the contact with Tahiti had corrupted the islanders, never revived. Tea, however, brewed from the homonymic *ti*-plant was permitted. Milk was never used, although nanny goats were plentiful. Perhaps its flavor degenerates as a result of Polynesian grazing, or it may be that something in the Polynesian constitution finds it repellent; in any event, the natives esteem neither cows nor goats for their lactic glands.

Beechey thus describes a rather special meal prepared for him and the other officers visiting the island.

"The smoking pig, by a skillful dissection, was soon portioned out to every guest, but no one ventured to put its excellent qualities to the test until a lengthened Amen, pronounced by all the party had succeeded an emphatic grace delivered by the village parson. 'Turn to' was the signal for attack, and as it is convenient that all the party should finish their meal about the same time, in order that the one grace might serve for all, each made the most of his time. In Pitcairn's Island, it is not deemed proper to touch even a bit of bread without a grace before and after it, and a person is accused of inconsistency if he leaves off and begins again. So strict is their observance of this form, that we do not know of any instance in which it has been forgotten. On one occasion I had engaged Adams in conversation, and he incautiously took the first mouthful without having said the grace; but before he had swallowed it, he recollected himself, and feeling as if he had committed a crime, immediately put away what he had in his mouth, and commenced a prayer.

"Welcome cheer, hospitality, and good humour, were the characteristics of the feast, and never was their beneficial influence more practically exemplified than on this occasion, by the demolition of nearly all that was placed before us. With the exception of some wine we had brought with us, water was the only beverage. This was placed in a large jug at one end of the board, and when necessary, was passed round the table—a ceremony at which, in Pitcairn's Island in particular, it is desirable to be the first partaker, as the gravy of the dish is invariably mingled with the contents of the pitcher: the natives who prefer using their fingers to forks, being quite indifferent whether they hold the vessel by the hands or the spout."

One characteristic of a Pitcairn meal which caused considerable disappointment among the officers of the *Blossom* was the separation of the sexes. The women, as in Tahiti, never ate with the men, but took their meal afterwards. The officers had to be content to chat with the women who served them, standing behind their chairs brushing the flies away with whisks. To anyone accustomed to traditional Tahitian manners such a scene would be distinctly familiar.

The most important activity on Pitcairn as in other communities is getting a living. But the inhabitants of this island are more fortunate than the majority of mankind, for with moderate toil they reap rich harvests from the land and by what many men regard as a sport they garner food from the sea. The plantations on Pitcairn are situated on the rolling plateau that constitutes the roof of the island. In the early days of the colony, before there were enough men to till the fields, the women also shared the burdens of agricultural labor.

It is unfortunate that no description has come down to us of the details of Pitcairn agriculture. It would have been of interest to know more than we do of the agricultural techniques that sailors could evolve for raising food plants unfamiliar to them. One might reasonably assume that English seamen despite their calling would perhaps have had a little knowledge of the husbandry of English foodstuffs, but they could have known nothing of the cultivation of the Polynesian plants which constituted the crop on Pitcairn. On the other hand, the natives would certainly have been well acquainted with the methods of raising such plants as the taro and the *kumara*.

It is, however, clear that the agriculture of the islanders was primitive and that the foods were crude. Hoe culture appears to have been prevalent. Such refinements as subsoil ploughing were unknown. Fertilizer, however, in the form of seaweed had become a necessity after a couple of decades of intensive cultivation. Many fields yielded two crops a year, but since the soil was not carefully replenished or allowed to lie fallow it tended to become exhausted in later years.

The principal crops raised included yams, taro, and *kumara* (sweet potato). Planted in September, the yams usually matured by April or May. The taro, grown from young shoots, required somewhat special treatment. Aside from these plants, the island also produced the following foods which served as a welcome variety: breadfruit, cocoanuts, plantains, bananas, pumpkin, watermelons, peas, *yappai*, sugar cane, ginger, and turmeric. After relations with the world were established in the early part of the nineteenth century, a great variety of food plants were imported to the island to furnish a richer supply of vegetables. One other plant infamous in the annals of the island, the *ti*-plant, was extensively cultivated for its root and leaves. The root yields a sweetish liquor, like molasses, and the leaves were used both as fodder for goats and hogs and as food wrappers.

Fishing, like agriculture, was chiefly carried on by the men, although the women sometimes joined them. Usually once or twice a week, a day would be devoted to angling. To the nonfisherman the technique and lore of catching fish may seem the same the world over. But such is by no means the case. The Polynesian fisherman had evolved numerous specializations and a body of piscine knowledge that differ sharply from European methods and lore. In Polynesia, the extraordinary development of these traditions culminated in the famous "nights of the moon," a kind of almanac that guided the Polynesian angler. By following the "nights of the moon" he knew when and where to seek for certain fish.

On the other hand sailors, such as the mutineers, must have entertained rather definite notions about the best method of capturing fish. And such Tahitian developments as fish-spearing and stone fish-traps must have appeared strange to them. Unfortunately, few details are known of the fishing methods practised on Pitcairn before European contact.

It is known, however, that the first settlers made fish-hooks, presumably of European type, from the *Bounty's* iron. Fishing lines also were made on the island and even continued to be preferred by the islanders to later European importations, since their own product had less tendency to twist in deep water. The Pitcairn Islanders adopted the Tahitian method of spearing fish, both because of its appeal as a sport and because of its effectiveness in the hand of an expert. To this day they are fond of catching fish in this manner. The spear tipped with five prongs was a type borrowed directly from the Tahitians. Polynesians also lent the torch which attracted the fish and made them fall easy prey to a sure and deft hand. I can find no mention on Pitcairn of nets or stone fish-traps, both common in Polynesia. The rocky coast and precipitous shore may well account for the absence of the latter.

The common varieties of fish caught at Pitcairn were cod, gray mullet, red snapper, and a kind of mackerel. The agile women often captured squid and crawfish among the rocks on the shore.

The nautical skill of the Pitcairn Islanders is eminently appropriate to a people descended from British seamen and Polynesian women. They inherit from both sides traditions of maritime prowess. When the settlement was discovered in 1808, the islanders already possessed a native craft in the form of a dug-out canoe light enough for two men to handle. The *Quarterly Review*, quoting Folger, referred to a "double canoe," but aside from this single mention I have found no other indication that the Polynesian outrigger principle was in use. Unfortunately, Folger's own statement does not elaborate on the type of canoe he saw, and we do not know whether or not the outrigger was adopted by the Pitcairn Islanders. It is certain, however, that the type of craft first employed was a dug-out with or without an outrigger. Perhaps this was made as are those of the present time in two longitudinal sections joined along the keel and caulked with a resinous substance extracted from the banyan tree.

The skill with which these frail craft were handled astonished all visitors. Landing at Pitcairn when there is a bit of weather requires expert judgment and experience. Says Captain Freemantle, "The landing is particularly hazardous; it being rarely that a ship's boat ought to land. The natives are very clever with their canoes and will land in almost any weather."

In addition to these pursuits, the island men were accustomed to hunt the goats and hogs which after a few years had multiplied until they overran the island and created havoc in the plantations. To control the breeding of these animals the islanders resorted to keeping the males penned but permitting the females to run loose. Somewhat later, when barter with whale ships assumed considerable proportions, these wild goats and hogs became a valuable source of fresh meat for sailors weary of salt beef.

But life on Pitcairn was not exclusively devoted to agriculture, hunting, fishing, *tapa*-making, and household duties. Even though the islanders exhibited a reluctance in the company of strangers to engage in levity or light amusement, they were capable of frivolous pursuits. When Beechey pressed them to put on an entertainment, they complied but not without much giggling and shyness. The dance, Beechey concluded, was rarely enjoyed, but to entertain him the islanders organized one. A large room was prepared, and the performers "glowing beneath a blazing string of *doodoee* nuts" were arranged along one side of the chamber. Along the other side were ranged the musicians under the direction of Arthur Quintal who was seated on the ground before a large gourd. With his toes he worked a piece of musical wood (*porou*) and he beat the gourd with two sticks in his hands. With her hands Dolly beat a rapid tattoo on another gourd which had a longitudinal slit at one end. A third musician provided the bass on the copper fishkettle of the *Bounty*. The time was excellent and the coördination of the musicians perfect. To this rhythm, three adult women danced with shy reluctance, "as they consider such performances an inroad upon their usual innocent pastimes," adds Beechey. The dance, a decorously abridged version of a Tahitian one, was merely a kind of shuffling of the feet and a simple figure executed by passing each other, the whole being accompanied by snapping fingers.

During the performance Beechey remarked that some of the spectators were overcome by amusement, and that shyness paralyzed others from rising to join the dancers. Nor did this terpsichorean effort continue long, "from an idea," Beechey observes, "it was too great a levity."

Nor did the Englishmen's attempts to entertain the islanders have any apparent success. One of the officers brought out his violin and offered to play some tunes in order to stimulate the dancing, but the island women declined to respond. Nevertheless, the violinist presented a specimen of his art, but the performance, though well executed, did not produce the anticipated effect. "They had not yet arrived at a state of refinement to appreciate harmony, but were highly delighted with the rapid mo-

tion of the fingers, and always liked to be within sight of
the instrument when it was played. They were afterwards heard to say, that they preferred their own simple
musical contrivance to the violin." The unfavorable picture of the musical tastes of the Pitcairn Islanders drawn
by Beechey was further confirmed when they showed
no aptitude or desire to learn another tune than the single
one to which they sang all psalms and hymns.

However, I think that Beechey did the islanders an
injustice in his judgment of their capacity for music and
of their attitude toward the lighter diversions. No doubt,
before distinguished visitors they had a natural desire,
fostered by their religious training, to pretend to a
greater sanctity than they usually maintained. But shyness in the presence of strangers proved more effective
as a damper on gaiety. From Miss Young's descriptions
of a celebration held years later, it is clear that modified
forms of the Tahitian dance survived, indicating a continuous tradition. She speaks of the ancient Tahitian
ihara and *uri* which were known in her day.

As for the musical reactions of the islanders, it is difficult to measure innate musical sense. We must remember
that unaccustomed music often receives an ungracious
welcome even in cultivated musical centers. Later visitors reversed Beechey's judgments. They found the islanders singing intricate part songs. Carleton, in 1850,
declared himself amazed at their aptitude for choral singing. Indeed, the praise of the young and susceptible
Fortescue Moresby is fulsome. "They sang two hymns
in magnificent style; and really I have never heard any
church singing in any part of the world that could equal
it, except at Cathedrals."

Swimming was a favorite sport among both sexes. The
feat of swimming around the island, a circuit of about
seven miles, was common. One of their water sports, surf
riding, was of Polynesian origin. "To have a slide" meant
taking a surf board about three feet long, shaped like a
canoe with a small keel, which the swimmer held before

him as he dove into the sea. Swimming out from the shore, they would wait for a heavy sea. Then lying prone on the board, they were carried on the crest of the wave at a terrific speed hard on to the rocky shore. But just before disaster seemed inevitable, the rider would nimbly leap to his feet.

The younger part of the population was fond of kite flying, which was practised both in Tahiti and England, and they also found diversion in an undescribed game played with a ball.

But it was not only on these forms of activity that the mark of Tahiti or England was stamped. We find that even the domestic relations of the sexes also bore traces of the origins of the colony. In Tahiti, at the period of its discovery, although the women occupied positions of authority and enjoyed considerable freedom, they retired to an inferior status at meals. In Polynesia, women suffered ceremonial disabilities as well. They could not enter the sacred *marae* and in the Marquesas were forbidden to touch a canoe, so that Melville records with surprise that the female visitors had perforce to swim out to the ship carrying their vestments in one hand.

The only vestige evident on Pitcairn of the conventional status of Polynesian women cropped out in the aforementioned refusal of Pitcairn women to eat with the men, even at the invitation of their British visitors. The ceremonial concomitants were, of course, lost on Pitcairn where *maraes* were not held in reverence or canoes sacred. The rationalization of this custom on Pitcairn was drawn from Biblical sources. Man, said the islanders, was made first and ought, therefore, on all occasions to be served first. But this tradition did not reflect a genuinely inferior position of the women in the social structure of the island. In fact, the women, like their Tahitian ancestresses, took a leading part in social activities and did not allow themselves to be oppressed. They shared the labor with the men, even working in the fields before marriage. John Adams was said to oppose early mar-

COURTESY OF TEMPLETON CROCKER

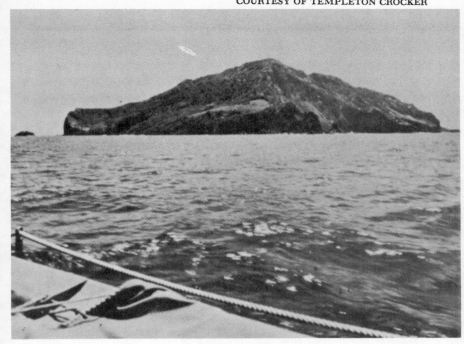

1   Pitcairn Island.

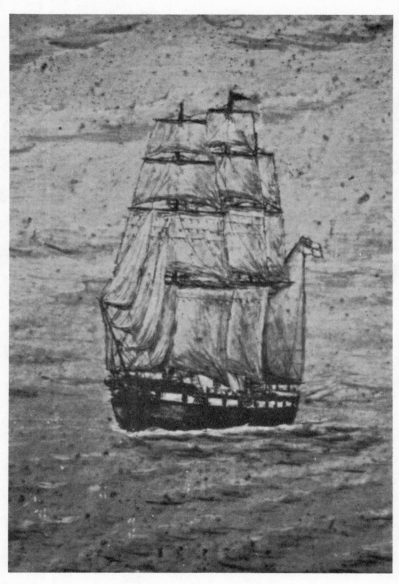

Drawing of the *Bounty*.

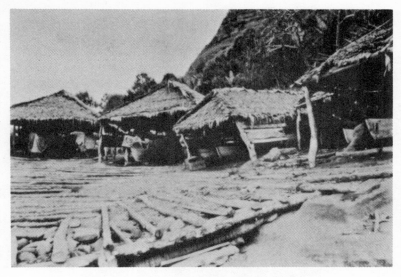

3a   Housing the Long-Boat at Bounty Bay.

3b   Fishing Dugouts and Long-Boats.

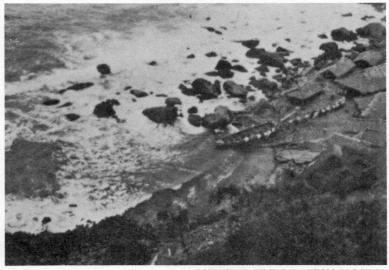

COURTESY OF TEMPLETON CROCKER

COURTESY OF TEMPLETON CROCKER

Adamstown, Pitcairn Island.

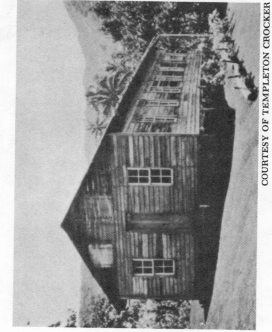

The Village School.

5b

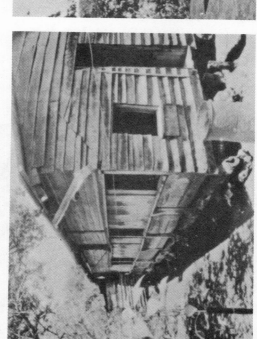

The Island's Oldest House.

5a

COURTESY OF TEMPLETON CROCKER

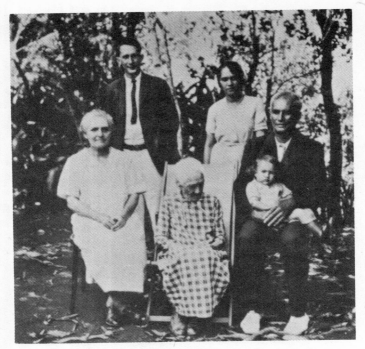

6a   Four Generations of Pitcairn Islanders.

6b   School Interior.

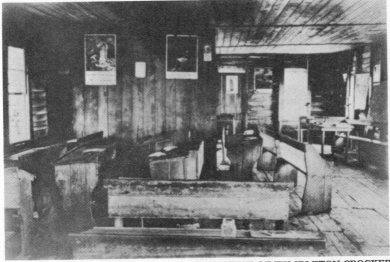

COURTESY OF TEMPLETON CROCKER

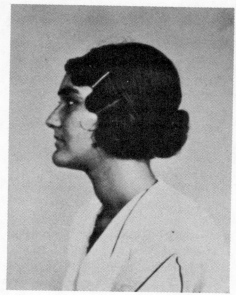

7a

Representing Pitcairn's Younger
Generation.

Burley Warren—the Author's Host
on Pitcairn.

7b

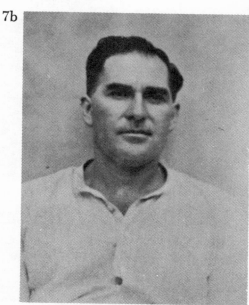

COURTESY OF TEMPLETON CROCKER

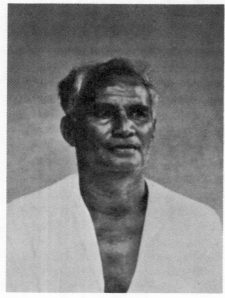

8a

Parkins Christian, Great-Great-
Grandson of Fletcher Christian.

Mary Ann McCoy—the Oldest
Woman on Pitcairn.

8b

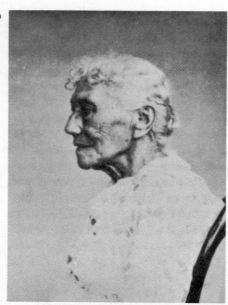

COURTESY OF TEMPLETON CROCKER

riages for this reason, since the colony was deprived of a necessary worker when a girl married. "When once they become mothers," said Adams, "they are less capable of hard labour, being obliged to attend to their children." And Captain Pipon observed, "One may conclude they would be prolific." Later when a more formal governmental machinery was organized, the equality of women was recognized by granting them full rights along with the men in voting for administrative officers of the island. This, let it be remembered, was at a time when European women still labored under medieval disabilities.

The effects of accident are obvious in the social organization of the Pitcairn community. The orgy of violence which accompanied the founding of the colony resulted in reducing the population to a handful of Tahitian women, their twenty-five children by the mutineers, and a solitary man, John Adams. The children, rendered fatherless while they were still infants or young children, had come to look on Adams as their father, their teacher, and their guide. In fact, the colony was like a large family with a patriarch ruling its destiny. We know the startling series of events which created this situation. It was unique and it had unique consequences. The community on Pitcairn was an indigenous growth, pruned by massacre and trained by circumstance to grow around John Adams.

Unlike the material aspects of the community which had been shaped while the mutineers were still living, the social and governmental life changed its character as the children grew older, developing a pattern like nothing in Tahiti or England. It grew into a framework which accident had created and as its tender tissue hardened it preserved the design of its mold like a Chinese cricket gourd. The absence of a code of laws or a crystallized tradition did not make any the less effective the conditioning of Pitcairn life. All the children were raised together, the distinctions between "my" mother and "your" mother were vague as they often are in Polynesia, and the parenthood of the one surviving man, John Adams, was extended to serve all the mites of humanity who were growing up in a strange world that was the most normal they could imagine.

Under such circumstances, it never occurred to the islanders to consider a machinery of self-government necessary while Adams was still living. Having been trained in infancy to accept his dicta unquestioningly, they continued to do so even after reaching adult years. And to the day of his death, John Adams ruled the colony. He might have justly said, if he ever glorified his community by calling it a state, *"L'état, c'est moi."* As a patriarch, he was just and kind, eager to do what was best for the common good, and as a leader, he was strict with himself in maintaining a standard for the conduct of his charges.

A true picture of Pitcairn social and family relationships would, of course, have to include the occasional difficulties, the rare disputes, and the infrequent bitternesses. The islanders were human. But the surprising thing is not the fact that such disagreements arose, but that they arose so seldom. The community, by universal testimony of its visitors, was remarkably harmonious and coöperative. The report of a Pitcairn idyll had elements of truth. "Adams assured his visitors that they were all strictly honest in all their dealings, lending or exchanging their various articles of livestock or produce with each other, in the most friendly manner; and if any little dispute occurred, he never found any difficulty to rectify the mistake or misunderstanding that might have caused it, to the satisfaction of both parties." Brodie contributed this description: "Quarrels and swearing were unknown amongst the islanders, who are as one large family bred up together; they are, in point of fact, all more or less related to each other, and look upon each other more as brothers and sisters than anything else. The children appear to be more nursed by their relations than by their mothers, which makes it often difficult to distinguish the married from the unmarried."

In times of stress or affliction, the entire population was always ready to render assistance, and this readiness reflected the warm ties of affection that bound the colony together. It was customary to wander into a neighbor's house as freely as into one's own. But unlike more sophisticated folk they deemed it a wrong to carry slander or gossip from house to house. Their homogeneity was so pronounced that it was a source of irritation to some visitors who were unsuccessful in extracting secret intimacies concerning the islanders.

Such a social pattern, common origin, and intimate family relationship inevitably led to a complementary attitude towards personal property. A Pitcairn Islander felt free to borrow a tool or a book from his neighbor without formal permission. But real property was not so loosely held. On arriving at Pitcairn, the mutineers had divided all the island, except the village and the common, into nine equal shares: one for each Englishman. The Tahitian men received no land, since their position was little better than that of servants. These allotments, held privately, were inherited equally by all the children of the family. The system eventually led to glaring discrepancies and hardships. After several generations the members of prolific families found themselves in possession of scraps of a divided and redivided estate, whereas the children of smaller families had considerable holdings. Indeed, the situation became acute enough to form a barrier to the marriage of some of the young people who could neither support a family on their inheritance nor sell their labor.

Not only was the land held privately, but the very rocks on the shore were also in the possession of various families. These rocks were of value for fishing and for the collection of sea salt which was an important element in the island economy.

In addition to personal and private property, certain

properties were held in common. The village and the green were owned jointly by all the community. But of greater interest in illustrating the foresight of the islanders was the general reserve supply of food and other articles maintained by the community. Food and other requirements were issued on account to any individual in need of them, to be repaid later. Or for an article in the common store which he lacked an islander might exchange something from an abundance in his own supply. Salt for fresh provisions, and vegetables and fruit for poultry, were typical exchanges.

We turn now to another aspect of Pitcairn life which developed in response to local conditions, *i.e.*, education. To use this dignified word for the informal instruction that the children received, carries perhaps too great a connotation of fixed curricula and prescribed training. It is true that, after the arrival of Buffett and Nobbs, a school was established and a regular system of education inaugurated, but at this period—the first thirty-five years of the colony—the education of the children had not yet reached such comparative perfection.

The responsibility of imparting instruction in reading and writing fell upon Young and Adams. Young had had a good education, but unfortunately he died in 1800, soon after undertaking the task. This left Adams with the duty of instilling the rudiments into tender minds. He could hardly have been more ill-fitted for the position of schoolmaster. Adams learned to write only near the end of his life, and indeed always read with difficulty. But persistence won out, and the children were able eventually to decipher the Bible. Some few principles of arithmetic completed the course.

After the arrival of Buffett and Nobbs in the second decade of the nineteenth century, the school system acquired greater formality as well as enhanced efficiency. To accommodate the steadily increasing number of scholars a schoolhouse was erected under Nobbs' direction. Attendance was by this time compulsory for all chil-

dren between the ages of six and sixteen. It is worthy
of note that compulsory and universal education, such as
it was, existed on this isolated scrap of land long before
it was ever enforced in most of the civilized lands of the
day. In fact, the islanders enacted a law to this end. The
enactment also required that the children be able to repeat the alphabet before entering school. Mr. Nobbs held
school from 7 a.m. to noon (the hours were changed at
various times) on all days except Saturdays and Sundays. The tax to support the school system was one
shilling per child per month. Since the sale of provisions
to an occasional passing ship provided the only source
of revenue, money was scarce. The canny island legisla-
tors therefore provided a list of equivalents which might
be accepted if shillings were not available.

One barrel of yams	8 shillings
One barrel of sweet potatoes	5 shillings
One barrel of Irish potatoes	12 shillings
3 good bunches of plantains	4 shillings
One day's labor	2 shillings

To insure the salary of the schoolmaster, it was also
provided that a parent could not escape the tax by removing his child from school. The tax was imposed for
each child within the age limits whether or not he or
she attended classes. Mr. Nobbs must have been in considerable demand as a godfather, since he was in the
habit of instructing his godchildren without charge.

The curriculum about 1850, although later than the
period under consideration, is not without interest. Each
day began and ended with "prayer and praise." Mon-
days and Tuesdays included a recital of weekly tasks, a
reading of Holy Scriptures, writing, arithmetic, and class
spelling. Wednesdays were devoted to history and geography. Thursdays were a repetition of the fundamentals
of the first two days. But Friday was the busiest day of
the week. On this day the scholars were asked to tran-
scribe words together with their meanings from Walker's

dictionary; hymns and other devotional and moral poetry were read for their edification; Watts' and the Church Catechism were repeated; and finally "arithmetical tables" and "emulative spelling" completed the full day.

Under such tuition the islanders acquired a facility in the fundamentals. Visitors, on whose reports we must depend, were lavish in their praise of the progress achieved by the Pitcairners. To illustrate the literacy of some of them I have culled bits from a letter too long to quote in full. It was from a Pitcairn Island woman to Admiral Moresby soon after the removal to Norfolk. She writes: "I cannot express my joy on receiving the kind letter you sent me by the *Iris,* and I heartily thank you for the scolding you gave me, and I only wish it was from your own dear lips. . . . And now I must tell you about our new home. . . . When we first came on shore everything looked strange to us, but it did not last long. Some of our people like Pitcairn best, but I think Norfolk Island is much better. We have such beautiful houses and gardens, which give lots of employment to keep them clean, and we have milked the cows and made butter. We have our men employed in the field, and I assure you they have enough to do. Norfolk Island is a much healthier climate than Pitcairn, although it is colder. We do not go so thinly clad as formerly, and I believe we are improving in everything; in fact, we are having everything after the English fashion. It is a great advantage for us to be so near the colonies; for we can easily get what we want. . . .

"The report you heard about our young men going to Sydney for wives is false, for there are many already engaged, and they are still preferring their countrywomen. . . . Dear, good, little Forty (Fortescue Moresby) has again come to see us. . . . Old times, and old associations and recollections, came vividly to my mind, and I did, in a measure, live over again a few of those happy hours spent at dear little Pitcairn. If you could only fancy to yourself a road some three and a half miles in length, with only two solitary persons upon it at first, and then one, and another, and another, and so on until half the population was hanging around, kissing and shaking hands, and expressing their joy in a thousand different ways, you may form some idea of Forty and his retinue, from his landing at the back of the island to the settlement. The delight at meeting was mutual. We were delighted, and so was Forty; but he had the worst of it— he saw and can learn for himself how all his Pitcairn friends are; but we, poor things, had to press him with a thousand and one questions concerning our very dear friends of the *Portland*. He was, I am sure, bewildered with the shower of anxious questions heaped upon him, and by the time he went to bed his patience must have been severely taxed. . . ."

In one respect I would hazard the guess that most prophets would have been wrong had they attempted to forecast the future of the Pitcairn colony from the circumstances surrounding its founding and from the characters of the founders themselves. Nor was there anything in the cultural background of the settlers or in the nature of the Pitcairn environment to foreshadow the spiritual characteristics of the mutineers' descendants. Most people would have predicted a dire end for the nascent population. Indeed, the feeling that the Pitcairn Eden was not a logical outcome of the planting of cutthroat mutineers was partially responsible for the great interest the civilized world showed in the news of its discovery.

After Staines and Pipon in 1814 greeted the Pitcairn youths on their coming out to the ship, they proceeded to quiz the young men, impatient to learn what they could of the island.

QUESTION: "Have you been taught any religion?"
ANSWER: "Yes, a very good religion."
QUESTION: "In what do you believe?"
ANSWER: "I believe in God the Father Almighty," and so on through the whole of the belief.

QUESTION: "Who first taught you this belief?"

ANSWER: "John Adams says it was first by F. Christian's order, and that he likewise caused a prayer to be said every day at noon."

QUESTION: "And what is the prayer?"

ANSWER: "It is: I will arise and go to my Father, and say unto Him, Father, I have sinned against Heaven, and before Thee, and am no more worthy of being called thy son."

QUESTION: "Do you continue to say this every day?"

ANSWER: "Yes, we never neglect it."

From this it is evident that Fletcher Christian had planted the first seed of religious observance on the island. How much of John Adams' subsequent zeal sprang from Christian's example, it is impossible to say. It is traditional that Young, too, before his death in 1800, had begun to impart religious instruction to the children. This Adams continued. Another tradition, previously mentioned, has it that Adams had several visions in which the fury of hell was depicted so vividly that he came to realize the necessity of saving the young Pitcairn Islanders from such a fate.

But whatever impulse may have moved him, the fact remains that Adams was the principal religious mentor of the community. To his congregation he was able to read chapters from Holy Writ, and for guidance in ritual he referred to a prayer book salvaged from the *Bounty's* library. So eager did Adams become to follow the letter as well as the spirit, that coming upon a reference to Ash Wednesday and Good Friday and recalling from a remembrance of things past that these were fast days, he decreed that Wednesday and Friday of every week be observed by abstinence from food. After John Buffett's arrival, the unnecessary regimen for these days was pointed out. Influenced perhaps as much by the strain under which his docile disciples had been laboring as by the error of his calculations, Adams was persuaded to give up Wednesday as a weekly fast day. He could not, however, bring himself to relinquish Fridays also. Habit had become too strong, and until his death the Friday of each week was scrupulously set aside as a day of fasting.

One of the observances most carefully maintained among the islanders was the saying of grace before and after every meal. Staines' and Pipon's youthful visitors from the island piously and distinctly pronounced, "For what we are going to receive the Lord make us truly thankful," before partaking of the food offered them. This simple and sincere grace made a deep impression on the Englishmen. Beechey, in a passage already quoted, observed the faithful adherence to the same custom.

John Adams was nominally an adherent to the Church of England, but since his acquaintance with ecclesiastical ritual was very limited we must conclude that the version of that Church's articles of faith and ritualistic practices that he attempted to foster among his charges was a very inadequate reproduction. The following is the dignified prayer preserved in his own quavering script, which he used for the Lord's Day Morning.

> *Suffer me not O Lord to waste*
> *this day in Sin or folly*
> *But Let me Worship thee with*
> *much Delight teach me to know*
> *more of thee and to Serve thee*
> *Better than ever I have Done Before,*
> *that I may Be fitter to Dwell*
> *in heaven, where thy Worship and*
> *Service are everlasting   Amen.*

After the arrival of Buffett in 1823, the conduct of the religious welfare of the islanders was entrusted to him. Nobbs' arrival in 1828 brought another and more permanent change. Nobbs by virtue of his superior education and greater ambition replaced Buffett and introduced services more nearly like those of the Church of England. The reader may remember that eventually

Nobbs was taken to England where he was ordained a priest after some months of instruction. But this takes us to a later period when the original adjustments of Pitcairn life were undergoing modifications.

Beechey's account is the only nearly complete one for this early period, and we must rely on him for our information concerning the details of the religious observances during these first three decades of the colony's history. It is impossible to know how much was the result of Buffett's influence, for he had already been settled on the island about two years at the time of Beechey's visit.

Each family both in the morning on rising and in the evening at sunset assembled for hymn-singing and family prayers. Again, before retiring, the family was accustomed to collect in the main room of the house for the same purpose. In addition to these collective pious observances, each individual offered up a private prayer before going to sleep. On the Sabbath the entire day was given over to devotion: prayers, reading, and meditation. No work of any kind was permitted. Beechey attended the church on Sunday and discovered that Adams read the prayers and Buffett the lessons. Hymns preceded the service. He observed that the congregation showed close attention, even the children evincing "a seriousness unknown in the younger part of our communities at home."

The loyalty of the islanders to their sovereign was scrupulously displayed by prayers for his welfare offered during the litany. "Adams," comments Beechey, "fearful of leaving out any essential part, read in addition all those prayers which were intended only as substitutes for others." The sermon which followed was delivered by Buffett who repeated it three times in order that none of it be "forgotten or escape attention." Finally the service was completed by the singing of hymns first by the adults and then by the children.

All told, the community assembled five times on Sundays, for religious purposes. Such a plethora of devotional exercises argues either a very sincere belief, fostered and cultivated by Adams, or a substitute for the absence of a more varied social life. It may have occurred to the reader from the anecdotes previously quoted that a strong taint of sanctimony flavored all this hyper-religiosity. And as far as one can judge from miscellaneous accounts, such an impression seems justified by the actions and words of a few of the later islanders. It would have been a natural result, it seems to me, of the hyperbole showered upon them by their visitors for their simple and sincere faith. Pride in worship and eagerness to inspire a repetition of praise are an insidious pair of human traits. But at this period, the islanders were still fresh in their contact with the world, and their devotions must be regarded as sincere and free from cant.

All christenings and marriages on the island were performed by Adams. Only one ring existed, and this Adams used for each couple whom he joined in holy wedlock. With a religious training and tradition borrowed directly from England, it would naturally follow that such a socio-religious institution as marriage would also be derived from the same source and that the paganism of a Tahitian marriage would not be tolerated. The license traditional among Polynesian youths before marriage was abhorrent to the islanders.

The foregoing outline is illustrative of a culture adjustment which spontaneously flowered from the grafting of one culture on another. It has been my purpose to emphasize in this chapter only the first view we are vouchsafed of the island and its life, leaving to the following chapter a description of the present-day Pitcairn Islanders. And it has been my aim to indicate what the Pitcairn Islanders, through the media of their mothers and fathers, adopted from their culture-heritage, why these particular customs, manners, or objects were selected, and, finally, how they responded to situations which were novel and which required original solutions. Certain clusters of culture traits were borrowed from either Tahiti or England because of the dichotomy of sex. All the women were Tahitian, and most of the men, notably all of the dominant ones, were English. We should expect that such a division of cultural background, when associated with sex, would inevitably mean that the occupations of the women would be borrowings from Tahiti and that the activities of the males would be influenced by English usage. Such a simple explanation, however, does not always hold water. It is true that cooking, *tapa*-making, and like activities were merely Tahitian transferals. But the exigencies of life on Pitcairn, its lack of the necessities with which to reproduce English implements, and its exotic character enforced a different pattern upon the masculine contributions than we might have anticipated. The better to appreciate the significance of Tahiti and England in developing the characteristic life of the first generation of Pitcairn Islanders, I have prepared the following table. For each culture trait on which I have sufficient evidence to make a judgment I have indicated its principal source.

	TAHITIAN	ENGLISH	ORIGINAL
The Household Arts:			
Underground oven	x		
Food preparation	x		
Tapa-making	x		
Use of calabash	x		
Dress style	x		
Hats	x		
Houses:			
Building materials		x	
Structure		x	x
Roof thatch	x		
Arrangement			x
Household equipment:			
Furniture		x	
"Linens"	x		
Lighting	x		

	TAHITIAN	ENGLISH	ORIGINAL
Fishing:			
Gear		x	
Methods	x	x	
Boats	x		x
Agriculture:			
Tools		x	
Methods	x	x	
Family life			x
Social life:			
Social organization			x
Separation of sexes at meals	x		
Position of women			x
Dance	x		
Music	x	x	
Surf-riding	x		
Kite-flying	x	x	
Private ownership of land		x	
Common fund			x
Education		x	
Religion		x	x

Summarizing the situation by this method, it becomes apparent that the Tahitian contributions outweighed the English. For reasons already mentioned this is not unexpected: Pitcairn is more like Tahiti in its resources; the Tahitian women coming from a simpler plane of life were more efficient in adapting their culture to its new home; the Englishmen conditioned by specialization and hindered by the absence of the necessary materials were less able to draw upon their own background for contributions to their new existence.

But the most unexpected findings of this survey concern the relatively large number of original adaptations to the exigencies of Pitcairn life which this handful of people developed on a pinhead of land. Merely to list some of them is impressive: the original architecture, the modified Tahitian canoe, the patriarchal social organization, the development of a community chest from which an individual could draw and by which inequalities in production could be equalized, the position of women, which in spite of certain Tahitian conventions, permitted them greater freedom than was customary in the age and allowed them equal franchise and inheritance rights, and, finally, a simple but personal faith that evolved from a crystallized, conventional religious system.

In their small way and without placing on their frail structure the weight of a top-heavy analogy, these developments of culture integration and fertility on Pitcairn are consistent with the conclusions of students of culture who have found that culture contacts are prolific in producing new combinations and original contributions. As race-crossing in nature reshuffles the genes and opens new possibilities for gametic pairings that result in a richer variety in the offspring, so the impact of cultures may, and often does, produce evidences of originality even under unfavorable circumstances.

THEY EAT THE APPLE

Over a century has elapsed since the days I have been describing in the last chapter—one hundred years of immense consequence to the Pitcairn colony. In the beginning came the whalers. A dribble at first, only a ship every other year. Then the numbers increased until 1846, when forty-nine ships in a single year called at Pitcairn —an average of almost one a week. In these ships came the articles of the civilized world: pots, pans, tools, cloth, knives, forks, plates, books, and pictures. And with their coming, the few simple, homemade manufactures of the islanders departed.

Less tangible but more profound in their consequences, however, were the subtler influences of English and American ideas and attitudes. These have tended to convert a simple, carefree people into a very self-conscious one. I don't mean to imply a generally unpleasant quality. Strangely enough, for a community unaccustomed to the attention of the world, the Pitcairn Islanders behaved extremely well under the spotlight of public notice. And among the present-day islanders, there are a large number of well-poised, self-contained individuals whose demeanor is full of dignity. But the naive charm of unspoiled children has vanished. And one does encounter islanders who are unpleasantly eager to impress the visitor with their sophistication or who are too anxious to reflect the standards of the outside world—

with a conspicuous lack of success. Fortunately they are few, even though the impression they make lingers in the memory.

But European and American contacts were not the only forces remolding Pitcairn life. The population increased by leaps and bounds. Birth control was unheard of during the early days on Pitcairn, and huge families were produced generation after generation. Population pressure grew to the point where release was sought, first in the abortive and disastrous movement to Tahiti and then in the mass hegira to Norfolk Island. But this concentration of inhabitants had other consequences; the old patriarchal order became inadequate, and the value of private property was enhanced.

Still another significant influence on the community was exerted by the newcomers to the colony—the three Englishmen in the 1820's: Evans, Buffett, and Nobbs; and later the three Americans: Warren, Coffin, and Clark. These men brought in new ideas and foreign methods.

Even though whaling contact declined after the middle of the last century until Pitcairn returned to an isolation almost as profound as in the beginning, nevertheless the changes wrought were fixed, and today life on Pitcairn is different from what it was a century ago.

But all things are relative. While Pitcairn was undergoing its modification, the world of America and Europe was experiencing even more radical innovations and alterations. Therefore, today Pitcairn remains as relatively simple to the modern world as its prototype of a century ago did to the early nineteenth century voyagers.

The first thing visitors to Pitcairn notice about the inhabitants is that they wear European clothes. Why the traveler should be mildly disappointed by such a costume is not difficult to explain. The sentimental voyager likes to see native people in no clothes at all or in picturesque garb. But the experienced traveler in Polynesia knows that practically all the natives now take pride in their imported clothing and that *tapa* is a thing forgotten.

Fortunately for the Pitcairn Islanders, they can secure cast-off clothes from passing ships. But to the despair of the women most of these are male garments. Nevertheless, the women have another source of supply. Friends of the colony in England and America occasionally dispatch bundles of clothing which are distributed to the various families. One woman on the island made a comment that will strike every woman as pathetic. She told me that she had never had a new dress or enjoyed the feminine ecstasy of selecting a dress for herself. But conditions are not quite as desperate as this sounds. Money earned from the sale of curios sometimes permits a housewife to order material by mail. The children, of course, are clothed in hand-me-downs retailored to suit their diminutive proportions. Jewelry was rarely displayed during our visit. Homemade necklaces of seeds are common, but they are usually reserved as gifts to visitors. Occasionally a frangipani flower is stuck behind the ear, but wreaths are never worn although I saw some made.

Sewing by hand and by machine is a general accomplishment since the nondescript clothing received on the island usually requires revamping. The few antiquated sewing machines I saw often served a number of families. The art of dressmaking was introduced by foreign women. In whaling days, wives of the skippers sometimes took long voyages and Pitcairn was often a favored spot at which to deposit, until the return trip, a wife who either had become fatigued by the privations endured on a whaler or had become *enceinte* and required the ministrations of her own sex. Such occasional visitors, usually New England women, introduced not only sewing but other household and culinary arts. These culture-bearing functions have in more recent times been the by-products of the visits of missionaries and their wives. Two articles of local dress are, however, still manufactured on Pitcairn. These are the hats nicely woven from bleached pandanus leaves and the slippers made of canvas and rope soles, like the canvas shoes of Southern France.

Having read the old descriptions of Pitcairn life, I was immediately struck, on landing, by another change. The snug, fitted houses of the first settlers were no longer in evidence. They had with a few exceptions been destroyed around 1857 or 1858 by a shipwrecked crew who had dismantled them during the absence of the entire community on Norfolk Island. With the timbers taken from these sturdy houses, the desperate sailors constructed a boat in which they reached Tahiti. Other houses, replacing these, were then built on more conventional models and I was successful in discovering vestiges of only a few of the previous habitations. But the remodeled structures, built to suit the altered needs and standards of their present occupants, still retained enough of the features described by Beechey to make their discovery a distinct delight.

Nowadays Pitcairn dwellings are frame houses on whose walls rough boards are laid in overlapping courses like huge clapboards. The roofs are covered by corrugated iron and the interior is covered with fitted planks like match boards. The windows are furnished with glass. One story high, these dwellings by accretions often acquire a careless shabby charm. The unpainted exterior weathers to a rich brown and gray that harmonize well with the deep red brown of the soil and the mature greens of the foliage.

The interiors lack any regular plan, each house having its own arrangement. Usually there is a living room, a dining room, and a varying number of bedrooms. A few living rooms are decorated with wall paper, now tattered, but most of them are modestly and neatly painted either white or blue. The floors are covered with wide hand-sawn boards.

The kitchens are always in an attached shed where the ovens and fireplaces are kept, the remaining outbuild-

ings consisting of a privy and storage or work sheds.
Plumbing, of course, does not exist. Water is carried by
hand from a spring or more often from a stone-lined
vat. Most houses have such storage tanks where the rain
water is conducted by a flue from the corrugated iron
roof.

The lumber used in construction is cut and dressed on
the island. A rough elevated platform serves as a mill.
The sawyer lays the logs on this structure, standing on
the openwork scaffold, and with the aid of an assistant,
saws out planks which are later trimmed to the purposes for which they are designed.

Hammers, saws, chisels, planes, nails, and other house-
building equipment are imported. The ancient *Bounty's*
anvil which has rung to blows of generations of Pitcairn
mechanics is used now mainly for repair work and as an
historic monument. Its adamantine back no longer serves
for beating out homemade tools.

The furniture of the Pitcairn home is a mixture of late
nineteenth-century importations and of native manufacture. Chairs, tables, old harmoniums, and bureaus from
England and America have flooded the island, making
the living rooms and bedrooms look as though they had
been furnished from an unpretentious suburban attic.
The only note of distinction is the heavy sea chests,
products of native craft. Burley Warren, adept in handling wood, has in his house beds which he made himself. Unadorned and sturdy, they added a peasant
quality to an interior otherwise notable only for its
gimcrackery.

Needless to add, the other household paraphernalia,
linens, dishes, cutlery, are all cheaper varieties of well-
known articles. As means of illumination the *doodoee* nut
has now been superseded by lamps and kerosene. And
the drums and musical wood have been replaced by the
victrola, several of which blare raucous music from ancient, scratched records.

I was struck by a curious lack of any innate decorative

impulse. An occasional print, a picture from an illustrated magazine, or an illuminated text sometimes adorns
a wall. But neither on the exteriors nor in the interiors of
their dwellings do the islanders apply any native art.
This absence of aesthetic development has a curious
parallel in the relative inferiority of both the English
among European peoples and the Tahitians among the
Polynesians in graphic or plastic expression.

In the kitchen, perhaps more than in any other department of Pitcairn life, one still may see the lingering influence of Tahiti. It is true that flour, once unknown, has
brought in the use of bread and the oven. Each kitchen
possesses a large squarish chamber built of stone and set
up on a support. A coat of cement makes it air-tight, and
with an iron door added it becomes a satisfactory oven.
The old underground oven, though not used as widely
as it once was, has not yet completely lost favor. An open
fireplace and an iron pot-rest, however, remain the principal apparatus for cooking food.

When first partaking of a Pitcairn meal, the foreign
visitor tends to confine his choice to those dishes most
like the ones to which he is accustomed at home. His
selection would be based indubitably on aesthetic considerations. *Pillihai,* the most characteristic of Pitcairn
dishes, is not a confection designed to make the mouth
water. It looks heavy and soggy, and it is. But its flavor
is not unpleasant after several trials. The island recipe
requires either bananas and *kumara* (sweet potato) or
taro. The *kumara* or taro is grated on a peculiar grid
which consists of a flat stone deeply scored by crossing
lines, thus leaving stony elevations that reduce the vegetable to small fragments. Cocoanut milk, from the grated
meat, is added to the bananas and *kumara,* and the resulting doughy mass is baked in a shallow pan and
served cold. *Pillihai,* I suppose, once took the place of
bread, and it remains a favorite even though bread is
now available. Another native preparation, arrowroot
pudding, contains cubes of pineapple.

The Pitcairn table is heavily laden with food, mostly of vegetable origin. The more recent additions to the vegetable resources of the island include potatoes, cabbage, squash, manioc (cassava), carrots, beets, corn, onions, and radishes.

Being observant Seventh Day Adventists, the more devout eat only vegetables, although some weaker vessels occasionally succumb to temptation and consume fowl, fish, and goat-meat. Pork, however, once the principal flesh food, is now regarded as an unworthy food. All the pigs, it is said, were killed so that the temptation to eat their succulent flesh might be removed. One wonders if a huge pork banquet was prepared from this slaughter— the last porcine orgy.

Fruits such as oranges, lemons, limes, pineapples, bananas, watermelon, grapes, wild strawberries, rose apples, breadfruit, passion fruit, melons, custard apples, pawpaws, mangoes, and guavas include recent importations and are numerous and very good. Bananas are sometimes hastened in their ripening by being buried for forty-eight hours between layers of pandanus nuts covered by earth.

Even to this day the islanders abhor intoxicants. None were to be seen, and no one privately dropped a word that a wee drop might be good for the health. As a matter of fact, the islanders are as abstemious in respect to drink as to food. The standard bearers of the community disapprove of coffee and tea, confining themselves instead to pure water or "tea" steeped from bran husks. Since milk is not particularly relished the goats are not milked. Cows do not exist on the island at all, although well-meaning friends have several times shipped cattle to Pitcairn. Eggs are a staple food.

The meals I ate on Pitcairn were varied and except for the native dishes mentioned above were prepared in a manner similar to our own. Soups, boiled and baked vegetables, and, for my benefit, roasted goat-meat, fowl, and baked fish were on the menu. Pie—an odd New England touch—was a favorite dessert.

As in most communities the principal activities of the men are directly concerned with getting a living, the chief Pitcairn occupations being agriculture and fishing. The upland plateau is devoted to the former activity, although small gardens are also found on the lower reaches of the island near the settlement. In consequence of divisions of inheritance, the plantations have been cut up into a large number of individual plots which from a distance present a pleasant pastoral design of a kind familiar in many agricultural areas. Since no horses or other suitable beasts of burden exist on Pitcairn, plowing and harrowing are unknown. Spading and hoeing are the agricultural methods employed, and fertilizing with sea weed used to be practised and may still be in use.

Fishing, on the other hand, has become less important as a means of livelihood. The methods already described are still used, although hooks and lines are no longer made locally. One of the commodities most in demand from the store of the *Zaca* was fishing tackle. With a couple of men to each little dugout, the native fishermen cruise the coast in pursuit of the red snapper, rock cod, tuna, 'cuda (barracuda), and kingfish. Many of the local names for fish are still Tahitian in origin: *faafaia, upapa,* and *manue.* The last named is always caught by spearing. *Pickpick* and *whistlin'* and *dotter* are Pitcairn names for varieties of fish I could not identify. Shellfish, however, are not gathered by the islanders, since that form of sea life is not approved by the dietary regulations of their church.

In this connection mention should be made of the islanders' boats. Besides the light dugouts, they have some heavy whale boats of which I counted at least four. Both types are made by the natives and are worthy of high praise. Sometimes they carry sails. The dugout is mainly used for fishing since it can be easily managed by one or two men. It is usually eighteen to twenty feet long and thirty to thirty-four inches wide. It has a narrow keel and a flat bottom. The wood employed in its fabrication is obtained from the *doodoee*-nut and the *toonena* tree.

The dory, on the other hand, is modeled after the whale boats which were used by the whalers of the last century. The frame is constructed of native *purau* wood, and imported pine is employed for the planking. The oars for the big boats are imported, but those for the dugouts are made locally. In these sturdy craft the men make voyages of ninety miles to Henderson Island for the *miro*, a kind of wood favored for cabinet work. I have already commented on the ease and skill with which these heavy boats are maneuvered. Perhaps unfortunately, we had no opportunity to see the skill of the Pitcairn men put to a really severe test, since the weather was unusually fine during our visit. Nevertheless, what the natives regarded as a mill pond seemed to me to be fraught with numerous hazards, and I was grateful for their experience and their prowess. For protection against the weather the boats are housed in sheds on the beach. They form a clump of picturesque, thatch-roofed structures that are the first to greet the eye on "entering" Bounty Bay.

Besides these occupations, one finds the men engaged in a variety of chores. The goats tethered to the house post or penned in an enclosure must be fed and the *ti*-plant leaves gathered as fodder. The chickens have to be cared for and their eggs gathered. Ducks and turkeys are raised. Wood for the kitchen fire must be replenished and expeditions made to the wooded hill-slopes for timber. Coming down the steep hill-paths, I would frequently see an islander with his specially constructed, underslung wheelbarrow heaped high with knotty lengths of firewood. Then there are the repairs to the house that require attention and odd jobs that are too numerous to list.

The making of sugar or, rather, molasses is an intermittent activity. The press with its four huge spokes is housed under a huge open shed where the sugar cane is pressed and a thick molasses extracted. Lumber-cutting is carried on in quantity only when a house is under construction.

About once a year each family organizes an expedition to Tauma on the opposite side of the island where it boils salt day and night for two weeks. Great stacks of wood are piled high to keep the fires constantly banked. Sea water is let into wide shallow pans beaten out of corrugated iron and as the water evaporates in steam a deposit of salt is left behind encrusted on the pan.

Finally, the spare moments of the day are devoted to the turning, carving, inlaying, and polishing of wooden objects: cups, boxes, walking sticks, and other curios that are made to be sold on passing ships. The early accounts of the islanders mention this craft. On an occasion briefly noted in a previous chapter, an elegantly inlaid box with drawers was sent as a birthday gift to Queen Victoria. Small hand lathes are used for turning the cups. At intervals I would catch a glimpse of Burley busy at his work bench, cutting thin strips of orange wood for inlay and polishing the red *miro*. This last is a species of wood of very tough texture, once common on the island, but now almost exhausted.

After finishing their household duties, the women, too, have their moments of leisure, during which they occupy themselves plaiting hats and baskets. Pitcairn women plait baskets as countrywomen used to knit socks—automatically. With hardly a glance at their work and without interrupting their conversation, they deftly twist and turn the long fringe of pandanus fibers until the finished basket seems miraculously to flower from its own strands. In spite of their skill in basketry, mat-weaving is not carried on today. I was struck by the designs on the baskets which I learned were rather recent adoptions and not native inventions.

The constructive talents of the islanders are most ambitiously embodied in their public buildings which take three principal forms, aside from the tithe house, the boat-houses, and the sheds that house the smithy and cane press. The most imposing is, fittingly, for so religious a people, the church. It stands firmly rooted despite its sagging lines, which are due both to settling and to a slight departure from the true in the original construction. It is a two-story building with a rectangular ground plan. I had no opportunity to measure its dimensions, but some conception of its size may be formed by the fact that each side is long enough to accommodate eight windows on each story. A modest porch adorns the façade and leads into a small hall with a staircase on each side. Both floors are fitted out as meeting rooms for religious services, but the first floor is the principal one and is somewhat more pretentiously decorated. A series of round wooden pillars extends down the center aisle, on either side of which are arranged the pews— simple, unpainted, wooden benches. The pulpit stands on a rostrum on one end of which is the reed organ that supplies music during services. Hanging on the wall back of the pulpit is a huge map indicating the centers of Seventh Day Adventism throughout the world. On the side wall there is a print of a Melanesian black bearing the name: "James of New Hebrides," and below the portrait is the legend: "174 natives are now employed by us." Presumably in missionary endeavors. The light blue pigment with which the walls and the pillars are painted, adds a touch of color to the room. The upper hall, equal in size, is similar to the lower one.

Outside the church door a bell hangs from a wooden crossbar supported by two uprights. Its resonant and peremptory voice calls the inhabitants not only to church, but summons them for various other group activities such as road-work, public assembly, and manning the boats, or for any emergency that requires the people's effort or voice. Each duty has its allotted number of strokes so that the purpose for which the bell is tolled is immediately known to the entire settlement.

About a hundred feet away from the church stands the courthouse which, with the church, forms the opposite sides of a square that occupies a terrace overlooking the road about six feet below. Along the road side of the square is a long bench where one may sit while waiting for church or assembly. Here the islanders are accustomed to linger for a little gossip after services. The fourth and inner side of the square is formed by a denuded terrace on which perches the house of the recently deceased Philip Coffin, an American settler from Nantucket. This square is the community center of Pitcairn.

The courthouse is but one story high and smaller than the church, yet sufficiently commodious to seat all the adults. A veranda runs along almost its entire length. The interior is roughly finished, with one end partitioned off by wooden bars behind which the postmaster functions. During our visit the recovered rudder of the *Bounty* was visible here through the bars. As in the church, rows of backless benches provide the seating accommodations.

Just outside the door is the community bulletin board. Here was posted the list of voters eligible to cast a ballot for the candidates whose names were recorded alongside.

The third of the public buildings is the schoolhouse. Like the other two community structures, it is of relatively recent date. Standing apart from the church and courthouse, it is without exterior distinction. The interior is a large open room about fifty feet long, equipped with benches for the students and table-desks for the masters. The walls are hung with religious texts.

The social organization of Pitcairn, as far as I could judge in a brief visit, has undergone considerable changes, though it preserves a distinct flavor reminiscent of earlier descriptions. The patriarchal system of John Adams' day was, after all, the product of peculiar circumstances which could not well survive as conditions became more normal. As the children grew to maturity, mated, and produced offspring of their own, the natural tendency to split up into separate family units was not only desirable but necessary. Consequently, after Adams' death a system of family units was fully formed, ready to be released from the restraints of the patriarchate.

It must not be assumed from this that the young couples chafed under Adams' rule. On the contrary, the combined power of custom and of Adams' kindness and concern for the common weal was sufficient earnest in the minds of the islanders of his right to assume authority. As a matter of fact, the harmony of the Pitcairn Islanders was one of their greatest charms. More practically, it was one of the prerequisites to a tolerable life on so constricted an island. At present the inhabitants form family groups just as among us with, however, somewhat greater intimacy between the various families. This closer cohesion is natural. Not only do the islanders live in a geographically tight settlement where privacy is not easily maintained, but they all own a common origin, have a common tradition, and by constant inbreeding share the same ancestors.

Family life is consequently very informal. Young Edward, seeing a light in John's and Mary's house as he passes, just drops in and without a word sits down, may or may not join the conversation and may as unceremoniously depart. Similarly, Henry may decide on the spur of the moment to invite himself to a meal in progress at David's house. A place is made for him at once, without surprise and without question.

Under these circumstances, secrets, family or personal, are not easily concealed. The transgressor is known, and he (sometimes she) must suffer the judgment of the community. Some laxity or, by a kinder name, tolerance tempers this group control. A noticeable change has affected the sex morality of the community. The days when the virtue and chastity of Pitcairn women were recognized as inviolable by the hard-boiled crews of whaling ships have disappeared. Illegitimacy in the early part of the nineteenth century was unknown except in a couple of instances. All this has changed in the last fifty years. Practically 25 per cent of births at present are illegitimate and a considerable number of the permanent unions are not legitimatized, even though they may have produced large broods of children. The evidence of greater sexual freedom is shown by comparing the age of the women at marriage with their age at the birth of their first child (see Chapter 10). It is to some extent a distortion to consider some of these births illegitimate even when the parents have not been legally married. Extra-legal unions, as permanent as the legal variety, have been contracted, and are regarded as just as binding in the eyes of the community. Such marriages might well be considered as an expression of a community change in procedure and not as evidence of an alteration in attitude towards sex. But besides these respectably "illegal" matings there are many examples of a roving taste in sex relationships. The older members of the community are well aware of the change occurring among the younger people, and they lament the breakdown of the older *mores* in terms that seem very familiar. Not even Pitcairn has escaped the problem of the "younger generation."

Family life on Pitcairn is generally very harmonious. I know of only one exception. Divorce in a legal sense does not occur among the islanders, although in one or two instances a working agreement was reached by which the partners in marriage were able to lead their own lives.

Despite the greater publicity of family life than that to which we are ordinarily accustomed, it would be erroneous to conclude that no privacy exists at all. In practice it is usual to find each family carrying on its functions as a unit without undue inspection from the neighbors. Besides the biological and social cohesion of the family, there is, of course, the economic and the religious. The land is inherited through the family, and the labors of the family are devoted to its own maintenance.

As for the religious functions, each family conducts prayers together. In this rite, it is usual for the wider circle of the family to join forces, that is to say, grandpa and grandma, with all their married children and grandchildren, may congregate for hymn-singing, reading the Bible, and the joint offering of prayer.

I was interested to find that a disconcerting remnant of Tahitian custom—the separation of the sexes during meals—had vanished. Captain Beechey would no longer be annoyed by the absence of the ladies from the table, were he to visit Pitcairn now. And his younger officers would be able to continue their enjoyment of island beauty even during the meals. There is no recognition of any social or political distinction between the sexes. Nor is the position of women economically disadvantageous. They inherit property on equal terms with the men.

Land, as has always been the case on Pitcairn, is privately owned and may be disposed of as the owner sees fit. This also applies to houses and personal property, although in practice real estate transactions are very rare. Public property includes the church, the courthouse, the schoolhouse, the roads, the spring, and—take note—the boats. I consider this last an interesting extension of the limits of public property. If one speculates why this should be so, the size of the whale boats and the necessity of large crews to handle them immediately suggest the corollary of group ownership whenever the social pattern favors such a solution. The small dugouts, manageable by one or two men, are, on the contrary, the property of individual families.

Education has made vast strides on Pitcairn since the days when John Adams laboriously framed with hesitating lips the Biblical words by which he instructed the young in the mysteries of reading. A commodious building now houses the forty-four school children of Pitcairn. They have four teachers and are provided with textbooks which have been sent out to the island. The master of the school is Roy Clark. His father, Lincoln Clark, while a cabin boy was wrecked in 1881 on Henderson, an uninhabited island near Pitcairn. When he was rescued by a passing ship, he left his shipmate, Philip Coffin, an American like himself, behind on Pitcairn. Lincoln Clark returned to the United States, married, and begat a son. In 1906, after the death of his wife, Clark determined to return to Pitcairn which persisted in his memory as an island paradise. After some difficulty, Clark and his sixteen-year-old son, Roy, landed on Pitcairn. The father married an island woman and sired another family. Roy very easily adjusted himself to Pitcairn life and now with increasing years has taken on the responsibilities of a leader of the community. As elder, he conducts religious services, and because of his superior education in American schools he has been appointed schoolmaster. For his services in the school, Roy Clark receives £3 quarterly. The three other teachers are Pitcairn Islanders, educated in the island school. One has a quarterly stipend of £2 while the other two, of whom one is a woman, receive £1 10s. The general running expenses of the school are provided by church funds.*

According to Clark, my informant with regard to the school system, the curriculum reaches the level of the fourth grade in New Zealand. Reading, writing, and arithmetic are the principal studies, and history, geography, and kindred subjects are taught to the older pupils.

All children between six and sixteen years of age are required to attend school. On the whole, in the opinion of the master, the children are neither very eager nor apt pupils. But this opinion is based on a limited teaching experience. Evidence on the other side cites one of the island boys, Richard Christian. Eager to pursue his education, he left Pitcairn for New Zealand where he en-

---

* Since my visit to Pitcairn some changes in the educational system have taken place, and new teachers have replaced those I knew.

tered college, and, according to a report received by his parents, was doing satisfactory work.

As part of the education of the islanders the influence of their reading matter is enormous. Newspapers somewhat out of date but none the less acceptable are secured from passing ships. Books, frequently of a religious character, are received from abroad. And numerous magazines of the popular American variety and of the illustrated English type are often seen in the houses of the island. All these help to form a picture of world activities which has a more than ordinary appeal for the Pitcairn Islanders. They are interested in world events and eagerly questioned us on the possibility of another world war.

Their favorite reading has naturally kindled a desire in many of the young men to see the world. A surprising number have been off the island, voyaging mostly to New Zealand and Australia, though Polynesia also has come within their orbit. Some of the more ambitious and enterprising have established themselves permanently abroad. It was difficult to obtain accurate estimates of the number who have migrated, but twenty-odd would probably include all living emigrants.*

After school hours Pitcairn children have a variety of games and amusements. They fly kites much like ours but with banana-bark tails. Tops are easily manufactured by sticking the stiff midrib of the cocoanut leaf through a *doodoee* nut. It is spun like a spindle by a quick twist across the palms of the opposed hands. Swimming is a favorite sport of the children, but rarely of the adults. And surfing by lying prone on a small board is likewise a diversion of the young, as well as the more formal game of cricket. On New Year's Day there is an annual boat race—an occasion for considerable rivalry and merriment.

I frequently have been asked what the Pitcairn Islanders do in case of illness. They do exactly what any

* The number living off the island today is very much greater.

very isolated doctorless community does. They have a variety of home remedies, native herbs, infusions of ginger and of the *ti*-plant, and a small supply of standard pharmaceuticals. A few of the more skilful islanders are summoned when their services are required. If the complaint is a minor one and easily diagnosed, there is ordinarily no difficulty, but for serious illnesses nature takes its course, and the patient dies or recovers. They see the working of Providence when the surgeon of a passing ship can be secured for an ailing islander. Cases demanding surgery are, if possible, reserved for the ministrations of a ship's physician. Acute attacks of illness such as appendicitis find the islanders completely helpless. Fortunately these are rare.

The presence of Dr. George Lyman as physician on the *Zaca* was a great boon to the islanders who lost no time in making use of his presence. He was besieged by the elderly sufferers from chronic conditions common to old age and by the possessors of warts, encysted splinters, benign tumors, and such like, eager for minor surgical operations. On the whole, he found the islanders very healthy and free from any endemic diseases. The ailments for which he was consulted are of a kind that might occur in any random lot of Europeans of equivalent ages. His diagnoses included high blood pressure, cancer, osteomyelitis, fibroma, asthma, arthritis, varicose veins, arteriosclerosis, and tuberculosis.

Recently the islanders have been able to repair their dental defects. A New Zealand dentist, Cooze by name, has settled temporarily on the island. His membership in their church brought him into contact with them, and he determined to visit the island in search of health. Equipped with a rather primitive dental instrumentarium, Mr. Cooze has found a rich field for its use. He has furnished most of the islanders with sets of false teeth which not only have improved their appearance but also have increased their masticatory efficiency.

The tradition of piety for which Pitcairn was famed

has continued in full flower, even though to some the flower may seem slightly overblown. The naive and un-adorned faith of the fathers has been replaced by a more self-conscious observance of religious rites. I do not wish to suggest that the islanders are insincere, for that would be utterly untrue. After witnessing their moving devotions no one can doubt the conviction that fills their hearts. But it seemed to me that religion had become formalized and, in some of its observances, mechanical.

The theological tenets held universally by the islanders are those of Seventh Day Adventism. The reader will recall that Pitcairn received a visit from John I. Tay in 1886, after the inhabitants had absorbed a box of Seventh Day Adventist literature which had been sent before his arrival. The community was baptized in a body, and Seventh Day Adventism replaced the faith of their fathers exactly a century after the landing of the mutineers on Pitcairn.

Among the articles of faith of Seventh Day Adventism to which the islanders, as devout believers, adhere is the belief in the imminent second coming of Christ. For that reason reports appear in the press at more or less regular intervals that the Pitcairn Islanders have ceased to cultivate their plantations from the conviction that Christ is due on a date close at hand. The islanders expressed to me a mild resentment at these misinformed rumors. But being the victims of more than one distorted news story, they have learned to adopt a resigned attitude towards the newspaper clippings they receive concerning themselves. I have already mentioned another precept they all obey faithfully: abstinence from pork.

The Sabbath on Pitcairn is celebrated, according to the custom of the church, on Saturday by three long services. Sabbath school at 7:30 in the morning, services again at 11 a.m., and young people's service at 3:30 in the afternoon. On the Sabbath I spent at Pitcairn there was in addition a quarterly business meeting held at 7:30 in the evening. Besides these Sabbath services, church meetings are also conducted during the week. Family prayers complete the list of formal religious observances.

Tithes constitute a final and interesting feature in the religious life of the islanders. Most of them are punctilious in their contributions which ordinarily take the form of garden produce. Money obtained from the sale of curios is also frequently added to the regular tithe. The fruits and vegetables received are stored in a small wooden building known as the tithe house. Except for a small proportion sold to passing ships, these perishable articles of food merely rot away.

Managing the affairs of their church as well as the temporal concerns of the island has given the islanders excellent training in the technique of democracy. Just as the town meeting in New England was one of the closest approaches to true democracy, so the community meetings for church affairs and for governmental matters on Pitcairn are genuine expressions of the popular mind. Accustomed to rise and state their views, both the men and the women are clear and forceful speakers, undisturbed by public attention. Self-government dates back a century. Up to the time of Adams' death in 1829, there was no formal machinery of any kind for self-government. It is said that Adams, foreseeing a troubled future without his established and accepted control, urged the adoption of some sort of mechanism for self-government. Nothing, however, was done until the tragi-comic dictatorship of Joshua Hill awoke the islanders to the necessity of a formal government to protect their rights. After the removal of Hill, Captain Elliott, H.M. sloop *Fly*, established a form of government that permitted the islanders to conduct their affairs with decorum and legality.

It was provided that a chief magistrate be elected annually on the first day of the year. Only a native of Pitcairn Island was eligible for office. The candidate receiving the greatest number of votes, cast by every islander and every resident of five years' standing, over the age of eighteen, was to be duly appointed to the office. The duties of the office were to exercise the chief authority on the island and to settle all differences which might arise between various members of the community. In these functions the chief magistrate was advised and assisted by the council, consisting of two members, one elected by the islanders, the other appointed by the chief magistrate. The officials were answerable in the fulfilment of their vows to the commanding officers of visiting British men-of-war.

The following oath was a solemn part of the induction into office. "I solemnly swear, that I will execute the duties of magistrate and chief ruler of Pitcairn's Island, to which I am this day called on the election of the inhabitants, by dispensing justice and settling any differences that may arise, zealously, fearlessly, and impartially; and that I will keep a register of my proceedings, and hold myself accountable for the due exercise of my office to Her Majesty the Queen of Great Britain, or her Representative. So help me God."

Continuing the history of the present government on Pitcairn, we are indebted to Brodie for the contents of the code of laws which existed in 1850. He cites ten regulations besides a number of other rulings by which the island theoretically was governed. Aside from defining the conduct and the prerogatives of office, they exposed what were matters of public concern and what in the opinion of the natives required formal regulation. It is interesting to note that the increasing number of American ships calling at Pitcairn had brought about the substitution of dollars for shillings in the currency of the island and in the value of fines. The first law stated precisely the duties of the chief magistrate. He was to convene the public on occasions of complaint and after hearing both sides to commit the affair to a jury. He was to levy all fines and direct all public work. Only with the sanction of the people might he assume power or responsibility beyond that which was assigned to his office.

The second law concerned dogs. The owners had to pay a fine of a dollar and a half if their pet was found chasing goats; a dollar to be given the owner of the goat and a half dollar to the informant. The latter reward might have been a temptation to abuse, but we have no record of the existence of professional informants. Full damages, however, were exacted from the owner of the dog if the goat were killed.

Cats were regarded highly on Pitcairn. The third law protected them by imposing corporal punishment on children up to ten years, if they were guilty of killing a cat. If the offender were older, from ten to fifteen, he had to pay a fine of twenty-five dollars. This time the informer was to be rewarded by half the proceeds. The offense became a very expensive luxury for anyone over fifteen, since the fine was then raised to fifty dollars.

Unpenned swine must have constituted a definite hazard to agriculture since their rooting habits could easily undo the hard labor of months. Therefore, the owner of a plantation was entitled to keep a pig caught trespassing on his property or to collect damages from its owner if he had actually caught the animal *flagrante delicto*.

The law regulating education has already been given in full.

A number of laws were grouped together under "miscellaneous." They ruled that an islander desiring to cultivate any lands had to give proper notice of such intention. To prevent waste the wood left over after completion of a house had to be turned over to the next man who began a similar undertaking. The cutting of timber was so carefully controlled that people had to get permission to fell trees on their own property. The slaughter of "white birds" was punished by the fine of one dollar for each bird killed. Birds killed to provide delicacies for the sick were excepted.

The malicious, if there were any, were severely fined on Pitcairn. "There shall be no bringing up things that are past to criminate others, with a view to prevent justice with the case before the magistrate," runs the law.

Reckless cutting of the *miro* and the *purau*, the principal timber on the island, had already so decimated the supply that special steps were taken to protect these trees from further wasteful destruction. Accordingly, it was forbidden to cut the *miro* or the *purau* except for building purposes. Nor could the more cunning attempt to circumvent this regulation or seek to lay up a supply against a future shortage, for the law expressly provided that on the third year from the time a person began to cut wood for a house, he had to build it. But if the house is not begun, then the authorities may confiscate it for the benefit of the next builder.

Landmarks are important in defining the boundaries of private property, and on Pitcairn the magistrate was instructed to inspect them at least once a year, replacing all those destroyed.

Frequent reference has been made in this book to the lively intercourse with whaling ships in the middle decades of the last century. Although the simplicity and kindness of the Pitcairners were completely disarming and the crews on the vast majority of these vessels behaved towards the islanders with respect and affection, nevertheless it was necessary to regulate the mutual relationships. The sale of spirits was absolutely forbidden ashore, and no one was permitted to bring any on land except for medicinal purposes. Women were not to go aboard on any occasion except with the permission of the magistrate who had to watch over them if he were to be aboard himself. In his absence aboard, he was to appoint four men to protect them.

The value placed on the *Bounty's* anvil is stressed by the special law framed for its protection. If anyone, taking the public anvil or the public sledge hammer from the smithy, should lose it, he was to get another and, in addition, pay a fine of four shillings. This fine apparently has never been imposed, and the original anvil is still in its place.

In addition to these formally recognized laws there were, according to Brodie, a number that were unwritten but none the less effective. They were concerned with trespassing fowl, pigs, and other livestock, and with the regulation of fishing for squid or fish from certain rocks, the fishing rights of which were held as private property in certain families. "Carving upon trees is forbidden," ruled another commandment. Apparently the cutting of initials and true-lover's knots on tree trunks was considered an insidious custom, and parents, regarding such pledges as dangerous, actively discouraged their continuance. A practice long established among the Pitcairn Islanders was the appeal to the commanding officers of British men-of-war for final adjudication in disputes they were unable to arrange themselves.

Although many of these laws are still in force, others have become dead letters. The actual machinery of government has undergone a series of further modifications and changes which, however, have not affected the simple democratic character of the administration of public affairs. Alterations in the customs of the islanders have made these changes necessary. The additional laws, adopted since 1850, reflect this change in manners. Breaches of behavior, once too rare to merit specific control, are now covered by legal regulation and reprimand.

Most of my information on the present form of Pitcairn government is derived from the *Book of Records of Pitcairn Island*, which is worth a short digression before returning to the subject of modern government on Pitcairn. This volume is the lineal descendant of the famous record that preceded it: *The Pitcairn Island Register*. The Society for Promoting Christian Knowledge has performed a service to Pitcairn enthusiasts by publishing the complete *Register* which previously had been known only from inadequate quotations by Brodie and others. Started by John Buffett soon after his arrival in 1823 and continued by Nobbs, the *Register* contains the annals of the colony from the arrival of the *Bounty,* in 1790, to 1854. It was fortunate that Adams was still living when Buffett arrived, for the latter was thereby able to secure first-hand information about the happenings on the island previous to his own arrival. If for no other reason, we must at least be grateful to John Buffett because he preserved an invaluable record.

The book of records now maintained on Pitcairn contains the laws and regulations by which the islanders are governed; sections devoted to the registry of births, marriages, and deaths; lists of brands and other marks of ownership; and a roster of the British warships which have visited the island since 1860. Unfortunately the expansive style of Nobbs was not maintained, and thus the record is mainly one of fertility without the relief of such incidents as lent color to the old *Register.* The present *Book of Records* was begun soon after the return to Pitcairn and has been kept faithfully ever since, each chief magistrate being responsible for its maintenance during his tenure of office.

To return to the government of Pitcairn, the *Register* reveals that on January 1, 1893, after a conference of the principal men with Captain Rookes of H.M.S. *Champion* in October, 1892, the assembled community decided to adopt a modified system of self-rule. Conceiving that certain unnamed abuses might be corrected if a larger number of islanders were directly responsible for the welfare of the colony, they adopted a new plan that provided for a parliament of seven empowered "to legislate, to plan for the public good, to execute all decisions of the court, and to see that all public demands are attended to without unnecessary delay." In addition there were a president as the chief executive officer, a vice president, a secretary, and a judge from whose decisions one might appeal to the parliament. The complete code of laws will be found in Appendix A.

The new laws in the code of 1850 reflect the changes

in insular behavior. These additional regulations lead us to conclude that illicit sex relations have increased noticeably since that former era of innocence. There are legal provisions for illegitimacy, penalties for fornication and adultery, fines for peeping. Unhappily, we find that libel, slander, theft, wife-beating, assault, and carrying of weapons required specific enactments. It would, perhaps, be overweighting these regulations to conclude that the islanders had reverted to the practices of their mutineer ancestors. That was not the case, but I think it does suggest that the idyllic days of sweetness and light were slightly overcast by a cloud of human nature.

The marriage laws of the island also were put under the control of the parliament whose permission henceforth was needed by those wishing to marry. No legal provision was made for divorce.

The parliamentary system endured for a decade, and then in 1904 the machinery was again overhauled. There have been no major changes since. The president, vice president, and parliament were scrapped, and their places were taken by a chief magistrate, a council, two assessors, and two committees, one for internal and one for external affairs. The chief magistrate is not to hold office in the church during his term. As highest authority on the island, he is to be aided by a council composed of the two assessors and the chairman of the committees for internal and external affairs. The committee for internal affairs consists of a chairman elected annually by the people and of two members designated by the chief magistrate. The companion committee for external affairs was similarly constituted, but the body languished for want of function and was later dropped. The assessors' chief duty was to preside together with the chief magistrate at all litigations involving more than £5. Smaller sums were dealt with by the magistrate alone or at his invitation with an assessor. The office of secretary, provided by the previous system, was maintained. The details of these various offices may be found *in extenso* in Appendix A.

The laws revised at this date were similar to those previously described, with, in some cases, further provisions to cover the greater variety of misdemeanors developed since 1893. Abortion, for example, is officially recognized for the first time as a crime and anyone guilty of inducing it was liable to imprisonment. Quarantine laws were also enacted, for Pitcairn not being a recognized port of call had no way of dealing with visiting ships.

To provide for the imprisonment of those convicted of serious crimes, the community has built a prison. Fortunately, it remains untenanted most of the time, although during my visit it had one occupant who was being held for trial on a charge of wife-beating. However, the carefully itemized regulations for the treatment of prisoners seemed to have been in abeyance, for the man was a prisoner only in the loosest sense of the term.

One of the duties of the committee for internal affairs is the direction of the public work. Pitcairn Islanders are fortunate in that they pay no taxes in the form of money. In lieu of taxes, seven days of labor is exacted yearly from every man over eighteen and under sixty. These days are devoted to road-making, repair of public buildings, work on the boats, and other tasks for the common good.

The committee also has jurisdiction over brands. With goats grazing at will and chickens wandering about the village it is necessary to have marks to distinguish mine from thine. This is accomplished by branding. Each family has its special brand which is registered in the *Pitcairn Island Book of Records*.* I counted 63 goat brands, which usually are various forms of ear-slitting; 90 for chickens, mostly different combinations of toe-cutting; and 127 letters and combinations of letters for marking trees. Linens are sometimes lettered with the indelible juice of the alligator-pear seed. The corner to be marked is held tightly over the seed and a needle or pin is stuck through into the seed. The juice stains the cloth in the desired pattern.

* See Appendix B.

"ANOTHER LANGUAGE"

Among themselves the Pitcairn Islanders speak a dialect incomprehensible to English or Polynesian ears. In conversation, however, with English or American visitors they use a familiar English spoken with a peculiar accent. Some of the men who have been to New Zealand or Australia have brought back a slightly British intonation as well as a few of the slang phrases common in that part of the Empire. But the stay-at-homes who are linguistically less stylish enunciate with a softness and a slur that is rather more pleasing than the recently imported variety of intonation.

All this goes to show that language is as much a cultural phenomenon as the construction of a house or the manufacture of *tapa*. It may be modified by cultural contact or borrowed or dropped just like any other item in the culture equipment. And in this instance, were the history of Pitcairn's settlement unknown, it might reveal the diverse origins of the community. It is a matter for regret that no previous visitor left any accurate notes on Pitcairnese, to distinguish it from its mother tongues, or bothered to record their impressions of its character. Such data would have been invaluable for comparison with the present-day dialect.

To understand the genesis of the Pitcairn dialect, we must return once more to the beginnings of the colony, to a group of men speaking no Tahitian and to a group of women speaking no English. No doubt the mutineers, like modern travelers in Tahiti, picked up a handful of native words such as *maitai, tamaa,* and *pape* (or its classical predecessor, *vai*), and imagined that they knew the language. And no doubt the Tahitian ladies in their innocence accepted such words as "goddam," and others less printable, as English fit for their use. But no one knows exactly in which medium—English or Tahitian— the mutineers and their ladies communicated: perhaps they developed a bastard language. My own guess is that the women spoke much more English than the mutineers did Tahitian, especially if we remember that the English, despite Norman Douglas, are proverbially bad linguists, and have, according to the French, forced the world to speak their language by their inability to use another.

Certainly, the tenacious loyalty of the English to their native language may be inferred from the fact that, despite the elimination of all the men save Adams, the children grew up speaking English. We have on record the astonishment of Folger, Shillibeer, Staines, and Pipon at the excellent English in which they were addressed by the Pitcairn youths who came out to greet their ships. It would be strange, however, if nothing remained of the Tahitian tongue, considering the eight or nine women who survived with Adams. They surely must have lapsed into the more familiar Tahitian when talking to their children. Nevertheless, I am aware of only one passing literary reference to the general use of Tahitian by the islanders. This suppression of Tahitian seems to me a reversal of expectation. Not only do we usually think of mothers as teaching their offspring the rudiments of language, but where the women so outnumbered the one surviving man who had no English companion to exercise and to keep agile his mother tongue, we might logically expect the natural influence of the maternal language would have predominated. But the fact remains that English was spoken by the Pitcairn children, and spoken well; and that Tahitian, if spoken at all, was so little in evidence that most of the visitors fail even to mention its use.

I first discovered that a dialect was in use among the descendants of the mutineers when I found that traces of it were still preserved on Norfolk Island among the older inhabitants. But I could recover only very little of it there. On Pitcairn, where the community has been much more isolated, Pitcairnese still flourishes, the children hardly speaking any other form of English than this to which they are bred, and the adults frequently lapse into it when they are not on their company manners. After the ear becomes accustomed to the intonation and the type of vocal changes characteristic of the speech, it becomes easy to leap to the meanings behind the queer distortions of common English words.

In many ways the dialect seems as if it had its origin in the efforts of the mutineers to teach the Tahitians the English language. The grammatical breakdown suggests this, as well as the elisions of sounds. I find that it is a common tendency for most of us when confronted with a foreigner, who has little understanding of English, to shout a horribly debased kind of English, as though bad grammar and a loud voice could render the language intelligible. (Listen to a customer in a Chinese laundry.) But whatever its precise origin, the Pitcairn dialect today consists of mispronounced English and Tahitian words with a spattering of coined words, the whole employed in a degenerate English syntax.

I append here a list of common words and expressions. Not having special linguistic knowledge, I was unable to record what I heard in the approved phonetic symbols. The list is not very ample, but I gathered what I could during intervals between other more pressing work.

PITCAIRN WORD LIST

solen: the last; *es (a) solen,* it is finished, there is no more. This word is probably derived from "sole one."

a little sullen: a little child.

illi-illi: used to describe a rough sea. The derivation is obviously from hilly, and the intensifying reduplication is a common usage in Tahitian and Polynesian in general.

tai-tai: Tahitian word meaning tasteless and, by transference, without charm when applied to people. This word also survives among the Norfolk Islanders, but it has vanished from modern Tahitian.

boney-boney: very thin. This is a nice example of Pitcairn adaptations: an English word reduplicated in Polynesian fashion with a distinction all its own.

I kawa: I don't know. *Kauaka = Kauraka,* meaning do not, occur in Tahitian. The loss of the second *k,* a phenomenon common in Polynesian, would produce a word like *kawa.* Another Tahitian word: *Kaore,* a negative adverb, also suggests *kawa.*

plān: banana, plantain. Apparently a contraction of plantain.

Es stolly: It's a story, or in more brutal manner, it's a lie. *You tallin' stolly* is a similar usage.

(a)bout you bin: Where have you been? I assume that this is descended from "whereabouts have you been?"

(a)bout you gwan: I sometimes seemed to hear this as *"bout you gowin?"* "Whereabouts are you going?"

almos' daid for tired: This needs no explanation.

lebby: Leave it alone; let it be, which can easily become *lebby* if repeated frequently without knowledge of the words in the phrase.

(d)ā: the definite article the, or sometimes the demonstrative that. For example, *gen a bed,* would mean alongside the (that) bed.

not sah: It is not so.

what a way to maik it: How do you do (make) it? This, too, can be traced simply to "what's the way to make it?"

cah fetch: can't be done.

no fet: used of things that don't fit.

huppa: bad or inefficient.

I starten: I'm starting or I'm going.

I nor believe: I don't think so.

mono-mono: very good. Here again is an example of re-duplication. *Mona* means sweet in Tahitian and in the related Tuamotuan.

soffa: softer.

fwhut you ally come yah: Why do you come here? Such a phrase recalls a dialect rather familiar to us.

fut you ally comey diffy and do daffy: Why do you come and behave that way? I think the reader can easily reconstruct "do this way and do that way" from *diffy and do daffy.*

I see yawl-ey scows segoin' out (d)a big ship: I see your boats going out to the big ship (the *Zaca* in this case).

See (d)a ship come to een: See the ship come close to land.

su'pa fai: all broken up. *Pofa'i* in Tahitian signifies to break off.

fut: What?

morga: thin.

hem: them, those as in *"hem orange on ā tree segrowin' big."*

naaway: to bathe or swim. *By you gwin naaway:* where are you going to swim? *Naue* is a Tahitian word meaning to leap or dive into water.

Los' bawl: lost ball, also used for a ship which passes by without stopping.

Thems aketch plenteh gott: They have caught many goats.

cocknut: cocoanut.

I'sa roll: I've fallen.

side: place; for example: *Up a side, Pugy'sa roll,* which would signify, Up at that place, Pugy fell down.

gingsa: ginger.

walley: valley.

Yousa heway me: You have heaved me away.

I'sa dona school: I've finished school.

Eeno: no.

You loy: You lie.

Wha you pick up ā, boy: Where did you learn that, child?

Stay-well-out: Remain where you are.

I tella you: I'm telling you.

ruma in the night: torch fishing. In Tahitian *rama* means to fish by torch light.

tolly: a kind of wood or tree.

boat of lanterns: used to describe boat-racing crews because the men's faces, covered with perspiration, shine like lanterns.

Tomolla ha tudder one: day after tomorrow.

Tomolla ha tudder one ha tudder one: second day after tomorrow.

Ā two junk torch: two-cell electric torch.

Bin tak hold: wrestled.

Aint account un: doesn't count.

Want a beak for eat it: You need a beak to eat it, therefore used for something unpalatable.

Want a tongs for eat it: has same significance as the above.

Es important es: One is assuming airs.

Dunt climb hem tree, bair you fall off: Don't climb that tree, lest you fall off.

Fus': first.

I don't know, too, myself: I don't know either.

O'er yanna: over yonder.

Come yare: Come here.

maolo: to break.

I'sa frettin': I'm fretting.

Foo you want da: Why do you want that?

Ka 'bout: I don't know where. Compare with *I kawa.*

What thing you want: What do you want?

From der way: from that way.

Nautical words and phrases are frequently employed.

"All hands," "grub," "sing out," "pull away," are among those in more common use. I overheard one sentence that was a puzzle until the light was furnished by one of the islanders. *"See ā twiss horn billeh foh pugy's,"* meant nothing to me at first except that someone's attention was being directed to some object. On inquiry I discovered that the literal translation is, "See that twisted horned billy goat of Pugy" (nickname for Edwin Christian). OtLer sentences after the adjustment is made to the Pitcairn accent were less difficult. *"You'sa daid," "You'sa dirty dawg," "You'sa daid as a hatchet, growin' fahs,"* need no commentary.

One of the peculiarities of the Pitcairn speech is the elision of the letter *r*. Even where I have written it in, I have done so not because the sound was distinct but because doing so suggested the English word more easily.

I wish it were possible to indicate the drawl and the rhythm of Pitcairn speech. It is these that give it a special character, and transmute the caricatured words into a cadence.

IV. BIOLOGICAL

10

ANGLO-POLYNESIAN

The biological experiment that blind circumstances have created on Pitcairn offers a rare opportunity for the investigation of the laws of heredity. Accident, that arbiter of events, deposited on deserted and almost unknown Pitcairn men of one race and women of another, and there accident yielded to nature. The forces thus joined were allowed to resolve themselves as surely as though they had been active chemicals in a test tube. Isolation has preserved the results.

In most communities of racially mixed origin there are usually to be discovered serious obstacles, often veritable barriers, in the path of the inquiring seeker after the laws of heredity. For example, the mixture may be so ancient that its exact composition is lost in the fogs of antiquity, and the investigator can merely prove what is already known: that race mixture has occurred. Or the social *mores* of the contracting parties may be such that parentage is systematically concealed. Or again, the half-caste population may take no interest in genealogical pursuits, and the history of their blood lines thus may be lost. These are some of the conditions which combine to give a genealogical blank. For the geneticist it is of prime importance to know precisely what elements have entered into the making of a given hybrid, when it occurred in terms of generations, what crossbreeding has occurred since the original cross, and, finally, the matings in each generation. Otherwise the conclusions derived from such studies become circular, and the investigator returns to the point from which he started.

But knowledge of the family tree is not the only desideratum, nor is its absence the only drawback. Such studies are facilitated if the parental groups are sufficiently distinctive to present clear-cut differences which may then be followed in the progeny with greater ease. Miscegenation between closely allied stocks produces complex and blurred results by virtue of overlapping characters and genetic similarities. Greater differences, therefore, between the parents clarify the consequences of mixture in the offspring.

In addition to genealogical *lacunae* and the confusion of genetic similarities, another factor frequently mars the perfection of most mixed groups as subjects for research. In the crossings of races that show marked physical differences or in cases where deep prejudice exists the partners of such unions are often unrepresentative or socially inferior members of one or both groups. It would, of course, be naive to assume that this is always the case. Where slave populations exist or where native mistresses have a recognized position, the reverse does occur, but the fact remains that the evils which are popularly assigned to the mingling of blood may with greater justice be attributed to the quality of the blood which produced the hybrid. It stacks the cards, to say the least, against the half-caste to attribute any defect in his heritage to the irregularity of his breeding.

But the social matrix of the problem has wider implications, important as these are. The social, economic, and, therefore, environmental background of the half-caste is almost always inferior to the best in the possession of one of his ancestral stocks, and frequently it is worse than the average to be found in both. The social stigmata attached to those unfortunates of mixed blood are often almost insupportable and may engender at their worst unfortunate physical and psychological consequences.

On Pitcairn none of these handicaps to the study of race mixture exist. The genealogical history of the islanders is well known from the mutineers and their consorts to the present generation. When new blood has been added, as it has been at various times, that too was recorded. Fortunately Buffett began, and Nobbs preserved, the *Register* in which, from the beginning of the colony, every birth, marriage, and death was entered. But with all this official recording, the question naturally arises whether illegitimacy may not be present here as elsewhere and thereby vitiate the results based on the official pedigrees. No doubt that little monkey running up and down the branches of a family tree can do considerable damage.

I frankly admit that this is something to give one pause. However, we can do some checking, the more tactful, perhaps, the better. I already had in my records of the Pitcairn Islanders several cases of illegitimacy. And during my visit I was able to secure considerably more information on the subject. Several of the islanders, wishing to keep the record straight, and appreciating my reasons for inquiries of so intimate a nature, gave me valuable information which coincided not only with each other's but with the official record book. I am unwilling to boast that I have detected every case of illegitimacy which has ever occurred on Pitcairn, but I feel confident that very few have escaped me. The credit goes not to me but to my informants who, moved by a sense of duty and honesty, confided in me only after the greatest internal struggles. I should add that in a settlement as intimate as Pitcairn, instances of irregularity had only to exist to be known.

Nor can the quality of the ancestry of the Pitcairn Islanders be questioned. Christian came from an ancient, respected, and influential Manx family. Edward Young was the nephew of a baronet. Quintal, McCoy, Adams, and Mills, the other four mutineers who founded families, were ordinary seamen of the working class. They were stout, hearty sailors, fit enough to endure the rough life of the sea. Their record as mutineers certainly is not above reproach, but neither were they without provocation. Their faults may have been serious, but they were, at least, positive and aggressive ones. It is recorded that the men of the *Bounty* were a superior lot, hand-picked for the job. I would rate the men as a good average lot, with a touch of the gentry thrown in. The other white men who joined the colony and commingled their blood with that of the mutineers, were likewise men of simple but sound origins. Nobbs, if the tradition is to be trusted, even laid claims to a left-handed aristocratic lineage. I emphasize these social criteria, not from any profound conviction that the best blood is concentrated in the upper classes, but to show that on the European side the ancestry of the Pitcairn Islanders is not derived from a degenerate or a depressed class.

Of the Tahitian women little is known. One or two had excellent connections, and all of them were raised in favorable conditions and belonged to a stock famous for its physical beauty. The fact that these women readily formed liaisons with the *Bounty's* crew does not argue their depravity or socially inferior status. The more than liberal ideas of the Tahitians and the almost divine repute of the white man were sufficient to account for the ease with which the sailors established these connections.

Finally, the Pitcairn Islanders, unlike other half-caste populations, have never had to eat the bitter bread of social or economic prejudice. Isolated on their fertile island, they are free of the usual disabilities under which half-castes ordinarily labor. They have an abundance of food, nutritious and varied. They are inferior to no one. In other words, they have been allowed to develop in an environment that is wholesome and in a manner dictated by their innate capabilities.

In the remainder of this chapter I shall describe some of the physical characteristics of the Pitcairn Islanders in terms of their ancestral stocks. I have followed the usual statistical procedures and have calculated the average or mean for each measurement. There were sixty-two adult men and sixty-two adult women in my total series of islanders, but in the following the males only are considered, since the comparative data for males are better. It must be kept in mind that these means represent a hypothetical Pitcairn Islander. No one individual would conform in all respects to these averages. But, on the other hand, the mean does indicate the value that covers the greatest number of cases.

Stature is a measurement subject to certain fluctuations directly correlated with environmental conditions. It has been found, other things being equal, that stature increases with improved economic status, the general assumption being that nutrition, among other factors, is mainly responsible for this phenomenon. Eschewing, therefore, the elevated statures of the English upper classes and the depressed ones of the population at the other end of the socio-economic scale, we may take 172 cm. as representative of the average Englishman. Somewhat less than this was the mean stature of the six mutineers who left progeny on Pitcairn. Taking their individual heights from the Admiralty records, I obtained an average of 170.6 cm. Tahitians are also of good stature, the men averaging about 171.4 cm. There is, therefore, but little difference in stature between the English and Tahitians. This would lead us to expect among the Pitcairn Islanders an average stature in close agreement with those of their parent stocks. If we contrast the descendants of the mutineers and the Tahitian women with the racial stocks from which they have sprung, we discover that they are taller. The male descendants of the mutineers living on Norfolk have an average height of 174.0 cm., the Pitcairn men of 173.0 cm. Moreover, this excess, though small, was once much greater. In 1825 the children of the first generation born on Pitcairn were measured by Beechey's surgeon who obtained an average of 177.8 cm., the tallest man being six feet one-quarter inch, and the shortest five feet nine and one-eighth inches.

In animal and plant experimental genetics the production of hybrids often leads to an increase in size and vigor. Such a phenomenon is technically called heterosis or hybrid vigor, and it is used extensively in the cultivation of seed corn for commercial purposes. On Pitcairn we find a human analogy to the lower forms in the increased size of the hybrid islanders. Some diminution in stature, it is true, may be noted in the present generation—the fourth, fifth, and sixth from the original cross, but it still remains greater than that of either English or Tahitian.

In the dimensions of the vault of the head there is a marked difference between the two branches of the colony. The Norfolk Island males have longer and wider heads than their relatives on Pitcairn. It must be remembered, however, that the two colonies have had a separate existence for about seventy-five years and that little of the Nobbs-Buffett-Evans heritage is represented on Pitcairn. Moreover, considerable new blood has been added to the Norfolk strain since the 1860's. Pitcairn, on the other hand, has received Warren, Coffin, and Clark.

Since I have already dealt with the Norfolk Islanders in another place, I shall confine my remarks to the Pitcairn Islanders. Their average head length of 189.6 mm. is almost identical with the head lengths of the Tahitians —188.01—and is very much smaller than English averages which range from 193 to 198, according to the group. We may conclude, therefore, that in the length of head the Tahitian heritage is dominant. The reverse is true for the head width. For this trait we find that the Pitcairn mean of 152.04 mm. falls into English group range—150 to 155—and far below the Tahitian average of 159.6 mm. The resulting cephalic index, the percentage of head width in relation to head length, of the Pitcairn Island men is intermediate between English and Tahitian.

The minimum frontal diameter is a measurement taken on the forehead. It is the minimum distance between the bony ridges which, rising from the outer corners of the eyebrows, pass upwards and backwards along the margins of the forehead. One of the most characteristic features in the architecture of the Tahitian face is the constriction of the brow, as defined above, in relation to the face width which is very great.

Let us compare the Pitcairn Island men with their ancestral stocks for this trait. The minimum frontal diameter is only 100 mm. in width which is even narrower than the equivalent feature among the Tahitians, who average 104.0 mm. Compared to the English, the gulf is even wider, for their mean is well over 106.0 mm. The face width, on the contrary, reveals a different line-up. Compared with the Tahitians the English have narrow slab-sided faces. For the latter the average is about 138–139 mm., for the former 145.7 mm. The Pitcairn Islanders, with a face width of 138.5 mm., are identical with the English. Thus the English width of face is dominant. But the minimum frontal diameter of the Pitcairners offers a puzzle, since it is unlike either parent stock, being much narrower even than that of the Tahitians. The anomaly may be explained in this wise. The proportions between the face and brow width among the Pitcairn Islanders are distinctly characteristic of Tahitians— that is, a brow relatively narrow compared with the face width. But since they have inherited a narrow face from their English ancestors, the brow, in maintaining the proportions of the Tahitian type, has had to remain much narrower than either racial average.

In height of nose, measured from the nasal root to the juncture of the nasal septum and the lip, there does not appear to be any difference between the ancestral stocks. The slight differences which exist are not great enough to exceed the large personal error involved in taking this difficult measurement. In the nose width, however, there is a definite contrast between the broadish Tahitian nose and the narrow English one. The width of the former is 43.4 mm. compared to 35–36 mm. among the English. The Pitcairn mean of 38.5 mm. is roughly intermediate. Its somewhat closer approximation to the English average may well be the effect of the additional Anglo-American blood which has reached the island since its settlement.

These few measurable features are enough to illustrate the general character of the Pitcairn heredity. The others exhibit a similar pattern. The Pitcairn Islanders reveal in their sum total a mosaic of characters, some borrowing their colors from Tahiti, others from England, with an occasional patch where the colors have run to produce a blend.

If we examine the less tangible characteristics of the Pitcairn inhabitants, we find a different pattern. I shall treat here only skin color, eye color, distribution and color of hair, nasal bridge and profile, and lip thickness.

The skin color we see in the people about us is the resultant of a number of factors: the actual amount of pigment matter in the dermis, the thickness of the epidermis, the vascularity of the skin, and the surface quality of the tissue. The precise effects of these various factors are not known nor can we, by present methods, measure them in any satisfactory and objective fashion. In lieu, therefore, of any dependable quantitative analysis of the complex phenomenon of skin color, we must, until better methods are devised, content ourselves with a rough approximation by using a color scale which gives us a rating in a graduated series. To secure the most reliable rating it is customary to observe an unexposed part of the skin, usually the inner side of the upper arm. Among the Pitcairn Islanders the determinations of skin color for this area are as follows:

VON LUSCHAN SKIN COLOR SCALE	MALES No.	MALES Per cent	FEMALES No.	FEMALES Per cent
3	7	11.29	5	8.06
7	14	22.58	14	22.58
8	7	11.29	4	6.45
9	10	16.13	5	8.06
10	12	19.35	22	35.48
11	3	4.84	4	6.45
12	5	8.06	7	11.29
13	1	1.61		
14	1	1.61		
17	1	1.61	1	1.61
18	1	1.61		

Numbers 3, 7, and 8 correspond to skin colors most frequent among north Europeans. Tahitians, however, range from numbers 10 to 22, with most of them clustering around 10 and 16–18. The Pitcairn Islanders overlap both English and Tahitian. None are as dark as the darker Tahitians and relatively few are as fair as the fair English. This kind of distribution is typical when a character is the resultant of a number of genetic factors. It is sometimes called, erroneously, blending inheritance.

Pitcairn men are somewhat lighter in hair color than the women. The males have 68.5 per cent with black hair, 29.6 per cent with dark brown, and 1.9 per cent with light brown. The females fall into the same categories, but with 78.6 per cent having black hair, 19.6 per cent dark brown, and 1.8 per cent light brown. One adult individual had blonde hair, but unfortunately he was not available for inclusion in this series. A number of the children were fair-haired, but since we are dealing only with mature subjects they must be omitted, for hair color being correlated with age darkens on maturity. Evidently the factors producing blonde hair are present among the Pitcairn Islanders but their heritage from Tahiti, where the hair is predominantly black, is sufficiently prepotent to prevent any widespread appearance of blondness.

Hair color among the English varies widely in the different districts of the British Isles, but on the whole the majority have brown hair of various shades. Compared to the English, the Pitcairn Islanders are much darker. Whereas the English have only about 5 per cent with black hair the Pitcairn Islanders of both sexes have 73.5 per cent. The Tahitians, whom the Pitcairners resemble more closely in this respect, are 80–90 per cent blackheaded.

The eye color of the Pitcairn Islanders is of particular interest because of the patent contrast between the parental stocks. Tahitians are without exception browneyed. A small minority of them, about 15 per cent, have what might be described as light brown eyes; the remainder have deep brown. No unmixed blue eyes occur in pure-blooded Tahitians, except in an occasional albino. The English, on the contrary, are endowed with a large share of the genes which produce blue or mixed blue eyes. The percentage of blue eyes, however, varies in the different areas, but in all the blue-eyed factor or factors is generally distributed. The following table presents the average percentages of the various eye colors among British and Americans of British origin.

	LIGHT	INTERMEDIATE	BROWN
Old Americans ♂	23.8	59.7	16.5
Old Americans ♀	20.0	60.0	20.0
England, Scotland, and Wales	53.3	15.2	31.5

The "lights" include only blue or gray eyes, the "intermediates" hazel, blue-brown, or gray-brown eyes, and the "browns" only pure light or dark brown eyes. Remembering that the Tahitians are 100 per cent brown, let us examine the distribution of eye color among the Pitcairn Islanders.

	LIGHT	INTERMEDIATE	BROWN
Pitcairn men	6.45	64.51	29.03
Pitcairn women	4.84	37.09	58.06

We note first of all that the women of Pitcairn are darker-eyed than the men; 58 per cent have brown eyes compared with only 29 per cent among the males. It is tempting to link up this sex difference with the fact that the women by virtue of their sex resemble their Tahitian ancestresses more closely than their English sires. This is technically known as sex-linked inheritance. Unfortunately we cannot, on the basis of Pitcairn material, draw such a conclusion. In a perfect experiment, we might have crossed not only Englishmen and Tahitian women but also have reversed the sexes to mate English women with Tahitian men. The progenies of such matings properly controlled would have yielded data designed to answer queries whose solution must wait on other data. Nevertheless, the Pitcairn array of eye colors and their frequencies do illustrate in human heredity several well-known principles of genetics. If we allow DR or intermediate to represent the gene pattern among the Englishmen, and DD or pure brown the genetic formula for the Tahitian women, the expectations after several generations of unselected matings would be these:

	LIGHT	INTERMEDIATE	BROWN
Theoretical expectations	6.25	37.50	56.25
Actual distributions:			
Pitcairn males	6.45	64.51	29.03
Pitcairn females	4.84	37.09	58.06

We see in this table that the Pitcairn women fit the theoretical expectations as perfectly as one might expect in a small sample of sixty-two women. The men also agree with the expectation for "light" but have a very much higher proportion among the intermediates and a much smaller among the browns. The eye color among the women therefore shows a dominance of the brown over the blue, whereas for the men there appears to be an additional factor operating to modify the expected dominance of brown pigment.

Another phenomenon of considerable importance is also illustrated by these figures. It is sometimes termed the conservation of the genes. The genes are minute protein molecules which bear the substance of heredity from one generation to another. Both male and female sex cells carry approximately equivalent arrays of genes that unite on fertilization. If the genes for a specific character differ, one or the other may "dominate." This does not mean that this "recessive" gene is lost. It will reappear in later generations. Blue eyes in this case, although generally a recessive character, have once more recurred in a proportion determined by the concentration of genes for blue eyes in the population.

The nose contributes a very special character to the face. This feature among Tahitians is, as we have remarked previously, moderately wide. It is also predominantly straight in profile, 83 per cent being so classified, with 11 per cent having concave profiles and 6 per cent convex. In spite of its tendency to breadth and fleshiness the Tahitian nose is not low at the bridge like the African. As a matter of fact 76 per cent have noses of medium height; only 19 per cent have low-bridged noses, while 5 per cent have high noses. The effect of a low-spreading nose is created, however, by the great width of the bony bridge which conceals its moderate elevation.

The English nose, unfortunately, has never been described to my knowledge in comparable terms. We are all familiar, however, with the narrow, constricted, and high-bridged nose common among the British. Both convex and straight profiles are numerous, but concave outlines appear less frequently.

In comparing the Pitcairn nose with the English, it is necessary to rely on data obtained from an Old American series, since they are absent for the English themselves.

Of the Pitcairn Islanders 66 per cent have convex nasal profiles, 31 per cent straight, and 3 per cent concave. This is a distribution quite different from the Tahitian and, judged by Old American standards, very close to the English. The following table confirms this.

	CONVEX	CONCAVO-CONVEX	STRAIGHT	CONCAVE
Old American ♂	42.0	27.3	22.0	8.7
♂ Pitcairn	66.13		30.65	3.23
♂ Tahitian	6.1		82.93	10.97

Without quoting the actual figures, I may add that the Pitcairn women, like the men, resemble the English in this feature.

Unfortunately, information on the elevation of the nasal bridge is not even available for Old Americans. But a comparison of the Pitcairn Islanders with Tahitians shows that the former are definitely divergent in their greater elevation of the bony nasal ridge. Only 8 per cent of the men have low bridges and 47 per cent have high ones, whereas among Tahitians as many as 19 per cent have low bridges and only 5 per cent high.

For the thickness of the lips, likewise, no adequate English data exist. The Tahitian series of males provides only 1 per cent with thin lips, 88.0 per cent with medium, and 11.0 per cent with thick. The Pitcairn men equal and even surpass their Tahitian relatives in the number having thick lips—15.7 per cent. And at the same time 43 per cent of the Pitcairn men show thin lips, a percentage far in excess of the Tahitian. It is obvious, therefore, that in lip thickness the contributions of both stocks are well represented and neither dominates. However, a contributory factor to the refinement of the lip demands mention. The general loss of teeth so prevalent among the Pitcairn Islanders has caused, by the removal of the supporting structure, the lips to collapse, with a consequent appearance of a greater thinness than they might otherwise manifest.

The Pitcairn Islanders are dental unfortunates. Not one adult woman out of sixty examined had a complete set of teeth, and nineteen had all the teeth missing. Thirty-seven, or roughly 61 per cent, had lost ten or more teeth. The men are somewhat better off. I actually found five men out of sixty who still had full dentures. Eight had become edentulous and thirty-one, or about 52 per cent, had lost ten or more teeth. It is difficult to account for this dental condition. The diet appears to be adequate, although no investigation of the chemistry of the food was undertaken. The same situation prevails on Norfolk where more meat and fish are consumed. It is true that the English have notoriously bad teeth which may be an important factor in the shocking dental degeneracy on Pitcairn. Its English origin is supported by the case of Edward Young, one of the mutineers, who had already lost his incisor teeth at the age of twenty-four. Since the incisors are ordinarily among the most resistant teeth, Young's loss suggests either fisticuffs or a congenital defect. If the latter hypothesis is true, it is not difficult to see that the close inbreeding practised on Pitcairn might spread and intensify the defect among all the population.

We may sum up the heredity of the Pitcairn Islanders by saying that they show in their traits evidence of both their English and Tahitian ancestry. Some of them are, in their physical expression, more influenced by the English heritage, some more by the Tahitian, and others appear to be intermediate. Each one is a varying mixture of both. It is true that on the whole the features of the islanders are definitely English, but familiarity reveals a number of individuals who favor the Tahitian side.

During the course of my investigations I made a subjective rating of a number of men and women, according to their general appearance and, I quickly add, not one was sufficiently Tahitian in appearance to be able to pass as such, whereas a number of the islanders might readily escape detection in an English community. Of course, this preponderance of the English type is natural, for all the new additions to the colony have been of English stock. But to return to my ratings, each individual was classified as strongly, moderately, slightly English; or intermediate; or slightly, moderately, strongly Tahitian. Here are the results for fifty men and fifty-one women.

	MALES	FEMALES
Strongly English	12	6
Moderately English	8	5
Slightly English	13	8
Intermediate	11	14
Slightly Tahitian	3	13
Moderately Tahitian	3	5
Strongly Tahitian	0	2

I have already mentioned the darker complexions of the Pitcairn women. Perhaps this fact influenced me in recording a stronger Tahitian trend among the women, even though I tried to preserve a balanced judgment based on all the traits.

In a mixed population such as the Pitcairn Islanders, one might normally expect to find an increased variability. The potentialities contributed by both ancestral stocks should expand the range of the various characters among the hybrids. Actually the Pitcairn Islanders show no evidence of such a phenomenon. The statistical expression of the variability inherent in a series is measured by the standard deviation. The standard deviations of the Pitcairn Islanders are in some cases smaller than those of the English or Tahitians, in many they are the same, and in only one or two are they significantly greater. I can offer in explanation of this reversal of expectation only the suggestion that the inbreeding which has occurred among the Pitcairn Islanders has led to a greater homogeneity than exists in most mixed groups. The extent of inbreeding will be discussed in the next chapter.

11

BREEDING AND INBREEDING

Vital statistics are the bookkeeping of a population. They reveal the present state of affairs, uncover past trends, and cast up a balance, favorable or otherwise. And in this instance they provide invaluable data pertinent to the problems of race mixture.

The population figures relating to the Pitcairn Islanders presented in the following pages were derived from the previously mentioned *Book of Records of Pitcairn Island* where each birth, death, and marriage occurring on Pitcairn is entered or is supposed to have been entered. I have actually found remarkably few discrepancies or omissions. From internal evidence I have, however, been forced to assume that some of the births and deaths in the first years after the return to Pitcairn were omitted either inadvertently or because the infant died soon after birth, and the recorder, not foreseeing the needs of a future investigator, felt no compulsion to register such ephemeral additions to the colony. It is my belief that the register is sufficiently complete to yield trustworthy results. It also agrees very closely with the genealogical tables drawn up from independent sources.

One of the most remarkable facts about the population of Pitcairn is its prodigiously rapid increase. The following table illustrates this growth up to 1856, when the entire community was transported to Norfolk Island.

YEAR	TOTAL	MALES	FEMALES
1808	35		
1814	40		
1825	66	36	30
1839	106	53	53
1840	108	53	55
1841	111	54	57
1842	112	53	59
1843	119	59	60
1844	121	60	61
1845	127	65	62
1846	134	69	65
1847	140	72	68
1848	146	74	72
1849	155	76	79
1852	170		
1853	172	85	87
1855	187	92	95
1856	193	94	99

In 1858 sixteen returned to Pitcairn. In 1864 twenty-six more joined the previous lot who meanwhile had increased somewhat. There were, therefore, in 1864 about forty-five souls on Pitcairn. Seventy years later, in 1934, I found the colony increased to about two hundred, and to more than two hundred and twenty-five, including those who had emigrated to foreign lands. In these seventy years the population has multiplied itself by at least five times. Meanwhile on Norfolk the population had grown so rapidly that by 1924 there were over six hundred inhabitants. Unfortunately, the census of Norfolk includes the foreign residents, so that the actual number of descendants of the mutineers can be less exactly determined than is the case on Pitcairn. Thus in the course of one hundred and forty-five years the six mutineers who lived long enough to produce offspring have a living progeny well exceeding eight hundred on Norfolk and Pitcairn and which might easily number one thousand if all the wanderers were included. A prodigious spectacle of human breeding!

The present composition of the population living on the island is as follows:

	MALES	FEMALES
Under 18	36	27
18–44	44	38
45–64	18	24
65–86	3	9
Total	101	98

It is commonly observed in population analyses that females survive to greater ages than males. The Pitcairn Islanders are no exception to this rule. We find between the ages of sixty-five to eighty-six that the females outnumber the males three to one, and between the ages of forty-five to sixty-four the proportion of women to men is four to three. In the earlier ages, however, the males are more numerous than the females.

Actually, from 1865 to 1933 there have been 165 male to 139 female births, or 118.7 males to 100 females. This sex ratio at birth among the Pitcairn Islanders is much higher than is ordinarily expected. From 1841 to 1916, in England and Wales, the sex ratio at birth varied from 103.5 to 105.2. In Sweden, during the course of over one hundred and fifty years, the sex ratio at birth has been maintained at about 105 or 106. But the higher mortality among the males generally alters the ratio until, in the middle period of life and in old age, the women become more numerous than the men. This phenomenon we find repeated on Pitcairn. On Norfolk Island in 1924 I found a group of twenty-four survivors of the original migration, the youngest being sixty-five years old and the oldest ninety-five. Of these twenty-four, fifteen were females and nine males. It is sometimes offered in explanation of the preponderance of aged women that the greater hazards of male occupations take a greater toll on life, but unless these hazards are also to be blamed

for weakening those males who survive it is difficult to see
why the death rate should continue to be greater among
males even during the decades of retirement from active
life. There appears to be no escape from the conclusion
that man is the weaker vessel.

The extraordinary increase in the population of Pitcairn suggests that in the not far distant future the island may again be overpopulated and that once more
the compact little community may by sheer necessity be
forced to cast off another daughter colony. Pitcairn is
only slightly more than two miles long and a little more
than one mile wide. Only a limited part of its precipitous
surface is suitable for agriculture. Were the principles
of Malthus known to them they would be only too real
to the Pitcairn Islanders, who, however, do not appear
to be disturbed excessively by the prospects of the
crowded future. But before drawing too gloomy a conclusion from the past it would be wiser to inquire into
the present trends of population replacements. In the following paragraphs, therefore, I shall set forth some of
the results of various calculations I have computed from
the vital records of the island. These, I think, may throw
some light on the future of the Pitcairn population, in so
far as it is possible to illuminate the future at all.

If the births and deaths are arranged by decades, they
show the following results:

DECADE	BIRTHS	DEATHS	INCREASE
1864–1873	36	5	31
1874–1883	38	12	26
1884–1893	49	21	28
1894–1903	42	5	37
1904–1913	49	27	22
1914–1923	45	21	24
1924–1933	45	21	24

These figures seem to indicate that although the births
have increased in number with the increase in population, the deaths have more than kept pace. This fact re-

sults in the net increase of population becoming progressively smaller. The decade 1894–1903 does show a sudden increase in population gain, but it is significant that it was not as a consequence of a more pronounced fertility but because of a temporary reduction in the number of deaths.

To demonstrate this decline in population increase in another manner, I shall give the percentages that each decade's increase represents of the total population. Unfortunately I have no official census figures for these periods, but if each decade's increase is added in turn to the preceding decade's total, a figure near to the actual population will be achieved. For example, there were about forty-five islanders in 1864. During the next decade to 1873 there were thirty-one more births than deaths, which would mean that by 1873 the population reached a total of seventy-six. This method of computation would, it is true, make the present population 237, whereas it is actually only two hundred.

The discrepancy, however, is not entirely the fault of the calculations but of emigrations that have removed some of the islanders to New Zealand, Australia, San Francisco, and Bridgeport, Connecticut. If the discrepancy were distributed evenly and subtracted from each decade's increase, the resulting figure would probably be near the truth, at least not sufficiently wide of it to alter the significance of the comparison I wish to draw. It would require much grosser errors in my figures than I believe they contain to affect materially the steady progressive decline in the rate of growth of Pitcairn's population. Here are my approximations to the successive rates of growth.

YEAR	ESTIMATED POPULATION	ACTUAL INCREASE	PER CENT INCREASE
1864	45		
1874	71	31	43.66
1884	92	26	28.26
1894	115	28	24.35
1904	147	37	25.17
1914	164	22	13.41
1924	183	24	13.11
1934	202	24	11.88

The high rate of increase in the first decade may be in part the consequence of the abnormal age composition of the little band that repopulated the island. There were very few old people, and a relatively large number of the inhabitants in their active child-bearing period. But the steady decline of the ratio of population replacement since 1884 seems to indicate a falling birth rate or an increasing death rate.

By the same method we may determine the percentage of deaths to the estimated population.

YEAR	PER CENT DEATHS
1874	7.04
1884	13.04
1894	18.26
1904	3.40
1914	16.46
1924	11.48
1934	10.40

These mortality percentages from 1874 to the present do not explain the previously noted decline in the rate of increase. It is necessary, therefore, to seek another cause for the decline in the rate of population increase. In order to test whether or not the birth rate in Pitcairn has declined, I have calculated the average number of children borne by the women who are listed according

to the year of their birth. The following table includes
all the women, regardless of their sex history.

BIRTH YEAR OF MOTHER	NUMBER OF WOMEN	AVERAGE NUMBER OF CHILDREN PER FEMALE
1790–1814	2	5.5
1815–1839	5	11.4
1840–1864	12	6.8
1865–1889	31	4.2
1890–1914	33	2.4

In the next table I have eliminated all the women except those who reached the age of forty-five and were
married up to that age. It is needless to add that the
age at marriage varied.

BIRTH YEAR OF MOTHER	NUMBER OF WOMEN	AVERAGE NUMBER OF CHILDREN PER FEMALE
1790–1814	1	6.0
1815–1839	5	11.4
1840–1864	8	8.0
1865–1889	20	5.0
1890–1914	2	2.5

A comparison of these two tables reveals that the character of the sex life of the women does play a part in
their fertility. The women who have married or mated
and have remained so to the end of their child-bearing
period are definitely more fertile than those who have led
more irregular lives. But both these tables reveal a similar trend—a decline in fertility. From the extraordinary
child-bearing capacity capable of producing an average
family of 11.4 the decline has been constant and definite.
The rate for the last group of women is inconclusive,
being based, in the first table, on women who are still
in their active child-bearing period and, in the second,
on only two women who had reached the age of forty-
five. Nevertheless, it is unlikely that the fertility rate for
the women born between 1890–1914 will equal that of
the preceding group.

Some idea of the magnitude of these averages may be obtained by comparison with the figures for the population of the United States. For American women the estimated average number of offspring for completed families varies according to State from 2.33 to 4.13.

The decline in fertility among the Pitcairn Islanders has a counterpart in the fertility records of the Norfolk Islanders. In my study of the Norfolk Islanders I obtained the following figures.

	NUMBER OF MATINGS	NUMBER OF CHILDREN PER MATING
Original cross	6	4.17
First generation	9	7.44
Second generation	38	9.10
Third generation	77	5.39
Fourth generation	26	2.96

In the next table the average ages of the females are given at the time of their first marriage.

YEAR OF BIRTH	NUMBER	AVERAGE AGE AT FIRST MARRIAGE
1815–1839	3	15 years 3 months
1840–1864	11	21 years 10 months
1865–1889	27	22 years 11 months
1890–1914	24	20 years 3 months

The numbers are few, but as far as they are reliable the generation of women who had the magnificent child-bearing proclivities capable of producing an average of 11.4 children also appear to have married at an earlier age than their descendants. The averages for the succeeding generations are all considerably greater, and show only slight differences from 1840 on. The explanation may be that the fewer possible mates in the earlier days resulted in all the girls being rushed into matrimony as soon as it was decently possible. No later bride equaled the record of one girl born in the 1815–1839 generation. She married at the age of 14 years and 2 months. Even more remarkable was her contemporary, Maria Christian, whose record belongs with Norfolk Island statistics. Maria Christian was born in 1815, married at fourteen years of age, produced twenty-five children including twins, and survived three husbands! Such was the stuff of that fabulous generation.

The figures of the preceding table should be compared with those below which record the average age of the women at the birth of their first child.

YEAR OF BIRTH	NUMBER	AVERAGE AGE AT BIRTH OF FIRST CHILD	
1815–1839	4	17 years	1 month
1840–1864	12	22 years	9 months
1865–1889	29	20 years	10 months
1890–1914	26	19 years	9 months

This table includes all the women who have given birth to a child whether with benefit of clergy or without. These averages, therefore, compared with those for age at marriage, reveal that the morality of the islanders as well as the birth rate has undergone changes. Apparently girls born after 1865 were rather impatient.

Although the famous generation of 1815–1839 leads its successors, nevertheless we find that the later generations, from 1865 on, show a secondary tendency towards a younger age at the commencement of child-bearing. If we take the age at first childbirth as an index of fertility it would appear that the latest generation has suffered no recent decline. Even though such an assumption might be tenable, there are too many other factors involved to make this as natural a conclusion as it might seem at first glance. The recent tendency toward earlier age at the birth of the first child may well be the consequence of a relaxation in sex *mores*.

This difficult question of fertility can be approached

in still another way. For the following table I have calculated the average age for the women at the birth of
the last child. It is, of course, to be understood that only
those women are included who enjoyed a married life
up to at least the age of forty-five. Practically all, however, lived in a connubial state to a greater age than this.

YEAR OF BIRTH	NUMBER OF WOMEN	AVERAGE AGE AT FINAL PARTURITION
1790–1814	1	45 years
1815–1839	4	42 years 5 months
1840–1864	8	36 years 6 months
1865–1889	19	34 years 10 months

Taking these figures at their face value, it is clear that
the period of fecundity was not only of longer duration
in the earlier generations, but that it ceased sooner in
the more recent generations. It is true that the numbers
for the first two generations are very scanty indeed, but
it may be pointed out that of the five women included
in the first two generations the youngest was thirty-nine
at the birth of her last child and the oldest forty-five
years and five months. Three of these five had children
when past the age of forty-four. Contrast this with the
fact that in succeeding generations not a single woman
whose record I have been able to find had a child after
her forty-fourth birthday. Actually the oldest was forty-
three years and six months. Most of the women in the
last two generations ceased their child-bearing during or
before their thirties.

I have been discussing the women without any reference to the men in this important phenomenon of child
production. In the following table I have analyzed the
data for the Pitcairn males from the standpoint of the
age at birth of first child, regardless of marital state.

YEAR OF BIRTH	NUMBER	AVERAGE AGE AT BIRTH OF FIRST CHILD
1815–1839	4	20 years 8 months
1840–1864	12	22 years 10 months
1865–1889	24	22 years ½ month
1890–1914	23	25 years

The men show a progressive and uninterrupted increase in age before assuming their procreative functions. This is quite unlike the situation among the females who, in the more recent generations, tended to start childbearing at an early age.

I intended tabulating the males by age at the birth of the last child in order to provide comparable data with those for the females, but I soon had confirmed what I suspected might be the truth. The age of the men at the birth of their last child was conditioned by the age of their wives. This was made all the clearer by several instances in which philandering men whose wives had long ceased to bear children were able at rather advanced ages to produce illegitimate offspring by younger women. It did not, therefore, appear to be a safe procedure to estimate the duration of the procreative powers of the men by examining their ages at the birth of their final offspring.

This discussion of the birth rates and the child-bearing ages of the Pitcairn Islanders leads to the conclusion that the rate of population increase has declined. Not only do the women produce fewer children but they now cease to bear them at all at a younger age than they formerly did. It is impossible to predict how far this drying up of fertility will continue, but it is at least clear that the island will not become overpopulated in the immediate future. In fact, the present birth rate hardly suffices to maintain the existing population and any further drop would lead to a decline. Such a prediction might come as a shock to the Pitcairn Islanders, who are accustomed to believe that their island is headed for serious overpopulation. So potent, indeed, is this belief that, aside from a natural reluctance to seeing strangers settle among them, they have always resisted the invasion of eager would-be immigrants on the ground that the island is hardly spacious enough to accommodate their own future requirements.

It is tempting to speculate on the cause of the decline in the birth rate of the Pitcairn Islanders. There are at least three obvious explanations which will occur to the reader, according to his training or bias. It is possible to argue that the high birth rate of the first generations was a perfect illustration of the hybrid vigor which is released when genetic lines are crossed, and that the subsequent decline in physiological vigor is the result of inbreeding and the exhaustion of the forces of hybrid vigor. There is much to be said for this view. Among another hybrid group, the Rehobother Bastards of South Africa, who were carefully studied by Eugen Fischer, there was no discernible diminution of a marked fertility even after five or six generations. Inbreeding, however, has been a relatively rare factor in the marriages of the Rehobother Bastards.

But the situation is rather more complex than at first appears. For example, it is conceivable that medical reasons may be causing the decline in birth rate on Pitcairn. Unfortunately no opportunity was available to determine the extent of gonorrhea or other venereal diseases among the population, for it is well known that gonorrhea is important among the causes of infertility. And it might be pointed out that the beginning of a marked decline in birth rate coincides with the breaking down of sex morality. During the second half of the last century the islanders began to find the old rigidity of conduct irksome. Under such circumstances it does not take many infections from the maritime world to spread its poison throughout a tiny population. Anyone familiar with the tobogganlike decline of the birth rate among Polynesians knows how significant the introduction of venereal disease can be—a fact that was brought forcefully to my attention on many occasions. And I have also been able to record the extraordinary improvement in the birth rate of Nuku Hiva when enlightened efforts were made to combat gonorrhea.

Finally, there is a less probable explanation but one that cannot be entirely overlooked. It is obvious that the contraceptive devices and techniques known and employed in Europe and America are not readily available to the Pitcairn Islanders, but some information may well have seeped through into the island.

From 1858 to 1934 three hundred and twenty births occurred on Pitcairn. Of this total nine were twins, giving a proportion of 1 to 35.6. The frequency of twin to normal births is usually around 1 to 80, although this proportion has been found to fluctuate among various peoples from 1:60 to 1:250. But I know of no population where the frequency of twins is as high as here. I am not acquainted with any reliable data on the phenomenon among Tahitians, but my observations do not lead me to believe that twinning is more frequent among them than among the English. It is not inconceivable that inbreeding has increased the chances for multiple births among the Pitcairn Islanders.

During the period from 1864 to 1934 inclusive there were recorded in the *Book of Records* the deaths of 114 native islanders. The following list gives the various causes assigned for the deaths and the frequency under each category.

Accident 19
Lockjaw 4
Internal injury and old age ... 1
Spinal injury 1
Consumption 12
Pneumonia 2
"Flu" and old age 1
Typhus 12
Old age 7
Paralytic stroke and old age ... 1
Dysentery 5
Heart trouble 3
Dropsy 3
Asthma and dropsy 1
Fever 3
Childbirth 3
Convulsions 2
Whooping cough 2
Stomach and intestinal trouble 1
"Disease through whole body" 1
Amenorrhea 1
Craniotomy 1
Stillborn 2
"Inherited fever" 1
Not stated .... { 16 adults
                            { 9 infants

TOTAL 114

It hardly needs mentioning that the above causes of death possess doubtful value; nevertheless, the list does provide several facts of great interest. The number of deaths by accident is relatively large, comprising 16.7 per cent of the total. And if to these nineteen cases of death by accident we add the deaths by internal injury, by spinal injury, and by lockjaw (two of these were specifically stated to have acquired lockjaw from a splinter), the total of twenty-five would amount to 21.9 per cent of all deaths.

Whatever doubt may surround the other attributed causes of death, there can be no question of those by accident. They include many who were washed from rocks, some who fell from cliffs, others accidentally shot, two who were crushed by a boat, and similar victims of work and play. This large total speaks volumes for the hazards of life on Pitcairn.

Tragedy rates but a few lines in the records. On March 28, 1898, Andrew Stevens Christian, son of Francis and Eunice Christian, aged ten years and two months, was sent by his mother to climb a banana tree and gather its fruit. "He remained longer than he should," runs the account, "and, failing to answer his mother's repeated calls, she sent two of his young sisters to look and see what was the matter. Arriving at the place, they found him dead, with the banana tree lying across his body."

The twelve deaths recorded as caused by typhus occurred in 1893, "having been communicated by means of the wrecked ship *Bowdon*, lost on Oeno reef." Death by "craniotomy" was the fate of little Anderson Warner, "age about 1 hour." "Fracture of the skull due to partial craniotomy rendered necessary to save the mother's life," says the recorder. Newborn Nelly Dolly Warren died on March 26, 1911. "Cause mother being sick with fever in child birth, child also inherits the fever for few hours then died."

Among those listed under deaths were seventeen infants who died when less than one year old, and two stillborns. Not including the two stillborn infants, it appears that one in every six deaths was that of an infant less than one year old. Stated in another way, the infant mortality under one year was about fifty-six per thousand births. This is not an excessively high rate, even when compared with corresponding rates in Europe and America. In fact, it is remarkably low for a population lacking the attentions of a medical man.

If for no other reason, inbreeding among the Pitcairn Islanders would make them worthy of serious study. The limited number of families with which the colony began and the fact that only a few strangers have joined the community forced an intense form in inbreeding on passing generations. So many people believe inbreeding to be fatal to the health of families given to its practice that it has become almost an eleventh commandment: Thou shalt not marry thy cousin. Any closer blood relationship, of course, is incestuous and held in horror. Nor is this fear of inbreeding completely irrational. Numerous enough instances of cousin marriages which have led to disastrous results suggest that such a prohibition is more than an empty taboo. Inbreeding will increase very considerably the chances of the appearance of a latent defect—if there is a defect latent in the stock. But if the genetic line is sound, there should theoretically be no unpleasant consequence from cousin marriage. In fact, mice and other laboratory animals have been brother-sister mated for generations without producing an unnatural number of defectives. Moreover, there have been historic examples of brother-sister matings in Egyptian dynasties and among the Peruvian Incas which have been successful. And in many primitive societies, where cousin marriage has been a general and ancient custom, it has not inevitably led to degeneration.

The carefully preserved records of Pitcairn make it possible to draw up a family tree for each individual, and from a study of these genealogical tables we can derive an exact idea of the amount of inbreeding which has occurred in the Pitcairn ancestry of every islander. It can be easily imagined how rapidly these ancestral lines become exceedingly intricate and how difficult it would be, after five or six generations, to describe all the complicated interrelationships adequately. I have, therefore, attempted to obtain for each of my adult subjects a simple index which would express the exact degree of inbreeding. To do this I have carried each individual back to the generation of the mutineers and divided the total number of ancestors theoretically possible for that generation into the actual number found. For example, to state a case in its simplest terms, if a subject is in the fifth generation from the mutineers, he has thirty-two possible ancestors in the mutineers' generation. Now, if by actual count there are only twenty different ancestors, indicating a number of cousin marriages, then twenty divided by thirty-two gives an inbreeding index of .625 or 62.50 per cent.

Brother-sister mating in a family previously outbred would give an index of 50.00 per cent, and first-cousin marriage an index of 75.00 per cent. Previous inbreeding in such cases would, of course, lower the index. In the following table I have listed by decades the average index of inbreeding among my adult Pitcairn subjects, male and female.

	NUMBER	AVERAGE INDEX OF INBREEDING
1850–1859	4	84.38 per cent
1860–1869	7	91.07 per cent
1870–1879	15	86.67 per cent
1880–1889	22	70.87 per cent
1890–1899	26	71.36 per cent
1900–1909	26	61.96 per cent
1910–1916	23	51.53 per cent

These figures indicate a very rapid increase in inbreeding to the point where the index is practically the same as that for the offspring of a brother-sister marriage. It should, however, be noted that an index of 51.53, such as is found for the youngest subjects, is not really equivalent to an index of 50.00 for brother-sister marriage. In the former, part of the reduction comes from the doubling of ancestors five, six, or seven generations removed, while the latter reaches back only two generations. The closer to the subject's generation the doubling takes place the more intense is the inbreeding, although the index gives no measure of this. Nevertheless, it is clear that inbreeding among Pitcairn Islanders is extremely close.

One subject had an index of 25.56. In his family tree Fletcher Christian appeared seven times, Edward Young six times, John Mills three times, William McCoy three times, Matthew Quintal three times, John Adams once, and John Buffett once. This inbred young man is a healthy islander and shows no obvious stigmata of his restricted ancestry.

The rise in the average index for the decade 1860–1869 is caused by the fact that of the seven individuals born in that period four were the children of Samuel Warren, a Providence, R. I., man, who settled on Pitcairn.

It has, no doubt, occurred to the reader that the increase in inbreeding is a function both of the succession of generations and of the limitation in the numbers of the original founders. The advance of each generation doubles the possible number of ancestors for a given level. If the number of individual ancestors remains constant at that level, then the inbreeding increases proportionately to the number of generations. Unless new blood is added to the Pitcairn mixture, each successive generation will become statistically more inbred. Genetically, however, the increase in population provides an opportunity for variation and diversification of ancestral lines.

All this leads to the question whether or not the highly inbred mating of the Pitcairn Islanders has debilitated the stock. Physically, the islanders are robust and healthy. Their medical record is good, with no evidence of degenerative diseases peculiar to them. Abnormalities of physical structure are practically nonexistent on Pitcairn. As for the birth rate, it is not incontestable that inbreeding has brought about the decline I have already mentioned. Other causes might more plausibly be invoked to explain it. The only general defect I know of among the Pitcairn Islanders which may be attributed to inbreeding, is the degeneration of their dentitions.

The mental and psychological qualities of the islanders tend rather to elude exact measurement. I had no time to administer psychological tests, even if there were any adequate for the special environment in which the Pitcairners live. I have, therefore, only subjective impressions, and these are perhaps biased in favor of the islanders. Actually I knew of only two or three who were distinctly below par mentally—a small proportion in a group of two hundred. Several were dull but able to manage their affairs efficiently enough. The rest seemed to me to fit into the average range of intelligence.

As I think back to the individuals I knew on Pitcairn, I am impressed by the relatively large number of men such as Parkins Christian, Fred Christian, Edgar Christian, Norris Young, and Arthur Herbert Young and of women such as Mary Ann McCoy, Ada Christian, Margaret Lucy Christian, and Harriet Warren, who possessed qualities of leadership or traits of personality that raised them above the level of their neighbors. All in all, therefore, I can only conclude that inbreeding, as far as my evidence goes, has not caused degeneration among the Pitcairn Islanders. To that extent, this confirms the results of experimental inbreeding, that it is the presence of latent defects which makes inbreeding a dangerous thing and not any mysterious punishment consequent to the process itself.

V. DIURNAL

PITCAIRN DIARY: 1934-1935

This is a chapter out of a diary. At the end of each day, after hours of work, and full of fatigue, I tried to keep a record of the events of the day. They were intended merely as notes around which to fill in memories, but in the hope that they may add a significant stroke to the picture I have tried to paint of Pitcairn life I shall quote pertinent sections.

December 24. Up at 5:30. Slept rather well. After shaving, had tea and bread which were specially prepared for me, since the custom here is to breakfast at about eleven. The kindness and thoughtfulness of Eleanor and Burley are very touching. I hate upsetting their routine, but they insist they don't mind.

Kept saying "good-morning" to the numerous passers-by. The paths are close to the house so that anyone who passes by gets an intimate view of the interior and its occupants. A little after seven the bell rang to summon the men to the boats. It was the *Ruahine* arriving. The women snatched up their baskets, the men grabbed their fruit packed the night before and their wooden curios. I found myself alone in the house, even the children, excited by the event, have departed, and at last the village is quiet.

I went up to the courthouse—just in case someone left behind might come. I wrote for a while, and then a woman, lean in the Pitcairn mold and with hard round eyes and a high-reaching curving nose, came along and we gossiped. She spoke in a soft slurring voice. She—the islanders in general—were glad to welcome us. They enjoyed the change. No, we were no trouble at all. It was a pleasure. She hoped the people would come forward. They were inclined to be a bit shy.

Then Roy Clark arrived. He came to the island in 1906 with his father, Lincoln Clark. Roy was only sixteen years old at the time. His father had been wrecked on Oeno years before, together with Philip Coffin, a Nantucket sailmaker. Coffin married a Warren girl on Pitcairn and remained, but Clark returned to his home in California. He was a mere boy at that time—I think he was cabin boy. Years later, after his wife's death in California, he decided to return to the island with his son, Roy. Lincoln died a few years ago, leaving a Pitcairn family, and Roy has become one of the islanders. He is a leader in the church and teaches school for which services he receives £3 per quarter. Has married a daughter of Philip Coffin, but is childless. Showed me his house, the oldest of the island, formerly the home of Thursday October Christian. Part of the frame is original and nearly a hundred years old, but the interior has been extensively altered. It was interesting to see the old-type construction, with the sliding shutters, the wall boards set horizontally, edge to edge, in slots. The great squared uprights are exposed and the planks fitted between them. Roy has promised to add to my Pitcairn word list.

Later I returned again to the courthouse. George arrived from the *Zaca* on his way to visit the Miss Ross who is ill. T. C. came ashore also and is collecting insects. I had breakfast at eleven o'clock and then returned to the laboratory-courthouse, taking Burley with me. I commenced my examinations with him and, having made a beginning, worked steadily until almost five, seeing, in all, seventeen of the islanders. Had only one interruption when the bell rang to call the people for the division of biscuits and flour which had been pre-

sented to them on the *Ruahine*. Each family representative brought a tin, a pail, or some other container, deposited it on the veranda of the courthouse, and then
retired to the community bench to await the just ap-
portionment. A couple of men, appointed by the council
and chief magistrate, distributed into equal shares the
ship's biscuits and flour so that each family received its
proper share. Each family, regardless of its size, gets the
same amount.

A "missionary" meeting is held every Monday night,
but I wasn't able to attend.

December 25. Christmas Day! and up at 5:30 with
the dawn. Very tired after a tumultuous evening. It was
well after eleven before I got to bed. After supper last
night we watched the rockets sent up from the *Zaca* in
honor of the occasion. We stood at the windows looking
across the tree-tufted slope falling below us sharply into
the sea. The air was purplish blue and soft. The children
enjoyed the display and the grown-ups, too. Then David
Young, Eleanor's father, came in to visit. We all sat
around the rough homemade table, covered with a white
cloth. I had a chair but the others sat on benches. David's face was beautifully illuminated by the lamp. He
has a face like Lincoln's—craggy and hollow—and the
bony elevations, picked out by the light, cast heavy
shadows in the deep excavations of his face. His eyes
appeared to be looking out of deep caverns. I began asking him about land, government, fishing, and other Pitcairn matters. Parkins came in and joined us. I had just
begun to get some interesting dope from them both when
we noticed through the window that someone was approaching with a lantern. It was Parkins' wife. She
wouldn't come in, but insisted that Parkins come out to
her. After a minute, he politely excused himself and disappeared. We were all a bit apprehensive, for Mrs.
Christian's voice sounded decidedly disturbed. I knew
that my presence had caused her guarded manner.

About ten minutes later, the calm induced by a dull

lamp and a dark night was shattered into bits by the clang of the bell giving the call to man the boats. Burley, Eleanor, and I ran out into the night. I was terrified for fear that some dire thing had happened to the *Zaca* and that they had signaled for a boat. It was pitch dark —black—and I couldn't see but could only hear figures scurrying about. Electric torches began flashing like fireflies and excited voices increasing like a dread chorus. The feeling became very tense. Little groups became distinguishable as my eyes grew accustomed to the dark. I asked what the matter was. I discovered that a woman had been so seriously beaten by her husband that she was unconscious. They wanted to send a boat for Dr. Lyman.

Some of the men started for the landing place. Burley and I followed, my feet stumbling over the indistinct, rutted lane. Half way to the descent, we suddenly stopped. The men stood around indecisively—some local difficulty I couldn't fathom. Burley seemed reluctant to be mixed up in the affair. Nothing was done and after about ten minutes Burley and I returned. I hesitated about offering my services lest the islanders be embarrassed at my knowing more than was necessary concerning something of which they were rather ashamed. Everyone seemed very distraught, and Burley kept muttering "oughter kick his arse," evidently referring to the wife-beater. It was then about 9:40 and I turned in since apparently I could do nothing.

About an hour later I was wakened out of a sound sleep by George Lyman, Parkins, and Burley. Parkins had gone out after all and brought George ashore. I got up and hurriedly dressed. George and I started off for the injured woman's house. We stumbled along in the dark tortuous paths, chasing the long legs of Parkins. We found a crowd around the house and the living room full of people—like mourners at a funeral. The poor woman was in the bedroom, her mother and son hovering over her. She was unable to speak, was suffering intensely, and was almost unconscious except for the agony twitching the muscles of her face. She had stiffened into an unconscious state some time earlier and had been out for over half an hour. George examined her and found that she was suffering from some cerebral pressure. She was made as comfortable as possible. When I could be of no more assistance to George, I returned once more to Burley's and back to bed.

Early this morning George appeared for a cup of tea. The patient is a bit better. At 6:30 I was up to the courthouse ready for work, but the annual election was going on. It seems as though all the island group activities are concentrated disastrously for my work. Men and women were everywhere scribbling on ballots which consist of bits of paper. Both sexes over eighteen vote on Pitcairn. The votes were being counted by two men seated at a table on the veranda of the courthouse.

In spite of the turmoil occasioned by the balloting I was able to get under way with Mr. Cooze, who kindly volunteered to act as my assistant and secretary. Examined thirteen. Knocked off at eleven for breakfast and shortly after noon was back at work again. Meanwhile I had secured a list of twenty men who hadn't appeared and I asked Parkins to round them up. He was kind enough to do so and until nearly five o'clock I continued without interruption, adding thirteen more to the total.

I went aboard the *Zaca* for Christmas dinner. Sea was rougher, and we found it a bit hazardous clambering aboard as the boat bobbed up and down in the swell. The islanders who had come out sat around on the deck, and we played the victrola to amuse them. They asked if we had any religious music. Unfortunately, or perhaps fortunately, we had none. Then they offered to sing to us, which they did—hymns—in great vibrant voices that went out in rolling waves of sound. After they had returned to their boats, they sang again, before casting off, a song entitled "Goodbye," which Parkins boomed out was a Pitcairn song.

It was interesting to watch their faces while they were on board. Parkins with his dark skin, tall, hard, lean figure—very distinguished, masterful, and slow-speakin', but with a humorous twinkle that lights up his face so reminiscent of Tahiti. Arthur Young, shorter, with a high, beaked, red-tipped nose, a small chin, and a high bony head. He looks like an old-time professor caught out on the farm. Some of the others are like old New England tars. Still others like cockneys and a few like half-castes. Most of the men are lean and wiry, with big knobby feet and bony toes, thin hard legs, and great hairy chests. Heavy face hair is common. A recurrent type has a high, curving nose with a very small chin, even further reduced by the early loss of teeth. Exaggerated specimens of the type are Charles Young and his brother, Edwin.

The women, also, are apt to become bony and withered in middle age. There is only one who might be called the "village idiot," but he is quite able to take care of himself. In fact, he displays occasional amusing insight. A few others are not very bright, but it is difficult to make just estimates. There are shyness before strangers, a feeling of awkwardness in the presence of yachting magnificence, diffidence towards the confident, and lack of education. In spite of these handicaps it is wonderful that fine, self-possessed, and poised personalities like Parkins Christian, Arthur Young, David Young, Edgar Christian, Norris Christian, Harriet Warren, Louisa Christian, and Edith Young develop. The newer blood has not added anything noticeably superior to the population. In fact, the finest individuals appear to be those from the purest Pitcairn strains. It is regrettable that the original population were not kept unadulterated.

After our visitors left, we sat down to a grand Christmas dinner. A huge turkey and all the additions, concluding with a real plum pudding. Florence Jaques had remembered way back in September to purchase a set of little novelty figures, one for each of us. I received a nice, friendly radio greeting from Dick back in New York. The Stock Exchange seems another world from here. Mr. Cooze gave George, Templeton Crocker, and me each an ancient stone adze as Christmas presents. They were all turned over to me as the anthropologist. These relics of a former population are occasionally discovered. In the course of many years a large number have been found, but most of them have disappeared again as gifts to passing friends. Kenneth has written an interesting paper on the evidences of a former Polynesian settlement. Stone adzes and chisels in great number all show clear relationships with standard Polynesian types. The mutineers discovered a ruined *marae* (sacred enclosure) and a *tiki* on Pitcairn. Perhaps these extinct Polynesians were an offshoot from Mangareva which, after all, is only about 300 miles distant—a mere nothing to Polynesians who never flinched at 1000-mile-long voyages.

December 26. The late Christmas dinner made it impossible to go ashore last night to my discomfort, for I got little sleep on account of the roll. It was not until about nine o'clock this morning that a boat finally came out from shore to fetch me. James, George, and I, besides some of the crew, went ashore in the first boat. It seems peculiar getting into open boats as big as these. They are about thirty-seven feet long with a nine-foot beam and are manned by fourteen oars. The seats are so wide that two oarsmen and a couple besides can sit on each one without undue crowding. The old *Mahina-i-te-Pua* that Kenneth, Ua, and I sailed about 2500 miles in the Tuamotus five years ago was only twenty-five feet long, and she was decked in and had a cabin containing four bunks and the engine.

When the boats come alongside, the islanders all turn their faces up eagerly, and looking down on them from the deck is as though one were gazing down into a sea of supplicants.

Arrived at Burley's to find "breakfast" being prepared.

Although we had already eaten, it was necessary to do so again. Before eating, however, T. C. and I went off to find the Pitcairn register. I had arranged to make use of it to copy the data I need in analyzing the vital records. T. C. has kindly volunteered to lighten my chores, by copying the register for me. After breakfast, I commenced work, and from 10:30 in the morning until after five in the afternoon, had no let-up. I examined and measured twenty-four.

Toshio set up his camera and photographed all comers. I am anxious to get as complete a photographic record of the island and its inhabitants as possible. Toshio has agreed to relieve me of the burden of photography so that I may devote myself uninterruptedly to my job.

The blood groupings have not yet been started, but we hope to get that organized a little later.

Supper tonight consisted of cow peas, chicken stuffed with pieces of potato and beef, gruelly soup made of rice and macaroni, tomatoes, cucumbers, *pillihai, kumara,* tea, and bread. After supper David Young, his sister Edith, and a number of others came in and talked until 8:30. They have gone now and it is very still and peaceful as I write. Burley is sitting on the chest and the calm of fatigue has settled on him. Eleanor is plaiting a basket for me to take as a souvenir. One of the boys is watching me very studiously, while the other two are fooling on the settee in the corner.

December 27. Not much to relate for today. Merely another full day of work. I only moved from the courthouse for meals. The day began at 5:30—I'm amazed at my unwonted early rising—and work ceased with the daylight at 6 p.m. I had breakfast today at Parkins' and a good one it was. There was square pumpkin pie, but its shape detracted no whit from its goodness. Cow peas, salad, sliced tomatoes, cucumbers, potatoes, and chicken. No tea or coffee served in that house! The chicken was for my benefit, for Parkins and his family are all strict vegetarians. Parkins was characteristic. I never tire of

watching him. He is very deliberate as he shifts his bulk
slowly. Sprawling or towering over the table, he naturally focused all attention, as he told in his slow drawling
bass voice of his experiences on Tahitian schooners.

Parkins and Arthur Young were shipmates in their
youth on Tahitian trading schooners. Quite a number of
the older men have served aboard ships in their younger
days and are familiar with the remote coral atolls in the
Tuamotus. Parkins told a long yarn about an adventure
on one of the schooners in a storm, during which he defied the captain's authority and saved the schooner. He
narrated a number of other stories about his sailing
days on the trading schooners. Has no respect for the
"drunken pigs" who captain them.

Parkins' humor is rather naive. When the first mate of
the *Zaca* came in, Parkins offered him some oranges.
John took one. Then very seriously and with effort Parkins drawled, "Ah wou'd'n eat that one." John replied,
"Well if you wouldn't maybe I shouldn't," and was
about to return the fruit. Parkins, still very serious, "No,
I wou'd'n eat that one, but maybe I would eat one like
it," and with that chuckled as he took one for himself.
The other day when Chapin, who was botanizing, said,
"That's a funny flower," Parkins asked, "What, did it
laugh?"

Examined thirty-three today—a record. There are only
about thirty or so adults now left to do. I have arranged
with Roy Clark to have all the school children assembled
one morning.

After supper tonight, went with Burley and Eleanor
to the school tea which is given for the children in celebration of the close of school and the beginning of vacation. All day as I worked I watched the activity around
the courthouse. Long planks set on barrels and boxes to
be used as tables were erected in the open square between the church and the courthouse. When we arrived
on the scene, after our supper, about thirty-odd children
and assorted adults were sitting at the tables, wander

ing about and eating out of nondescript plates and tins.
Great piles of light brown buns and thick crumbly slices
of bread were stacked at intervals along the board. Huge
tin sugar-basins, tureens of soup, etc. The women moving around to see that everyone was amply served, themselves munching a bun. I was invited to join the feast.

After everyone had eaten his fill, the tea things were
removed and the tables dismantled and put out of the
way. The adults all retired to the long bench facing the
square and the children, under the direction of Roy and
his assistant teachers, were lined up by sex and by size.
They looked like children on exhibition day at school.
The lamps and lanterns which were now lit, made the
littlest tots seem very wistful. They sang a number of
songs, then deployed into drill formation and executed
various exercises at which one or two seemed a bit uncertain. I liked the informality and the enthusiasm of the
adults who were enjoying it all very much, helping the
songs a little by humming softly. But it was a funny and
touching scene. A kind of brave attempt. This little human striving suddenly finding expression on a tiny speck
of land with countless miles of ocean all around it. It
suddenly became incredibly fragile and as defenseless as
an ant hill.

The formal exercises over, the hurly-burly of the released children drowned everything else. The children,
in various kinds of garments, were yelling and playing
in the light provided by lanterns, open kerosene flares,
and electric torches. A wandering spear of light from a
torch would pick out for a moment some wildly excited
child playing with all its heart. The grown-ups remained
seated on the bench, talking and watching the children.
It was not really very romantic, but it was pleasant as a
household of playing children can sometimes be—vigor-
ously domestic. But up above on the terracelike bank
tenuous cocoanut palms, leaning gracefully, made a
singularly entrancing pattern against a misty night-blue
sky.

There is perhaps too much of a suggestion of shanty white about these islanders—the not quite neatly built houses, the cast-off clothing, the necessarily makeshift furniture, the air of utilizing the junk shop—which makes them too close to our seamy side to be truly romantic. One has constantly to be whipping the imagination with scenes from the *Bounty* or with glamorous names like John Adams or story-book ones like Thursday October Christian to keep from forgetting that these are Pitcairn Islanders. And yet their kindness is very touching. And I have a great affection for inarticulate Burley and Eleanor. And the clean brown paths carefully besomed each Friday, the terraced village, the cocoanut-bole-lined roads do make a nice picture. The fault lies with civilization. We have taken away their fresh, crackling *tapa* and offer only discarded clothing in its stead, we have shown them the uses of tin and destroyed the beauty of thatch, we have sent them our broken-down furniture and displaced their simple benches.

December 28. Did twenty more today. Most of the afternoon I spent with Mary Ann McCoy, a gentle old maid who was in the lot that went to Norfolk and with the first of the pilgrims who came back to the sacred island. I met her the first day. She held my hand in her quavering, feeble fingers and with an aged voice that seemed about to break into tears spoke of her pleasure in welcoming us. She is blind and moves about slowly and cautiously; her face lit with a smile is held slightly forward; and her manner is one of faith in those around her. I gave her the book that Norman Hall had entrusted to me and she was very pleased to receive it, though she sadly remarked that she could never read it herself. She is the old lady that Norman Hall quotes, but her promise is perhaps too ambitious, for she doesn't remember all the genealogies—that is too much to expect. But it is phenomenal what she does recall. I rarely found her mistaken. Her memory, as in many old people, has to run on its own way without too much interference, for then she loses the thread and must retrace. Therefore I had to listen to all her anecdotes about missionaries, etc., to cull the facts that I needed. We started by listing the first families to return and tied them on to the genealogies I had collected on Norfolk in 1923–24. The effort after a while was tiring for Aunt Ann, and I decided to adjourn the session for another time.

Today being Friday, the day before the Pitcairn Sabbath, it is called "preparation day." Food is gathered and cooked for tomorrow, the village paths are swept clean, the fallen leaves and refuse are burned, and all the necessary cleaning and scrubbing are done, for on Sabbath no one must labor. Everywhere I saw the women sweeping the paths and making great piles for burning, and indoors I found Eleanor too busy cooking to be bothered by anything else.

During dinner tonight as Burley, Eleanor, the three boys, and I all sat eating, there came the faint sound of singing. Burley recognized the direction and decided that it was coming from the throats of the island men on the *Zaca*. It sounded well coming over the blue Pacific and up the green slope of the hill. We could distinguish the words, "When twilight comes stealing over the sea." The other day when I was aboard, they had sung in great lusty and heavy voices that vibrated like organs.

Figured out today that there are exactly thirteen foreigners resident on Pitcairn. Six in the Cooze family: Mr. and Mrs. Cooze, three children, and Mr. Cooze's father, all New Zealanders; Dick Fairclough and his sister Jessie Westall who are from Birmingham, England; the Misses Aggie and Harriet Ross, retired spinsters from New Zealand; Roy Clark from California, and married to a Pitcairn girl; Adella (Schmidt) Young, the daughter of a Danish father and a Chilean mother. Old Mr. Schmidt had sent Adella to Pitcairn from Mangareva when she was little in order that she might go to school and learn English. When she grew up, Adella married Arthur Young, a *Bounty* descendant. Finally, there is a very recent and, to my knowledge, the only Polynesian addition since the original cross. This is a young Mangarevan girl, Aunoa, whom Andy married while visiting Mangareva, where he had gone with Norman Hall on the ill-fated *Pro Patria*. Thus of all these only three have added new blood to the permanent population. The known additions since the original cross are the following: Evans, Buffett, Nobbs, Warren, Coffin, Butler, Clark, Adella Schmidt, and the recent Mangarevan girl. Besides these, there has been some miscegenation not officially recognized, and several others took their wives and families when they left the island.

After dinner tonight we followed the usual Friday-night custom of Burley and of Eleanor. We joined Eleanor's family at her brother Andrew's. Andrew is the wireless operator. He has constructed a wireless set by following a book of instructions, and, having taught himself the code, is now able to pick up messages within a radius of fifty miles and can prepare the islanders for the arrival of steamers.

There gathered at Andrew's his father David and his mother Kitty, his aunt Edith and her husband and two sons, his brother and sister-in-law, his wife and three children, besides ourselves. Aunt Ann also came down from her little house, blindly tapping her way and carefully shuffling her feet encased in outsize men's shoes. We all sat around the room, some on goatskins on the floor, others on chairs and benches. We were twelve adults and eight children, gathered for family prayers. We began with a hymn. Then Andrew read a passage from the Old Testament, followed by an eloquent prayer couched by Edith in fine Biblical style. This was succeeded by the singing of hymns again—about half a dozen old favorites were sung. A particular favorite would be called for by someone and the whole party would oblige. Aunt Ann sat through it all with a beatific expression which became even more ecstatic when a hymn she had requested was sung. During these services various people slipped in for a few minutes and as quietly out again.

When the sound of our singing ceased, we could hear similar hymns from other houses where identical family groups were gathered.

Had a talk with Aunt Ann after the singing. She told me that originally all the houses were built of the wood, called *miro* on Pitcairn. It is a very hard, resistant wood and still sound in the houses, even in those parts of them that date back to the earliest days of the community. During the absence of the people on Norfolk, Captain Knowles, who had been shipwrecked on Oeno, that graveyard for ships, landed on Pitcairn. To secure timber he tore down most of the old houses and with the planks built a cutter which he sailed to Tahiti. Aunt Ann remembered that when the first lot returned to Pitcairn they found the scribblings of the sailors on their slates left behind in the schoolhouse. There was one name that seemed to have remained imbedded in her memory—John Armitage. She also informed me that Peter Butler was shipwrecked in the *Khandeish* on Oeno. Peter left twin daughters, one of whom is now the wife of Parkins Christian. Coffin and Clark were wrecked in 1881 on Henderson Island. Coffin remained, but Clark returned to California, but in 1906 came back to the island with his son, Roy. The latter is now married to Hyacinth May, the daughter of his father's old shipmate.

December 29. Up later than usual this morning—6 a.m. But I was ready for Sabbath school when the bell rang at 7:30. I decided to sit through all the services in order to be able to observe the manner with which they are conducted on the island.

There are two assembly rooms in the church, one on the ground floor and another identical in size and similar in decoration on the floor above. The Sabbath school service began as a general meeting held downstairs. The church was crowded. Practically every able-bodied man, woman, and child attended. The service commenced with hymns. A prayer was offered by Fred Christian, assistant elder. Fred is a Titan, with a voice which seems to well up from the bottom of his entire six feet six inches. In vibrant 'cello tones he uttered his prayer in the ever-moving and hypnotic words of the Old Testament. Then followed a reading by Fred from some Seventh Day Adventist missionary literature. It contained an appeal for funds to help build a boat for the missionaries laboring in Melanesia. This being the thirteenth Sabbath since the last missionary drive, he collected the sum of £8 10s for this "thirteenth Sabbath offering." I was astounded that a congregation of only about 178 poor islanders were able to roll up such a figure. It made me rather hot to think of dragging the few hard-earned pence from these people to aid in work of doubtful efficacy. While the collection was being taken, the congregation sang a tune with the *andante* words "dropping, dropping, hear the pennies dropping," and ending with "every one for Jesus." I should like to believe that.

After the collection had been taken, the congregation divided itself into five classes, each of which retired to its own accustomed place. Several gathered in opposite corners of the upstairs meeting room. One went outdoors for its lessons. Leaving the Sabbath school to its various preceptors and preceptresses I departed to call on old Vieder Young whom I had been too busy heretofore to visit, and who, being incapacitated by a gangrenous foot, could not come to see me. Vieder was born in 1850 and has a fair memory of his visit to Norfolk. He was six at the time. He said that he didn't want to quit Norfolk, and he tried to run away as his family was about to depart. Poor youngster, he was caught on the road and carried back to his anxious parents. I was struck by the strong resemblance between Vieder and his sons Charles and Edwin. The two latter, however, are like feebler copies of the old man. They are smaller and their faces are more whittled. Vieder and his second wife, Louisa, and I worked together checking some of the genealogical data that I had arranged.

Early breakfast today in order to be ready for the eleven o'clock services. The bell rang out imperatively just as we had finished our pre-prepared meal. This time the services were in the upstairs room and were principally attended by adults, though there was a good sprinkling of children. As before, the meeting began with hymns, then a passage was read from the Scriptures. After Roy had finished his reading he called on five of us, among them myself, to rise and read designated verses. When Roy called out my name I was completely surprised and rose to read, fumbling for the chapter and verse. I felt as I did years ago when I read in class. My sensations when I had finished, a mixture of relief and desire to do it over again better, were the same as then.

Roy, being the elected elder, now proceeded to deliver his text and his sermon, based on the significance of the communion which was about to be taken. The lack of professionalism lent an air of sincerity and devotion to the preacher who acquitted himself acceptably. After the services two young men went forward to receive trays of biscuits which were passed around, then a native wine poured into tiny glasses was distributed. Burley took his wine eagerly, picking a brimming glass. Leaning towards me, he whispered with an implied smacking of lips, "It's goo-od wine." It was really terrible stuff.

After finishing the rite of communion, the men all rose and retired to the anteroom, closing the doors after them. I followed in mystification. As I stepped into the anteroom, which is really the platform at the head of the stairs, I saw a pile of white enameled basins and pitchers and a stack of hand towels. The men divided into two equal groups, the members of the one providing themselves with towels, basins, and pitchers of water; those in the other group removing their shoes and rolling up their trouser legs. The former, pairing off with the latter group, proceeded to wash the feet of their partners.

After the feet had been washed and dried, the men reversed positions and repeated the performance. This was the foot washing ceremony—the symbol of humility. It was done in utmost seriousness. It was deeply impressive.

Then back again to another prayer, more hymns, and dismissal. I was feeling rather warm by that time and glad to get out into the open.

In the afternoon Cooze came to call and I listened to an exposition of Seventh Day Adventism. The chief tenets of the faith appear to be the celebration of the Sabbath on Saturday, the belief in the imminent second coming of Christ, and the observance of dietary laws that forbid pork and scaleless fish and recommend a strictly vegetarian regimen. This all sounds remarkably like the beliefs of the Jews. Cooze takes his Bible literally. He argued the superiority of a vegetable diet by citing that the ancient Hebraic patriarchs lived immeasurably longer lives before they ate from the fleshpots of Egypt. I did not point out that in all likelihood the ancient patriarchs ate plenty of flesh as do most nomadic herders, or that "fleshpots" sometimes referred to other forms of sustenance, or that in agricultural Egypt vegetables perhaps were more abundant than they were in Judaea.

Tiring of this theological monologue, I suggested visiting John Adams' grave, which Aunt Ann told me is near the site of Adams' house. Therefore the grave must also be near where the original village stood. We found the grave on the further outskirts of the present village. It is marked by a simple headstone on which is inscribed:

SACRED
TO THE MEMORY OF
MR. JOHN ADAMS
WHO DIED MARCH 5TH 1829
AGED 65 YEARS.
IN HOPE

Three other graves alongside Adams' are marked by anonymous boulders and are the resting places of some of the women in Adams' family. All around is a thick mass of lantana and various brambles which makes it impossible to explore the terrain. All one could see was that it was flat land and rather extensive.

At 3:30 in the afternoon there was another service— the young people's—which was a repetition of the earlier ones.

Had supper this evening at David Young's. Family prayers followed. It was while we were sitting in the living room comfortably talking that the bell rang again— 7:30 and time to attend the church business meeting. There is such a meeting every quarter, but this, it being the last quarter of the year, was the most important. As usual the session opened with the singing of a hymn. No gathering of Pitcairners is decent without the chanting of a hymn. The next item was the reading of the various committee reports. As each committee was called, the chairman rose, walked to the front of the congregation, and delivered his or her report, reading from manuscript. There were reports on the distribution of missionary literature to passengers and crew of passing steamers, reports on church attendance, on the Sabbath school, on the young people's society, etc., etc. But one that interested me very much was concerned with the tithes. The tithes committee listed an extraordinary amount of foodstuff turned in for the benefit of the church. Each householder is conscientious in this duty. There is a special tithe house for the storage of the fruit of the land, but being able to sell only very small quantities to occasional ships, a vast amount of the stuff rots and is thrown away. Nevertheless, no one thinks of reducing the tithes to a smaller fraction.

Another report that I found full of interest was the statement of the financial affairs of the church. During the preceding year the sum of £240 odd was collected from this tiny community. It seems extraordinary to me. The only apparent source of money income is from the sale of curios and small quantities of fruit to the steamers.

Edith told me that one-tenth of this goes for the support of the church, aside from good-will, freewill, and thank offerings. Some individuals gave as much as £6 and £8. Most of this money is sent to the church in New Zealand for the support of the faith. It astonishes me that the population gives so lavishly. It is sincere giving, for they deprive themselves of many necessities in order to swell the fund. Of course, there is a strong pride in their record, and the letters of praise from their church, no doubt, supply a recompense.

All the reports were accepted by vote. Then Fred Christian rose to propose changing the hour of Sabbath school from 7:30 a.m. to 10:00 a.m. Fred, his six feet six rising to its full height and his deep bass filling every cranny of the room, argued that the later hour would allow the people more time in which to prepare their lessons. This proposal seemed to start a mild tempest. Excited figures kept popping up on all sides. Each in turn argued pro or con. Arthur Young heartily seconded the idea because his digestion had suffered as a result of the disruption of his meal times caused by the inconvenient hour. Others preferred the earlier hour for the sake of the children. It was cooler in the early morning. Those who spoke did so with admirable poise and brevity. A vote favored the present hour of 7:30.

After the business meeting Parkins brought up the question of the luncheon which the islanders were giving the *Zaca's* party on the morrow. Details were discussed. As gently as he could, he asked the parents to keep their children within bounds. Seizing the opportunity to speak to the entire adult population, I asked permission to address them. It was granted, and I spoke briefly for myself and the others on the *Zaca*, thanking them all for the hearty and affectionate welcome they had offered us.

After meeting, Arthur asked me to breakfast at his home on the next day. I accepted with pleasure. On arriving home again, we received some visitors. Edith and her family dropped in. Again I got busy with my word list. Edith was less shy than the others about giving me real Pitcairn words and expressions. I found Eleanor more reticent from a feeling of shyness and of reluctance to inspire mirth or contempt for their dialect. When she saw that my interest was real and not designed for humor she became more communicative.

Edith is very keen and has a fine sense of humor. She has derived considerable amusement from the passengers on the steamers. Invariably when she goes out and speaks to them, they look on her as a strange kind of creature. She said she felt as though she were being inspected very carefully. From the tag ends of their memories the passengers seem to recall that Pitcairn is the island whose people were regenerated after a sinful conception, that the Pitcairners are the pattern of virtue and godliness. But their impertinence is truly extraordinary. Edith said that these ten-minute acquaintances asked the most intimate questions which they themselves would deeply resent from another. Most frequently the tourist ladies wished to know "if the people on Pitcairn *really* live without sin." To this inquisition Edith usually responded with infinite good nature that the Pitcairn people are merely human like othér folks. I've never been able to determine exactly why quite decent people automatically become insufferable the moment they start traveling. Perhaps it is because subconsciously they metamorphose the new and the strange into the inferior and, as a corollary, a note of condescension creeps in.

December 30. Have been here a week today. Roy Clark was as good as his word, for this morning at six the school bell rang to assemble all the scholars. I hastened over to the schoolhouse. The forty-odd children of school age were outdoors in the yard playing. They ranged from little tots about six to almost grown-up boys and girls. And a fine lot of children. I worked hard and steadily for about three hours, seeing each child in turn. It was an enormous help to have the routine organized

this way. As I finished with one, Roy would have another
ready to step forward so that no time was lost.

After my school work, I called on Vieder again, both
to add him to my series, thus completing it, and to
dredge more genealogical minutiae from his memory.
Chatted with Vieder until I saw the *Zaca* crowd appearing on the road below the porch. When I saw their
familiar faces, I had a curious feeling as though I had
been away on a visit all this time.

T. C. went off to copy from the *Register,* George to
see his various patients, and the others to their special
occupations. At ten I hied me to Arthur Young's to
breakfast. The women were still occupied in its preparation when I arrived, so I waited in the living room talking to young Ray, Arthur's son. The house is very neat
and clean and better furnished than most. The walls are
painted a pleasant blue. There was a victrola which Ray
was operating to produce dreadful music from ancient,
scratched discs. The rest of the furniture consisted of a
native-made but nicely polished table, a sofa, and several
sturdy, simple chairs. A number of family photographs
and decorative pictures on the walls. We ate a very nice
breakfast out of doors, served by Arthur's handsome
daughter.

From Arthur's I went to Edgar Christian's to relieve
T. C. on the copying. At 12:30 I returned to meet
George. By one o'clock we had our apparatus set up for
blood-grouping and ready for finger-sticking.

Outside in the square there was a hammering and a
pounding. Tables were being set up for the dinner in our
honor. At the inner side of the square under an overhang-
ing bank the men had started fires on which the food
was cooking. The entire business seemed to be in the
custody of the males. Above the tables an awning of sail-
cloth was stretched. A constant stream of people bearing
bread, pies, roast chicken, and other edibles. This great
concourse of the inhabitants enabled us to gather sixty-
five subjects on short order. The first few were dubious

about having their fingers pricked. But that wore off when they discovered that it didn't hurt. They were all very curious to see their blood under the microscope.

At four o'clock we all sat down to the dinner. All of the *Zaca's* crew that could be spared were on hand. The central table was reserved for us. T. C. sat at the head and Parkins on his right. Several men and women hovered at our backs, leaning over our shoulders to brush off the flies with leafy twigs. It reminded me of Beechey's account of the fly-brushing activity of Pitcairn ladies of over a century ago. The usual blessing was sung instead of spoken. The food was very abundant and good. Potatoes, chicken, fish, roast goat, salad with cocoanut-milk dressing, pineapple, sweet potatoes, *pillihai*. I recognized Mrs. Parkins Christian's contribution by the square shape of the delicious pumpkin pie. After the meal was over the islanders gave three cheers for the *Zaca*, a compliment which we of the *Zaca* returned. It all ended with a graceful speech by T. C. and the singing of the "Star Spangled Banner" and "God Save the King."

December 31. Had a final session with Aunt Ann McCoy today. The dear old lady was in her bedroom when I arrived, and she asked me to wait in her minute sitting room while she changed her dress. During the process, I could observe her quarters. It is a tiny one-story house divided into two halves, one of which is a sitting room, the other subdivided into a bedroom and a kind of storeroom. The sitting room contains a table, an easy chair on one side of it, a couple of other chairs, a chest of drawers, and a sea chest—all scrupulously neat and clean.

Aunt Ann deprecated the behavior of the younger generation. She felt that they had lost the moral fiber of their ancestors. "Since the *Acadia* was wrecked here," she informed me, "the young people have changed." "If only the parents would train their children in the way they should go," she lamented. And she added, referring to the parental attitude towards the sins of their children,

"But they make light of it." "Loose conversation leads to sinful behavior" was another of her comments.

The Polynesian inheritance cannot be blamed for this "sinful behavior," for among the worst offenders are those with the most European blood.

Aunt Ann and I went over long charts which I had constructed and checked all the names I had recorded. It was a tedious job, and I was glad when it was completed. As I was about to leave, Aunt Ann produced a basket and a string of seed beads as a gift to me. I was extremely touched.

After leaving Aunt Ann's I sketched and photographed Norris Young's house, since it shows along its façade and on one side the old type of construction. The heavy, sinuous logs of *miro* are still sound. Unfortunately the interior has been entirely altered. A kind of match boarding now covers the inner walls.

At eleven o'clock, had another session with the register, copying until one o'clock by which time my hand had succumbed to writer's cramp. I had arranged to meet George at 1:30 at the courthouse where we again set up a laboratory for blood-groupings.* We made good progress, raising our samples from sixty-five to eighty-two. During a lull when the supply of subjects was temporarily exhausted, I started down the road to get blood samples from Aunt Ann and Vieder Young who were unable to get up to the courthouse. As I left Aunt Ann's holding a test tube containing a few drops of blood in a saline solution, I met Eldon Coffin running hard down the lane, his face and arms glistening with sweat, yelling as he ran, "Ray's a hit. Ray's a hit." He was leaving a wake of excited women drawn to the lane by his shouts. Ray is the seventeen-year-old son of Arthur Young. Apparently from Eldon's hurried account he and Ray were out hunting goats near Tautama on the other

---

*The results of our examination of the blood groups will appear later in a technical report on the Pitcairn Islanders.

side of the island. One of the shots from Eldon's gun had ricocheted from the bole of a tree and hit Ray. Some of the women immediately recalled that Adella, Ray's mother, hadn't wished him to go off hunting that morning. And an unexpressed but pregnant moral was implied. A group of men had already started on the run to fetch Ray back to his home. Along the village lane little groups of excited women were discussing the accident and anxiously awaiting Ray's arrival. George had been informed and his reassuring presence was the subject of much congratulation.

About a quarter of an hour after Eldon's frantic announcement, Ray appeared leaning on a couple of men, but walking. He had started to crawl toward the village as soon as Eldon had left him, and the rescue party found him well on the way home. I saw him stretched out on the floor of his home. He had been hit by a .22 long shot, the bullet having lodged in his right buttock. George, having prepared him for the ordeal, began probing for the bullet with no success at first. It was necessary to make an incision and a local anaesthetic and additional instruments had to be sent for aboard the *Zaca*. During the wait, Ray was moved to the sofa and made comfortable. When the necessities arrived, George continued his search and finally found the bullet close to the skin but about eight or ten inches from its point of entry. It was a nice operation.

The circumstances under which it was imperative to work were most primitive. A crowd of the islanders gathered around to watch, and another larger one sat outside waiting for the removal of the shot which was then passed eagerly from hand to hand.

We had planned to board the *Zaca* at five in the afternoon in order to sail early in the morning, but the accident interfered with these plans. Ray wasn't finally sewn up until about 7:30. George and I had to spend the night ashore since it was too late to go out to the *Zaca*, and moreover George wished to see his patient once more before departing.

January 1, 1935. My day commenced when George came in at 5:15 and woke me up. It was as lovely a day as have been all the others since our arrival. This perfect weather makes for easy landing and has been a never-failing topic of conversation. Ours has been the longest visit by a ship in the memory of the present inhabitants.

While George went off to make his rounds, I remained behind to do a bit of writing and to take a few photographs. On his return we both went to see how Ray was progressing. We found him in excellent condition. Arthur gave George and myself canes as presents. Later Edith arrived with another. George has been loaded down with gifts from grateful patients who have no other means of showing appreciation.

At Burley's until 8:15 waiting for the men to start down to the boats. Most of the men and some of the women were preparing to go out to the *Zaca*. The women are very excited about the visit to the yacht since they haven't been out since our arrival. On the way down we bade those who were remaining a fond good-bye. Met old Frank Christian who was waiting at the edge of the cliff to give me a couple of pairs of island canvas slippers. He also lent me an ancient photograph of his father, Thursday October Christian. Those who were not coming along remained on the cliff to watch our descent and to wave farewell.

The launching of the boats was uneventful. It was a wrench to watch the island recede. I had had ten happy busy days. The islanders had taken us to their hearts so completely that it was easy to become somewhat sentimental about parting.

More than seventy islanders, men and women, came out to the *Zaca* in two whale boats and in two canoes, or scows as they are called. They filled the decks and sat about everywhere. We took parties of them in relays to inspect belowships.

Burley and Eleanor clung to me and I showed them my cabin where we sat for a while. Burley gave me a beautifully inlaid collar box, a puzzle box, a cigarette box, and a basket of fruit. Eleanor had two baskets for me. We said our private good-byes, Eleanor silently weeping and Burley gripping my hand and his voice husky. My own voice and eyes were in a similar condition.

We then went back on deck where the ship's victrola was being played. But the islanders preferred to make their own music, singing "Happy New Year" and a number of other songs.

It is customary to have an annual boat race on New Year's, but our visit had upset their plans. But when the men discovered that we would have enjoyed watching a boat race, they quickly organized an impromptu affair. The two boats were quickly filled with the rowers. The race was from the shore to the *Zaca*. It was exciting and well done.

After the rowers were back on board again and had regained their breath, they once more broke into song. This time they started with "We Shall Meet by the River" and continued to sing hymn after hymn until all the general favorites had been exhausted. Parkins finally gave the word, and the departure began. The anchors of the *Zaca* were hauled aboard, and the engines began to throb and black clouds to pour out of the exhaust pipes. Then as the *Zaca* and the boats drew apart, the islanders once more lifted up their voices in song. Our parting view was of boat-loads of natives standing up to pour their voices into the air.

VI. POSTSCRIPT

13

PRESENT AND FUTURE

It is now more than a generation ago since I last saw Pitcairn Island. For some years I kept in fairly close touch with its affairs, for the islanders are excellent correspondents and write to a wide circle of friends. The war broke this connection, but nevertheless news trickled out and I would hear from time to time of the course of events.

The war years were hard on the islanders, not that they were in want or hunger, but because they were cut off from their friends and from the supplies that they had come to depend upon. Such things as glass for windows, sheets of corrugated metal for roofs, nails, needles, clothing were unobtainable. One does not realize how important these things become until one has to find substitutes for them.

The war also brought a profound effect on the size of the population. The need for labor in New Zealand created opportunities that appealed to some of the island families who migrated chiefly to Auckland, where a small colony was settled. This was brought to my attention by Mr. H. E. Maude, who through his official duties in Fiji had developed an interest in the history of Pitcairn and knew of mine. Although I had planned to visit this tiny outpost of Pitcairn during my visit to New Zealand in 1949, the affairs of the scientific meeting I was attending interfered and I did not see any of my old friends.

It was not until 1958 that I again saw one of the islanders. Parkins Christian, whom I have already described in some detail, suddenly arrived in New York as a delegate to an International Congress held by the Seventh Day Adventists. Before he left for Ohio where the Congress was to be held, I managed to see him and catch up on news of the island. He was much amused by the newspaper reporters who, he said, seemed to think he had never worn shoes and were disappointed that he remained self-possessed among the wonders of New York. It would have perhaps startled his interviewers to know that he had traveled more widely than some of them and had visited the cities of New Zealand and Australia. I discovered from Parkins and again from a fellow islander who visited New York still more recently that the emigration begun during the war has continued and that the population on Pitcairn is now down to less than 150. The educational opportunities for their children to be found in New Zealand, aside from obvious economic advantages, attract some of the families; and now that a tiny beachhead is established there the chances are that a certain proportion of the population will continue to be drawn off in the future. The fears of overpopulation under these circumstances need not trouble them any longer.

Whether this interesting people will survive as a distinct population either on Pitcairn or elsewhere is open to question. It is highly probable that the New Zealand branch will continue to siphon off more of the islanders who, inevitably, it seems to me, will become absorbed into the New Zealand population.

Even if some islanders remain on Pitcairn, their chances of survival become increasingly precarious as they are reduced in number, for the hazards to the survival of a small isolated population become proportionately great.

APPENDIX A

From the *Book of Records* of Pitcairn Island*

*Form of oath to be administered to witnesses in court,
by the Judge.*

(*The witness, standing before the judge, is told by the
judge to lift up his right hand and take the oath. The
judge then administers the following oath.*)
"You (*here the judge mentions the full name of the
witness*) do hereby solemnly swear before God, that
in the case now before the court, you will tell the
truth, the whole truth, and nothing but the truth."
"Do you thus swear?"
(*Witness answers, "I do"*).
(*Judge says, "So help you God"*).
On the arrival of H.B.M.S. "Champion," October 3,
1892, Capt. Rookes, her commander, at a meeting with
the principal members of the community suggested some
changes in the form of government, to what had, until
then, been followed.

* Words within double parentheses (( )) were crossed
out in original records.

His suggestion was thankfully received and heartily adopted, and accordingly, on January 1, 1893, the voters assembled, and the suggestion was carried into effect, seven members being nominated to form a parliament, and from among those seven, the following officers were elected, viz. a president, a vice-president, two judges and a secretary.

RESOLUTION.

Whereas, We have witnessed in the past, that, thro' lack of strength and firmness, on the part of the government officers, some evil has resulted, and,

Whereas, we believe that a larger number of officers would tend to make a stronger government, and that plans for the public welfare would be executed with better success, therefore,

Resolved, That we heartily endorse the plan of having a government consisting of a parliament of seven, with power to legislate, to plan for the public good, to execute all decisions of the court, and to see that all public demands are attended to without unnecessary delay.

DUTIES OF THE OFFICERS.

The President.

1st. It shall be the duty of the president to preside at all sessions of the parliament, and at all assemblies of the regular voters.

2nd. To order and to see that all acts of the parliament, and all laws, are properly executed.

Vice President.

The duty of the vice president shall be to perform the duties of the president in his absence.

Secretary.

The secretary shall be charged with the custody of all papers, and documents of every description belonging to the parliament, and shall, at each meeting, make a true record of all the actions of the said parliament. Beside this, he shall act as treasurer, to hold all public funds subject to the order of the parliament.

Judge.

The judge shall preside at all sittings of the court, and shall decide cases brought before the court, according to the letter of the law, and to appoint all sessions of the court, and its adjournment.

Court of Appeals.

Should either party in a case before the court be dissatisfied with the decision of the judge, said party may appeal to the parliament, a legal quorum of which shall constitute a final court of appeals. The parliament, however, may refuse a case tried by the judge, if, in their estimation, the case has been fairly tried and justly decided.

NOTICE.

1. All fines are so decided according to the discretion of the court.
2. Any fine, a draft of the same, when paid in work, shall be eight hours a day.
3. All fines paid in cash, must be in either English or American coin.

LAWS AND REGULATIONS.

Law One.

No one shall be allowed to assemble the court without a good evidence or satisfactory proof against an opposing party or parties, without laying himself open to punishment. Anyone so offending shall be fined sixpence an hour for that time.

Law Two.

Refusal to obey any of the lawful orders of the court shall be punishable by a fine of from one to five pounds sterling.

Insulting the court will be regarded as a grave offence.

Law Three.

No one shall call in question any preceding case that has passed the investigation of the court to prevent the course of justice.

Anyone so offending shall pay a fine within £1 to £4 sterling.

Law Four.

Any two persons convicted of the crime of fornication shall pay a fine of within £4 to £20. Should said crime result in offspring, the father shall support the child as long as it lives. ["Needs supporting," the original wording.]

Further, anything coming from the father to support his illegitimate child, as long as it lives with the mother, shall be sent to the mother thro' the hands of the parliament.

Law Five.

Any persons convicted of the crime of adultery, shall be punished by paying a fine within £10 to £25.

Law Six.

If two persons of the opposite sex, one, or both of whom, at the time shall be legally married, shall associate together in secluded places or otherwise, on terms of intimacy not consistent with his, or her, marriage vows, or in a manner to cause separation from his, or her,

husband or wife, they shall on conviction be fined within
£2 to £10.

Any person or persons aiding or abetting them in this
crime shall pay the same amount.

It shall be lawful for the court to punish the crime of
adultery ((by banishment)) from the island as well as
fining the parties.

Law Seven.

It shall be unlawful for two persons of the opposite
sex to associate together at such times and in such places
as shall tend to create scandal, or to endanger the morals
of the rising generation by their evil example. Further,

It shall be unlawful for any householder to allow any
such persons who may have thus offended, to meet at
his, or her, house, or premises, to further their evil designs without fear of discovery. Fine from £1 to £3
sterling.

Law Eight.

It shall be unlawful for anyone of the opposite sex to
intentionally remain near the place where the women
and girls do their washing.

Anyone so offending, shall pay a fine of from £2 to
£4.

Law Nine.

It shall be unlawful for any persons to raise a fake report against his neighbor out of malice or revenge.

Whoever is convicted of such offence, shall pay a fine
of, from 10 to 20 shillings.

Law Ten.

Whoever is convicted of stealing, shall be fined within
£1 to £10. The stolen property also shall be made
good.

Law Eleven.

Parents shall be responsible for property stolen by their children, (for the purpose of supporting their families, or otherwise) from the age of 16 years and under.

Law Twelve.

Should any person or persons bring forward any charges against anyone, said charge or charges having a month previous to the time of its being made known to the parliament, and produced for the sake of malice or revenge, such person or persons must be punished as the case is determined upon by the court.

Law Thirteen.

Any man who shall beat, or in any way abuse his wife, shall pay a fine of within £1 to £15.

Law Fourteen.

Any person, in a quarrel, striking his opponent with the fist, or with any kind of weapon, shall pay a fine of from £1 to £6.

Should the blow be returned, save in a case of self-defence, both parties shall pay the same fine. Any one is at liberty to defend himself.

Law Fifteen.

It shall be unlawful for any person to carry concealed weapons, or to appear before the court or parliament with deadly weapons on their person.

The fine for this law is £1 to £10.

Law Sixteen.

Any person or persons after this date, 24 September 1884, maliciously wounding, or causing the death of a cat, without permission, will be liable to such punishment as the court will inflict. Further, Any person, or persons aiding, or abetting in the aforesaid misdemeanor, will also be convicted under the same indictment. Should any dog, going out with his master, fall in with a cat, and chase him, and no effort be made to save the cat, the dog must be killed for the first offence. Fine 10 shillings.

Cats in any part of the island doing anyone damage, must be killed in the presence of one of the members of parliament.

Law Seventeen.

It shall be unlawful for any person or persons to treat cruelly, or to beat in an unmerciful manner, their fellow beings, or animals of whatever kind, to injure them or in any way to inflict pain. First violation of the law punishable by reprimand of the court. Subsequent violations by fine of from 12 to 40 shillings.

Law Eighteen.

Should any man's fowls do damage to his neighbor's property, the owner of the fowls must take them away. The owner of the plantation must first notify his neighbor concerning his chickens and if he refuse to remove them, the owner of said plantation shall be at liberty to shoot them.

Law Nineteen.

Any person or persons going after fowls in any part of the island, must call one or more of the other parties who have chickens in the same direction. Should any of the parties refuse to go, they must bear whatever damage may be done.

Anyone found going without consulting any of the said parties, is amenable to a fine of from 4 to 20 shillings.

Law Twenty.

Should any dog be found killing fowls or eating eggs, he is to be killed for the first offence.

Law Twenty-one.

Shooting goats from the bend of the ridge at White Cow's Pen inland toward Ante Valley, and following the same line up to William's Block, and across to the head of McCoy's Valley, Taro Ground and so on throughout the entire boundary line for goats, is strictly prohibited.

Fowls may be killed with bullets if found in the place allotted to goats.

Discharging of bullets from firearms anywhere within the village, is not allowed, except it be into the air, or into the sea. First offence reprimand. Second offence eight shillings.

Law Twenty-two.

Threatening the life of any person or persons will be regarded a great crime. Any such threats will be punishable by the decision of the court.

Law Twenty-three.

It shall be unlawful for any one to land from ships, drugs of any kind without first getting permission from the president. Anyone found doing so shall be punished. Further,

It may be lawful for parents to treat their own children in case of sickness with any kind of medicine that may alleviate their pain, or give relief. But no one will understand that he is at liberty to treat, or give any dose of medicine, unless it be one of his own family, without first getting license from the president. If anyone be found so doing, he shall be severely punished, as the court shall decide.

Law Twenty-four.

Any person or persons going to the sugar mill, and eating the sugar cane which belongs to another after it has been cut and brought there, and that without the permission of the owner of said sugar cane, shall be submitted to whatever punishment or fine the judge may see fit to impose upon him.

Law Twenty-five.

From henceforth (April 6, 1896) no person or persons are allowed to bring cocoanut or cocoanuts from 'TOtherside unless accompanied by one or more of the members of parliament, on the first week of every month, on Sundays, (unless otherwise arranged thro' unforeseen circumstances) and, further,—

No one, while at the above named place will be permitted to use cocoanuts from other persons trees, without first obtaining permission from the owner or owners, thereof.

All cocoanuts needed for cooking while stopping at 'TOtherside must be gathered in the presence of one of the members of parliament.

Law Twenty-six.

All the men, and the boys from the age of 14 years and upward, to whatever age the parliament may think proper to limit, are to be employed in the public work on the island, whenever their services are required.

Law Twenty-seven.

Any person, or persons, calling at, or passing by, places where public work is being done, or where persons are filling appointments made by the judge, president, or parliament, staying around, meddling, or interfering with them in their business, and thus hindering work, or in any way causing trouble, must be submitted to whatever penalty the judge may think fit to impose.

Law Twenty-eight.

No one is allowed to pay *gratis*, without first consulting with the court in regard to the matter.

Law Twenty-nine.

Whoever shall do any action which, though it has not been mentioned above,—is contrary to the decency, peace and good order of the Island, shall be punished by a fine not exceeding ——

Law Thirty.

Reports from children under the age of 14, will be noticed. Also, offenders under that age, when found guilty of glaring misdemeanors, will have punishment meted out to them by the parliament.

Law Thirty-one.

The use of bows and arrows, rifles, revolvers, or fire-arms of any description, by children under the age of 14 years, is strictly prohibited.

Marriage Laws.

ARTICLE 1. The solemnization of marriage shall be wholly under the direction of the parliament.

ARTICLE 2. The president of the parliament shall, by virtue of his office, be authorized to perform the marriage ceremony. In his absence, the acting vice-president shall have the same authority.

ARTICLE 3. Any ordained minister of the Gospel or an ordained local church elder, may perform the marriage ceremony when authorized to do so by the parliament.

Laws as Revised in 1904

Administration as laid down by His Majesty's Deputy Commissioner B. F. Simons.

The chief magistrate (who must not be a church officer) as the representative of the people will be elected by them annually.

He will be the chief official authority on the island and as such, will take general cognizance (knowledge of judicial notice) of the affairs of the island in the manner herein provided for. He will preside over and be assisted by a council composed of two assessors and the chairman of the committee for dealing with the Internal and External affairs of the Island hereinafter mentioned. This council, presided over by the chief magistrate, will deal with, and decide upon any question or any differences of opinion that may arise in connection with, or between, the committee((s)) above mentioned, or in any other matters affecting the well being or the welfare of the community.

Should it at any time be necessary, this council is authorized through the Chief Magistrate to submit to the Deputy Commissioner for the consideration of His Majesty's High Commissioner for the Western Pacific, any suggestions or questions affecting the local laws or regulations—either in regard to their amendment, their execution, their extension or otherwise; but no such suggestions or amendments can be carried into effect pending the written authority of the Deputy Commissioner.

A committee composed of a chairman elected annually by the people and of two members elected annually by the Magistrate in council, will be charged with the Internal and External affairs of the Island—such as cultivation, branding and care of animals, poultry and matters of a like nature. This committee is empowered to draw up local regulations for the furtherance of their duties which will become law on being approved and promulgated by the Chief Magistrate in Council.

The deliberations of this committee will be entered into a book kept by the Government Secretary which must be submitted to the Chief Magistrate once a month for his approval and signature.

A similar committee appointed and composed in the manner mentioned in the preceding paragraph will be charged with the External affairs of the Island, such as the disposal and shipment of produce, the working of vessels owned by the Islanders etc. etc. This committee will deliberate (weigh in the mind) on the question of produce suitable for export, the rearing of pigs and other animals for commercial purposes etc. and will submit its views for the consideration of the officers charged with the Internal affairs of the Island. The proceedings of this committee will be entered into a book kept by the Government Secretary which must be submitted to the Chief Magistrate once a month for his approval and signature.

Local Registrar and Government Secretary.

A capable Government Secretary must be elected annually by the people. This officer will keep a record of all cases tried in the Local Court of Justice. He will see that proper minutes of the deliberations (act of weighing in the mind) of the Chief Magistrate in Council are kept. He will also record the proceedings of the Committees charged with the Internal ((and External)) affairs of the Island and submit them from time to time to the Chief Magistrate as provided for. He will undertake the official correspondence of the Chief Magistrate and see that copies of the same are kept and properly filed in the archives of the Island. This officer will further deal as directed by the Chief Magistrate with the communications of the Deputy Commissioner and see that they are correctly filed for easy reference together with any documents affecting the public affairs of the Island.

The Government Secretary will also act under the direction of the Chief Magistrate, as Government Treasurer. In this capacity he will be responsible for the disbursement (pay out) of Public Funds and will see that correct a/cs with vouchers (a paper that concerns a receipt) and receipts are carefully kept.

The Government Secretary will each half year, prepare returns of cases tried before the Court, of the deliberations of the Chief Magistrate in council and of the proceedings of the Committee((s)) for Internal ((and External)) affairs for transmission to the Deputy Commissioner for the consideration of the High Commissioner for the Western Pacific.

In the event of the death of the Chief Magistrate during his term of office, a person to fill the vacancy for the rest of the term may be elected by the council. A vacancy in the Council may be filled on the nomination of the Chief Magistrate.

Judicial.

The Chief Magistrate who is the chief judicial authority will impartially and strictly enforce the local laws and regulations in force. In both civil and criminal matters in which justice can be met by a fine not exceeding £5, or by imprisonment not exceeding one week, the Chief Magistrate will act alone. In all other cases he will be assisted by two Assessors, members of his council, elected annually for the purpose.

In cases tried before the Chief Magistrate with Assessors, in the event of a difference of opinion between them, the combined voices of the Assessors will prevail, but the punishment to be awarded will be determined by the Chief Magistrate alone.

Civil and criminal matters of a serious character for which punishment is not provided for in the local laws and regulations must be dealt with by His Majesty's High Commissioner's Court for the Western Pacific at Pitcairn Island.

Local Court of Justice at Pitcairn Island.

The court will be opened for the administration of Justice on the Monday of the second and fourth weeks of each month and will be presided over by the Chief Magistrate with or without Assessors as may be necessary.

LOCAL LAWS AND REGULATIONS AT PITCAIRN ISLAND.

1. Summons and orders of the Court are to be obeyed immediately. Any infringement of this regulation will be deemed Contempt of Court and will be punished accordingly, either by imprisonment for 24 hrs. or by a fine of 20/ according to the decision of the Court.

2. Any person convicted of seducing a girl under the age of 14 yrs. will be liable to a fine of £20, with or without imprisonment, not to exceed one month. Any person convicted of being the father of an illegitimate child will be fined £5 and will be called upon to pay 2/ per week for the maintenance of the child until it arrives at the age of 14 yrs.

3. The question of Adultery and Rape (Violation by force) cannot be dealt with by the local Court. Such matters must be referred to the High Commissioner's Court for the Western Pacific.

4. If two persons of opposite sex one or both of whom are legally married to other persons shall be found in adultery or shall associate together in secluded places for the purpose of acting in a manner not consistent with his or her married vows, or for the purpose of committing carnal offenses, they shall on conviction be fined from £5 to £10 each, independent of any action which may be taken subsequently under paragraph 3. Any persons aiding or abetting in the offence referred to above are subject to like penalties on conviction.

5. Unmarried persons of either sex congregating together in such a manner as to cause scandal or to endanger the morals of the younger members of the com-

munity, will upon conviction be fined from £2 to £5. Further any householder or other person conniving (to wink at) at the offence mentioned in this paragraph will upon conviction be liable to similar penalties.

6. Any male person intentionally loitering about the places where the women do their washing will upon conviction be fined from 10/ to 40/.

7. Any person ((defaming)) slandering another in a spirit of malice or revenge, will, on conviction, be fined from 10/ to 20/. In cases of a gross or serious character recourse (application as for help) may be had to the High Commissioner's Court for the Western Pacific.

8. Any person over the age of 14 yrs. convicted of theft will be punished by either a fine not exceeding £20, or imprisonment not exceeding one month, or both, and the stolen goods must be returned or made good. Offences under this paragraph, which, either on account of the value of the property involved, or the gravity and circumstances of the case, cannot be dealt with locally, will be tried in the High Commissioner's Court for the Western Pacific.

9. Parents instigating their children under the age of 14 yrs. to steal produce or other goods, will on conviction, be dealt with under the provisions of paragraph 8; the children so offending will be admonished by the Chief Magistrate on the first offence; for the second or subsequent offence they will receive from 3 to 12 strokes with a cane, according to the age and health of the child and to other circumstances. Children under the age of 14 yrs. convicted of theft under circumstances other than those above mentioned, will, for the first offence, receive from 3 to 12 strokes of cane. For a second or Subsequent offence, they will be imprisoned from 3 to 7 days. In both instances the parents or guardians of the child so offending will be called upon to return the goods stolen or to pay the value of the same to the owners.

10. Any person committing a breach of the peace, such as striking or abusing his wife, striking any person either

with his fist or with any weapon, save in self defence, and all other offences not provided for that may disturb the peace of the community, shall on conviction be fined from 10/ to £5, according to the gravity (seriousness) of the offence. An habitual disturber of the peace may be dealt with in the High Commissioner's Court for the Western Pacific.

11. Firearms, or other weapons may not be carried by any person under the age of 14 years. Persons over that age will be permitted to carry firearms for shooting purposes on obtaining a license from the Chief Magistrate, the charge for which will be for three months 2d, for six months 3d, for one year 6d. Licenses may not be transferable. Any person convicted of carrying firearms, concealed or otherwise, without a license will be fined £2.

Any person coming into Courthouse while the Court is sitting with arms on his person will be fined £1 for contempt of Court.

12. All regulations promulgated by the Chief Magistrate, on the recommendation of the Committees charged with the Internal ((and External)) affairs of the Island, relating to the preservation of cats, cruelty to animals etc. depredation (to destroy) caused by fowls and dogs, the shooting of goats and chickens and matters of a similar nature, are to be strictly adhered to. Any infringment of these regulations ((both)) as regarding Internal ((and External)) affairs will be punished by a fine of from 5/ to £1 at the discretion of the Court.

13. Firearms must not be discharged within the precincts of the village except as authorized under the provisions of the preceeding paragraph.

14. Threats against the life of any person or persons will be dealt with under paragraph 10 and are subject to like penalties. All persons meddling, interfering or hindering other persons in their employment will be charged with committing a breach of the peace and will also be dealt with under the provision of paragraph 10.

15. Abortion is a serious crime and is punishable by a

lengthy term of imprisonment. Any such cases occuring on Pitcairn Island must be brought to the notice of the Deputy Commissioner who will deal with them under the provisions of His Majesty's Order in Council. The Chief Magistrate will not fail to keep himself informed of any such cases or suspected cases, and will immediately act as directed above. Further, in order to prevent the misuse of imported drugs, the Chief Magistrate will, alone, authorize a competent person to import ordinary and simple medicines for the use of the Islanders. The person selected for this duty will exercise his discretion in the issue of such drugs, bearing in mind that any misuse of the privilege accorded to him will be severely dealt with by His Majesty's High Commissioner's Court for the Western Pacific.

16. All men and boys over the age of 14 years are renumeration (reward & recompense) when required, should circumstances permit. It is to be clearly understood, however, that if in the opinion of the Committee((s)) charged with the Internal affairs of the Island, the crops or produce will suffer by the employment of the men as above mentioned, that their services are to be dispensed with until a more fitting occasion.

It could be arranged, however, that such men willing to carry on the Public Work of the Island should be permitted to do so by the said Committee provided that the interests of their respective plantations do not suffer in the meanwhile. In any case it will be the duty of the Chief Magistrate to support the Internal interests of the Community equally with those appertaining to Public Work. Prisoners may be employed on Public Work.

17. The evidence of children may be accepted provided that such children are of a sufficient age to understand the nature of an oath or the nature of the deposition (act of determining) they are called upon to make.

18. All fines and penalties levied (collected) in cash are to be held at the disposal of His Majesty's High Commissioner for the Western Pacific.

Persons unable to pay cash fines or penalties may be permitted to work out the same in the service of the Public departments at the rate of 5/ per day, provided that outside of the Sabbath day, the said person is allowed one day per week for the care of his own plantation or interests.

19. Foreigners, should they visit and reside on Pitcairn Island at any time, should be made acquainted with the laws and regulations governing the Island. No one except His Majesty's High Commissioner for the Western Pacific, or, under certain circumstances, the Deputy Commissioner is legally empowered to deport a person from the Island.

20. No alcoholic liquors are to be imported into the island by the islanders except such as may be required for medical purposes and then only under the written permission of the Chief Magistrate. Other residents and foreigners may from time to time import sufficient for their personal use with the written sanction of the Chief Magistrate. These persons, however, are prohibited from selling or disposing of the same, or any portion of the same, to the natives of the Island under the penalty of a fine not exceeding £10 for the first offence, and a similar fine with imprisonment not exceeding one month for a second or subsequent offence. Smuggling will be punished by similar penalties and the liquors confiscated.

21. In the event of the death of a person under suspicious circumstances, the Chief Magistrate assisted by his council, will enquire into the matter, examine witnesses and take down evidences and submit the same, together with his covering report, for the consideration of the Deputy Commissioner.

22. No punishments, pains, or penalties, other than those above provided for can be imposed by the Chief Magistrate. Cases of a grave and serious character will be dealt with by His Majesty's High Commissioner's court for the Western Pacific at Pitcairn Island.

23. These Laws and Regulations will come into force on

and from Thursday the 19th day of May 1904 but are
subject to the concurrence and revision of His Majesty's
High Commissioner for the Western Pacific.

Read at the close of law 16.

Prisoners may be employed on Public Work.
No. 24 and 25 of the Local Laws are found on page 93
of this book.

REGULATIONS MADE BY CAPT. GARNIT, APPROVED BY R. T. SIMONS.

Constant disputes having arisen as to the control of
the boats, in the future the boats are to be under the control of the committee for Internal ((External)) affairs
who will not only require the men for manning them, but
will requisition men for keeping them in order, a certain
number of hours each week.
24. It having been brought to the notace of the Deputy
Commissioner that theft accompaned by burglary is a
frequent occurance on Pitcairn Island, it is hereby enacted that when there is a suspicion that goods stol-
((l))en are secre((c))ted in one or other of the islanders houses a written warrant may be issued by the Chief
Magistrate for the ((serch)) search of the said houses
by the court policeman, and cases are to be tried in the
High Commissioner's court for the Western Pacific.
25. No Pitcairn Islander shall board a passing ship untill
it has been definitley ascertained that no sickness of any
kind exist on board.

INSTRUCTIONS IN REGARD TO THE YEARLY ELECTION OF GOVERNMENT OFFICIALS.

a. Every native born inhabitant of the island who has attained the age of eighteen years shall be qualified to vote
at the election of government officers. Foreigners may

take part in election and local affairs provided that the community is willing.

The Chief Magistrate and the two assessors must always be natives of Pitcairn Island.

b. Within the first five day after the twentieth of December in each year the Chief Magistrate and Government Secretary shall prepare a register of all persons qualified to vote at the election of government officers.

This register shall be signed by the Chief Magistrate and committed to the care of the Government Secretary.

c. The register so prepared shall be called the Register of voters and shall be used at the election of government officers and shall continue to be used untill superseded by a revised registere. And no person shall be entitled to vote at any election whose name is not upon the register of voters. Candidates for the ((office)) post of Government officers shall be nominated in public meeting by the community. Such nomination shall be publicalty notified not less than four days before the day fixed for the election.

d. On a day within 5 days after the 25 of December of each year and at a place and hour of which forty eight hours public notace shall be given by the Chief Magistrate the persons desirous of voting at the election shall repair to the place so notified for the holding thereof and ((and)) there severally (each by itself or taken singly) tender their names to the Recorder (that is the government secretary), who shall be appointed (approved by the Deputy Commissioner) by the Deputy Commissioner to be recorded in favour of the particulars candidate for the posts of Government officers for whom they shall severally (separatly) desire to vote.

e. The Recorder shall be provided with a book in which he shall before the election is held enter each in a separate column the names of the candidates for election. And the particular post for which each has been nominated. And upon a vote being tendered him he shall then and there record the name in the sight of the person who tender it.

f. At nine oclock in the forenoon of the day of election the votes when given shall be counted by the person appointed to receive and record them and the names of the successful candidate by him publically notified.

g. All government officers for the year shall be elected at one and the same time.

Local Laws no 24 and 25 continued from page 90.

Local Laws 24. It having been brought to the notice of the Deputy Commissioner that theft accompanied by burglary is a frequent occurence on Pitcairn Island it is hereby enacted that when there is suspicion that goods stolen are secreted in one or other of the Islanders houses, a written warrant may be issued by the Chief Magistrate for the search of the houses by the Court Police man. such cases are to by tried in the High commissioners court for the W.P.

25. No Pitcairn Islander should board a passing ship until it has been definitly ascertained that no sickness of any kind excists on board.

R. T. Simon's

H.M.S. Deputy Commissioner
for Pitcairn Island
12 of June 1903
Pitcairn Island

Regarding Prosecution in Police cases.

In the case of a criminal action where there is no prosecutor and it is necessary for the public morals that the case should come into court, the Chief Magistrate should detail the constable or some one outside the case altogether to prosecute in court.

The Chief Magistrate should not prosecute himself as he is judging the case.

Payment for fines may be received in arrowroot or

fungers at the discretion of the Chief Magistrate when the culprit states he is not able to pay in money.

VAUGAN LEWIS
Captain. R.N.
A Deputy Commissioner for the Western Pacific.

Pitcairn Island
7th July. 1909.

Prison Rules.

1. Prisoners are not allowed to communicate with any one outside the prison. And no communication is to take place between prisoners, whilst in their cells.
2. Nothing whatever is allowed to be passed in or out of the prison without permission of the jailer.
3. No food is allowed between meal hours.
4. Prisoners are to keep clean the inside of the prison, and outside near the prison under the supervision of the jailer.
5. No visitors are allowed to visit prisoners without a written permit from the Chief Magistrate and that visit to take place between 4 and 6 P.M. on —— of each week, the visit not to extend beyond 30 minutes. Bible workers may visit at any time providing they have their permit from the Chief Magistrate.
6. Prisoners are not allowed to write letters and no writing material is to be passed in or out of the prison without having been read by the jailer.
7. No one is allowed near the prison unless on business.
8. Prisoners misbehaving themself will be liable to extra imprisonment or loss of food as the court may decide.

VAUGAN LEWIS
Captain R.N.
Deputy commissioner for the Western Pacific.

Prison Routine

hours

6.0   A.M.   Rise—clean out cells, and wash.

6.30 ⎫
to   ⎬   "   Walking exercises—20 paces up and down
7.30 ⎭   with an interval of 4 paces between each
             prisoner.

7.30.   "   Return to large room.

8.30   "   Breakfast (clean large room)

9.15   "   Muster for labour. Road making & stone
            breaking, wood cutting, digging, etc.

Noon.   Return to large room.

1.00 P.M. Muster for labour.

4.0   "   Return to large room and wash.

4.30   "   Tea, clear up large room and remain there.

7.50   "   Prepare bedding and return to their cells.

8.0   "   Lock up cells.

VAUGAN LEWIS
Captain R.N.

Deputy commissioner for the Western Pacific
7th July 1909.

March 15th 1915.

Extract from the Deputy commissioner at
Papeette, Tahitei, last communication for 1913.

It is suggested that before any outside person should
be allowed to come and reside on Pitcairn Island that
he should have the permission of the Deputy commissioner to come. And also that before coming he should
deposit with the Deputy commissioner a sum of money,
the money to be forfeited should he have an illegitimate
child while resident in Pitcairn. If he should marry the
money to be returned to him.

H. A. RICHARD. *Deputy Commissioner*
Papeette.
Tahiti.

no.2. It having been pointed out to me that there is no authority for the detention of an accused persons in serious cases which have to be reported to the High Commissioner's Court it is my direction the Chief Magistrate and assessors is authorized to ensure the necessary confinement.

E. S. S GAUNT

21 July. 1906

Captain and senior Naval Officer

no. 3. Minutes of council of 22nd February 1905, show that it was decided to ask the Deputy Commissioner to extend no. 16, of the local laws so as to allow of the women being employed roofing public buildings.

I am in favour of this, exempting women three month's gone with child, but it is not a matter of urgency and can await the decision of the Deputy Commissioner.

Internal
((Ex))ternal Committe's Regulations

1. The boat and boat house and public trading will be under the control of the ((external)) internal committee who will require men for manning as well as for keeping them in order. ((from the Internal Committee)) [Note: The next sentence is marked "Left Out."] The committee will deal with all affairs from boathouse to ship and ship to boathouse.

2. Suitable men will be appointed ((yearly)) by the committee to act as traders ((and tally)).

3. Public interest will be given preference over private, an exception being made in regard to tithe produce.

4. Goods obtained from passing vessels &c. will be retained for the use of public departments if so needed.

5. a. To Captains
Feb 16th 1917 Should the acting committee consider it best for no women passengers to be in the boats when working for their purpose the coxswain or whoever in

charge of such boats are to submit to the acting committee.

b. That in the matter of overloading and in regard to the carrying or not of any person other than the actual members of the crew, and the Com. representative you are being responsible, in the case of accident, you* shall have full authority whenever the necessity exist, such as bad weather, leaky boats, &c. But in all ordinary circumstances the arrangement of the ((Ex))ternal [Note: Changed to Internal] Committee shall stand, and whenever possible as many as two places are to be available for ((surf)) ship missionaries should such wish for passage.

c. You shall receive a list of public stuff in your boat and you will be responsible for the same until handed over to the committee's representatives. All stuff is in your charge as long as it is in your boat.

d. If on board ship you consider it unsafe to remain longer, the committee's representative and passangers will always be ready to leave at your request; your crew being always subject to your instruction.

In case of emergency, and in cases in which it is not possible to consult a member of the committee for whose purpose the boats are being used ((you)) any capable man [Note:† the words "any capable man" are inserted later in pencil] will act as seem best under the circumstances.

On Sabbath days one boat only will go off to calling ships in the following order—Ella May Longboat, Adelia May clew boat, Surprise Life boat [Note‡: The proper names are inserted later] Any member or crew wishing to be excused from conscientous reasons can make arrangements with the captain of his boat.

[NOTE: The following two sentences are marked "Left

---

* ("You" is inserted in pencil later.)
† Erasure and last three words inserted later in pencil.
‡ The names inserted later.

out."] No public trading will be conducted by the committee on such dys.

Repairs and alterations to the boats will be effected by the ((Ex))ternal Committee.

It will be the duty of the captains to report to the committee whenever his boat need attention. Captains of boats will have the right to work with the boat builders on their own boats. Small jobs such as repairing of clits, leathering oars etc. will be attended to by the captain and crew.

6 a. To coxswains: Boat's cargoes will be discharged by the watches of the boats in turn under the instruction of the coxswain.

b. The care of the boats when laying along side vessels will devolve upon the crew who will perform this duty in turns under the instruction of the coxswain.

No one who has been left in charge or partial charge of a boat will leave such boat without the sanction of the coxswain.

7. Any person stealing or inciting others to steal or committing any other misdemeanor on board passing ships will be prosecuted before the Local Court by the ((External)) Internal Committee. [Note: The word anyone is later inserted before the word Internal. viz. "by the anyone Internal Committee."]

INTERNAL COMMITTEE REGULATIONS

1. a. All persons liable for public work shall assemble at the Court house within 15 minutes after the ringing of the bell.

b. Men unable from sickness or other reasons to answer the call to public work shall send written notace to the Chairman of the Internal Committee.

c. Any neglect of public work authorized by the Committee; such as sweeping of the road, or neglect to render prompt obediance to lawful demand of overseer will be deemed an offence against these Regulations.

2. a. Any persons using public property shall sweep and

put in order the buildinds and return tools etc. to their appointed places in good order.

b. Refuse from the mill house must be carried beyond the first row of cocoanut tree.

c. The throwing of rubish such as cane or arrowroot refuse ect. in any of the public roads is prohibited.

d. Firewood may be split on public roads when necessary, but persons so doing must clean up the roads after they have finish.

3. a. Any person destroying or interfearing with public property will be prosecuted.

b. Suitable men will be appointed by the Committee to keep the water works in good order and to advise the Committee of any work necessary not within their line of duty.

4. a. No sea bathing will be allowed within the village unless bathers are clothed from neck to knee. Village limits mean from Rocks to Landing inclusive.

b. Bathers in any other parts of the Island must be similarly clothed where there are the two sexes. Cases of immergences are excusable.

5. a. Cruelty, birds ect. is forbidden. The word cruelty means the giving of unnecessary pain or torment.

b. No wild cats, or sparrow are to be destroy except as the Committee may direct.

c. The Noddy may be killed from ((Dec.)) Feb 1 to July 31 and the White birds from Jan 1 to July 31 only.

6. a. ((Goats)), Pigs, horses ((or cows)) will not be allowed to run loose. Any of the above mentioned animals found straying may be driven to the Magerstraits house where the owner shall pay the sum of 1/ before receiving his animal. Half of the above amount is to be given as a reward to the person secureing the straying animal.

7. Any animal or bird, except ((goats)), horses, ((cows)), committing a second depredation the owner having been warned of the first offence may be destroyed. ((Goats)), ((cows)) or horses, committing a

second depredation the owner thereof shall be fined from 5/ to £1 in addition to making good the damage to the one despoiled.

[Note: The two following rules regarding dogs are marked Ammended].

Dogs chasing goats may be killed for the first offence, in the act anywhere. Dogs destroying chickens without their masters must be killed for the first offence.

8. a. The shooting of goats will be allowed outside the following boundaries only: From the bend of the ridge at White Cow pen inland, toward Outer Valley following the same line to William's Block, across the head of Mc-Coys Valley and Taro Ground, from thence along the ridge to the head of Paavala Valley, Itie and Mr. Nobbs cocoanuts. No one is allowed to shoot goats anytime and anywhere on the island for shot.

b. That outside these boundaries bullets may be fired into the air sea and earth only.

c. Persons carlessly shooting with fire arms bows and arrows or throwing stones across the public roads will be prosecuted.

9. a. The committee will appoint suitable men to act as goat masters. One of whom, or of the committee, must either brand or witness the branding of all kids and goats. [Note: The entire last sentence is marked Left out].

b. No one shall chase or catch kids or goats without the sanction of one of the goat masters.

c. No one shall kill kids or goats unless accompanied by two other men. [Note: This sentence is marked Left out].

d. The ears of kids and goats killed must be shown to one of the committee, or goat masters, and to the Gov.-Sec. to be recorded. [Note: This sentence is marked Left out].

10. a. Each family on the Island shall not keep more than ((six)) four breeding nanies.

b. This Reg. was changed by R. T. Simons Dep. Commissioner in the year 1907.

[Note: Original version—]: Families not residing on the Island but expecting to return may have not more than three breeding nannies kept for them the committee being informed of the caretaker's name.

[Note: Altered version—]: Families not residing on the Island have the same privelage to keep four breeding nannies just the same as those on the Island the committee being informed of the caretaker's name.

c. Goats suffering from "Big Bubby" must be either isolated or killed unless heavy with kid; when the goat masters may allow it to remain untill after kiding.

11. a. Persons intending to kill fowls outside village limits shall first give notice to those owning fowls in the same vacinety.

b. [Note: Marked Left out]: Persons killing, selling or in any manner despose of fowls or turkey must present the legs to some one of the members of the government.

12. No one shall plant or erect buildings within one yard of the boundaries of their lands without the written consent of the owner of the adjoinin lands.

13. a. Children under 14 years of age are forbidden to light fires on land except under the supervision of an adult.

b. Any persons lighting fires on lands within five yards of the bounderies without permission of the owner of the adjoining lands; or leaving the fire before it is out, will be held responsible for any damage done by the fire.

14. a. Cocoanuts at Tedside will be gathered under the supervision of one of the committee on such days only as the committee shall appoint.

b. In case of necessity cocoanuts may be picked anytime for drinking purposes.

c. Cocoanuts elsewhere may be picked anytime in company with ((two)) three owners of the same patch.

d. From this date the 4th of May 1914 the gathering of Fungers will be considered as a regulation of the Internal committee, the chopping of sticks bearing fungers for firewood is also prohibited.

Amendment

9. Any person or persons wanting to catch goats must give notice to the Committee and the Committee are to see to the catching of said goats, as decided by the committee.

Amendment

Reg. no 11. Any person or persons killing chickens, if they eat it, they must let the owners or the Chief Magistrate know about it, if they take it in payment for their property.

Amendment

Reg. No 7 Dogs Apr. 1st 1924.

Dogs destroying chickens or goats, the owner of such dogs pay damage for first offence, for second offence the dog or dogs are to be killed. Dogs biting any person without cause are to be killed for first offence.

APPENDIX B

Some Registered Family Brands Used on
Pitcairn Island

From the *Book of Records* of Pitcairn Island

———

Family Brands in Goats
[Note: Selected at random]

THURSDAY CHRISTIAN. Right ear forked. Left ear split.

WM. G. CHRISTIAN. Right ear forked. Two slits in left.

JAMES CHRISTIAN. Both ears split. Back piece on right cut off.

EDWARD CHRISTIAN. Both ears split. Both pieces behind cut off.

PHILIP C. COFFIN. Both ears split. Front piece on left and back piece on right cut off.

VIEDER YOUNG. Right ear cut off. Left ear forked (*nannie*).
Split both ears (*wether*).

[Note: In all about 63 goat brands are recorded]

FAMILY BRANDS IN CHICKENS
[Note: Selected at random]

ROBERT BUFFETT. Right short toe behind, left short toe inward.

FREDDIE WARREN. Left long toe.

BURLEY WARREN. Two behind toes inside on left leg.

BENJAMIN YOUNG. Inward and long toes on right.

About 90 chicken brands are recorded.

FAMILY BRANDS IN TREES
[Note: Selected at random]

ALICE BUTLER.	AY
THURSDAY O. CHRISTIAN.	IX
MABEL WARREN.	XII
JAMES WARREN.	XV
ALPHONSO CHRISTIAN.	A+
GERARD CHRISTIAN.	AN
FRED CHRISTIAN.	HM
VIOLA YOUNG.	▷◁
ANDY WARREN.	EN.

Over 125 tree brands are recorded.

PUBLISHED SOURCES

The following list is appended for those readers who wish to explore the principal sources of information concerning the *Bounty* and the colony on Pitcairn.

BARROW, SIR JOHN. *The Eventful History of the Mutiny and Piratical Seizure of H. M. S. Bounty.* London: 1831. Also in reprints.

BEECHEY, CAPT. F. W. *Narrative of a Voyage to the Pacific and Bering Strait.* London: 1831.

BELCHER, LADY. *The Mutineers of the* Bounty *and Their Descendants in Pitcairn and Norfolk Islands.* London: 1870.

BLIGH, LIEUT. WILLIAM. *A Narrative of the Mutiny on H. M. S. Bounty.* London: 1790.
A Voyage to the South Sea. London: 1792.

BRODIE, WALTER. *Pitcairn Island and the Islanders in 1850.* London: 1851.

FRYER, JOHN. *Journal* (with Bligh, W. *Voyage of the* Bounty's *Launch*). London: 1934.

LUCAS, SIR CHARLES. *The Pitcairn Island Register Book.* London: 1929.

MOERENHOUT, J. A. *Voyages aux Îles du Grand Ocean.* Paris: 1837.

MORRISON, J. *Journal of James Morrison,* boatswain's mate of the *Bounty.* London: 1935.

MURRAY, REV. T. B. *Pitcairn: The Island, the People, and*

the Pastor. First published in 1853 and repeatedly re-published.

RUTTER, OWEN. *The Court-Martials of the* Bounty *Mutineers*. Edinburgh: 1931.

SHAPIRO, H. L. *Descendants of the Mutineers of the* Bounty. Bishop Museum, Honolulu: 1929.

SHILLIBEER, LIEUT. J. *A Narrative of the* Briton's *Voyage to Pitcairn Island*. London: 1818.

YOUNG, ROSALIND AMELIA. *Mutiny of the* Bounty *and Story of Pitcairn Island, 1790–1894*. Oakland, California: 1894.

INDEX

ABOUT THE AUTHOR

HARRY L. SHAPIRO is Chairman of the Department of Anthropology and Curator of Physical Anthropology at The American Museum of Natural History. He is also Adjunct Professor of Anthropology at Columbia University. Born in Boston, Massachusetts, in 1902, he graduated *magna cum laude* in 1923 from Harvard University, where he also received his A.M. and Ph.D.

Dr. Shapiro's major research has been in the fields of physical anthropology, human biology, and the study of race mixture and population. He has been particularly interested in the South Pacific, having conducted studies in Norfolk Island, Tahiti, the Marquesas, and Hawaii. The Hall of the Biology of Man, which opened at The American Museum of Natural History in 1961, was conceived and supervised by Dr. Shapiro.

A Thaw Fellow and Tutor in Anthropology at Harvard from 1924 to 1926, he was appointed Research Professor at the University of Hawaii from 1930 to 1935, began teaching at Columbia University in 1938, and has been professor there since 1942.

A Fellow of the National Academy of Sciences, Dr. Shapiro is also a member of the American Anthropological Association (of which he was president in 1948), the American Association of Physical Anthropology, the American Eugenics Society (of which he is president), and the American Ethnological Society. He was formerly chairman of the Anthropology Section of the New York Academy of Sciences.

Dr. Shapiro's books include: *The Heritage of the Bounty* (1936), *Migration and Environment* (1939), *Race Mixture* (published by UNESCO in 1953), *Aspects of Culture* (1957), and *The Jewish People, A Biological History* (1961); he has edited *Man, Culture, and Society* (1956).